Mosby

St. Louis Baltimore Boston Carlsbad Chicago Minneapolis New York Philadelphia Portland
London Milan Sydney Tokyo Toronto

Mosby
Dedicated to Publishing Excellence

A Times Mirror Company

Publisher: Geoff Greenwood
Editor: Robert Hurley
Developmental Editor: Lauranne Billus
Associate Developmental Editor: Marla Sussman
Editorial Assistant: Jori Matison
Project Managers: Christopher Baumle, David Orzechowski
Senior Production Editor: Stacy M. Loonstyn
Production Editor: Susie Coladonato
Designer: Carolyn O'Brien
Manufacturing Manager: William A. Winneberger, Jr.

Third Edition

Printed in the United States of America
Composition by Maryland Composition
Printing/binding by Maple Vail Book Manufacturing Group

Mosby–Year Book, Inc.
11830 Westline Industrial Drive
St. Louis, Missouri 63146

International Standard Book Number 0-8151-2135-0

97 98 99 00 01 / 9 8 7 6 5 4 3 2 1

Associate Editors

Paul W. Flint, M.D.
Associate Professor
Department of Otolaryngology-Head and Neck Surgery
Johns Hopkins University School of Medicine
Baltimore, Maryland

Bruce H. Haughey, M.B., Ch.B.
Associate Professor
Department of Otolaryngology-Head and Neck Surgery
Washington University School of Medicine
Director
Division of Head and Neck Surgical Oncology
Barnes-Jewish Hospital
St. Louis Children's Hospital
St. Louis, Missouri

K. Thomas Robbins, M.D.
Professor and Chairman
Department of Otolaryngology-Head and Neck Surgery
University of Tennessee College of Medicine
Director
Head and Neck Oncology Program
Memphis, Tennessee

J. Regan Thomas, M.D.
Professor and Chairman
Department of Otolaryngology-Head and Neck Surgery
St. Louis University School of Medicine
Director
The Facial Plastic Surgery Center
St. Louis, Missouri

Contributors

Paul J. Abbas, Ph.D.
Professor
University of Iowa
Iowa City, Iowa

George L. Adams, M.D., F.A.C.S.
Professor and Head
Department of Otolaryngology
University of Minnesota
Minneapolis, Minnesota

David Albert, M.B., B.S., F.R.C.S.
Pediatric Otolaryngologist
Hospital for Sick Children
London, United Kingdom

James Alex, M.D.
Assistant Professor
Section of Otolaryngology
Director
Division of Facial Plastic and Reconstructive Surgery
Yale University School of Medicine
New Haven, Connecticut

Eugene L. Alford, M.D., F.A.C.S.
Assistant Professor
Department of Otorhinolaryngology
Baylor College of Medicine
Department of Dermatology and Division of Plastic Surgery
The Methodist Hospital and St. Luke's Hospital
Houston, Texas

New York, New York

George Gordon Blozis, D.D.S., M.S.
Professor Emeritus
Ohio State University College of Dentistry
Consultant
Dayton Virginia Medical Center
Columbus Children's Hospital
Columbus, Ohio

Allan C. D. Brown, M.B., Ch.B., F.R.C.A.
Associate Professor
Departments of Anesthesiology and Otorhinolaryngology-Head and Neck Surgery
University of Michigan Medical School
Director
The Difficult Airway Clinic
University of Michigan Medical Center
Ann Arbor, Michigan

Carl M. Allen, D.D.S., M.S.D.
Professor
Oral and Maxillofacial Pathology
Ohio State University
College of Dentistry
Columbus, Ohio

Mário Andrea, M.D., Ph.D.
Head and Chairman
Department of Otolaryngology
Faculty of Medicine
Lisbon, Portugal

Douglas Backous, M.D.
Otology, Neurotology and Skull Base Surgery
Virginia Mason Medical Center
Seattle, Washington

Shan R. Baker, M.D.
Professor of Otolaryngology
Chief, Division of Facial Plastic Surgery
University of Michigan Medical School
Ann Arbor, Michigan

Thomas Balkany, M.D., F.A.C.S., F.A.A.P.
Hotchkiss Professor and Vice-Chair

Robert W. Dalley, M.D.
Associate Professor
Department of Radiology
University of Washington Medical Center
Seattle, Washington

Terence M. Davidson, M.D.
Professor
Department of Head and Neck Surgery
Associate Dean for Continuing Medical Education
University of California, San Diego, School of Medicine
San Diego, California

Larry E. Davis, M.D.
Professor of Neurology and Microbiology
University of New Mexico School of Medicine
Chief
Neurology Service
Albuquerque Veterans Administration Medical Center
Albuquerque, New Mexico

Antonio De La Cruz, M.D.
Clinical Professor
Department of Otolaryngology-Head and Neck Surgery
University of Southern California
Director of Education
House Ear Institute
Los Angeles, California

Steven R. DeMeester, M.D.
Assistant Professor
Department of Cardiothoracic Surgery
University of Southern California University Hospital
Los Angeles, California

Lawrence W. DeSanto, M.D.
Professor and Chairman Emeritus
Department of Otolaryngology-Head and Neck Surgery
Mayo Clinic
Scottsdale, Arizona

Leigh Anne Dew, M.D.
Resident Physician
University of Utah
Salt Lake City, Utah

Oscar Dias, M.D., Ph.D.
Assistant Professor
Department of Otolaryngology
Faculty of Medicine
Lisbon, Portugal

Robert A. Dobie, M.D.
Chairman and Thomas Walthall Folbre Professor
Department of Otolaryngology-Head and Neck Surgery
University of Texas Health Science Center
San Antonio, Texas

Timothy D. Doerr, M.D.
Department of Otolaryngology-Head and Neck Surgery
Wayne State University School of Medicine
Detroit, Michigan

Larry G. Duckert, M.D., Ph.D.
Professor
Department of Otolaryngology-Head and Neck Surgery
University of Washington School of Medicine
University of Washington Medical Center
Seattle, Washington

Newton O. Duncan, III, M.D.
Clinical Assistant Professor
Departments of Otorhinolaryngology and Pediatrics
Baylor College of Medicine
Co-Director
Texas Pediatric Otolaryngology Center
Houston, Texas

David W. Eisele, M.D.
Associate Professor
Department of Otolaryngology-Head and Neck Surgery
Johns Hopkins University School of Medicine
Director
Division of Head and Neck Surgery
Johns Hopkins Hospital
Baltimore, Maryland

Charles N. Ellis, M.D.
Professor and Associate Chair
Department of Dermatology
University of Michigan Medical School
Chief
Dermatology Service
Veterans Affairs Medical Center
Ann Arbor, Michigan

Jane M. Emanuel, M.D., F.A.C.S.
Assistant Professor
Department of Otolaryngology and Human Communication
Creighton University School of Medicine
Staff Otolaryngologist
Boys Town National Research Hospital
Omaha, Nebraska

Emily J. Erbelding, M.D., M.P.H.
Assistant Professor
Johns Hopkins University School of Medicine
Baltimore, Maryland

Ramon M. Esclamado, M.D.
Associate Professor
Department of Otolaryngology
Director
Division of Head and Neck Surgery
The Cleveland Clinic
Cleveland, Ohio

David N.F. Fairbanks, M.D.
Clinical Professor
Department of Otolaryngology
George Washington University School of Medicine
Sibley Memorial Hospital
Washington, D.C.

Michael L. Farrell, M.B.B.S., F.R.A.C.S.
Visiting Medical Officer
St. George Hospital
Liverpool Hospital
Sydney, New South Wales, Australia

Edward H. Farrior, M.D.
Clinical Associate Professor
University of South Florida
Tampa, Florida

Richard T. Farrior, M.D., F.A.C.S.
Clinical Professor
University of South Florida School of Medicine
Tampa, Florida
Clinical Professor
University of Florida School of Medicine
Gainesville, Florida

Willard E. Fee, Jr., M.D.
Edward C. and Amy H. Sewall Professor and Chairman
Stanford University Medical Center
Stanford, California

Berrylin J. Ferguson, M.D.
Assistant Professor
Department of Otolaryngology
University of Pittsburgh School of Medicine
Director
Sino-Nasal Disorders and Allergies
University of Pittsburgh Medical Center
Pittsburgh, Pennsylvania

Paul W. Flint, M.D.
Associate Professor
Department of Otolaryngology-Head and Neck Surgery
Johns Hopkins University School of Medicine
Baltimore, Maryland

Arlene A. Forastiere, M.D.
Associate Professor
Department of Medical Oncology
Johns Hopkins University
Baltimore, Maryland

L. Arick Forrest, M.D.
Assistant Professor
Department of Otolaryngology
Ohio State University
University Hospital Clinic
Columbus, Ohio

James W. Forsen, Jr., M.D.
Instructor
Pediatric Otolaryngology
Washington University School of Medicine
St. Louis, Missouri

Howard W. Francis, M.D.
Assistant Professor
Johns Hopkins University
Assistant Chief of Service
Johns Hopkins Hospital
Baltimore, Maryland

John M. Fredrickson, M.D.
Lindburg Professor and Head
Department of Otolaryngology
Washington University School of Medicine
Director
Implantable Hearing Aid Development Program
St. Louis, Missouri

John L. Frodel, M.D.
Associate Professor and Director
Division of Facial Plastic Surgery
Department of Otolaryngology-Head and Neck Surgery
John Hopkins University School of Medicine
Baltimore, Maryland

Nabil S. Fuleihan, M.D.
Chairman
Department of Otolaryngology-Head and Neck Surgery
Boston University Medical Center
Boston, Massachusetts

Ruth Gaare, J.D., M.P.H.
Academic Program Director
The Bioethics Institute
Johns Hopkins University
Baltimore, Maryland

Bruce J. Gantz, M.D.
Professor and Head
Department of Otolaryngology-Head and Neck Surgery
University of Iowa College of Medicine
Iowa City, Iowa

C. Gaelyn Garrett, M.D.
Assistant Professor
Department of Otolaryngology
Vanderbilt University Medical Center
Nashville, Tennessee

George A. Gates, M.D.
Professor
Department of Otolaryngology-Head and Neck Surgery
University of Washington School of Medicine
Director
Virginia Merrill Bloedel Hearing Research Center
Seattle, Washington

Scott M. Gayner, M.D.
Instructor in Otorhinolaryngology
Mayo Clinic
Rochester, Minnesota

Eric M. Genden, M.D.
St. Louis, Missouri

Douglas A. Girod, M.D.
Assistant Professor and Vice Chairman
Chief
Department of Otolaryngology
Veteran's Administration Medical Center
Kansas City, Missouri

Harvey S. Glazer, M.D.
Professor of Radiology
Washington University School of Medicine
St. Louis, Missouri

Jack L. Gluckman, M.D.
Professor and Chairman
Department of Otolaryngology-Head and Neck Surgery
University of Cincinnati
Cincinnati, Ohio

George S. Goding, Jr., M.D.
Associate Professor
University of Minnesota
Minneapolis Veterans Administration Medical Center
Minneapolis, Minnesota

W. Jarrard Goodwin, Jr., M.D., F.A.C.S.
Sylvester Professor and Chairman
Department of Otolaryngology
University of Miami School of Medicine
Director
Sylvester Comprehensive Cancer Center
University of Miami Hospitals and Clinics
Jackson Memorial Hospital
Miami, Florida

Michael P. Gorga, Ph.D.
Professor
Department of Otolaryngology and Human Communication
Creighton University School of Medicine
Director
Clinical Sensory Physiology Laboratory
Boys Town National Research Hospital
Omaha, Nebraska

H. Devon Graham, III, M.D., F.A.C.S.
Clinical Assistant Professor
Department of Otolaryngology-Head and Neck Surgery
Tulane University School of Medicine
New Orleans, Louisiana

Daniel O. Graney, M.D.
Associate Professor
Department of Biological Structure
University of Washington School of Medicine
Seattle, Washington

Steven D. Gray, M.D.
Associate Professor
University of Utah School Of Medicine
Primary Children's Medical Center
Alta View Hospital
Salt Lake City, Utah

William C. Gray, M.D.
Associate Professor
Department of Otolaryngology-Head and Neck Surgery
University of Maryland School of Medicine
Baltimore, Maryland

Roy C. Grekin, M.D.
Assistant Professor
Department of Dermatology
University of Michigan Medical School
Ann Arbor, Michigan

Andrew J. Griffith, M.D., Ph.D.
Chief Resident
Department of Otolaryngology-Head and Neck Surgery
University of Michigan Hospitals
Ann Arbor, Michigan

Kenneth M. Grundfast, M.D.
Professor of Otolaryngology and Pediatrics
Georgetown University School of Medicine
Washington, D.C.

Jerry Thomas Guy, M.D.
Clinical Professor of Medicine
Ohio State University
Director of Oncology
Park Medical Center
Regional Oncology Center at Park
Columbus, Ohio

Joseph Haddad, Jr., M.D.
Associate Professor and Vice Chairman
Department of Otolaryngology-Head and Neck Surgery
Columbia University College of Physicians and Surgeons
Director
Pediatric Otolaryngology-Head and Neck Surgery
Babies and Children's Hospital
New York, New York

Jeffrey R. Haller, M.D.
Assistant Professor
Division of Otolaryngology
University of Utah School of Medicine
Salt Lake City, Utah

Ronald C. Hamaker, M.D.
Physician
Head and Neck Surgery Associates
Indianapolis, Indiana

Ehab Y. Hanna, M.D.
Assistant Professor
Department of Otolaryngology-Head and Neck Surgery
University of Arkansas for Medical Science
Little Rock, Arkansas

Lee A. Harker, M.D.
Deputy Director
Boys Town National Research Hospital
Vice Chairman
Department of Otolaryngology and Human Communication
Creigton University School of Medicine
Omaha, Nebraska

Stephen G. Harner, M.D.
Professor of Otolaryngology
Mayo Medical School
Consultant, Department of Otolaryngology
Mayo Clinic
Rochester, Minnesota

Jeffrey P. Harris, M.D., Ph.D.
Chief of the Division of Head and Neck Surgery
University of California
San Diego, California

Donald F.N. Harrison, M.D., M.S., Ph.D., F.R.C.S.
Emeritus Professor
Departments of Laryngology and Otology
University of London
Royal National ENT Hospital
London, England

Bruce H. Haughey, M.B., Ch.B.
Associate Professor
Department of Otolaryngology
Washington University School of Medicine
Director
Division of Head and Neck Surgical Oncology
Barnes-Jewish Hospital
St. Louis Children's Hospital
St. Louis, Missouri

Gerald B. Healy, M.D.
Professor of Otology and Laryngology
Harvard Medical School
Otolaryngologist-in-Chief, Surgeon-in-Chief
Children's Hospital
Boston, Massachusetts

Arden K. Hegtvedt, D.D.S.
Assistant Professor
Department of Oral and Maxillofacial Surgery
Ohio State University
Columbus, Ohio

Jay P. Heiken, M.D.
Professor
Department of Radiology
Director
Abdominal Imaging
Co-Director
Body Computed Tomography
Mallinckrodt Institute of Radiology
Washington University School of Medicine
St. Louis, Missouri

David A. Hendrick, M.D.
Clinical Instructor
Veterans Administration Hospital
Denver, Colorado
Private Practice
Vail, Colorado

Hajime Hirose, M.D., D.M.Sc.
Professor
Department of Otolaryngology
School of Allied Health Sciences
Kitasato University and Univeristy Hospital
Sagamihara, Japan

William E. Hitselberger, M.D.
Neurosurgeon
St. Vincent's Hospital
Los Angeles, California

Henry T. Hoffman, M.D.
Associate Professor
Department of Otolaryngology
University of Iowa College of Medicine
Iowa City, Iowa

Lauren D. Holinger, M.D., F.A.C.S, F.A.A.P.
Professor
Department of Otolaryngology
Northwestern University School of Medicine
Head
Pediatric Otolaryngology
Children's Memorial Hospital
Chicago, Illinois

David B. Hom, M.D., F.A.C.S
Assistant Professor
Division of Facial Plastic and Reconstructive Surgery
Department of Otolaryngology-Head and Neck Surgery
University of Minnesota School of Medicine
Associate Physician
Department of Otoalryngology-Head and Neck Surgery
Facial Plastic Surgery
Hennepin County Medical Center
Minneapolis, Minnesota

Vicente Honrubia, M.D.
Professor and Director of Research
Division of Head and Neck Surgery
The Center of the Health Sciences
University of California
Los Angeles, California

John W. House, M.D.
Clinical Professor
Department of Otolaryngology
University of Southern California School of Medicine
House Ear Clinic
Los Angeles, California

Andrew F. Inglis, Jr., M.D.
Associate Professor
Department of Otolaryngology
University of Washington
Children's Hospital and Medical Center
Seattle, Washington

Robert K. Jackler, M.D.
Professor of Otolaryngology and Neurological Surgery
University of California Medical Center
San Francisco, California

John R. Jacobs, M.D.
Professor
Department of Otolaryngology and Radiation Therapy
Wayne State University School of Medicine
Director
Head and Neck Cancer Program
Karmanos Cancer Center
Detroit, Michigan

Ivo P. Janecka, M.D., F.A.C.S.
Director, Longwood Skull Base Program
Departments of Otolaryngology, Neurosurgery and Plastic Surgery
Harvard Medical School
Boston, Massachusetts

Pawel J. Jastreboff, M.D.
Professor
Department of Surgery and Physiology
University of Maryland School of Medicine
Director
University of Maryland Tinnitus and Hyperacusis Center
Baltimore, Maryland

Virginia W. Jenison, M.A.
Clinical Instructor
Department of Otolaryngology-Head and Neck Surgery
Washington University School of Medicine
St. Louis, Missouri

Herman Jenkins, M.D.
Professor
Baylor College of Medicine
Houston, Texas

Calvin M. Johnson, Jr., M.D.
Director
Hedgewood Surgical Center
New Orleans, Louisiana

Jonas T. Johnson, M.D.
Professor and Vice Chairman
Department of Otolaryngology
Director
Division of Head and Neck Oncology and Immunology
University of Pittsburgh School of Medicine
Pittsburgh, Pennsylvania

Timothy M. Johnson, M.D.
Assistant Professor
Department of Dermatology, Otolaryngology, Surgery
University of Michigan
Director
Cutaneous Surgery and Oncology Unit
Ann Arbor, Michigan

Kim Richard Jones, M.D., Ph.D.
Assistant Professor
Division of Otolaryngology-Head and Neck Surgery
University of North Carolina School of Medicine
University of North Carolina Hospitals
Chapel Hill, North Carolina

Sheldon S. Kabaker, M.D., F.A.C.S.
Associate Clinical Professor
Division of Facial Plastic Surgery
Department of Otolaryngology
University of California
San Francisco, California

Joel C. Kahane, M.D.
Professor
Director
Anatomical Sciences Laboratory
School of Audiology and Speech-Language Pathology
University of Memphis
Memphis, Tennessee

Michael Kaliner, M.D.
Clinical Professor
George Washington University School of Medicine
Medical Director
Institute of Asthma and Allergy
Washington Hospital/George Washington University
Washington, D.C.

William J. Kane, M.D.
Assistant Professor
Department of Plastic and Reconstructive Surgery
Mayo Clinic
Rochester, Minnesota

Dan H. Kelly, Ph.D.
Associate Professor
Department of Otolaryngology-Head and Neck Surgery
University of Cincinnati College of Medicine
Voice Pathologist
Barrett Cancer Center
ENT Voice Center
Cincinnati, Ohio

Eugene B. Kern, M.D.
Professor
Department of Otorhinolaryngologic Surgery
Endicott Professor of Medicine
Mayo Medical School
Mayo Clinic
Rochester, Minnesota

Robert C. Kern, M.D.
Assistant Professor
Northwestern Medical School
Northwestern Memorial Hospital
Chicago, Illinois

Maurice Morad Khosh, M.D.
Assistant Clinical Professor
Department of Otolaryngology-Head and Neck Surgery
Columbia University School of Medicine
St. Luke's/Roosevelt Hospital Center
New York, New York

S. Khosla, M.D.
Resident
Department of Otolaryngology
Washington University School of Medicine
St. Louis, Missouri

Paul R. Kileny, Ph.D.
Professor
Department of Otolaryngology
University of Michigan Medical School
Director
Audiology and Electrophysiology
University of Michigan Health Systems
Ann Arbor, Michigan

Sam E. Kinney, M.D.
Clinical Associate Professor
Department of Otolaryngology-Head and Neck Surgery
Case Western Reserve University
Head
Section of Otology and Neurotology
Cleveland Clinic Foundation
Cleveland, Ohio

Wayne Martin Koch, M.D.
Associate Professor
Department of Otolaryngology-Head and Neck Surgery
Johns Hopkins University and Hospital
Baltimore, Maryland

James A. Koufman, M.D.
Director
Center for Voice Disorders
Professor
Department of Otolaryngology
Bowman Gray School of Medicine
Wake Forest University Medical Center
Winston-Salem, North Carolina

Frederick K. Kozak, M.D., F.R.C.S.C.
Assistant Professor
University of British Columbia
Pediatric Otolaryngologist
B.C. Children's Hospital
Vancouver, British Columbia, Canada

Eric H. Kraut, M.D.
Professor of Medicine
Ohio State University
Arthur James Cancer Hospital Research Institute
Columbus, Ohio

Dario Kunar, M.D.
Instructor
Department of Otolaryngology-Head and Neck Surgery
Johns Hopkins University School of Medicine
Baltimore, Maryland

Ollivier Laccourreye, M.D.
Department of Otolaryngology-Head and Neck Surgery
Laennec Hospital
University of Rene-Descartes
Paris, France

Paul R. Lambert, M.D.
Professor, Director
Division of Otolaryngology-Neurology
Department Otolaryngology-Head and Neck Surgery
University of Virginia Medical Center
Richmond, Virginia

George E. Laramore, M.D., Ph.D.
Professor
Department of Radiation Oncology
University of Washington
Vice Chairman
Department of Radiation Oncology
University Medical Center
Seattle, Washington

Peter E. Larsen, D.D.S.
Associate Professor
Oral and Maxillofacial Surgery
Ohio State University
College of Dentistry
Columbus, Ohio

Daniel M. Laskin, D.D.S., M.S.
Professor and Chairman
Department Oral and Maxillofacial Surgery
Medical College of Virginia
Virginia Commonwealth University
Director
Temporomandibular Joint and Facial Pain Research Center
Richmond, Virginia

Richard E. Latchaw, M.D.
Professor
Department of Radiology and Neurosurgery
Chief, Interventional Neuroradiology Section
University of Miami School of Medicine
Miami, Florida

Susanna Leighton, B.Sc., F.R.C.S. (Orl)
Pediatric Otolaryngologist
Hospital for Sick Children
London, England

Donald Leopold, M.D.
Associate Professor
Johns Hopkins University
Department of Otolaryngology-Head and Neck Surgery
Baltimore, Maryland

Greg R. Licameli, M.D.
Assistant Professor
Director of Pediatric Otolaryngology
Department of Otolaryngology-Head and Neck Surgery
University of Illinois at Chicago
Chicago, Illinois

William H. Liggett, Jr., M.D., D.M.D., D.M.S.C.
Senior Clinical Fellow in Medical Oncology
Johns Hopkins School of Medicine
Baltimore, Maryland

Raleigh E. Lingeman, M.D.
Betty Morgan Professor
Department of Otolaryngology-Head and Neck Surgery
Indiana University School of Medicine
Indianapolis, Indiana

Neal M. Lofchy M.D., F.R.C.S.C.
Clinical Instructor
Rush Medical College
Rush-Presbyterian-St. Luke's Medical Center
Chicago, Illinois

Jeri Logemann, Ph.D.
Ralph and Jean Sundin Professor
Department of Communication Sciences and Disorders
Professor
Departments of Head and Neck Surgery and Neurology and Dental Prosthetics
Northwestern University Medical School
Director
Speech, Voice and Swallowing Service
Northwestern Memorial Hospital
Chicago, Illinois

Brenda L. Lonsbury-Martin, Ph.D.
Chandler Professor
Director of Research
Department of Otolaryngology Research Laboratories
University of Miami Ear Institute
University of Miami School of Medicine
Miami, Florida

Rodney P. Lusk, M.D.
Associate Professor
Department of Otolaryngology
Washington University School of Medicine
Otolaryngologist-in-Chief
St. Louis Children's Hospital
St. Louis, Missouri

Joseph P. Lynch, III, M.D.
Professor
Department of Internal Medicine
Division of Pulmonary and Critical Care Medicine
University of Michigan Medical Center
Ann Arbor, Michigan

Anna Lysakowski, Ph.D.
Assistant Professor
Department of Anatomy and Cell Biology
University of Illinois
Chicago, Illinois

Richard L. Mabry, M.D.
Professor
Department of Otorhinolaryngology
University of Texas Southwestern Medical Center
Dallas, Texas

Michael R. Macdonald, M.D., F.R.C.S.C.
Chief
Division of Head and Neck Surgery
Alameda County Hospital
Oakland, California
Director
Aesthetic Surgery Center
San Francisco, California

Eileen M. Mahoney, M.C., U.S.A., M.D.
Pediatric Staff
Otolaryngology Section
Brook Army Medical Center
Fort Sam
Houston, Texas

Robert H. Maisel, M.D.
Professor
Department of Otolaryngology
University of Minnesota
Chief
Department of Otolaryngology-Head and Neck Surgery
Facial Plastic Surgery
Hennepin County Medical Center
Minneapolis, Minnesota

Patrizia Mancini, M.D.
Policlinico Umberto
Ear Nose and Throat Department
University "La Sapienza"
Rome, Italy

Lee M. Mandel, M.D.
Co-Director
Head and Neck-Facial Plastic Surgery Associates of South Florida
Plantation, Florida

Scott C. Manning, M.D.
Associate Professor
Department of Otolaryngology-Head and Neck Surgery
University of Washington School of Medicine
Chief, Pediatric Otolaryngology-Head and Neck Surgery
Children's Hospital and Medical Center
Seattle, Washington

Lawrence J. Marentette, M.D.
Associate Professor
Director
Cranial Base Program
Department of Otolaryngology
University of Michigan
Ann Arbor, Michigan

James E. Marks, M.D.
Radiation Oncologist
Missouri Baptist Medical Center
St. Louis, Missouri

Bernard R. Marsh, M.D.
Professor
Department of Otolaryngology-Head and Neck Surgery
Johns Hopkins University
Johns Hopkins Hospital
Baltimore, Maryland

Michael Marsh, M.D.
The Holt-Krock Clinic
Ear, Nose and Throat
Fort Smith, Arkansas

Glen K. Martin, Ph.D.
Professor
Department of Otolaryngology
University of Miami Ear Institute
Miami, Florida

Robert H. Mathog, M.D.
Professor and Chairman
Wayne State University
Harper Hospital
Detroit, Michigan

Douglas E. Mattox, M.D.
Professor and Head
Department of Otolaryngology-Head and Neck Surgery
Emory University
Atlanta, Georgia

Ernest L. Mazzaferri, M.D., F.A.C.P.
Professor and Chairman
Ohio State University
Columbus, Ohio

Thomas V. McCaffrey, M.D., Ph.D.
Professor
Mayo Medical School
Consultant
Department of Otorhinolaryngology
Mayo Clinic
Rochester, Minnesota

Robert A. McCrea, Ph.D.
Associate Professor
Department of Pharmacological and Physiological Sciences
University of Chicago
Chicago, Illinois

Timothy M. McCulloch, M.D.
Associate Professor
Department of Otolaryngology-Head and Neck Surgery
University of Iowa College of Medicine
Iowa City, Iowa

Thomas J. McDonald, M.D., M.S., F.A.C.S., F.R.C.S. Irel.
Professor
Department of Otolaryngology
Mayo Medical School
Chairman
Department of Otorhinolaryngology
Mayo Clinic and Foundation
Rochester, Minnesota

John T. McElveen, Jr., M.D.
Head
Otology-Neurotology
Carolina Ear and Hearing Clinic
Director
Carolina Ear Research Institute
Raleigh Community Hospital
Rex Hospital
Wake Medical Center
Raleigh, North Carolina

Trevor J.I. McGill, M.D.
Associate Professor
Department of Otolaryngology
Harvard Medical School
Clinical Director of Otolaryngology
The Children's Hospital
Boston, Massachusetts

W. Frederick McGuirt, Sr., M.D.
Professor
Department of Otolaryngology
Bowman Gray School of Medicine
Wake Forest University
Winston-Salem, North Carolina

Christine M. Menapace, M.A.
U.S. Clinical Manager
Symphonix Devices, Inc.
San Jose, California

Saumil N. Merchant, M.D.
Assistant Professor
Department of Otology and Laryngology
Harvard Medical School
Massachusetts Eye and Ear Infirmary
Boston, Massachusetts

Charles A. Miller, Ph.D.
Assistant Research Scientist
Department of Otolaryngology-Head and Neck Surgery
University of Iowa
Iowa City, Iowa

Lloyd B. Minor, M.D.
Associate Professor
Department of Otolaryngology-Head and Neck Surgery
Johns Hopkins University
School of Medicine
Baltimore, Maryland

Mahmood Moosa, M.D.
Clinical Fellow In Endocrinology
Ohio State University, College of Medicine
Ohio State University Medical Center
Columbus, Ohio

Jeffrey Morray, M.D.
Professor
Department of Anesthesiology and Pediatrics
University of Washington School of Medicine
Director
Department of Anesthesia and Critical Care
Children's Hospital and Medical Center
Seattle, Washington

Michael R. Morris, M.D., F.A.C.S.
Staff Otolaryngologist
Moore Regional Hospital
Pinehurst Surgical Clinic
Pinehurst, North Carolina

John B. Mulliken, M.D.
Associate Professor of Surgery
Harvard Medical School
Director
Craniofacial Center
Division of Plastic Surgery
The Children's Hospital
Boston, Massachusetts

Craig S. Murakami, M.D.
Associate Professor
Department of Otolaryngology/Head and Neck Surgery
University of Washington School of Medicine
Seattle, Washington

Alan D. Murray, M.D.
Assistant Professor
Department of Otorhinolaryngology
University of Texas Southwestern Medical Center
Attending Physician
Children's Medical Center of Dallas
Dallas, Texas

Charles M. Myer, III, M.D.
Professor
Department of Otolaryngology and Maxillofacial Surgery
University of Cincinnati College of Medicine
Professor
Department of Otolaryngology and Maxillofacial Surgery
Children's Hospital Medical Center
Cincinnati, Ohio

Eugene N. Myers, M.D.
Professor and Chairman
Department of Otolaryngology
University of Pittsburgh School of Medicine
University of Pittsburgh Medical Center
Pittsburgh, Pennsylvania

Robert M. Naclerio, M.D.
Professor and Chief
Otolaryngology-Head and Neck Surgery
University of Chicago Pritzker School of Medicine
Chicago, Illinois

Joseph B. Nadol, Jr., M.D.
Walter Augustus Lecompte Professor and Chairman
Department of Otology and Laryngology
Harvard Medical School
Chief of Otolaryngology
Massachusetts Eye and Ear Infirmary
Boston, Massachusetts

Philippe Narcy, M.D.
Professeur of Otorhinology
Universite Paris VII
Chief
Department of Pediatric Otorhinolaryngology
Hopital Robert Debre
Paris, France

Julian Nedzelski, M.D., F.A.C.S. (C)
Otolaryngologist in Chief
Sunnybrook Health Science Centre
Professor and Chairman
Department of Otolaryngology
University of Toronto
Toronto, Ontario, Canada

H. Bryan Neel, III, M.D., Ph.D.
Professor and Past Chairman
Mayo Medical School
Consultant
Mayo Clinic
Rochester, Minnesota

Brock D. Ridenour, M.D.
Assistant Professor and Director
Facial Plastic Surgery Division
Washington University School of Medicine
Barnes-Jewish Hospital
St. Louis, Missouri

K. Thomas Robbins, M.D., F.R.C.S.C., F.A.C.S.
Professor and Chairman
Department of Otolaryngology-Head and Neck Surgery
University of Tennessee, Memphis College of Medicine
Director
Head and Neck Oncology Program
Memphis, Tennessee

William D. Robertson, M.D.
Professor
Department of Radiology
University of Washington Medical Center
Seattle, Washington

Robert A. Robinson, M.D., Ph.D.
Professor
Department of Pathology
University of Iowa College of Medicine
Iowa City, Iowa

J. Thomas Roland, Jr., M.D.
Assistant Professor
Department of Otolaryngology
New York University School of Medicine
Bellevue Hospital
Manhattan VA Medical Center
New York, New York

Anne M. Rompalo, M.D.
Associate Professor
Johns Hopkins University School of Medicine
Johns Hopkins Hospital
Baltimore, Maryland

Richard M. Rosenfeld, M.D., M.P.H.
Associate Professor
Department of Otolaryngology
SUNY Health Science Center at Brooklyn
Director of Pediatric Otolaryngology
University Hospital Brooklyn and The Long Island College Hospital
Brooklyn, New York

Jay T. Rubinstein, M.D., Ph.D.
Assistant Professor
Department of Otolaryngology-Head and Neck Surgery and Physiology and Biophysics
University of Iowa
Iowa City, Iowa

Stephen J. Salzer, M.D.
Clinical Instructor in Surgery
Department of Otolaryngology
Yale University School of Medicine
New Haven, Connecticut

Peter A. Santi, Ph.D.
Professor
Departments of Otolaryngology and Neuroscience
University of Minnesota
Minneapolis, Minnesota

Clarence T. Sasaki, M.D.
Charles W. Ohse Professor
Yale School of Medicine
New Haven, Connecticut

Gordon H. Sasaki, M.D.
Chief, Plastic Surgery Section
St. Luke Medical Center
Pasadena, California

Steven D. Schaefer, M.D.
Professor and Chair
Department of Otolaryngology
New York Medical College
Chair
Department of Otolaryngology
New York Eye and Ear Infirmary and Affiliated Hospitals
Valhalla, New York

David Arthur Schessel, M.D., Ph.D.
Assistant Professor
Department of Otolaryngology and Neurosurgery
George Washington University
Assistant Professor
George Washington University Hospital
Washington, D.C.

David E. Schuller, M.D.
Professor and Chairman
Department of Otolaryngology
The Ohio State University
Director
Arthur G. James Cancer Hospital and Research Institute
Columbus, Ohio

Timothy A. Scott, M.D.
Private Practice
John Muir Hospital
Walnut Creek, California

Roy B. Sessions, M.D.
Professor and Chairman,
Department Otolaryngology-Head and Neck Surgery
Georgetown University
Washington, D.C.

Larry R. Severeid, M.D.
Clinical Assistant Professor
University of Wisconsin-Madison Medical School
Gunderson Clinic
LaCrosse, Wisconsin

Robert V. Shannon, Ph.D.
Head
Department of Auditory Implants and Perception
House Ear Institute
Los Angeles, California

Stanley M. Shapshay M.D., F.A.C.S.
Professor
Department Otolaryngology-Head and Neck Surgery
Tufts University School of Medicine
Otolaryngologist-in-Chief (Chairman)
Tufts-New England Medical Center
Boston, Massachusetts

Pramod K. Sharma, M.D.
Oncologic Surgery Fellow
Department of Otolaryngology
Ohio State University Medical Center
Columbus, Ohio

Clough Shelton, M.D., F.A.C.S.
Associate Professor
University of Utah, School of Medicine
Salt Lake City, Utah

Neil T. Shepard, Ph.D.
Associate Professor
Department of Otolaryngology
University of Michigan Medical School
Director
Vestibular Testing Center
University of Michigan Hospital and Clinics
Ann Arbor, Michigan

David A. Sherris, M.D.
Assistant Professor
Mayo Medical School
Senior Associate Consultant
Mayo Clinic
Rochester, Minnesota

Kevin A. Shumrick, M.D.
Associate Professor
Department of Clinical Otolaryngology
University of Cincinnati College of Medicine
Director
Division of Facial Plastic and Maxillofacial Trauma
University Hospital
Cincinnati, Ohio

Kathleen C.Y. Sie, M.D.
Assistant Professor
Department of Otolaryngology-Head and Neck Surgery
University of Washington School of Medicine
Children's Hospital and Medical Center
Seattle, Washington

Robert W. Seibert, M.D.
Professor
Department of Otolaryngology-Head and Neck Surgery
University of Arkansas for Medical Sciences
Chief, Pediatric Otolaryngology
Arkansas Children's Hospital
Little Rock, Arkansas

Marilyn J. Siegel, M.D.
Professor
Department of Radiology and Pediatrics
Washington University School of Medicine
St. Louis, Missouri

Patricia Silva, M.D.
Clinical Assistant Professor
Department of Radiology
University of Miami School of Medicine
Miami, Florida

Jonas Singer, M.D.
Visiting Professor
Mallinckrudt Institute of Radiology, St. Louis Program
Alton Memorial Hospital
Alton, Illinois

Margaret W. Skinner, Ph.D.
Professor
Director of Adult Cochlear Implant Program
Department of Otolaryngology-Head and Neck Surgery
Washington University School of Medicine
St. Louis, Missouri

Richard J.H. Smith, M.D.
Professor and Vice-Chairman
Department of Otolaryngology-Head and Neck Surgery
University of Iowa College of Medicine
Head
Division of Pediatric Otolaryngology
Director
Molecular Otolaryngology Research Laboratories
Iowa City, Iowa

Gordon B. Snow, M.D.
Professor and Chairman
Department of Otolaryngology-Head and Neck Surgery
Free University Hospital
Amsterdam, Netherlands

Robert C. Sprecher, M.D.
Assistant Professor
Departments of Otolaryngology and Pediatrics
Rainbow Babies and Children's Hospital
Case Western Reserve University
Cleveland, Ohio

Steven J. Staller, Ph.D.
Clinical Studies Manager
Cochlear Corporation
Englewood, Colorado

Robert B. Stanley, Jr., M.D., D.D.S.
Professor
Department of Otolaryngology-Head and Neck Surgery
University of Washington School of Medicine
Chief
Department of Otolaryngology-Head and Neck Surgery
Harborview Medical Center
Seattle, Washington

Patricia G. Stelmachowicz, Ph.D.
Professor
Department of Otolaryngology and Human Communication
Creighton University School of Medicine
Director, Audiological Services
Boys Town National Research Hospital
Omaha, Nebraska

Laura M. Sterni, M.D.
Fellow
Division of Pediatric Pulmonary
Johns Hopkins Children's Center
Baltimore, Maryland

Susan Strauss, M.D.
Assistant Professor
University of Washington
Children's Regional Hospital and Medical Center
Seattle, Washington

Barbara S. Stroer, M.A.
Assistant Professor
Department of Communication Disorders
Fontbonne College
St. Louis, Missouri
Coordinator of Audiology Services
St. Joseph Institute for the Deaf
Chesterfield, Missouri

James Y. Suen, M.D.
Professor and Chairman
Department of Otolaryngology-Head and Neck Surgery
University of Arkansas for Medical Sciences
University Hospital of Arkansas
Little, Arkansas

Gordon W. Summers, D.M.D, M.D.
Department of Otolaryngology-Head and Neck Surgery
Providence Medical Center
Portland, Oregon

Neil A. Swanson, M.D.
Professor and Chair
Department of Dermatology
Professor
Department of Otolaryngology-Head and Neck Surgery
Oregon Health Sciences University
Portland VA Medical Center
Lagacy Emmanuel Medical Center
St. Vincent's Hospital
Portland, Oregon

Jonathan M. Sykes, M.D.
Associate Professor
Facial Plastic Surgery
Department of Otolaryngology/Head and Neck Surgery
University of California, Davis, Medical Center
Sacramento, California

M. Eugene Tardy, Jr., M.D.
Professor
Department of Clinical Otolaryngology
Director, Division of Facial Plastic Surgery
University of Illinois College of Medicine
Chicago, Illinois

Steven A. Telian, M.D.
Associate Professor
University of Michigan Medical Center
Ann Arbor, Michigan

Fred F. Telischi, M.D.
Assistant Professor
Department of Otolaryngology
University of Miami Ear Institute
Miami, Florida

Jeffrey E. Terrell, M.D.
Assistant Professor
University of Michigan Medical Center
Ann Arbor, Michigan

Stanley E. Thawley, M.D.
Associate Professor
Department of Otolaryngology
Washington University School of Medicine
Chief Adult Division Department of Otolaryngology
Barnes-Jewish Hospital
St. Louis, Missouri

J. Regan Thomas, M.D.
Professor and Chairman
Department of Otolaryngology-Head and Neck Surgery
St. Louis University School of Medicine
Director
The Facial Plastic Surgery Center
St. Louis, Missouri

James N. Thompson, M.D.
Dean
Wake Forest University
Bowman Gray School of Medicine
North Carolina Baptist Hospital
Winston-Salem, North Carolina

R. David Tomlinson, Ph.D.
Associate Professor
Departments of Otolaryngology, Physiology, and Medicine
University of Toronto
Toronto, Ontario, Canada

Dean M. Toriumi, M.D.
Associate Professor
Division of Facial Plastic and Reconstructive Surgery
Department of Otolaryngology-Head and Neck Surgery
University of Illinois College of Medicine
Chicago, Illinois

Joseph B. Travers, Ph.D.
Associate Professor
Department of Oral Biology
Ohio State University College of Dentistry
Columbus, Ohio

David E. Tunkel, M.D.
Associate Professor
Department of Otolaryngology-Head and Neck Surgery and Pediatrics
Johns Hopkins University School of Medicine
Director
Division of Pediatric Otolaryngology
Johns Hopkins Hospital and Outpatient Center
Baltimore, Maryland

Mark L. Urken, M.D., F.A.C.S.
Professor and Chairman
Mt. Sinai School of Medicine
Mt. Sinai Medical Center
New York, New York

Thierry Van Den Abbeele, M.D.
Chef de Clinique
Faculte de Medecine Bichat
Assistant
Service D'or Pediatrique
Hopital Robert Debre
Paris, France

Isaäc van der Waal, D.D.S., Ph.D.
Head
Department of Oral Maxillofacial Surgery Pathology
Professor
Department of Oral Pathology
Hospital of the Free University
Amsterdam, Netherlands

Mark A. Varvares, M.D.
Instructor
Department of Otolaryngology and Laryngology
Harvard Medical School
Massachusetts Eye and Ear Infirmary
Boston, Massachusetts

David L. Walner, M.D.
Assistant Professor
Rush-Presbyterian St. Luke's Medical Center
Chicago, Illinois

Harrison G. Weed, M.D.
Assistant Professor
Department of Internal Medicine
Ohio State University College of Medicine
Arthur G. James Cancer Hospital and Research Institute
Columbus, Ohio

Mark S. Weinberger, M.D.
Clinical Instructor
University of Illinois at Chicago
Fellow
Facial Plastic and Reconstructive Surgery
University of Illinois Eye and Ear Infirmary
Chicago, Illinois

Gregory S. Weinstein, M.D.
Assistant Professor
Department of Otorhinolaryngology-Head and Neck Surgery
University of Pennsylvania
Philadelphia, Pennsylvania

Ralph F. Wetmore, M.D.
Associate Professor
Department of Otorhinolaryngology-Head and Neck Surgery
University of Pennsylvania School of Medicine
Children's Hospital of Philadelphia
Philadelphia, Pennsylvania

Ernest A. Weymuller, Jr., M.D.
Professor and Chairman
Department Otolaryngology-Head and Neck Surgery
University of Washington School of Medicine
Seattle, Washington

Brian J. Wiatrak, M.D.
Associate Professor
Department of Surgery and Pediatrics
University of Alabama School of Medicine
Chief of Pediatric Otolaryngology
Children's Hospital of Alabama
Birmingham, Alabama

Gregory J. Wiet, M.S., M.D.
Fellow
Department of Pediatric Otolaryngology
University of Arkansas for Medical Sciences
Arkansas Children's Hospital
Little Rock, Arkansas

Ewain P. Wilson, M.B., B.Ch.
Assistant Professor
Director, Head and Neck Surgical Oncology
West Virginia University School of Medicine
Morgantown, West Virginia

Franz J. Wippold, II, M.D.
Associate Professor
Mallinckrodt Institute of Radiology
Washington University School of Medicine
Barnes-Jewish Hospital
St. Louis Children's Hospital
St. Louis, Missouri

Gregory T. Wolf, M.D.
Professor and Chair
Department of Otolaryngology
University of Michigan Medical School
Ann Arbor, Michigan

Gayle Ellen Woodson, M.D., F.A.C.S., F.R.C.S.C.
Professor
Department of Otolaryngology-Head and Neck Surgery
Director
Voice Disorder Clinic
University of Tennessee
Memphis, Tennessee

Audie L. Woolley, M.D.
Assistant Professor
Division of Otolaryngology-Head and Neck Surgery
University of Alabama School of Medicine
Birmingham, Alabama

Eiji Yanagisawa, M.D.
Clinical Professor
Department of Otolaryngology
Yale University School of Medicine
New Haven, Connecticut

Charles D. Yingling, Ph.D.
Director
Neurophysiologic Monitoring Service
University of California San Francisco Medical Center
San Francisco, California

Christine Yoshinaga-Itano, Ph.D.
Associate Professor
Department of Speech, Language, and Hearing Sciences
University of Colorado, Boulder
Boulder, Colorado

George H. Zalzal, M.D.
Associate Professor
Department of Otolaryngology and Pediatrics
George Washington University
Chairman
Department of Otolaryngology
Children's National Medical Center
Washington, D.C.

David S. Zee, M.D.
Departments of Neurology, Otolaryngology-Head and Neck Surgery and Ophthalmology
Johns Hopkins University School of Medicine
Baltimore, Maryland

S. James Zinreich, M.D.
Associate Professor
Johns Hopkins Medical Institution
Baltimore, Maryland

Teresa A. Zwolan, Ph.D.
Director and Assistant
Cochlear Implant Program
Research Scientist
University of Michigan Medical Center
Ann Arbor, Michigan

Preface

Otolaryngology—Head and Neck Surgery was created to fill the needs for a contemporary, definitive textbook on the specialty of otolaryngology-head and neck surgery. The scope of the third edition is a testimonial to the tremendous expansion of knowledge in this specialty. Our desire is to record this expansion in a retrievable fashion so that these volumes become indispensable reference works. The third edition builds on the success of the past two editions. The reader will note new algorithms and boxed lists which serve to enhance learning.

The field of otolaryngology-head and neck surgery is represented in all of its diversity; the extensive interrelationship of its various components provided the skeleton for the table of contents. These volumes are intended as a detailed reference text and not as a surgical atlas: a definitive work, not an introductory overview. It is designed for residents and practitioners alike. We hope that our quest to document significant and up-to-date information in the specialty has been successful.

Another of our goals throughout the pages of this textbook is to acknowledge all those who have contributed to the specialty. Since significant medical expertise has no geographic boundaries, there are contributors from countries all over the world. Recognizing the unique aspects of pediatric otolaryngology-head and neck surgery, the editors have created an additional volume edited by Mark A. Richardson. This freestanding resource meets the global criteria of the comprehensive textbook.

To ensure continuity at the editorship level, Drs. Paul Flint, Bruce Haughey, K. Thomas Robbins, and J. Regan Thomas have assumed associate editorship roles in this expanded effort. It is hoped that the ecumenicism which combines the effort of all the contributors will further the excellence of those now associated with otolaryngology-head and neck surgery and provide the foundation for continued progress by the generations to follow. This third edition builds on the success of the first two. It is more comprehensive, is of broader scope, and continues the tradition established 11 years ago.

Acknowledgments

The editors of these volumes wish to acknowledge the individuals who have contributed immeasurably to the successful completion of our task; most specifically, the contributors to these many pages. These authors were specifically selected by the editorial board to ensure the presence of the most contemporary thinking on their respective topics. The expertise of all of these individuals provides for this book's infinite potential.

In addition, we wish to thank all the employees at Mosby–Year Book, Inc. This is a truly first rate organization. Special mention should be made of the efforts of Robert Hurley and Lauranne Billus for this current edition as well as those of Anne Patterson and Carol Trumbold, so instrumental in the past success. Most certainly those who contributed time, words, and expertise to this edition should be thanked collectively as well as individually.

Acknowledgments

I would like to acknowledge my father for enabling me to survive comfortably during my seemingly endless years of education. As well, my wife, Jane, and my family who have recognized the importance of and supported the mission that resulted in, this resource for Otolaryngology Head and Neck Surgery. I would also like to acknowledge the students and residents who are a constant source of motivation and the patients who served as the fuel that energized this project. Through their coping with illness we are constantly aware that our search for resolution of illness must continue.

Charles W. Cummings

Once again, it has been great fun working with my co-editors. As this is my last contribution as co-editor, I will miss the fellowship which has grown over the years. I thank the authors for their excellent work and our Mosby colleagues for their diligence and professionalism. Foremost, I thank my partner, Alix, and with love, I dedicate my contribution to her and our children, Kristin, Lisa, and Erik.

John M. Fredrickson

Scientific knowledge is fleeting; part of what we know today is true, and part soon will be disproven or rendered obsolete. Galen was as right in his day as we are today. The authors of volume four have done a superb job of expressing today's knowledge. I thank them for that and for responding to my suggestions and prodding. Thanks are also extended to Dr. Patrick Brookhouser at Boy's Town National Research Hospital for his encouragement and support. My contribution to this volume is dedicated with love to my wife, Jill, my mother, my late father, and to Elizabeth, Robert, and Alexa.

Lee A. Harker

I would like to dedicate my contribution to these volumes to my wife, Barbara, and our children, Sharon, John, and Ann, for their encouragement and support throughout this lengthy endeavor; and to my parents, William and Ruby Krause, who committed so much more of their lives to their children. I would like to thank my administrative secretary, Linda Edberg Diebold, for her effort, her patience, and the very considerable skill with which she assisted on this project.

Charles J. Krause

It has been a special opportunity to continue to be involved with the original authors who have demonstrated tremendous dedication to maintaining the highest standards for this textbook. All of the students, residents, fellows, and patients certainly provide a strong motivation to be actively involved in life-long learning activities. But Carole, Becky, and Mike have continued to be my strongest supporters. My involvement is dedicated to them as an expression of my love as well as to my parents, Daniel and Elsie, who instilled in me the enjoyment of learning. I would also like to express appreciation for the excellent support and patience provided by Debra O. Parker, administrator of our head and neck oncology program, as we jointly worked to meet the numerous deadlines.

David E. Schuller

This volume represents the cooperative efforts of many who we think have created a sum greater than any of its component parts. My special thanks go to the senior editors, Drs. Cummings, Fredrickson, Harker, Krause, and Schuller for the opportunity to participate in their reference work in otolaryngology and their guidance in editorship. Also, the individual contributors who have provided so much time and work to produce this volume and without whom it would not exist. The editorial staff, including Bob Hurley, Lauranne Billus, Marla Sussman, Jori Matison, Susie Coladonato, and Stacy Loonstyn who kept me and the volume on track. Especially my wife Ellen, daughters Caroline and Abigail, who are a never ending source of inspiration and support, and my mother and father who enabled me to pursue medicine and otolaryngology as a career.

Mark A. Richardson

Volume Two
NOSE

PARANASAL SINUSES

SALIVARY GLANDS

ORAL CAVITY/OROPHARYNX/NASOPHARYNX

SKULL BASE

Volume Five
PEDIATRIC OTOLARYNGOLOGY

COLOR PLATES
Anatomic:

Color plates:

Chapter 1

General Considerations

Mark A. Richardson

The specialty pediatric otolaryngology within the realm of otolaryngology is helping to bridge the gap between a surgical discipline and pediatric medicine. This trend began with pediatric surgery, was followed by pediatric anesthesiology, and is continuing with ophthalmology, urology, and other surgical subspecialties.

Almost every surgeon practices pediatric otolaryngology at times: the cancer surgeon who treats childhood lymphomas, the otologist who corrects aural atresia, and the facial plastic surgeon who deals with children's nasal fractures are all involved in the care and treatment of pediatric head and neck disorders. An estimated 25% to 50% of a general otolaryngologist's practice may be related to pediatric problems. Consequently, the subspecialty of pediatric otolaryngology is becoming increasingly important in training programs. Learning about the special problems facing children, the approach to treatment in this population, and special considerations related to diagnosis and surgical management is a vital part of any otolaryngology residency. The development of neonatal and pediatric intensive care units has led to an increased demand for management of disorders encountered in this population, including intubation trauma, bronchoesophagology, infectious diseases, and congenital malformations.

One difference between pediatric and adult medicine is that although the patient is being treated, the parents must also be included in the initial evaluation. Both the parents and the child must have confidence in the surgeon, must understand the procedures being performed, and in many cases, must supply the history related to the illness. Complicating this situation is the fact that explanations, questions, and rapport must be directed to two very different levels of maturity.

Physiologic differences between infants, children, and adults have occupied major research efforts and complete textbooks. The following introductory comments are meant to point out the differences among neonates, infants, children, and adults and should be used as a starting point for further investigation.

RESPIRATORY SYSTEM

Control of ventilation

Observations of neonatal control of ventilation are difficult to interpret. The intervention necessary to obtain measurements, such as the placing of a mask on the face or a tube into the larynx, may itself induce a change in the ventilation. In addition, the use of measurements of ventilation to assess respiratory drive is based on the assumption that the respiratory muscles are performing optimally to convert this drive into work—and that may not be the case in neonates or infants.

The newborn's muscles are subject to fatigue, a tendency that is determined by the types of muscle fibers present. In preterm infants, less than 10% of the fibers in the diaphragm are type I (i.e., slow twitch, highly oxidative, fatigue-resistant). In full-term infants, 30% of these fibers are type I, and the percentage increases to 55% (approximately the adult level) during the first year of life. The preterm infant is thus prone to ventilatory muscle fatigue, a predisposition that disappears progressively with advancing maturity. Changes that occur during changing sleep states also affect ventilation. Preterm infants spend 50% to 60% of the time in rapid eye movement (REM) sleep, during which intercostal muscle activity is inhibited and paradoxic movement of the soft chest wall occurs. This lack of intercostal activity is compensated for by an increase in diaphragmatic activity, much of which is wasted when the ribs move paradoxically and which may lead to diaphragmatic fatigue.

Control of ventilation, which involves biochemical and reflex mechanisms, is at least partially developed in healthy, full-term neonates. The ventilatory response to increased concentrations of carbon dioxide is proportionately similar to that of adults; however, ventilation relative to body mass is greater for any given partial pressure of carbon dioxide (Pco_2), reflecting a higher metabolic rate. The response of preterm infants to a specific inspired carbon dioxide level is less than that in adults. Newborns are also sensitive to changes in arterial oxygen tension. Administration of 100% oxygen decreases ventilation, indicating the existence of chemoreceptor activity.

Many factors modify the ventilatory response of newborns to hypoxia, including gestational and postnatal age, body temperature, and sleep state. Preterm and full-term infants younger than 1 week of age who are awake and normothermic usually demonstrate a biphasic response: ventilatory depression preceded by a brief period of hyperpnea. Hypothermic infants respond to hypoxia with ventilatory depression without initial hyperpnea. This depression of ventilation is thought to be caused by the central effects of hypoxia on the respiratory center. The peripheral chemoreceptors that are shown to be active in newborns are presumably unable to maintain a significant influence over this response. Infants may be even less responsive to hypoxia during REM sleep. During non-REM sleep, however, increased ventilation is sustained. The arousal response to hypoxia during sleep is not seen in newborns but normally develops over the first few weeks of life. Infants older than 1 week demonstrate hyperpnea in response to hypoxia, probably because of the maturing of chemoreceptor function. Hypoxia that occurs during sleep usually results in awakening. During hypoxia the ventilatory response to carbon dioxide is depressed in newborns, in contrast to that in infants and adults.

Reflexes arising from the lung and chest wall are probably more important in maintaining ventilation in newborns, primarily determining the respiratory tidal volume. Periodic breathing, which consists of rapid ventilation alternating with periods of apnea, occurs in many preterm and some full-term infants and is thought to result from incoordination of feedback loops controlling ventilation. During episodes of periodic breathing, arterial Pco_2 level is above normal but heart rate does not change significantly.

Periodic breathing seems to have no serious physiologic consequences and usually ceases by 6 years of age. Some preterm infants demonstrate far more serious and indeed life-threatening episodes of apnea. These episodes commonly exceed 20 seconds and are accompanied by bradycardia. Apneic episodes may represent an example of the failure of the response to hypoxia. Because many apneic episodes occur during REM sleep, ventilatory muscle fatigue as well as an impaired chemoreceptor response to hypoxemia may be etiologic factors. Usually stimulation of the infant easily terminates apneic episodes. The incidence of apneic episodes is decreased by therapy with aminophylline, which provides central stimulation, or by the institution of continuous positive airway pressure, which causes increased activity of lung and chest wall reflexes.

Laryngospasm

A laryngeal adductor response can be elicited in juvenile animals with stimulation of fibers of the superior laryngeal nerve. Coupled with apnea, tachycardia, and hypertension, this response is remarkably similar to the clinical entity of laryngospasm and is termed the *laryngeal chemoreflex* (LCR). The LCR can be stimulated by acid, base, and pressure but is most sensitive to water and is ablated by saline. Experimentally, the LCR can cause death in susceptible animals, which may have implications for sudden infant death syndrome (SIDS). Deaths attributed to SIDS have diminished as a result of a change in the recommended sleeping position from prone to supine. A proposed mechanism is the elimination of rebreathing causing hypercarbia, a factor that is known to potentiate the LCR.

Lung volumes

In full-term infants, total lung capacity is approximately 160 ml, with functional residual capacity at about half this volume. Tidal volume is approximately 16 ml, and dead space volume is about 5 ml. In proportion to body size, all of these volumes are similar to the values in adults; however, any increase in dead space is much more significant when related to the small volumes in infants. In contrast to the static lung volumes, alveolar ventilation is proportionately much larger in newborns (100 to 150 ml/kg of body weight) than in adults (60 ml/kg of body weight). This high alveolar ventilation in infants results in a much higher alveolar: functional residual capacity ratio of 5 : 1 compared with 1.5 : 1 in adults. Consequently, the functional residual capacity is a much less effective buffer in infants, so that changes in the concentration of inspired gases are much more rapidly reflected in alveolar and arterial levels.

The total surface area of the air–tissue interface of the alveoli in infants is small (2.8 m^2). When this area is related to the metabolic rate for oxygen, infants (who are dependent on a smaller air–tissue interface: oxygen metabolic ratio than adults) have a reduced reserve capability for gas exchange. This difference may have significance if congenital defects interfere with lung growth or if the lungs become damaged. The remaining healthy lung tissue may be inadequate to sustain life.

Respiratory rate

In newborns approximately 37 breaths per minute has been calculated to be the most efficient respiratory rate; and this is close to the rate observed in healthy newborns. Full-term infants are similar to adults, requiring approximately 1% of their metabolic energy to maintain ventilation; the oxygen cost of breathing is 0.5 ml per 0.5 l of ventilation. Preterm infants have a higher oxygen cost of breathing (0.9

ml/0.5 l), which is greatly increased if the lungs are diseased. This increased "cost" of respiration also necessitates higher caloric and nutritional demands.

Ventilation–perfusion relationships

Ventilation and perfusion are imperfectly matched in neonatal lungs. The normal arterial oxygen tension in a newborn infant breathing room air is about 50 mm Hg. The tension increases to 70 mm Hg by 24 hours of age. The high alveolar–arterial oxygen difference in infants is also caused by persisting anatomic shunts and the relatively high closing volume (Table 1-1).

CARDIOVASCULAR SYSTEM

Newborn heart and cardiac output

In healthy neonates the thickness of the right ventricle exceeds that of the left wall; this preponderance is evident in the electrocardiogram, which shows an axis of up to 180° during the first week of life. After birth the left ventricle enlarges disproportionately. At approximately 6 months of age, the adult ventricular size ratio is established. During the immediate newborn period the heart rate is between 100 and 170 beats per minute and the rhythm is regular. As the child grows, the heart rate gradually decreases (Table 1-2).

Sinus arrhythmia is common in children. All other irregular rhythms should be considered abnormal. Systolic blood pressure is approximately 60 mm Hg in full-term newborns, and diastolic pressure is approximately 35 mm Hg. These pressures vary considerably, however, increasing by 10 to 15 mm Hg if clamping of the umbilical cord is delayed or if the cord is stripped. In either case the pressures fall to normal limits within 4 hours. Preterm infants have lower blood pressures (as low as 46/25 in a 750-g baby).

The myocardium of newborns contains less contractile tissue and more connective tissue than exists in the adult heart. Consequently, neonatal ventricles are less compliant when relaxed and generate less tension during contraction. Because the low compliance of the relaxed ventricle tends to limit the size of the stroke volume, the cardiac output of newborns is rate-dependent; bradycardia is invariably accompanied by reduced cardiac output. The autonomic innervation of the heart is incomplete in newborns, with a relative lack of sympathetic elements. This may further compromise the ability of the less contractile neonatal myocardium to respond to stress.

Blood volume

Blood volume varies considerably during the immediate postnatal period, depending on the amount of blood drained from the placenta before the cord is clamped. Delay in clamping or stripping the cord, as mentioned previously, may increase the blood volume by over 20%, resulting in transient respiratory distress. Conversely, fetal hypoxia during labor causes vasoconstriction and a shift of the blood to the placental circulation. Thus asphyxiated neonates may be hypovolemic.

The response to hypovolemia and restoration of the blood volume is of great importance to the surgeon because significant blood loss often accompanies surgery in newborns. Withdrawal of blood during exchange transfusion has been demonstrated to cause a progressive parallel decline in systolic blood pressure and cardiac output. Reinfusion of an equal volume of blood restores these parameters to their original values. Changes in arterial blood pressure are thus proportional to the degree of hypovolemia. A newborn's capacity to adapt the intravascular volume to the available blood volume is very limited, perhaps as a result of less efficient control of capacitance vessels. The baroreflexes of infants, especially preterm infants, are not fully active, further compromising the response to hypovolemia.

The infant's systolic arterial blood pressure is closely related to his or her circulating blood volume. Blood pressure is therefore an excellent guide to the adequacy of blood or fluid replacement during anesthesia, a fact that has been amply confirmed by extensive clinical experience.

Response to hypoxia

Because of a high metabolic rate for oxygen, hypoxemia can develop rapidly in neonates, in whom the first observed response is usually bradycardia. During surgery the anesthesiologist should treat any episode of unexplained bradycardia by immediately ventilating the patient with 100% oxygen. During hypoxemia pulmonary vasoconstriction occurs and pulmonary artery pressure increases more than in adults. Changes in cardiac output and systemic vascular resistance

Table 1-1. Arterial oxygen tension (Po_2) in healthy infants and children

Age	Po_2 room air
0-1 week	70
1-10 months	85
4-8 years	90
12-16 years	96

Table 1-2. Heart rate (beats/minute)

Age	Average	Range
Newborn	120	100-170
1-11 months	120	80-160
2 years	120	80-160
4 years	100	80-120
6 years	100	75-115
10 years	90	70-110

in infants also differ from those in older children and adults. During hypoxemia in adults the principal response is systemic vasodilatation, which, together with an increased cardiac output, helps to maintain oxygen transport to the tissues. Fetuses and some neonates respond to hypoxemia with systemic vasoconstriction. During fetal life this vasoconstriction directs more blood to the placenta. After birth, however, this response may reduce cardiac output, thereby further limiting oxygen transport and forcing the heart to work harder. In infants, early and pronounced bradycardia (in response to hypoxia) may be caused by myocardial hypoxia and acidosis.

Neonates exposed to hypoxemia suffer pulmonary and systemic vasoconstriction, bradycardia, and a decrease in cardiac output. Rapid intervention is necessary to prevent this state from proceeding to cardiac arrest.

Blood volume and oxygen transport

Neonatal blood volume is approximately 80 ml/kg at term and about 20% higher in preterm infants. The hematocrit is approximately 60%, and the hemoglobin content is 18 to 19 g per 100 ml. The values for blood volume, hematocrit, and hemoglobin content vary from infant to infant, depending on when the umbilical cord is clamped. Little change in these values occurs during the first week of life, after which the hemoglobin level starts to fall. This change occurs more rapidly in preterm infants.

Approximately 70% to 90% of the hemoglobin present at full-term birth is of the fetal type. The affinity of fetal hemoglobin for oxygen is greater than that of adult hemoglobin. Thus fetal hemoglobin combines with more oxygen but releases it less readily in the tissues than does adult hemoglobin. Adequate oxygen transport to the tissues of newborn infants therefore demands a higher hemoglobin concentration. Less than 12 g per 100 ml constitutes anemia, and higher levels are very desirable in hypoxic states. Correction of anemia by blood transfusion is indicated if the infant requires oxygen therapy or is experiencing apneic episodes.

During the first weeks of life the hemoglobin and hematocrit levels decline steadily as a result of early suppression of erythropoiesis with improved tissue oxygenation and a progressive increase in blood volume. This physiologic anemia in infancy reaches a low point at 2 to 3 months of age, with a hemoglobin level of 9 to 11 g per 100 ml. By this time the fetal hemoglobin content has been largely replaced by adult hemoglobin, and as a result oxygen delivery at the tissues is improved. Provided nutrition is adequate, the hemoglobin level then gradually increases over several weeks to 12 to 13 g per 100 ml, which is maintained during early childhood.

FLUIDS AND FLUID MANAGEMENT

Operative and postoperative fluid management in children should follow the same principles used in adults: replacement of maintenance requirements and correction of any existing deficits. Physiologic differences among neonates, infants, older children, and adults make fluid administration more critical. Because of their small intravascular volume (70 to 80 ml/kg), children can essentially become dehydrated or excessively hydrated very easily. Compartmentalization of total body water varies with age; electrolyte composition remains relatively stable.

	Na+	*K+*
Intracellular	10 mEq	150 mEq
Extracellular	140 mEq	4.5 mEq

Deciding the maintenance requirements for any child can be based on relatively simple formulae, which vary according to metabolic and physical activity. The basis for water utilization in caloric expenditure under normal conditions at bed rest is the following:

0 to 10 kg	100 cal/kg
10 to 20 kg	50 cal/kg
>20 kg	20 cal/kg

(Increase 12% for each degree centigrade above normal and increase 0% to 50% for varying increased activity or metabolic rate.)

The calculation of water loss per calorie can be based as follows:

Urine	55 ml/100 cal
Insensible loss	
via lungs	15 ml/100 cal
via skin	30 ml/100 cal
Adding up to	100 ml/100 cal

Therefore, with milliliters proportional to calories, the following correspondences exist:

1 to 10 kg	100 ml/kg
10 to 20 kg	50 ml/kg
>20 kg	20 ml/kg

As an example, following are maintenance water requirements for a 17-kg child at bed rest with normal temperature and metabolism:

first 10 kg = 10 kg × 100 ml/kg = 1000 ml
second 7 kg = 7 kg × 50 ml/kg = 350 ml
Total 1350 ml
maintenance water requirement every 24 hours

Following are maintenance electrolyte requirements:

3 mEq Na+/100 ml H_2O
2 mEq K+/100 ml H_2O

Discussion of complex deficits has not been undertaken in this chapter; in most cases these problems require pediatric medical assistance.

PAIN MANAGEMENT

It is commonly believed that newborns and infants do not experience pain because of their immature nervous systems and that they do not have any memory of pain if it does take place. We now know that the neurophysiologic pathways for nociception are developed in premature babies and that newborns respond to noxious stimuli with well-categorized behavioral and physiologic changes suggestive of substantial stress and distress.

Pain certainly is both a sensory and an emotional experience that may be altered by various psychologic factors. These factors may be specific for each individual based on the individual's expectations and past experiences. It is clear that many of the procedures performed in the office, and certainly in the surgical suite, will induce pain in children. A management plan must be used in order to reduce this pain. Efforts to reduce stress, anxiety, and fear, which commonly amplify the pain experience, can be expected to decrease the distress associated with acute or chronic pain. In patients of the appropriate age, relaxation techniques such as guided imagery, breathing techniques, and hypnosis may diminish the emotional component of pain.

Nonnarcotic analgesics such as oral acetaminophen in doses ranging from 10 to 15 mg/kg every 4 hours are useful in patients of all ages. In older children and adolescents, ibuprofen (4 to 8 mg/kg per dose every 6 hours) and naproxen (5 to 7 mg/kg every 8 to 12 hours) may be more effective than acetaminophen. Ketorolac is a newer nonsteroidal antiinflammatory agent with excellent analgesic properties that can be used in children. Ketorolac has been shown to prolong bleeding time and should be used with caution when hemostasis is a significant concern.

Narcotic analgesics are indicated for moderate to severe pain in patients of all ages; however, optimal use requires consideration of the needs of individual patients. Neonates require special care in the administration of narcotics. They have diminished ventilatory responses to hypoxia and hypercarbia; and they also have pharmacokinetic differences, including prolonged elimination half-life, diminished clearance, and increased permeability of the blood–brain barrier. The use of oral narcotics for postoperative pain may be safe when used in the appropriate dosages and if signs of toxicity are monitored carefully. In certain instances, when available, patient-controlled anesthesia can be used as it is in adults. This permits adolescent inpatients to self-dose pain and provides improved pain control.

SEDATION

The use of sedation for outpatient examinations, including computed tomography scanning, magnetic resonance imaging, and audiologic evaluations, is becoming increasingly common. Although this in itself is not dangerous, preparations should be made in advance for complications secondary to the use of sedation. In a patient with large tonsils and adenoids, a simple agent such as chloral hydrate may produce intermittent obstructive apnea requiring active airway management. The use of midazolam, diazepam, or other more potent sedative agents may produce apnea or respiratory depression requiring positive-pressure ventilation with oxygen. Any office or radiologic suite that uses sedation to facilitate examinations of children should use appropriate monitoring equipment and be prepared for the resultant complications if they occur.

REFERRAL SOURCES

Pediatric patients are referred to otolaryngologists in a variety of ways, such as members of a family previously treated, as friends of other patients who are satisfied with services the physician has provided, or as referrals from other physicians. By far the most common referral source is pediatricians. Pediatric medicine is a specialty that legitimately considers itself to be the child's advocate. This specialty has also earned the respect given to any group representing a special body of knowledge within the field of medicine. The pediatrician may serve as a consultant for preoperative planning or postoperative management for children with complicated illnesses, such as endocrine or other metabolic disorders; for psychiatric problems related to that particular patient, or for interfamily difficulties that may affect the patient's reaction both to surgery and the hospital experience.

A delineation of duties should always be established between the otolaryngologist and the referral source. Although all of those involved must understand that the surgeon is ultimately responsible for the care of any patient undergoing surgery, a decision to proceed with surgery should always be accepted by the parent as well as by the referral source. Difficult situations can sometimes arise when the patient or parents have been led to believe that a certain surgical procedure will be performed before they have discussed the issue with the surgeon. In these cases, how a decision has been made must be explained clearly and logically; all parties must clearly understand the steps leading to that logical conclusion. Mutual respect, open lines of communication, and a sincere desire to do what is best for the patient should allow for the best possible result from the management of any pediatric head or neck disorder.

PATIENTS

Children are certainly different from adults, not only in age but in maturity, shyness, and other factors. All children, however, should be shown the same rights, dignity, and respect given to adults. The first thing the author tries to establish when entering the examination room is a rapport with the child, not by approaching him or her immediately but by an introduction to the parents and the child in a friendly and open manner. Whether the patient is a neonate or an adolescent, he or she needs to sense or understand that the physician is not someone who is going to inflict pain or punishment but instead someone who is going to help him or her feel better. Once an introduction has been made, the patient can generally be involved in a conversation regarding siblings, pets, or activities at home—putting the patient further at ease and allowing the physician to continue the examination. Seeing the physician involved with the child also puts the parents at ease and allows them to be comfortable during their initial contact with the physician. The child is always examined with a parent in the room and, in the case of an infant or young child, sitting on the parent's lap if possible. Parents are sometimes asked at the request of the patient to leave the room, although that is unusual. Most children are more secure with family present.

The physician continues to engage the child in conversation during the examination, explaining in advance everything that is going to happen to him or her in a clear and straightforward way. If a particular portion of the examination is uncomfortable or unpleasant, delaying it until the end is preferable. In some cases the child may be excessively frightened or crying, and completing an examination may be impossible. If this is the case, and the child is old enough to reason with or remember the experience, the preferred approach is usually to ask the parents to return with the child at another time to try and repeat the examination. If the patient is an infant or young child, proceeding with the examination as speedily as possible is preferred.

Quickness and experience allow for a brief but relatively complete examination without undue stress on the child or parent. Restraining an older child who may be traumatized by a forceful examination is wrong and could be dangerous. In these cases, sedation may be used to complete the examination if necessary.

PARENTS

The parents of an ill child are already under a dramatic amount of stress, and dealing with them can sometimes be difficult. A great deal of experience is required to be able to allay parents' fears and misconceptions regarding the nature of their child's illness and surgery, if surgery will be performed. Fortunately, in most cases a referral source has named a physician as an expert who can deal with their child's problem. In addition, at the initial meeting with the parents and child, establishing a rapport with the child quickly fills the parents with additional confidence in the specialist's skills.

Allowing additional time is advisable when dealing with new patients and their parents so that complete explanations can be given as to the nature of the illness, the prognosis, the way in which surgery is technically performed, and the expected outcome. The child is allowed to stay in the room during this explanation to allay any fears that he or she might have regarding an upcoming hospitalization. During this discussion it is important to remember that the anesthesiologist or other consultant should represent the final word within the realm of his or her specialty.

At the end of the meeting the parents should clearly understand and agree with the need for surgery. This is easily accomplished in emergency situations in which choices are limited, but in elective cases it may be more difficult for parents to commit their child to a procedure that undoubtedly carries some associated risk. The guilt over making such a decision can be difficult to overcome, and the surgeon must not place him- or herself in the position of persuading the parents to allow their child to undergo surgery. All preexisting notions about any upcoming surgery are colored by a friend's or relative's experience, and the surgeon must understand that experience to combat any misconceptions that might arise about the procedure. Urging patients to consider a decision at home and to call back if they want to schedule surgery is advisable.

Congenital abnormalities

When dealing with children who have congenital abnormalities or sensorineural hearing loss, the otolaryngologist must be very careful in approaching the parents so as not to present information that is contradictory to what they have already been told by their primary care provider. Most parents of a child with a congenital abnormality have unexpressed guilt related to their child's maldevelopment, which can lead to anger, confusion, and denial on their part.

Explaining as clearly as possible the origin of any abnormality, its eventual prognosis, and the fact that quick and easy solutions are generally not available is important. Parents should understand that problems must be faced as they arise, and difficulties encountered must be shared with the physician and other healthcare professionals; the physician, as a consultant, will thus be able to correct or help the parents adapt to their child's difficulty.

At one time genetic counseling was routinely advised for all children with congenital abnormalities. The feeling today is that genetic counseling should be offered only to parents who desire it. Other than speaking in general terms of the inheritable nature of sensorineural deafness, cleft palate, or whatever the problem, the physician should not force the parents to face information that they do not wish to acknowledge. The denial phase is related to their eventual acceptance of the child's problem; once they have adapted to the child's abnormality, the parents are much more receptive to genetic counseling.

The parents should understand that any developmental or hereditary abnormality generally requires a team of physicians or healthcare professionals to evaluate and manage. In addition to a surgeon's expertise, a child with a cleft lip or palate will need speech therapy, audiometric evaluations, and dental care to provide for optimal remediation. For more complex craniofacial abnormalities, additional team members (e.g., a neurosurgeon or plastic surgeon) are required in addition to the pediatrician or developmentalist. These individuals can help to ensure that appropriate milestones are being reached.

HISTORY

The history is generally obtained from the child's parent. Hearing how events occurred in the parent's own words is important, starting with the first symptom or problem. To accept the diagnosis made by another physician is all too easy and unfortunately is sometimes wrong. Further questioning of the parents and child may elicit additional specifics regarding the illness. Parents are generally extremely astute regarding the symptoms that their child develops during the course of an illness, and their comments should be taken at face value and not be disregarded. Also, children may have difficulty expressing their complaints but should be believed until their symptoms can be properly defined.

It is also important to obtain a general family history as well as a history of any diseases or illnesses affecting the patient's siblings. Information regarding the pregnancy and delivery of the child should be obtained along with (if possible) some insight into any family stresses or school problems that might be influencing the child's psychosocial development.

PHYSICAL EXAMINATION

After the surgeon has established him- or herself as a nonthreatening person, the physical examination is often accomplished quite easily. Otoscopy is generally managed without difficulty, especially after the physician explains that the otoscope is merely a light used to look in the ears. Sometimes insufflation is used to check the movement of the tympanic membrane; this should not cause any discomfort or pain. Nasal examination is accomplished with the otoscope and a speculum larger than the traditional nasal speculum, which is a fearful object to some children. The oral examination is best accompanied without a tongue depressor, although a tongue depressor may be necessary to view the posterior pharynx in some patients. Palpation of the neck can be accomplished without significant discomfort, and any notation of masses or tenderness can be made. During the examination further observation of the child's facial features can be made, making sure that the ears appear normal, no preauricular pits or other fistulas are present, the eyes are symmetric, and no apparent hypertelorism or heterochromic iris exists. Additional aspects to check are that the external nose appears to be within normal limits, that the child is breathing adequately through the nose and does not seem to be a chronic mouth-breather, that no abnormalities exist within the palate, that there are no dental abnormalities, and that the patient seems to be breathing easily and without stridor. Auscultation of the neck and chest is generally performed, and any obvious deformities of the extremities, abdomen, and so forth are searched for. The otolaryngologist certainly concentrates the physical examination on the particular area of interest, which is the head and neck; however, a general physical examination should be performed in a brief but complete manner.

SPECIAL CONSIDERATIONS

Microscopic examination of the ear

On the initial visit, every patient is subjected to a microscopic examination of the ear. Details regarding the condition of the tympanic membrane, its movement, and the presence of any fluid or infection can be determined more accurately by the otomicroscope than by any other means. It is also the best means available to assist the physician in cleaning debris and wax from the ear to allow for more complete visualization. Most children permit microscopic examination of the ear once they are told that the machine to be used is merely a light with a magnifying glass. Again, the parents sit next to the child during this examination and, in some cases, help to hold the child's hands or head still so that the examination can be accomplished without difficulty. Parents can generally hold infants sufficiently still to permit microscopic examination.

For an 18-month-old baby who is difficult to restrain, a papoose board is sometimes necessary. Continuing to allow the parents to hold the head still and to comfort the child should he or she be nervous or frightened is advisable. Larger children who cannot be restrained successfully on a papoose board should be asked to return for another examination when they have been desensitized to it. Sedation is not usually successful but may be tried in certain cases. A general anesthetic may be needed for complete examination and evaluation.

The suction used to clean the ear is sometimes especially frightening to young children, and rather than using a suction, the physician sometimes finds it less traumatic to use a cotton wisp to absorb any discharge present in the ear. In all cases, extreme care must be taken because once the ear is injured, the examination cannot continue.

Flexible endoscopy

The small-caliber flexible endoscope (2.2 mm) is often used in pediatric practice for the evaluation of stridorous infants or children with voice disorders or speech problems. Although in some cases a mirror can still be used in older children and adolescents, performing an adequate laryngeal examination with a mirror in younger children is very difficult. The flexible endoscope permits visualization of the larynx in young infants and children and also allows a dynamic view of the pharynx, velum, and hypopharynx, adding a new dimension to the evaluation and treatment of disorders affecting these structures. This instrument has proved invaluable in the assessment of tracheal and endotracheal tube placement because it can be placed through the lumen of all but the smallest tubes.

In infants and young children, anesthesia can be obtained easily with either lidocaine gel or 2% lidocaine drops placed in the nose with an eyedropper. The nose must first be examined to make sure no septal deviation or obstruction lesion exists that would prevent the passage of a small telescope. Using cocaine in young children is not advisable because of its variable absorption rate. In infants cocaine can produce unwanted symptoms of irritability and nervousness.

Parents should be carefully cautioned that after anesthesia has been obtained in the nose and pharynx, the child should not eat or be fed for approximately 30 to 40 minutes and after that should try eating slowly. Sedation is not generally necessary for this examination; instead, the endoscope can usually be used quickly on infants without serious stress or other poor consequences. For neonates, who may require some restraint, a towel may be used to bundle the infant or someone may have to hold the infant's head still. In children 3 years of age or older, a careful explanation of what is about to happen, with assistance from the parents, is generally all that is necessary to complete the examination successfully. For uncooperative patients, the practitioner must decide whether to proceed.

Complications using the flexible endoscope in the examination of children are rare; however, an emergency cart should be available in the examination space for intubation or emergency therapy should it become necessary. Having instruments for intubation and resuscitation of small children nearby is certainly reasonable in the examination and treatment of childhood disorders, in case of any catastrophic event that necessitates ventilation, administration of drugs, or cardiac stimulation.

The flexible endoscope has proven to be invaluable in the evaluation and management of pediatric patients who have undergone endoscopic sinus surgery. These small endoscopes allow for visualization of the surgical site and the interior of the maxillary sinus without the need for sedation. This examination permits an assessment of healing and functional status of the sinus that is not easily attainable with rigid endoscopes or general anesthesia.

Needle biopsy

The fine-needle aspiration technique used to evaluate neck or facial masses is just as useful for children as for adults. If a cytopathologist is available and interested in reading specimens, the adjunctive value in diagnosis can sometimes prevent the need for an open biopsy. Children are quite frightened of needles or other sharp objects; however, a 22- or 23-gauge needle can usually be passed into a neck or facial mass without complication. The procedure is carefully explained to the child, and the child is restrained if needed. EMLA cream (Astra Pharmaceuticals, Westborough, Mass) is applied under an occlusive dressing for 20 minutes. (This mixture of 2.5% lidocaine and 2.5% prilocaine is very effective in reducing discomfort at an injection site.) The area is prepared with a povidone–iodine solution, and the needle, with a 10-ml syringe, is placed into the mass while the syringe is aspirated. The sample obtained within the needle core is placed on a glass slide, which is then wiped on another slide and placed in a fixative. An adhesive bandage is used to cover the puncture wound. The procedure is generally no more traumatic than obtaining a blood sample and should be explained in those terms to parents.

Audiology

Every child can be tested for hearing loss. Pediatricians or other referral sources, who tend to delay early diagnosis and referral, often overlook this fact. Parents are generally acute observers, however. If their child does not seem to hear, or somehow seems different from other children, the physician should give credence to their thoughts and suggestions and obtain a hearing test for that particular child.

Using brainstem evoked response audiometry is certainly not a necessity for every surgeon. If children comprise a large proportion of the patients seen, however, visual-response audiometry is very helpful, in addition to routine audiometric evaluation and tympanometry, for the testing of children. Infants 6 months of age or older can be behaviorally conditioned to respond visually to stimuli at certain sound levels. These responses are extremely reliable and can be used in experienced hands to determine the level of hearing and the need for further diagnostic testing. The use of otoacoustic emissions to determine baseline hearing levels has been used in statewide screening programs and is increasingly used as a standard evaluation process in infants and children.

Early identification of hearing loss in children is of utmost importance for safeguarding their eventual verbal and language abilities. Current efforts are directed toward universal screening of all newborns. Maintaining a high-risk register of infants and children who are at risk for hearing loss may aid the practitioner and parents in identifying children who may have a hearing loss and who would benefit from early intervention.

Functional disorders

Somatization of stress within childhood and adolescence is not uncommon. Every child who is evaluated with a complaint is assumed to have an organic basis for his or her problems. In some cases, however, it can clearly be determined that a functional disorder exists; and although an organic cause may stimulate the chief complaint, there is no problem at the time of examination. In cases of hearing loss in which the Stenger test is positive or in which the patient is aphonic yet has mobile vocal cords, direct confrontation is not advisable. Instead, a search should be undertaken for causes of the complaint in the family, school, and extracurricular activities. Sometimes relying on the primary care provider, school counselor, or other counselor to delve completely into the situation is preferable, although the parents must always be informed as to the nature of the child's complaint and its possible causes.

PREPARATION FOR HOSPITALIZATION AND SURGERY

Once the decision to proceed with hospitalization or surgery has been made, the child and parents must be emotionally prepared in order to achieve a successful result. Having already discussed the surgery in factual terms, the surgeon has laid important groundwork for that preparation. The surgeon or a nurse familiar with all aspects of the procedure should undertake careful explanation of all details of the hospitalization. Admission to the hospital, venipuncture, injections, withholding of food and drink, transport to the operating room, and induction of anesthesia must all be discussed to allay any fears or misconceptions in the child.

A tour of the hospital, including the patient stay areas and operating rooms, and an introduction to nurses and other staff is helpful in eliminating fear in a child who is coming to the hospital. Special films and booklets are also valuable in reducing the concern about an upcoming hospitalization. The parents must be encouraged to be truthful, to the best of their ability, about any upcoming surgery. It is important for the physician to communicate enough about a hospitalization or surgery to both the parents and the child so that questions may be answered completely.

The Hospital

A children's hospital is a great asset, providing a team of physicians, nurses, and other staff who can best handle a hospital stay or surgery for pediatric patients. Children's hospitals are an important resource, and every surgeon involved in pediatric practice should support them. If there is no facility for children in the area, a search for the hospital best able to provide care and support for pediatric patients should be undertaken. The hospital must be able to provide services that make the patient's experiences as comfortable as possible and also allow for the greatest safety in the patient's preoperative, surgical, and postoperative management.

The concept of a team of professionals who deal strictly with pediatrics is not new; it is, however, one that is becoming increasingly accepted as the standard of care. When complications arise, as they inevitably do in the course of medical practice, having support facilities and personnel available to handle the needs promptly is vital.

Selecting anesthesia

Pediatric anesthesia is a subspecialty in itself. Reaching a degree of proficiency for delivering anesthesia to young children requires considerable time and experience. The younger the infant and the more complex the problem that must be dealt with, the more specialized are the techniques that must be used. Without question, some anesthesiologists are better trained and more comfortable in dealing with the challenging aspects of pediatric anesthesia. Reliance on those individuals benefits both the patients and the surgeon.

Local anesthesia is generally not used in young children because of their inability to understand the need for painful injections. The short attention span of most children makes them unlikely to remain still and quiet. The use of sedation for extended periods of time in elective procedures is probably not advisable unless support personnel can monitor the child carefully and ensure that he or she does not develop sequelae related to the sedative being given.

One notable exception is the use of iontophoresis for myringotomy. Iontophoresis, which is generally a safe technique, is at least 90% effective in cooperative children for achieving adequate local anesthesia of the tympanic membrane so that a myringotomy or tube placement can be accomplished without too much difficulty. It cannot be accomplished through an infected or markedly thickened eardrum, and it should not be used in a child who is unable to hold still or cooperate for a microscopic examination. The 4- to 5-year-old patient is generally the youngest child for whom this procedure can be performed. Having the parents remain next to the child and provide support can make all the difference in the ultimate success of the procedure. Obviously, the surgeon must have confidence in his or her technical ability to perform a myringotomy without injuring the external canal, because anesthesia is obtained only in the eardrum.

Postoperative management

The most important aspect in postoperative management is having the parents and child well prepared for the effects of surgery and the recuperative period with clear, well-detailed instructions as to normal and abnormal occurrences, level of activity, diet, and other details. Without detailed teaching and written instructions, postoperative management of even simple problems is confusing to the parents who are concerned about the postoperative difficulties their child may encounter. Knowing what to expect is the single most important factor that enables the patient to recover from a surgical procedure without multiple phone calls from the parent and excessive concern from both parties.

It has been clearly demonstrated that when children have to remain hospitalized for either medical or postsurgical treatment, the presence of their parents makes the hospital stay less fearsome and less troublesome to them. If possible, arranging for a parent to stay with the child during the hospital admission can provide the security necessary for a rapid recovery. Without question, the briefest possible hospital stay is best for the child and least expensive for the parents.

Short-stay surgery is being used extensively to manage the procedures in pediatric otolaryngology that require minimal inhospital care. Myringotomies, tonsillectomies, adenoidectomies, and minor ear surgery can easily be performed in a short-stay surgical suite, allowing for early discharge from the hospital and recuperation at home.

Remembering that modifications in surgical technique should occur in the management of pediatric problems is important. Dressing changes, suture removals, and postoperative manipulations should be kept to a minimum so as not to provoke fear and discomfort in a child who must undergo minor procedures. Sometimes sedating the child is necessary for removal of packing or sutures, a precaution that is certainly unnecessary in adults. It is reasonable then to plan ahead at the time of surgery and to use absorbable sutures, dressings that need to be removed only once, and few manipulations.

SUMMARY

Because each child is an individual, every child's care should also be special and individually tailored. The extra effort required to learn different techniques and approaches is necessary for physicians who are interested in providing excellent care to children.

SUGGESTED READINGS

Avery ME and others: Ventilatory response to inspired carbon dioxide in infants and adults, *J Appl Physiol* 18:89, 1963.

Bodegard G and others: Control of respiration in newborn babies. I. The development of the Hering-Breuer inflation reflex, *Acta Paediatr* 58:567, 1969.

Bryan AC, Bryan MH: Control of respiration in the newborn, *Clin Perinatol* 5:269, 1978.

Children's Hospital and Medical Center: *Selected handouts for housestaff*, ed 14, Seattle, 1990-1991, Childrens' Hospital and Medical Center.

Cook CD and others: Studies of respiratory physiology in the newborn infant. III. Measurements of mechanics of respiration, *J Clin Invest* 36:440, 1957.

Filston HC: *Surgical problems in children: recognition and referral*, St Louis, 1982, Mosby.

Gans S: *Surgical pediatrics: non-operative care*, New York, 1980, Grune & Stratton.

Graff TD and others: The ventilatory response of infants to airway resistance, *Anesthesiology* 27:168, 1966.

Graham GR: Circulatory and respiratory physiology of infancy and childhood, *Br J Anaesth* 32:97, 1960.

James LS, Rowe RD: The pattern of response of pulmonary and systemic arterial pressures in newborn and older infants to short periods of hypoxia, *J Pediatr* 51:5, 1957.

Ledbetter MK, Homma T, Farhi LE: Readjustment in distribution of alveolar ventilation and lung perfusion in the newborn, *Pediatrics* 40:940, 1967.

Nelson NM: Neonatal pulmonary function, *Pediatr Clin North Am* 13:769, 1966.

O'Brien RT, Pearson HA: Physiologic anemia of the newborn infant, *J Pediatr* 79:132, 1971.

Raffensperger J: *Swenson's pediatric surgery*, ed 4, New York, 1980, Appleton-Century-Crofts.

Ravitch MM and others: *Pediatric surgery*, ed 3, Chicago, 1979, Mosby.

Rigatto H: Apnea, *Pediatr Clin North Am* 29:1105, 1982.

Rowe MI, Marchildon MB: Physiological considerations in the newborn surgical patient, *Surg Clin North Am* 56:245, 1976.

Steward DJ: *Manual of pediatric anesthesia*, Edinburgh, 1985, Churchill Livingstone.

Wallgren G, Barr M, Rudhe U: Hemodynamic studies of induced acute hypo- and hypervolemia in the newborn infant, *Acta Paediatr Scand* 53:1, 1964.

Wallgren G, Hansen JS, Lind J: Quantitative studies of the human neonatal circulation. III. Observations on the newborn infant's central circulatory responses to moderate hypovolemia, *Acta Paediatr Suppl* 179:43, 1967.

Chapter 2

Developmental Anatomy

Daniel O. Graney
Kathleen C.Y. Sie

For discussion purposes, most descriptions of the neck divide the anatomy into triangles. To the student this may seem a futile, pedantic exercise in geometry. However, the use of triangles is simply an organizational device that manages the volume of anatomic detail in the neck by parceling it into reasonable study units. When an incision is made over the carotid triangle, surgeons can predict the structures they will encounter in precise order. Similarly, the embryologic correlates of the triangles are important in understanding the development and differential diagnosis of certain masses in the various triangles of the neck.

The term *triangle* initially connotes a planar form (i.e., a flat structure). In the anatomy of the neck, however, the triangles are three-dimensional spaces that should be visualized as shallow triangular boxes. These boxes have not only three sides but also a roof (top) and floor (bottom). The next step is to define the contents of the box. As will be described, most of the triangles are three-dimensional spaces bounded by bone and muscles, with distinct fascial layers forming the roof and floor of the space. In general terms the triangular space contains blood vessels, nerves, lymphatic vessels, and lymph nodes. With this somewhat contrived schema, the organizational problems of the neck anatomy can be greatly simplified.

This chapter begins with descriptions of the posterior triangle and the subdivisions of the anterior triangle. There is also a description of the root of the neck that relates the anatomy of the two major triangles to the radical neck procedure. The chapter concludes with a discussion of the embryology of the branchial arches and the pharyngeal pouches and their contribution to various masses in the neck.

POSTERIOR TRIANGLE

The posterior triangle of the neck is bordered by the sternocleidomastoid muscle, the anterior border of the trapezius muscle, and the middle third of the clavicle (Fig. 2-1). Specific layers of deep fascia form the floor (medial wall) and roof (lateral wall) of the triangle. An understanding of the fascial relationships in the neck is important, not only because of the boundary relationships but also because fasciae form planes that provide routes of surgical access or pathways for hemorrhage and abscess formation. For this reason a brief discussion of the fascial planes is necessary before proceeding with the anatomy of the posterior triangle.

Fascia

One of the earliest lessons in anatomy is that there are two types of fascia in the body: the superficial fascia and the deep fascia. In the region of the abdominal wall, the superficial fascia consists of two layers: a fatty layer (Camper's fascia) and a deeper, membranous layer (Scarpa's fascia). The deep fascial layer of the abdominal wall is not subdivided but simply envelopes the abdominal muscles. In the neck the superficial fascia is very thin and is not divided into layers, whereas the deep fascia is divided into three layers.[5] The names of these layers vary among authors, resulting in a somewhat chaotic terminology. Regardless of the terminology used, however, the divisions are arbitrary at best. A simple approach can provide a workable solution for either the anatomist or the surgeon.

Superficial cervical fascia

The superficial layer of cervical fascia is a single layer underlying the skin. It is usually thin, except in obese indi-

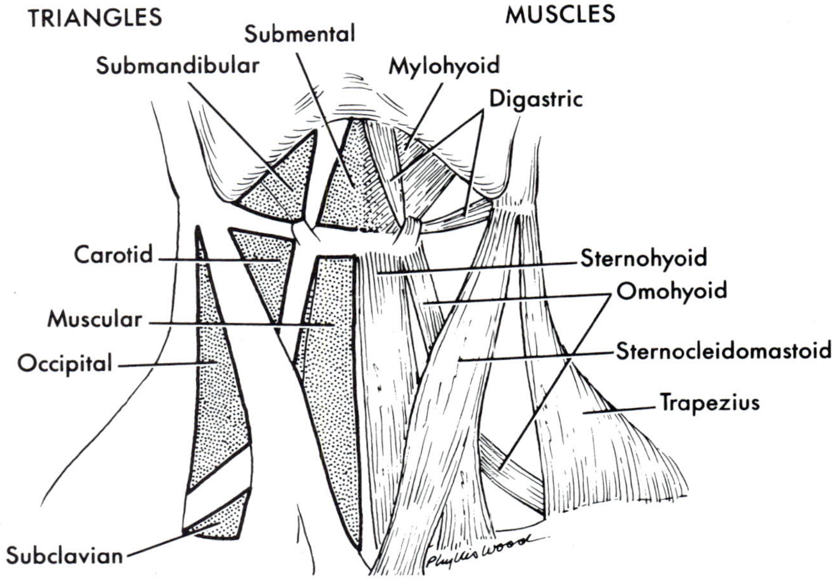

Fig. 2-1. The triangles of the neck and their boundaries.

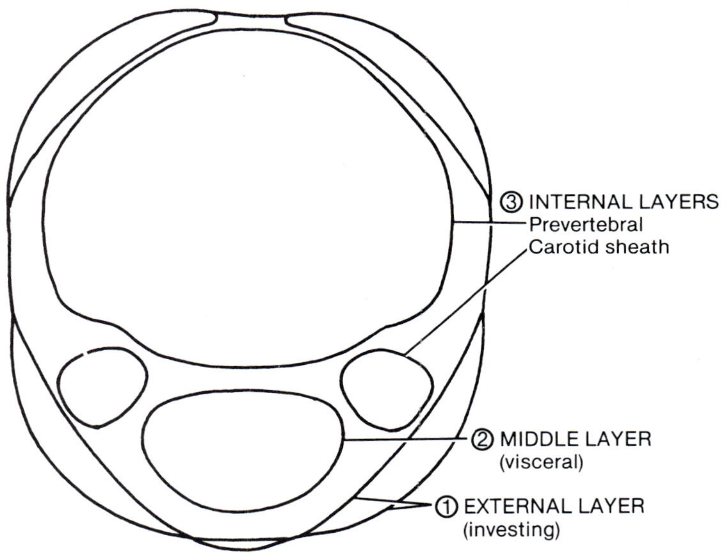

Fig. 2-2. Divisions of the deep cervical fascia seen in transverse section at the level of cranial nerve VII.

viduals, in which case it is thickened by adipose tissue. The primary surgical significance of the superficial layer is that it provides a fascial pad that protects underlying structures when a skin incision is made. In exceptionally lean individuals, however, the paucity of this layer may not protect the underlying structures (e.g., the accessory nerve), so the surgeon should be wary when operating on such individuals.

Deep cervical fascia

The deep fascia is divided into the external, middle, and internal layers. These layers are best illustrated when the neck is viewed in cross-section (Fig. 2-2). The external layer of deep fascia underlies the platysma muscle and completely invests or encircles all of the superficial neck structures. For these reasons the external layer is also known as the superficial, or investing, layer of deep fascia. In the region of the sternocleidomastoid and trapezius muscles, it splits and envelopes the individual muscles. A middle layer of fascia encloses the visceral structures of the neck (the trachea and esophagus); hence the synonym for the middle layer is the *visceral fascia.*

The third, or internal, layer of deep fascia surrounds the deep muscles of the neck and cervical vertebrae (Fig. 2-3). This layer is also known by its descriptive term, the *preverte-*

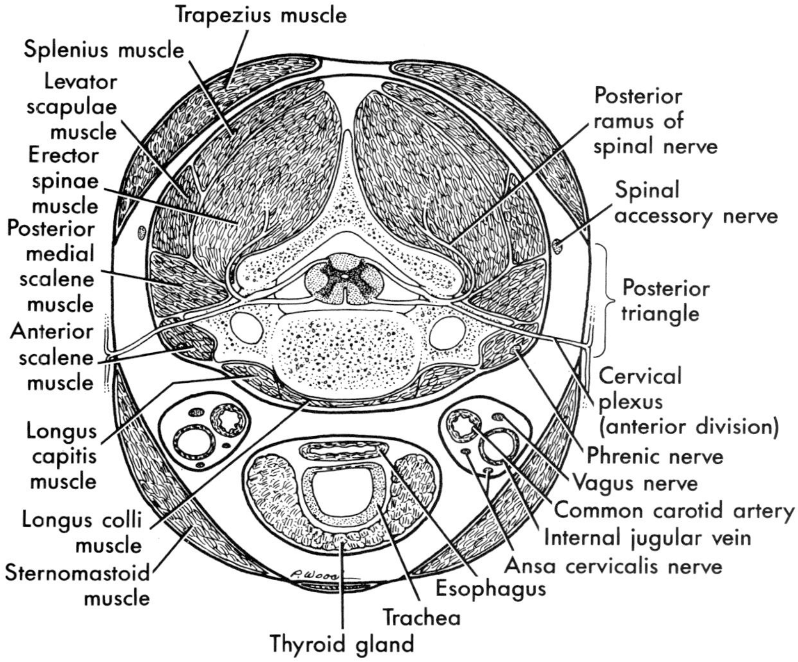

Fig. 2-3. Structures contained by the deep cervical fascia seen in transverse section at the level of cranial nerve.

bral fascia (although *paravertebral fascia* would have been a more appropriate term). The muscles enclosed by the prevertebral fascia include (1) the deep muscles of the neck (cervical aspect of the erector spinae); (2) the levator scapulae; (3) the scalenus anterior, medius, and posterior; and (4) the longus colli and longus capitis muscles, which lie on the anterior aspect of the cervical vertebrae. The latter pair of muscles serve as flexors of the vertebrae and, in the case of the longus capitis muscle, assist in flexion of the skull. The scalenus group underlies the prevertebral fascia in the region of the transverse processes of the cervical vertebrae. The anterior tubercles of the transverse processes provide the origin for the scalenus anterior muscle, whereas the posterior tubercles provide the origin for the scalenus medius and posterior muscles. Continuing posteriorly, in order, are the levator scapulae and deep cervical muscles already noted.

The internal layer of the deep fascia is described by some authors as enveloping the carotid and jugular vessels. Hence the carotid sheaths are included as part of the definition of this layer. An effective means of visualizing the spatial relationships of these layers of fascia is to examine a cross-section of the neck. This view not only is informative in defining the three layers of deep fascia but also serves to relate them to the posterior triangle of the neck (see Fig. 2-3). If one places a finger over the middle of the posterior triangle (i.e., between the trapezius and sternocleidomastoid muscles), it is evident that the roof (lateral wall) of the triangle is formed by the superficial layer of deep fascia. Palpation deeper into the triangle brings the tip of the finger into contact with the prevertebral fascia that forms the floor of the posterior triangle and invests the prevertebral muscles. If the superficial layer of the deep fascia is incised and a finger inserted into the space exploring anteriorly between the sternocleidomastoid and prevertebral muscles, one encounters the carotid sheath. This is a surgical approach to the retropharyngeal area or carotid vessels.

Contents of the posterior triangle

The major contents of the posterior triangle are the cutaneous branches of the cervical plexus, the accessory nerve (cranial nerve [CN] XI), two arterial branches of the thyrocervical trunk, and an abundant number of lymph nodes associated with the veins of the region.

Cutaneous branches of the cervical plexus

The sensory branches of the cervical plexus contained within the posterior triangle are four cutaneous nerves, which supply the skin of the head and neck from the area of the posterior scalp to the supraclavicular region. These nerves are the lesser occipital nerve, the great auricular nerve, the anterior cutaneous nerve of the neck, and the supraclavicular nerve (Fig. 2-4). The first three of these nerves contain cervical segments C-2 and C-3 and the supraclavicular nerves C-3 and C-4. The topographic relationships of these nerves and their distribution to the skin are illustrated in Figure 2-5. The important landmark for the cervical nerves is the accessory nerve at the point where it enters the posterior triangle from under the cover of the sternocleidomastoid

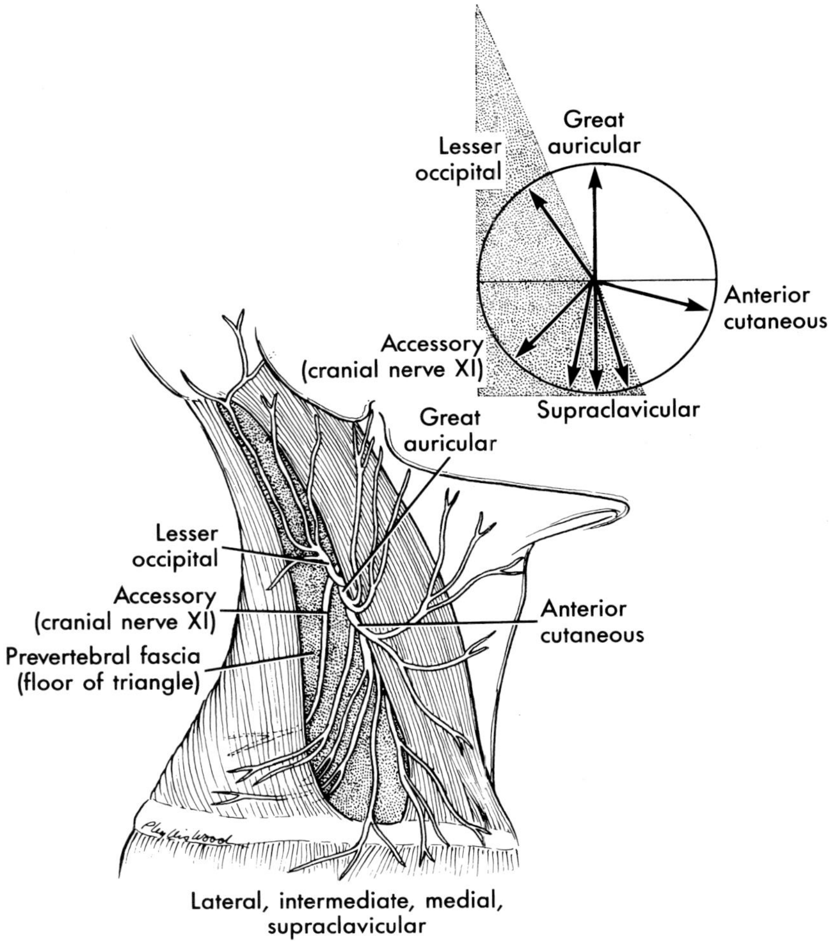

Fig. 2-4. Nerves of the posterior triangle seen on the right side of the neck.

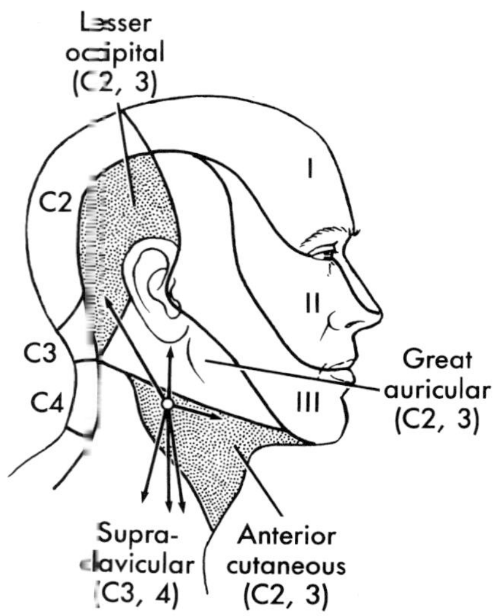

Fig. 2-5. Distribution of the cutaneous branches of the cervical plexus.

muscle. If this point is viewed as the center of a clock's face, the cervical nerves mimic the clock's hands pointing in different directions (see Fig. 2-4, *inset*). For example, on the right side the lesser occipital nerve is approximately at the 11 o'clock position, the great auricular nerve is at the 12 o'clock position, and the anterior cutaneous nerve is at the 3 o'clock position. The supraclavicular nerves consist of three or four bundles of filaments scattered between the 5 and 7 o'clock positions. Continuing this analogy, the accessory nerve can be seen to traverse the posterior triangle along the line of the 8 o'clock position until it enters the deep surface of the trapezius muscle. The accessory nerve serves in this manner as a focus for organizing the pathways of the cutaneous nerves as well as for emphasizing CN XI as a motor nerve in the posterior triangle.

Accessory nerve

The accessory nerve supplies both the sternocleidomastoid and trapezius muscles; however, in the posterior triangle the only fibers remaining in the nerve are those destined for the trapezius. The accessory nerve should be preserved whenever possible because paralysis of the trapezius muscle has devastating effects on shoulder joint function. The range of shoulder abduction is diminished by at least 50% when scapular rotation is impaired because of a trapezius palsy.

The accessory nerve is the only motor nerve in the posterior triangle. However, if the prevertebral fascia is incised, it is possible to encounter the motor nerves of the deep cervical muscles, the phrenic nerve, or the brachial plexus. With regard to its innervation of the sternocleidomastoid and trapezius muscles, CN XI is in fact a spinal nerve. Cell bodies of the motor neurons innervating these muscles lie near the ventral horn in the upper cervical spinal cord, in the region of segments C-2 through C-4. The axonal fibers exit the anterolateral portion of the cord as a series of fine filaments before becoming bundled as a nerve fiber within the subarachnoid space of the vertebral canal. The nerve ascends in the subarachnoid space, enters the posterior fossa through the foramen magnum, and joins with the cranial root of the accessory nerve before existing the skull via the jugular foramen. As the nerve descends the neck adjacent to the carotid sheath, motor or sensory filaments may join the nerve directly from segments C-2 through C-4.[6] After crossing the deep surface of the sternocleidomastoid muscle, the nerve enters the posterior triangle, as already described.

Arterial branches

The major arteries of the posterior triangle are the suprascapular and transverse cervical arteries, which are located in the supraclavicular fossa near the base of the triangle. These arteries are derived from the thyrocervical trunk of the subclavian artery at the medial border of the scalenus anterior muscle and cross the muscle and the fossa transversely to course deep to the sternocleidomastoid muscle. Ascending and descending branches of the transverse cervical artery are usually described. The descending branch is of interest because it divides into a superficial branch that parallels the accessory nerve and a deep branch that parallels the nerve to the rhomboid muscle. The suprascapular artery, after crossing the fossa, is directed toward the suprascapular notch, where it supplies the posterior scapular muscle.

In addition to the transverse cervical and suprascapular veins that parallel the course of the arteries, the posterior triangle contains the external jugular vein. This vein enters the triangle after crossing the superficial aspect of the sternocleidomastoid muscle in company with the great auricular nerve. The vein courses inferior to the base of the supraclavicular fossa, where it may anastomose with small vessels before entering the subclavian vein near the junction with the internal jugular vein.

ANTERIOR TRIANGLE

The anterior triangle of the neck is complementary to the posterior triangle and is bounded by the sternocleidomastoid muscle, the body of the mandible, and the midline of the neck. This space can be further subdivided into smaller triangular units, such as the submandibular triangle, described in Chapter 64, and the carotid and muscular triangles, which are included in this discussion (see Fig. 2-1).

Carotid triangle

The carotid triangle is bordered by the posterior belly of the digastric muscle, the superior belly of the omohyoid muscle, and the midportion of the sternocleidomastoid muscle. The roof (lateral wall) of the carotid triangle is bounded by the superficial layer of deep fascia, whereas the floor (medial wall) is formed by the prevertebral fascia of the vertebral column and the visceral fascia covering the pharynx and larynx. The contents of the carotid triangle are the carotid sheath structures. These include the common carotid artery with its internal and external branches, the last four CNs (IX, X, XI, and XII), and the ansa cervicalis. In the carotid triangle only a small branch of CN IX is left to supply the carotid sinus, because its main portion left the sheath to enter the posterior third of the tongue. CN XI, which is also in the upper portion of the carotid sheath, enters the sternocleidomastoid muscle at the apex of the carotid triangle, where the posterior belly of the digastric muscle crosses the sternocleidomastoid muscle. The vagus nerve travels the entire length of the carotid sheath between the internal jugular vein and the carotid artery. Whereas the CNs just mentioned lie in the posterior aspect of the carotid sheath, CN XII lies in the anterior aspect of the sheath. At the level of the hyoid bone, CN XII courses anteroinferiorly to pass deep to the posterior belly of the digastric muscle onto the surface of the hyoglossus muscle before entering the substance of the tongue.

The major focal point of the triangle is the bifurcation of the common carotid artery (Fig. 2-6). The internal carotid artery ascends the neck without branching. The external carotid artery provides several branches, many of which are important landmarks. The external carotid artery has anterior branches, posterior branches, and terminal branches.

The three anterior branches are common. In ascending order they are the superior thyroid, lingual, and facial arteries. In some individuals the lingual and facial arteries form a common lingual–facial trunk. Another important variation is the origin of the superior thyroid from the common carotid rather than the external carotid artery. The latter variation is important because the external carotid artery is occasionally ligated (e.g., for management of chronic epistaxis). If the superior thyroid artery is used as a landmark for the external carotid artery in patients with this particular anatomic variation, it is possible to inadvertently ligate the common carotid instead of the external carotid artery.

The posterior branches of the external carotid are the occipital and posterior auricular arteries. The occipital artery is noteworthy for its small sternocleidomastoid branch, which supplies the sternocleidomastoid muscle. The origin of this small artery hooks around CN XII as it courses anteroinferiorly and prevents it from ascending further in the neck. Thus

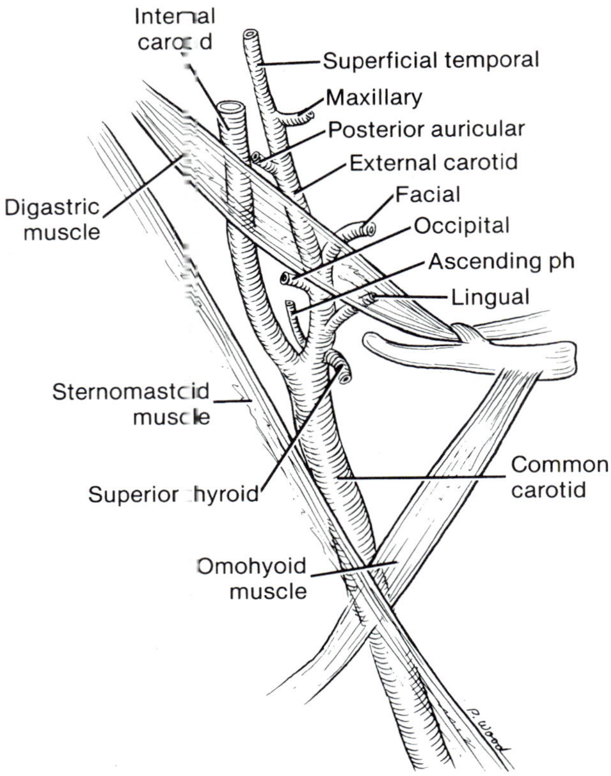

Fig. 2-6. Arterial branches of the carotid triangle.

the sternocleidomastoid artery can be used to trace the position of CN XII. Similarly, the sternocleidomastoid artery enters its muscle near the point of CN XI, thus also providing a means of locating the accessory nerve.

Ansa cervicalis

The ansa cervicalis is part of the cervical plexus. Its essential role is to supply the infrahyoid muscles: the sternohyoid, sternothyroid, and omohyoid (Fig. 2-7). C-1 nerve fibers enter the hypoglossal nerve and travel as far as the occipital artery. At this point the hypoglossal nerve curves anteroinferiorly, but C-1 fibers descend the neck to form the branch of CN XII, termed the *superior root of the ansa*. Fibers from C-2 and C-3 form an inferior root, which descends the carotid sheath on the surface of the internal jugular vein before turning anteroinferiorly to join the superior root. The ansa "loop" is thus formed by the union of the two roots of the ansa.

At the origin of the superior root of the ansa, some C-1 nerve fibers do not follow the superior root but rather continue in the hypoglossal nerve transversely across the neck, before leaving CN XII to supply either the thyrohyoid or the geniohyoid muscle (see Fig. 2-7). In summary, all four of the infrahyoid, hyoid, or "strap" muscles are supplied by the ansa. In addition, one suprahyoid muscle, the geniohyoid, is also supplied by the C-1 fibers that have continued in route with the hypoglossal nerve. Except for proprioceptive fibers carried within the ansa, it is a motor nerve.

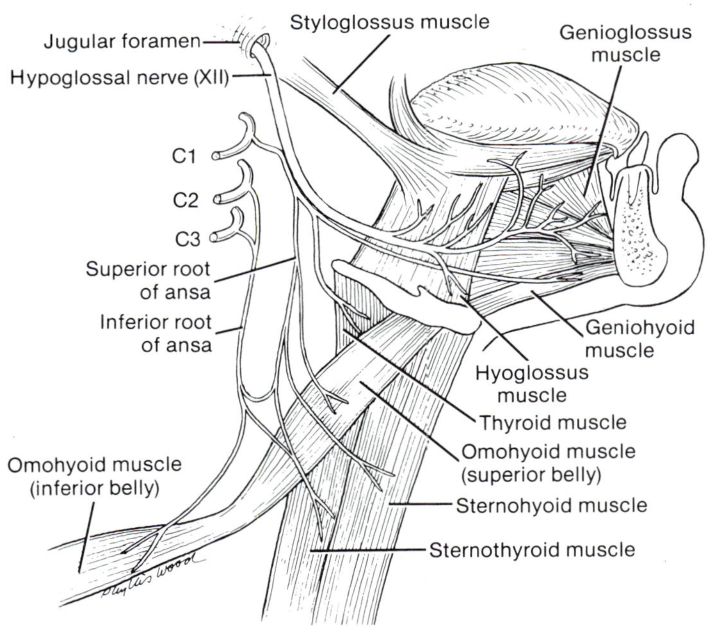

Fig. 2-7. Distribution of the ansa cervicalis and the hypoglossal nerve (cranial nerve XII).

At this point in the discussion, two major groups of nerves of the cervical plexus have been discussed: the ansa cervicalis (principally motor) and the sensory (cutaneous) branches of the posterior triangle. Two other groups of fibers comprise the cervical plexus. One is composed of motor filaments from cervical roots 3 and 4 supplying the levator scapulae muscle and located deep to the prevertebral fascia. The other is the phrenic nerve, which is derived from cervical segments C-3, C-4, and occasionally C-5. This nerve supplies motor fibers to the diaphragm and sensory fibers to the region of the central tendon of the diaphragm.

ROOT OF NECK

The boundaries of the root of the neck are somewhat ill-defined. Its base is the plane of the thoracic inlet and can be traced from the manubrium laterally along the first rib and then posterosuperiorly to the transverse process of C-6 (Fig. 2-8). For the purposes of this chapter the root of the neck is divided unilaterally by the midline into a pyramidal space—bounded laterally by the scalenus anterior muscle, inferiorly by the first rib, and medially by the tracheoesophageal tract and midline. Its contents include the great vessels emerging from the mediastinum, principally the subclavian

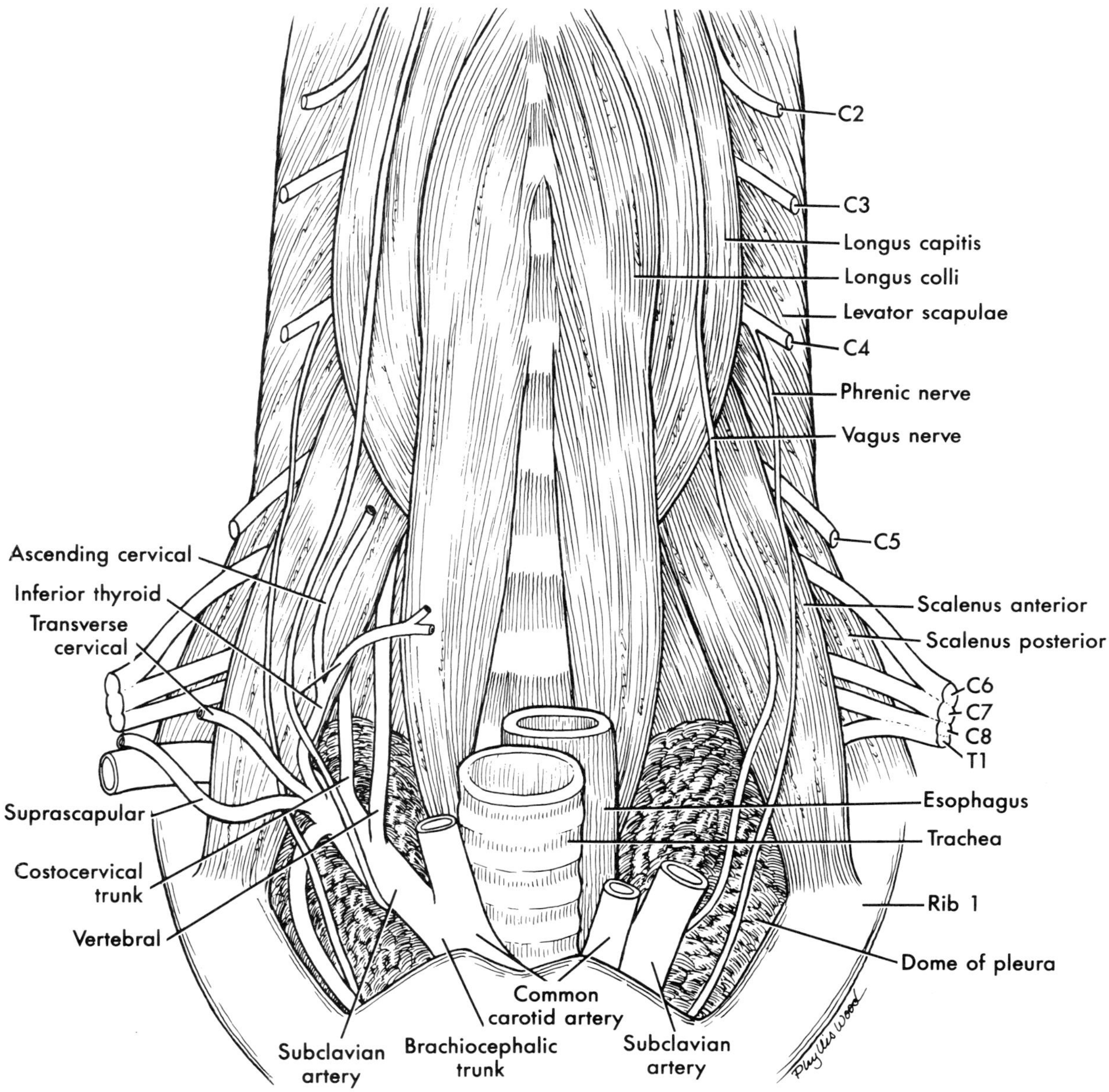

Fig. 2-8. Root of the neck and subclavian artery. *T1,* First thoracic foot; *Rib 1,* First rib.

and common carotid arteries, brachiocephalic vein, vagus, and sympathetic trunk. As the great vessels traverse the thoracic inlet from the mediastinum, their course is divided by the scalenus anterior muscle. The subclavian vein crosses anterior to the muscle, whereas the subclavian artery courses between the cleavage plane of the scalenus anterior and scalenus medius muscles. In this region the subclavian vessels usually divide into three parts: the first part proximal to the scalenus, the second part posterior to the scalenus anterior muscle, and the third part between the lateral border of the scalenus and the lateral edge of the first rib.

The majority of the vascular branches arise from the first portion of the subclavian artery. The first branch of the subclavian artery is normally the vertebral artery, which ascends the root of the neck between the scalenus anterior and longus colli muscles to enter the foramen processus transversus of C-6. Next is the thyrocervical trunk, which normally has four described branches: a small ascending cervical artery, which supplies the prevertebral muscle region; the inferior thyroid artery coursing to the inferior pole of the thyroid gland; the transverse cervical artery; and the suprascapular artery. The latter two have already been described in relation to the posterior triangle of the neck. Two branches arise from the inferior surface of the subclavian artery: the costocervical trunk and the internal thoracic artery, which descends over the suprapleural fascia into the mediastinum and anterior chest wall. There are multiple variations of these vessels; for details one should consult Daseler and Anson.[3]

Other important structures of this region are the major nerves. On the right side the vagus nerve lies in the posterior aspect of the carotid sheath and gives off its recurrent laryngeal branch at the level of the first rib. The recurrent branch circles the lateral aspect of the subclavian artery to cross medially and enter the tracheoesophageal groove. On the left side, the recurrent nerve arises from the vagus nerve at the aortic arch and hooks posteriorly around the ligamentum arteriosum. It then enters the tracheoesophageal groove, ascending the mediastinum and neck until it enters the larynx at the level of the cricoid cartilage.

In the most posterior part of the root of the neck, against the longus colli muscle, the sympathetic trunk ascends from the mediastinum following the prevertebral space to the level of C-2, where the superior cervical sympathetic ganglion is located. The inferior cervical ganglion lies close to the level of C-7, and sometimes a middle sympathetic ganglion is described at approximately the level of C-4.

This region is of particular importance during radical neck surgery, because the deep dissection is usually begun by detaching the sternocleidomastoid muscle from its attachments to the manubrium and clavicle. This exposes the carotid sheath and its contents and opens up the posterior and anterior triangles. As the dissection proceeds, the internal jugular vein is mobilized, exposing the carotid artery and its branches, which have been left in place. Because the *en bloc* mass of the internal jugular vein and sternocleidomastoid muscle is mobilized superiorly, it is important to leave the prevertebral fascia intact. In this manner the fascia provides a protective veil over the brachial plexus, phrenic nerve, sympathetic trunk, and motor nerves to the deep cervical muscles. When the prevertebral fascia is exposed, two muscles—the scalenus anterior and the longus capitis—serve as important landmarks for the spinal nerves. As the nerves emerge from the intervertebral foramina, they lie in a groove on the transverse process of the cervical vertebrae. If the vertebrae and prevertebral muscles are envisioned as being enclosed in a cylinder of prevertebral fascia, the logical conclusion is that the spinal nerves must penetrate this fascia to reach superficial structures in the neck (see Fig. 2-3). With these guidelines it is possible to identify cervical nerves C-1–4 at the lateral border of the longus capitis, and the roots of C-5–T-1 can be identified at the lateral edge of the scalenus anterior (see Fig. 2-8).

At this point in the radical neck dissection, the cutaneous nerves of the posterior triangle are encountered at their origin from the spinal nerves, and the surgeon has returned to the anatomic relationships of the posterior triangle.

LYMPHATIC DRAINAGE OF THE HEAD AND NECK

As discussed earlier, the deep fascia of the neck has outer, middle, and inner layers. This same rule might be applied to the lymphatic drainage of the head and neck. This plan is similar to one described by Last.[9] The superficial layer might be thought of as an outer circle of superficial or regional lymph nodes, the middle layer as a visceral layer of nodes draining the viscera of the neck such as the larynx and pharynx, and the deep circle of nodes composed of the paired carotid sheaths containing the internal jugular vein and deep cervical lymph nodes. The deep cervical lymph nodes are tributaries for both the superficial and visceral circles of lymph nodes.

Superficial lymph nodes

The superficial lymph nodes may be thought of as a circle of nodes beginning on the face and extending posteriorly to the occipital area of the scalp. The efferent lymphatics of these nodes drain inferiorly along the major veins of the face and scalp. On the anterior face, buccal nodes in the cheek and facial nodes along the path of the facial vein drain inferiorly across the mandible, into the submandibular triangle, and to submandibular nodes. Inferior to the mandible the superficial circle is composed of submandibular and anterior cervical lymph nodes. Sublingual nodes adjacent to the tongue receive afferent lymphatics from the anterior part of the face, particularly the lower lip and tip of the tongue, and then drain superficially on the neck to deep cervical nodes approximately at the level of the omohyoid muscle. The lymphatics from these nodes then enter the plexus of lymphatics in the carotid sheath, follow the internal jugular vein, and connect with other deep cervical nodes.

In the more posterior portion of the face (in the region

of the parotid), afferent lymphatics begin in the scalp along the path of the superficial temporal vessels and drain inferiorly to parotid nodes in the superficial aspect of the parotid gland. Efferent lymphatics from parotid nodes course inferiorly along the common facial vein and then to the deep cervical nodes. Posterior to the ear, retroauricular and occipital nodes follow their major channels to the deep cervical nodes of the internal jugular vein.

The general rule is that the more anterior regions of the face have a more rapid lymphatic drainage to the lower portion of the neck because there is a sparser chain of nodes to traverse before entering the deep cervical nodes. In contrast, the deeper and more posterior portions of the face usually have a more complicated chain of lymphatic nodes and channels and thus require more time before reaching the jugular lymph chain.

Deep cervical lymph nodes

The deep cervical lymph nodes are a series of nodes that parallel the course of the internal jugular vein from the base of the skull to its terminus at the brachiocephalic junction. Most of the nodes are closely associated with the vein within the carotid sheath and lie deep to the sternocleidomastoid muscle. Two particular areas are notable. One is the region where the posterior belly of the digastric muscle crosses the internal jugular vein; it is usually the site of one or more palpable lymph nodes, termed the *jugulodigastric nodes*. Similarly, another large node or series of small nodes exists at the junction of the superior belly of the omohyoid and sternocleidomastoid muscles, termed the *jugulo-omohyoid nodes*. Efferent lymphatics from the deep nodes enter the internal jugular trunks, which ultimately enter the venous system at the jugulosubclavian angle.

LYMPHATIC DRAINAGE OF THE PHARYNX AND LARYNX

The upper portion of the pharynx, the nasopharynx, drains directly to the upper deep cervical lymph nodes along the jugular chain. The oropharynx and particularly the tonsil drain through the parapharyngeal spaces to the region of the midportion of the jugular and particularly the jugulodigastric nodes. Some books describe the jugulodigastric nodes as the "tonsillar nodes." The region of the hypopharynx and larynx drains principally along the vascular pedicles of the hypopharynx and larynx. The upper portion of the larynx from the false cord drains along the superior laryngeal vessels to deep cervical nodes on the internal jugular vein near the bifurcation of the common carotid artery. The lower half of the larynx (from the true cords inferiorly) drains along the interior laryngeal vessels to nodes about the pretracheal region and eventually to deep nodes near the base of the internal jugular vein.

CLASSIFICATION OF THE CERVICAL LYMPHATICS

Nomenclature of the cervical lymphatics historically has been inconsistent. As the focus of oncologic surgery has shifted from radical extirpation to functional preservation, it has become more important to standardize the classification system for the cervical nodes. The American Academy of Otolaryngology–Head and Neck Surgery, along with the American Society of Head and Neck Surgery, has developed a standardized classification scheme for the cervical lymphatic system and for neck dissections.

The groups of lymph nodes are designated as levels I through VI. Level I includes nodes in the submental and submandibular triangles. Level II includes the upper jugular nodes located around the superior third of the jugular vein and spinal accessory nerve extending from the carotid bifurcation or hyoid (inferiorly) to the skull base (superiorly). The anterior and posterior boundaries of this nodal group are the lateral border of the sternohyoid muscle and the posterior border of the sternocleidomastoid muscle, respectively. Level III includes the middle jugular nodes around the middle third of the jugular vein extending from the carotid bifurcation superiorly to the omohyoid or cricothyroid notch inferiorly. The anterior and posterior boundaries are the same as for level II. Level IV includes the lower jugular group surrounding the jugular vein from the omohyoid muscle to the clavicle. The anterior and posterior borders are the same as in levels II and III. Level V is the posterior triangle group consisting of the nodes surrounding the lower half of the spinal accessory nerve and the transverse cervical artery, including the supraclavicular nodes. The anterior boundary is the posterior border of the sternocleidomastoid muscle, and the posterior boundary is the anterior border of the trapezius muscle. Level VI includes the anterior compartment group surrounding the visceral structures of the neck from the hyoid superiorly to the sternal notch inferiorly. The lateral boundary on either side is the medial aspect of the carotid sheath. This space crosses the midline and includes the perithyroidal, paratracheal, and precricoid nodes as well as the nodes along the recurrent laryngeal nerve.[16] The terminology for neck dissection is discussed in Chapter 95.

EMBRYOLOGY OF THE HEAD AND NECK

The development of many structures in the head and neck is intimately related to either the branchial arches or the pharyngeal pouches (Fig. 2-9). These are transient embryonic structures that undergo substantial remodeling so that their original embryonic form is essentially unrecognized in adults. The derivatives of these structures are nevertheless important to adult morphology; hence, aberrations in branchial arch development may produce significant malformations of the adult anatomy.

BRANCHIAL ARCHES

At 5 weeks of age the area of the future face and neck of the embryo consists of five or six pairs of finger-like masses of tissue named the *branchial arches*. Prominent in lateral profile (see Fig. 2-9), these masses are aligned transversely to the plane of the neck and are separated by the branchial clefts. The surface of the arches and

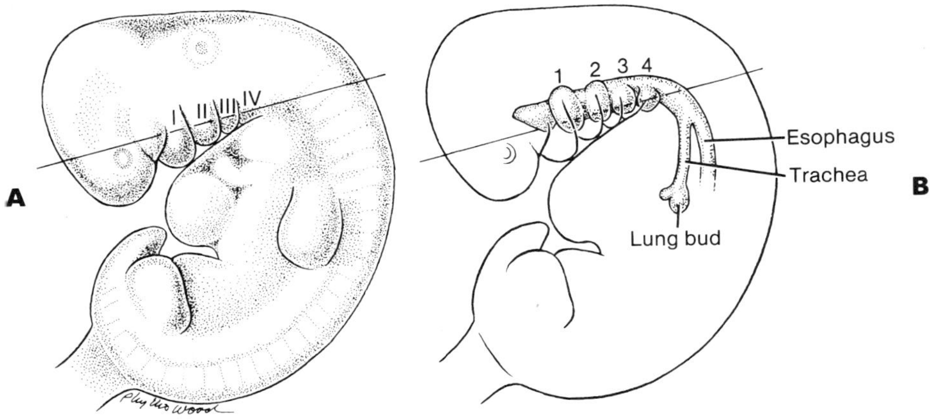

Fig. 2-9. **A,** Branchial arches. **B,** Pharyngeal pouches.

clefts is lined by ectoderm, with mesodermally defined tissues contained within the branchial arches. The tissues underlying the region of the clefts are thin because of the close approximation of outpouchings from the foregut region, called *pharyngeal pouches* (see Fig. 2-9). The derivatives of the arches and pouches are different because of the embryonic germ layers contained within the branchial arch (the mesoderm), whereas the pharyngeal pouches are composed of endoderm. Because of the differences in the embryonic germ layers, a generalization can be made that in adults the derivatives of the branchial arch will be structures composed of muscle, bone, or similar mesodermal derivatives, whereas the derivatives of the endodermal pharyngeal pouch will be glandular or associated with the digestive tract.

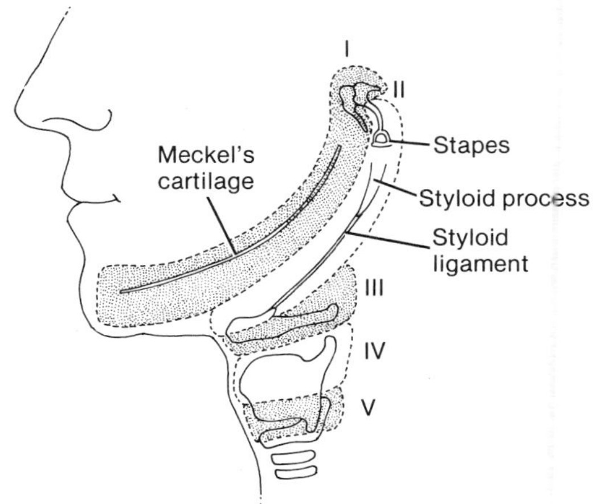

Fig. 2-10. Skeletal derivatives of the branchial arches.

DERIVATIVES OF THE BRANCHIAL ARCHES

In the early phase of branchial arch development the mesodermal mass of the arch forms a bar of cartilage, which remodels into bone, cartilage, or other connective tissue elements in adults. Similarly, the adult musculature of the face and neck also develops from the mesoderm of the arches.

Skeletal derivatives

The proximal portion of the first branchial arch cartilage (Meckel's cartilage) is remodeled and contributes to the formation of the ramus of the mandible (Fig. 2-10). The distal part of the cartilage withers, and the body of the mandible is formed from intramembranous bone. Other structures formed by the proximal part of the cartilage are the sphenomandibular ligament, anterior malleolar ligament malleus (except the manubrium, which is formed from the second arch), and the incus (except for its long process, which is also formed from the second arch).

The cartilage element in the second branchial arch (Reichert's cartilage) forms bony structures proximally and distally, but its central portion withers during development, leaving a fibrous band—the stylohyoid ligament—in the adult. Proximally, the second branchial arch cartilage forms the styloid process, manubrium of the malleus, long process of the incus, and stapes, except for the stapes footplate, which is mostly derived from the otic capsule.[1,18] Distally (anteroinferiorly), the second arch cartilage forms a portion of the body of the hyoid and the lesser cornu of the hyoid bone. In adults, the path of the embryonic second arch cartilage can be traced from the styloid process to the stylohyoid ligament, ending at the lesser cornu of the hyoid bone (see Fig. 2-10).

The remaining portions of the hyoid bone (i.e., the body and greater cornu) are formed by cartilage elements derived from the third branchial arch. The cartilaginous elements of the fourth, fifth, and sixth arches contribute to the formation of the thyroid, cricoid, arytenoid, corniculate, and cuneiform laryngeal cartilages.

Muscle derivatives

The muscles formed from mesodermal elements in the first branchial arch include the muscles of mastication: temporalis, masseter, and medial and lateral pterygoid. In addition, the tensor tympani, tensor veli palatini, anterior belly of the digastric, and mylohyoid muscles are also derived from first arch mesoderm.

Muscles formed from mesoderm in the second branchial arch include all of the muscles of facial expression from the region of the scalp inferiorly to the platysma muscle in the neck. In addition to those muscles, grouped as the muscles of facial expression, the posterior belly of the digastric, the stylohyoid, and the stapedius muscles are also derived from second arch mesoderm.

Only one muscle is formed from mesoderm in the third branchial arch. This is the stylopharyngeus muscle, a small muscle that aids in elevating the pharynx during swallowing. The muscles of the fourth, fifth, and sixth arches include those that form the pharynx and larynx. Pharyngeal muscles include the superior, middle, and inferior constrictor muscles. In addition, the mesodermal elements from these branchial arches also form the striated muscle composing the upper half of the esophagus. The inferior part of the esophagus is usually composed of smooth muscle derived from the splanchnic mesoderm of the primitive foregut.

Laryngeal muscles derived from mesodermal elements in the fourth, fifth, and sixth arches include the extrinsic muscle of the larynx, the cricothyroid, and all of the intrinsic muscles associated with movement of the arytenoid cartilage and true and false vocal folds.

Innervation

Because of the proximity of the developing branchial arches to the brainstem, each branchial arch receives motor or sensory innervation from an adjacent CN. A comparable parallel to this pattern occurs in the trunk, where a muscle is derived from the myotome region of a somite and receives its innervation from the adjacent segmental spinal nerve. In both cases, regardless of where the primordial muscle cell migrates, it retains its primary embryonic innervation. After each arch receives its CN innervation, the adult pattern is established regardless of its future migration onto the back of the head or base of the neck.

The nerve of the first branchial arch is the trigeminal nerve, which supplies motor innervation to all of the muscles derived from the first arch. In addition, sensory innervation is provided not only over the region of the mandible via the third division of the trigeminal nerve but also over the maxillary process of the first arch and the frontal nasal process via the second and first divisions of the trigeminal nerve.

The nerve of the second branchial arch is the facial nerve, which supplies motor innervation to all of the muscles derived from this mesoderm. Other than a small sensory branch of CN VII, which may supply part of the external auditory meatus, there is no sensory distribution of CN VII to ectoderm.

CN IX supplies the only muscle derived from the third arch (the stylopharyngeus muscle). As will be seen in the next section, however, CN IX also supplies sensory innervation to parts of the pharynx associated with this region.

The vagus nerve and the cranial part of the accessory nerve supply the muscles derived from the third through sixth branchial arches. Originating in the nucleus ambiguus of the medulla, the axonal processes of these nerves descend in the vagus nerve after exiting the skull via the jugular foramen. Specifically, the pharyngeal constrictors are supplied by the pharyngeal branch of the vagus and the transitional portion of the pharynx and esophagus via its recurrent laryngeal branch. In addition, the superior and recurrent laryngeal nerves supply the muscles and mucosa of the larynx.

Pharyngeal pouches

The pharyngeal pouches are lateral outpouchings of the foregut or region of the primitive pharynx (see Fig. 2-9). At the extreme lateral wall of each pharyngeal pouch the endodermal lining contacts the ectodermal epithelium of a branchial cleft (Fig. 2-11). Thus the branchial clefts are named in relation to the pharyngeal pouch with which they are apposed. The endodermal epithelium lining either the branchial arch or the pharyngeal pouch contributes to the formation of specific elements of the pharynx in adults.[8]

The first pharyngeal pouch becomes elongated and incorporated into the temporal bone to form the epithelial lining of the middle ear (Fig. 2-12). The most lateral portion of the pouch, along with the first closing plate of the first branchial cleft, forms the tympanic membrane (see Fig. 2-12). From this relationship it is clear that the external auditory canal is nothing more than a remodeling of the first branchial cleft (Fig. 2-13).

The endodermal layer of the second pharyngeal pouch forms the epithelial lining of the palatine tonsil, whereas underlying mesenchymal elements contribute to the formation of the tonsillar tissue itself (see Figs. 2-12 and 2-13).

The region of the third pharyngeal pouch is subdivided into superior and inferior portions. The superior portion forms cells that eventually differentiate into the inferior parathyroid gland (see Fig. 2-12). The inferior portion of the third pouch forms thymic tissue, which eventually migrates into the neck and mediastinum to form the thymus (Fig. 2-14).

The endoderm of the fourth pharyngeal pouch forms the superior parathyroid gland. The adjacent area is variably named as the fifth or sixth pouch or the ultimobranchial body (see Fig. 2-13), which is subsequently infiltrated by cells migrating from the neural crest region. These cells are eventually incorporated into the thyroid gland and become the parafollicular cells (C cells) responsible for the secretion of calcitonin.[11,12]

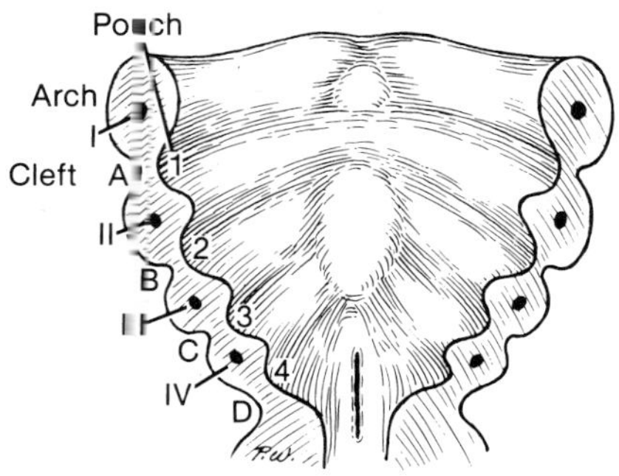

Fig. 2-11. Relationships of the branchial arches, clefts, and pouches in the floor of the mouth; stage I.

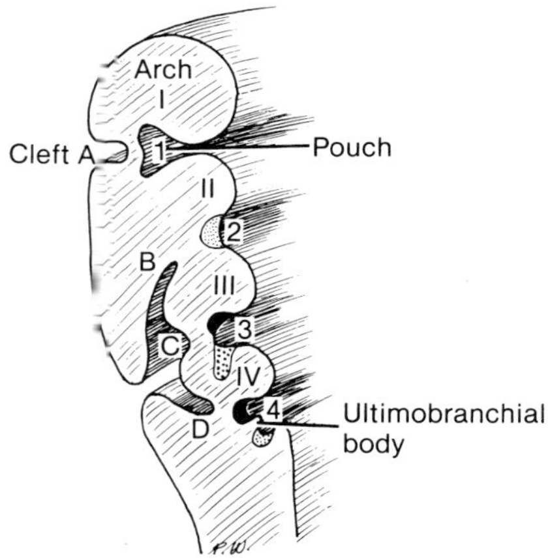

Fig. 2-12. Derivatives of the pharyngeal pouches and formation of the cervical sinus; stage II.

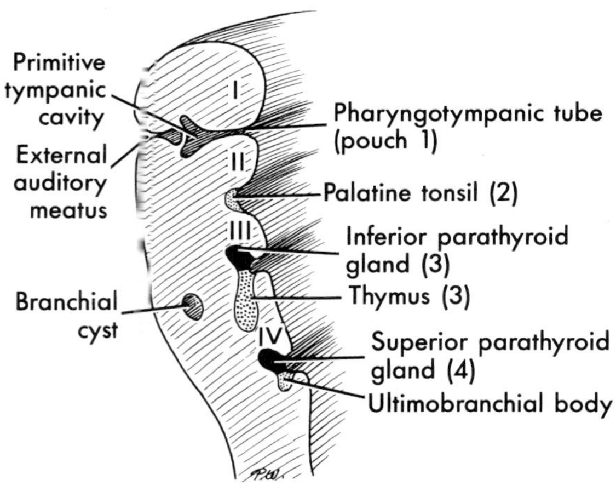

Fig. 2-13. Maturation of the pharyngeal pouches; stage III.

Branchial cleft remnants

The first branchial cleft becomes part of the external auditory canal, but the remaining branchial clefts are remodeled and normally do not form derivatives identifiable in adults.

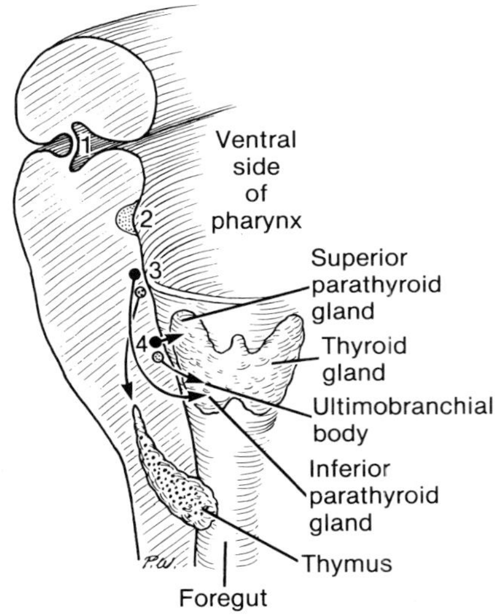

Fig. 2-14. Migration of the pharyngeal derivatives into the neck; stage IV.

However, the complicated morphodynamics of the branchial arch region seem to predispose this area to abnormalities, which range from minor cysts to major orofacial malformations. The clinical terminology of the various branchial abnormalities is confusing. Part of this confusion results from the clinical spectrum of these anomalies (i.e., they may present as a cyst, sinus, or fistula). A cyst has no communication with the body surface; a sinus communicates with a single body surface, either the skin or the pharynx; and a fistula communicates with two body surfaces. A cystic dilation of the tract may be associated with either a sinus or a fistula. The terms *branchial cleft* and *branchial pouch* are often used interchangeably, even though they refer to distinct structures. Occasionally, the term *groove* is used instead of pouch or cleft.

Craniofacial syndromes related to branchial arch structures

Hemifacial microsomia is thought to be related to a vascular injury in the region of the stapedial artery that results in microtia and mandibular hypoplasia.[14] Patients with hemifacial microsomia often have associated aural atresia. Mandibulofacial dysostosis (Treacher Collins syndrome) is related to bilateral abnormalities of the first and second branchial arches. This syndrome is characterized by lid colobomata, downslanting palpebral fissures, hypoplastic zygoma and mandible, and malformations of the external ear.[7] Other syndromes related to dysmorphogenesis of the first and second branchial arches include oculoauricular vertebral dysplasia (Goldenhar's syndrome) and branchio-otorenal syndrome.

Abnormalities of the first branchial cleft

Aberrant development of the first branchial cleft may lead to the formation of a cervical cyst or sinus in the region of the ear. Work[20] and Aronsohn and others[2] emphasized the difference in the embryogenesis of preauricular cysts versus cysts of the first branchial cleft. Preauricular cysts or pits occur anterior to the external auditory canal, usually superior to the region of the tragus. In essence, they are inclusion cysts related to fusion of the ectodermal hillocks on the first and second branchial arches during formation of the auricle.[10]

In contrast, true first branchial cleft abnormalities are duplications of the membranous part of the external auditory canal, and they present clinically as cysts, sinuses, and fistulas. Work[20] classified these abnormalities into two types: type I, of ectodermal origin, involves only the membranous part of the canal; and type II involves both ectoderm and mesoderm because there is also duplication of cartilage. As cystic masses or sinus tracts they may involve the parotid gland and CN VII (this is particularly true of type II), or they may lie inferior to the ear, in the superior neck.

Abnormalities of the second through fourth branchial clefts and pouches

During closure of the cervical sinus lying between the second branchial arch and the epipericardial ridge, ectoderm may become trapped, resulting in a future inclusion cyst (see Figs. 2-12 and 2-13). These are the more familiar branchial cleft cysts or sinuses, which lie in the lateral neck, anterior to the sternocleidomastoid muscle. As such, they may overlie the carotid or muscular triangles of the neck. The fistulous forms of these abnormalities are surgically challenging because they may extend from the superficial area of the neck near the clavicle superiorly to the bed of the palatine tonsil. The course of the tract through the deep part of the neck usually lies between the internal and external carotid arteries. The pathway of this tract is easily explained on an embryologic basis. The medial wall of the cervical sinus is the region of closing plates 2 to 4 (see Fig. 2-12). A fistulous pathway breaking through into the pharynx will penetrate one of these closing plates and thus enter into either the tonsillar bed (the second), the thyrohyoid membrane (third), or pyriform sinus or cricothyroid membrane (fourth).

Third branchial cleft sinuses, which communicate with the pharynx, travel deep to the carotid artery system in their superior extent. Thymopharyngeal cysts represent third branchial cleft remnants. As congenital cystic lesions of the neck, these are easily confused with lymphatic malformations. Remnants of the fourth branchial pouch, or pyriform sinus fistulas, may present as recurrent suppurative thyroiditis and are usually located on the left side of the neck.[17] These lesions may be associated with parathyroid, thymic, or thyroid tissue. Isolated branchial arch remnants may present as subcutaneous cartilaginous tags along the anterior border of the sternocleidomastoid muscle.

Midline lesions of the neck

Thyroglossal duct cysts and dermoids are the most common midline lesions of the neck in children and are often difficult to distinguish clinically. Thyroglossal duct cysts derive from persistence of the embryonic thyroglossal duct, anywhere between the foramen cecum and the thyroid gland. Because of the attachments to the base of the tongue, thyroglossal duct remnants will move superiorly in the neck when the patient protrudes his or her tongue. The thyroglossal duct remnant may contain ectopic thyroid tissue. Occasionally the cyst contains all of the functioning thyroid tissue. Because of the potential for permanent hypothyroidism after surgical excision, many authors advocate routine preoperative assessment of the thyroid.[13,15]

Ultrasound of the neck provides information regarding the consistency of cystic lesions and can also be used to assess for the presence of thyroid tissue in its normal position lower in the neck. Ultrasound examination is easily tolerated by children but does not provide functional information. Radionuclide thyroid scans provide functional information regarding thyroid tissue. There is a possibility of malignancy, usually arising from thyroid tissue, within these lesions. Surgical excision is the management of choice. Thyroglossal duct remnants often involve the central part of the hyoid, necessitating removal of the midportion of the hyoid to minimize the risk of recurrence.[19]

Another midline developmental abnormality of the neck is the midline cleft. The clinical presentation of this abnormality varies from an area of subcutaneous absence of midline tissue, presenting as a bluish area in the midline of the neck, to a midline vertical band. The vertical band becomes more restrictive with growth of the child and may interfere with mandibular excursion. Management involves excision of the band and Z-plasty.

The otolaryngologist must be familiar with the developmental anatomy of the neck. A working knowledge of neck anatomy and embryology is critical in diagnosing and managing patients effectively.

REFERENCES

1. Anson BJ, Donaldson JA: *Surgical anatomy of the temporal bone and ear*, ed 2, Philadelphia, 1973, WB Saunders.
2. Aronsohn RS and others: Anomalies of the first branchial cleft, *Arch Otolaryngol Head Neck Surg* 102:737, 1976.
3. Daseler EH, Anson BJ: Surgical anatomy of the subclavian artery and its branches, *Surg Gynecol Obstet* 108:149, 1959.
4. Godin MS and others: Fourth branchial pouch sinus: principles of diagnosis and management, *Laryngoscope* 100:174, 1990.
5. Grodinsky M, Holyoke EA: The fascias and fascial spaces of the head, neck and adjacent regions, *Am J Anat* 63:367, 1938.
6. Haymaker W, Woodhall B: *Peripheral nerve injuries*, ed 2, Philadelphia, 1953, WB Saunders.
7. Jones KL: *Smith's recognizable patterns of human malformation*, ed 4, Philadelphia, 1988, WB Saunders.
8. Langman J: *Medical embryology*, ed 4, Baltimore, 1981, Williams & Wilkins.
9. Last RJ: *Anatomy: regional and applied*, ed 6, Edinburgh, 1978, Churchill Livingstone.
10. Minkowitz S, Minkowitz F: Congenital aural sinuses, *Surg Gynecol Obstet* 118:801, 1964.
11. Pearse AGE, Carvalheira AF: Cytochemical evidence for an ultimobranchial origin of rodent thyroid C cells, *Nature* 214:929, 1967.

Box 3-1. Intraoperative monitoring standards

Continuous presence of qualified anesthesia personnel in the operating room
Continuous evaluation of:
- Oxygenation
  - Inspired oxygen concentration with an oxygen analyzer
  - Blood oxygenation with a pulse oximeter
- Ventilation
  - Qualitative assessment: chest excursion, observation of the reservoir bag, auscultation of breath sounds
  - Quantitative assessment with end-tidal CO_2 analysis
  - A low-pressure disconnect alarm when mechanical ventilation is used
- Circulation
  - Continuous electrocardiogram
  - Arterial blood pressure at least every 5 minutes
  - At least one of the following: palpation of pulse, auscultation of heart sounds, intraarterial blood pressure monitoring, ultrasound peripheral pulse monitoring, or pulse plethysmography
- Body temperature

Box 3-2. Indications for preoperative laboratory testing at Children's Hospital and Medical Center, Seattle

Hematocrit
- Any infant born prematurely who is less than 6 months of age
- Any child in whom significant blood loss is expected

Electrolytes
- Any patient with chronic renal failure
- Any patient on diuretic therapy

Sickle cell screen
- Any black patient not previously screened

Pregnancy test
- Any sexually active teenager not using contraception

In addition the use of pulse oximetry alone or in combination with capnography has reduced the relative frequency of adverse respiratory events compared with adverse cardiovascular events, perhaps because pulse oximetry and capnography are more effective in preventing respiratory events than cardiovascular events.[6]

3. The use of subspecialty-trained pediatric anesthesiologists for the care of infants and children has been suggested to be associated with improved outcomes,[36] although this contentious claim is difficult to prove.[64]

Current estimates of anesthetic mortality vary widely, depending on the definition of anesthetic death. However, in ASA Physical Status 1 and 2, pediatric outpatients' demise from an anesthetic-related cause is very rare, perhaps as low as 1 in 50,000 cases. Thus, parents of otherwise healthy children can be reassured that outcomes in modern-day pediatric anesthesia are excellent.

PREOPERATIVE ASSESSMENT

Preanesthesia clinics

The recent emphasis on cost containment has forced many changes in the practice of pediatric anesthesia over the past decade. More and more patients with increasing severity of illness are being operated on as outpatients, forcing preoperative contact between anesthesiologists and their patients and families into a very few minutes. Preoperative anesthesia clinics have developed in response to these changes.

The preanesthesia clinic was originally aimed at medically complicated patients but can and should be more widely used. The clinic visit affords the opportunity—in a relaxed setting—for the anesthesiologist to take a history; perform a physical examination; obtain necessary laboratory tests; and inform the family about the anticipated procedures, including nothing-by-mouth (NPO) times, premedication, anesthetic induction and maintenance, and postoperative pain management techniques. Anesthetic risk can be discussed, with ample time for patients and their families to ask questions. A trained clinic nurse can educate the child and family about the impending surgical visit and discuss family and patient fears and concerns. The costs of operating an anesthesia clinic relate primarily to nursing personnel, as the physician costs are generally considered to be part of the global anesthesia fee. Justification of these costs can be made on the basis of facilitation of movement of patients into the operating room on the day of surgery as well as on patient and staff satisfaction.

Medical assessment

Necessary preoperative information includes a review of the patient's body systems, response to previous anesthetics, current medications, allergies, recent illnesses, (including upper respiratory infections [URIs]) and family history of problems with anesthesia. The physical examination concentrates on airway anatomy, including the mouth, jaw, teeth, and neck, as well as chest and heart auscultation. Laboratory tests are obtained as indicated by the child's condition rather than as a routine. For example, a preoperative blood count is a low-yield test that is probably not cost-effective, given the low incidence of anemia in children younger than 18 years of age.[26,80] Situations in which preoperative laboratory tests should be considered are shown in Box 3-2.

A number of medical conditions may modify preoperative preparation or intraanesthetic or postanesthetic management. Therefore, patients with these conditions make excellent candidates for preanesthesia clinic visits.

Upper respiratory infection

The decision of whether to anesthetize a child with a URI is recurrent in pediatric anesthesia. In making this decision, it is helpful to know the risks involved. Deterioration in pulmonary function occurs during a URI, including a decrease in flow rates such as forced expiratory volume in 1 second (FEV_1),[67] decreased mucociliary clearance,[49] and increased airway reactivity.[19] Resolution of these abnormalities can take up to 6 weeks.

These changes in pulmonary function have other clinical correlates. McGill, Coveler, and Epstein[57] reported on 11 cases (no denominator) of intraoperative atelectasis identified by chest radiography in children anesthetized within 4 weeks after a URI. Children with a URI may be at increased risk for postoperative desaturation,[15] croup, or airway obstruction. Conversely, a prospective series of nonintubated children undergoing myringotomy failed to show a difference in perioperative complications between asymptomatic children and children with URI symptoms.[95]

Other factors must also be considered. Do the symptoms result from allergy rather than infection? How severe is the URI? A child with fever, cough, malaise, and myalgias may be at higher risk than a child with mild rhinorrhea. How elective is the surgery? How much inconvenience would result for the family from cancellation or postponement? How often is the child symptom-free? Given the frequency of URIs in some children and the time required for resolution of pulmonary function abnormalities, it may be difficult to find a disease-free interval. Will the surgery reduce the frequency of URIs in the future?

Frequently, the decision seems to involve more art than science. In equivocal cases, a leukocyte count and a chest radiograph may be helpful.[83] Measurement of the child's hemoglobin saturation while breathing room air may identify some at-risk children but is not very sensitive. Unfortunately, no combination of historical features, physical findings, or laboratory tests can define the child at risk. A discussion of the potential risks and benefits with the parents will allow them to participate in the decision-making process. Good communication between the anesthesiologist and the otolaryngologist is essential for establishing some consistency in approach.

Infants born premature

In the early 1980s, a high incidence of apnea was reported following administration of general anesthesia in the first few months of life to children who had been born prematurely (37 weeks gestational age or younger).[47,93] The risk probably extends to approximately 55 weeks of postconceptual age and is inversely related to both postconceptual and postgestational age as well as hematocrit.[11]

Although the etiology of apnea is unknown, most episodes are central in origin; however, nearly one third are associated with airway obstruction.[43] Halothane blunts the ventilatory response to carbon dioxide and hypoxia, even in subanesthetic concentrations,[40] thus accentuating preexisting abnormalities of respiratory control that may result in an apneic event. Although apnea has been reported after general, spinal,[13] and caudal[101] anesthesia, one prospective series has suggested the incidence is lower following regional techniques without adjunctive sedation than after either general or regional anesthesia with intravenous sedation.[104] Administration of caffeine may also lessen the incidence of postoperative apnea.[103]

Elective procedures should be postponed until premature infants are 55 weeks of postconceptual age, at which time the incidence of apnea is less than 1%.[11] Following nonelective procedures on children at risk for postoperative apnea, cardiorespiratory and pulse oximetry monitoring should be performed for 12 to 24 hours; monitoring should be continued until at least 12 apnea-free hours have elapsed.

Asthma

A history of asthma in a child is important to the anesthesiologist because good preoperative preparation and careful intraoperative anesthetic management can usually prevent serious episodes of bronchospasm. History of severity (i.e., current medication, recent wheezing history, past need for emergency room visits or hospitalization) correlates well with intraoperative risk. A thorough physical examination, including chest auscultation, is necessary to rule out active bronchospasm. Elective surgery should not be performed in the presence of active wheezing. In a child with active wheezing, pulmonary function testing, especially FEV_1, may be useful for documenting the extent of obstructive disease and the potential for reversal with bronchodilators. Improvement in expiratory flow rates after a trial of bronchodilators suggests that adjustments in bronchodilator therapy before elective surgery may be beneficial.[39] A variety of bronchodilator compounds are available for preoperative and intraoperative use, including β_2 agonists, corticosteroids, xanthine derivatives, and anticholinergics.[39] Nebulized β_2 agonists such as albuterol are the most commonly used agents in the perioperative period because of ease of administration, good efficacy, and low incidence of side effects.

Intraoperatively, the most common cause of bronchospasm in susceptible patients is instrumentation of the airway under light planes of anesthesia.[84] Both general and regional anesthetic agents can be used to obtund airway reflexes. Lidocaine (1 to 2 mg/kg) can be sprayed into the trachea or given intravenously to prevent reflex-induced bronchospasm.[16] Although most inhaled anesthetics prevent or ameliorate bronchospasm, halothane remains the time-honored drug of choice. Halothane increases bronchial caliber and pulmonary compliance, decreases pulmonary resistance, and improves gas exchange during active bronchospasm.[8,23] Extubation of the trachea while the patient is under surgical planes of anesthesia, followed by a slow, smooth emergence, minimizes the risk of bronchospasm. Careful attention must be paid to airway patency until the child is awake.

Cystic fibrosis

Early diagnosis and antibiotic treatment have improved the health and survival of children with cystic fibrosis (CF); currently, nearly 50% of CF patients are over the age of 18 years. More than 90% of children with CF develop pansinusitis and 20% develop nasal polyps, which may require surgery. A child with CF presents a significant challenge to the pediatric anesthesiologist; malnutrition, dehydration, and pulmonary insufficiency are all potential concerns. In a recent series, 13% of patients with CF had some anesthetic complication.[44]

Preoperative evaluation of patients with CF is important in minimizing postanesthetic morbidity. The severity of pulmonary disease can be quantitated with historical features (e.g., degree of exercise intolerance and amount of sputum production) and a thorough physical examination (e.g., respiratory rate, work of breathing, quality of breath sounds, and skin color). Patients with evidence of significant disease should have oximetry and arterial blood gas analysis as well as an electrocardiogram and echocardiogram to screen for right ventricular dysfunction (cor pulmonale). If the patient is cooperative, pulmonary function tests may help to quantitate the degree of pulmonary compromise and serve as a baseline to assess the impact of preoperative therapy.

In patients with significant pulmonary disease, a preoperative "tune-up" may help prevent perioperative complications. A regular program of chest physiotherapy includes chest percussion and postural drainage. Sputum samples are sent for culture and sensitivity, and the patient receives an aminoglycoside and synthetic penicillin until culture results are available. The patient is well hydrated to avoid inspissation of secretions. Patients not taking oral vitamin K supplements are given enteral vitamin K. Many of these patients are emotionally labile and require psychologic support before surgery.

If a general anesthetic is required, halothane is useful because it allows rapid induction and emergence from anesthesia, is potent enough to allow administration of high-concentration oxygen, and is bronchodilating. If premedication is required, a benzodiazepine can be given with minimal risk of respiratory depression. An anticholinergic can be given if desired; the concern about excessive drying of secretions has not been a significant clinical problem. An endotracheal tube is usually placed to deal with the most commonly reported complications, which include copious secretions, airway irritability, and compromised oxygenation.[44] Ventilation is usually assisted or controlled to prevent intraoperative loss of lung volume and subsequent atelectasis. All delivered gases are humidified and intravenous hydration is maintained to facilitate clearance of secretions. Tracheal suctioning is performed as necessary. At the end of the procedure, the trachea is extubated once the patient is awake and breathing spontaneously.

Diabetes mellitus

The key to successful anesthetic management of a child with diabetes mellitus is careful administration of dextrose and insulin and frequent monitoring of blood glucose. Knowledge of the patient's daily insulin type and amount and the resulting blood glucose is important to the anesthesiologist. A normal diet and insulin regimen should be maintained up to the day of surgery. Diabetic children should be scheduled as the first surgery of the day. One of several approaches can be taken in the management of glucose and insulin[91]:

1. On the morning of surgery, half of the usual insulin dose is given as regular insulin (onset in 30 minutes, peak effect in 2 to 4 hours, duration of action 6 to 8 hours) after an intravenous infusion of 5% dextrose in 0.45% normal saline is established at 1500 ml/m^2/day. Serum glucose levels are monitored frequently before and after surgery and are maintained between 100 and 250 mg/dl with a sliding scale of regular insulin until the patient is eating and can resume his or her usual insulin regimen.
2. On the morning of surgery, a continous infusion of insulin and glucose is initiated (1 to 2 units of insulin per 100 ml of 5% dextrose). Adjustments can be made in the ratio to maintain blood glucose in the desired range.
3. For procedures that are brief and will allow oral intake in the recovery room (e.g., myringotomy), no insulin and no glucose are given. These cases should be scheduled as the first of the day. When oral intake is reinitiated, 40% to 60% of the usual daily insulin dose is given subcutaneously, and blood glucose is monitored carefully.

Appropriate use of nonsedating antiemetics in the postoperative period allows this group of patients to return to oral intake as soon as possible.

PREPARATION FOR ANESTHESIA

Psychologic preparation

Fears about hospitalization are common among children, including fear of separation, pain, loss of control, and even death. Many of these fears are age-dependent[98] (Table 3-1). Awareness of these developmental stages allows the anesthesiologist to anticipate the needs of any given child. For children old enough to comprehend, details of the anesthetic and surgical experience should be presented in age-specific language.[42] Children given specific information before surgery have been shown to be less anxious than children given only general information.[17] Movies or videotapes can help

Table 3-1. Age-specific concerns of children

Age	Specific concerns
Infant (6-18 months)	Separation anxiety
Toddler (1-2 years)	Fear of strangers, loss of mastery of the environment
Preschool (2-5 years)	Separation anxiety; difficulty distinguishing reality from fantasy; fear of pain, mutilation
School age (6-12 years)	Fear of the unknown, loss of control, autonomy, pain, mutilation
Adolescent (13-18 years)	Precarious sense of self; fear of pain, mutilation, loss of control, autonomy

From Orr RJ, Lynn AM: *Curr Rev Clin Anesth* 12:29, 1991.

Table 3-2. Recommended nothing-by-mouth times

	Fasting time (hours)	
Patient age	**Solids (includes breast milk and formula)**	**Clear liquids**
Younger than 6 months	4	2
6-36 months	6	3
Older than 36 months	8	3

Adapted from Coté C: In McGoldrick KE, editor: *Ambulatory anesthesiology: a problem-oriented approach,* Baltimore, 1995, Williams & Wilkins

children and parents cope with the mysteries of hospital routines.[35]

Premedication

The choice of premedication is based on the age and specific needs of the patient. The usual goals of premedication are to reduce anxiety and ease separation from parents. Because most children fear needles, oral or rectal administration of sedatives is preferred to intramuscular injection. Children younger than 8 months of age generally do not need premedication and separate easily from their parents. Children 8 months to 2 to 3 years of age may not accept oral premedication well; these patients may do better with rectal administration of either a barbiturate such as methohexital (20 to 30 mg/kg of a 10% solution)[48] or a benzodiazepine such as midazolam (0.5 to 1.0 mg/kg).[81] While midazolam administration usually results in drowsiness and even euphoria, methohexital often results in complete loss of consciousness and must be treated as the induction of anesthesia, with careful attention to vital signs and airway patency.

Children 3 to 4 years of age and older usually accept oral premedication well. Midazolam (0.5 mg/kg up to a 20-mg total dose), mixed in a flavored syrup and administered 10 to 20 minutes beforehand, usually smoothes the induction of anesthesia and has become the most popular of the sedative–hypnotics for premedication in children.[58] Midazolam is usually well tolerated, although an occasional decrease in saturation or blood pressure may be observed. In addition, emergence delirium may occur and require reversal with intravenous flumazenil (1 to 3 μg/kg).

Anticholinergic agents may be desirable when copious airway secretions are a concern or when vagal tone from airway manipulation may produce decreases in heart rate and cardiac output. In children younger than 6 months of age, halothane is more likely to cause bradycardia and a significant reduction in cardiac output than in older children. In this age group and with this anesthetic agent, the routine use of anticholinergic agents can prevent these changes.[60] Atropine (0.02 mg/kg) or glycopyrrolate (0.01 mg/kg) given intravenously at the time of induction can obviate the pain of an intramuscular injection.

Nothing-by-mouth orders

To minimize the risk of aspiration of gastric contents during the induction of anesthesia, an adequate period of fasting must be maintained. Traditionally, both food and fluids have been withheld after the midnight before surgery. However, a prolonged period of fasting is uncomfortable for children, is unpleasant for the family, and risks depletion of intravascular volume. It has recently been recognized that administration of clear liquids to children 2 to 3 hours before induction does not increase gastric residual volume or acidity compared with a more prolonged fast.[86] In addition, morbidity and mortality due to aspiration of gastric contents in children is exceedingly rare.[69] Thus fasting guidelines have been liberalized in recent years (Table 3-2). Nevertheless, it is important when giving these instructions to parents to emphasize the safety issues involved in order to maximize compliance and avoid unnecessary delays in the start of the procedure.

INDUCTION TECHNIQUES

Anesthesia can be induced by mask inhalation of a potent vapor in oxygen with or without nitrous oxide (inhalation induction), by injection of a sedative–hypnotic agent through an intravenous catheter (intravenous induction), or by intramuscular injection. As much as possible, this choice is given to children; younger children tend to fear needles and prefer an inhalation induction, whereas older children and teenagers usually accept an intravenous induction.

Parental presence

With increasing frequency, parents are expressing a desire to be present at the time of their child's anesthetic induction.[29] Although parental motives vary, most hope that their child's anxiety will be less if one or both parents are present. Hospitals tend to support this request as a marketing tool. Some hospitals have induction areas outside the sterile envelope of the operating room. If not, parents can be dressed in cover gowns and escorted into and out of the operating room for the induction.

Studies examining the impact of parental presence have had variable results, with some showing no significant impact,[34] some showing a decrease in patient anxiety,[27,87] and others showing an increase in patient anxiety.[110] Parents with a high anxiety level seem to have a negative impact on their child during induction. As there is no evidence that patient safety is compromised with the parents present at induction, the majority of anesthesiologists surveyed are in favor of this practice.[77] Thus it is likely that the trend will continue. Parents should be thoroughly educated about what to expect and how they can best help their child. They must agree to leave the induction area immediately when instructed to do so. Highly anxious parents should be encouraged not to participate.

Inhalation induction

Until recently, halothane was the agent of choice for inhalation induction because of its lack of pungency. The recently introduced agent sevoflurane is even less pungent and is replacing halothane as an induction agent in many pediatric centers. A small amount of scented liquid (e.g., bubblegum, watermelon, root beer) applied to the inside of the mask disguises the odor of the anesthetic agent and improves the patient's acceptance of the technique. Noise in the room should be kept to a minimum during anesthesia induction. The anesthesiologist can tell the child a soothing and entertaining story that directs the child's thoughts away from the reality of the situation. As the concentration of anesthetic agent is increased rapidly, most children lose consciousness in less than 1 minute. The parents, if present, can be ushered out at this point, and an intravenous drip is started in preparation for the balance of the procedure.

Intravenous induction

Intravenous induction requires the presence of an intravenous catheter and thus is reserved for older children or teenagers, children with a preexisting intravenous drip, children who need a rapid-sequence induction because of a full stomach, or children who object to an inhalation induction.

Eutectic mixture of local anesthetics (EMLA) cream is a mixture of lidocaine and prilocaine that penetrates intact skin and, when applied for 45 minutes or more, significantly decreases the pain associated with an intravenous insertion.[31] The reliability of EMLA is increased if it is applied for at least 1 hour. EMLA should be used with caution in children younger than 3 months of age or in children receiving other medications that may induce methemoglobin because of the risk of methemoglobinemia.[20] Plasma concentrations of lidocaine and prilocaine are well below the toxic level[20] but may be higher in children with traumatized or inflamed skin.

The most common agent for intravenous induction is thiopental, an ultra–short-acting barbiturate that produces sleep in healthy, unpremedicated children within 1 minute of administration of 5 to 6 mg/kg.[10] This drug can produce hypotension and must be used with caution in hypovolemic patients or patients with poor myocardial contractility.

An alternative intravenous induction agent is propofol, an alkylphenol that, because of poor solubility in water, is formulated as a 1% solution in a white soybean oil, egg licithin, and glycerol emulsion. Propofol is highly lipophilic and rapidly redistributes throughout body compartments with a distribution half-life of about 2 minutes and an elimination half-life of about 30 minutes. The dose for induction of anesthesia varies with age[71]; infants 1 to 6 months of age require about 3 mg/kg, whereas older children require about 2.5 mg/kg. The major advantages of propofol are a rapid, clear-headed recovery with minimal associated nausea and vomiting. The major disadvantage is pain on injection, particularly into small veins.[105] Lidocaine (0.5 to 1.0 mg/kg) administered before or during propofol injection may decrease the incidence of pain. Propofol may cause hypotension, apnea, and desaturation. Another disadvantage is its cost compared with pentothal. Propofol is also used for anesthesia maintenance as an intravenous infusion of 100 to 200 μg/kg/min. Propofol has minimal analgesic properties, however, and must be combined with a narcotic or other analgesic to provide a complete anesthetic.

Rapid-sequence induction

Patients with a full stomach are at increased risk for aspiration of stomach contents during induction of anesthesia. Patients who require full-stomach precautions include those who have not fasted for an adequate period, those with gastrointestinal obstruction, and trauma patients whose gastric motility is depressed. Patients are preoxygenated with 100% oxygen by mask then given an induction dose of sedative and a muscle relaxant, usually succinylcholine (2 mg/kg). Manual pressure is applied over the cricoid in an attempt to seal the esophagus and prevent passive regurgitation.[88] Pressure is not released until the endotracheal tube is in place and the cuff, if present, is inflated.

Intramuscular induction

Ketamine is a derivative of phencyclidine with potent analgesic and amnestic properties when given in the recommended doses of 1 to 3 mg/kg intravenously or 5 to 10 mg/kg intramuscularly. Ketamine is very useful as an intramuscular induction agent in children who are combative or unable to cooperate with a standard inhalation or intravenous induction, often because of mental retardation or emotional handicaps. Because ketamine has sympathomimetic properties, it does not cause hypotension as does thiopental and thus is an excellent choice for anesthetic induction in hypovolemic patients. Ketamine may be the intravenous induction agent of choice in patients with reactive airways[9] because it increases circulating catecholamines and causes relaxation of tracheal smooth muscle. Other uses include burn dressing changes and suture removal.

Ketamine tends to produce copious secretions and should be accompanied by atropine or another antisialogue. The incidence of postoperative vomiting may be as high as 30%. Intraoperative and postoperative dreams and hallucinations have been reported,[106] more often in older than in younger children and less often when other sedative–hypnotic agents are used.

ANESTHESIA MAINTENANCE

Inhalational agents

Nitrous oxide

Nitrous oxide is the most widely used anesthetic agent in children and adults. Its popularity is due to its low solubility resulting in rapid uptake and distribution, its lack of odor, and the fact that it does not cause cardiovascular depression. Although it allows the delivery of lower concentrations of other anesthetic agents, nitrous oxide itself is not very potent. Consequently, it must be delivered in high concentration to have an analgesic and hypnotic effect, thereby limiting the concentration of oxygen that can be delivered; it is not useful in patients who require high concentrations of oxygen. There is a thirty-fourfold difference in the blood–gas coefficients of nitrogen (0.013) and nitrous oxide (0.46); thus nitrous oxide will enter air-filled cavities faster than nitrogen can leave. In a fixed cavity like the middle ear, the result is an increase in pressure. Nitrous oxide may represent a hazard in patients with previous reconstructive middle-ear surgery.[72] During tympanoplasty, the tympanic membrane graft can be lifted off by the middle-ear pressure generated by nitrous oxide. Thus nitrous oxide should be limited to 50% concentration and turned off 15 minutes before the closure of the middle ear[65] or even avoided entirely.[73]

Halothane

Halothane is the most commonly used potent inhalational agent for infants and children because of its acceptance by patients, ease and rapidity of induction, reliable depression of airway reflexes, potent bronchodilation, rapid awakening, and long safety record. Because it is a potent agent, it can be delivered with a high concentration of oxygen. Halothane also has well-recognized side effects, the knowledge of which usually allows titration of the dose to minimize the risk of complications:

1. Halothane decreases minute ventilation and tidal volume, resulting in an increase in arterial CO_2 tension.[45] Controlled or assisted ventilation is therefore indicated in small children and infants.
2. Halothane is a direct myocardial depressant, perhaps more so in the neonatal myocardium than in the adult.[66] In addition, halothane tends to decrease heart rate both by a direct depressant effect on the sinoatrial node and by inhibiting baroreceptor function.[102] This is particularly detrimental in newborns, whose cardiac output is linearly related to heart rate because of low ventricular compliance. Thus, during administration of halothane to newborns and infants, strict attention to vital signs is critical; the dose is reduced when cardiovascular depression is deemed to be clinically significant.
3. Halothane sensitizes the myocardium to the effects of catecholamines and elevated CO_2 tension, resulting in the frequent occurrence of ventricular arrhythmias such as ventricular premature contractions and, rarely, ventricular tachycardia. Such arrhythmias usually resolve with reduction of the CO_2 tension, administration of lidocaine (1 mg/kg), or a change in anesthetic agent from halothane to isoflurane or sevoflurane, which do not have the same propensity to sensitize the myocardium.
4. Halothane increases cerebral blood flow in a dose-dependent manner and is relatively contraindicated in patients with elevated intracranial pressure. Reduction of arterial CO_2 levels partially ameliorate this effect.
5. Halothane is a trigger agent for malignant hyperthermia and should be avoided in susceptible patients.
6. Halothane, at least in adults, has been associated with a postoperative form of hepatitis, usually after repeated exposures. The incidence in children is perhaps as low as 1 in 200,000 cases compared with 1 in 6000 adult cases.

Isoflurane

Isoflurane offers no advantage over halothane for the pediatric otolaryngology patient. It is more pungent and not nearly as well accepted by children during as inhalation induction. It also tends to stimulate rather than obtund airway reflexes. Although isoflurane increases rather than decreases heart rate, and therefore may have some advantage over halothane for use in newborns, it is still a myocardial depressant and causes dose-related decreases in cardiac output in newborns and infants of the same magnitude as those caused by halothane.[66] It is a good alternative to halothane when ventricular arrhythmias develop.

Sevoflurane

Sevoflurane is a valuable addition to the anesthesiologist's armamentarium for several reasons: first, it is less pungent than halothane, and even better tolerated during inhalation induction. Second, it has a blood/gas partition coefficient that is similar to that of nitrous oxide, so induction and emergence times are shorter than with halothane. Finally, it may be associated with less cardiovascular depression than is halothane, although additional studies are needed before a conclusion can be drawn.

Sevoflurane has several disadvantages. Its offset is so rapid that without adjunctive administration of narcotics the perception of and response to pain may be accentuated. In addition, sevoflurane is approximately 10 times more expensive than halothane, which is a significant issue in a time of cost containment. Sevoflurane has assumed a role as an induction agent and a maintenance agent for very short procedures, but it is generally replaced by halothane following induction for longer procedures.

Intravenous agents

Narcotics

Morphine sulfate. Morphine is the most frequently used narcotic in children. The usual intravenous dose is 0.1 to 0.2 mg/kg; the dose may need to be reduced in critically ill children. The half-life after intravenous administration is approximately 3 hours in older children but is significantly longer in infants as a result of diminished clearance.[52] The major side effect is respiratory depression, resulting from diminished tidal volume and respiratory rate. Many believe that newborns are at higher risk than older children for respiratory depression, although it is unclear whether this reflects a difference in pharmacokinetics or pharmacodynamics. Infusions of morphine at rates of 10 to 30 mcg/kg/hr have been described; these dosage rates result in good analgesia without significant respiratory depression.[51] Morphine also causes histamine release and can cause significant hypotension when given as a bolus, particularly in hypovolemic patients.

Fentanyl. Fentanyl is the most commonly used supplement to anesthesia in children. Although the usual intravenous dose is 1 to 2 mcg/kg, doses up to 100 mcg/kg have been given to cardiac surgery patients with minimal cardiovascular depression.[108] Preterm and full-term newborns have variable and prolonged clearance, probably because of reduced hepatic blood flow.[56]

The effect of low-dose fentanyl is terminated largely by redistribution, resulting in a rapid reduction in clinical effect. Because fentanyl is highly lipophilic, however, higher or repeated doses result in drug accumulation; clearance then becomes dependent on metabolism,[94] and the clinical effect, including respiratory depression, may last for hours. Chest-wall rigidity has been reported following rapid fentanyl administration, although the etiology of this problem is unclear. Bradycardia may occur due to increased vagal tone.

Meperidine. Meperidine is a commonly used narcotic that has been reported to cause less histamine release than morphine when given to adults, although this reaction has not been carefully studied in children. The usual intravenous dose is 1 to 2 mg/kg, although reduced doses should be given to critically ill patients. The half-life is just under 4 hours.[54] Meperidine has been used to reduce postoperative shivering, with a concomitant reduction in oxygen consumption and CO_2 production.[53] Meperidine is relatively contraindicated in patients with seizure disorders; seizures have been reported secondary to accumulation of the metabolite normeperidine.

Muscle relaxants

Succinylcholine. Succinylcholine is the only depolarizing relaxant used in children. Because 90% of an intravenous dose is rapidly hydrolyzed in the plasma by pseudocholinesterase, patients with deficient or reduced levels of pseudocholinesterase have a prolonged effect from succinylcholine. With the advent of intermediate-acting nondepolarizing relaxants, the use of succinylcholine for routine surgical procedures is declining, primarily due to side effects relating to its depolarizing mode of action. However, it remains the most rapid-acting of all muscle relaxants and is still indicated for use in rapid-sequence inductions and in treatment of laryngospasm. Intravenous administration of 1.5 to 2.0 mg/kg achieves 95% twitch depression in 40 seconds,[59] resulting in excellent intubating conditions. Succinylcholine can also be given intramuscularly (4 to 5 mg/kg) if the intravenous route is unavailable, although the clinical effect is delayed in onset, depending on perfusion to the area of deposition.

The side effects of succinylcholine are numerous. Some degree of increase in masseter muscle tone is common and in some cases is extreme enough to mimic true trismus.[96] This is an important distinction to make because as many as 50% of patients with trismus after succinylcholine are biopsy-positive for susceptibility to malignant hyperthermia.[68] Succinylcholine can also cause bradycardia from an increase in vagal tone. The decline in heart rate is usually transient and if not is responsive to intravenous atropine; occasionally, true asystole is seen. Hyperkalemia can be seen as a result of depolarization of the myoneural junction; increases of serum potassium of 0.5 mEq/l occur even in normal children.[24] Life-threatening hyperkalemia after succinylcholine administration can occur in children with burns, tetanus, paraplegia, encephalitis, crush injuries, and neuromuscular disease.[24] Myoglobinemia occurs in approximately 40% of children anesthetized with halothane who are given succinylcholine, an effect that can be partially attenuated with a prior dose of a nondepolarizing agent to prevent fasciculations. A series of cardiac arrests has recently been reported in boys, presumably with previously undiagnosed muscular dystrophies, who were given succinylcholine and developed massive muscle breakdown and potassium release.[78] In 1994, in response to these reports, the manufacturer placed a warning on the package insert cautioning the practitioner about the routine use of succinylcholine.

Intraocular pressure increases after succinylcholine administration whether or not fasciculations occur; this is due to contraction of the extraocular muscles.[14] Thus succinylcholine is relatively contraindicated in patients with open eye injuries.

For the reasons stated above, many pediatric anesthesiologists have abandoned the routine use of succinylcholine except for rapid-sequence inductions and laryngospasm.

Nondepolarizing muscle relaxants. A variety of nondepolarizing muscle relaxants are available. These agents vary

Table 3-3. Approximate doses, onset times, and recovery times for commonly used muscle relaxants

	ED95 (mg/kg)		Onset times* (minutes)		Recovery time to 95% of control	
	Infants	Children	Infants	Children	Infants	Children
Mivacurium	NA	0.115	NA	1.5	NA	18
Rocuronium	NA	0.300	NA	1.3	NA	42
Atracurium	0.150	0.260	NA	3.8	25	25
Vecuronium	0.028	0.045	1.5	2.4	73	35
Pancuronium	0.05	0.06	2.5	2.5	50	50

ED95—Estimated dose to produce 95% neuromuscular blockade; NA—Not available.
* Time to maximal blockade.

according to dose, speed of onset, and duration of action. As shown in Table 3.3, the pharmacologic properties of these drugs may be different in infants than in older children. The choice is generally made on the basis of duration of the surgical procedure. None of the nondepolarizing agents, even rocuronium, produce good intubating conditions as rapidly as succinylcholine. In addition, at the higher doses required to produce paralysis in less than 1 minute, duration of action is prolonged.

EMERGENCE FROM ANESTHESIA

The decision of whether to extubate a patient while he or she is awake or under surgical planes of anesthesia depends on a number of factors. Deep extubations are smoother and facilitate rapid turnover. Also to be considered, however, are the patient's age, airway anatomy and underlying disease, the presence of blood or secretions in the airway, the presence of a full stomach, and environmental factors (e.g., the ability of the postanesthesia care unit [PACU] staff to manage an obstructed airway and the availability of an individual able to reintubate a patient if necessary). Deep extubation is preferred in patients with asthma or in those for whom coughing would be contraindicated. Factors that favor awake extubation include a full stomach, age less than 6 months, difficult airway anatomy, copious blood or secretions in the airway, or a predisposition to apnea. Systematic comparisons of awake versus deep extubation have revealed that patients extubated while awake have lower saturations (probably because of coughing during emergence), but there is no difference in overall morbidity or mortality.[70,74] It appears that either technique can be performed safely; the anesthesiologist should have both approaches in his or her armamentarium and, using clinical judgment, choose the one that best fits the situation.

POSTOPERATIVE MANAGEMENT

Nausea and vomiting

Nausea and vomiting can result in an unpleasant recovery from surgery and anesthesia as well as a delayed discharge from the PACU. The incidence of nausea and vomiting in pediatric anesthesia is variable, depending on the type of surgery and the type of anesthetic used. Tonsillectomy and middle-ear surgery may be associated with an incidence of vomiting as high as 70%.[21] The use of narcotics and perhaps nitrous oxide increases the risk of nausea and vomiting. By contrast, propofol reduces the incidence of vomiting compared with halothane in children undergoing adenotonsillectomy.[97]

Several antiemetics have been found to reduce the incidence of postoperative nausea and vomiting. Metoclopramide (0.1 to 0.15 mg/kg), a short-acting drug that speeds gastric emptying but also has central antiemetic effects, has been shown to be effective and without significant side effects in children following tonsillectomy.[21] Droperidol is an effective antiemetic in doses from 5 to 75 μg/kg; however, when higher doses are used, sedation and extrapyramidal side effects may be seen.[50] Ondansetron, a long-acting, nonsedating drug used frequently in chemotherapy patients, is also effective in tonsillectomy patients[90] but is expensive. Doses of 50 μg/kg have been found to be as effective as 100-μg/kg doses.[100] In a recent comparative study of children undergoing outpatient tonsillectomy, the frequency of inhospital emesis was 16% in patients given ondansetron and 30% in the droperidol group.[89] One approach is to use metoclopramide as a first-line drug and use the more expensive ondansetron as a backup. However, ondansetron's additional cost may be justified by shorter recovery times.

An inexpensive but effective method of reducing the incidence of nausea and vomiting is to withhold oral fluids in the postoperative period until the child asks for them, as forced oral fluids increase the incidence of vomiting and delay discharge.[85]

Postintubation croup

In children up to approximately 8 years of age, the subglottis is the narrowest portion of the airway and may be the source of postoperative airway obstruction because of mucosal swelling. A reduction in the reported incidence of postintubation croup from 1% in 1977[41] to 0.1% more recently (1991)[46] may result from using proper-size, non–

tissue reactive tubes that allow an air leak around the tube at 25 cm H_2O or less.

Racemic epinephrine (0.5 ml in 2.5 to 3 ml of normal saline) nebulized in oxygen is the management of choice for postintubation croup; the effect is thought to result from vasoconstriction of the subglottic mucosa. Because symptoms can recur within 2 to 4 hours, the child should be observed before being sent home. If frequent and repeated treatments are necessary, hospital admission should be considered. Dexamethasone (0.3 to 0.5 mg/kg) may also be tried,[55] although its effect is slow in onset if at all.

Pain management

The theory that children, particularly neonates, perceive pain less acutely and therefore do not need pain medication is no longer accepted.[2] Assessing degree of pain in preverbal children is problematic, although visual analogue scales may be helpful. Intravenous opioids, whether given by bolus, infusion, or patient-controlled analgesia, are the mainstay of therapy for severe pain.[109] Children 10 years of age and older, and some mature 8- to 10-year-olds, do well with patient-controlled anesthesia, tend to use less total drug, and have a better feeling of control than with traditional methods of administration.

Milder degrees of pain can be handled with nonopioid analgesics. Acetaminophen (10 to 15 mg/kg every 4 to 6 hours to a maximum dosage of 4 g/24 hours) alone or with codeine (0.5 to 1.0 mg/kg) is useful for children who can take oral medications. Rectal acetaminophen can also be given, although doses of approximately 35 mg/kg are necessary to achieve equivalent serum levels as 10 to 15 mg/kg given orally.[32] Ketorolac is a nonsteroidal antiinflammatory agent that has potent analgesic properties, which may be equivalent to those of morphine,[99] without the respiratory depression or nausea associated with opioids. However, ketorolac requires 30 to 45 minutes for onset and may be associated with a higher incidence of bleeding because of effects on platelet function.[22]

ANESTHETIC CONSIDERATIONS FOR SPECIFIC PROCEDURES

Rigid bronchoscopy

Anesthesia for rigid bronchoscopy presents a significant challenge for the pediatric anesthesiologist for several reasons. First, bronchoscopy is most often indicated for diagnosis and management of children who are younger than 1 year of age, predominantly because of congenital defects (Table 3-4)[107]; this is relevant because anesthetic risk appears to be highest in this age group.[7,75] Second, patients who require bronchoscopy often present with difficult airway anatomy or with compromised oxygenation and ventilation; these factors may predispose them to intraoperative problems. Finally, the need to share the airway with the endoscopist demands effective two-way communication and coordination to ensure a smooth anesthetic and to prevent complications. Thus the importance of communication between anesthesiologist and endoscopist in preoperative planning and intraoperative management cannot be overstated.

Table 3-4. Diagnosis according to age in children undergoing bronchoscopy for airway obstruction

	Younger than 1 year (%)	1 to 3 years (%)	Older than 3 years (%)
Congenital defects*	43	8	3
Acquired defects†	12	13	15
Normal findings	4	1	1
Total	69	22	19

Modified from Wiseman, Sanchez, and Powell: *J Pediatr Surg* 27:1294, 1992.

* Laryngomalacia, tracheolmalacia, bronchomalacia, vocal cord paralysis, vascular ring, hemangioma, cysts.

† Subglottic stenosis, papillomatosis, infection (tracheitis, epiglottitis).

Anesthetic technique may be modified depending on the age and suspected diagnosis of the child, the underlying impairment of oxygenation and ventilation, the estimated duration of the procedure, and the training and experience of both the endoscopist and the anesthesiologist. Once the anesthesiologist has performed a history and physical examination and has reviewed pertinent laboratory values, a discussion with the endoscopist should ensue. Of particular importance is the choice of spontaneous versus controlled ventilation, which influences the choice of drugs for premedication and maintenance of anesthesia, including muscle relaxants.

The choice of anesthetic agents and techniques is often diagnosis-driven. In evaluating a patient with stridor or other evidence of a compromised lumen, spontaneous breathing allows dynamic assessment of the pathophysiology. Anesthesia can be induced with either intravenous (sodium thiopental, ketamine, or propofol) or inhalation (sevoflurane or halothane) agents with oxygen, although inhaled rather than fixed agents are preferred when high-grade obstruction of the upper airway is suspected because their effect is more readily reversed. Nitrous oxide must be used with caution in patients with compromised oxygenation and is contraindicated in patients with air trapping because of the risk of lung overinflation.

Once the patient can tolerate laryngoscopy, the airway can be sprayed with 4% lidocaine, which provides local anesthesia to the larynx and trachea and reduces the requirement for halothane or other anesthetic agents. Lidocaine doses up to 7 mg/kg have been proven safe if administered over 15 minutes.[1] Intravenous lidocaine (1 to 2 mg/kg) is helpful[3] but is not as effective as properly administered topical anesthesia.

Use of the Storz pediatric bronchoscope and rod lens telescope permits good visualization of the airway while oxygen with or without an inhaled anesthetic is delivered via the side-arm attachment. However, if the 2.5-, 3.0-, and 3.5-mm internal-diameter bronchoscopes are used, there will be increased resistance to breathing. In combination with anesthetic agents that depress respiration, this increased resistance may result in compromised ventilation and oxygenation during spontaneous breathing.[76] The telescope should be removed periodically to allow the child to breathe without the resistive load. Constant communication between the anesthesiologist and the endoscopist is essential.

When spontaneous ventilation is not necessary, lighter planes of anesthesia (i.e., lower concentrations of halothane) with less associated cardiovascular depression can be provided through the use of adjunctive administration of short-acting muscle relaxants. Alternatively, propofol can be used adjunctively with airway topical anesthesia and a muscle relaxant. Propofol has the advantage that it can be given continuously during the procedure, resulting in a more constant level of anesthesia than can be achieved with halothane, which may be interrupted repeatedly. The choice of muscle relaxant can be made on the basis of anticipated duration of procedure: mivacurium (0.2 to 0.3 mg/kg) for procedures lasting 15 to 30 minutes, vecuronium (0.1 mg/kg) for procedures lasting 30 minutes to 1 hour (except for newborns and infants), and pancuronium (0.1 mg/kg) for procedures lasting more than 1 hour.

During removal of a foreign body, close communication between the anesthesiologist and the endoscopist is essential. Adequate relaxation of the upper airway and glottis reduces the risk that the foreign body will be lost when it is pulled out of the airway with the grasping forceps and the bronchoscope. If the foreign body is lost in the trachea, total airway occlusion can occur. If prompt removal is not possible, the foreign body should be pushed into either mainstem bronchus to allow one-lung ventilation.

In 1967, Sanders described a system in which oxygen at 50 to 60 psi was directed down the bronchoscope in intermittent bursts.[82] Although the device is usually successful at both oxygenating and ventilating patients, a number of potential problems exist. Because room air is entrained by the Venturi effect, hypoxemia may be seen in some patients. Peak inflation pressures and flow rates are influenced by the driving pressure, diameter and shape of the bronchoscope, diameter and length of the injector, and angle from the axial line of the bronchoscope. Because of their smaller diameter, pediatric bronchoscopes tend to have lower flow rates and higher inflation pressures than adult bronchoscopes. Low tidal volumes may occur in patients with poor lung compliance. Due to the higher inflation pressures, pneumothorax or pneumomediastinum may occur.[92] Finally, blood or particulate matter in the airway may be forced distally by high-pressure bursts.

Hypoxemia and CO_2 retention are the most frequent complications of bronchoscopy; it is the rare bronchoscopy procedure that escapes at least mild degrees of either or both. Early detection and prompt intervention usually result in resolution without incident. Thus, pulse oximetry monitoring is mandatory. Monitoring of ventilation with capnography is impossible during bronchoscopy because of dilution of expired gas with high fresh gas flows. Thus it is imperative to leave the chest uncovered to allow observation of chest movement. A precordial stethoscope is also useful to auscultate breath sounds. Pneumothorax, although rare, must be kept in mind if acute deterioration of ventilation and oxygenation occurs, particularly if accompanied by a decrease in lung compliance and blood pressure. A portable chest radiograph should be obtained if the index of suspicion is high. Ventricular premature beats are also frequent and usually reflect light levels of anesthesia and CO_2 retention during halothane administration. Return to normal sinus rhythm usually occurs with a reduction in the CO_2 tension, an increase in the anesthetic depth, administration of intravenous lidocaine (1 mg/kg), or a change to another anesthetic agent.

Bronchospasm can also occur during bronchoscopy, particularly in patients with a history of reactive airway disease. Frequently, bronchospasm results from instrumentation of an inadequately anesthetized airway, particularly if the bronchoscope is in contact with the carina. Removal of the instrument and deepening the anesthetic topically or systemically usually resolves the problem. If not, administration of a β sympathomimetic agent such as aerosolized albuterol (0.05 to 0.15 mg/kg in 5% solution) or subcutaneous terbutaline (3 to 5 μg/kg) is indicated.

When the examination is complete, the bronchoscope is removed and bag-and-mask ventilation with 100% oxygen is instituted. An endotracheal tube may be inserted if the patient is apneic; if blood, secretions, or difficult anatomy make the airway tenuous; or if the patient has a full stomach. If not, the patient may be awakened without an endotracheal tube, as long he or she is closely observed by qualified personnel until airway reflexes have returned.

Adenotonsillectomy

Although still a common surgical procedure, adenotonsillectomy has become less common in the past decade as the indications for this surgery have changed. With more effective antimicrobial therapy, the percentage of patients with recurrent infection as the indication for surgery has declined, and the percentage of patients with obstructive symptoms has increased; currently, nearly 30% of tonsillectomies are performed to remove obstructions.[79] With this change has come a greater appreciation that adenotonsillar hypertrophy may lead to obstructive sleep apnea (OSA) (Box 3-3) and, in the extreme, to cor pulmonale. Because of the need to prevent cor pulmonale in patients with OSA, the adenotonsillectomy population has become younger; 60% of children operated on for obstruction are younger than 8 years of age.[79] Of children younger than 3 years of age who require tonsillectomy, 81% have an obstruction.[79]

Sedative premedication should be used with caution in

Box 3-3. Features of obstructive sleep apnea

Cessation of air flow for at least 10 seconds despite continuing ventilatory efforts
Five or more episodes per hour of sleep
A decrease of at least 4% in oxyhemoglobin saturation
Arousal associated with increasing ventilatory efforts
Excessive daytime sleepiness

From *The international classification of sleep disorders: diagnostic and coding manual,* Rochester, Minn, 1990, American Sleep Disorders Association.

children with OSA because these children are sensitive to both the sedative and the ventilatory depressant effects of sedative–hypnotic drugs. An inhalation induction is most common, with careful monitoring and attention to airway patency, which can often be improved with jaw thrust or the addition of continuous positive airway pressure during spontaneous breathing.

Intubation can be accomplished either with the patient under deep inhalational anesthesia or following administration of a short- or intermediate-acting nondepolarizing muscle relaxant. A Ring-Adair-Ellwyn tube is generally used because of the low profile it provides under the self-retaining mouth gag. Careful monitoring of breath sounds is necessary because the tube can become obstructed or dislodged during placement, opening, and removal of the gag.

Anesthesia is usually provided with a volatile agent, most often halothane, combined with nitrous oxide and oxygen. Muscle relaxants may be used but are generally not necessary. Titration of supplemental narcotics helps provide a smooth anesthetic and emergence but must be done cautiously, if at all, in patients with OSA. If desired, narcotics may be withheld until emergence in the PACU. The decision about timing of extubation is left to clinical judgment, as previously discussed. Patients with OSA are usually extubated while awake whereas patients without OSA can be extubated deep. If a deep extubation is chosen, thorough pharyngeal suctioning, placement of an oral airway, and lateral, head-down positioning allow blood and secretions to drain cephalad and prevent aspiration, laryngospasm, and airway obstruction.

Occasionally, reoperation is required for persistent hemorrhage, sometimes hours or even days after the original procedure. Careful assessment of intravascular and erythrocyte volume are mandatory, as is intravenous rehydration prior to anesthesia induction. Patients requiring reoperation have full stomachs and are candidates for rapid-sequence induction. Awake intubation should be considered if airway anatomy is distorted.

Most adenotonsillectomies can be performed on an outpatient basis, as long as the patient is monitored closely for at least 6 hours following surgery.[25] Most anesthesiologists have recommended overnight hospitalization following adenotonsillectomy in patients with OSA. However, a recent study that found improvements in polysomnograms in patients with mild OSA the night after adenotonsillectomy suggests that hospitalization is necessary only for high-risk patients.[28] At particular risk are children younger than 3 years of age with OSA, as this age group has a higher incidence of airway complications and delayed oral intake.[79] Other conditions that increase risk include cerebral palsy, seizure disorders, congenital heart disease, and prematurity.

Laryngeal surgery

Like bronchoscopy, laryngeal surgery is challenging for the anesthesiologist because the airway is shared with the surgeon and because the surgery is often performed on infants with congenital laryngomalacia, laryngeal clefts or webs, vocal cord disorders, or laryngeal tumors. Other common indications are acquired subglottic stenosis and recurrent laryngeal papillomatosis.

Several techniques allow the surgeon and the anesthesiologist to occupy the airway simultaneously. One is the *spontaneous ventilation technique*, which is useful when the surgeon needs to assess airway dynamics.[5,30,38] The concentration of halothane, delivered to the oropharynx by a side port attached to the suspension layngoscope, must be high enough to prevent coughing or layryngospasm but not so high as to cause significant cardiovascular depression or apnea. Adjunctive agents such as propofol or narcotics may be used to reduce the need for high concentrations of halothane. Thorough topical anesthesia with 4% lidocaine delivered either by atomizer or by syringe with a metal or plastic introducer needle, provides additional anesthesia and may also reduce the required halothane concentration. Premedication with intravenous atropine helps to maintain heart rate and cardiac output if high concentrations of halothane are necessary. Scavenging is performed by a vacuum hose attached to the stabilizing support of the laryngoscope (Fig. 3-1). Propofol and a narcotic may be used in lieu of halothane or with lower concentrations of halothane (provided that good topical anesthesia has been performed) to reduce operating room pollution.

The spontaneous ventilation technique has been very useful for children with recurrent papillomatosis. Because most of these children are older than 1 year of age, halothane-induced myocardial depression is not as likely as in an infant. The surgeon can proceed with the laser device in an unhurried manner. For children who become psychologically sensitized by frequent needs for laser removal, the smell of halothane can become abhorrent. The sequence of EMLA cream followed by an intravenous start (sometimes with a butterfly needle) and then a propofol anesthetic may prove to be more tolerable for family, child, and physician alike.

The *apnea technique* may be preferred if spontaneous ventilation is not necessary and if the anesthesiologist is uncomfortable with the unprotected airway. Anesthesia is provided with a combination of a muscle relaxant, high-

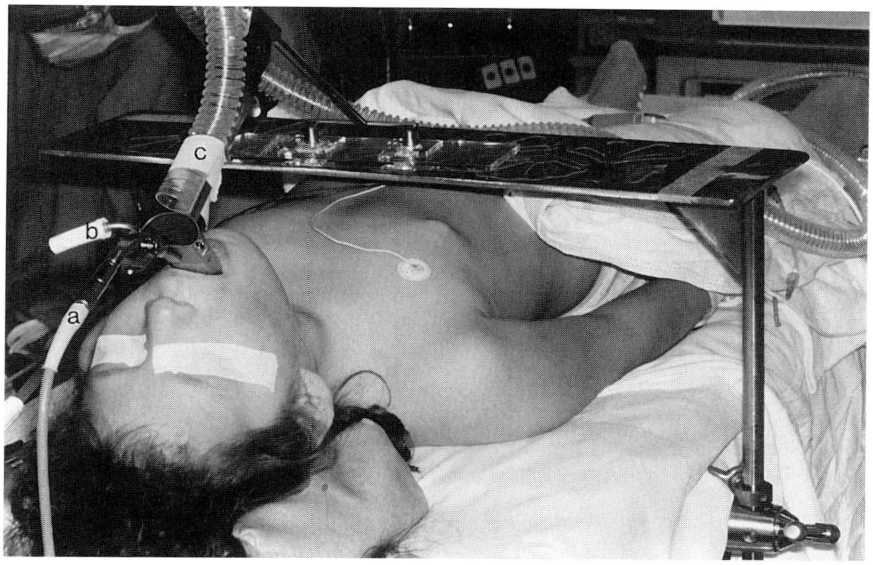

Fig. 3-1. A child anesthetized for laryngeal surgery. Attached to the suspension laryngoscope are a fiberoptic light source *(a)*, a fresh gas source for insufflation *(b)*, and a vacuum hose for scavenging of anesthetic agents *(c)*.

concentration oxygen, and halothane or propofol. Topical anesthesia is provided to the airway prior to intubation. After the suspension laryngoscope is set up, the tube is removed and the surgeon proceeds while the patient is apneic. The tube is replaced when the pulse oximeter indicates decreasing saturation, with a threshold established by the team. Repeated reintubation and ventilation are performed until the procedure is completed. The potential for CO_2 retention is high, particularly if only short periods of ventilation are used between periods of extubation and apnea.

Supraglottic jet ventilation incorporates the use of an intravenous anesthetic such as propofol with a muscle relaxant. After topical anesthesia is provided to the airway, the suspension laryngoscope is introduced and a jet ventilating device is attached. The characteristics and potential risks of this technique are as discussed in the section on rigid bronchoscopy.

Finally, it is possible to place a small *endotracheal tube* around which the surgeon works, although this frequently proves to be awkward. An endotracheal tube is now available for use in larger children. This tube has a small bore that the surgeon can work around, allows ventilation of the lungs, and will not burn in response to laser contact.[33]

REFERENCES

1. Amitai Y, Zylber KE, Avital A: Serum lidocaine concentrations in children during bronchoscopy with topical anesthesia, *Chest* 98:1370, 1990.
2. Anand KJ, Hickey PR: Pain and its effects in the human neonate and fetus, *N Engl J Med* 317:1321, 1987.
3. Baraka A: Intravenous lidocaine controls extubation laryngospasm in children, *Anesth Analg* 57:506, 1978.
4. Beecher HK, Todd DP: A study of deaths associated with anesthesia and surgery, *Ann Surg* 140:2, 1954.
5. Benjamin B, Lines V: Endoscopy and anesthesia in noninfective airway obstruction in children, *Anaesthesia* 27:283, 1972.
6. Cheney FW: The changing pattern of anesthesia-related adverse events, *ASA Newsletter* 60:10, 1996.
7. Cohen MM, Cameron CB, Duncan PG: Pediatric anesthesia morbidity and mortality in the perioperative period, *Anesth Analg* 70:160, 1990.
8. Colgan FJ: Performance of lungs and bronchi during inhalation anesthesia, *Anesthesiology* 26:778, 1965.
9. Corssen G and others: Ketamine in the anesthetic management of asthmatic patients, *Anesth Analg* 51:588, 1972.
10. Coté C and others: The dose response of intravenous thiopental for the induction of general anesthesia in unpremedicated children, *Anesthesiology* 55:703, 1981.
11. Coté CJ and others: Postoperative apnea in former preterm infants after inguinal herniorrhaphy, *Anesthesiology* 82:809, 1995.
12. Coté CJ and others: A single-blind study of pulse oximetry in children, *Anesthesiology* 68:184, 1988.
13. Cox RG, Goresky GV: Life-threatening apnea following spinal anesthesia in former premature infants, *Anesthesiology* 73:345, 1990.
14. Craythorne NWB, Rottenstein HS, Dripps RD: The effect of succinylcholine on intraocular pressure in adults, infants and children during general anesthesia, *Anesthesiology* 21:59, 1960.
15. DeSoto H and others: Changes in oxygen saturation following general anesthesia in children with upper respiratory infection signs and symptoms undergoing otolaryngological procedures, *Anesthesiology* 68: 276, 1988.
16. Downes H, Gerber N, Hirshman CA: IV lignocaine in reflex and allergic bronchoconstriction, *Br J Anaesth* 52:873, 1980.
17. Edwinson M, Arnbjornsson E, Ekman R: Psychological preparation program for children undergoing acute appendectomy, *Pediatrics* 82: 30, 1988.
18. Eichhorn JH: Prevention of intraoperative anesthesia accidents and related severe injury through safety monitoring, *Anesthesiology* 70: 572, 1989.
19. Empey DW and others: Mechanisms of bronchial hyperreactivity in normal subjects after upper respiratory tract infection, *Am Rev Respir Dis* 113:131, 1976.
20. Engberg G and others: Plasma concentrations of prilocaine and lidocaine and methaemoglobin formation in infants after epicutaneous application of a 5% lidocaine-prilocaine (EMLA), *Acta Anaesthesiol Scand* 31:624, 1987.
21. Ferrari LR, Donlon JV: Metaclopromide reduces the incidence of vomiting after tonsillectomy in children, *Anesth Analg* 75:351, 1992.

22. Gallagher JE, Blauth J, Fornadley JA: Perioperative ketorolac and postoperative hemorrhage in cases of tonsillectomy and adenoidectomy, *Laryngoscope* 105:606, 1995.
23. Gold MI, Han YH, Helrich M: Pulmonary mechanics and blood gas tensions during anesthesia in asthmatics, *Anesthesiology* 27:216, 1966.
24. Gronert GA, Theye RA: Pathophysiology of hyperkalemia induced by succinylcholine, *Anesthesiology* 43:89, 1975.
25. Guida RA, Mattucci KF: Tonsillectomy and adenoidectomy: an inpatient or outpatient procedure? *Laryngoscope* 100:491, 1990.
26. Hackmann T, Steward DJ, Sheps S: Anemia in pediatric day surgery patients: prevalence and detection, *Anesthesiology* 75:27, 1991.
27. Hannallah RS, Rosales JK: Experience with parent's presence during anesthesia induction in children, *Can Anaesth Soc J* 30:286, 1983.
28. Helfaer MA and others: Polysomnography after adenotonsillectomy in mild pediatric sleep apnea, *Crit Care Med* 24:1323, 1996.
29. Henderson MA, Baines DB, Overton JH: Parental attitudes to presence at induction of paediatric anaesthesia, *Anaesth Intensive Care* 21:324, 1993.
30. Herbert WI, Cohen SR, Thompson JW: Anesthetic management of microlaryngeal laser surgery in children: apneic technique anesthesia, *Laryngoscope* 98:347, 1988.
31. Hopkins CS, Buckley CJ, Bush GH: Pain-free injection in infants: use of a lignocaine-prilocaine cream to prevent pain at intravenous induction of general anesthesia in 1-5 year old children, *Anaesthesia* 43:198, 1988.
32. Houck CS and others: Pharmacokinetics of a higher dose of rectal acetominophen in children, *Anesthesiology* 83:A1126, 1995.
33. Hunsaker DH: Anesthesia for microlaryngeal surgery: the case for subglottic jet ventilation, *Laryngoscope* 104(65 suppl):1, 1994.
34. Kain ZN and others: Parental presence during induction of anesthesia: a randomized controlled trial, *Anesthesiology* 84:1060, 1996.
35. Karl HW and others: Preanesthetic preparation of pediatric outpatients: the role of a videotape for parents, *J Clin Anesth* 2:172, 1990.
36. Keenan RL and others: Bradycardia during anesthesia in infants: an epidemiologic study, *Anesthesiology* 80:976, 1994.
37. Keenan KL, Boyan CP: Cardiac arrest due to anesthesia: a study of causes, *JAMA* 253:2373, 1985.
38. Kennedy MG, Chinyanga HM, Steward DJ: Anesthetic experience using a standard technique for laryngeal surgery in infants and children, *Can Anaesth Soc J* 28:561, 1981.
39. Kingston HGG, Hirshman CA: Perioperative management of the patient with asthma, *Anesth Analg* 63:844, 1984.
40. Knill RL, Gelb AW: Ventilatory responses to hypoxia and hypercapnia during halothane sedation and anesthesia in man, *Anesthesiology* 42:244, 1978.
41. Koka BV and others: Postintubation croup in children, *Anesth Analg* 56:501, 1977.
42. Korsch BM: The child and the operating room, *Anesthesiology* 43:251, 1975.
43. Kurth CD, LeBard SE: Association of postoperative apnea, airway obstruction, and hypoxemia in former premature infants, *Anesthesiology* 75:22, 199 .
44. Lamberty JM, Rubin BK: The management of anaesthesia for patients with cystic fibrosis, *Anaesthesia* 40:448, 1985.
45. Lindahl SGE, Charlton AJ, Hatch DJ: Ventilatory responses to rebreathing and carbon dioxide inhalation during anaesthesia in children, *Br J Anaesth* 57:1188, 1985.
46. Litman RS, Keon TP: Postintubation croup in children, *Anesthesiology* 75:1122, 1991.
47. Liu LMP and others: Life-threatening apnea in infants recovering from anesthesia, *Anesthesiology* 59:506, 1983.
48. Liu LMP, Goudsouzian NG, Liu PL: Rectal methohexital premedication on children: a dose comparison study, *Anesthesiology* 53:343, 1980.
49. Lourenco RV and others: Abnormal deposition and clearance of inhaled particles during upper respiratory viral infections, *J Clin Invest* 50:62, 1971.
50. Lunn DV and others: Low-dose droperidol reduces postoperative vomiting in paediatric day surgery, *Br J Anaesth* 74:509, 1995.
51. Lynn AM, Opheim KE, Tyler DC: Morphine infusion after pediatric cardiac surgery, *Crit Care Med* 12:863, 1984.
52. Lynn AM, Slattery JT: Morphine pharmacokinetics in early infancy, *Anesthesiology* 66:136, 1987.
53. Macintyre PE, Pavlin EG, Dwersteg JF: Effect of meperidine on oxygen consumption, carbon dioxide production, and respiratory gas exchange in post anesthesia shivering, *Anesth Analg* 66:751, 1987.
54. Mather LE and others: Meperidine kinetics in man: intravenous injection in surgical patients and volunteers, *Clin Pharmacol Ther* 17:21, 1975.
55. Maze A, Block E: Stridor in pediatric patients, *Anesthesiology* 50:132, 1979.
56. McClain DA, Hug CC: Intravenous fentanyl kinetics, *Clin Pharmacol Ther* 28:106, 1980.
57. McGill WA, Coveler LA, Epstein BS: Subacute upper respiratory infection in small children, *Anesth Analg* 58:331, 1979.
58. McMillan CO and others: Premedication of children with oral midazolam, *Can J Anaesth* 39:545, 1992.
59. Meakin G and others: Dose response curves for suxamethonium in neonates, infants and children, *Br J Anaesth* 62:655, 1989.
60. Miller BR, Friesen RH: Oral atropine premedication in infants, *Anesthesiology* 67:A491, 1987.
61. Moller JT and others: Randomized evaluation of pulse oximetry in 20,802 patients I. *Anesthesiology* 78:436, 1993.
62. Moller JT and others: Randomized evaluation of pulse oximetry in 20,802 patients II. *Anesthesiology* 78:445, 1993.
63. Morray JP and others: A comparison of pediatric and adult anesthesia closed malpractice claims, *Anesthesiology* 78:461, 1993.
64. Morray JP: Implications for subspecialty care of anesthetized children, *Anesthesiology* 80:969, 1994.
65. Munson ES: Transfer of nitrous oxide into body air cavities, *Br J Anaesth* 46:202, 1974.
66. Murray DJ, Forbes RB, Mahoney LT: Comparative hemodynamic depression of halothane versus isoflurane in neonates and infants: an echocardiographic study, *Anesth Analg* 74:329, 1992.
67. O'Connor SA and others: Changes in pulmonary function after naturally acquired respiratory infection in normal persons, *Am Rev Respir Dis* 120:1087, 1979.
68. O'Flynn RP and others: Masseter muscle rigidity and malignant hyperthermia susceptibility in pediatric patients, *Anesthesiology* 80:1228, 1994.
69. Olsson GL, Hallen B, Hambraeus-Jonzon K: Aspiration during anaesthesia: a computer-aided study of 185,358 anaesthetics, *Acta Anaesthesiol Scand* 30:84, 1986.
70. Patel RI and others: Emergence airway complications in children: a comparison of tracheal extubation in awake and deeply anesthetized patients, *Anesth Analg* 73:266, 1991.
71. Patel DK and others: Induction dose of propofol in children, *Anaesthesia* 43:949, 1988.
72. Patterson ME, Bartlett PC: Hearing impairment caused by intratympanic pressure changes during general anesthesia, *Laryngoscope* 85:399, 1976.
73. Perrault L, Roussea P: Problem of gas diffusion into the middle ear during anaesthesia for tympanoplasty, *Can Anaesth Soc J* 28:136, 1981.
74. Pounder DR, Blackstock D, Steward DJ: Tracheal extubation in children: halothane versus isoflurane, anesthetized versus awake, *Anesthesiology* 74:653, 1991.
75. Rackow H, Salintire E, Green LT: Frequency of cardiac arrest associated with anesthesia in infants and children, *Pediatrics* 28:697, 1961.
76. Rah KH, Salzber AM, Boylan CP: Respiratory acidosis with the small

Storz-Hopkins bronchoscope: occurrence and management, *Ann Thorac Surg* 27:197, 1978.
77. Roman DEM, Barker I, Reilly CS: Anesthetists' attitudes to parental presence at induction of general anaesthesia in children, *Anaesthesia* 48:338, 1993.
78. Rosenberg H, Gronert GA: Intractable cardiac arrest in children given succinylcholine, *Anesthesiology* 77:1054, 1992.
79. Rothchild MA, Catalano P, Biller HF: Ambulatory pediatric tonsillectomy and the identification of high-risk subgroups, *Otolaryngol Head Neck Surg* 110:203, 1994.
80. Roy WL, Lerman J, McIntyre BG: Is preoperative hemoglobin testing justified in children undergoing minor elective surgery? *Can J Anaesth,* 38:700, 1991.
81. Saint-Maurice C and others: Better acceptance of measures of induction of anesthesia after rectal premedication with midazolam in children: comparison of a placebo-controlled study, *Anaesthetist* 36:629, 1987.
82. Sanders RD: Two ventilating attachments for bronchoscopes, *Del Med J,* 39:170, 1967.
83. Sane SM and others: Value of preoperative chest x-ray examinations in children, *Pediatrics* 60:669, 1977.
84. Schnider SM, Papper EM: Anesthesia for the asthmatic patient, *Anesthesiology* 22:886, 1961.
85. Schreiner MS and others: Should children drink before discharge from day surgery? *Anesthesiology* 76:528, 1992.
86. Schreiner MS, Treibwasser A, Keon TP: Ingestion of liquids compared with preoperative fasting in pediatric outpatients, *Anesthesiology* 72:593, 1990.
87. Schulman JL and others: A study of the effect of the mother's presence during anesthesia induction, *Pediatrics* 39:111, 1967.
88. Sellick BA: Cricoid pressure to control regurgitation of stomach contents during induction of anesthesia, *Lancet* 2:404, 1961.
89. Splinter WM and others: Ondansetron is a better prophylactic antiemetic than droperidol for tonsillectomy in children, *Can J Anaesth* 42:848, 1995.
90. Splinter WM and others: Oral ondansetron decreases vomiting after tonsillectomy in children, *Can J Anaesth* 42:277, 1995.
91. Stevens A, Roizen MF: Patients with diabetes mellitus and disorders of glucose metabolism, *Anesth Clin North Am* 5:339, 1987.
92. Steward DJ: Percutaneous transtracheal ventilation for laser endoscopic procedures in infants and small children, *Can J Anaesth* 34:429, 1987.
93. Steward DJ: Preterm infants are more prone to complications following minor surgery than are term infants, *Anesthesiology* 56:304, 1982.
94. Stoeckel H, Hengstmann JH, Schuttler J: Pharmacokinetics of fentanyl as a possible explanation for recurrence of respiratory depression, *Br J Anaesth* 51:741, 1979.
95. Tait AR, Knight PR: The effects of general anesthesia on upper respiratory tract infections in children, *Anesthesiology* 67:930, 1987.
96. Van Der Spek AFL and others: Increased masticatory muscle stiffness during limb muscle flaccidity associated with succinylcholine administration, *Anesthesiology* 69:11, 1988.
97. Ved SA and others: Vomiting and recovery after outpatient tonsillectomy and adenoidectomy in children, *Anesthesiology* 85:4, 1996.
98. Vistainer MA, Wolfer JA: Psychological preparation for surgical pediatric patients: the effect on children's and parents' stress responses and adjustment, *Pediatrics* 56:187, 1975.
99. Watcha MF and others: Comparison of ketorolac and morphine as adjuvants during pediatric surgery, *Anesthesiology* 76:368, 1992.
100. Watcha MF and others: The dose-response relationship of ondansetron in preventing postoperative emesis in pediatric patients undergoing ambulatory surgery, *Anesthesiology* 82:47, 1995.
101. Watcha MF, Thach BT, Gunter JB: Postoperative apnea after caudal anesthesia in an ex-premature infant, *Anesthesiology* 71:613, 1989.
102. Wear R, Robinson S, Gregory GA: The effect of halothane on the baroresponse of adult and baby rabbits, *Anesthesiology* 56:188, 1982.
103. Welborn LG and others: High-dose caffeine suppresses postoperative apnea in former preterm infants, *Anesthesiology* 71:347, 1989.
104. Welborn LG and others: Postoperative apnea in former preterm infants: prospective comparison of spinal and general anesthesia, *Anesthesiology* 72:838, 1990.
105. Westrin P: The induction dose of propofol in infants 1-6 months of age and in children 10-16 years of age, *Anesthesiology* 74:455, 1991.
106. Wilson RD, Traber DL, Evans BL: Correlation of psychologic and physiologic observations from children undergoing repeated ketamine anesthesia, *Anesth Analg* 48:995, 1970.
107. Wiseman NE, Sanchez I, Powell RE: Rigid bronchoscopy in the pediatric age group: diagnostic effectiveness, *J Pediatr Surg* 27:1294, 1992.
108. Yaster M: The dose response of fentanyl in neonatal anesthesia, *Anesthesiology* 66:433, 1987.
109. Yaster M, Deshpande JK: Management of pediatric pain with opioid analgesics, *J Pediatr* 113:421, 1988.
110. Yeman TA, Nelson W: Parental presence at induction: do the parents make a difference? *Anesthesiology* 77:A1167, 1992.

Chapter 4

Characteristics of Normal and Abnormal Postnatal Craniofacial Growth and Development

Frederick K. Kozak

Volumes of literature have been written on facial growth and development and entire academic careers have been spent researching various concepts and theories. Searching through the written literature can be overwhelming. This chapter provides the reader with a place to begin to study facial growth and development and reviews major changes in growth from birth to late adolescence. *Growth* refers to an increase in size, whereas *development* indicates an increase in complexity of structure and function.

In order to understand the abnormal, one must first comprehend the normal. To accomplish this, this chapter is divided into two parts. The first part provides a brief review of the main theories of postnatal craniofacial growth and the characteristics of normal postnatal facial growth and development. The second part reviews abnormal facial growth and development through several clinical examples that are relevant to pediatric otolaryngology. Embryology of the head and neck is covered in Chapter 2 of this volume.

THEORIES OF CRANIOFACIAL GROWTH

Postnatal facial growth appears to be a complex, multifactorial phenomenon. It is clear from the resemblance of children to their parents in both facial structure and soft-tissue development that genetic factors play a significant role in basic facial pattern. However, ''environmental'' factors most certainly influence facial growth. These factors can range from intercellular influences to biomechanical forces (i.e., physical forces acting on bone). This essentially is Wolff's law (1870), which states that ''changes in the function of a bone are attended by alterations in its structure.''[110] Bone is a tissue that responds to the stresses placed on it; bone remodels.

The genetic and environmental control mechanisms of postnatal facial growth and development are poorly understood. The three main theories of postnatal facial growth control are the genetic preprogrammed theory, the cartilage-mediated growth theory, and the functional matrix hypothesis. Following is a brief review of these theories, none of which is fully satisfactory.

Genetic preprogrammed theory (growth sites)

Early theorists believed that the sizes and shapes of bones were genetically determined within their cells and that sutural patterns were therefore predetermined. Because bone size and shape are defined by sutures in the head, they theorized that the position of sutures limits and controls the expansion of bones. Baume[7] described ''growth centres'' as a place of endochondral ossification with tissue-separating force, resulting in an increase of skeletal mass, and ''growth sites'' as regions of periosteal or sutural bone formation and modeling resorption that are adaptive to environmental influences.[96] The cells of the sutures grew into the void left as the bone segments pulled apart from the tissue-separating force. In other words, growth sites are where growth literally takes place and growth centers are areas where genetically predetermined growth takes place. This theory was tested by experiments involving suture removal and transplantation, and the conclusion was that sutures are not primarily responsible for growth.[82] This theory is no longer accepted as correct.

Cartilage-mediated growth (Scott)[103]

In 1953, Scott theorized that the cartilage of the nasal septum "is an extension of the cartilage of the cranial base."[103] In its growth the cartilage of the nasal septum separates the facial bones from one another and from the cranial portion of the skull and allows growth to take place at the sutures by the ordinary mechanism of surface deposition. He held that the nasal septum, along with the mandibular condyles and synchondroses (otherwise known as cephalic cartilages) are growth centers. As the nasal septum grows, it puts tension on the sutures of the nasomaxillary complex, thereby displacing it forward and downward with resultant growth occurring at pressure-related growth sites. Tension occurring in the maxillary sutures causes new bone growth when the sutures are pulled apart. Therefore, suture growth is passive and secondary.

Latham[67] theorized that a septomaxillary ligament (connection between the septum and maxilla) in the fetus causes the maxilla to be pulled forward by the septum as the maxilla grows. It is unknown whether this ligament plays a role in postnatal growth, and experimentation related to the role of the nasal cartilage in this concept is unknown. Animal experimentation involving removal of septal cartilage shortly after birth[80] or secondary to trauma seems to result in midface hypoplasia, but such experiments cannot clearly prove that the cartilage removal causes the growth deficiency. Cartilage seems to play some role that has not yet been precisely determined.

The functional matrix hypothesis (Moss)

Moss[83,84] described the most fundamental dictum of the functional matrix hypothesis as follows:

> "The origin of all skeletal units, all of their subsequent changes in size, shape and location and their subsequent maintenance and being, are always, and without exception, secondary, compensatory and mechanical obligatory responses to the morphogenetically and temporally prior and primary alterations of the operational (functional) demands of their specifically related functional matrices."

Put more succinctly, "bones do not grow, they are grown."[81]

The basic premise of this theory is that bone and cartilage do not regulate their own growth. This theory proposes that craniofacial bony growth occurs as a reaction to or in response to the functional matrix surrounding it. A functional matrix consists of the cells that comprise muscle, soft tissue, teeth, glands, and nerves as well as the functioning volumes of various cavities associated with the head and neck region (e.g., nasal, orbital, oral, pharyngeal and neurocranial). A feedback system exists between the functional matrix and the bone and cartilage involved. Growth of cranial size occurs in response to growth of the brain, growth of the bony orbits occurs in response to the size of the orbit, and growth of the facial bones occurs in response to growth of the surrounding soft tissues. There is a resultant enlargement of the associated cavities of the head and neck because of the functional demands of the airway, breathing, and eating "spaces." The craniofacial bones are in a dependent relationship to the surrounding soft tissues. Critics state that Moss' theory explains what happens during growth but does not explain how it happens. Moss' theory is quite useful in clinical practice because it allows separate assessment of each functional unit in the craniofacial skeleton (i.e., brain–cranium, eye–orbit, jaws (mandible)–mastication, nasomaxillary complex and associated airways–respiration and the ear/hearing–temporal bone). The functional matrix operates within the genetic constraints of the cells and tissues involved.

Facial growth involves intimate morphogenic and biomechanical relationships among all of its component tissue parts, each influenced by, and in turn influencing, the other. A fundamental principle is that no part is developmentally independent or self-contained.[33]

At this time, all theories of growth control mechanisms are speculative, with strengths and faults in each. Further research is required before any definite conclusion can be made.

BONE GROWTH CONCEPTS

Osteogenesis

A review of bone formation is required for a discussion of craniofacial growth. The initial step in osteogenesis is the laying down of primary or woven bone. Primary bone is immature bone defined by random orientation of collagen fibers and is temporary except in a few locations such as the tooth sockets and sutures of the cranial bones. Primary bone generally either becomes secondary (lamellar) bone or is removed to leave bone marrow cavities. Secondary bone differs from primary bone in that its collagen has an orderly pattern and there is an increased number of osteoblasts. Osteogenesis occurs through intramembranous ossification in mesenchyme and endochondral ossification in preexisting cartilage.

Intramembranous bone formation

During intramembranous bone formation, mesenchymal cells differentiate into osteoblasts and accumulate in the area where bone is laid down. The osteoblasts begin to produce osteoid, which consists of collagenous fibers and a homogeneous matrix that is primary bone. Secondary bone replaces the primary bone through ossification of the osteoid.

Endochondral bone formation

In endochondral bone formation there is simultaneous removal of cartilage and subsequent formation of bone. Endochondral bone formation is more complex than intramem-

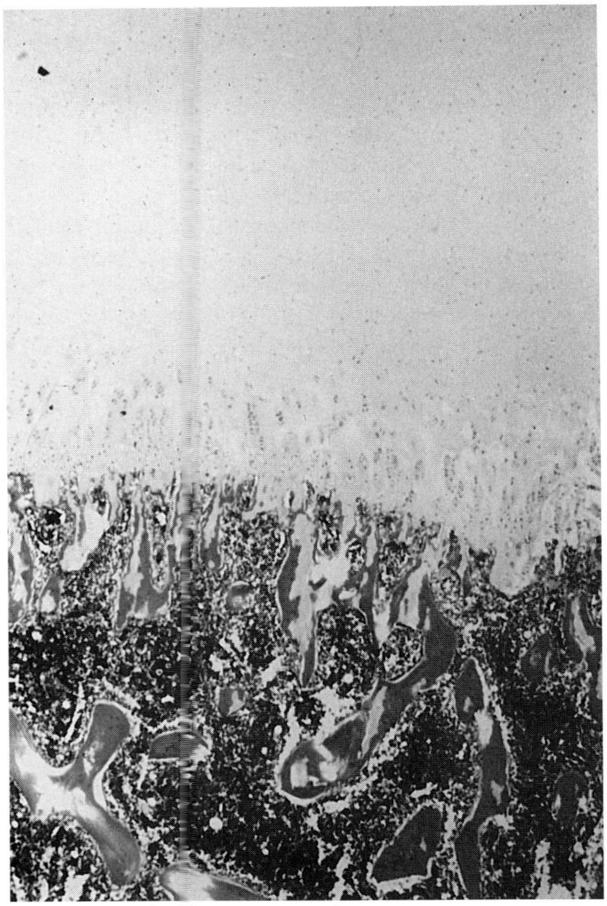

Fig. 4-1. Endochondral bone formation at an epiphyseal plate.

branous bone formation. Various zones exist in active endochondral bone formation, including the zones of reserve cartilage, proliferating cartilage, hypertrophic cartilage, calcified matrix, and resorption. The hypertrophic cartilage cells enlarge, and the surrounding matrix becomes calcified. A separate collar of bone forms around the circumference of the center of this cartilage bar. This is periosteal or, more precisely, perichondral bone. A vascular bud migrates into the cartilage and a primary marrow cavity forms. Meanwhile, activity at the various zones continues. Erosion of the cartilage takes place at the two ends of the expanding primitive marrow cavity, and bone forms on the spicules of the cartilage at the erosion front. The epiphyseal plate of long bones allows simpler visualization of this process (Fig. 4-1).

This descriptive review of bone formation can be supplemented by a molecular review of bone formation.[34]

REMODELING AND DISPLACEMENT

Enlow[99] described the two basic types of growth movement: remodeling and displacement. This concept pertains to both bone and the surrounding soft tissues in the craniofacial complex. Remodeling involves changes in the size and shape of bone, the joining of separate bones and how they fit together, the adaptation intrinsically and extrinsically of these newly joined bones, and finally the relocation of these bones, each influenced by their overall enlargement. Displacement is the process whereby a space is created between bones as they enlarge. Resorption and deposition are ongoing in bones throughout the craniofacial complex during growth as part of the remodelling and displacement processes.

According to Rodan,[101] "bone formation and bone resorption are finely regulated processes, controlled by local and systemic factors, carried out by a family of different interacting cells which communicate via cytokines, cell contacts and elaboration of matrix which feeds back on cellular behavior."

FACIAL CHANGES DURING NORMAL GROWTH AND DEVELOPMENT

General

The faces of infants and children clearly differ from those of adults. Matching an infant's photograph with that of the corresponding adult photograph is challenging because of the changes that occur with growth and development of the craniofacial region. A baby's face is pudgy and round, relatively wide, and vertically short; the nose is small; the eyes appear relatively far apart; and there is a prominent forehead.

Infants have a large head relative to their body size. Their facial complex, which includes the nasomaxillary complex and mandible, is much smaller than the calvaria and basicranium (Figs. 4-2 through 4-4). With growth and development of the facial complex come changes in the size ratio of the cranium to the face. In infants the cranium : face ratio is approximately 3 : 1, whereas in adults it is approximately 2 : 1 (see Fig. 4-4).

With growth, increasing demands are made on the respiratory and masticatory systems. As part of the growth of the facial complex, the nose, mandible, and maxilla increase in size—resulting in the larger, coarser features of the adult face in comparison with the child's (see Fig. 4-3). The facial complex increases in size relative to the cranium; similarly, body size increases relative to head size to result in normal adult body and head proportions (Fig. 4-5).

Craniofacial regions of growth

The craniofacial complex can be divided into three regions: (1) the neurocranium, which is further divided into the calvaria and basicranium; (2) the nasomaxillary complex; and (3) the mandible. Figures 4-2 and 4-3 show the changes that occur in the craniofacial complex from birth to adulthood. In the embryonic human skull there are 110 ossification centers, many of which fuse to result in 45 bones in the neonatal skull and ultimately 22 bones in the young adult skull.[110] Table 4-1 notes the changes in size of various

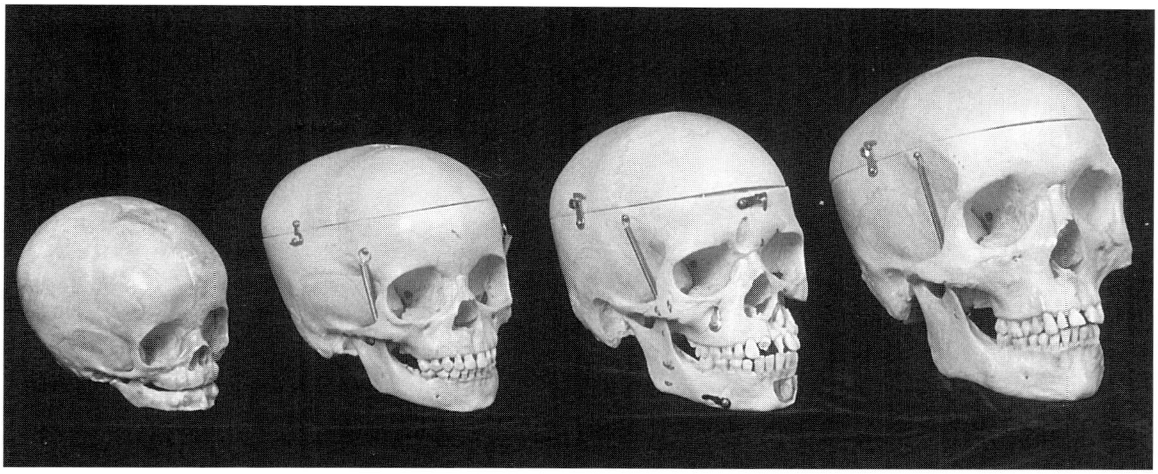

Fig. 4-2. The skulls of an infant (approximately 8 months of age), a 5- to 6-year-old, a 10- to 12-year-old, and an adult. Note the bony craniofacial changes with increasing age.

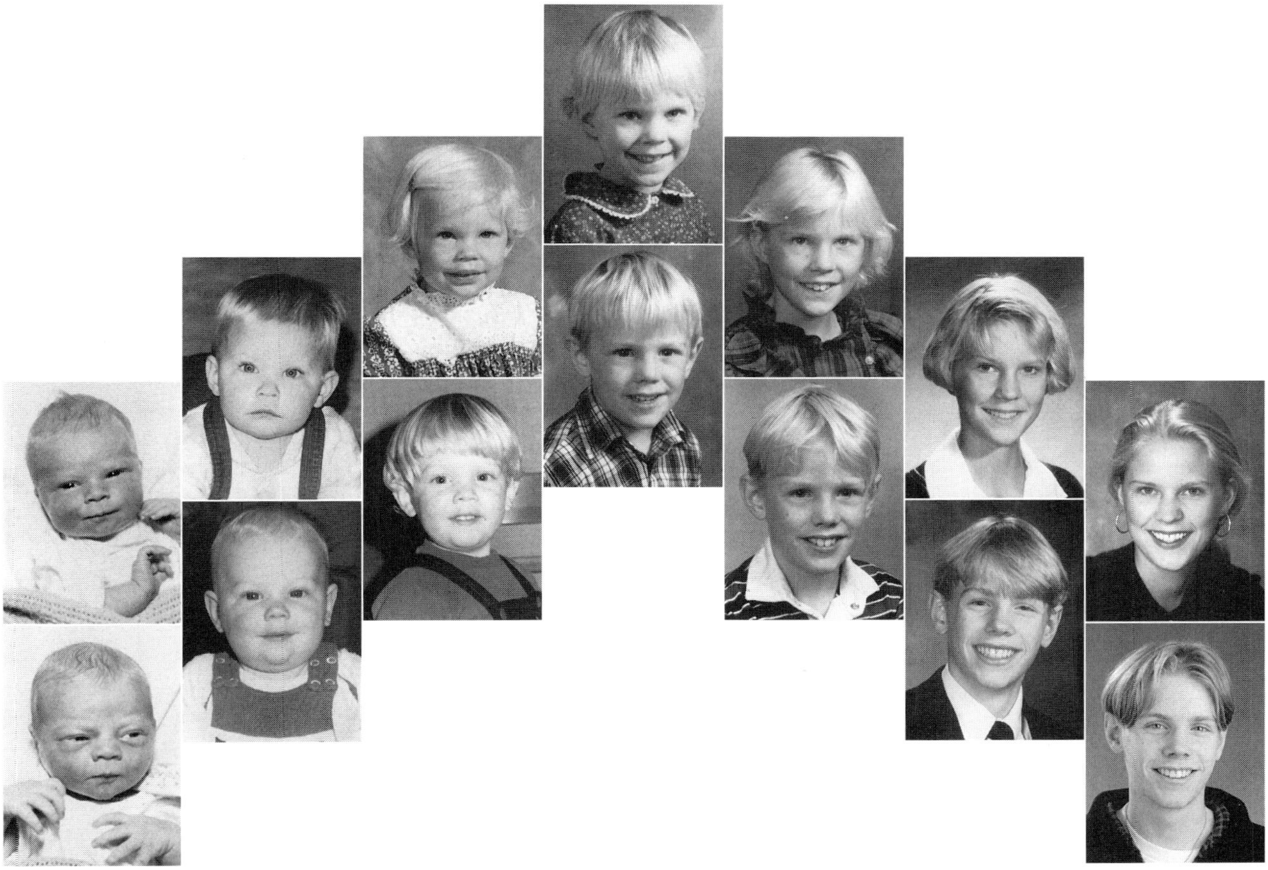

Fig. 4-3. Siblings from birth to adulthood demonstrating changes in the craniofacial complex with growth and development. The female is shown at birth, 10 months, 2.5 years, 6 years, 10 years, 14 years, and 18 years of age. The male is shown at birth, 7 months, 2 years, 5 years, 9 years, 15 years, and 19 years of age.

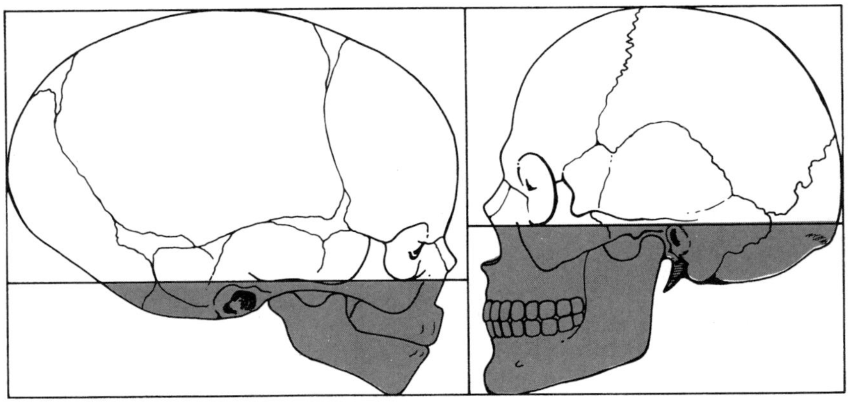

Fig. 4-4. Changes in the size ratio of the cranium to the face with growth and development. In the newborn the cranium:face ratio is approximately 3:1, whereas in adults this ratio is approximately 2:1. (From Proffit WR and others: *Contemporary orthodontics,* ed 2, St. Louis, 1993, Mosby.)

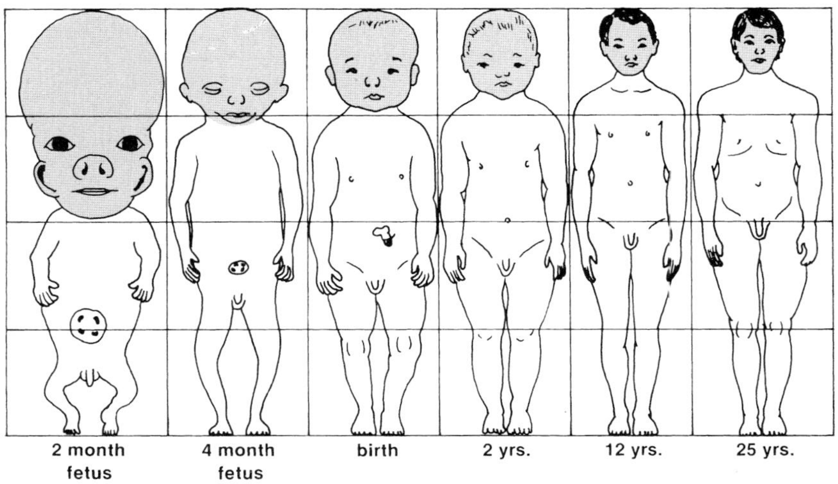

Fig. 4-5. Schematic drawing noting the changes in body proportions during normal growth and development. (From Proffit WR and others: *Contemporary orthodontics,* ed 2, St. Louis, 1993, Mosby.)

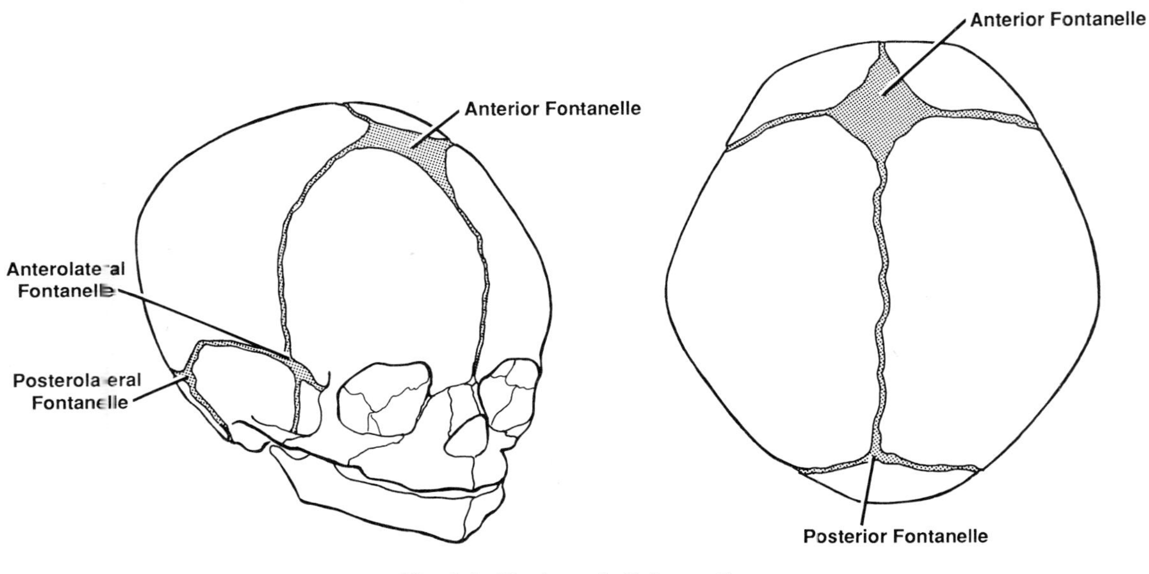

Fig. 4-6. Newborn skull fontanelles.

Table 4-1. Normal craniofacial growth and development*

Growth aspect	Age/development
Neurocranium growth	Birth/25% of ultimate growth
	6 months/50% of ultimate growth
	2 years/75% of ultimate growth
	10 years/95% of ultimate growth
Facial skeletal growth	10 years/65% of ultimate growth
Neurocranium: face size ratio	Birth/8:1
	2 years/6:1
	5 years/4:1
	Adult/2.1-2.5:1
Brain size	Birth to adulthood/3.5× increase
Fontanelle closure	3 months after birth/Anterolateral
	Second year of life/Posterolateral
	2 months after birth/Posterior
	Second year of life/Anterior
Orbits	2 years/50% of ultimate growth
	7 years/100% of ultimate growth
Inner ear	6 months of *fetal* life/Full adult size
Brain weight	Full-term infant/25% of eventual weight
	6 months/50% of eventual weight
	2 years/80% of eventual weight
	10 years/almost eventual weight
Postnatal brain growth	1 year/60% of ultimate growth
	2 years/80% of ultimate growth
	8 years/95% of ultimate growth
	Minimal growth continues to at least age 25 years
Facial height (males)	Birth/40%-61% of ultimate growth
Upper facial height	1 year/63%-86% of ultimate growth
	3 years/72%-90% of ultimate growth
	5 years/82%-100% of ultimate growth (mean, 89%)
Total facial height	Birth 38%-45% of ultimate growth
	1 year/50%-66% of ultimate growth
	3 years/66%-78% of ultimate growth
	5 years/68%-82% of ultimate growth (mean, 77%)
Facial dimension	3 months/equivalent to 40% of adult
	2 years/equivalent of 70% of adult
	5 years/equivalent of 80% of adult
Foramen magnum	1 year/80% of transverse adult size
	1 year/74% of sagittal adult size
Skull base (basion–nasion)	Birth/56% of adult length
	2 years/70% of adult length
	10 years/90% of adult length
	⇒ prechordal part contributes 75% of the postnatal length and parachordal (basioccipital) contributes to 25%
Dentition eruption	8 months-2.5 years/primary teeth
	6 y-20 years/permanent teeth
Maxillary antrum height	Birth/20%
	7 years/50%
	10 years/55%
Bizygomatic width	Birth/60%
	3 years/80%
	5 years/82%
	10 years/85%
Cranial width	Birth/65%
	3 years/85%
	5 years/92%
	10 years/95%
Cranial length	Birth/60%
	3 years/85%
	5 years/90%
	10 years/95%

* Refs. 13, 31, 32, 48, 57, 59, 75, 92, 96, 110, 113, 115.

anatomic sites that take place during growth and development from infancy to adulthood.

NEUROCRANIUM (CALVARIA = ROOF AND BASICRANIUM = FLOOR)

Calvaria

The calvaria comprises the frontal, parietal, and parts of the temporal, occipital, and sphenoid bones. These bones are formed via intramembranous ossification, with the exception of noncalvarial parts of the occipital, temporal, and sphenoid bones, which are formed through endochondral ossification. These bones are initially separated by fontanelles, which develop into sutures early and then finally fuse in adult life (Fig. 4-6).

As the child's brain grows, the calvarial bones are displaced. This displacement theoretically results in the deposition of new bone on the sutural edges. Growth of bone is seen on both the internal and external tables of the calvaria; this also results in an expanded medullary space. Significant thickening occurs from infancy to adulthood. The ascendancy (dominance) of the neurocranium over the facial complex during the early stages of life is clearly related to the inordinately early development of the brain.[75] The majority of calvarial growth is completed by 4 years of age (Fig. 4-7).

Basicranium

Growth of the cranial base creates space for the enlarging brain and oronasal structures with their associated airway. The basicranium grows more slowly than the neurocranium. At birth and at 10 years of age the cranial base is 63% and 95% of its ultimate size, respectively.[75] The basicranium is comprised of parts of the occipital, temporal, sphenoid, and ethmoid bones. The occipital, temporal, and sphenoid portions form through endochondral ossification. The ethmoid and inferior nasal concha form solely by intramembranous bone formation.

In the midline, synchondroses are present (Fig. 4-8). These synchondroses remain after the chondrocranium (cartilage precursor of the basicranium) has ossified. During childhood, the spheno-occipital synchondrosis is the principal growth cartilage of the basicranium and its growth persists into early adolescence.[33,97] Other synchondroses of the basicranium are the sphenoethmoidal, intersphenoidal, sphenofrontal, and frontoethmoidal synchondroses, all of which play a minimal role in postnatal growth. The synchondroses have zones similar to those in the epiphyseal cartilage of long bones. However, there are two directions of growth that result in elongation of the basicranium until its ultimate ossification occurs (Fig. 4-9).

The development of ossification center sutures and synchondroses in the chondrocranium were recently chronicled throughout childhood through computed tomography (CT). These data can provide standards for skull-base maturity. In

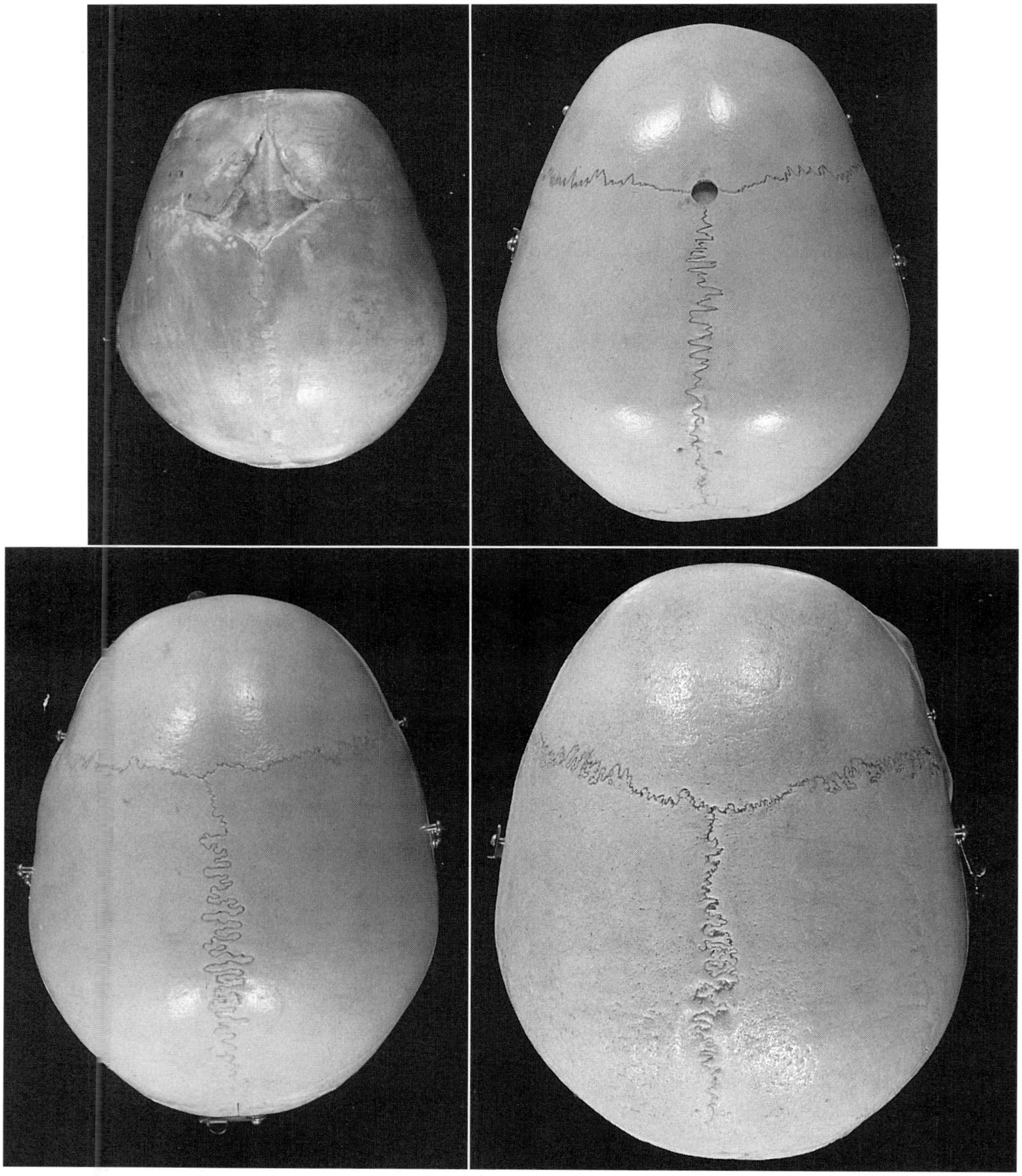

Fig. 4-7. Top view of skulls showing the shape change that occurs from infancy to adulthood. Shown are infant (approximately 8 months of age), 5- to 6-year old, 10- to 12-year-old, and adult skulls.

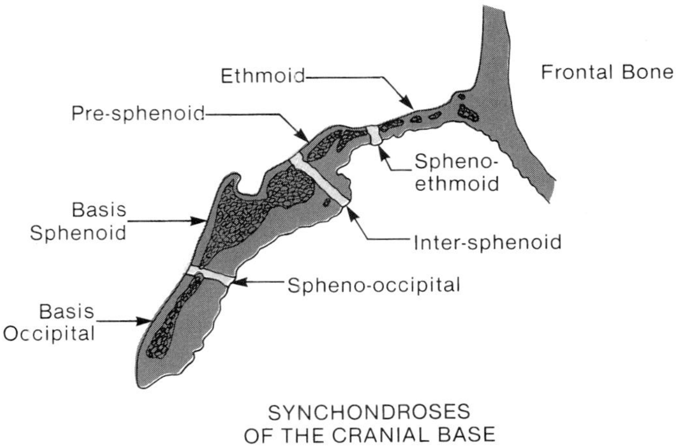

Fig. 4-8. Diagrammatic representation of the synchondroses of the cranial base, showing the location of these important growth sites. (From Proffit WR and others: *Contemporary orthodontics*, ed 2, St Louis, 1993, Mosby.)

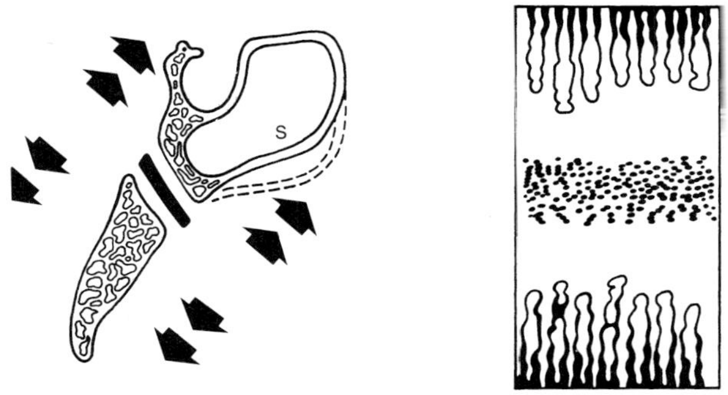

Fig. 4-9. Diagrammatic representation of growth at the intersphenoid synchondrosis. A bank of immature proliferating cartilage cells is located at the center of the synchondrosis, whereas a band of maturing cartilage cells extends in both directions away from the center; endochondral ossification occurs at both margins. Growth at the synchondrosis lengthens this area of the cranial base. (From Proffit WR and others: *Contemporary orthodontics*, ed 2, St Louis, 1993, Mosby.)

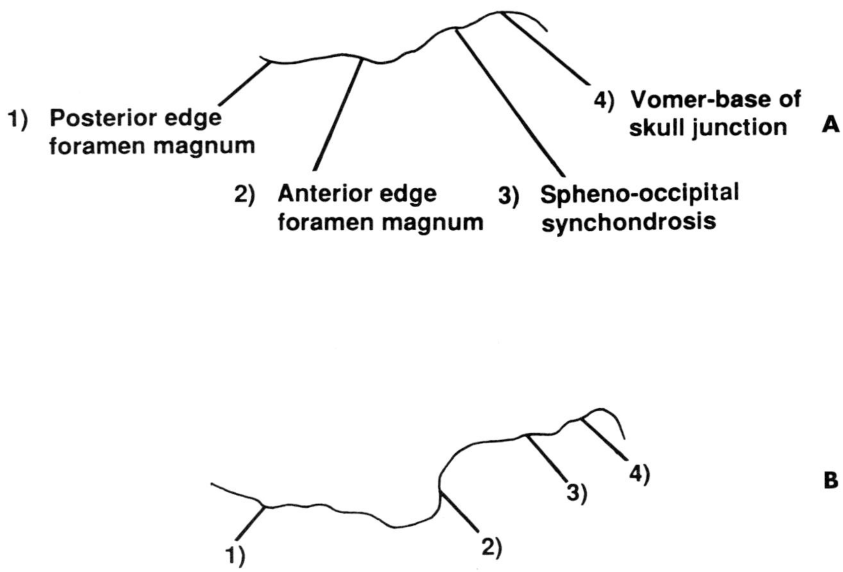

Fig. 4-10. Flexion of the cranial base. With growth there is a more convex superior or flexed appearance from infancy to adulthood. **A,** Infant. **B,** Adult.

addition, postnatal normal CT variants and magnetic resonance imaging assessment of the cranial base have been characterized.[72,73]

In newborns and infants the cranial base is quite flat. With growth into childhood there is a more convex superior or flexed appearance, which enlarges further during adolescence and adulthood. The spheno-occipital synchondrosis becomes more flexed as the maxillary portion of the nasomaxillary complex moves toward the foramen magnum and moves under the anterior cranial fossa (Fig. 4-10). Components of the cranial base can be seen more clearly in older pediatric skulls than in infant skulls. The foramen magnum approaches adult size and the primary dentition has erupted by 3 years of age. By 8 years of age the occipital bone has fused around the foramen magnum, and the secondary dentition is erupting. The major difference between the adolescent and adult skull is fusion of the spheno-occipital synchondrosis. Fusion of this synchondrosis begins at approximately 15 years of age for boys and 12 or 13 years of age for girls on the cerebral surface, ossification on the external aspect is complete by age 20[110] (Fig. 4-11). The chondrocranium–basicranium is a junction between both the neurocra-

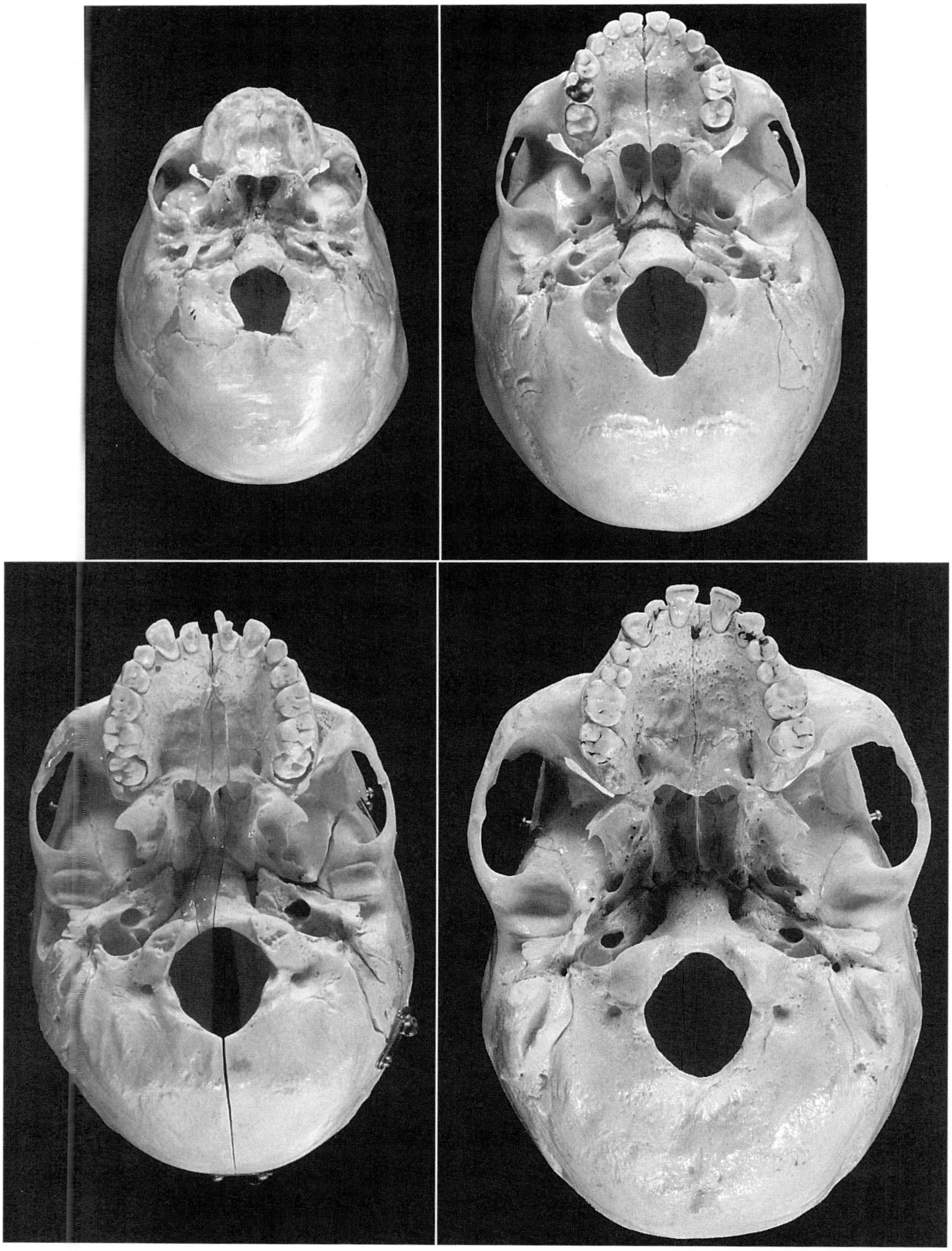

Fig. 4-11. Basal extracranial skull views of an infant (8 months of age), a 5- to 6-year-old, a 10- to 12-year-old, and an adult. Components of the cranial base are more clearly seen in the older skull. Note the open spheno-occipital synchondrosis in the 5- to 6-year-old skull and that the most posterior molar on the right side of the photograph is not the patient's and was falsely inserted.

nial and facial complex bones. Its alteration affects not only neurocranial and skull growth but also facial morphology.[97]

Nasomaxillary complex

The nasomaxillary complex develops through intramembranous ossification. It includes the nasal, lacrimal, maxillary, zygomatic, pterygoid, and vomer bones.

The nasomaxillary complex is displaced forward and downward from the cranial floor (basicranium) as a result of growth of the associated soft tissues. New bone growth occurs at sutural contact surfaces on both sides of the suture, with a resultant increase in the size of both bones involved (Fig. 4-12). Bone is added at the frontal maxillary, zygomaticotemporal, zygomaticosphenoidal, zygomaticomaxillary, ethmoidomaxillary, frontoethmoidal, nasomaxillary, nasofrontal, frontolacrimal, palatine, and vomerine sutures. There is constant interaction between the basicranium and the nasomaxillary complex. Rotatory displacement is caused by the downward and forward growth of the middle cranial fossa, resulting in greater or lesser amounts of displacement and remodeling growth in the posterior and anterior parts of the maxilla, depending on the biomechanical forces involved.[33]

The anterior surface of the maxilla is an area of significant resorption (Fig. 4-13). Even though bone is being resorbed here, the maxilla is still growing forward. This is a good example of remodeling and displacement (Fig. 4-14). Growth and development of the nasomaxillary complex is shown in Fig. 4-15. Vertical nasomaxillary growth occurs at the frontomaxillary, frontozygomatic, frontonasal, ethmoidomaxillary, and frontoethmoidal sutures as a result of orbital and nasal growth.

The orbits are quite large at birth because of their relationship with the globe, which are linked to cranial growth. Orbital remodeling is quite complex; 50% of postnatal orbital growth is achieved by 2 years of age, and it is almost complete by age 7.[75] The superior aspect of the orbit in toddlers is similar to that in adults, although the inferior aspect differs. The floor of the nose is almost at the level of the inferior orbital rim in infants and then the distance progressively increases to be significantly lower in adults. The eyes in the adult face are not much farther apart than those in a child's. According to Enlow and Hans,[33] however, "because of the larger nose, higher nasal bridge, increase in the vertical facial dimension and the widening of the cheekbones, the eyes of

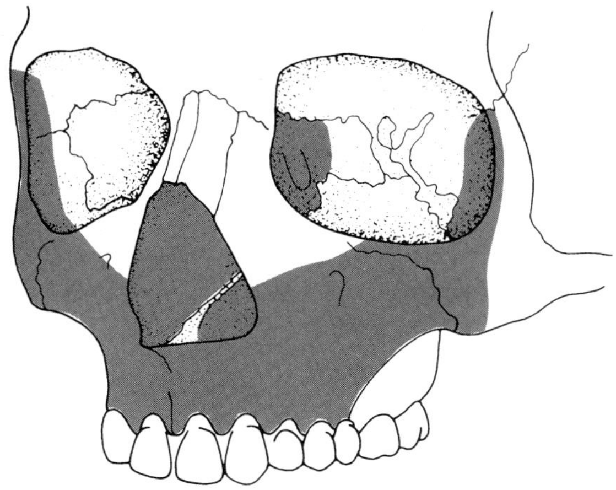

Fig. 4-13. As the maxilla is carried downward and forward, its anterior surface tends to resorb. Resorption surfaces are shown in *pink.* Only a small area around the anterior nasal spine is an exception. (From Proffit WR and others: *Contemporary orthodontics,* ed 2, St. Louis, 1993, Mosby.)

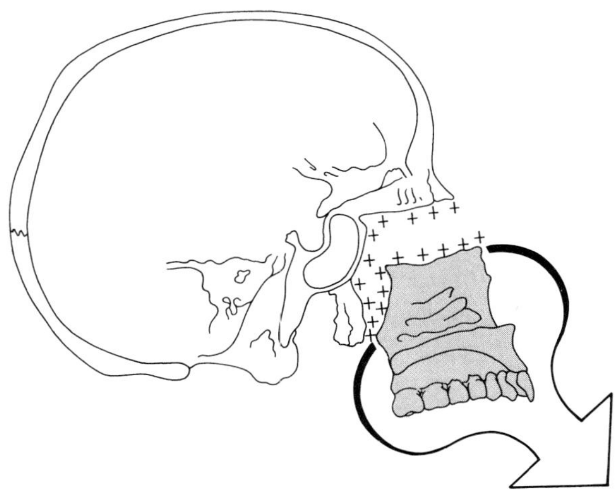

Fig. 4-12. As growth of the surrounding soft tissues translates the maxilla downward and forward, opening of space at its superior and posterior sutural attachments, new bone is added on both sides of the sutures. (From Proffit WR and others: *Contemporary orthodontics,* ed 2, St. Louis, 1993, Mosby.)

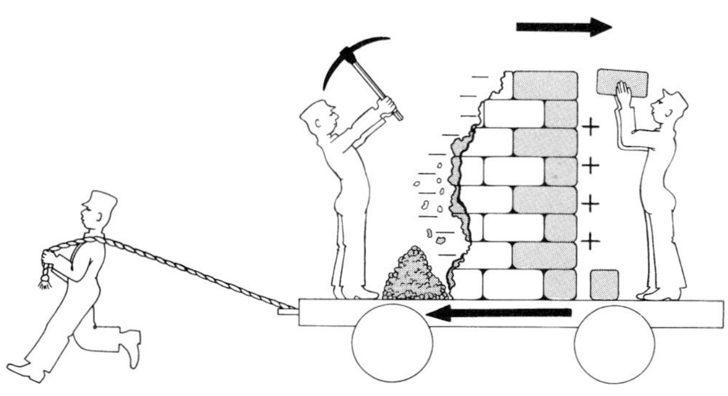

Fig. 4-14. Surface remodeling of a bone in the opposite direction to that in which the bone is being translated by growth of adjacent structures creates a situation analogous to this cartoon, in which the wall is being rebuilt to move it backward at the same time the platform on which it is mounted is being moved forward. (From Proffit WR and others: *Contemporary orthodontics,* ed 2, St. Louis, 1993, Mosby.)

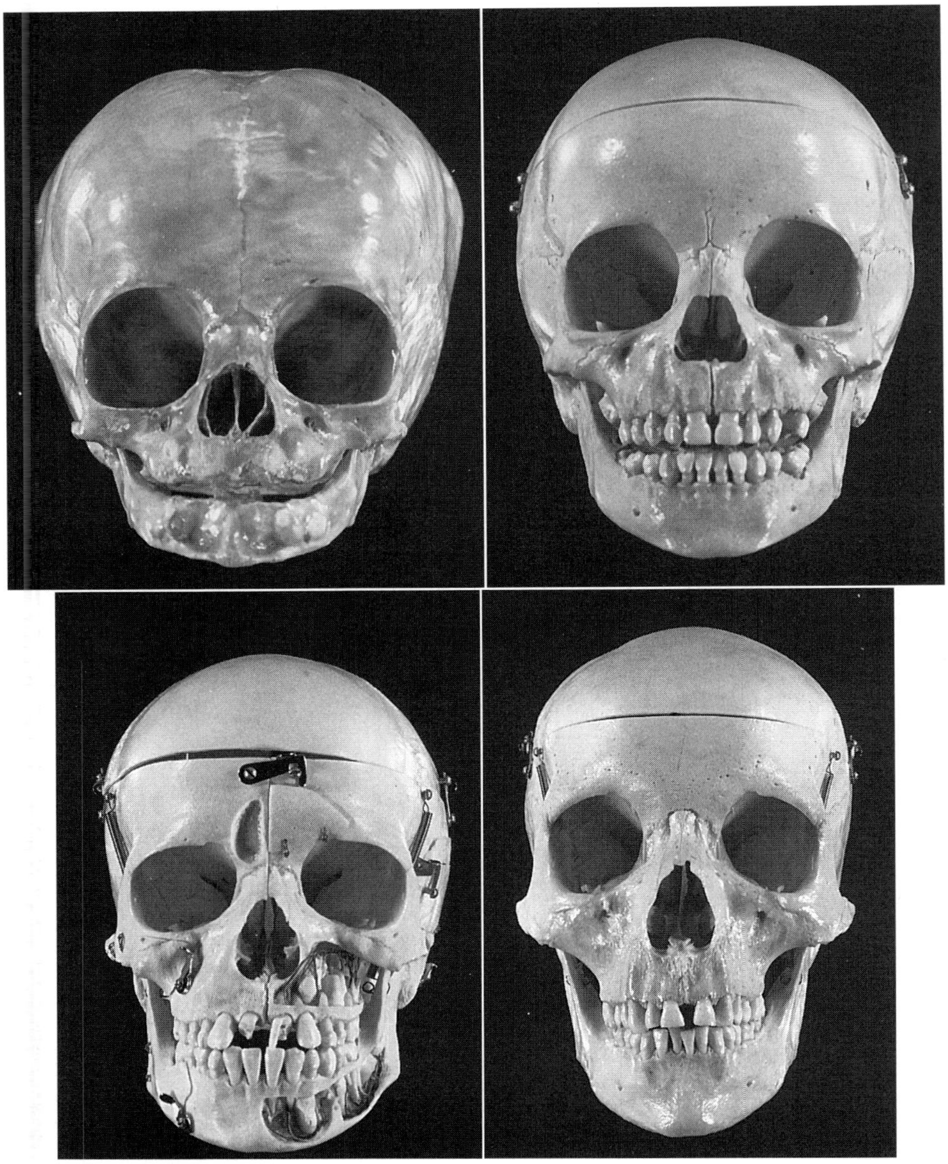

Fig. 4-15. Anterior view of infant (8 months), 5- to 6-year-old, 10- to 12-year-old, and adult skulls. Note the overall change of skull shape and the facial complex to cranium ratio, the relationship of the orbits to the floor of the nose, nasomaxillary and mandibular growth, and dental changes.

the adult appear much closer together.'' The main contribution to the widening face is from the lateral expansion of the zygomaticomaxillary sutures and the intermaxillary suture growth. Eruption of the primary and secondary teeth results in an increase in the size of the maxilla. As the maxilla moves downward and forward and secondary teeth erupt, the maxillary sinuses increase in size as well.

Mandible

The mandible forms in relation to the first branchial cartilage, otherwise known as Meckel's cartilage. Meckel's cartilage is interesting in that it is not replaced by bone. Instead, membranous bone forms lateral to Meckel's cartilage, and Meckel's cartilage then disappears[3] (Fig. 4-16). At birth, the mandible is comprised of two bones with the symphysis menti between them. This suture closes by 1 year of age, after which the majority of mandibular growth occurs posteriorly.

Resorption anteriorly and deposition posteriorly result in the overall growth of the mandible (Fig. 4-17). Although the condyles are a major site of growth, they are not a master growth center as previously thought.

There is a variation of endochondral bone growth at the articular contact portion of the condyle. The main contribution of condylar cartilage is to provide regional adaptive growth by maintaining the condylar area in a proper anatomic relationship with the temporal bone as the whole mandible is simultaneously being carried downward and forward.[33] The mandible grows by enlarging and widening in response to the increase in size of the muscles of mastication and an enlarging oropharynx, which accommodates the concomitant growth of the nasomaxillary complex. The ramus grows posteriorly and at the same time increases the interramal dimension along with the laterally expanding cranial floor. The coronoid processes grow superiorly and buccally, with the anterior edges of the rami being continually resorbed in the process. The condyles grow posteriorly, superiorly, and laterally (Fig. 4-18). Even though it is a single bone, Sperber[110] described the mandible functionally as six skeletal subunits. These subunits are the alveolar, coronoid, and angular bones, the condylar process, and the chin, all of which are attached to the ''body'' of the mandible. Moss' concept of functional matrices then influences the growth of each subunit (teeth–alveolar unit, action of the temporalis muscle–coronoid process, masseter and medial pterygoids–angle and ramus, lateral pterygoid–condylar process, perioral muscles, tongue, and expanding oropharyngeal cavity–entire mandible).

The infant mandibular arch is U-shaped, whereas the adult arch is more V-shaped (Fig. 4-19). The gonial angle (angle between the ramus and the body) is more obtuse in infants than in adults (Fig. 4-20). Mandibular growth has two specific growth spurts. The first occurs between 5 and 10 years of age and the second occurs between 10 and 15 years of age.[79] Growth in mandibular width is completed

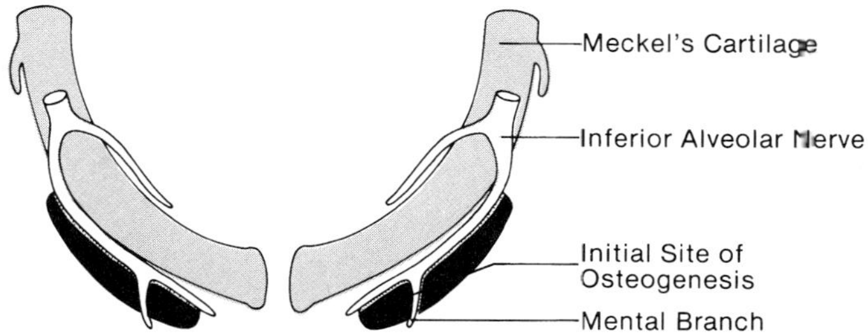

Fig. 4-16. Diagrammatic representation of the relation of the initial bone formation in the mandible to Meckel's cartilage and the inferior alveolar nerve. Bone formation begins just lateral to Meckel's cartilage and spreads posteriorly along it without any direct replacement of the cartilage by the newly forming bone of the mandible. (From Proffit WR and others: *Contemporary orthodontics,* ed 2, St. Louis, 1993, Mosby.)

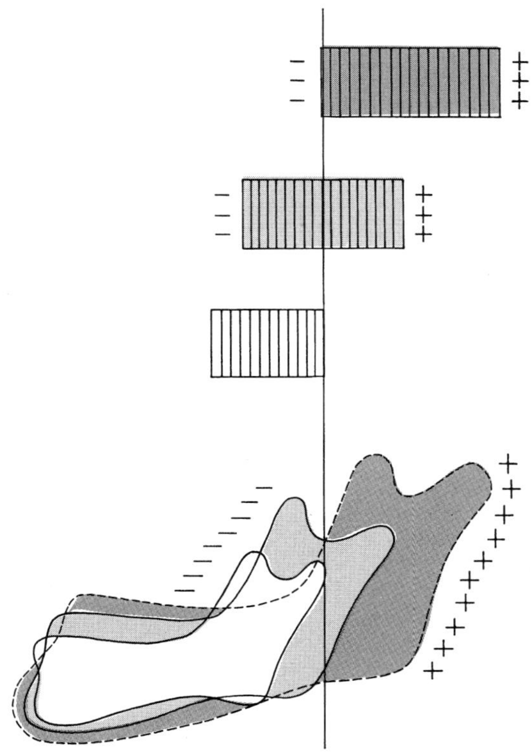

Fig. 4-17. As the mandible lengthens, the ramus is extensively remodeled—so much so that the bone that is at the tip of the condylar process at an early age can be found at the anterior surface of the ramus some years later. Given the extent of surface remodeling changes that occur, it is an obvious area to emphasize endochondral bone formation at the condyle as the major mechanism for growth of the mandible. (From Proffit WR and others: *Contemporary orthodontics,* ed 2, St. Louis, 1993, Mosby.)

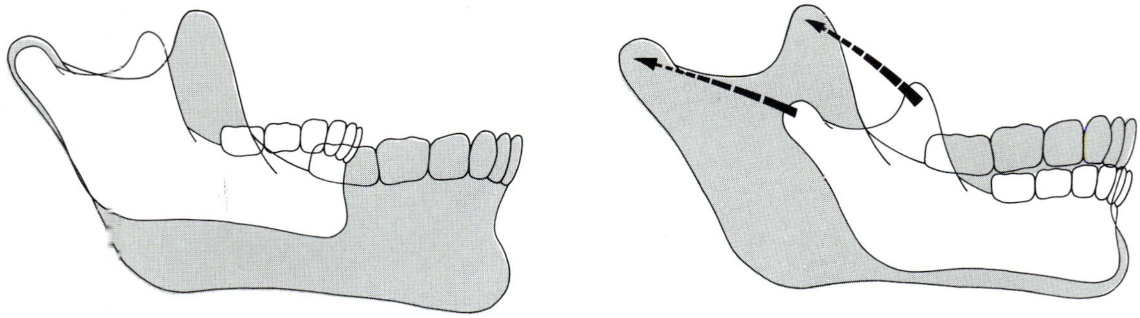

Fig. 4-18. Mandibular growth, as viewed from the perspective of vital staining dyes. Note there are minimal changes in the body and chin area, while there is exceptional growth and remodeling of the ramus, moving it posteriorly. The correct concept of mandibular growth is that the mandible is translated downward and forward and grows upward and backward in response to this translation, maintaining its contact with the skull. (From Proffit WR and others: *Contemporary orthodontics*, ed 2, St Louis, 1993, Mosby.)

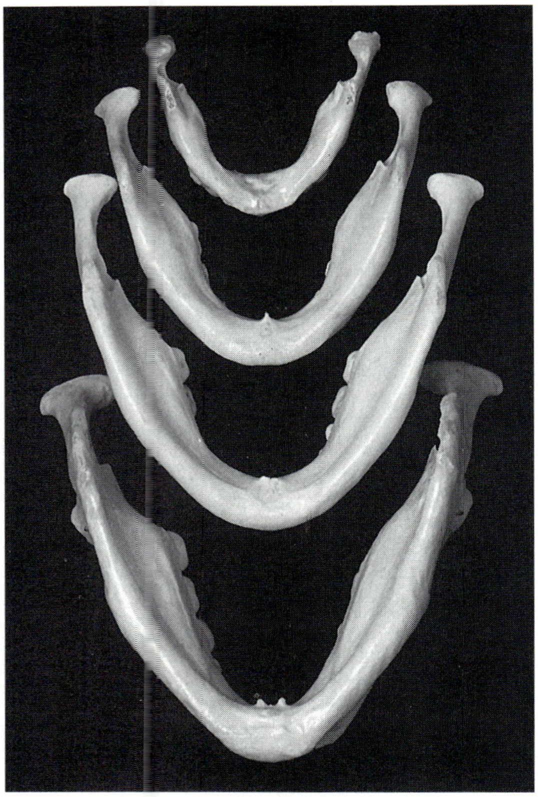

Fig. 4-19. With mandibular growth the U shape of the infant mandible changes to more of a V shape, as seen in the adult.

during early adolescence, length 2 to 3 years after menstruation in females and approximately 4 years after attainment of sexual maturity in males, and height in the late teens in females and early twenties in males (Fig. 4-20).

Internal and external rotational changes of the mandible occur during growth and, of course, in conjunction with rotational changes in the maxilla (Fig. 4-21). Bjork and Skieller[12] described this in detail using metallic implants. Miller and Kerr[79] supported their finding but used a digitizer program to follow longitudinal cephalograms in a number of patients. Overall mandibular growth is not uniform and steady because corpus length and ramus height grow in an irregular pattern.[29,128] Jaw rotation influences the degree of tooth eruption.

Craniofacial cephalometric and anthropometric studies are abundant in the literature, and normative data are available. A review of these topics is beyond the scope of this chapter; however, these measurements may be used to assist in the interpretation of optimal growth and development in the clinical situation.[4,35-39,96]

ABNORMAL FACIAL GROWTH AND DEVELOPMENT

Asymmetry of the human face is well recognized as a normal finding and in fact is an intrinsic facial characteristic. According to Ferrario and others, "the skeletal structures show a greater degree of asymmetry than their soft tissue drape."[41] Age is certainly one factor that influences asymmetry. Melnik[77] found that the left side of the face was larger at 6 years of age, whereas the right side of the face was larger at 16. There is disagreement in the literature regarding the degree, side, and localization of normal facial asymmetry, although some authors believe that this is due to methodologic differences.[41] Normal facial asymmetry involves many subtle differences that are not readily apparent to the viewer. Conversely, abnormal facial asymmetry is typically quite obvious.

Our culture is obsessed with physical attractiveness, which to a large extent is based on facial symmetry and what is perceived to be "normal." Langlois[66] found that the preference for attractive persons is evident early in life and involves all age groups and races. As a result, individuals

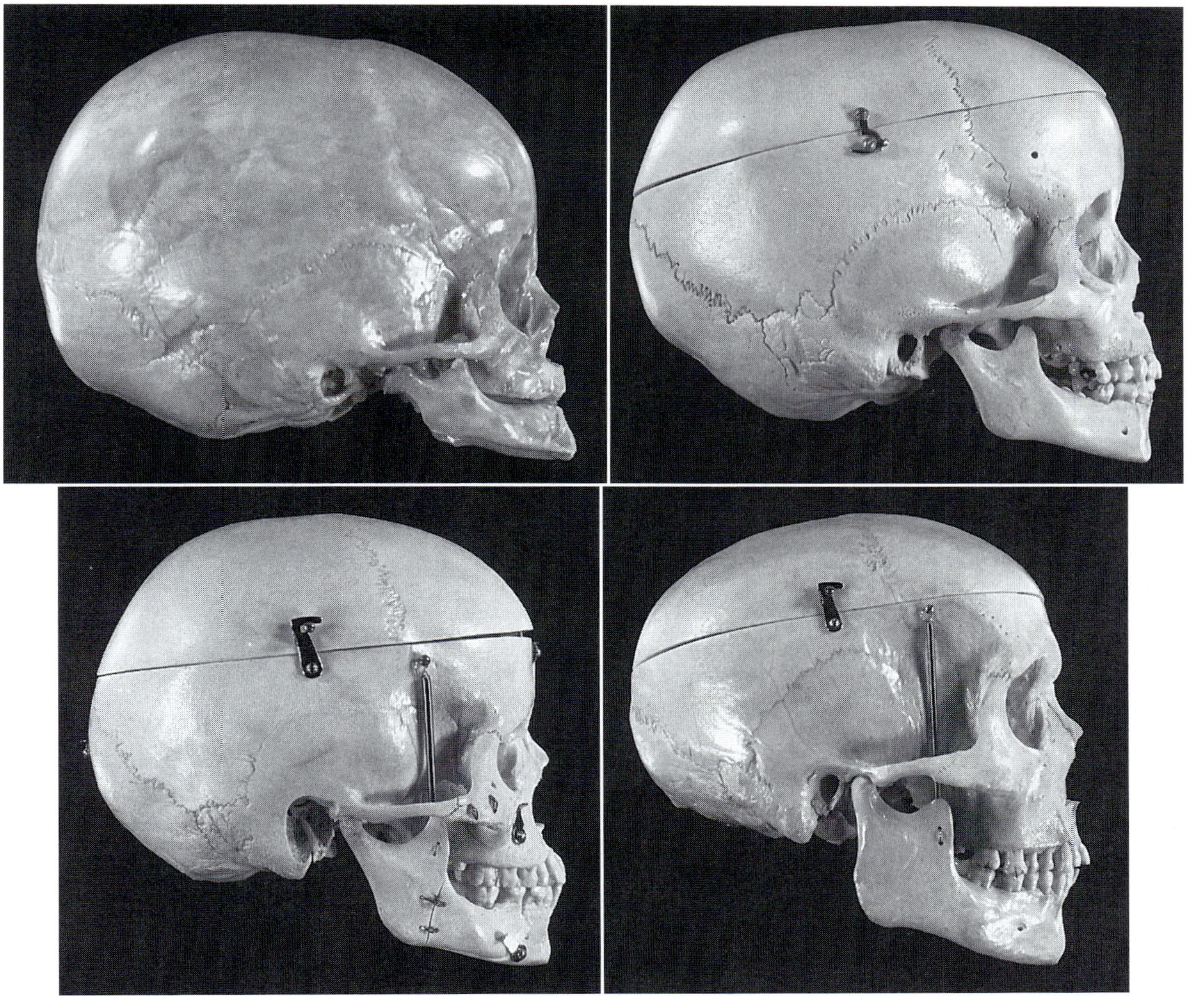

Fig. 4-20. Lateral view of the infant (8 months), 5- to 6-year-old, 10- to 12-year-old, and adult skull. Note the gonial angle of the mandible is more obtuse in the infant. The overall change in size of the mandible over time is dramatic.

who appear divergent "from the norm," with or without intellectual impairment, are viewed differently in our society.

Abnormal facial growth and development and the resultant characteristics arise from numerous etiologies. The following describe some examples seen in pediatric otolaryngology, with the focus on various aspects of craniofacial abnormalities.

Robin sequence (Pierre Robin syndrome)

The combination of micrognathia, cleft palate, and glossoptosis is known as the Robin sequence (Fig. 4-22). Previously known as Pierre Robin syndrome, it is now known that this condition does not meet the criteria for a syndrome with a single identifiable etiology but that there is etiologic heterogeneity. Cohen[21] proposed that "etiologic heterogeneity suggests pathogenetic heterogeneity in Robin sequence."

There are various definitions of the Robin sequence, including the presence or absence of a cleft palate, glossoptosis, and airway difficulty. These varying definitions have caused confusion in the literature. The Robin sequence can be classified as either isolated (nonsyndromic) or in association with a syndrome (syndromic). Shprintzen[107] found that approximately 20% of patients had isolated Robin sequence, with the remaining 80% of cases associated with various syndromes. The primary clinical implications of this condition are airway obstruction and feeding difficulty. Anatomically, the larynx is under the base of the tongue in patients with micrognathia and glossoptosis, making direct laryngoscopy or intubation difficult and occasionally impossible.[10] Cleft palate and respiratory difficulty can hamper feeding and contribute to failure to thrive.

Whether the Robin sequence is isolated or associated with a syndrome has very significant implications with respect to mandibular growth. A common error made by physicians

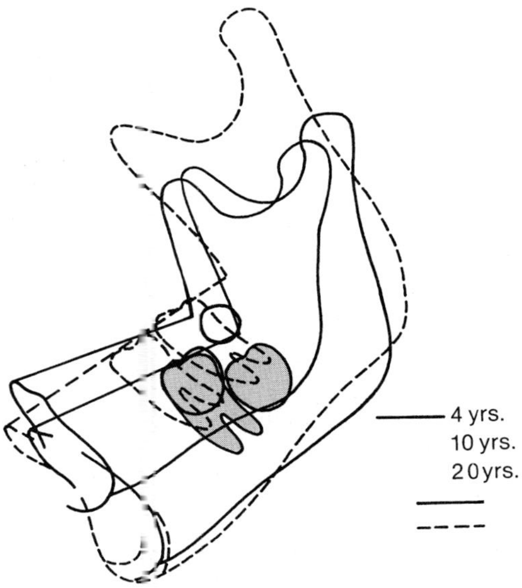

Fig. 4-21. Superimposition on implants for an individual with a normal growth pattern showing surface changes in the mandible from ages 4 to 20 years. For this patient there was a −19° internal rotation but only a −3° change in the mandibular plane angle. Note dramatic remodeling in the area of the gonial angle, with a net resorption over this period. This surface remodeling or external rotation compensates for, and conceals the extent of, the internal rotation. (From Bjork A, Skiller V: Normal and abnormal growth of the mandible: a synthesis of longitudinal cephalometric implant studies over a period of 25 years, *Eur J Orthod* 5:1, 1983.)

is to convey to the family of a newborn with Robin sequence that the child's mandible will reach relatively normal size within a couple of years.[108] If the Robin sequence is associated with a known syndrome (primary error or nondeformational cause) such as Treacher Collins or Stickler syndrome, mandibular hypoplasia will persist throughout the patient's life unless surgical intervention is undertaken. In these cases, postnatal catch-up growth does not occur.

If the Robin sequence is isolated, however, with the etiologic pathogenesis related to deformation, then catch-up growth does occur. Pruzansky[94] believed that postnatal growth potential should be included in the analysis of differences between malformed mandibles and that ''some mandibles are capable of considerable postnatal recuperations.''

It was once thought that upon completion of growth the mandibles of patients with Robin sequence would be of essentially normal size. Pruzansky[94] noted that such patients' mandibles differed from the normal mandible in that ''the gonial angle was more obtuse, the condyle extended distally from the ramus, and ramus to body proportions were deviant because of the greater reduction in body length.'' He also noted that these features persisted from infancy into adulthood. The mandible appears to grow faster than normal in affected patients during the first few months of life, resulting in alleviation of breathing problems and feeding difficulty in many patients. Not all patients are so fortunate, however, and numerous measures have been advocated to assist the patient, from positioning to subperiosteal tongue release to tracheostomy.*

Even in the isolated Robin sequence, full or complete catch-up growth does not occur (see Fig. 4-22 *A, B*). Figueroa and others[43] performed a retrospective longitudinal cephalometric study analyzing size, growth, and the relation of the mandible, tongue, and airway in isolated nonsyndromic Robin sequence infants. They found that the increased mandibular growth rate in these infants was significant but did not reach values seen in healthy infants. There was a significant difference in the craniofacial variables between healthy patients and those with the Robin sequence. Their study supported the concept of ''partial mandibular catch-up growth.'' They also discussed an unpublished study from their institution in which adolescent patients with Robin sequence were compared with healthy children. Results indicated that craniofacial dimensions, including the maxilla, mandible, and airway, were smaller in Robin sequence patients. Laitinen and Ranta[64] and Laitinen[65] found the dental arches at birth of patients with Robin sequence (isolated or possibly syndromic) and those of patients with isolated cleft lip and palate to be equal; by 6 years of age, the dental arches in patients with Robin sequence were smaller than isolated cleft palate arches, which in turn were smaller than those in children without clefts.

The U-shaped cleft palate in Robin sequence and its mode of development are different from those of the usual V shape seen in primary defects (see Fig. 4-22, *C*). Hanson and Smith[55] hypothesized that with micrognathia the posteriorly displaced tongue is interposed between the palatal shelves. The palatal shelves do not close, resulting in less posterior growth of the soft palate and subsequently the U-shaped cleft palate. That is, the small mandible causes the tongue to be placed abnormally in the posterior portion of the oral cavity, in between the palatal shelves, and the subsequent lack of closure and growth of the palatal shelves and the lack of growth of the soft palate result in the U-shaped defect.

Robin sequence is relatively common, occurring in approximately 1 in 8500 births. Prevalence is confusing, however, because of the isolated/syndromic differentiation. The most important issue in these patients is first to ensure an adequate airway and feeding, then to determine whether there is an associated syndrome in order to communicate to the family the degree of intervention that will likely be needed.

Down syndrome (trisomy 21)

Down syndrome (trisomy 21) is the most common malformation syndrome Fig. 4-23. It occurs in approximately 1 in 650 live births, and there is a greater prevalence with increasing maternal age. These individuals, who have an extra copy of the genetic material on chromosome 21, have

* Refs. 10, 27, 85, 105, 107, 109.

A

B

C

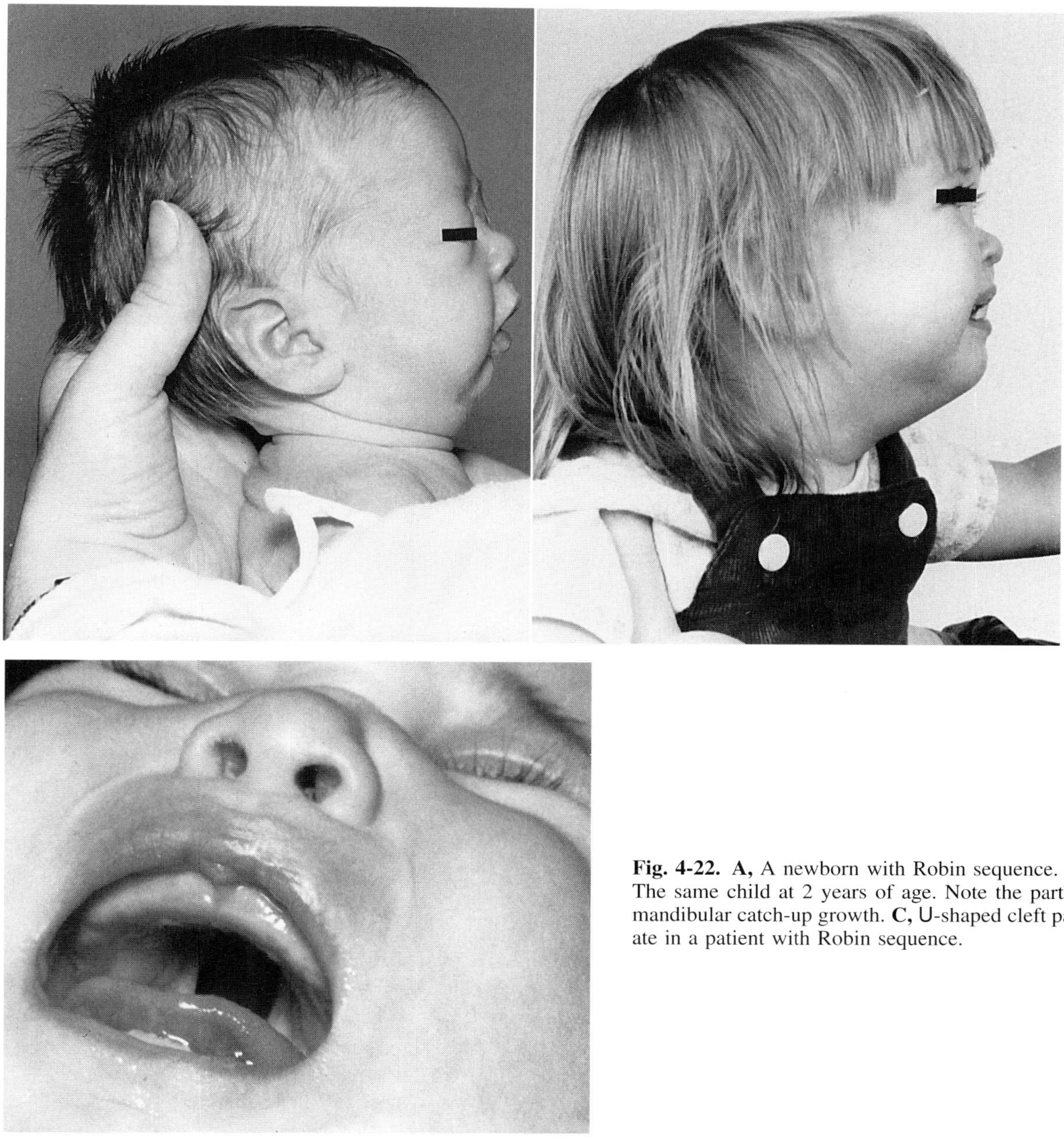

Fig. 4-22. A, A newborn with Robin sequence. **B,** The same child at 2 years of age. Note the partial mandibular catch-up growth. **C,** U-shaped cleft palate in a patient with Robin sequence.

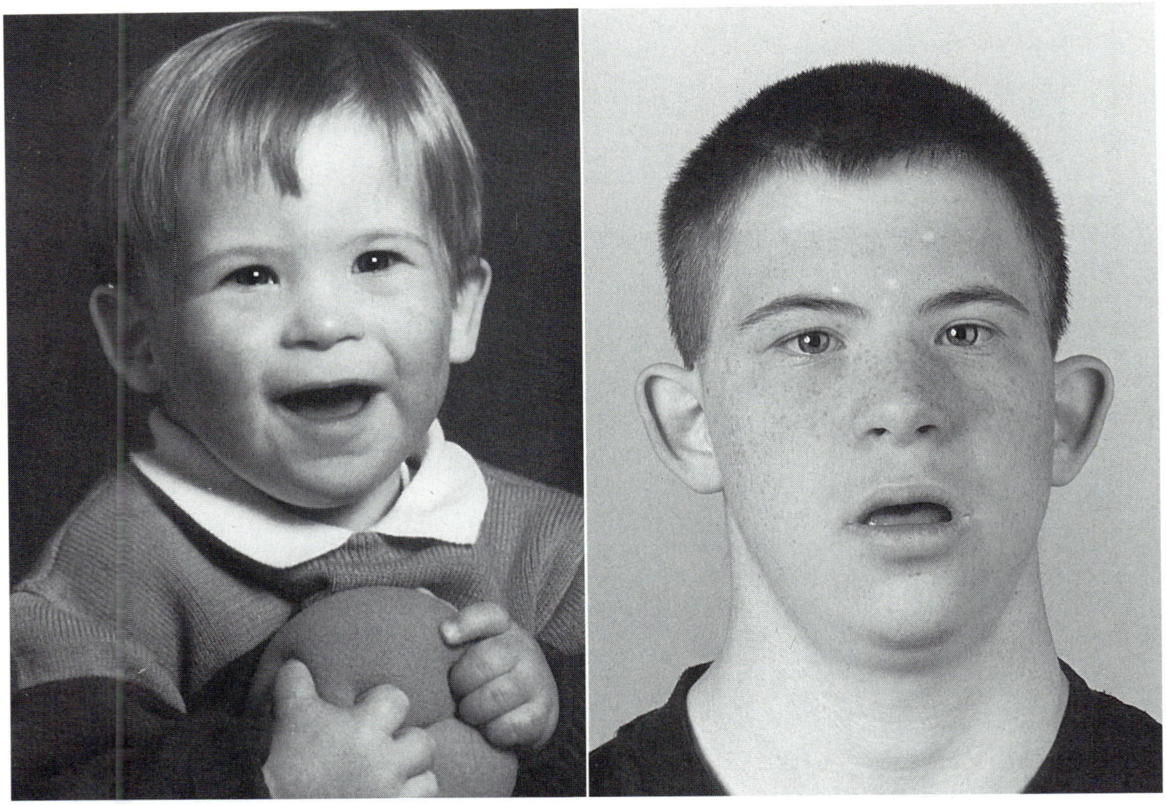

Fig. 4-23. **A,** A 2-year-old male with Down syndrome (trisomy 21). **B,** The same child at 14 years of age.

Box 4-1. Craniofacial features of Down syndrome

- Brachycephaly
- Flat occiput
- Upslanting palpebral fissures
- Epicanthic folds
- Short, small nose
- Abnormal, small ears
- Short neck
- Midface hypoplasia
- Large, fissured lips
- Large, fissured tongue
- Dental abnormalities

a very characteristic appearance.[46,62] There are over 100 different physical signs in Down syndrome. The main features, in addition to intellectual deficit, are the craniofacial physical characteristics listed in Box 4-1. These characteristics make individuals with Down syndrome appear significantly different from the rest of the population. Pueschel and Pueschel[95] extensively reviewed the biomedical concerns of Down syndrome patients, including growth and development. The specific dysmorphic facial features of Down syndrome, outlined in Box 4-1 can be further classified into five main regions: skull, midface, mandible and oral manifestation, ears, and eyes. The growth changes in each of these regions are reviewed here.

Skull

The majority of patients with Down syndrome have brachycephaly. Head breadth (largest lateral diameter of the head) and head length (measured from the nasion to the largest length across the occiput) were found to be essentially normal in the first 6 months of life when compared with healthy children.[100,117] At 6 months and 1 year, however, the mean values were less by 1 SD for head breadth and 2 to 3 SDs for head length. The greater difference in head length versus head breadth suggests that cranial growth is more reduced at the cranial base than in the area of the calvaria. In 1979, Hamill[54a] determined that head circumference is smaller in individuals with trisomy 21; however, this is thought to be a reflection of overall body size. When head circumference is plotted against body-length ratios, these values are found to be within normal range. Head circumference is related to intracranial or brain growth, whereas cranial base growth is probably under the same control as total body growth. The occiput also is found to be flat, which is

Box 4-2. Craniofacial findings in mandibulofacial dysostosis (Treacher Collins syndrome)[46,62]

Eyes

Antimongoloid slanting of palpebral fissures
Lower-lid coloboma
Partial to total absence of lower eyelashes

Ears

Auricular malformations with or without tags and preauricular blind fistulas
Stenosis or atresia of the external-ear canals
Middle-ear and ossicular abnormalities

Face

Malar hypoplasia (hypoplastic zygomatic bones) and nonfusion of the zygomatic arches
Flat frontal nasal angle
Hypoplastic supraorbital rims and ridges
Narrow nares and hypoplastic alar cartilages
Tongues of hair onto cheeks

Mandible oral region

Mandibular hypoplasia and severe hypoplasia of the mandibular condyle
Microstomia
High, narrow, or cleft palate
Dental abnormalities

especially noticeable in the profile view. Allanson and others[2] obtained 21 craniofacial anthropometric measurements from patients with trisomy 21 between the ages of 6 months and 61 years of age. Their data were compared with normal known standards and were in agreement with previous studies involving craniofacial findings in Down syndrome. The authors specifically mention brachycephaly, round face, and small ears but add that underdevelopment of the maxilla in comparison with the mandible also occurs. They found that as age increases, maxillary growth is reduced in comparison with mandibular growth, resulting in a change from the usual round face seen in infants to the more oval shape seen in older patients (see Fig. 4-23 *A, B*).

Sperber[110] indicated that the reduced cranial base results in an increased angulation due to loss of the flattening effect of the growth of the spheno-occipital synchondrosis. In a skull of normal or reduced capacity an increase in the basal angle is highly suggestive of Down syndrome.[17] This results in a dished deformity of the midface, accentuated by the large neurocranium. The anterior fontanelle is late to close and the so-called "third fontanelle," an open saggital suture in the region of the parietal bone, is present.[19] A metopic suture is quite common in Down syndrome patients.

Midface

Benda[8,9] noted a deficiency in postnatal development of the nasal bones, the ethmoid, and the maxilla that results in continuance of the fetal proportions of the face in individuals with Down syndrome. He also noted that hypoplastic or even absent paranasal sinuses also contribute to midface hypoplasia. Shapiro and others[104] found that Down syndrome patients have narrower and shorter palates. The deficiency in palatal length, in comparison with healthy individuals, was so great in the patients from their study (age range, 7 to 1[illegible] years) that they could distinguish between a Down syndrome patient and a healthy individual based on this dimension alone. Palatal vaults were previously thought to be abnormal (higher in trisomy 21 patients), but Shapiro and others confirmed that they are within the normal range.[104] Smaller nasal bones appear to contribute to the saddle nose/small nose of trisomy 21 patients.[110] Interorbital distance is reduced, and the mandible is more obtuse.[44] The angle between the base of the skull and the hard palate is less acute than normal in patients with trisomy 21, and the nasopharynx is generally small because of soft tissue encroachment.

Sperber[110] theorized that the neural crest tissues involved in facial bone formation, (including the nose) either "may be deficient in number, may not complete migration to their destination, or fail in their inductive capacity or cytodifferentiation." The generalized retardation in midfacial growth along with the underdevelopment of the sinuses in patients with trisomy 21 results in the overall poor development and flat facial profile of the midface.

Ears

Individuals with Down syndrome have long been recognized to have small ears. The ears are frequently small and boxlike and can be low set with abnormal overlapping or folding of the helix. Aase, Wilson, and Smith[1] noted that "of all the anthropomorphic measurements studied, the longitudinal dimensions of the pinna fell furthest below the expected norm at all age levels studied." This finding was usually greater than 2 SD below the norm in newborns to 1-year-olds and 1 SD in patients older than 1 year of age. External-ear canal narrowing is extremely common, and middle-ear abnormalities exist.[5,114] The mastoid abnormalities in Down syndrome are mainly hypoplasia and sclerosis.[41] These abnormalities may have an inflammatory etiology from increased problems of middle-ear pathology secondary to eustachian tube dysfunction. Generalized hypotonia in Down syndrome may affect the tensor veli palatini muscle, resulting in eustachian tube dysfunction.

Mandible and oral manifestations

The oral manifestations in individuals with Down syndrome are outlined in Box 4-1. Thickened and fissured lips as the patient advances in age, a large, fissured tongue (possibly related to a relatively small oral cavity), and various dental abnormalities are very common in these patients.* After 16 or 18 years of age, progressive mandibular prognathism may occur and is believed to be related to the large tongue in a small oral cavity.[47]

Eyes

Using radiographic methods, Gerald and Silverman[44] described narrowing of the interorbital distance in patients with Down syndrome and concluded that this orbital hypotelorism is the skeletal substrate for the characteristic face of these patients. Cohen and others[20] agreed that ocular hypotelorism is true when measured; however, they also noted that the illusion of hypertelorism exists in trisomy 21 patients because of the characteristic epicanthic folds and low nasal bridge. Other factors that contribute to the illusion of hypertelorism include exotropia, narrow palpebral fissures, dystopia canthorum, and widely spaced eyebrows that contribute to the perception of hypertelorism. In Down syndrome, epicanthic folds appear to result from underdevelopment of the nasion.[8] An alternate theory is that the epicanthic folds result from an abnormal distribution of the orbicularis oculi muscle, with some fibers passing circularly in front of the tendon rather than inserting wholly into the ligament.[113]

Abnormal and poor growth in Down syndrome

No specific gene or genes on chromosome 21 have been identified to contribute to our understanding of how the many phenotypic findings arise in Down syndrome. However, it is postulated that a dosage effect occurs because of the extra chromosome. No growth-regulating genes have been mapped on chromosome 21, but Pueschel and Pueschel[95] postulate that ''gene coding for growth-regulating proteins may play a part in the growth retardation observed in individuals with Down syndrome.'' According to this theory, the extra chromosome 21 is responsible for the abnormal embryogenesis of the fetus with Down syndrome and somehow the balance in the growth process is altered. Further studies in the molecular biology of growth and development will ultimately delineate this unknown.

Achondroplasia

Achondroplasia is the most common of the chondrodysplasias. A full description of this disorder of bone formation can be found in Jones,[62] Gorlin, Cohen, and Lovin,[46] and OMIM.[86]

Achondroplasia is an autosomal dominant disorder, with the majority of cases representing a new mutation. Bone formed from cartilage is abnormal due to a mutation in the fibroblast growth factor receptor-3 *(FGFR-3)* gene, which is located at 4p16.3.[101a,105a] Two different point mutations have been found in the *FGFR-3* gene of patients with achondroplasia, and both lead to the substitution of an arginine residue for a glycine at position 380 of the mature protein, which is in the transmembrane domain of *FGFR-3*.[86] In addition to the gene being expressed in cartilage, *FGFR-3* transcripts are present in fetal and adult brains (which have the highest levels of any tissue). This may indicate that the effects of the gene involve calvaria content as well as skeletal cartilage, leading to true megalencephaly.[27a,86] The exact process leading to the phenotypic appearance is unclear.

Individuals affected by this disorder have short stature secondary to rhizomelic shortening of the limbs as well as abnormalities of a number of other bones, including the lumbar spine, carpals, metacarpals, phalanges, and pelvis (Fig. 4-24, *A*). The characteristic facial appearance of achondroplasia results from early spheno-occipital closure, a short cranial base, a small foramen magnum, and resultant megalocephaly with frontal bossing, sunken bridge of the nose, and midfacial hypoplasia (Fig. 4-24, *B*). In addition, the eustachian tube is shortened. Head growth is normally rapid in the first 6 months of life in patients with achondroplasia.[54]

It is postulated that the genetic defect in achondroplasia leads to reduced growth of the occipital bones, resulting in the small foramen magnum.[57] Premature fusion of the associated synchondroses could also explain the abnormal foramen magnum configuration. Measurement of the foramen magnum may identify individuals at risk for possible neurologic complications in achondroplasia. Basilar kyphosis is present, with the angle between the ethmoidal plane and clivus reduced to 85° to 90° (normal angle, 110° to 120°).[102] The clivus is vertical, and the sphenoid sinus frequently extends into it.[25] The sella may be small and abnormally J-shaped.[6] The petrous portion of the temporal bone is very distorted, and the internal and external acoustic meatus and labyrinths are abnormally oriented. Interestingly, balance is not affected in these patients. Mastoid development is minimal.[25] The chondrocranium is short and narrow, as noted above. Dorst[31] noted that the midface is recessed in profile because the facial bones ''hang down'' from the chondrocranium. Articulation is normal.[102] The mandible is not affected by the genetic mutation but appears disproportionately large. Class 3 dental occlusion is common. Surgical correction via standard craniofacial procedures and nasal bone grafting improve the cosmetic appearance if this is desired.[6,29]

Mandibulofacial dysostosis (Treacher Collins syndrome, Franceschetti syndrome)[116]

Mandibulofacial dysostosis (MFD), also known as Treacher Collins syndrome, is a rare malformation syndrome with a very characteristic appearance[116] (Fig. 4-25). The craniofacial abnormalities in MFD are outlined in Box 4-2, and the syndrome is covered in detail elsewhere.[46,62,86]

Mandibulofacial dysostosis is a rare autosomal dominant condition with complete penetrance and variable expression. Sixty percent of cases are spontaneous new mutations. The gene was first localized to chromosome 5q32-33.1 by linkage analysis and was subsequently identified by positional cloning. The identification of mutations in the *TCOF1* gene

* Refs. 16, 18, 22, 23, 60, 95.

A

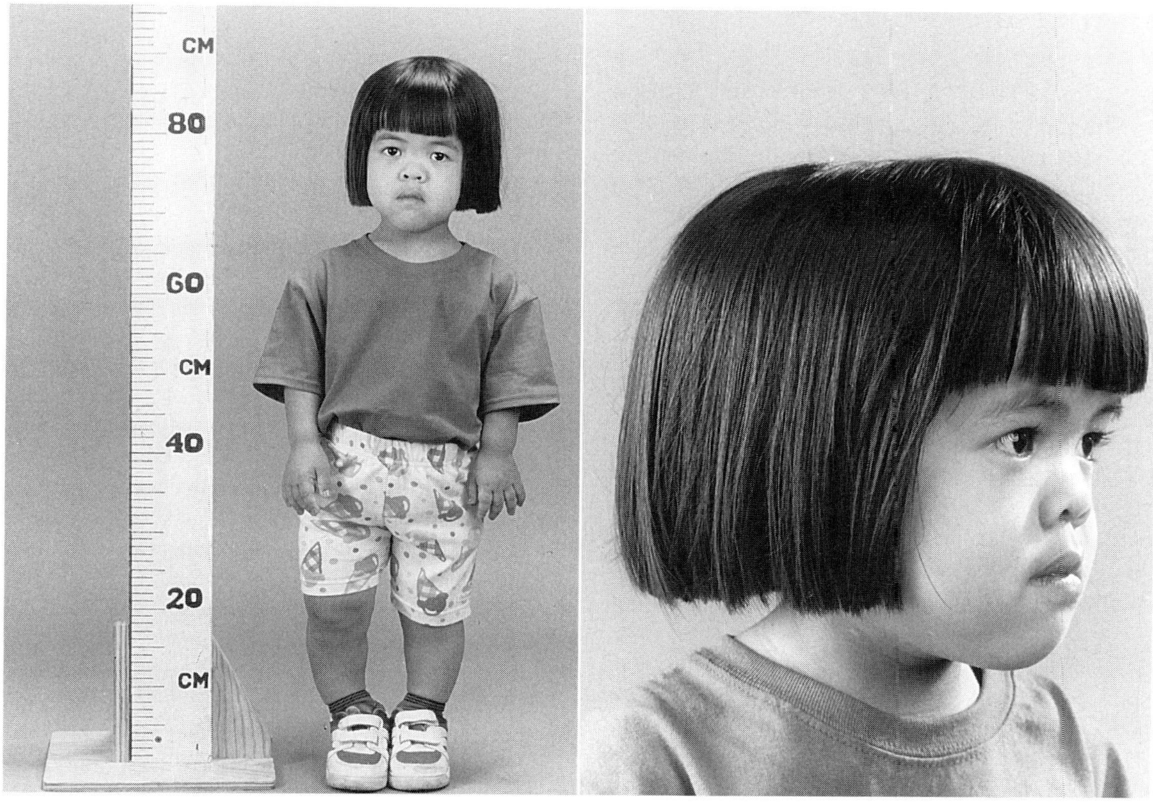

B

Fig. 4-24. **A,** A 6-year-old female with achondroplasia. **B,** The characteristic facial appearance of achondroplasia: frontal bossing, sunken bridge of the nose, and midfacial hypoplasia. The normal mandible appears larger than usual.

A

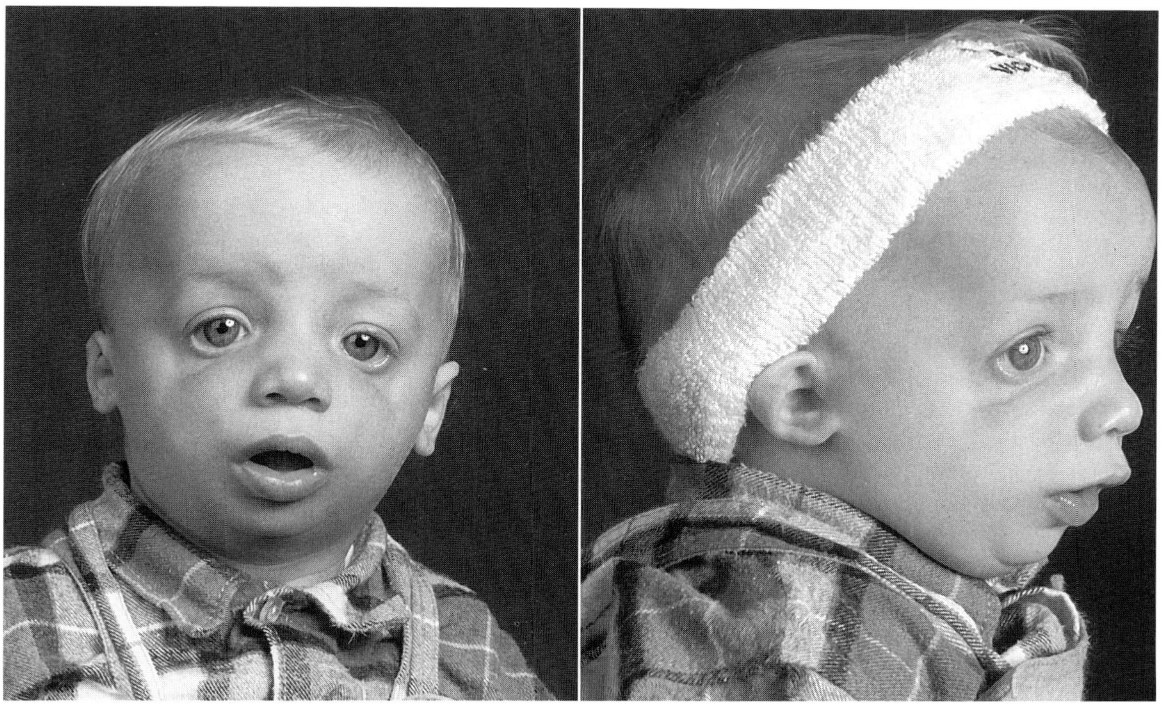

B

Fig. 4-25. **A,** Characteristic facial appearance of a 10-month-old child with mandibulofacial dysostosis (Treacher Collins syndrome). **B,** Oblique view of same patient. Note the absent external ear canal, which is bilateral, and the headband, which holds bone-conduction hearing aids.

(also referred to as the *TREACLE* gene) in five different families confirmed the causative nature of this gene in MFD. Its function is unknown. At present, linkage analysis or mutational analysis can be undertaken to identify affected family members who may exhibit only mild phenotypic features of this syndrome.

Marsh and others[74,75] provide an exhaustive, outstanding review of the cranial dysmorphology in MFD, both from the literature and from three-dimensional re-formation imaging from CT scans. From a clinical standpoint, pharyngeal hypoplasia in individuals with MFD is significant because it makes these patients prone to airway difficulty both early in life and later in life. Pharyngeal hypoplasia existed in all 11 patients with MFD reviewed by Shprintzen.[106] In fact, patients with a mild or incomplete phenotype were equally at risk. Shprintzen recommended nasopharyngoscopy and anterior posterior roentgenography to aid in the diagnosis. With growth there is an increase in basilar kyphosis exacerbating the problem. MFD patients reported in the literature have responded to craniofacial surgery to alleviate their apnea.[24,61]

Patients with MFD have an abnormal acute cranial base that is 2 to 3 SDs below normal.[107] Peterson-Falzone and Figueroa[90] reviewed the longitudinal measurements of cranial base angulation in 24 patients with MFD. They showed an increase in the flexure of the cranial base angle over time, with more than 50% falling into the kyphotic range, confirming previous reports of this finding in the literature. The authors attribute the increasing flexion to intracranial resorption and extracranial bony apposition as described by Enlow.[32,33] They speculate that the increased flexion may be greater in MFD because the clivus resorbs to a greater degree during cranial base development. This may be due to a disproportion between normal brain mass in individuals with MFD and the reduction in facial height and the association with the anterior cranial base.

Deficient growth of the spheno-occipital and intersphenoidal synchondroses also plays a role in the formation of the abnormal cranial base. Kreiborg and Dahl[63] studied craniofacial growth in two children with MFD. Progressive basilar kyphosis occurred in both children, and the authors hypothesized that bending took place at the sphenofrontal suture. They felt that this, along with abnormal growth of the mandible, led to impairment of the airway, that the calvaria appeared to rotate backward and downward in relation to the anterior cranial base, and that the sphenofrontal suture acted as a joint. They also concluded that the abnormal growth of the mandible occurred at the condyle, which is in agreement with Enlow's[32,33] work. This study is also consistent with previous findings of hypoplasia of the greater wings of the sphenoid and pterygoid plates.

The mandible in MFD is hypoplastic. The gonial angle (ramus to body angle) is obtuse. The condyles are hypoplastic or completely absent. Antegonial notching (the concavity on the inferior border of the mandible anterior to the ramus–body junction) has been described as characteristic of MFD, distinguishing it from other syndromes that involve the mandible. These features have been presented from studies of lateral cephalograms, longitudinal roentgencephalometric analyses using metallic implants, and a review of dry skulls.[11,26,93] Grayson, Bookstein, and McCarthy[99] disputed this conclusion, although their methods did not employ classic cephalographic landmarks. They believed that complex craniofacial deformities require assessment from more than just conventional methods of measurement.[50]

Moss' functional matrix theory involves the concept that the mandible exhibits plasticity as it relates to the functional matrix with which it is involved, namely the anatomic features related to respiration and feeding. The relationship between the abnormal mandible seen in MFD and its functional matrix (respiration and feeding) in the context of Moss' functional matrix hypothesis in experimental form would be helpful to better understand how the abnormal mandible functions in affected patients.[81-84]

Arvystas and Shprintzen[4] used 12 patients ranging in age from 3 to 22 years (mean age, 10 years, 4 months) as a sample population of MFD. A number of cephalometric analyses were undertaken. They concluded that ''the characteristic appearance of the face in Treacher Collins syndrome (MFD) is a product of the distinctive relationship between the abnormal basicranium, the dysmorphic mandible, and anomalous maxillary-malar complex. The anterior displacement of the temporomandibular joint, the short ramus, short mandibular body, synthesis distortion, and displaced maxilla all result in the appearance so characteristic of this syndrome.''[4]

Craniofacial surgery for patients with Treacher Collins syndrome is mandatory when problems with the airway become life-threatening or are so severe as to compromise the individual. Previously, onlay techniques and soft-tissue augmentation were employed. However, craniofacial surgery using osteotomies and advancement techniques appears to assist in the orientation of subsequent growth in a more normal direction and to enlarge the airway at the same time. This results in both cosmetic and functional improvement.

As patients with MFD grow, their abnormally formed bones also grow, maintaining their original anatomy. ''As they are malformed, so shall they grow.''[91] Some researchers believe that the facial appearance of MFD individuals may improve during childhood growth.

Nasal obstruction and dentofacial growth

There is controversy in the literature regarding the role that nasopharyngeal obstruction plays with regard to dentofacial growth and development. Two schools of thought pre-

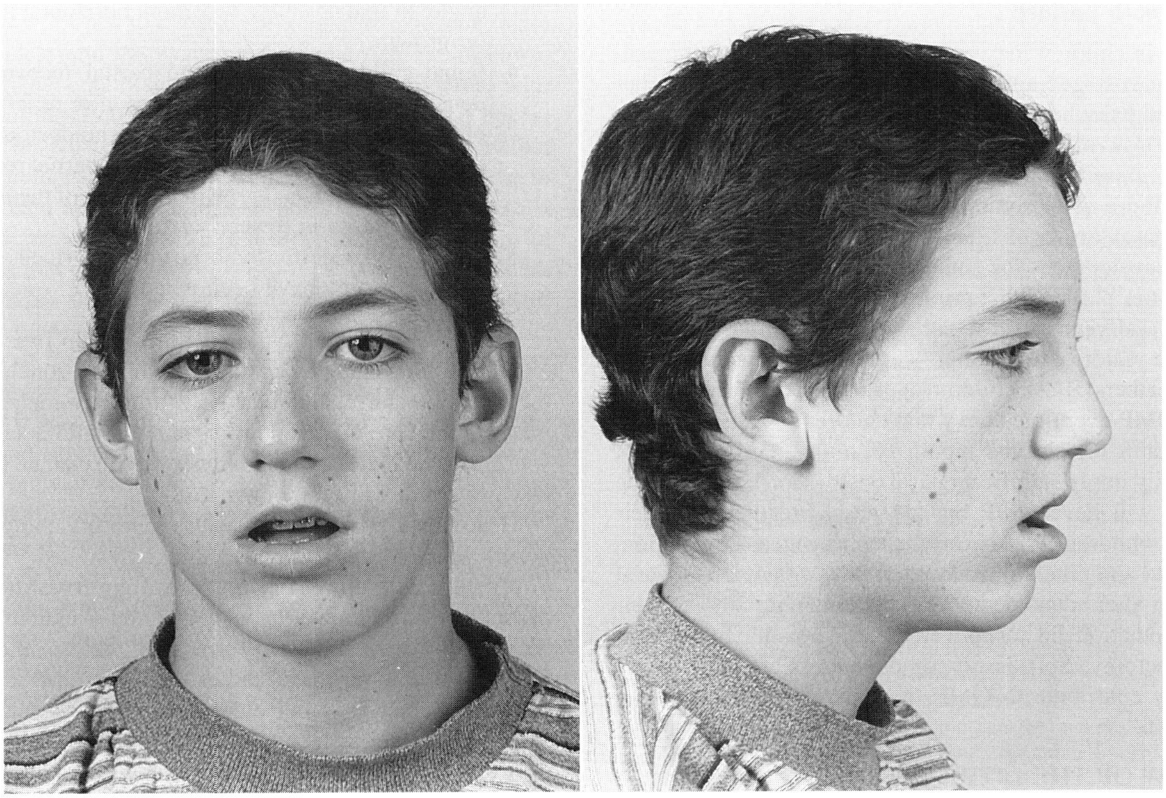

A B

Fig. 4-26. **A** and **B,** Typical "adenoid facies" in a 14-year-old child. Note the long face, open-mouth posture, short upper lip, larger lower lip, small nose, and dull facial expression.

vail: one in agreement that nasal obstruction plays a role and the other that it does not.[120]

Nasal obstruction results in increases in both nasal flow resistance and nasal power (rate of energy required to move air through the nose) such that the child may be forced to switch to mouth breathing. When mouth breathing, the child has an open-mouth posture (OMP)—the mandible and tongue are displaced downward and backward, and the head is tilted backward. It has been hypothesized that OMP affects the direction of jaw growth and the interaction of the teeth both horizontally and vertically. Stress from the suprahyoid muscles and the platysma are thought to influence growth on the lower aspect of the mandible. Sperber[110] makes reference to Moss' functional matrix hypothesis, noting that the nasal cavity may also influence growth of the face. Enlarged adenoids in young children are one of the most common causes of nasal obstruction and may result in the typical "adenoid facies" (narrow, increased facial height, protruding teeth, open lip/mouth posture, short upper lip and larger lower lip, small nose, high vaulted palatal arch, and the appearance of a vacant or dull facial expression; Figure 4-26. However, the cause-and-effect relationship of nasal obstruction and this facial morphology has not been substantiated; there also may be a degree of heredity involved.[110]

It should be noted that the term "mouth breathing" is in fact a misnomer, as most individuals are oronasal breathers. Complete mouth breathing is unusual, and Ung and others[121] reported only 2 of the 49 children they studied to be 100% mouth breathers. In fact, the accurate determination of respiratory mode (oral, nasal, or oronasal breathing) remains elusive, leading to significant difficulties in researching the effect of nasal obstruction on facial growth. The nasal valve area also may play a significant role in nasal obstruction. Ung and others found that the breathing modes of growing children varied on different days of testing. Hairfield, van Devanter, and Shapiro[53] concluded that "the variation in respiratory mode we observed may make it impossible to identify clear cause-and-effect relationships regarding upper airway function on facial development." The lack of normative data on nasorespiratory breathing and problematic measurement of respiratory mode must be kept in mind when reviewing the literature regarding implications of nasal obstruction on facial growth and development.

22. Cohen MM Sr, Cohen MM Jr: The oral manifestations of trisomy G1 (Down syndrome), *Birth Defects Orig Article Series.* VII:241, 1971.
23. Cohen MM, Arvystas MG, Baum BJ: Occlusal disharmonies in trisomy G (Down syndrome, mongolism), *Am J Orthod* 58:367, 1970.
24. Col-menero C and others: Sleep apnea syndrome associated with maxillofacial abnormalities, *J Laryngol Otol* 105:94, 1991.
25. Crawford DB, Ensor RE, Dorst JP: *The chondrocranium in achondroplasia.* In Bosma JF, editor: *Development of the basicranium,* DHEW Pub No (NIH) 76-989:301, Bethesda, 1976, US Department of Health, Education, and Welfare.
26. Reference deleted in pages.
27. Delorme R-P, Larocque Y, Caouette-Laberge L: Innovative surgical approach for the Pierre Robin anomalad: subperiosteal release of the floor of the mouth musculature, *Plast Reconstr Surg* 83:960, 1989.
27a. Dennis JP, Rosenberg HS, Alvard EC Jr: Megalencephaly, internal hydrocephalus and other neurological aspects of achondorplasia, *Brain* 84:427, 1961.
28. Denny AD, Gingrass DJ, Ferguson DJ: Comprehensive correction of the craniofacial deformity in achondroplastic dwarfism, *Ann Plast Surg* 29:550, 1992.
29. Dibbets JMH, de Bruin R, Van der Weele LT: *Shape changes in the mandible during adolescence.* In Carlson DS, Ribbens KA, editors: *Craniofacial growth during adolescence,* Craniofacial Growth Series, Monograph No. 20, 1987.
30. Dixon MJ and others: Narrowing the position of the Treacher Collins syndrome locus to a small interval between three new microsatellite markers at 5q32-33.1, *Am J Hum Genet* 52:907, 1993.
31. Dorst JP: Changes of the skull during childhood. In Newton TH, Potts DG: *Radiology of the skull and brain,* St Louis, 1971, Mosby.
32. Enlow DH: *Normal craniofacial growth.* In Cohen Jr MM: *Craniosynastosis: diagnosis, evaluation and management,* New York, 1986, Raven Press.
33. Enlow DH, Hans MG: *Essentials of facial growth,* Philadelphia, 1996, WB Saunders.
34. Erlebacher A and others: Toward a molecular understanding of skeletal development, *Cell* 80:371, 1995.
35. Farkas LG and others: Growth patterns in the orbital region: a morphometric study, *Cleft Palate Craniofac J* 29:315, 1992.
36. Farkas LG and others: Growth patterns of the nasolabial region: a morphometric study, *Cleft Palate Craniofac J* 29:318, 1992.
37. Farkas LG, Munro IR: Anthropometric facial proportions in medicine, Springfield, Ill, 1987, Charles C Thomas.
38. Farkas LG, Posnick JC, Hreczko TM: Anthropometric growth study of the head, *Cleft Palate Craniofac J* 29:303, 1992.
39. Farkas LG: Accuracy of anthropometric measurements: past, present and future, *Cleft Palate Craniofac J* 33:10, 1996.
40. Ferguson MWJ: Craniofacial malformations: towards a molecular understanding, *Nat Genet* 6:329, 1994.
41. Ferrario VF and others: Distance from symmetry: a three-dimensional evaluation of facial asymmetry, *J Oral Maxillofac Surg* 52:1126, 1994.
42. Fields HW and others: Relationship between vertical dentofacial morphology and respiration in adolescents, *Am J Orthod Dentofacial Orthop* 99:147, 1991.
43. Figueroa AA and others: Mandible, tongue, and airway in Pierre Robin sequence: a longitudinal cephalometric study, *Cleft Palate Craniofac J* 28:425, 1991.
44. Gerald BE, Silverman FN: Normal and abnormal interorbital distances, with special reference to mongolism, *Am J Roentgenol* 95: 154, 1965.
45. Glass RBJ, Yousefzadeh DK, Roizen NJ: Mastoid abnormalities in Down syndrome, *Pediatr Radiol* 19:311, 1989.
46. Gorlin RJ, Cohen Jr MM, Levin LS: *Syndromes of the head and neck,* ed 3, New York, Oxford, 1990, Oxford University Press.
47. Gosman SD, Vineland NJ: Facial development in mongolism, *Am J Orthod* 37:332, 1951.
48. Graber TM: *Orthodontics: principles and practice,* Philadelphia, 1972, WB Saunders.
49. Grayson BH, Bookstein FL, McCarthy JG: The mandible and mandibulofacial dysostosis: a cephalometric study, *Am J Orthod Dentofacial Orthop* 89:393, 1986.
50. Grayson BH and others: A comparative cephalometric study of the cranial base in craniofacial anomalies: tensor analysis, *Cleft Palate Craniofac J* 22:75, 1985.
51. Gross AM and others: A longitudinal evaluation of open mouth posture and maxillary arch within children, *Angle Orthod* 64:419, 1994.
52. Gross AM and others: Open-mouth posture and maxillary arch width in young children: a three year evaluation, *Am J Orthod Dentofac Orthop* 106:635, 1994.
53. Hairfield WM, van Devanter DM, Shapiro PA: An improved method for airway assessment in children, *Am J Orthod Dentofac Orthop* 106: 298, 1994.
54. Hall JG and others: Head growth in achondroplasia: use of ultrasound studies, *Am J Med Genet* 13:105, 1982 (letter).
54a. Hamill PV and others: Physical growth: National Center for Health Statistics percentiles, *Am J Clin Nutr* 32:607, 1979.
55. Hanson JW, Smith DW: U-shaped palatal defect in the Robin anomalad: developmental and clinical relevance, *J Pediatr* 87:30, 1975.
56. Hartgerink DV, Vig PS: Lower anterior face height and lip incompetence do not predict nasal airway obstruction, *Angle Orthod* 59:17, 1989.
57. Hecht JT and others: Computerized tomography of the foramen magnum: achondroplastic values compared to normal standards, *Am J Med Genet* 20:355, 1985.
58. Houston WJB: Mandibular growth rotations: their mechanisms and importance, *Eur J Orthod* 10:369, 1988.
59. Hoyte DAN: A critical analysis of the growth in length of the cranial base, *Birth Defects Orig Article Series,* XI:255, 1975.
60. Jensen GM, Cleall JF, Yip ASG: Dental alveolar morphology and developmental changes in Down's syndrome (trisomy 21), *Am J Orthod Dentofacial Orthop* 64:607, 1973.
61. Johnston C and others: Obstructive sleep apnea in Treacher Collins syndrome, *Cleft Palate J* 18:39, 1981.
62. Jones KL: *Smith's recognizable patterns of human malformation,* ed 5, Philadelphia, 1997, WB Saunders.
63. Kreiborg S, Dahl E: Cranial base and face in mandibulofacial dysostosis, *Am J Med Genet* 47:753, 1993.
64. Laitinen SH, Ranta RE: Cephalometric measurements in patients with Pierre Robin syndrome and isolated cleft palate, *Scand J Plast Reconstr Hand Surg* 26:177, 1992.
65. Laitinen SH: Sizes of dental arches in children with the Pierre Robin syndrome and isolated cleft palate aged from 0.2 to 6 years, *Scand J Plast Reconstr Hand Surg* 27:285, 1993.
66. Langlois JH: *The origins and functions of appearance-based stereotypes: theoretical and applied implication.* In Eder RA, editor: *Craniofacial anomalies,* New York, 1995, Springer-Verlag.
67. Latham RA: Maxillary development and growth: the septo-premaxillary ligament; *J Anat* 107:471, 1970.
68. Linder-Aronson S, Woodside DG, Lundstrom A: Mandibular growth direction following adenoidectomy, *Am J Orthod Dentofacial Orthop* 89:273, 1986.
69. Linder-Aronson S: Normalization of incisor position after adenoidectomy, *Am J Orthod Dentofacial Orthop* 103:412, 1993.
70. Linder-Aronson S: Adenoids: their effect on mode of breathing and nasal airflow and their relationship to characteristics of the facial skeleton and the dentition, *Acta Otolaryngol Suppl (Stockh)* 265:1, 1970.
71. Linder-Aronson S: *Nasal respiratory function in craniofacial growth.* In McNamara JA Jr, editor: *Nasal respiratory function in craniofacial growth,* Craniofacial Growth Series, Monograph No. 9, 1979.
72. Madeline LA, Elster AD: Suture closure in the human chondrocranium: CT assessment, *Radiology* 196:747, 1995.

73. Madeline LA, Elster AD: Postnatal development of the central skull base: normal variants, *Radiology* 196:757, 1995.
74. Marsh JL and others: The skeletal anatomy of mandibulofacial dysostosis (Treacher Collins syndrome), *Plastic Reconstr Surg* 78:460, 1986.
75. Marsh JL, Vannier MW: *Comprehensive care for craniofacial deformities*, St Louis, 1985, Mosby.
76. McNamara Jr JA: Influence of respiratory pattern on craniofacial growth, *Angle Orthod* 51:269, 1981.
77. Melnik AK: A cephalometric study of mandibular asymmetry in a longitudinally followed sample of growing children, *Am J Orthod Dentofacial Orthop* 101:355, 1992.
78. Miller JDR, Capusten BM, Lampard R: Changes at the base of skull and cervical spine in Down syndrome, *J Can Assoc Radiol* 37:85, 1986.
79. Miller S, Kerr WJS: A new look at mandibular growth: a preliminary report, *Eur J Orthod* 14:95, 1992.
80. Moss MC: *The role of the nasal septal cartilage in midfacial growth.* In McNamara Jr JA, editor: *Factors affecting the growth of the midface,* Craniofacial Growth Series, Monograph No. 6, 1976.
81. Moss ML: *Growth and development of the craniofacial complex: an epigenetic viewpoint.* In Goodrich UT, Hall CD, editors: *Craniofacial anomalies: growth and development from a surgical perspective*, New York, 1995, Thieme.
82. Moss ML: Growth of the calvaria in the rat: the determination of osseous morphology, *Am J Anat* 94:333, 1954.
83. Moss ML: *The functional matrix.* In Kraus BS, Riedel RA, editors: *Vistas in orthodontics*, Philadelphia, 1962, Lea & Febiger.
84. Moss ML: The primacy of functional matrices in orofacial growth, *Dent Pract* 19:65, 1968.
85. Olson TS and others: Early home management of patients with Pierre Robin sequence, *Int J Pediatr Otorhinolaryngol* 20:45, 1990.
86. *OMIM (on-line) Mendalian inheritance in man*, No. 100800, No. 154500; http://www3.ncbi.nlm.nih.gov/Omim/
87. Oulis CJ and others: The effect of hypertrophic adenoids and tonsils on the development of posterior crossbite and oral habits, *J Pediatr Dent* 18:197, 1994.
88. Reference deleted in pages.
89. Paul JL, Nanda RS: Effect of mouth breathing on dental occlusion, *Angle Orthod* 43:201, 1973.
90. Peterson-Falzone SJ, Figueroa AA: Longitudinal changes in cranial base angulation in mandibulo-facial dysostosis, *Cleft Palate J* 26:31, 1989.
91. Poswillow D: The etiology and pathogenesis of craniofacial deformity, *Development* 103(suppl):207, 1988.
92. Proffit WR and others: *Contemporary orthodontics*, ed 2, St Louis, 1993, Mosby.
93. Pruzansky S, Richmond JB: Growth of the mandible in the infants with micrognathia, *Am J Dis Child* 88:29, 1954.
94. Pruzansky S: Not all dwarfed mandibles are alike, *Birth Defects: Original Articles Series* 5:120, 1969.
95. Pueschel SM, Pueschel JK: *Biomedical concerns in persons with Down syndrome*, Baltimore, 1992, Paul H. Brookes Publishing Co.
96. Ranly DM: *A synopsis of craniofacial growth*, Norwalk, Conn, 1988, Appleton & Lange.
97. Ricciardelli EJ: Embryology and anatomy of the cranial base, *Clin Plast Surg* 22:261, 1995.
98. Reference deleted in pages.
99. Reference deleted in pages.
100. Roche AS, Seward FS, Sunderland S: Growth changes in the mongoloid head, *Acta Pediatr* 50:133, 1961.
101. Rodan GA: Introduction to bone biology, *Bone* 12:S3, 1992.
101a. Rousseau F and others: Mutations in the gene and coding fibroblasts growth factor receptor-3 in achondorplasia, *Nature* 371:252, 1994.
102. Rubin P: *Diseases involving modeling of the physis.* In Rubin P, editor: *Dynamic classification of bone dysplasias*, Chicago, 1964, Mosby.
103. Scott JH: The cartilage of the nasal septum, *Br Dental J* 37, 1953.
104. Shapiro BL and others: The palate in Down's syndrome, *N Engl J Med* 276:1460, 1967.
105. Sher AE: Mechanisms of airway obstruction in Robin sequence: implications for treatment, *Cleft Palate Craniofac J* 29:224, 1992.
105a. Shiang R and others: Mutations in the transmembrane domain of FGFR3 cause the most common genetic form of dwarfism, achondorplasia, *J Cell* 78:335, 1994.
106. Shprintzen R and others: Pharyngeal hypoplasia in Treacher Collins syndrome, *Arch Otolaryngol Head Neck Surg* 105:127, 1979.
107. Shprintzen RJ: Pierre Robin, micrognathia, and airway obstruction: the dependency of treatment on accurate diagnosis, *Int Anesthesiol Clin* 26:64, 1988.
108. Shprintzen RJ: The implications of the diagnosis of Robin's sequence, *Cleft Palate Craniofac J* 29:205, 1992.
109. Smith JD: Treatment of airway obstruction in Pierre Robin syndrome, *Arch Otolaryngol Head Neck Surg* 107:419, 1981.
110. Sperber GH: *Craniofacial embryology*, London, 1989, Butterworths.
111. Reference deleted in pages.
112. Reference deleted in pages.
113. Stricker M and others: *Craniofacial malformations*, New York, 1990, Churchill Livingstone.
114. Strome M: Down syndrome: a modern otorhinolaryngological perspective, *Laryngoscope* 91:1581, 1981.
115. Sullivan PG: *Skull, jaw and teeth growth patterns.* In Falkner F, Tanner JM, editors: *Human growth: a comprehensive treatise*, New York, 1986, Plenum Press.
116. The Treacher Collins Collaborative Group: Positional cloning of a gene involved in the pathogenesis of Treacher Collins syndrome, *Nat Genet* 12:130, 1996.
117. Thelander HE, Pryor HB: Abnormal patterns of growth and development in mongolism: an anthropometric study, *Clin Pediatr* 5:493, 1966.
118. Reference deleted in pages.
119. Tomer BS, Harvold EP: Primate experiments on mandibular growth direction, *Am J Orthod Dentofacial Orthop* 82:114, 1982.
120. Tourne LPM: The long face syndrome and impairment of the nasopharyngeal airway, *Angle Orthod* 60:167, 1990.
121. Ung N and others: A quantitative assessment of respiratory patterns and their effect on dental facial development, *Am J Orthod Dentofacial Orthop* 98:523, 1990.
122. Reference deleted in pages.
123. Vig PS, Showfety KJ, Phillips C: Experimental manipulation of head posture, *Am J Orthod Dentofacial Orthop* 77:258, 1980.
124. Warren DW, Hairfield WM, Dalston ET: Effect of age on nasal cross sectional area and respiratory mode in children, *Laryngoscope* 100: 89, 1990.
125. Wiedemann HR and others: *Atlas of clinical syndromes: a visual aid to diagnosis*, St Louis, 1989, Mosby.
126. Winter RM: What's in a face? *Nat Genet* 12:124, 1996.
127. Woodside DG and others: Mandibular and maxillary growth after changed mode of breathing, *Am J Orthod Dentofacial Orthop* 100:1, 1991.
128. Woodside DG: *Data from Burlington growth study.* In Salzman JA, editor: *Orthodontics in daily practice*, Philadelphia, 1974, JB Lippincott.

Chapter 5

Hemangiomas and Vascular Anomalies of the Head and Neck

Trevor J.I. McGill
James W. Forsen, Jr.
John B. Mulliken

Our understanding of vascular anomalies has been hampered by confusing terminology. Occasionally this confusion has led to improper diagnosis, illogical treatment, and misdirected research efforts (Fig. 5-1). This chapter is based on a biologic classification of vascular anomalies that was introduced in 1982 by Mulliken and Glowacki[33]; it divides the differential diagnosis of cervicofacial vascular anomalies into two categories: *hemangiomas* and *malformations*. Vascular malformations are then subdivided into slow-flow and fast-flow lesions. Management of these various types of vascular lesions also is described, based on current biologic and rheologic knowledge.

CLASSIFICATION

The clinical presentation of vascular anomalies is confusing because all lesions appear in the color spectrum of blue, pink, and red. Standard nosology of vascular anomalies offers an array of overlapping descriptive and histopathologic terms. Unfortunately, the same word has often been used to describe entirely disparate vascular lesions. For example, *hemangioma* is a generic term that has been used to describe various vascular lesions with distinctive natural histories and differing etiologies. The most common tumor of infancy is known as a *strawberry, capillary, cellular,* or *juvenile hemangioma*. This lesion typically undergoes rapid growth during infancy, followed by slow, invariable involution. Port-wine stain, a lesion that never regresses, also has been classified as a *capillary hemangioma*.[39,48] The term *cavernous hemangioma* has been used to describe lesions that involute, never involute, or rarely involute.[26,44] The hyphenated appellation *capillary-cavernous hemangioma* has further compounded the issue.

There can be no useful classification without properly defined terms. The biologic classification proposed by Mulliken and Glowacki[33] defines the cellular features of vascular anomalies and correlates them with clinical behavior. Correlative studies of surgical specimens and natural history demonstrate that there are two major categories of vascular anomalies in infancy and childhood: (1) *hemangioma*, a lesion that grows rapidly in early infancy, is characterized by endothelial proliferation and invariably undergoes slow regression (Fig. 5-2): and (2) *vascular malformation*, a lesion that is present at birth, is characterized by a normal rate of endothelial cell turnover and grows commensurately with the child. Malformations are structural anomalies, errors of vascular morphogenesis. It is clinically useful to separate the vascular malformations into ''slow-flow'' (capillary, venous, lymphatic, or combined forms) or ''fast-flow'' (arteriovenous fistula [AVF] and arteriovenous malformation [AVM]) lesions.

DISTINGUISHING CHARACTERISTICS: HEMANGIOMA VERSUS VASCULAR MALFORMATION

Clinical

Hemangioma is usually not seen at birth. Approximately one third of these lesions, however, will present as a reddish macule or telangiectasia. This lesion occurs more commonly

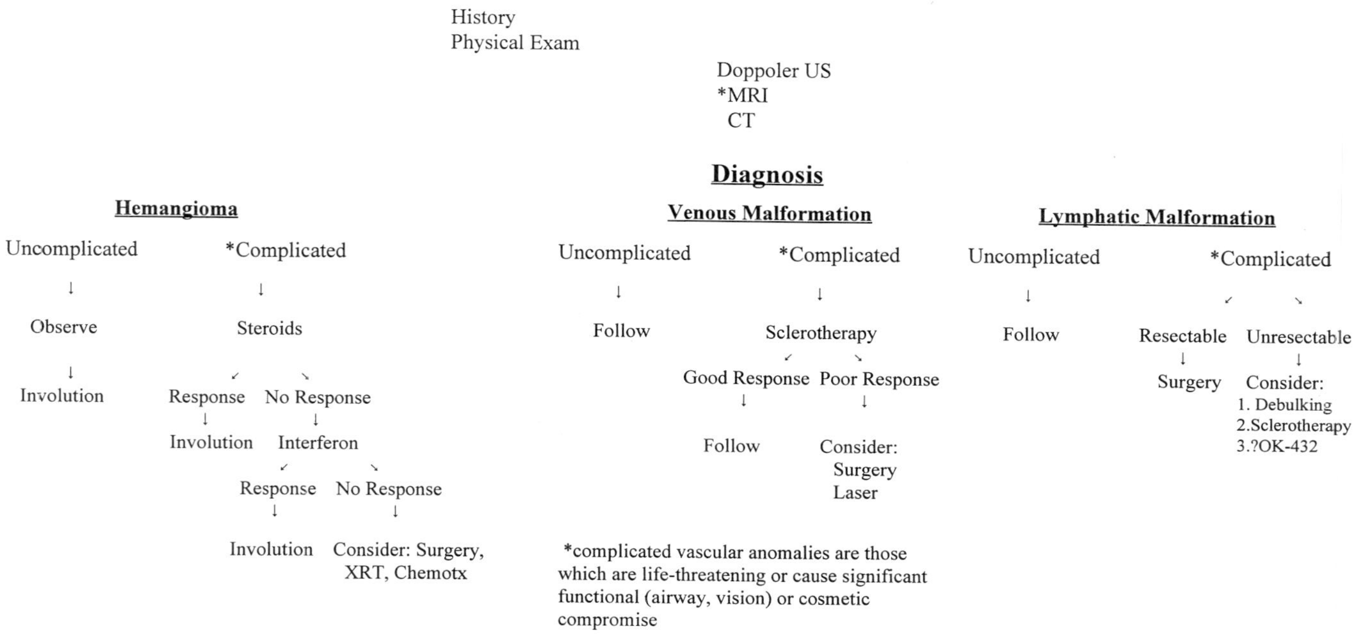

Fig. 5-1. Management algorithm of vascular anomalies.

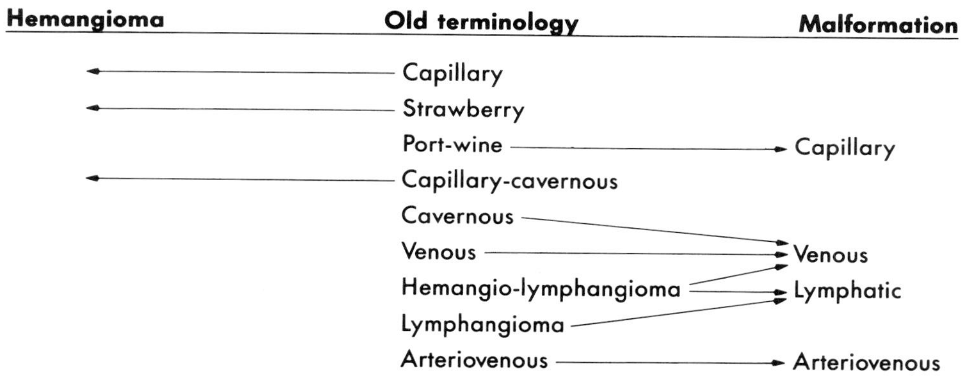

Fig. 5-2. Classification from old terminology to hemangioma or vascular malformation. (From Mulliken JB, Young AE: *Vascular birthmarks: hemangiomas and malformations*, Philadelphia, 1988, WB Saunders.)

in girls, with a ratio of 3 : 1.[32] This tumor also is more frequent in whites than in blacks. Clinically, hemangioma is characterized by a rapid postnatal growth (the proliferative phase) for the first 8 to 12 months of life, followed by a slow regression over 5 to 8 years (involutive phase) (Figs. 5-3 through 5-5).

Vascular malformations, by definition, are present at birth. Many are clearly seen in the nursery. Most lymphatic and many venous anomalies appear during infancy. Arteriovenous anomalies more commonly manifest later in childhood. A vascular malformation grows proportionately with the child, although the lesion may expand secondary to trauma, infection, hormonal changes, or embolic or surgical intervention.

Cellular

Hemangioma in its proliferating phase is composed of rapidly dividing endothelial cells forming syncytial masses with and without lumina (Fig. 5-6). Autoradiograms demonstrate this endothelial hyperplasia with incorporation of tritiated thymidine into replicating endothelial deoxyribonucleic acid (DNA).[32] Electron microscopic examination of proliferating hemangioma reveals multilamination of the basement membrane beneath the epithelium. Mast cells are signifi-

Eighty percent occur as an isolated lesion, whereas 20% are multiple hemangiomas.[29] The head and neck region of the body is the most commonly involved, followed by the trunk and extremities.[16] It is rare for an infant with a visceral hemangioma not to have multiple cutaneous lesions. Cervicofacial lesions may be associated with laryngeal and tracheal lesions.[19,20] Hemangioma is the most common tumor of infancy.

When hemangioma begins or extends into the superficial dermis, the cellular proliferation causes the skin to become raised with a vivid bright-red color. Most lesions will remain well circumscribed, measuring 0.5 to 5.0 cm in diameter, whereas some spread in a geographic fashion. Some hemangiomas proliferate in the lower dermis or subcutaneous tissue with little involvement of the superficial or capillary dermis. These lesions may be slightly raised. The overlying skin is smooth with a bluish hue; enlarged, radially draining veins are often a clue. In the past, these deeper lesions were erroneously called *cavernous* hemangiomas (Fig. 5-7). When a hemangioma involved both deep and superficial skin layers, it was called a *mixed* or *capillary-cavernous* hemangioma. In fact, histologic examination of hemangiomas with these morphologic appearances show that the proliferating endothelial cell pattern is remarkably consistent throughout the depth of the tumor.[32] The terms *capillary* and *cavernous* are therefore confusing and should not be used in clinical practice. It is more accurate to refer to a bright-red lesion as a *superficial* hemangioma, to designate a lesion with normal overlying skin as a *deep* hemangioma, or to describe a combination thereof.

In 95% of cases, a hemangioma can be distinguished from a vascular malformation based on clinical history and physical examination.[33] The hemangioma feels firm and rubbery and is difficult to compress compared with the readily compressible venous malformation. In certain instances it may be difficult to differentiate a deep hemangioma from a lymphatic or venous malformation in the head and neck region, particularly in the preauricular or cervical area.

Radiologic imaging

Notwithstanding the accuracy of clinical findings in head and neck vascular anomalies, there are times when imaging technology is needed for a precise diagnosis. The following techniques should be considered in this order: ultrasonography (with Doppler flow study), MRI, occasionally CT, and, if necessary, angiography. Ultrasonography is highly operator-dependent; however, in experienced hands it will differentiate slow-flow malformations (specifically venous or lymphatic anomalies) from hemangioma. MRI is more expensive but provides more information and is highly sensitive and specific[31] (Fig. 5-8). MRI shows the extent of involvement within tissue planes as well as flow characteristics. In either the proliferative or involutive phase,

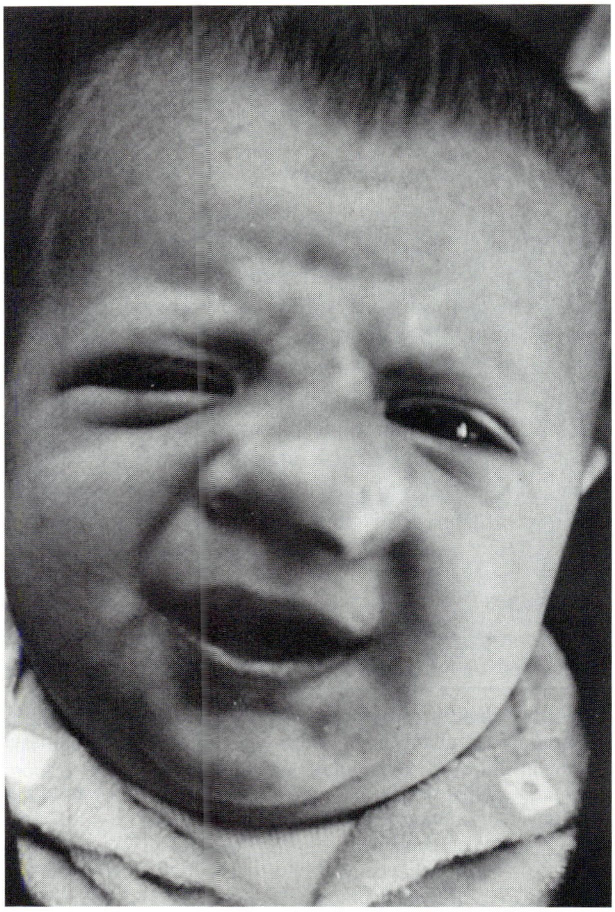

Fig. 5-7. A deep nasal hemangioma, which has erroneously been labeled *cavernous* in the past.

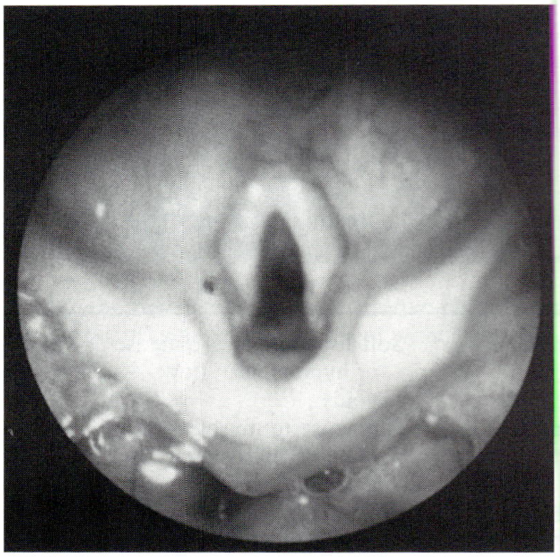

Fig. 5-8. Endoscopic appearance of a typical subglottic hemangioma on the posterolateral wall of the subglottic space on the left side.

hemangioma can be differentiated from AVM. Furthermore, slow-flow anomalies can be subcategorized as capillary, lymphatic, venous, or combined forms. The most difficult lesions to distinguish with MRI are lymphatic, venous, and lymphatovenous malformations. These, however, can usually be discriminated by administration of intravenous gadolinium and repetition of the T-weighted sequence.[31] CT with contrast enhancement may not distinguish slow-flow from fast-flow anomalies unless dynamic scanning is done. There may still be a place for CT evaluation of intraosseous vascular lesions. Angiography still has a well-deserved place in the diagnosis of vascular anomalies. Today it is usually part of management of an AVM by superselective embolization or is performed before surgical extirpation and reconstruction. Venous angiography is needed for sclerotherapy of venous malformations.

Complications

Obstruction

Visual. Obstruction of the visual axis by a hemangioma can result in deprivation amblyopia and failure to develop binocular vision. Even a small hemangioma of the upper eyelid may cause distortion of the growing cornea, producing refractive error and leading to astigmatic amblyopia.[41] Any infant with a hemangioma in the periorbital region should have a prompt ophthalmologic examination.

Subglottic hemangioma. Subglottic hemangioma is a potentially life-threatening lesion that usually presents after the first 6 weeks of life.[6,15,19,20] More than half of these infants have an associated cervicofacial cutaneous hemangioma.[15]

Clinically, these otherwise healthy patients present with the onset of biphasic stridor. With increasing size of the hemangioma there is reduction in the subglottic airway and the insidious onset of respiratory distress. In other cases, the child may first appear with a protracted episode of laryngotracheal bronchitis.[7] The child may be diagnosed with failure to thrive because of continued respiratory distress.

A lateral radiograph of the neck or a fluoroscopic study of the upper airway will show a smooth, usually posteriorly based round swelling in the immediate subglottic space. Diagnosis requires a direct laryngoscopy, which demonstrates the hemangioma as a smooth, easily compressible mass in the subglottic space[30] (Fig. 5-9). The subglottic hemangioma may occupy 20% to 80% of the subglottic space (Fig. 5-10). On rare occasions, it may extend circumferentially around the subglottic space. Biopsy of this lesion is not necessary for diagnosis. Further evaluation of the distal airway is important to rule out other hemangiomas.

Ulceration and bleeding

Local complications during the proliferative phase in infancy, such as ulceration and bleeding, may necessitate active management. When a hemangioma penetrates the epidermal basement membrane, ulceration or bleeding may

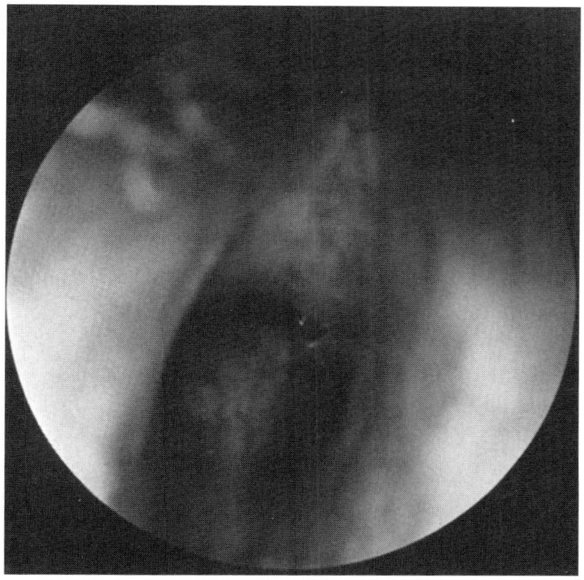

Fig. 5-9. Endoscopic view of a broad, posterior subglottic hemangioma occupying 80% of the airway.

occur. Bleeding is often sudden, punctate, and frightening. The parents should be taught how to compress the area with a clean pad, applying pressure for 10 minutes. Repeated bleeding is rare. If it does occur, a mattress suture may be indicated. Localized bleeding is usually not a manifestation of platelet-trapping coagulopathy (Kasabach-Merritt syndrome).

Ulceration is particularly common in hemangiomas of the lips. Secondary infection invariably accompanies ulceration. Superficial ulceration usually responds to daily cleansing and application of topical antibiotic ointment. Deeper ulceration may require dressings; these lesions often take several weeks to heal. Recurrent ulceration after healing is rare. Extensive or refractory ulceration may be an indication for pharmacologic therapy.

Alarming complications

Congestive heart failure. Congestive heart failure, a life-threatening complication of hemangioma, is typically seen with multiple cutaneous hemangiomas and with hemangiomatous proliferation within the viscera, typically the liver. High-output congestive heart failure also can occur with large cervicofacial hemangiomas. Despite multimodality treatment, the overall mortality rate is reported to be as high as 54%.

Platelet-trapping coagulopathy (Kasabach-Merritt syndrome). Kasabach-Merritt syndrome, the hematologic complication of hemangioma, was first documented in 1940.[24] It occurs early in the postnatal rapid-growth phase. Characteristically, the involved skin is deep red-purple, tense, and shiny. In large lesions there may be a central area of softness, suggesting intralesional bleeding. Petechiae and ecchymoses are seen overlying and adjacent to the hemangi-

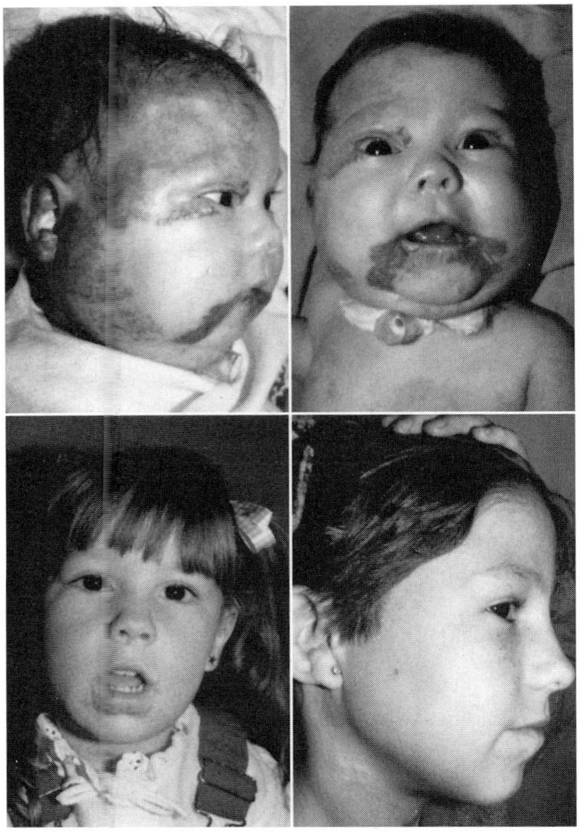

Fig. 5-10. **A,** A 6-month-old infant with an extensive proliferating hemangioma of the right cheek, lips, and oral cavity. **B,** This circumferential subglottic hemangioma in the same patient necessitated a tracheotomy. **C,** At 4 years of age, the patient was decannulated as the subglottic hemangioma involuted completely. There is still redundant tissue in the right cheek. **D,** The result following complete involution of the hemangioma when the patient was 9 years of age

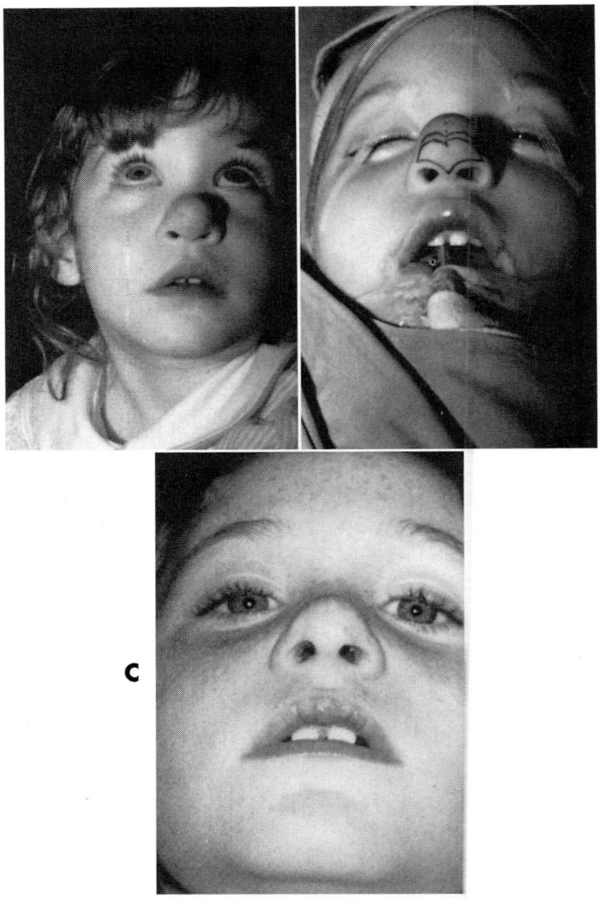

Fig. 5-11. **A,** A prominent involuting-phase hemangioma of nasal tip in a 5-year-old girl. **B,** Contour excision was undertaken for psychosocial reasons. **C,** Nasal contour 4 years after subtotal excision.

oma. Hematologic evaluation reveals a profound thrombocytopenia (2000 to 40,000/mm^3). Early on, the fibrinogen level is slightly low. In time, fibrinogen falls to trace levels, whereas prothrombin time and partial thromboplastin time become dangerously prolonged. There is a risk of acute hemorrhage in the gastrointestinal tract or the pleural, peritoneal, pulmonic, or central nervous systems. There also is the hazard of rapid expansion of the hemangioma secondary to intralesional bleeding, causing compression of a vital structure.

Management

Most hemangiomas in the head and neck region grow as small tumors and invariably regress, leaving inconsequential skin changes. Clinical studies confirm that complete resolution of hemangiomas occurs in over 50% of children by the age of 5 years and in over 70% by the age of 7 years, with continued improvement in the remaining children until 10 to 12 years of age.[4,44] Typically, the skin exhibits mild atrophy after involution, or it may have a wrinkled quality or a few telangiectatic vessels. The skin may be slightly more pale than normal skin. In summary, for the small hemangioma in an inconspicuous location, nothing should be done—*primum non nocere* (Fig. 5-11).

Laser excision for subglottic hemangioma

Not all infants with a subglottic hemangioma require management, especially those with a minimal lesion occupying less than 20% of the subglottic airway. The management of choice is watchful waiting until involution occurs. However, an adequate airway should be established with the onset of respiratory distress. Formerly, a tracheotomy was left in place for approximately 2 years until there was sufficient involution. Systemic corticosteroid therapy is a pharmacologic option.[8,18] Sixty percent of subglottic hemangiomas respond to corticosteroids. The usual dose is prednisone (2 to 3 mg/kg/day). A lower dosage or an alternate-day regimen may be continued for 4 to 6 weeks or longer.

The CO_2 laser is the therapeutic option in infants who fail to respond to corticosteroids. With general anesthesia, the subglottic hemangioma is exposed with an appropriate laryngoscope. An operating microscope coupled to a CO_2 laser is used to visualize the lesion. Jet ventilation with a Venturi apparatus is used to maintain oxygen while the infant is paralyzed. A CO_2 laser beam is used in the intermittent mode at a setting of 0.05 seconds at 20 watts. The laser is useful for treating eccentrically placed subglottic hemangiomas; often such a lesion can be removed in one operative procedure.[19,20,43] The rare circumferential subglottic hemangiomas should be removed in stages in an effort to prevent subglottic stenosis, or tracheostomy may become necessary.

Pharmacologic therapy for alarming complications

Corticosteroid. Since first reported in 1967, high-dose corticosteroids remain the premier pharmacologic agent for control of endangering hemangiomas.[52] The decision to proceed with drug therapy should be made early. There is emperic evidence that the young proliferating hemangioma is far more responsive to corticosteroid therapy than is a lesion in an older infant. The usual dosage is oral prednisone (2 to 3 mg/kg/day).[11] Intravenous corticosteroids may be used in infants with respiratory complications. There is no evidence, however, that the response is more likely or more profound with intravenous than with oral administration.

A responsive hemangioma exhibits signs of accelerated regression within several hours to days after beginning corticosteroid therapy. The signs are usually obvious (i.e., lightening of color, softening, and diminished growth). If there is no evidence of accelerated regression with prednisone at 2 to 3 mg/kg/day for 7 days, then the hemangioma must be considered unresponsive. Such a lesion will not respond to a higher dose, and the drug should be discontinued. If the lesion does respond, the dosage can be lowered slowly over several weeks, or the patient can be switched to alternate-day therapy. The duration and dosage of corticosteroid therapy depend on the tumor's location and maturity. Rebound growth may occur in a proliferative-phase hemangioma at a low steroid level. To minimize regrowth, the corticosteroid must be continued until the hemangioma is well into the involuting phase, usually at 8 to 10 months of age.

Intralesional corticosteroids should be considered for small protuberant hemangiomas on the face, particularly upper-eyelid and nasal-tip lesions. The dose is based on the size of the lesion and the infant's weight. The dose of triamcinolone and betamethasone should be no more than 40 and 6 mg, respectively, at each injection.[25,45] Usually one to five injections are necessary, spaced 4 to 6 weeks apart, to control the hemangioma.

The response rate is 30% to 60% with either systemic or intralesional corticosteroid administration.[2,13,25,45] The mortality rate for infants with platelet-consumption coagulopathy is 30% to 40% despite corticosteroid use.[12]

Interferon-α-2a. The antiangiogenic properties of interferon (IFN)-γ-2a were discovered fortuitously when the recombinant drug was used to manage patients with acquired immunodeficiency syndrome (AIDS). White and others[50] observed remarkable regression of pulmonary angiomatosis in a 7-year-old boy after IFN-γ-2a therapy. Orchard and others[38] and White and others[51] reported favorable responses to this drug in a small number of infants with Kasabach-Merritt syndrome. In the authors' institution a study of IFN-γ-2a therapy for endangering hemangiomas is in progress.[14] All 20 infants entered into the study have serious lesions that failed to respond to systemic corticosteroids. Most have shown resolution of their hemangioma after an average of 11 months of management. To date, there have been three deaths on this therapy. This preliminary study suggests that IFN-γ-2a be used in infants with life-threatening hemangiomas that do not respond promptly to corticosteroids and that this is the agent of choice for patients with Kasabach-Merritt syndrome. No serious side effects have been seen with the short-term use of this drug. Mild fever is seen in most patients, and several patients have developed spastic diplegia. Whether this is transient has not yet been determined.

Surgical therapy

Surgical excision during childhood is usually indicated for removal of the fibrofatty residuum or skin laxity that remains after complete regression of hemangioma. However, there are indications for earlier operative intervention. If a hemangioma is causing visual problems and is unresponsive to corticosteroid therapy, subtotal excision may relieve pressure on the developing cornea. Another example is early excision of an obstructing subglottic hemangioma using a CO_2 laser as discussed earlier. There are instances when the hemangioma is pedunculated and ulcerated. These lesions should be removed rather than waiting for involution to occur.

As the child with hemangioma reaches 2.5 to 3 years of age, he or she may evidence psychosocial problems. This is the age when a child first manifests a defined body or facial image. Children with facial hemangiomas are usually accepted by nursery school and kindergarten classmates. Problems are more likely to develop during the first grade, when the child is exposed to older classmates. This is a time for considering subtotal or possibly total excision of an involuting-phase hemangioma. Excision for psychologic indications should be carefully discussed, and often a psychologist can help with the decision. Excision also is a consideration when it is obvious that skin removal will be necessary in the future either because of color, quality, or contour, notwithstanding the final result of involution. The lip and nasal tip are psychologically sensitive foci of hemangiomas. Subtotal or contour excision may be beneficial during early childhood (see Fig. 5-11). As a general rule, subtotal or staged excision is the best approach. Caution should be taken for fear of causing late-contour deficiency or deformity. Residual fibrofatty tissue and skin can always be removed, often with local anesthesia, when the child is older.

VASCULAR MALFORMATIONS

Vascular malformations usually grow commensurately with the child. Each channel type, however, may change because of different pathophysiologic influences. Venous anomalies often expand because of hormonal changes such as puberty, pregnancy, antiovulants, or secondary to trauma. Lymphatic malformations typically enlarge with infection or intralesional bleeding. AVMs may enlarge in association with trauma, puberty, other hormonal changes, or after incomplete surgical excision. It is essential not to confuse these nonproliferative enlargements of vascular malformations with the proliferating phase of hemangioma.

Capillary malformation

Histology

The skin or mucosa involved with a port-wine stain contains abnormally dilated capillaries or venule-sized vessels in the superficial dermis.[35] The anomaly is present at birth and changes slowly with growth to a purple color in adulthood. Furthermore, the lesion may become raised and nodular with progressive vascular ectasia (Fig. 5-12).

Clinical features

Patients with port-wine stain within the V1 area alone or extending into the maxillary and mandibular regions are at serious risk for having choroidal and intracranial vascular anomalies (Sturge-Weber syndrome).[13] Children with dermal staining of the V2 or V3 general areas alone are not at increased risk. The capillary malformation in Sturge-Weber syndrome may involve the entire face and neck or trunk and distal extremities. The soft tissue is often hypertrophic, and skeletal overgrowth frequently occurs in the maxilla, particularly the alveolar region. Skeletal overgrowth may not be obvious at birth, but it is progressive throughout adolescence.

Cerebral angiography of patients with Sturge-Weber syndrome displays capillary, venous, and arteriovenous anomalies of the leptomeninges.[40] The anomalous circulation is responsible for the progressive degeneration and atrophy of the cerebral hemispheres.[27] Early diagnosis of intracranial anomalies can be made with single photon emission CT, positron emission tomography, or MRI. In time, serpentine calcifications may be seen in the temporal and occipital lobes. A 45% incidence of associated glaucoma occurs if the port-wine stain involves both the ophthalmic and maxillary divisions of the trigeminal nerve. Diagnosis is based on the presence of elevated intraocular pressure, increased corneal diameter, and typical defects in the visual fields.

Management

Laser therapy. Laser therapy is now the established management of choice for port-wine stains in both children and adults. Thermal thrombosis occurs within the port-wine stain, with resultant lightening of the stain and flattening of its surface. The efficiency of argon laser therapy can be predicted on the basis of age, stain color, and a preliminary biopsy.[35] The argon laser is used for adult patients.

The flashlamp pulsed tunable-dye laser is preferred for managing young children, patients with light-colored port-wine stains, and those whose skin is sensitive to heat[46,47] (see Fig. 5-12).

Surgical excision. In selected cases, it may be possible to surgically excise the port-wine stain and obtain primary closure by skin advancement or skin grafting. There are serious potential problems after excision and grafting, including scarred hypertrophy at the junction of the graft and normal skin and unpredictable pigmentation within the skin graft itself. Tissue expansion techniques also may be considered

A B C

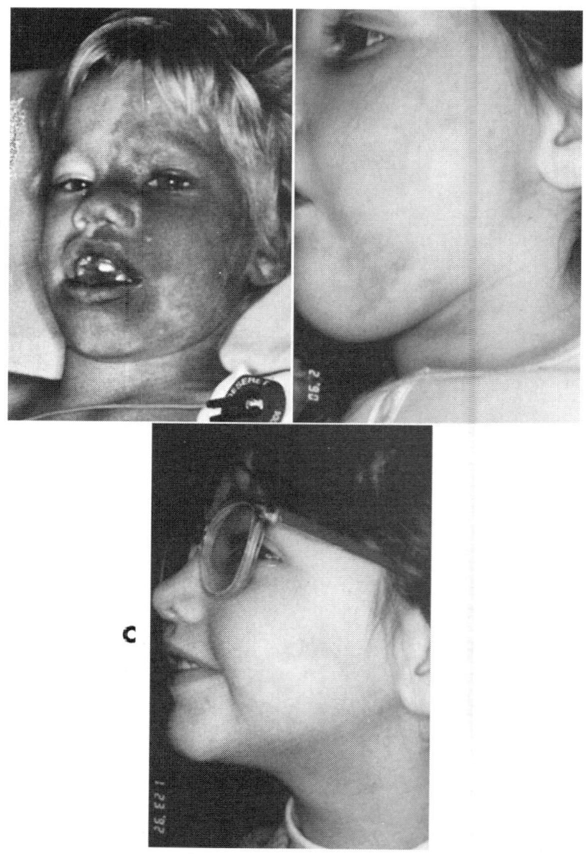

Fig. 5-12. A, A port-wine stain in the V1, V2, V3 dermatome with slight overgrowth of the lip and maxilla. **B,** Port-wine stain involving the cheek and neck in a 3.5-year-old child prior to laser treatment. **C,** Port-wine stain completely cleared by pulsed-dye laser system after seven treatments. (Courtesy of Dr. OT Tan.)

in removing a port-wine stain. Contour excision of the hypertrophied lip is often necessary.

Venous malformation

In the past, venous anomalies were erroneously termed *varicose* or *cavernous hemangiomas* or *lymphangiohemangiomas*. They are not hemangiomas at all but rather developmental anomalies of veins. Venous malformation usually occurs in pure form but may be combined as capillary or lymphatic anomalies.

Histology

Histologic examination shows dilated or ectatic vascular channels lined by normal endothelium. Thrombosis is common and is associated with dystrophic calcification, which is clinically and radiologically manifested as phleboliths.

Clinical features

Venous malformations can present in a variety of ways, ranging from an isolated skin varicosity or localized spongy mass to complex lesions infiltrating various tissue planes (Fig. 5-13). The overlying skin may be normal, or it may exhibit a bluish tinge caused by involvement of the dermis.

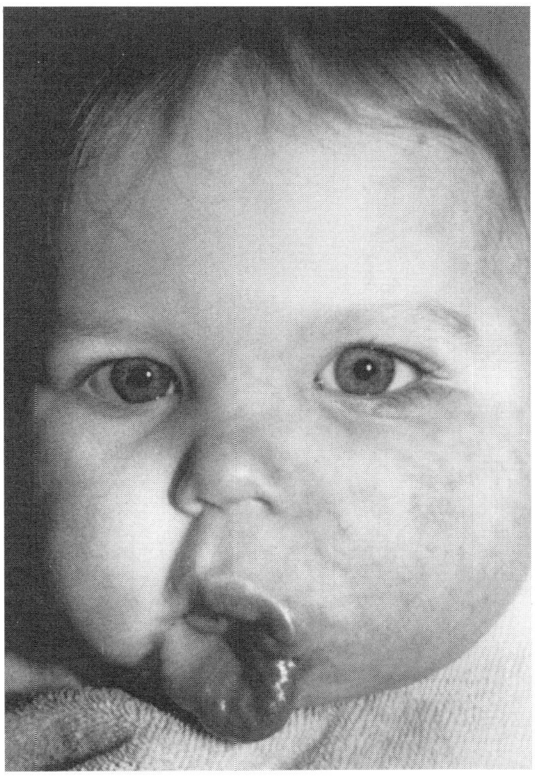

Fig. 5-13. An infant with a vascular anomaly of the right cheek and lips, present since birth. On palpation, the lesion is a soft, compressible, spongy mass that is nonpulsatile and slowly refills. This is a venous malformation. Management consists of sclerotherapy followed by contour excision of the lips.

Combined venous–lymphatic lesions often exhibit dermal lymphatic vesicles overlying the deep venous anomaly.

Venous anomalies are common in the skin and subcutaneous tissue of the head and neck region, particularly in the lips and cheeks. They may also be formed in skeletal muscle; intramasseteric lesions are the most common.[49] The clinical characteristic is a soft, compressible nonpulsatile mass with rapid refilling. Expansion will occur on compression of the jugular vein or Valsalva's maneuver or with the head in a dependent position. These lesions grow proportionately with the child and tend to expand following puberty, trauma, or attempted subtotal excision. Sluggish flow and stasis lead to phlebothrombosis, which presents clinically as recurrent pain and tenderness. Characteristic phleboliths can be palpated and seen on radiographic examination. Venous anomalies may also occur within the craniofacial skeleton and are most common in the mandible, less common in the maxilla, and rare in the nasal and cranial bones and zygomas. Mandibular venous anomalies may present with increased mobility of the teeth, expansion of the buccal cortex, or spontaneous bleeding.[23] The radiographic appearance of an intraosseous venous malformation is consistent: plain films demonstrate a localized hypolucency with a honeycombed, or *soap bubble* appearance.[42] Profile or tangential films show spicules of bone radiating in a sunburst pattern.

Management

Most venous malformations do not require any specific management apart from reassurance and an explanation of the natural history of the lesion.

Sclerotherapy. Direct injection of a sclerosing agent into the center of the soft-tissue venous malformation is an accepted mode of management. Sclerosing agents such as 95% ethanol or sodium tetradecyl sulfate (1% or 2%) are injected into the epicenter of the venous anomaly during occlusion of the arterial inflow and venous outflow. A skilled interventional radiologist is needed.

Surgery. Surgical resection is indicated for large or symptomatic venous anomalies. It is often advisable initially to shrink the venous malformation with sclerotherapy. Under most circumstances, total surgical extirpation is impossible, and a subtotal resection is indicated to reduce bulk and improve contour and function or relieve pain. Lesions of the jaw, nasal bones, and zygoma are managed by curettage and packing with a hemostatic agent.

Lymphatic malformation

Perhaps in no other category of vascular anomalies has nomenclature played such a perverse role as in lymphatic malformation. Most authors agree that these lesions are abnormalities of lymphatic development. Therefore, the term *lymphatic malformation* seems most appropriate. However, a persistent notion exists that these anomalies have the potential for neoplastic growth and recurrence after excision. This misconception is fostered by the old terms *cystic hygroma* and *lymphangioma*. In a strict semantic sense, the suffix *-oma* denotes a potential for growth by cellular mitosis. There is, however, little evidence that untouched lymphatic anomalies show increased cell turnover. Once transected, however, lymphatic malformation do indeed have a decided tendency to proliferate into the surgical scar.

Lymphatic malformations are uncommon congenital lesions that may occur throughout the body, although the head and neck region is the most common site. Most lymphatic malformations are seen at birth. There is equal frequency in both sexes and among all races.[17] Symptoms are related to the anatomic location of the malformation and the extent of involvement.

Histology

The classic lymphatic malformation consists of multiple dilated lymphatic channels lined by a single layer of flattened endothelium. The vessel walls are of variable thickness and are fibromuscular, with both striated and smooth muscle components. Collections of lymphocytes are common throughout the contained connective tissue. Hemorrhage within the cystic spaces is common, indicating recent or spontaneous trauma. The lesion may be a combined capillary–lymphatic malformation or a lymphatovenous malformation.[32,33]

Clinical features

Lymphatic malformation presents in diverse forms. Clusters of watery vesicles are common on the buccal mucosa, tongue, and conjunctiva. The vesicles often are red or black as a result of microscopic bleeding. There may be a generalized infiltration of the tongue, a common cause of macroglossia. Lymphatic malformation also is a common basis for macrocheilia, macrotia, macromala, and macrodontia.[33] The cystic variety, formerly called a *cystic hygroma*, occurs in the anterior and posterior triangles of the neck. This lesion consists of large, thick-walled cysts, with less infiltration of surrounding tissue. The more severe forms of lymphatic malformation extensively infiltrate throughout the head and neck, producing large deformities. This variety commonly involves the oral cavity, oropharynx, and preepiglottic space. Isolated supraglottic malformations, which are rare, usually occur and are associated with these extensively infiltrative lesions.

Lymphatic malformations are associated with hypertrophy of both bone and soft tissue. This is frequently seen as progressive distortion of the mandibular body, causing prognathism. Lymphatic malformations grow commensurately with the patient; however, a spontaneous, sudden, and rapid increase in size associated with infection or intralesional bleeding may occur. Spontaneous decompression or shrinkage of lymphatic malformation is extremely uncommon but may occur in cystic lesions of the lower neck.[33]

Lymphatic malformations can be divided into two management categories based on anatomic distribution, computerized imaging, and histologic findings.

Type I lymphatic malformations are located below the level of the mylohyoid muscle and involve the anterior and posterior cervical triangles. CT reveals ring-like margin enhancement with sharp demarcation of the cystic areas, which appear to be well circumscribed and discrete (Fig. 5-14). Histologically, type I malformations have large cystic structures without infiltration of the surrounding soft tissue. These malformations correlate most closely with the lesions formerly called *cystic hygromas* (Fig. 5-15).

Type II lymphatic malformations are found above the level of the mylohyoid muscle and involve the oral cavity, lip, and tongue. CT reveals isodense masses that are poorly defined and show obscured muscle and fatty planes. These lesions do not appear well circumscribed or discrete, and the ring-like enhancement seen in the type I lesions is notably absent. Histologic examination of type II lesions reveals smaller lymphatic channels with infiltration of the surrounding tissue.

Management

Therapeutic modalities such as repeated incision and drainage, aspiration, radiotherapy, and injection of sclerosing agents should be avoided. Surgical resection is the management of choice for control of this vascular anomaly. Appropriate surgical planning should be based on an under-

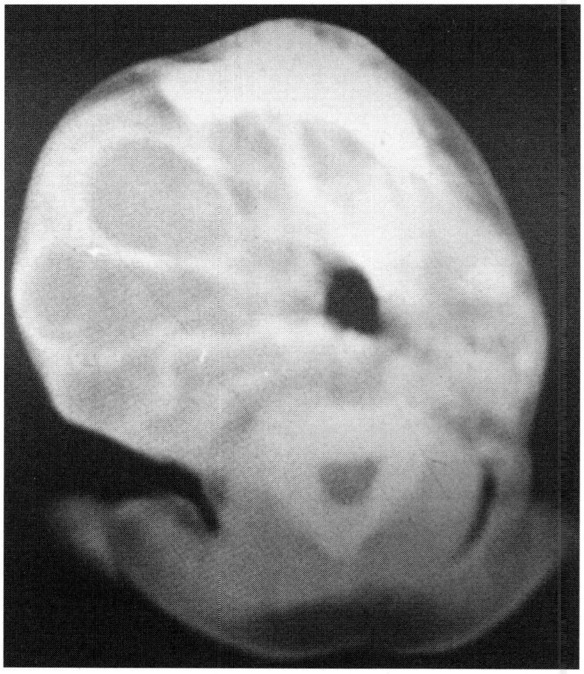

Fig. 5-14. Computed tomogram of a type I lymphatic malformation (formerly *cystic hygroma*) demonstrating large fluid-filled spaces with ring-like enhancement and sharp demarcation from the normal structure.

A

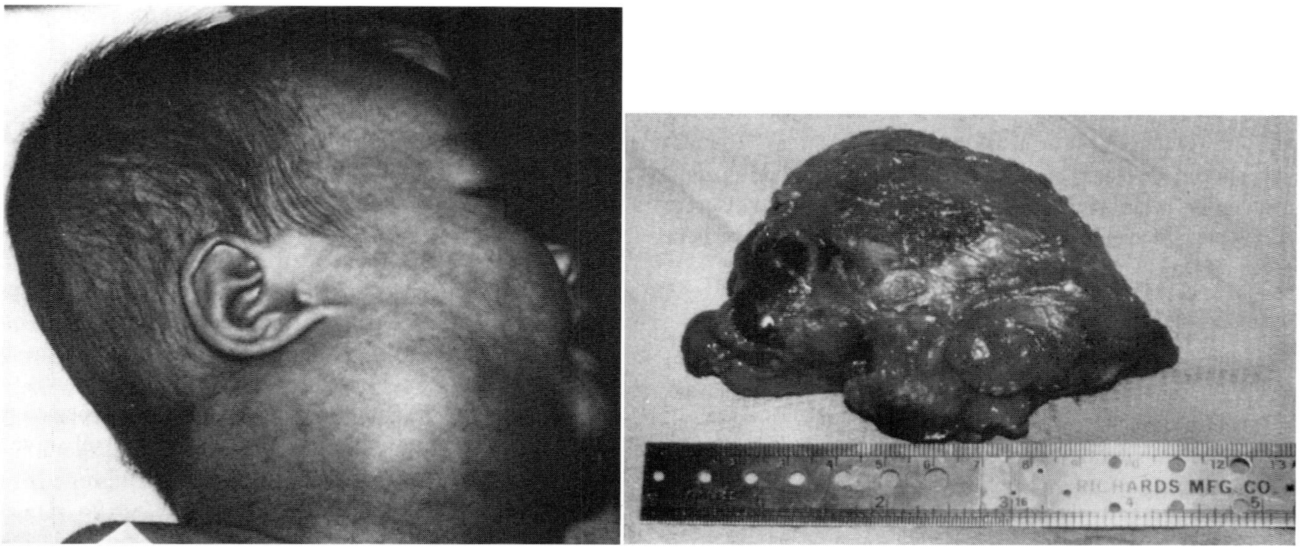

B

Fig. 5-15. A, A 6-month-old infant with a large cystic lymphatic malformation in the left anterior cervical triangle. This lesion was removed in toto. **B,** Surgical specimen.

standing of the two forms of lymphatic malformations and realistic expectations for each patient.

The physical examination of the patient and the preoperative imaging results are extremely important, bearing in mind the clinical significance of the typical infiltrative disease above the mylohyoid muscle. Photographic documentation is important because the care of many of these patients spans several years. Recalling the initial condition as well as interval results is helpful to the surgeon and family.

Surgical excision should be undertaken keeping in mind that lymphatic malformations are benign; therefore, complete and total resection of the lesion is not necessary and sometimes not possible. Aggressive resection is not warranted, nor is an excessively conservative approach condoned. The long-term psychologic and social ramifications of these malformations should not be underestimated.

Cold-knife dissection is often the modality of choice. Type I lesions are ideally removed in one procedure because repeated excisions are complicated by fibrosis and anatomic distortion. Because many of the type I lesions are resected fairly easily, surgical intervention can be carried out safely within the first 9 to 12 months of life.

Type II lesions are the most difficult to manage because there are no distinct tissue planes between the malformation and the normal structures. Because these lesions are not curable, the timing of intervention is less critical. Repeated procedures are necessary, and complete removal is almost impossible. Resection of lymphatic malformations before the age of 5 or 6 years is recommended. In planning such a procedure, restrictions should be set for the extent of dissection, duration, and acceptable blood loss.

Meticulous dissection is necessary because anatomic structures frequently are not in their normal position. Magnification and use of a nerve simulator are necessary. Disruption of the abnormal lymphatic channels frequently leads to prolonged wound drainage. Suction drains should remain in position for an adequate period to avoid reaccumulation of lymphatic drainage under the skin flaps.

The laser has a role in the management of these lesions. Use of the laser is reserved for disease that is not readily resectable by sharp dissection. Lesions involving the oral cavity and tongue are particularly amenable to CO_2 laser resection, as is involvement of the supraglottic region. The CO_2 laser may be helpful in localized lesions in the lip and buccal area. Neodymium:yttrium-aluminum-garnet laser has been relatively successful in controlling the vesicular lesions that are commonly found in the tongue.

Japanese researchers have recently described intralesional injection of OK-432, a lyophilized incubation mixture of group A *Streptococcus pyogenes*, as both primary and secondary management for lymphatic malformation.[36]

Special considerations

Airway obstruction. Airway obstruction caused by a cervical lymphatic anomaly and requiring intervention occurs primarily within the first 12 months of life. The lesion is usually an infiltrative lymphatic malformation involving the tongue, floor of the mouth, and preepiglottic space. A sudden increase in size demands immediate attention. Attempts at aspiration are unsuccessful. With progressive respiratory distress, evidenced by tachypnea and increasing chest retractions, orotracheal intubation becomes necessary. This procedure should be performed with the patient under general anesthesia, and it provides an opportunity for detailed examination of the oropharynx, hypopharynx, and su-

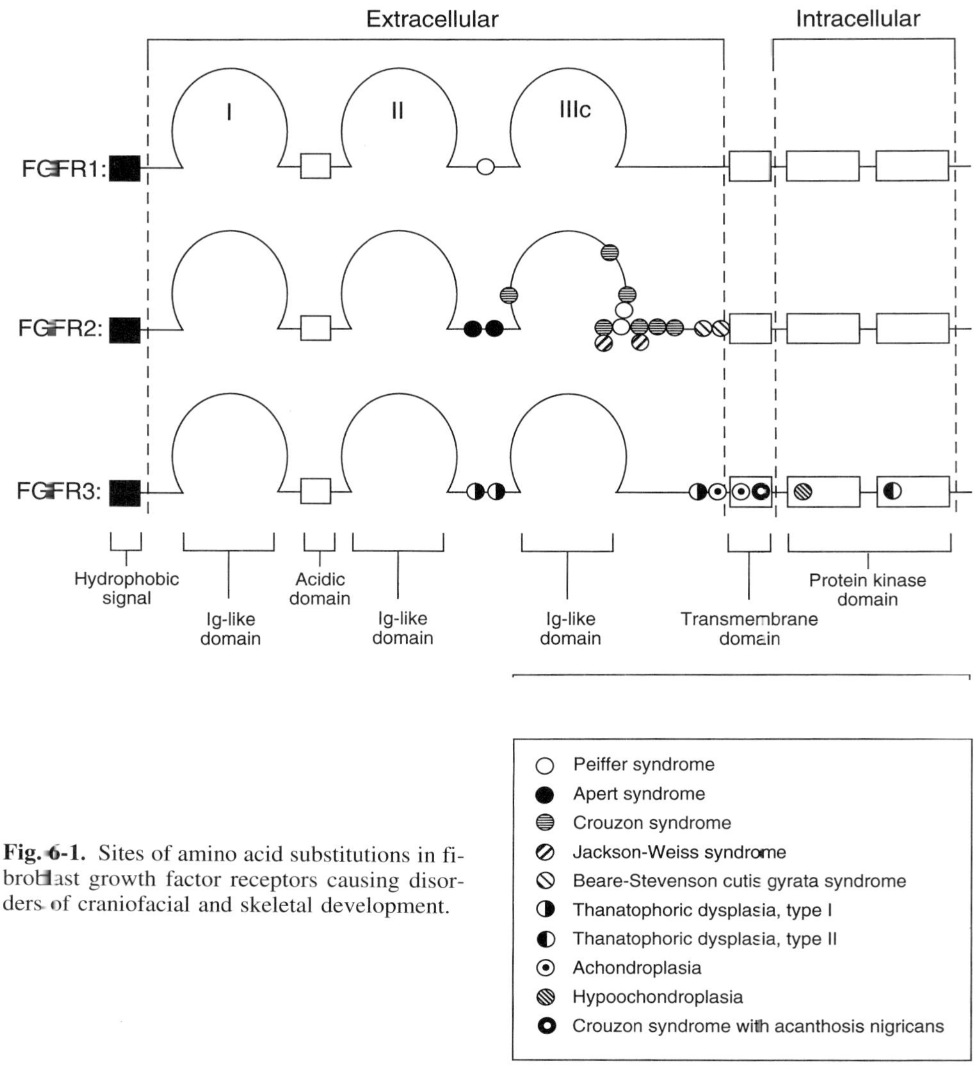

Fig. 6-1. Sites of amino acid substitutions in fibroblast growth factor receptors causing disorders of craniofacial and skeletal development.

opment of polymerase chain reaction (PCR) for rapid amplification and analysis of very small amounts of genomic deoxyribonucleic acid 23 (DNA) samples, and (2) discovery of highly polymorphic repetitive DNA sequences called microsatellites.[27] Microsatellites are polymorphic tandem repeats of di-, tri-, or tetranucleotides at reproducible sites throughout the genome. These highly informative molecular fingerprints are useful landmarks against which to map genes, inherited disorders, and other genetic loci of interest. Microsatellites are rapidly analyzed by PCR-based assays and have led to a rapid increase in the number of mapped and identified human disease genes within the past few years.

Many craniofacial disorders have been mapped (Box 6-1), including syndromic and nonsyndromic craniosynostoses, orofacial clefting syndromes, and other craniofacial disorders. The products of genes that have been identified appear to fall within one of three categories: transcription factors (*MSX2, GLI3, MITF, PAX3*), connective tissue structural proteins (type II and XI collagen, fibrillin-1); and growth factor receptors (fibroblast growth factor receptors [FGFRs] 1, 2, and 3; *PTC* and *FGDY* gene products).

The list of mapped and identified craniofacial disorder genes continues to grow at a rapid pace.

Craniosynostosis and the fibroblast growth factor receptors

Perhaps the greatest progress in craniofacial disorders has arisen from molecular genetic studies of craniosynostosis. Numerous craniosynostosis syndromes are caused by mutations in genes encoding transmembrane receptors for fibroblast growth factors (FGFs) (Fig. 6-1). Nine known FGFs act to stimulate any one of several mitogenic, differentiation, migration, or cell survival responses in the target cell.[29] FGFRs are composed of an intracellular tyrosine kinase enzymatic domain, a transmembrane domain, and an extracel-

Box 6-1. Genetic map locations of inherited craniofacial disorders

Disorder	*Location*	*Affected Gene (gene product)*
Apert syndrome	10q26	*FGFR2* (fibroblast growth factor receptor 2)
Branchio-oto-renal dysplasia	8q13.3	
Cleidocranial dysplasia	6p21	
Craniofrontonasal dysplasia	Xpter–p22.2	
Craniosynostosis, type 1	7p21.3–p21.2	
Craniosynostosis, Boston type (type 2)	5q34–q35	*MSX2* (homeobox transcription factor)
Craniosynostosis, Adelaide type (type 3)	4p16	
Crouzon craniofacial dysostosis	10q26	*FGFR2*
Crouzon syndrome with acanthosis nigricans	4p16	*FGFR3* (fibroblast growth factor receptor 3)
Faciogenital dysplasia	Xp11.21	*FGDY* (homology to *RAS*-like *RHO/RAC* guanine nucleotide exchange factors)
Greig cephalopolysyndactyly syndrome	7p13	*GLI3* (homology to zinc finger transcription factors)
Jackson-Weiss syndrome	10q26	*FGFR2*
Marfanoid-craniosynostosis syndrome	15q21.1	*FBN1* (connective tissue protein fibrillin-1)
Nevoid basal cell carcinoma syndrome	9q31	*PTC* (transmembrane protein)
Nonsyndromic cleft lip with or without cleft palate	6p24.3	
	19q13	
Nonsyndromic cleft palate	Xq21.3	
Noonan syndrome	12q22–qter	
Otopalatodigital syndrome	Xq28	
Pfeiffer syndrome	8p11.2–p11.1	*FGFR1* (fibroblast growth factor receptor 1)
	10q26	*FGFR2*
Pyknodysostosis	1q21	
Saethre-Chotzen syndrome	7p21	
Stickler syndrome, type I	12q13.11–q13.2	*COL2A1* (type II collagen, α_1 chain)
Stickler syndrome, type II	6p21.3	*COL11A2* (type XI collagen, α_2 chain)
Treacher Collins syndrome	5q32–q33.1	*TCOF1* (unknown function)
Van der Woude syndrome	1q32	
Velocardiofacial syndrome	22q11	
Waardenburg syndrome, type I	2q35	*PAX3* (paired box transcription factor)
Waardenburg syndrome, type IIA	3p14.1–p12	*MITF* (transcription factor)
Waardenburg syndrome, type IIB	1p21–p13.3	
Waardenburg syndrome, type III	2q35	*PAX3*

Adapted from Online Mendelian Inheritance in Man, OMIM (TM). Center for Medical Genetics, Johns Hopkins University, Baltimore, and National Center for Biotechnology Information, National Library of Medicine, Bethesda, Md, 1996.

lular domain. The extracellular domain contains three immunoglobulin-like domains, which are probably important for ligand binding and receptor dimerization. FGF-induced receptor activation is thought to be mediated by receptor oligomerization via conformational changes in the extracellular domain. It has been proposed that this oligomerization stabilizes interactions between the cytoplasmic regions of the adjacent receptors, leading to activation of the kinase activity. The genes encoding FGFs and FGFRs are evolutionarily conserved, underscoring their basic role in development and validating the use of animal models for human disorders caused by mutations in these genes.

Mutations in *FGFR1* and *FGFR2* are associated with craniosynostosis syndromes, which are inherited in an autosomal dominant fashion. Muenke and others[17] showed that a mutation in the extracellular domain of *FGFR1* is associated with some cases of Pfeiffer syndrome. However, Pfeiffer syndrome is genetically heterogeneous because some cases are associated with mutations of *FGFR2* but not *FGFR1*.[11,22] Furthermore, the Apert, Jackson-Weiss, and Crouzon syndromes are associated with mutations in *FGFR2* and are thus allelic with cases of Pfeiffer syndrome associated with mutations in *FGFR2*.[9,20,28] Finally, Beare-Stevenson cutis gyrata syndrome is also linked to mutations in the extracellular domain of *FGFR2*.[19] This syndrome causes craniosynostosis and craniofacial dysmorphism; skin, digital, and anogenital abnormalities; and early death. Thus, five craniosynostosis syndromes are associated with mutations in *FGFR2*.

In general, *FGFR2* mutations differ among the syndromes, although they are all located within or near the third immunoglobulin-like domain in the extracellular region of

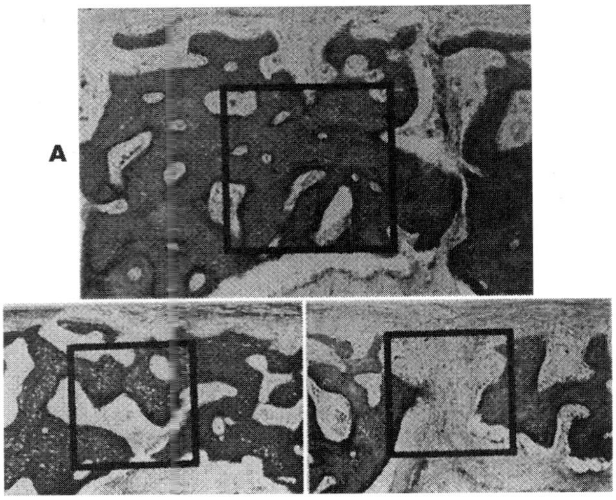

Fig. 6-2. Histopathology of human craniosynostosis. Photomicrographs of prematurely synostosed human coronal suture show **A**, complete; **B**, partial; and **C**, impending bony union. *Boxes* indicate areas previously occupied by sutural ligament. (From Kokich and others: *Cleft Palate J* 19:89, 1982.)

the receptor (Fig. 6-2). However, Rutland and others[22] observed that a cysteine-to-tyrosine/arginine mutation at amino acid 342 is associated with some cases of Crouzon syndrome and with some cases of Pfeiffer syndrome. This is surprising given the phenotypic dissimilarity between these syndromes and because both syndromes are familial. One explanation for this result is that another undetected polymorphism within the *FGFR2* gene may cause the variable expressivity of this particular mutation.

Interesting insights into sutural biology and craniosynostosis have arisen from observations of FGFR mutations in other disorders. Shiang and others[24] and Rousseau and others[21] independently showed that mutations in the transmembrane domain of *FGFR3* cause achondroplasia, an autosomal dominant condition characterized by premature fusion of long bone epiphyseal growth plates. Long bone epiphyses are histologically and functionally similar to synchondroses of the skull base because the synchondrosis is essentially two epiphyseal growth plates positioned back-to-back.[4] Analogous to achondroplasia, the primary defect in craniosynostoses caused by mutations in *FGFR2* may reside within the synchondroses, supporting the theory of Moss[16] that the primary defect is in the skull base.

Other disorders linked to mutations in *FGFR3* include hypochondroplasia and thanatophoric dysplasia.[25] Both syndromes resemble achondroplasia, although thanatophoric dysplasia also causes cloverleaf skull deformity secondary to craniosynostosis. In addition, *FGFR3* mutations have been observed in Crouzon craniosynostosis associated with acanthosis nigricans, an eruption of benign growths and hyperpigmentation occurring in the skin.[15] The correlation between mutation and clinical phenotype in these FGFR disorders should provide fertile ground for future investigations.

Genetically engineered animal models for craniofacial development

The molecular mechanisms of the FGFR diseases have been further characterized by targeted disruption of the *fgfr3* gene in mice. Mice heterozygous for the disrupted *fgfr3* gene (*fgfr3* +/−) had no phenotypic abnormalities, whereas homozygous mice with no functional *fgfr3* (*fgfr3* −/−) had increased length of the vertebral column and long bones and defects of the inner ear.[3] These results led to the proposal that *FGFR3* acts to limit osteogenesis and that *FGFR3* mutations in achondroplasia lead to constitutive activation (ligand activation) of the receptor. Analogous to *FGFR3* mutations in achondroplasia, *FGFR1* and *FGFR2* mutations may give rise to the autosomal dominant craniosynostosis syndromes by a similar gain-of-function mechanism. Theoretically, *FGFR1* and *FGFR2* mutations act via a dominant-negative mechanism, in which only one (dominant) copy of the mutation leads to a loss or decrease of function even in the presence of a normal gene copy. This question may be resolved by gene knockout experiments similar to those performed with *FGFR3*.

However, craniosynostosis may not be pathogenetically homogeneous. Craniosynostoses caused by mutations in genes other than the FGFRs may arise by different mechanisms. For example, Jabs and others[8] showed that a mutation in the homeobox gene *MSX2* is associated with nonsyndromic (Boston-type) craniosynostosis and that the murine homologue of this gene, which putatively encodes a DNA-binding transcription factor, is expressed in developing cranial sutures. Therefore, mutations in *MSX2* may directly affect the development and fusion of the cranial sutures, in support of Virchow's[26] theory that the suture is the site of the primary abnormality and the cranial base is affected secondarily.

Theories such as those of Virchow[26] or Moss[16] may be directly tested in animal models by engineering the mutations in human disorders into the homologous mouse genes. This has been accomplished with *MSX2*, in which the mutation found in Boston-type craniosynostosis was engineered into transgenic mice and found to cause precocious closure of cranial sutures and development of ectopic cranial bone.[12] Future studies of this animal model and those engineered with mutations from other craniosynostotic disorders should further elucidate the mechanisms of craniosynostosis and craniofacial development.

Understanding of the molecular mechanisms of craniofacial development and its associated disorders is just beginning. Early molecular identification of patients, perhaps even *in utero*, may allow early surgical or molecular interventions to circumvent later expression of the disease and its associated complications. These potential interventions may be tested beforehand in animal models, in which the specific genetic defect has been reproduced. These models will be ideal tools for developing such therapies in the future.

CLINICAL APPLICATIONS

Modern craniofacial surgery has evolved; pioneers in the field include Tessier and Obwegeser. The term *craniofacial* is descriptive of this branch of surgery, which deals with anomalies of the bones and soft tissues of the cranium and the face. In the purest sense, craniofacial surgery refers to procedures that combine an intracranial and extracranial approach to correct facial deformities. Techniques developed in craniofacial surgery are directly applicable to the expanding field of skull base surgery, particularly in the management of tumors of the anterior cranial fossa and infratemporal fossa. In the broadest sense, many management options are available depending on the age of the patient and the deformity. Patients with Treacher Collins syndrome may undergo bone grafting to malar and orbital areas to improve bony deficiencies caused by facial anomalies. At a later age, they may undergo orthognathic correction of maxillomandibular disharmonies. Similarly, patients with otomandibular dysostosis may require ramus reconstruction with costochondral grafts between the ages of 6 and 7 years, additional orthognathic corrections when in their teens, and soft-tissue augmentation later on. Patients with oral facial clefting require closure of the cleft and reconstruction of the underlying bony deficiencies at a very early age, followed by subsequent correction of orbital hypertelorism between the ages of 2 and 5 years, and finally, orthognathic correction of maxillary and mandibular deformities in their teens. Craniofacial surgery is useful for correcting congenital anomalies and acquired deformities caused by trauma or tumors of the cranial and facial bones.

Evaluation of patients with craniofacial deformities requires a team approach. The team usually consists of the craniofacial surgeon, neurosurgeon, oral and maxillofacial surgeon, speech pathologist, audiologist, pedodontist, orthodontist, prosthodontist, social worker, geneticist, pediatrician, and ophthalmologist. Other consultants may be added to the team as needed. Patients referred to a craniofacial clinic are seen by all members of the team at the same visit. At a subsequent team conference, each consultant makes recommendations, which are integrated into a comprehensive report by the team leader and presented to the patient's family and physician as a long-term management plan.

This chapter discusses the pathogenesis and evaluation of patients with congenital anomalies of the craniofacial skeleton and provides an overview of the management of these congenital anomalies. This requires a combined intracranial and extracranial approach to the upper facial skeleton.

PATHOGENESIS

Patients requiring craniofacial surgery usually present with multiple anomalies associated with syndromes, but these anomalies may occur as isolated events. Craniofacial anomalies can be categorized as (1) malformation, which is a morphologic defect of one or more organs resulting from intrinsically abnormal development; (2) deformation, which is an abnormal form or position of a part of the body caused by nondisruptive mechanical forces; or (3) disruption, which is a defect of an organ or region of the body resulting from a breakdown of or interference with originally normal development. Categorizing the craniofacial anomaly is helpful for planning long-term management and genetic counseling for the family. The various anomalies can be considered in regard to their different modes of presentation.

Craniosynostosis and craniofacial synostosis

Craniosynostosis is a premature fusion of a cranial suture. Craniofacial synostosis is an extension of this condition in which the sutures of the cranium fuse prematurely, as do those of the skull base and face. Craniosynostosis may be simple or multiple. Simple craniosynostosis refers to premature fusion of one suture of the calvarium. Multiple craniosynostosis involves more than one suture, such as both coronal sutures or coronal sutures and a lambdoid suture. Fusion of a cranial suture at birth is referred to as *primary craniosynostosis*; this has occurred *in utero*. In contrast, secondary craniosynostosis involves postnatal premature suture fusion, which can be caused by a ventriculoperitoneal shunt or sickle cell anemia.

Craniosynostosis may be isolated or syndromic. The isolated form is usually more limited in extent and severity. In isolated unilateral coronal craniosynostosis, for example, there is restriction of skull growth on the affected side and compensatory overgrowth along the ipsilateral lambdoid suture. The overall result is a retrusion of the forehead on the affected side and a bulging of the occiput on the same side. The deformities in multiple craniosynostosis are much more severe. Fusion of bilateral coronal and lambdoid sutures results in the deformity called *turricephaly* (tower skull), in which the skull is shaped like a tower and there is a significant risk of increased intracranial pressure and marked restriction on brain growth.

Many theories have been proposed about what causes primary craniosynostosis. Moss[16] believed that the abnormality centered in the skull base. He proposed that skull base deformity, in particular that of the sphenoid, results in premature fusion of calvarial sutures caused by transmission of abnormal forces from the skull base through the dura to the sutures themselves. Virchow[26] believed that the calvarial sutures themselves fused prematurely and that the skull base deformities were secondary to the calvarial deformity. Park and Powers suggested that the abnormality was centered in the mesenchymal cells in the embryo, which affected the calvarial and basilar sutures. Another hypothesis is that of fetal head constraint. Graham and others noted that in some cases of craniosynostosis, the mothers reported premature descent of the fetus into the pelvis.

Several conditions cause secondary craniosynostosis, including low cerebrospinal fluid pressure caused by a ventricular peritoneal shunt, thalassemia major, sickle cell anemia, and hyperthyroidism. It is important to classify the craniosynostosis because isolated nonsyndromal fusion has the best surgical outcome. Patients who have one suture fused and do not have a syndrome usually require only one surgical procedure to correct the craniofacial deformity. However, patients with multiple sutural fusions may require multiple surgical procedures. This distinction is important because the patient's family should be prepared for the possibility of multiple major procedures.

In contrast, craniofacial synostosis involves abnormalities of the sutures of the cranium, the face, and the cartilaginous growth centers (or synchondrosis) of the skull base. Patients with Apert syndrome manifest atypical facies, consisting of forehead retrusion with a wide skull, midface hypoplasia and retrusion, varying degrees of orbital hypertelorism, and exorbitism. Because both coronal sutures are fused, the forehead is retropositioned and patients have a short, wide skull (brachycephaly). The fusion of facial sutures, particularly of the skull base synchondroses, restricts downward and forward growth of the skull base and of the maxillae. Because of this restriction and the resultant lack of spatial movement of the midface, growth occurs primarily with deposition and resorption of bone in the midface. This produces the classical retromaxillism and micromaxillism found in Apert syndrome.

Orbital hypertelorism

Orbital hypertelorism is an increase in the actual interorbital distance. This can be measured by a PA cephalogram or axial computed tomography (CT) as the distance between the two anterior lacrimal crests (dacryon). The normal range for this distance is 18 mm in the newborn to 25 mm in the adult. Orbital hypertelorism is classified as mild (30 to 34 mm), moderate (35 to 39 mm), or severe (greater than 39 mm). The term *orbital hypertelorism* describes a physical finding and does not denote any specific syndrome; rather, it is found in many syndromes. Orbital hypertelorism may also be found in craniofacial anomalies that are not a part of a syndrome. These anomalies usually involve midline defects of the craniofacial skeleton, such as various nasofrontal, nasoethmoid, and nasoorbital encephaloceles in which there is a defect in the anterior cranial base, with the leptomeninges and brain extending into the nasofrontal and ethmoid complex. Hypertelorism in these cases is a result of a failure of midline fusion and is not associated with a specific syndrome. Hypertelorism associated with a syndrome is usually accompanied by marked widening of the ethmoid sinus complex.

Orbital hypertelorism may also be the result of a disruption, most frequently caused by amnionic bands. In these cases, although the midline structures have the potential to fuse normally and no syndrome is present, the hypertelorism is produced by a distracting force such as amnionic banding. The craniofacial clefting in these patients does not correspond to a failure along an embryologic line of fusion but rather is caused by a distracting extrinsic force.

Facial clefting

Cleft lip and palate are the most common forms of facial clefting. However, other clefts may arise in the craniofacial skeleton. These clefts may result from a failure of embryonic tissue migration or its failure to fuse. The ensuing facial cleft is the result of a malformation process. Facial clefting may also be the result of a deformation process; (e.g., in the Robin sequence, patients manifest micrognathia, glossoptosis, and palatal clefting). In this sequence, the clefting is theorized to be a result of the tongue lying between the palatal shelves, preventing fusion. Superior displacement of the tongue is a result of the retrodisplacement of the mandible caused by extrinsic compression. The Robin sequence is associated with many syndromes, including mandibulofacial dysostosis, Stickler syndrome, del 4q syndrome, fetal alcohol syndrome, amniotic band sequence, and CHARGE (coloboma, hearing deficit, choanal atresia, retardation of growth, genital defects [in men], and endocardial cushion defect). Tessier classified clefts involving the facial and the cranial skeleton. This classification relates to malformations along embryologic lines of fusion. Some facial clefts cannot be classified, nor can they be explained embryologically. These abnormalities are the result of disruptions.

A classic example of facial clefting is seen in Treacher Collins syndrome. This syndrome is autosomal dominant, with the patient exhibiting malar hypoplasia, antimongoloid slant of the eyes, decreased posterior height as a result of a short mandibular ramus, severe antegonial notching, and an open dental bite. In the most pronounced form of Treacher Collins syndrome, the facial skeleton exhibits clefts 6, 7, and 8 from the Tessier system. Clefts in these areas may extend through the inferior and lateral orbit and the arch of the zygoma, producing severe malar deficiency.

Disorders of branchial arches

Oculo-auriculo-vertebral spectrum

The oculo-auriculo-vertebral spectrum encompasses many craniofacial anomalies and several specific conditions that are frequently confused, including hemifacial microsomia, otomandibular dysostosis, Goldenhar's syndrome, and first arch syndrome. Because these syndromes vary widely in terms of degree and severity, they are referred to as *oculo-auriculo-vertebral spectrum*. In the mildest form, the patient may merely have a unilateral microtia; in severe forms, the mandibular ramus and the ear on the affected side, ipsilateral anophthalmia, and epibulbar dermoids may be absent. The incidence ranges from 1 in 3500 to 1 in 26,550 live births. The male to female ratio is 3:2. Two hypotheses explain this spectrum of deformities. Poswillo induced hematoma formation in the region of the ear of animal embryos. This resulted in destruction of the tissues of the ear and mandible and produced a condition similar to that in the human expression of the spectrum. Other theories suggest that changes in the neural crest cells result in a lack of development in the first arch area. Patients with this spectrum have at least microtia or another ear deformity. More than 50% of patients have facial asymmetry; when bilateral involvement is present, the deformity is always worse on one side.

Epibulbar dermoids and colobomas are common findings. In more severe cases, patients may manifest central nervous system disorders, including Arnold-Chiari malformation, hypocephalus, or agenesis of the corpus callosum. Additionally, pulmonary, renal, and cardiac anomalies have been reported. The Goldenhar complex includes fusion of cervical vertebrae in approximately 20% to 30% of cases. Cleft lip and palate have also been reported in these patients.

Mandibulofacial dysostosis

Mandibulofacial dysostosis, also known as Treacher Collins or Franceschetti-Zwahlen-Klein syndrome, is an autosomal dominant disorder with variable expression. Upper facial findings have been described in the section on orbital clefts. Branchial arch anomalies are associated with the syndrome. In addition to hypoplasia of the zygomas and other orbital and upper facial findings, there is a decrease in the height of the mandibular ramus and the gonial angle is more obtuse than normal. Significant antegonial notching may be present and is usually correlated with significant mandibular deficiency. Cleft palate may be found in approximately 35% of patients. The combination of upper facial clefting with malar and orbital abnormalities and mandibular deficiency makes mandibular facial dysostosis a relatively easy syndrome to recognize.

EVALUATION

Patients with congential craniofacial deformities should be evaluated by a multidisciplinary team, each member of which should be highly experienced. Because of multisystem problems in these patients, experts from several disciplines are necessary to evaluate and formulate an overall management plan. In the initial evaluation of patients with craniofacial deformities, it is important to list all of the known anomalies. A detailed family history is important. An attempt should be made to classify the collective group of physical findings into a known syndrome. If a syndrome is identified, the patient can be evaluated for other associated anomalies that may be unrecognized at the time of presentation. If the patient's condition cannot be classified into a known syndrome, the anomaly may be a sporadic one that is not genetically related. This information is important for patients and their families.

Radiographic evaluation of these patients should include skull films to evaluate sutures of the cranium for any evidence of craniosynostosis. Radiographs may be needed to determine bone age and to evaluate for syndactyly or abnormalities of bone metabolism. Three-dimensional CT (Fig. 6-3) may be obtained to evaluate the overall form of the cranium and face and to examine the skull base in relation to the basal and cranial sutures. If these is any fear of underlying central nervous system anomalies, magnetic resonance imaging (Fig. 6-4) can help rule out such deformities as corpus callosum agenesis, holoprosencephaly, or Arnold-Chiari malformation. In older children who are cooperative, lateral and PA cephalometric radiography is used routinely to evaluate the position of the facial bones in relation to each other and to the cranial base. Annual cephalometric

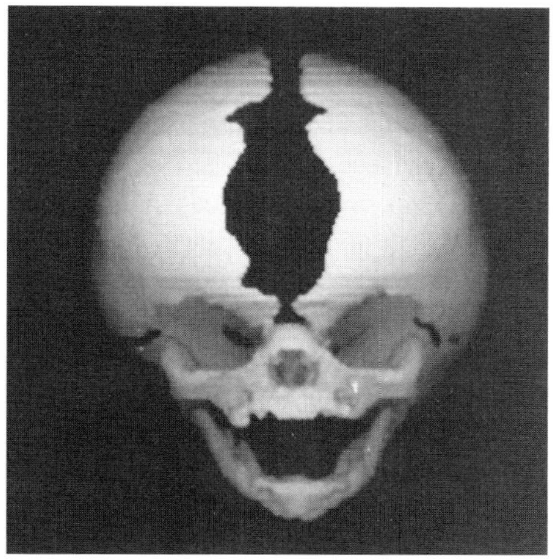

Fig. 6-3. Three-dimensional computed tomography scan of a patient with Apert syndrome. Note the underdeveloped maxilla, brachycephaly, and gapping metopic suture.

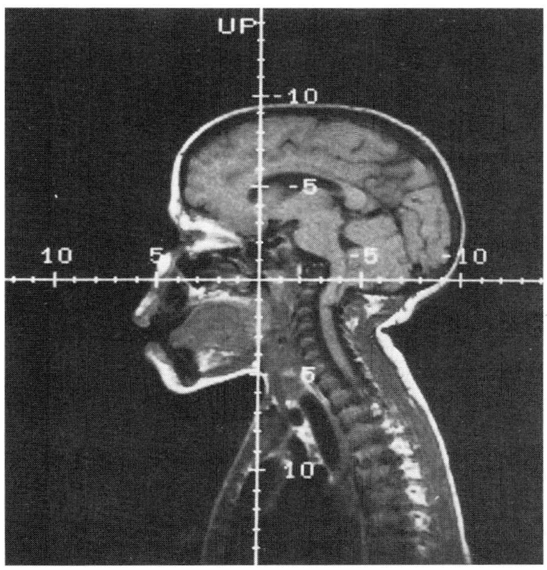

Fig. 6-4. Anterior basilar indentation of the brainstem at the craniocervical junction. There is partial herniation of the cerebellum posteriorly through the foramen magnum.

examinations are important to evaluate continued facial growth and development and to aid in the planning of orthognathic surgery and orthodontics. Dental casts are important for evaluating any existing malocclusion in older patients. The casts can be analyzed, and appropriate orthodontic management can be initiated. When patients require orthognathic surgery (e.g., Le Fort III osteotomy for a patient with Crouzon syndrome), the combination of cephalometric planning analysis with cast surgery allows the team to predict the final outcome.

Anthropometry is another way of evaluating the craniofacial skeleton and of following facial growth and development. This technique uses specific measurements of the facial skeleton, done externally with calipers. For example, bitemporal width measures the distance in centimeters between the two temporal fossa, and bizygomatic width measures the distance between the lateral aspect of the two malar prominences. Two measurements can be compared in a ratio that can provide information about the relationship of one structure to another. For example, if all measurements of the craniofacial skeleton except the bitemporal width are within normal limits, that abnormal finding can be compared with the other normal measurements. If the ratio of bitemporal to bizygomatic width is below the normal value, the craniofacial skeleton is too narrow in the bitemporal area, as occurs in trigonocephaly. This information can be used clinically to evaluate patients for surgery and to follow their facial growth and development. It also helps establish normative values for the various anthropometric measurements.

MANAGEMENT

The range of management modalities for patients with craniofacial deformities is extensive. These methods include closure of soft tissue clefts and subsequent bone grafting augmentation of deficient areas using bone grafts or soft-tissue flaps, various orthognathic and craniofacial osteotomies, and mandibular reconstructions. This chapter is limited to management modalities that involve combined intra- and extracranial approaches that are useful in dealing with the upper craniofacial skeleton.

Surgical approaches

The coronal approach offers the best exposure for surgery of the craniofacial skeleton. This involves a bicoronal incision with extensive dissection anteriorly above the pericranium. At a point approximately 2 cm above the supraorbital ridges, the pericranium is incised and subpericranial dissection is then carried down into the orbits. This preserves the supraorbital and supertrochlear nerves. The dissection medially can be carried down over the nasal bones and into the medial orbits, preserving the lacrimal sac. If necessary, the medial canthal ligaments can be detached, repositioned, and reattached toward the end of the procedure. Laterally, the dissection is carried down over the temporalis muscle through the superficial layer of the deep temporal fascia. The dissection proceeds inferiorly in this layer through the superficial temporal fat pad to the arch of the zygoma. Dissecting in this fashion allows the zygomatic arch to be approached from its superior aspect and deep to the frontal branch of the facial nerve. At this point, the periosteum of the zygomatic arch is incised superiorly, and subperiosteal dissection of the arch is accomplished with the frontal branch of cranial nerve VII being retracted laterally and protected by the superficial layer of the deep temporal fascia and the periosteum of the zygoma. Dissection along the zygoma is extended superiorly to connect with dissection of the frontal bone, and it proceeds circumferentially around the orbits, preserving the infraorbital nerves and detaching the lateral canthal ligaments. This approach allows total exposure of the cranium, orbits, zygomas, and nasoethmoid complexes. In some cases, the orbital floor may not be readily visualized through the coronal approach, so a transconjunctival-lateral canthotomy or subciliary incision may be necessary for further exposure. This may be particularly important for the correction of orbital hypertelorism when osteotomies are made through the floor of the orbit and through the face of the inferior orbital rim at the level of the infraorbital foramen.

Fronto-orbital advancement

After complete exposure of the craniofacial skeleton, the predetermined osteotomies are performed as required for correction of the deformity. In patients with craniofacial synostosis, the forehead and upper orbits are in a retruded position. Surgery is performed initially at 3 to 6 months of age to allow for suture release and normal brain growth. The most common osteotomy performed for this is the fronto-orbital osteotomy (Fig. 6-5). This consists of bifrontal craniotomy and upper orbital osteotomies involving the anterior cranial fossa, upper half of the orbits, the root of the nose, and the temporal fossa to include the greater wing of the sphenoid. After exposure of the anterior cranial fossa and bifrontal craniotomy, dura is dissected free from the roof of the orbits to allow access to perform the orbital osteotomies. Using a side cutting bone tool, osteotomies are created in the roof of both orbits and joined in the midline anterior to the crista gali, thereby preserving olfaction. The osteotomy at the root of the nose should angle from the intracranial side in an anterior and inferior fashion to avoid entering the nasal cavity, thus communicating that area with the epidural space. Laterally, the osteotomy continues from the orbital roof, through the sphenoid bone, into the temporal fossa and the middle cranial fossa. Tongue-and-groove osteotomy is created in the sphenoid wing and squamous portion of temporal bone to allow for adequate bone contact after frontal orbital bar advancement. After the tongue-and-groove is created, the osteotomy continues along the inferior portion of the temporal fossa, through the sphenoid bone, into the lateral wall of the orbit, and into the lateral orbital rim between the front of the frontozygomatic suture and the insertion of

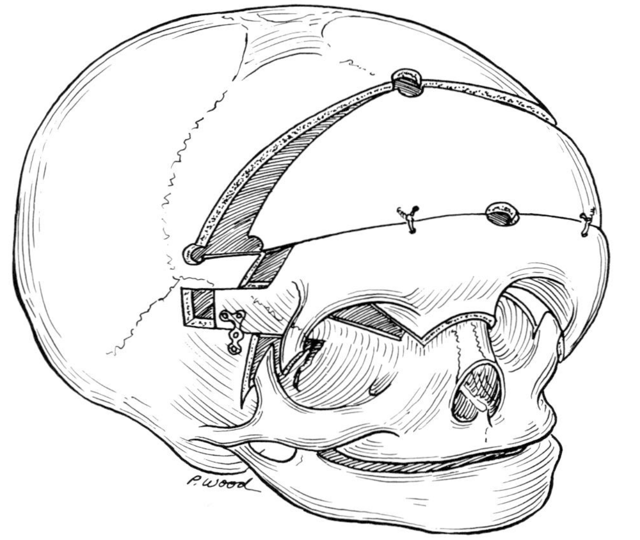

Fig. 6-5. Fronto-orbital advancement. Tongue-in-groove osteotomy in a temporal fossa allows for bone contact to ensure adequate healing. Osteotomy above the frontal suture prevents communication between the nasal cavity and epidural space.

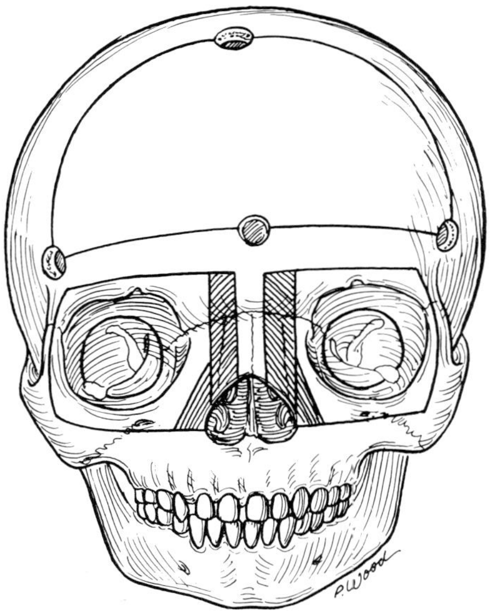

Fig. 6-6. Typical orbital hypertelorism correction. Paramedian excision of the ethmoid bones allows medial orbital translocation and preserves the septum and cribriform plate.

the lateral canthal tendon. Finally, an osteotoma is used to complete the bone cuts in the temporal fossa in the sphenoid wing. Care should be taken to control the osteotome so that only the wing of the sphenoid is separated. Deeper penetration of the osteotome can injure the structures of the infraorbital fissure and superior medially into the optic canal. At this point, the fronto-orbital bar is advanced or, if necessary, removed, remodeled, and replaced into the patient. Fixation is achieved in the temporal fossa with microplates. The lateral orbital rims are greenstick fractures so that smooth contour is achieved between the advanced fronto-orbital bar and the zygomas inferiorly. If necessary, onlay bone grafts may be placed in the nasal frontal suture area. However, with time and growth, bone deposits in this area, which is not a significant problem if bone grafts are not used.

Orbital hypertelorism correction

Similarly, orbital hypertelorism is corrected through a combined intra- and extracranial approach (Fig. 6-6). After a bifrontal craniotomy is done, periorbital osteotomies are made involving the four quadrants of the orbits. The bone cuts traverse the anterior cranial fossa and lateral orbital wall, through the orbital floor into the inferior orbital fissure, and medially through the medial orbital wall posterior to the posterior lacrimal crest. They then extend laterally into the inferior orbital fissure. Sagittal osteotomies of the lateral orbital rim are made. Additional osteotomies are made through the frontal bone, the nasal process of the maxilla medially, and the infraorbital rim at the level of the infraorbital foramen. If the cause of the deformity is an encephalocele, this needs to be resected before orbital mobilization is performed. If, however, there is a widened ethmoid block, paramedian resections of the nasal bone and nasal process of maxilla are done after the orbital osteotomies. These are followed by a complete ethmoidectomy to remove the widened intraorbital ethmoid block. Preservation of a midline strut of nasal septum and cribriform plate does not compromise olfactory function. After removal of aberrant intraorbital tissue, the orbits are translocated medially and secured in place with bone grafts and miniplates.

Monoblock correction

Monoblock facial advancement may be performed in children 4 to 6 years of age with severe midfacial and forehead retrusion, such as that in Crouzon or Apert syndrome (Fig. 6-7). In this procedure, a bifrontal craniotomy is performed, followed by upper orbital osteotomies involving the upper half of the orbits, root of the nose, and the temporal fossa. This is followed by a total midface mobilization achieved by disengaging the midface from the skull base with osteotomies extending down from the orbits through the posterior body of the maxilla into the pterygopalatine fossa, the pterygomaxillary suture, and the zygomatic arches. The nasal septum is also sectioned, and the midface is fractured with disimpacting forceps and mobilized anteriorly. After midface fixation with bone grafts and miniplates, the upper orbital complex is replaced and secured with plates and bone grafts. The forehead is remodeled and repositioned into its new forward position.

Oculo-auriculo-vertebral spectrum correction

Oculo-auriculo-vertebral spectrum requires extensive pre- and postsurgical orthodontic management. Because the syndrome involves first and second branchial arch anoma-

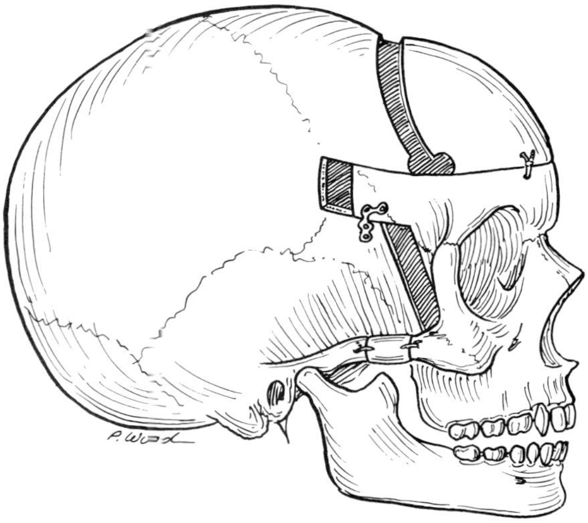

Fig. 6-7. Monoblock facial advancement. A modified Le Fort III osteotomy has been combined with fronto-orbital advancement. The maxilla and frontal bone have been positioned anteriorly in a patient with Apert syndrome who exhibited frontal and maxillary retrusion.

lies, the maxilla is secondarily deformed by the anomalous mandible. By correcting the mandible in the growing child, the maxilla can develop "catch up growth." Thus, the mandibular deformity can be minimized or eliminated by early mandibular surgical correction. Because this spectrum ranges from mandibular condylar hypoplasia to condylar and ramus agenesis, the skeletal correction differs among patients. Ideally, correction should be obtained in the mixed dentition: approximately between ages 7 and 9, before the pubertal growth spurt in the face. This will optimize maxillary growth. In patients with a mandibular condyle, mandibular ramus lengthening is recommended. This can be achieved through a high, carefully placed sagittal split ramus osteotomy that avoids the retromolar trigone or through an inverted L osteotomy that lengthens the mandibular ramus with an interpositional bone graft. Patients with complete absence of ramus and mandibular condyle are best managed by costochondral graft reconstruction. In either situation, a posterior open bite is created on the side of the deformity to allow vertical maxillary growth as the child develops. Maxillary surgery is not indicated in the growing child because the maxilla will grow to meet the inferiorly displaced mandible; Le Fort I osteotomy performed in the mixed dentition period will result in loss of permanent teeth. In the adult with maxillary mandibular deformity, the same mandibular principles can be applied to correction. However, a Le Fort I osteotomy is required to inferiorly displace the hypoplastic maxilla on the side of the deformity, which is stabilized with inner positional bone graft and plate fixation.

FUTURE

Much research is being done on the molecular biology of the various syndromes of the head and the neck. For example, disorders of mucopolysaccharide metabolism cause the facial features in Hurler syndrome. Inborn errors of bone metabolism may cause the facial deformities in craniotabular dysostosis. If the specific gene locus for the metabolic error can be identified, that gene can be altered, enabling metabolism to proceed in a normal fashion and, hopefully, lessening the outcome of the deformities caused by the metabolic disorder. Additionally, advances in fetal surgery may soon permit its practical use in humans. If craniofacial anomalies (e.g., craniosynostosis, facial clefting) are detected *in utero*, correction before birth may someday be possible.

REFERENCES

1. Bellus GA and others: A recurrent mutation in the tyrosine kinase domain of fibroblast growth factor receptor 3 causes hypochondroplasia, *Nature Genet* 10:357, 1995.
2. Reference deleted in pages.
3. Deng C and others: Fibroblast growth factor receptor 3 is a negative regulator of bone growth, *Cell* 84:911, 1996.
4. Enlow DH: *The facial growth process.* In Enlow DH, editor: *Facial growth,* ed 3, Philadelphia, 1990, WB Saunders.
5. Fairbairn LJ and others: Long-term in vitro correction of alpha-iduronidase deficiency (Hurler syndrome) in human bone marrow, *Proc Natl Acad Sci U S A* 93:2025, 1996.
6. Reference deleted in pages.
7. Hopwood JJ and others: Long-term clinical progress in bone marrow transplanted mucopolysaccharidosis type I patients with a defined genotype, *J Inherit Metab Dis* 16:1024, 1993.
8. Jabs EW and others: A mutation in the homeodomain of the human MSX2 gene in a family affected with autosomal dominant craniosynostosis, *Cell* 75:443, 1993.
9. Jabs EW and others: Jackson-Weiss and Crouzon syndromes are allelic with mutations in fibroblast growth factor receptor 2, *Nature Genet* 8: 275, 1994.
10. Reference deleted in pages.
11. Lajeunie E and others: *FGFR2* mutations in Pfeiffer syndrome, *Nature Genet* 9:108, 1995.
12. Liu YH and others: Premature suture closure and ectopic cranial bone in mice expressing *Msx2* transgenes in the developing skull, *Proc Natl Acad Sci U S A* 92:6137, 1995.
13. Reference deleted in pages.
14. Reference deleted in pages.
15. Meyers GA and others: Fibroblast growth factor receptor 3 (*FGFR3*) transmembrane mutation in Crouzon syndrome with acanthosis nigricans, *Nature Genet* 11:462, 1995.
16. Moss ML: The pathogenesis of premature cranial synostosis in man, *Acta Anat (Basel)* 37:351, 1959.
17. Muenke M and others: A common mutation in the fibroblast growth factor receptor 1 gene in Pfeiffer syndrome, *Nature Genet* 8:269, 1994.
18. Neufeld EF, Muenzer J: *The mucopolysaccharidoses.* In Scriver CE and others, editors: *The metabolic basis of inherited disease,* ed 6, New York, 1989, McGraw-Hill.
19. Przylepa KA and others: Fibroblast growth factor receptor 2 mutations in Beare-Stevenson cutis gyrata syndrome, *Nature Genet* 13:492, 1996.
20. Reardon W and others: Mutations in the fibroblast growth factor receptor 2 gene cause Crouzon syndrome, *Nature Genet* 8:98, 1994.
21. Rousseau F and others: Mutations in the gene encoding fibroblast growth factor receptor-3 in achondroplasia, *Nature* 371:252, 1994.
22. Rutland P and others: Identical mutations in the *FGFR2* gene cause

both Pfeiffer and Crouzon syndrome phenotypes, *Nature Genet* 9:173, 1995.

23. Saiki RK and others: Primer-directed enzymatic amplification of DNA with a thermostable DNA polymerase, *Science* 239:487, 1988.
24. Shiang R and others: Mutations in the transmembrane domain of FGFR3 cause the most common genetic form of dwarfism, achondroplasia, *Cell* 78:335, 1994.
25. Tavormina PL and others: Thanatophoric dysplasia (types I and II) caused by distinct mutations in fibroblast growth factor receptor 3, *Nature Genet* 9:321, 1995.
26. Virchow R: Uber den Cretinismus, namentlich in Franken, und uber pathologische schadelformen, *Verh Phys Med Gesellsch* 2:230, 1981.
27. Weber JL, May PE: Abundant class of human DNA polymorphisms which can be typed using the polymerase chain reaction, *Am J Hum Genet* 44:388, 1989.
28. Wilkie AOM and others: Apert syndrome results from localized mutations of FGFR2 and is allelic with Crouzon syndrome, *Nature Genet* 9:165, 1995.
29. Yamaguchi TP, Rossant J: Fibroblast growth factors in mammalian development, *Curr Opin Genet Dev* 5:485. 1995.

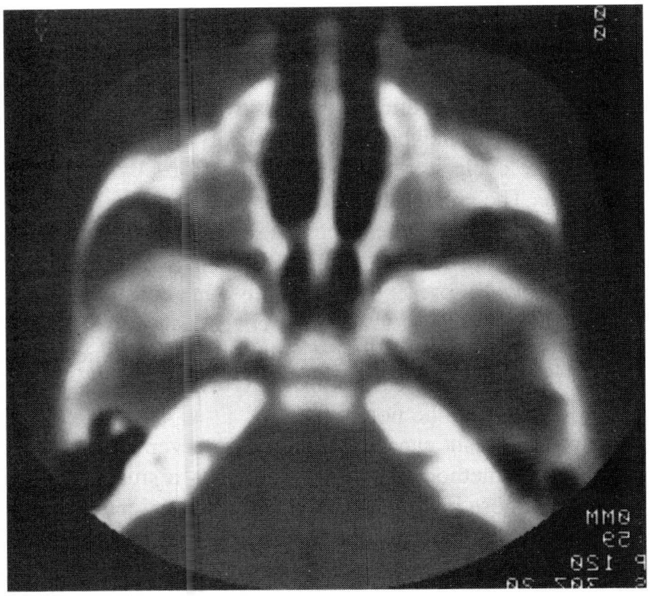

Fig. 7-3. Computed tomography of a patient with bilateral mixed bony-membranous choanal atresia.

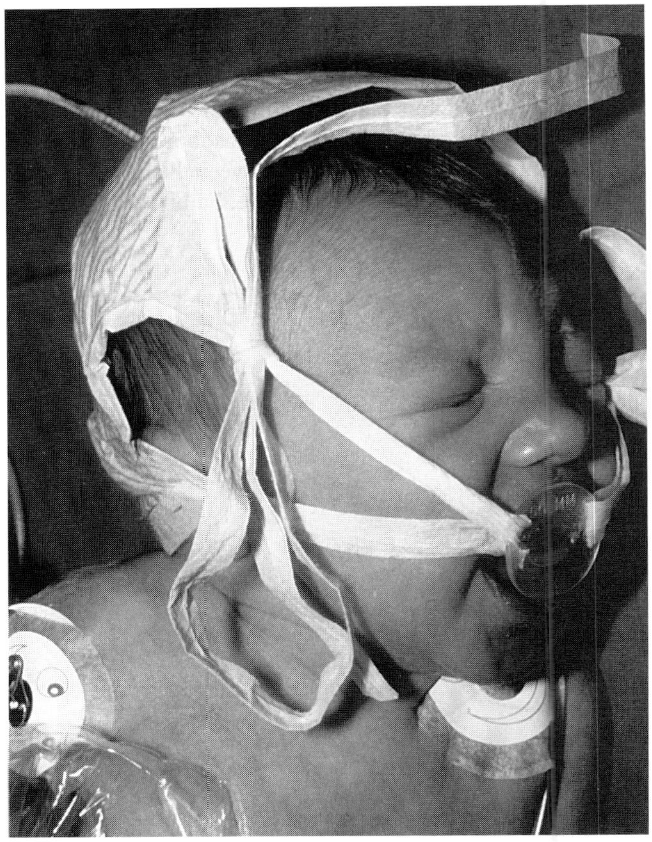

Fig. 7-4. A newborn with choanal atresia. An oral airway is secured by a surgeon's mask at the occiput.

the infant to breathe through the mouth with the aid of an indwelling oral appliance such as a McGovern nipple. A plastic oropharyngeal airway may be placed temporarily, although the infant cannot feed through this. A McGovern nipple serves the same purpose and can be used for gavage feeding. A McGovern nipple is an ordinary nipple with a single enlarged hole or two additional lateral holes. It is secured with ties or tape around the ears. Alternatively, a surgeon's mask may be used around the occiput to secure the oral airway or McGovern nipple (Fig. 7-4). In an emergency, the infant can be stimulated to cry; if this is unsuccessful, a finger can be inserted into the mouth until an airway is established. Endotracheal intubation usually is unnecessary unless the infant requires mechanical ventilation. With this method, the infant can be fed and the airway is protected while definitive management is delayed to allow time for a complete workup to rule out other anomalies. Because infants are obligate nasal breathers, bilateral choanal atresia is a much more urgent problem and, if not promptly recognized, can lead to severe asphyxia and death immediately after birth.

Surgical repair of choanal atresia includes transnasal, transpalatal, transantral, and transseptal approaches. Transpalatal approaches are traditionally reserved for older patients because of orthodontic growth and development may be interrupted.[21,22] Compared with the transpalatal approach, transnasal repair has been associated with a higher rate of restenosis and a need for serial dilations.[18,19] However, with the use of endoscopes, the operating microscope, and otologic instruments and drills via the transnasal approach, comparable results are achievable.[6,41] Although many methods are described, the key points are removal and shortening of the posterior bony septum and removal of the superior-lateral nasal wall and lateral pterygoid plate. Preservation of mucosal flaps for relining the lumen is very difficult.[6,41] Telescopic visualization can help assess surgical results intraoperatively.[33,34] Some physicians reserve transpalatal approaches for older patients, third time surgery, or other revision surgery. The incidence of dental occlusion is 50% in young patients undergoing transpalatal repair because of interference with palatal growth centers.[22] The transseptal approach can be used in older patients with unilateral atresia,[37] and the transantral approach is helpful in opening the posterior choanae into a common cavity with a maxillary sinus to prevent restenosis in cases of recurrent stenosis.[6] Stents are placed in these patients intranasally, secured with a circumseptal suture (Fig. 7-5), and left in place for 3 to 6 weeks. During this time, patients are given antibiotics against *Staphylococcus* and *Streptococcus* species. Patients are managed with antireflux drugs because gastroesophageal reflux can increase the incidence of granulations and stenosis.[3] Corticosteroids are not routinely used. Patients are followed closely with flexible endoscopic examinations and dilation with female urethral sounds as needed. This close follow-up and

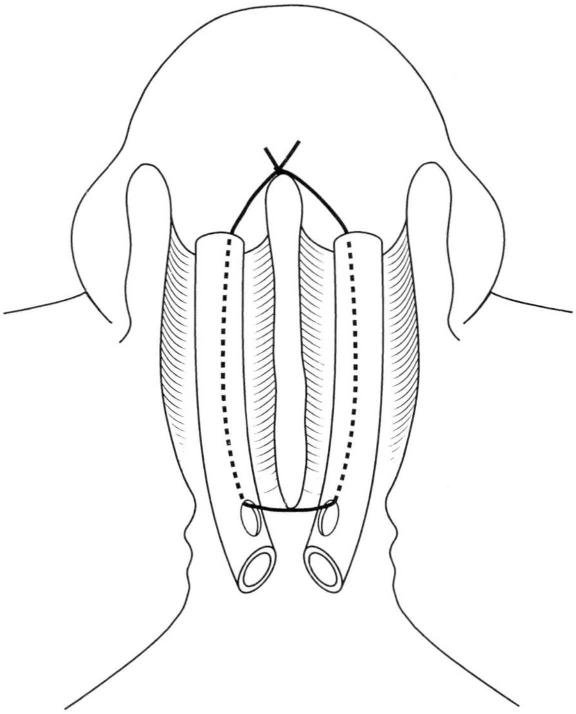

Fig. 7-5. Stents secured intranasally by circumseptal suture.

periodic dilation can prevent the development of a firm cicatricial scar band, which would necessitate revision surgery.[6,7]

PYRIFORM APERTURE STENOSIS

Pyriform aperture stenosis is a recently described anomaly that occurs secondary to bony overgrowth of the nasal process of the maxilla and typically presents in the first few months of life.[8,31,42] It most commonly occurs as an isolated anomaly, although it may be a forme fruste of holoprosencephaly.

The pyriform aperture is the narrowest portion of the nasal cavity, and very small changes in cross-sectional area may greatly increase nasal airway resistance and produce symptoms similar to bilateral choanal atresia. Epiphora is also commonly noted. Anterior rhinoscopy reveals a bony obstruction at the nasal vestibule that will not allow passage of a flexible endoscope (Fig. 7-6). Some patients also have a single central incisor. Diagnosis can be confirmed by CT, which shows bony narrowing of the pyriform aperture (Fig. 7-7). CT may also show the nasolacrimal ducts encased in the narrowed bony pyriform aperture. Mild cases may be handled with conservative management, including a McGovern nipple, gavage feedings, a home apnea monitor, and parental training in cardiopulmonary resuscitation. In more severe cases with significant nasal airway obstruction, respiratory distress, or failure to thrive, surgical correction is necessary via a transnasal or sublabial approach, taking care to preserve the nasolacrimal ducts and tooth buds. The sublabial approach is technically easier in the small nose of an infant. After preservation of the mucosa, the abnormal bone can be removed with drills and microscopic visualization. Usually, stents are left in place no longer than 1 week postoperatively. Patients should be given antibiotics while the stents are in place. Surgery does not seem to effect nasal or facial growth with follow-up to about 1 year.[1,8]

ENCEPHALOCELES AND GLIOMAS

Congenital midline masses can be divided into three major groups according to their tissues of origin. Neurogenic tumors include gliomas, encephaloceles, and neurofibromas. Dermoid cysts originate from ectoderm and mesodermal tissue, and hemangiomas arise from mesoderm. Congenital midline nasal masses are rare and occur in about 1 in 30,000 live births in the United States; they are more common in Asian populations, occurring in 1 in 6000 live births. Encephaloceles occur three times more often in males but have no familial tendency. Almost 40% of patients with these lesions have other associated anomalies.[27,30]

An encephalocele is a herniation of cranial contents through a defect in the skull. It may include meninges only, termed a *meningocele*, or it may involve brain and meninges, termed a *meningoencephalocele*. A glioma is thought to be an encephalocele that has lost the intracranial connection, although 15% remain attached to the central nervous system (CNS) via a fibrous stalk. Gliomas are composed of glial cells and fibrous and vascular connective tissue.[25,27]

During normal embryologic development, the prenasal space lies between the nasal and frontal bones and the cartilaginous skeleton. It extends from the nasal tip to the brain. The ectodermal anterior neuropore develops and fuses before the base of skull at about the third week of gestation. A space between the frontal and nasal bones, known as the *fonticulus frontalis*, completely fuses in the area of the future cribriform plate with the foramen caecum, separating the intracranial contents from the extracranial structures and nose. Failure of closure in this area may result in herniation of intracranial contents, producing an external or intranasal encephalocele. With faulty closure of the anterior neuropore, there may be no herniation but development of extracranial rests of CNS tissue, which form gliomas. These may remain attached to dura with a fibrous stalk. Any of these lesions can be associated with a cerebrospinal fluid (CSF) leak.[7,30]

Encephaloceles and gliomas generally have similar presentations because of their similar embryologic development. They are classified as occipital, sincipital (frontonasal), and basal. The most common are occipital lesions (75%). Sincipital masses are external lesions that are apparent at birth as subcutaneous masses over the nose, glabella, medial canthus, or lower forehead. Lesions can be further subdivided into three groups according to their location. Nasofrontal lesions protrude between the nasal and frontal bones, nasoethmoidal lesions along the side of the nose, and naso-orbital lesions bulge into the medial orbit. Patients may

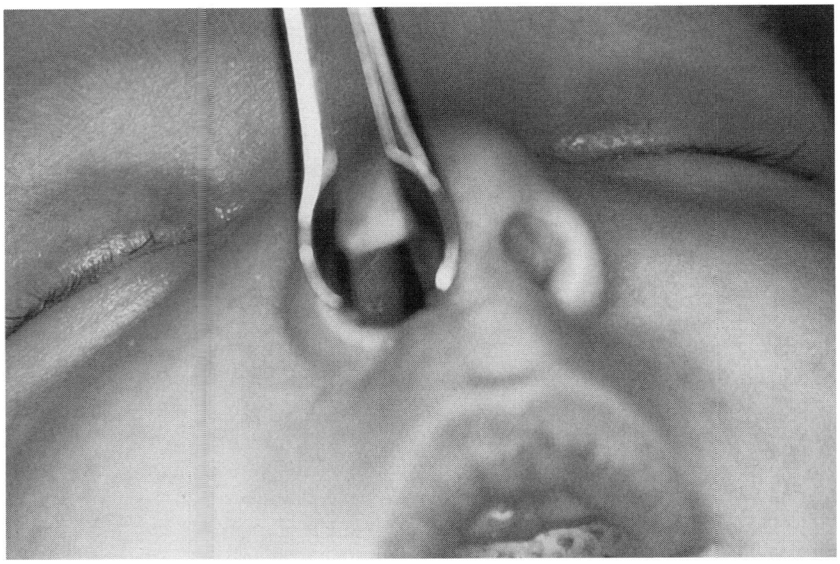

Fig. 7-6. A patient with pyriform aperture stenosis. Note the narrowed bony nasal valve.

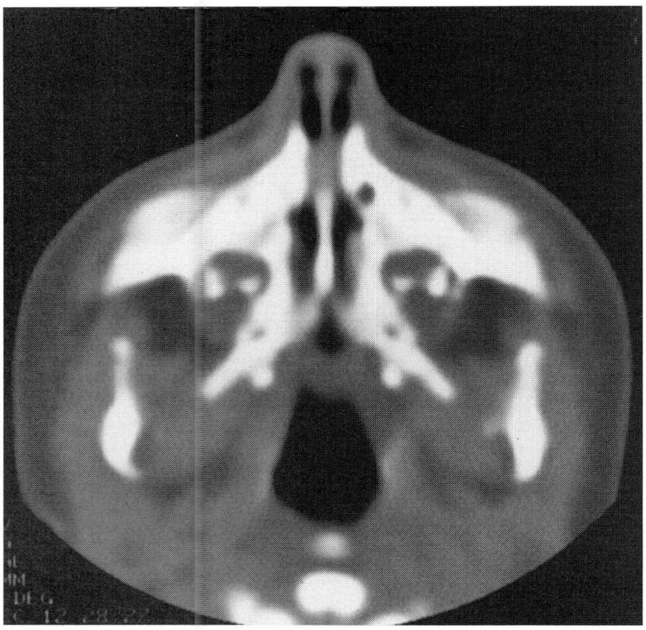

Fig. 7-7. Computed tomography of a patient with pyriform aperture stenosis. The anterior nasal valve is narrowed by abnormal bone.

have a widened nose, hypertelorism, or other midline CNS anomalies. Basal lesions are intranasal masses that are less common (about 10%) and may not be discovered until later in life when the child complains of nasal obstruction and discharge (Fig. 7-8 *A, B*). They may present as transethmoidal, sphenoethmoidal, transsphenoidal, or sphenorbital lesions. Encephaloceles tend to be bluish, soft, compressible masses that transilluminate and enlarge with crying. Manipulation of the mass should be avoided because of the risk of meningitis and because compression may cause somnolence or even seizures in some cases. Defects in the cranium are often visible or palpable with these lesions.[7,24,27]

Gliomas usually present at birth but may present at any age. They are typically reddish, firm, and noncompressible. They do not transilluminate, and the overlying skin may be covered with telangiectasias. A cranial defect is normally not appreciable with a glioma. Sixty percent of gliomas are extranasal, 30% intranasal, and 10% are both. A probe can usually be passed lateral but not medial to the intranasal encephalocele, whereas an intranasal glioma may arise from the lateral nasal wall. A Furstenberg test, in which the internal jugular vein is compressed, will usually cause an encephalocele to enlarge but not a glioma. Unilateral polyposis in children is very rare. If polyposis is seen, a sweat chloride test should be performed to screen for cystic fibrosis. Biopsy of a unilateral nasal mass should be avoided until a thorough workup is completed. Biopsy of an encephalocele may lead to CSF leak and meningitis.

Diagnosis is confirmed radiologically with midline nasal masses. The most commonly used studies are magnetic resonance imaging (MRI) and CT. CT better delineates the bony anatomy of the base of skull, whereas MRI more accurately represents soft-tissue connections to the CNS.[24,25]

After a thorough evaluation, definitive management is surgical. If an intracranial connection exists, neurosurgical consultation is mandatory. Most authors agree that encephaloceles should be managed in the first few months of life. This makes identification of the intracranial connection technically easier and allows more complete repair of the dural defect. The external component may be removed at the same time or delayed. Sometimes, removal of the external component becomes unnecessary. When removal is indicated, there are multiple surgical approaches, including lateral rhi-

A

B

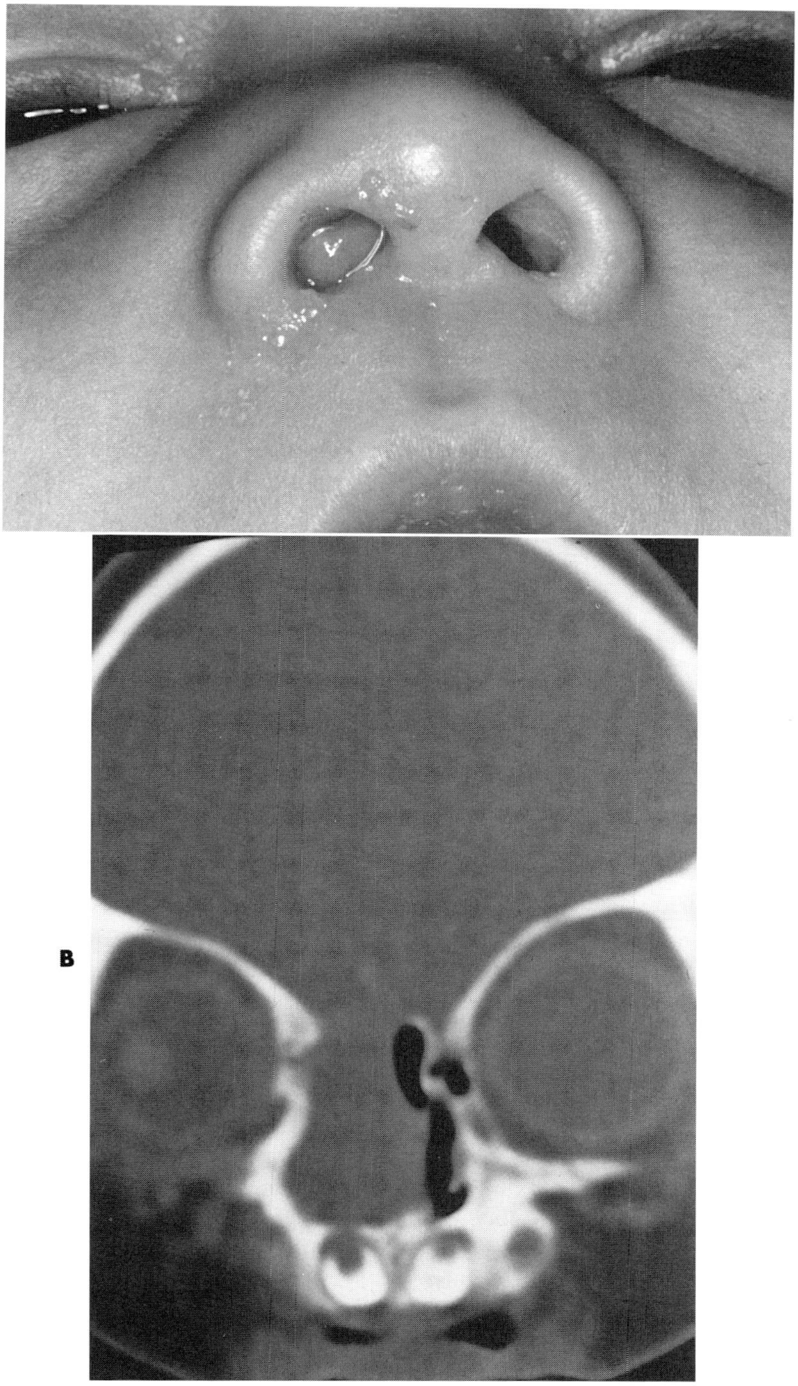

Fig. 7-8. A, A patient with unilateral intranasal encephalocele. **B,** Computed tomography of the same patient reveals a defect in the cribriform plate with unilateral encephalocele.

notomy, a transnasal approach, or a coronal flap approach for glabellar lesions.[27,30]

DERMOIDS

Dermoid cysts are masses that may contain skin, hair follicles, sebaceous glands, and sweat glands. They are different from epidermoids, which contain only epidermis and no elements of dermis. Unlike teratomas, which contain all three germinal layers, dermoids contain only ectoderm and mesoderm. Dermoids are the most common midline nasal mass. Nasal dermoids constitute about 1% to 3% of all dermoids and about 10% of those of the head and neck. Most lesions are present at birth, but patients may not develop symptoms that warrant attention by a physician until later in life when the lesions become infected or begin to drain. Most dermoid cysts occur sporadically, although rare familial associations have been reported. They may be associated with other anomalies of the nose (e.g., a bifid nasal septum), but association with other congenital anomalies is infrequent.[24,32]

Dermoids may be of similar embryologic origin to encephaloceles and gliomas. Faulty closure of the fonticulus frontalis may permit invagination of dermal elements between the developing nasal bones and cartilage. Dura herniating down through the defect may remain in contact with the epithelium. This can lead to many abnormalities, including dermal sinuses, dermal cysts, dermal fistulas, or dermoids with a continued attachment to the CNS. Another theory of origin is the prenasal space theory. This space between the developing nasal bone and deeper cartilage extends from the dura, along the midline, and to the tip of the nose. During development, a portion of the dura develops in close association with the skin of the nose. This normally separates and is retracted up through the foramen caecum, which then closes. Dura that remains in contact with skin as it retracts will result in a sinus or pit. A dermoid may be present anywhere along the prenasal space. The dermoid can also be pulled intracranially or left attached to the CNS by a fibrous stalk.[25,[illegible],32]

Dermoids may present externally as a firm, lobulated, and noncompressible mass with a negative Furstenberg test. They do not transilluminate. The most frequent presentation is a slow-growing cystic mass over the dorsum of the nose. They may present as a midline pit or deformity anywhere along the midline from the nasal tip to the glabella and may have hair protruding from the sinus opening. These lesions may become locally infected and present as an abscess with a history of previous incision and drainage. They may also be entirely intranasal. A lesion within the nasal septum will cause nasal obstruction. Slow expansion may also present as destruction of nasal bones or widening of the nasal bridge. There may be a connection with the CNS with an associated cranial defect. Dermoids should not be manipulated or biopsied until attachment to the CNS has been ruled out by radiologic study. Dermoids may also be entirely intracranial and present as any other intracranial mass with neurologic symptoms of compression.[24,32]

Nasal dermoids can be examined with plain radiography, including Caldwell or Waters views. However, to examine the anterior skull base for a defect or to determine CNS connection, CT or MRI is necessary. CT is good at defining the bony anatomy and may be more helpful to plan surgery in cases of encephaloceles. MRI can adequately delineate a CNS connection without exposing the patient to radiation. Obtaining both studies preoperatively may most accurately define the lesion and aid in planning surgical intervention (Fig. 7-9 *A*, *B*).[25,27]

Surgical excision of dermoid tumors prevents infection, expansion, and destruction of adjacent tissues. In cases with CNS connections, a neurosurgical consultation should be obtained and initial intracranial exploration undertaken. The external component can be excised immediately, can be excised in a delayed fashion, or rarely may not need excision at all. For a lesion with no intracranial connection, an elliptical incision can be made around the fistula tract and the tract is then followed and dissected out completely. Using a malleable probe or injecting the tract with methylene blue dye may be helpful in following the tract. It is important to leave no remnants. If the tract runs deep to the nasal bones, lateral rhinotomy may be performed to expose the septum and allow for complete dissection. Other transnasal approaches include lateral rhinotomy, open rhinoplasty, or an inverted-U incision. The open rhinoplasty approach offers the advantage of good cosmetic result, wide exposure with a good view of the cribriform plate, and better control of the medial osteotomies.[24,27]

HEMANGIOMAS

Hemangiomas are the most frequently occurring tumor in the head and neck in children. They may present anywhere in the head and neck. The subglottis and the nose are of particular concern to the otolaryngologist because of potential airway obstruction.

Hemangiomas are classified as capillary, cavernous, or mixed. These types often overlap within the same lesion. The most common hemangioma is the capillary type. These lesions typically present at birth and tend to enlarge fairly rapidly. Most resolve spontaneously during the first 18 months of life, and conservative management, if possible, is the guiding principle. Hemangiomas are thought to be a mesodermal rest of the vasoformative tissue, from which the vascular system develops. They are more a congenital malformation than a benign neoplasm.[27]

The imaging modality of choice for hemangiomas is MRI. MRI shows vascular tissue and helps rule out any connection with the CNS.

If surgical intervention is not necessary to provide an airway or improve feeding, observation is the best initial therapy. Many lesions resolve spontaneously, usually with superior cosmetic results. This is especially true of nasal

A

B

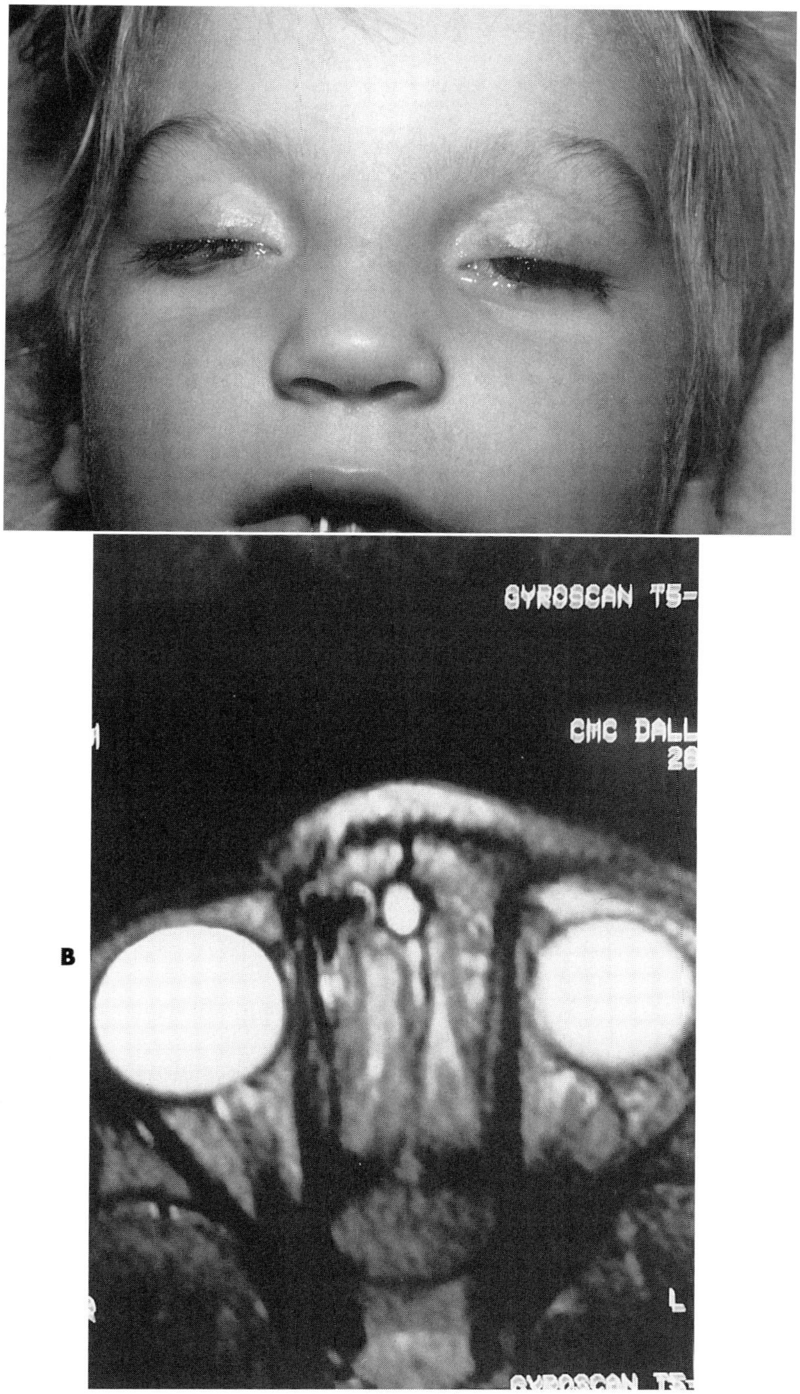

Fig. 7-9. A, A patient with a dermoid sinus at the glabella. A small hair (not shown) protrudes through the pit. **B,** Magnetic resonance imaging of the same patient reveals a small intracranial dermoid.

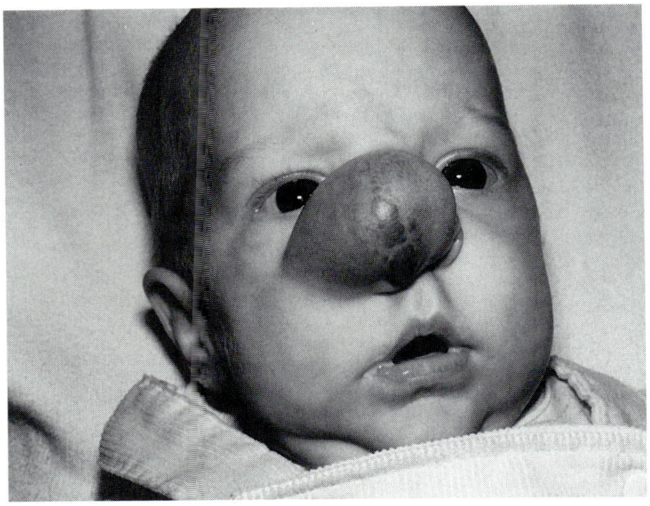

Fig. 7-10. A patient with a large nasal and facial hemangioma.

hemangiomas, for which surgical results are rarely cosmetically pleasing (Fig. 7-10). Parental pressure can be strong for intervention and it is important to give these patients close follow-up and psychologic support. The family can be counseled to expect rapid growth over the first several months followed by involution of the tumor over several months. The bulk of the tumor most commonly resolves within 18 months, and the remaining color may take a few years to fade. Noninvoluting lesions occur less commonly in infancy. These include port-wine stains, spider angiomas, salmon patches and true cavernous hemangiomas with adult type venous spaces. Lesions that do not show the characteristic growth pattern during early life are more likely to be noninvoluting hemangiomas. It may, however, be difficult to determine which lesions will spontaneously involute, even is biopsy is performed. Common practice is to reserve surgery for cases with airway or feeding difficulties, severe bleeding with ulceration, thrombocytopenia, cardiovascular decompensation, uncontrollable infections or abscesses, or questionable diagnosis.[43,44]

If the airway is stable, patients with subglottic hemangiomas may respond to high-dose corticosteroids. Young patients with severe airway obstruction may require tracheotomy for large obstructing lesions. Carbon dioxide laser can effectively manage these lesions, but care should be taken not to cause scarring that results in subglottic stenosis. The result after involution is very good in these patients at 2 to 3 years, so care should be taken not to cause an iatrogenic complication.

Other forms of management are discussed in the literature. Corticosteroids have been used by some authors to reduce the bulk of the tumor. The use of long-term corticosteroids is controversial because of their adverse sequelae. Corticosteroids are most effective when administered during the rapid growth phase of hemangiomas, and rapid regrowth may occur with discontinuation of the drug.[10,16] Radiotherapy has also been proposed as effective management. Although hemangiomas are very sensitive to radiotherapy, this approach should be avoided because of radiation-induced damage and scarring of surrounding tissue. Radiotherapy may also impair bone growth in the area and carries the additional risk of inducing other neoplastic processes later in life. In unusual circumstances, 1000 to 1500 rads are administered in small doses. Compressive dressings increase platelet counts and speed involution of the mass. This likely results from prolonged compression of vessels that narrow the lumens and result in stasis of blood flow with eventual thrombosis. Customized garments that apply pressure that does not exceed the arterial pressure should be used. This form of therapy for facial and especially nasal hemangiomas is not practical. Sclerosing agents, laser therapy, freezing, and cauterization have been used with limited success.[27]

CLEFT LIP-NASAL DEFORMITY AND NASAL CLEFTING

The appearance of the nose associated with a cleft lip or palate is very characteristic. The more severe the cleft, the more severe the nasal deformity. In the presence of a unilateral cleft, the affected side of the nose will have a medially and inferiorly rotated medial crura. This cartilage is very thin and weak and provides little structural support. The nostril is flat and flared secondary to the laterally displaced nasal ala, and the ala is also retrodisplaced as a result of maxillary hypoplasia. The tip of the nose appears uneven, bifid, wide, or boxy. The caudal septum and nasal spine are deviated to the noncleft side, and the base is widened. If the cleft is complete, the nasal floor will be missing. With a bilateral cleft lip and palate, the same defects are present. However, the columella is usually very shortened, and because the maxilla are bilaterally hypoplastic, there is a relative prognathism.[27,32,38]

Timing for surgical correction in these patients is somewhat controversial. It would seem most reasonable to postpone surgery until facial growth is complete. Because of social pressures, some cases may need earlier intervention. One approach is to correct the tip deformity at about age 6 years and postpone septal, bony, and upper lateral cartilage work until the child is fully grown. In infants in whom septal abnormalities cause nasal obstruction and respiratory distress, surgery is indicated at an early age. There are multiple surgical approaches for repair of this deformity. The initial lip repair alone can serve to lengthen the columnella and realign the alar base. Aligning the alveolar segments or using onlay grafts on the hypoplastic maxilla serves to correct the retrodisplacement of the ala and produce a stable nasal base. Medial and lateral osteotomies may be necessary to create a symmetrical dorsum. Many approaches are available to correct the lower lateral cartilages, the septal deflection, and the columellar deformity. Open rhinoplasty approaches provide wide exposure but should be reserved for older children because of their possible effect on nasal growth. Dermabrasion of the nasal and lip scars may be indicated as a final stage in reconstruction.[32,38]

Nasal clefting is a rare form of midline clefting commonly associated with hypertelorism and intracranial abnormalities. Nasal clefts can range from a small furrow in the nasal dorsum to an actual vertical division of the nose into two halves. Lateral clefts are defects in the nasal ala or lateral nasal wall area that may present as small notches in the alar rim or may involve the lacrimal duct and extend the entire length of the nose. The incidence of mental retardation and associated anomalies (e.g., hypertelorism, facial cleft, colobomas, encephaloceles, choanal atresia) increases with the severity of the anomaly.[24,27]

Many patients have no respiratory difficulty, and surgical intervention is cosmetic. The preoperative workup includes CT and MRI because many of these midline deformities are associated with abnormalities at the anterior base of skull and resultant encephaloceles. Surgical repair will likely require multiple stages and a team approach for adequate repair of more severe defects. Mild lateral clefts are managed with auricular cartilage grafts and local skin flaps.

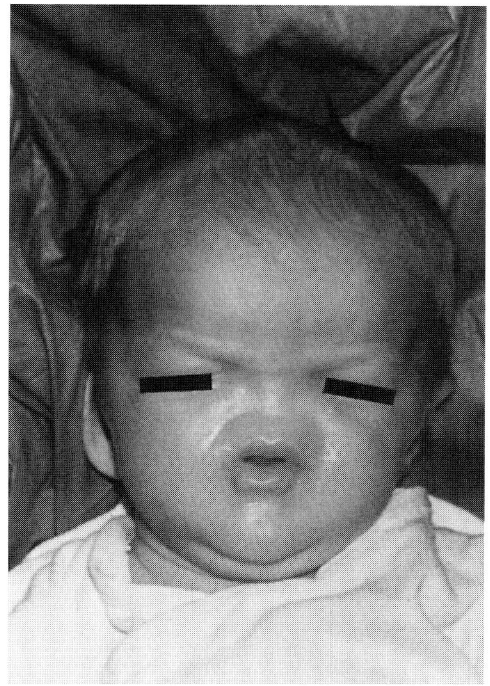

Fig. 7-11. Patient with congenital arhinia.

ARHINIA, POLYRRHINIA, AND PROBOSCIS LATERALIS

Complete congenital absence of the nose, or arhinia, is very rare; there are few case reports in the literature. This anomaly includes absence of the external nose and nasal airways, hypoplasia of the maxilla, a small high-arched palate, and hypertelorism (Fig. 7-11). It is usually sporadic and may occur as an isolated defect or in association with other anomalies. An infant with arhinia may or may not have associated CNS anomalies and can be of normal intelligence.[24]

Embryologically, arhinia or arrhinencephaly should be considered to be an anomaly of the spectrum of holoprosencephaly. The most severe malformation of this spectrum is cyclopia in which there is a single median eye and a single-chambered prosencephalon. Arhinia develops early in the fifth week of development when the nasal placode fails to invaginate to form nasal passages. As a result, no septum or sinus cavities develop and development of the external nose depends on prior development of nasal cavities and the nasal septum. Failure of these structures to develop results in arhinia. The associated ocular abnormalities are usually minor as the eye begins to form at an earlier stage. However, these infants can present with anophthalmia or hypoplasia of the orbits.[23,27]

Infants with arhinia may not have respiratory distress until they attempt to feed and become cyanotic. Older children learn to gulp food between breaths, which is referred to as canine eating and can be a serious social concern to these children. They also present with hyposmia and an obvious cosmetic deformity. Surprisingly, other than a nasal quality, the voice is fairly normal. The soft palate usually maintains normal contour and function although there is no basis for development of a competent velopharyngeal valve.[23]

Early management of these patients is with a cleft palate feeder or gastrostomy tube. A prosthetic nose can be used for reconstruction or until the child is older and can undergo definitive surgical repair. Surgery requires removing incisor teeth, creating an airway through the maxilla anteriorly, and releasing the high-arched palate. A split-thickness skin graft is placed over a stent and used to line this passage. As expected, restenosis is a problem, and long-term stenting with serial dilations is required. Reconstruction of the nasal pyramid is a multistaged procedure and may involve tissue expansion, bone or silicone implants, cartilage grafts, and local or regional flaps.[23,24]

Polyrrhinia, or double nose, is another rare anomaly. It is associated with pseudohypertelorism but has been reported as an isolated anomaly. The proposed embryologic mechanism suggests incomplete development of the frontonasal process, which results in separation of the developing lateral portions of the nose. The medial nasal processes and the septum are reduplicated, resulting in the appearance of a double nose.[27]

These patients usually present with a bilateral choanal atresia and require the same initial management. Surgical management includes correction of the atresia initially, and the nasal deformity is corrected by removing the medial portions of each nose and anastomosing the lateral portions in the midline.[24]

Proboscis lateralis presents as a tubular sleeve of skin attached to the inner canthus of the orbit and complete agenesis of the paranasal sinuses on the affected side. This lesion is commonly associated with other CNS abnormalities. The development of proboscis lateralis is uncertain. One theory is that the medial and lateral nasal processes and globular process are absent on the affected side. This results in the maxillary process of the affected side fusing with the globular and nasal processes of the opposite side.

Similar to other nasal anomalies, proboscis lateralis requires preoperative CT or MRI.[24,27] The tube of skin can be excised, and the affected side of the nose is reconstructed to form a nasal cavity. Stents and serial dilation are usually necessary long-term in this circumstance. One author reports limited success with rotating the tube of skin to reconstruct the affected side. It is pertinent, however, to preserve skin from this process to aid in the reconstruction. Bone and cartilage grafts are necessary for support. A prosthetic is a suitable alternative until facial growth is complete and reconstructive efforts can begin.

NASOLACRIMAL DUCT CYSTS

A nasolacrimal duct cyst is an abnormality in the newborn that may uncommonly lead to nasal obstruction and respiratory distress.[17,29]

Embryologically, the nasolacrimal duct system begins as a thickening of ectoderm. This thickening is buried in the mesoderm between the lateral nasal process and the maxillary processes. The duct begins to canalize from superior to inferior. At birth the inferior aspect of the duct has commonly not opened to communicate with the nasal passage. About 30% of full-term infants are born with nasolacrimal duct obstruction. When the proximal and distal aspects of the system are occluded, fluid accumulates and a cyst is formed.[17,29,45]

Patients can present with epiphora, nasal obstruction, and respiratory distress. Infants may have aspiration and difficulties with feeding because of their dependency on nasal breathing to feed. Unilateral cysts present as unilateral nasal obstruction and drainage. The obstruction resolves spontaneously by about 9 months of age in 85% of infants. Cysts that do not resolve spontaneously or cause respiratory distress require intervention.[17,29]

A nasolacrimal duct cyst is diagnosed with anterior rhinoscopy and identification of a cystic mass in the inferior meatus. CT confirms the diagnosis. The triad of a dilated nasal lacrimal duct, an intranasal cyst, and a cystic dilation of the lacrimal sac are classic CT findings.[45]

Management is usually surgical. Initial management includes nasal decongestants and feeding modifications. Indications for surgery include infection, feeding difficulties, and respiratory obstruction. Patients can be easily managed with transnasal marsupialization of the cysts using endoscopic sinus instruments. A carbon dioxide laser may be used, but endoscopic techniques are very successful.[29,45] It is wise to consult an ophthalmologist during the workup of these patients because intervention may be required intraoperatively for nasolacrimal duct probing and placement of nasolacrimal stents.

REFERENCES

1. Arlis H: Congenital nasal pyriform aperture stenosis, *Arch Otolaryngol Head Neck Surg* 118:989, 1992.
2. Bergstrom L, Owens O: Posterior choanal atresia: a syndromal disorder, *Laryngoscope* 94:1273, 1984.
3. Beste DJ, Conley SF, Brown CW: Gastroesophageal reflux complicating choanal atresia repair, *Int J Pediatr Otorhinolaryngol* 29:51, 1994.
4. Brown OE and others: The evaluation of choanal atresia by computed tomography, *Int J Pediatr Otorhinolaryngol* 12:85, 1986.
5. Brown OE and others: Bilateral posterior choanal atresia: a morphologic and histologic study and computed tomographic correlation, *Int J Pediatr Otorhinolaryngol* 13:125, 1987.
6. Brown OE, Pownell P, Manning SM: Choanal atresia: a new anatomic classification and clinical management implications, *Laryngoscope* 106:97, 1996.
7. Brown OE: Current management of pediatric nasal airway obstruction, *Curr Opin OTO-HNS* 3:402, 1995.
8. Brown OE, Myer CM, Manning SC: Congenital nasal pyriform aperture stenosis, *Laryngoscope* 99:86, 1989.
9. Castillo M: Congenital abnormalities of the nose: CT and MR findings, *Am J Radiol* 162:1211, 1994.
10. Cohen SR: Steroid treatment of hemangioma of the head and neck in children, *Ann Otolaryngol* 81:584, 1972.
11. Coniglio JU, Manzione JU, Hengerer AS: Anatomic findings and management of choanal atresia and the CHARGE association, *Ann Otol Rhinol Laryngol* 97:448, 1988.
12. Crockett DM and others: Computed tomography in the evaluation of choanal atresia in infants and children, *Laryngoscope* 97:174, 1987.
13. Dobrowski JM and others: Otorhinolaryngic manifestations of CHARGE association, *Otolaryngol Head Neck Surg* 93:798, 1995.
14. Duncan NO, Miller RA, Catlin FI: Choanal atresia and associated anomalies: the CHARGE association, *Int J Pediatr Otorhinolaryngol* 15:129, 1988.
15. Dunham ME, Miller RP: Bilateral choanal atresia associated with malformation of the anterior skull base, embryogenesis and clinical complications, *Ann Otol Rhinol Laryngol* 101:916, 1992.
16. Edgerton MT: The treatment of hemangiomas: with special reference to the role of steroid therapy, *Ann Surg* 517, 1975.
17. Edmond JC: Congenital nasolacrimal sac mucocele associated with respiratory distress, *J Pediatr Ophthalmol Strabismus* 28:287, 1991.
18. Reference deleted in pages.
19. Reference deleted in pages.
20. Fraser JS: Congenital atresia of the choanae, *BMJ* 2:1698, 1910.
21. Freng A: Congenital choanal atresia, *Scand J Plast Reconstr Surg* 12: 261, 1978.
22. Freng A: Growth in width of the dental arches after partial extirpation of the mid-palatal suture in man, *Scand J Plast Reconstr Surg* 12:267, 1978.
23. Gifford GH: Congenital absence of the nose and anterior nasopharynx, *Plast Reconstr Surg* 50:5, 1992.
24. Pashley NRT: *Congenital anomalies of the nose.* In Cummings CW and others, editors: *Otolaryngology–head and neck surgery,* St Louis, 1993, Mosby.
25. Harley EH: Pediatric congenital nasal masses, *Ear Nose Throat J* 70: 28, 1991.
26. Harner SG: The anatomy of congenital choanal atresia, *Otolaryngol Head Neck Surg* 89:7, 1981.

27. Hengerer AS: *Congenital malformations of the nose and paranasal sinuses*. In Bluestone CD, Stool SE, editors: *Pediatric otolaryngology*, vol 1, ed 3, Philadelphia, 1996, WB Saunders.
28. Hengerer AS, Strome M: Choanal atresia: a new embryologic theory and its influence on surgical management, *Laryngoscope* 92:913, 1982.
29. Hepler KM: Respiratory distress in the neonate, *Arch Otolaryngol Head Neck Surg* 121:1423, 1995.
30. Hughes GB: Management of the congenital midline nasal mass: a review, *Head Neck Surg* 222, 1980.
31. Hui Y, Friedberg J, Crysdale WS: Congenital nasal pyriform aperture stenosis as a presenting feature of holoprosencephaly, *Int J Pediatr Otorhinolaryngol* 31:263, 1995.
32. Jaffe BF: Classification and management of anomalies of the nose, *Otolaryngol Clin North Am* 14:989, 1981.
33. Kamel R: Transnasal endoscopic approach in congenital choanal atresia, *Laryngoscope* 104:642, 1994.
34. Lazar RM, Younis RT: Transnasal repair of choanal atresia using telescopes, *Arch Otolaryngol Head Neck Surg* 121:517, 1995.
35. Leclerc JE, Fearon B: Choanal atresia and associated anomalies, *Int J Pediatr Otorhinolaryngol* 13:265, 1987.
36. Liston SL: Stenting choanal atresia, *Laryngoscope* 90:1061, 1980.
37. McIntosh WA: Transseptal approach to unilateral posterior choanal atresia, *J Laryngol Otol* 100:1133, 1986.
38. Mulliken JB: Bilateral complete cleft lip and nasal deformity: an anthropometric analysis of staged to synchronous repair, *Plast Reconstr Surg* 96:9, 1995.
39. Pagon RA and others: Congenital heart disease and choanal atresia with multiple anomalies: the CHARGE association, *J Peds* 99:223, 1981.
40. Pirsig W: Surgery of choanal atresia in infants and children: historical notes and updated reviews, *Int J Pediatr Otorhinolaryngol* 11:153, 1986.
41. Richardson MA, Osguthorpe JD: Surgical management of choanal atresia, *Laryngoscope* 98:915, 1988.
42. Tavin E: Nasal pyriform aperture stenosis and the holoprosencephaly spectrum, *Int J Pediatr Otorhinolaryngol* 28:199, 1994.
43. Thompson HG: The Cyrano nose: a clinical review of hemangiomas of the nasal tip, *Plast Reconstr Surg* 155, 1979.
44. Wynn SK: Aesthetic reduction of ''Pinocchio''-nose hemangioma, *Arch Otolaryngol Head Neck Surg* 102:416, 1976.
45. Yee SW: Congenital nasolacrimal duct mucocele: a cause of respiratory distress, *Int J Pediatr Otorhinolaryngol* 29:151, 1994.

Chapter 8

Functional Endoscopic Sinus Surgery

Rodney P. Lusk

A large body of literature indicates that pediatric acute sinusitis and chronic sinusitis are associated with significant morbidity and healthcare costs. Chronic sinusitis among patients referred for evaluation has a peak incidence at approximately 3 years of age followed by a gradual tapering. It appears that as a patient matures, the incidence of sinusitis decreases for unknown reasons. Pediatric literature has focused primarily on the maxillary sinus because it is readily available to obtain cultures.[40,41,44,55-57]

Recent literature recognizes the importance of the ethmoid sinuses in the study of pediatric sinusitis.[55-58] The anterior ethmoid cells are involved nearly as often as the maxillary sinuses.[14,15,17,45]

It is difficult to determine the disease's course in any given patient; therefore, therapy should be individualized. Diagnosis is based on the reported symptoms and the physical examination, and it is confirmed through coronal computed tomography (CT). Medical management with broad-spectrum antibiotics to cover the β-lactamase–producing bacteria remains the therapeutic cornerstone. When medical management fails, surgery should be tailored based on the extent of the disease. If the ethmoid and maxillary sinuses are diseased, both are usually addressed at the time of surgery. Surgery should be used only as a last resort, and it should be as conservative as possible.

PATHOPHYSIOLOGY

Some variables that cause recurrent and chronic pediatric sinusitis are (1) inflammatory problems, such as upper respiratory tract infections and allergies; (2) mechanical obstructions, including adenoid hypertrophy, nasal polyps, foreign bodies, and choanal atresia; (3) systemic diseases, such as cystic fibrosis, immotile cilia syndrome, and immune deficiencies; (4) drug abuse; (5) mucosal irritants, such as cigarette smoke and air pollution; and (6) barotrauma as a result of air travel or diving.

The anterior ethmoids, frontal sinuses, and maxillary sinuses drain into a poorly defined area known as the osteomeatal complex. It is hypothesized that if this narrow channel is obstructed because of anatomic deformity or mucosal edema, the cilia do not function normally.[48,49] Secretions accumulate, and the patient is predisposed to recurrent or chronic sinusitis. Any inflammatory response can cause mucosal edema and result in obstruction of the sinus ostia. Inflammation may be the result of viral or bacterial infections, allergies, or other environmental factors (e.g., secondary smoke inhalation). The ostia are often located in nondependent positions, and clearing the secretions requires normal ciliary function.[11,12,34,50,62]

CT of the distribution of sinus disease in the ethmoid and maxillary sinuses showed the same amount of disease in the anterior portion of the anterior ethmoid cells and in the posterior portion of the anterior ethmoid cells. There was also the same amount of disease in the anterior and posterior ethmoid cells. However, comparing the anterior and posterior portions of the maxillary sinus reveals more disease in the anterior portion of the sinus (Fig. 8-1). This is consistent with obstruction at the natural ostium of the maxillary sinus and lends support to the theory that the primary cause of sinusitis is ostial obstruction.

Poor ciliary function is a significant underlying cause of acute and chronic sinusitis.[2,12,21] Messerklinger[34] noted that

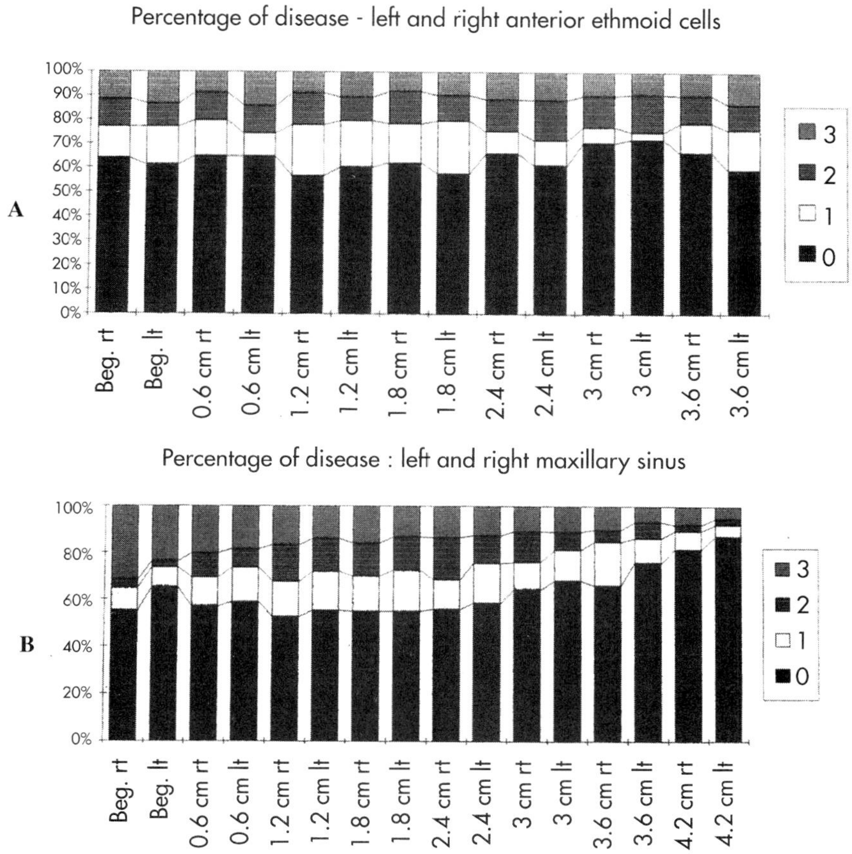

Fig. 8-1. Distribution of sinus disease in **A**, anterior ethmoid cells and **B**, maxillary sinuses at 6-mm intervals. *0*—Clear; *1*—Less than 50% disease; *2*—90% disease but without complete specification; *3*—Complete opacification.

when two mucosal ciliated surfaces come into close proximity, ciliary function and clearance are inhibited and result in secondary pooling of the secretions. Allergies are thought to be a risk factor for chronic sinusitis because inflammation causes destruction of the respiratory epithelium, ciliary dysfunction, stasis of secretions at the ostium, and subsequent infection of the involved sinus.[45,46]

Congenital anomalies that predispose patients to chronic sinusitis are readily identified on CT. Concha bullosa, seen in 16% of pediatric patients (Fig. 8-2, *A*), tends to occur in older children and is usually bilateral. In one study, paradoxical middle turbinates were found on the right side in 4% of children and on the left side in 4.5% (Fig. 8-2, *B*). The incidence of hypoplastic sinuses was 6.9%; infraorbital (Haller) cells were noted in 10% of patients (Fig. 8-2, *C*), and septal deviation was found in 10.4%.

The incidence and the role of esophageal reflux in sinusitis require further definition. Patients who fail to heal after surgery or who manifest excessive granulation tissue may have repeated trauma from gastric acids, thereby increasing scarring and mucosal edema. Figure 8-3 shows CT of a patient who failed multiple courses of antibiotics and surgical procedures for persistent maxillary sinusitis. Such patients are best diagnosed with a pH probe study and managed with antireflux regimens.

SIGNS AND SYMPTOMS

Symptoms of sinusitis vary significantly with the age of the patient and the severity of the infection. Young patients often have nasal congestion, cough, and anterior purulent rhinorrhea as primary symptoms. It is more common for patients to cough at night, but coughing during the day is thought to be a more reliable indicator of chronic sinusitis.[55] The exact cause of the cough and its association with chronic sinusitis remain unclear. Two theories correlate upper respiratory tract infections and cough. The first hypothesizes direct contamination of the airway by nasal secretions, which irritate the airway, causing cough.[1,32,39] The second hypothesizes that a reflex arc from the sinuses to the bronchi causes the cough.[1,3,19,36] Chronic sinusitis has been associated with exacerbations of coughing and bronchospasm in asthmatic patients, and there appears to be a correlation between upper

A

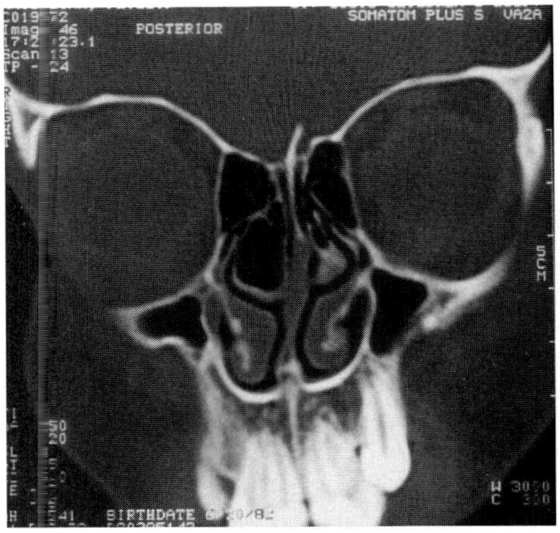

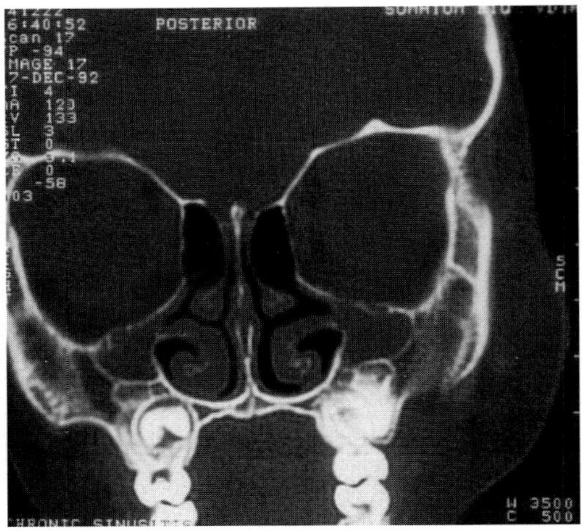

B

C

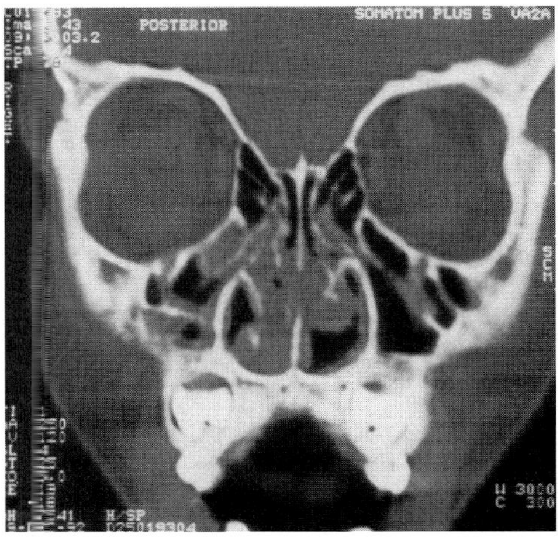

Fig. 8-2. Computed tomography reveals congenital anomalies. **A**, Concha bullosa of the middle turbinate. **B**, Paradoxical turbinates with hypoplastic maxillary sinuses. **C**, Infraorbital cells.

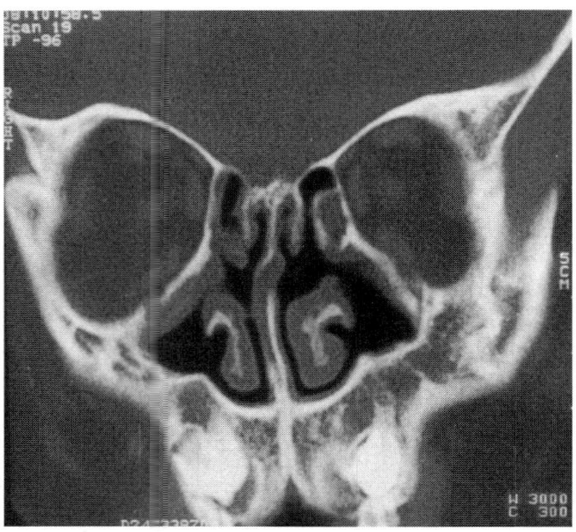

Fig. 8-3. Computed tomography of a patient with esophageal reflux and excessive scarring in the ethmoid sinus and at the ostium to the maxillary sinus.

respiratory tract disorders and the severity and course of asthma.[1]

Older children do not have anterior discharge as a primary symptom, but many complain of a sore throat or postnasal drip (rarely observed in the office because it is cleared by swallowing). In younger patients, anterior purulent rhinorrhea is often noted; low-grade fever is also a common complaint but is rarely documented in the office.

The most quantifiable and consistent symptoms are nasal airway obstruction, purulent nasal discharge, headaches, irritability, and day and night cough.

PHYSICAL EXAMINATION

Regardless of the method used, anterior rhinoscopy is all that can be accomplished in most pediatric patients. The otoscope, a familiar and usually nonthreatening instrument, is best for this purpose. The speculum of the otoscope is positioned beyond the vibrissae to visualize the middle meatus. This should be done with care because touching the septum causes pain and a child is less likely to be coaxed into further cooperation. Sinus disease may be present even though the middle meatus is clear.

The flexible scope can be used with uncooperative children and has the advantage of showing the anterior nose and the adenoid pad. The degree of adenoid obstruction is better assessed when it can be directly visualized with the flexible scope than when it is seen on CT or lateral plain radiography.

In a cooperative patient, the nose may be vasoconstricted and anesthetized for further examination. The most effective vasoconstrictor is 0.05% oxymetazoline; combined 1 : 1 with 4% lidocaine, it provides effective vasoconstriction and produces anesthesia of the nasal mucosa.[43] Purulence or crusting in the anterior nose should be noted. The color of the mucosa may be important. Erythematous mucosa is associated with inflammation or nasal corticosteroid sprays; if the nose is completely obstructed, the mucosa may appear bluish. The size of the inferior turbinates and whether they are causing obstruction should be noted. (However, obstruction may simply be part of the normal nasal cycle; if shrinkage is significant after vasoconstriction, the size is likely related to the nasal cycle.) The head is then extended, the middle turbinate is identified, and anterior septal deviation is noted. The turbinate is examined for evidence of polypoid mucosa or increased size as a result of concha bullosa. Attention is then directed laterally to identify the middle meatus, which is examined for narrowing, purulence, and polyps. Polyps are unusual in the nose of a child and suggest cystic fibrosis. If polyps are found, a sweat test should be performed.[10]

DIAGNOSIS

Differential diagnosis

Chronic sinusitis is difficult to diagnose. The first step is to ascertain whether the patient's symptoms are more consistent with recurrent upper respiratory tract infection or with recurrent acute sinusitis. This can usually be determined by paying close attention to a patient's history. If the patient is managed with antibiotics and the symptoms recur within just a few days, the most likely source of the problem is unresolved sinusitis. No data confirm when the infection is likely to become chronic, but many authors use 3 months as a clinical guideline.

Radiology

Plain film radiography

Plain film radiography has shown a lack of correlation with the findings noted at irrigation, sinoscopy, Caldwell-Luc operations, and coronal CT.[4,22,30,31] Findings are particularly misleading in children because the contents of small sinuses are not accurately depicted.

McAlister, Lusk, and Muntz[31] studied 70 children with chronic sinusitis to see if plain film radiography could identify patients who needed coronal CT. Plain film radiography and CT interpreted independently by pediatric radiologists and neuroradiologists showed no correlation in 74% of patients. The authors concluded that plain film radiography under- and overestimates the amount of disease on CT and was not a reliable screen for sinus disease. The authors believe, however, that plain film radiography has a place in the diagnosis of acute sinusitis in which air or fluid levels are commonly seen (Fig. 8-4).

Computed tomography

CT has become standard for diagnosing the extent and severity of chronic sinusitis. However, the optimal indications and timing have not been defined. The primary reasons for obtaining CT are to document the existence and extent of chronic sinusitis and to look for anatomic anomalies that could increase the risk of a complication. Other reasons include the need to document the disease for further medical therapy, to prove that sinusitis does not exist, to assess the cause of headaches, and to assess potential complications (e.g., subperiosteal orbital abscess formation.)

The presence of mucosal thickening on CT does not necessarily mean that the disease is chronic or that it requires surgical intervention. Lesserson noted that 41% of asymptomatic patients had some evidence of sinus disease, and Diament and others[9] concluded that there was only a 50% chance that opacification represents a sinus infection. To date, no studies correlate the amount of disease noted during surgery with the amount of disease on CT performed on the same day or a day before surgery.

The impossibility of assessing the chronicity of sinus disease with CT can be circumvented in part by using maximum medical management and assessing the amount of persistent disease. If the patient is not premanaged with antibiotics, there is the chance that the disease on CT will be interpreted as chronic and requiring surgery. In many cases, the disease may resolve with conservative management. Endoscopic sinus surgery should be considered as a last resort.

MICROBIOLOGY AND MEDICAL MANAGEMENT

Before surgery is considered as management for sinusitis, antibiotics directed toward the most common causative pathogens should be tried.

Bacterial studies

Few studies have ascertained the bacterial causes of pediatric sinusitis. Most have addressed the acute form of the disease. Bacteriologic studies of pediatric chronic sinusitis are based on tissue cultures rather than purulent secretions. In children, the lack of cooperation limits the ability to satisfactorily study the contents of the middle meatus.

Wald and others[59] found that acute sinusitis is caused primarily by *Streptococcus pneumoniae*, followed closely by *Moraxella (Branhamella) catarrhalis* and *Haemophilus influenzae;* anaerobes were not found often. Because the cultures were taken approximately 10 days after the onset of symptoms, viruses were rarely seen. Wald and others[59] believe that most acute sinus infections resolve spontaneously and that few progress to subacute infections. In

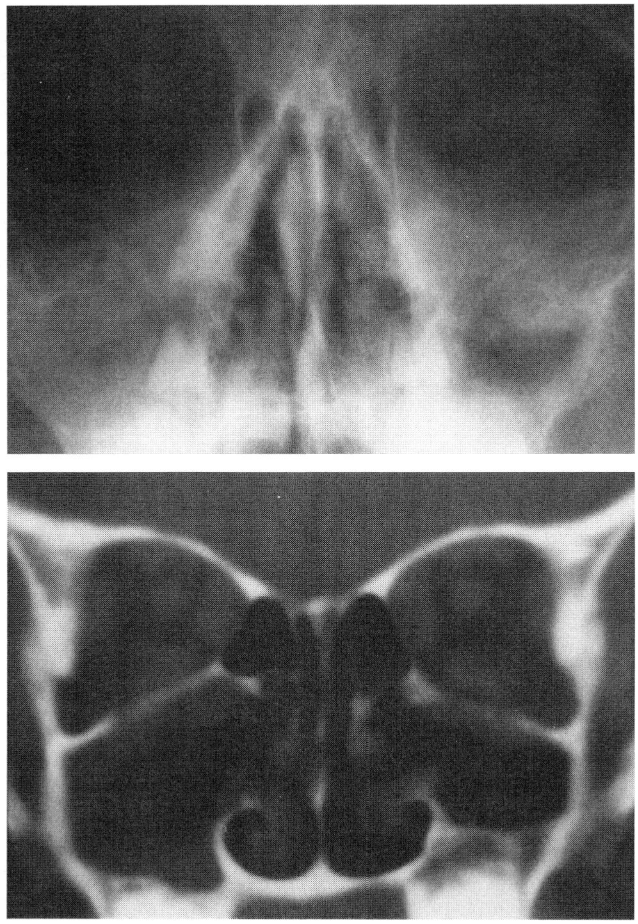

Fig. 8-4. **A**, Postoperative plain film radiography shows opacification of the right maxillary sinus and thickened mucosa of the left maxillary sinus. The ethmoid sinuses cannot be adequately assessed with this method. **B**, Computed tomography taken within 2 hours of the plain film radiography. Note that the ethmoid cells are clear, and the maxillary sinus shows truly thickened mucosa.

this study, the bacterial composition of subacute infections remained essentially the same as that of acute infections.

Brook[5] found increased anaerobic bacteria in patients who had symptoms that lasted longer than 3 weeks. The most common anaerobes were *Peptococcus, Peptostreptococcus*, and *Bacteroides;* the most common aerobes identified were α-hemolytic streptococcus and *Staphylococcus aureus*. Shapiro[49] evaluated 20 patients with cystic fibrosis and found *Pseudomonas aeruginosa, H. influenzae*, and α-hemolytic streptococcus to be the most common aerobes.

Using tissue cultures from the ethmoid bullae, Muntz and Lusk[35] found the principal isolated aerobic organisms to be α-hemolytic streptococcus (23%), *S. aureus* (19%), *M. catarrhalis* (7%), *S. pneumoniae* (7%), and *H. influenzae* (7%) (Table 8-1). They concluded that antibiotic therapy for chronic sinusitis should cover β-lactamase–producing organisms and have a special emphasis on *S. aureus*. The cultured anaerobic bacteria were sensitive to the antibiotics the patients were receiving at the time of surgery and were not cultured in high concentrations.

Antibiotic therapy

The mainstay of therapy for sinusitis continues to be appropriate antibiotics. Management of acute and recurrent sinusitis should be directed toward *S. pneumoniae, M. catarrhalis*, and *H. influenzae* because these bacteria account for approximately 70% of the bacteria that cause acute sinusitis. Currently, 75% of the *M. catarrhalis* and 30% of *H. influenzae* are β-lactamase producers. There also is an emergence of highly resistant strains of *S. pneumoniae*. This organism is a pathogen in children; the leading cause of minor bacterial upper respiratory tract infections (e.g., otitis media, pharyngitis, sinusitis), it may also cause more serious infections (e.g., life-threatening pneumonia, meningitis, sepsis).[61] Recently, resistant strains of *S. pneumoniae* have emerged in response to antibiotic use and perhaps because of day care

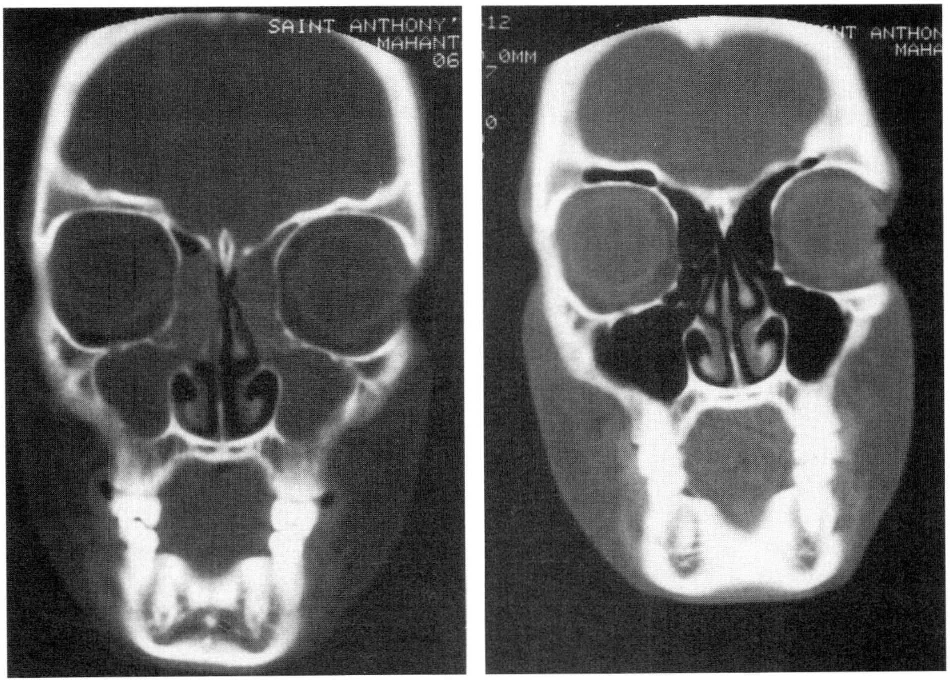

A B

Fig. 8-5. **A**, Computed tomography of a patient with acute sinusitis. **B**, Follow-up computed tomography of the same patient after 6 weeks of antibiotic therapy.

Table 8-1. Incidence of bacteria cultured from ethmoid bullae in children with chronic sinusitis

Bacteria	Incidence (%)
α-Hemolytic streptococcus	23
Staphylococcus aureus	19
Streptococcus pneumoniae	7
Haemophilus influenzae	7
Moraxella (Branhamella) catarrhalis	7
Corynebacterium species	5
Veillonella species	2
Streptococcus	2
Haemophilus parainfluenzae	1
Other	5

environments.[18,42,54] Of particular concern are strains that are resistant to multiple classes of antibiotics.

Amoxicillin with clavulanate potassium (40 mg/kg/day) extends coverage to these β-lactamase–producing organisms and to anaerobic bacteria. Erythromycin (30 to 50 mg/kg/day) with sulfisoxazole (150 mg/kg/day) gives good coverage for the spectrum of pediatric sinusitis. However, this combination should be administered four times a day, and it has a bitter taste. Another alternative is trimethoprim and sulfamethoxazole (1 tsp/10 lb body weight, twice daily), a combination of two folic acid antagonists. The disadvantages of this combination are that it is often hypersensitive to sulfa and its coverage of group A streptococcus is inadequate.[18]

The efficacy of cephalosporins is similar to that of penicillin. First-generation cephalosporins are not active against *H. influenzae* and therefore are not suitable for acute or chronic sinusitis. Among second-generation cephalosporins, cefaclor (20 to 40 mg/kg/day) is somewhat susceptible to the action of β-lactamase producers, and cefuroxime axetil (30 mg/kg/day) gives excellent coverage of bacteria associated with chronic sinusitis. It also has the advantage of twice-daily dosing and is now available as a liquid for young children. Other broad-spectrum antibiotics are available but have not been studied with sinusitis. No studies have used repeated aspiration to assess the efficacy of these drugs in pediatric sinusitis, nor has the appropriate duration of antibiotic therapy been systematically studied. Figure 8-5 shows the resolution of acute sinusitis after 6 weeks of antibiotic therapy. Typically the management of acute sinusitis lasts 10 to 14 days. If improvement is not significant, a different antibiotic and a longer course of management are appropriate. The standard management of chronic sinusitis appears to be 3 to 4 weeks of antibiotics, but this has not been evaluated in prospective studies. Although the efficacy of prophylactic antibiotics is clearly seen in some children with recurrent or chronic sinusitis, no studies have evaluated this, and the potential for developing resistant strains of bacteria has not been adequately assessed.

NONENDOSCOPIC SURGERY

The following nonendoscopic procedures have been advocated in the surgical management of chronic sinusitis in children, but critical information regarding their efficacy is not available.

Tonsillectomy and adenoidectomy

Numerous authors have noted that tonsillectomy and adenoidectomy do not uniformly correct all cases of sinusitis.[6,7,20,38,60] Adenoidectomy has not been efficacious in the management of chronic sinusitis.[37] However, children with large adenoid pads that cause nasal airway obstruction and stasis of secretions have been seen (Fig. 8-6). These secretions mimic the symptoms of chronic sinusitis. When the adenoid pad is removed, the symptoms often disappear. Some authors believe that these children did not really have chronic sinusitis. Cross and others[16] believe that a patent nasopharynx is essential for normal nasal physiology but do not believe that all sinusitis is cleared with an adenoidectomy. They reported that 57% of patients who underwent endoscopic surgery had had unsuccessful tonsillectomies and adenoidectomies. Therefore, it is not reasonable to insist that adenoidectomy is an essential first step in treating pediatric chronic sinusitis. However, it would seem prudent to remove a large obstructive adenoid pad as an initial attempt at surgical management. If symptoms persist, a more thorough investigation for chronic sinusitis should ensue.

Antral lavage

Antral lavage has been described as a diagnostic test and a therapeutic modality for recurrent and chronic sinusitis. In younger children, this procedure cannot be performed through the inferior meatus or without a general anesthetic because the floor of the maxillary sinus is insufficiently developed. The anterior wall of the maxillary sinus is thick, and the tooth buds increase the risk for canine antral lavage. One antral lavage is rarely successful, and several authors have recommended multiple lavages.[8,30,47,53] Because of the small size of the sinus, the need for a general anesthetic and multiple irrigations, and the fact that the ethmoid sinus is not addressed, antral lavage is not feasible for children.

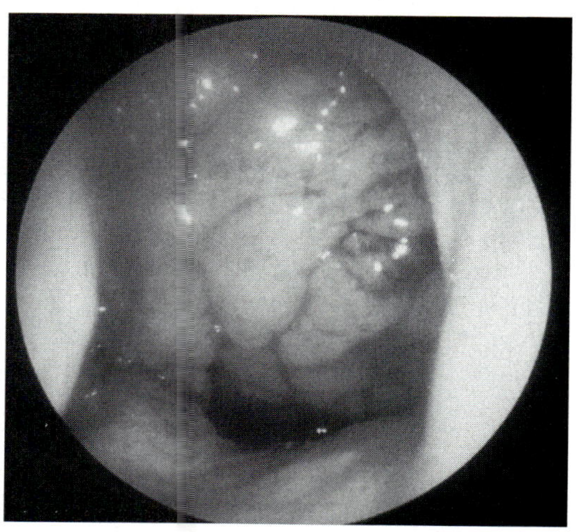

Fig. 8-6. Enlarged adenoid pad causing nasal airway obstruction.

Inferior meatal antrostomy (nasal antral windows)

Lund[28] found that in 45% of adults and in most children, inferior meatal antrostomies were closed at the time of reevaluation. The size of the antrostomy needed to be at least 1 × 0.5 cm to maintain patency, and the high closure rate is likely related to the inability to make the ostium large enough. In most pediatric patients, the inferior meatal autrostomy cannot be made large enough.

Another reason the inferior meatal antrostomy may not function is that cilia continue to carry secretions to the obstructed natural ostium, resulting in stasis of secretions. Muntz and Lusk[35] performed a retrospective evaluation of 35 children who had undergone bilateral inferior meatal antrostomies. They found that symptoms were not controlled in 60% of patients after 1 month and in 73% of patients after 6 months. This procedure has thus been abandoned as a primary surgical modality for managing chronic sinusitis in children. However, inferior meatal antrostomy may have a place in patients with ciliary dyskinesia, in which the cilia do not function normally and gravity may be a factor in improving the drainage of the sinus secretions.

Middle meatal antrostomy

An alternative method of ventilating the maxillary sinus is to open the natural ostium through the middle meatus. Kennedy and others[36] evaluated 117 patients and found 17% of middle meatal antrostomies difficult to perform. However, the ostium remained widely patent in 98% of the remaining cases. Identifying the natural ostium in children is often difficult because the uncinate process should be removed to identify the ostium. Clearing the maxillary ostium of obstruction appears to be the best mechanism for ventilating the sinus, and failure to open the natural ostium is the most prevalent cause of surgical failure. It also may be appropriate in patients with cystic fibrosis.

ENDOSCOPIC SURGERY

Endoscopic surgery has some distinct theoretical advantages when used in children. Messerklinger[33] described the principles for endoscopic sinus surgery, and the procedure was popularized by Kennedy and Stammberger.* Preservation of normal structures and mucosa is especially important in the pediatric population because the sinuses are small and still developing.

Most chronic sinusitis in children is located in the ethmoid and anterior maxillary sinuses. Therefore it makes

* Refs. 13, 23, 25, 26, 48, 49–52.

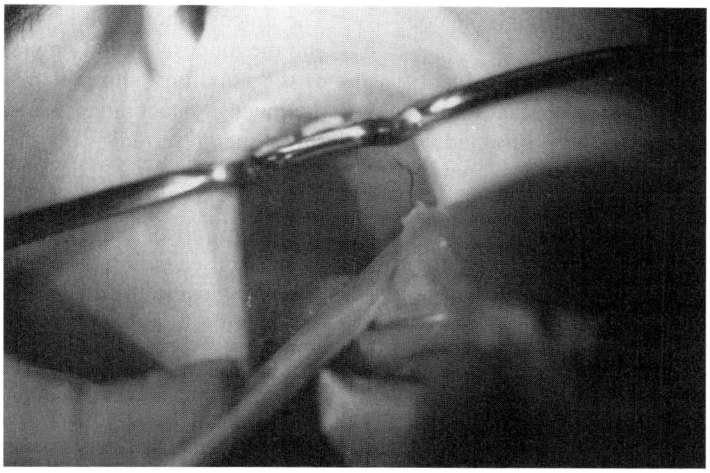

Fig. 8-7. Transoral sphenopalatine artery block.

sense to remove only the limited anterior disease by approaching the ethmoids and anterior maxillary sinuses directly through the middle meatus. In 113 patients who had signs and symptoms compatible with chronic sinusitis, 40% had no disease in the maxillary or ethmoid sinuses, 18% had disease in only the maxillary sinus, 12% had disease in only the ethmoid sinus, and 31% had disease in both sinuses. Thus the distribution of sinusitis is such that if a physician is going to manage the disease surgically, the ethmoid and maxillary sinuses should be opened.

Indications

Surgery should be considered only after appropriate medical management, including several courses of long-term (4 to 6 weeks) broad-spectrum antibiotics and probably nasal corticosteroid sprays, has proven unsuccessful. The patient should have had symptoms for several months. Surgery in a child who has had symptoms for less than 6 months is not recommended unless other factors are involved. To ensure that the disease is chronic, CT should show evidence of disease and be performed after a prolonged course of antibiotics. Indications for endoscopic ethmoidectomy and maxillary antrostomy need to be further refined.

Instrumentation

The Hopkins rod lens telescope is the most recent significant advance in instrumentation for surgery to manage sinusitis. This telescope was initially used for diagnostic work and gradually became a tool to assist in visualization of sinus operations. In adults, it is common practice to remove isolated anterior ethmoid disease and enlarge the maxillary ostium with endoscopic procedures.[23-26,48-50] The same techniques can be applied to children if smaller instruments and telescopes are used.

Technique

General anesthesia is required when this procedure is performed on children. The nasal cavity is vasoconstricted with 0.05% oxymetazoline and examined with a telescope. The authors use transoral sphenopalatine artery blocks with 0.5 ml of 1% lidocaine and 1 : 100,000 epinephrine because they cause additional vasoconstriction (Fig. 8-7). Usually an obstructive adenoid pad will already have been noted, and the decision about adenoidectomy will have been made preoperatively.

The pediatric nasal cavity is best examined with a 2.7-mm 0° telescope. The 0° telescope prevents distortion of the image and allows the nose to be examined with as little trauma as possible. It is difficult to roll the telescope into the middle meatus of a child in the manner described by Kennedy and others.[26] The best way to examine the middle meatus of children is to slightly displace the middle turbinate medially with a Freer elevator and insert the telescope into the middle meatus. Examination of the sphenoid recess in children is difficult even with a 2.7-mm telescope. Some authors recommend that the 4-mm telescope be used in almost all children, but a 2.7-mm telescope decreases trauma to the tissues and should be used more often.[16,27] With practice, the view is not restrictive and the light is adequate.

The uncinate process is identified and removed with a sickle knife or back-biting forceps. Either technique is satisfactory; however, if the patient has hypoplastic maxillary sinuses, the safest way to remove the uncinate process is with back-biting forceps (Fig. 8-8). The uncinate process is best removed with the seeker, and the residual mucosa around the uncinate process is best removed with a mechanical débrider. When all of the uncinate process is removed, the middle meatus is maximally opened, and the chance of trauma to the lateral surface of the middle turbinate is minimized. In other words, increased working space in the middle

parents stated that they would recommend the surgery to others. However, these results probably represent significant bias because the most satisfied parents were most likely to respond to the survey.

Duplechain, White, and Miller[10] found that the number of missed school days was significantly reduced in 88% of the children who had undergone endoscopic sinus surgery. They found endoscopic surgery to be safe, well tolerated, and effective in the pediatric population. In a retrospective study of 52 patients who were followed for an average of 21.8 months, Parsons and Phillips[37] found significant improvement in all symptoms after endoscopic sinus surgery.

The goal of endoscopic sinus surgery is to create a wider opening into the middle meatus to improve drainage. The most common procedure performed, constituting one third of the cases, is bilateral anterior ethmoidectomy and maxillary antrostomy; the second most common procedure is total ethmoidectomy and maxillary antrostomy. According to several surgeons, the degree of improvement is consistent in the 80% range.[10,16,27,29,37]

SUMMARY

Much work needs to be done on the natural history and cause of pediatric chronic sinusitis, but it is undoubtedly multifactorial. Children's immature immune systems and developing anatomies warrant a conservative approach because the situation may improve with maturation. Prospective assessment of the bacterial cause of chronic pediatric sinusitis and the efficacy of antibiotic therapy is needed. Greater understanding about the pathophysiology of sinusitis will allow better medical intervention and appropriate identification of children who require surgical intervention.

REFERENCES

1. Adinoff AD, Irvin CG: Upper respiratory tract disease and asthma, *Semin Respir Med* 8:308, 1987.
2. Afzelius BA, Gargani G, Romano C: Abnormal length of cilia as a possible cause of defective mucociliary clearance, *Eur J Respir Dis* 66:173, 1985.
3. Allison DJ and others: Effects of nasal stimulation on total respiratory resistance in the rabbit, *J Physiol (Lond)* 239:23, 1974.
4. Axelsson A and others: The correlation between the radiological examination and the irrigation findings in maxillary sinusitis, *Acta Otolaryngol (Stockh)* 69:302, 1970.
5. Brook I: Bacteriologic features of chronic sinusitis in children, *JAMA* 246:967, 1981.
6. Carmack JW: Sinusitis in children, *Ann Otol Rhinol Laryngol* 40:515, 1931.
7. Cleminson FJ: Nasal sinusitis in children, *J Laryngol Otol* 36:505, 1921.
8. Crooks J, Signy AG: Accessory nasal sinusitis in childhood, *Arch Dis Child* 11:281, 1936.
9. Diament MJ and others: Prevalence of incidental paranasal sinuses opacification in pediatric patients: a CT study, *J Comput Assist Tomogr* 11:426, 1987.
10. Duplechain JK, White JA, Miller RH: Pediatric sinusitis: the role of endoscopic sinus surgery in cystic fibrosis and other forms of sinonasal disease, *Arch Otolaryngol Head Neck Surg* 117:422, 1991.
11. Eavey RD and others: Kartagener's syndrome: a blinded, controlled study of cilia ultrastructure, *Arch Otolaryngol Head Neck Surg* 112:646, 1986.
12. Fontolliet C, Terrier G: Abnormalities of cilia and chronic sinusitis, *Rhinology* 25:57, 1987.
13. Friedman M and others: Difficult decisions in endoscopic sinus surgery, *Otolaryngol Clin North Am* 22:777, 1989.
14. Goodwin WJJ: Orbital complications of ethmoiditis, *Otolaryngol Clin North Am* 18:139, 1985.
15. Gross CW: The diagnosis and management of sinusitis in children: surgical management: an otolaryngologist's perspective, *Pediatr Infect Dis J* 4:S67, 1985.
16. Gross CW and others: Functional endonasal sinus surgery (FESS) in the pediatric age group, *Laryngoscope* 99:272, 1989.
17. Hawkins DB, Clark RW: Orbital involvement in acute sinusitis: lessons from 24 childhood patients, *Clin Pediatr (Phila)* 16:464, 1977.
18. Henderson FW and others: Nasopharyngeal carriage of antibiotic-resistant pneumococci by children in group day care. *J Infect Dis* 157:256, 1988.
19. Holtzman MJ and others: Effect of ganglionic blockade on bronchial reactivity in atopic subjects, *Am Rev Respir Dis* 122:17, 1980.
20. Hoshaw TC, Nickman NJ: Sinusitis and otitis in children, *Arch Otolaryngol* 100:194, 1974.
21. Karja J, Nuutinen J: Immotile cilia syndrome in children *Int J Pediatr Otorhinolaryngol* 5:275, 1983.
22. Kay NJ, Setia RN, Stone J: Relevance of conventional radiography in indicating maxillary antral lavage, *Ann Otol Rhinol Laryngol* 93:37, 1984.
23. Kennedy DW: Serious misconceptions regarding functional endoscopic sinus surgery, *Laryngoscope* 96:1170, 1986 (letter).
24. Kennedy DW, Kennedy EM: Endoscopic sinus surgery, *AORN J* 42:932, 1985.
25. Kennedy DW and others: Functional endoscopic sinus surgery: theory and diagnostic evaluation, *Arch Otolaryngol Head Neck Surg* 111:576, 1985.
26. Kennedy DW and others: Endoscopic middle meatal antrostomy: theory, technique, and patency, *Laryngoscope* 97:1, 1987.
27. Lazar RH, Younis RT, Gross CW: Pediatric functional endonasal sinus surgery: review of 210 cases, *Head Neck* 14:92, 1992.
28. Lund VJ: Inferior meatal antrostomy: fundamental considerations of design and function, *J Laryngol Otol Suppl* 15:1, 1988.
29. Lusk RP, Muntz HR: Endoscopic sinus surgery in children with chronic sinusitis: a pilot study, *Laryngoscope* 100:654, 1990.
30. Maes JJ, Clement PA: The usefulness of irrigation of the maxillary sinus in children with maxillary sinusitis on the basis of the Water's X-ray, *Rhinology* 25:259, 1987.
31. McAlister WH, Lusk RP, Muntz HR: Comparison of plain radiographs and coronal CT scans in infants and children with recurrent sinusitis, *Am J Roentgenol* 153:1259, 1989.
32. McLaurin JG: Chest complications of sinus disease, *Ann Otol Rhinol Laryngol* 41:780, 1932.
33. Messerklinger W: On the drainage of the normal frontal sinus of man, *Acta Otolaryngol (Stockh)* 63:178, 1967.
34. Messerklinger W: *Endoscopy of the nose*, Baltimore, 1978, Urban & Schwarzenberg.
35. Muntz HR, Lusk RP: Nasal antral windows in children: a retrospective study, *Laryngoscope* 100:643, 1990.
36. Nolte D, Berger B: On vagal bronchoconstriction in asthmatic patients by nasal irritation, *Eur J Respir Dis* 64:110, 1983.
37. Parsons DS, Phillips SE: Functional endoscopic surgery in children: a retrospective analysis of results, *Laryngoscope* 103:899, 1993.
38. Paul D: Sinus infection and adenotonsillitis in pediatric patients, *Laryngoscope* 91:997, 1981.
39. Quinn LH, Meyer OO: The relationship of sinusitis and bronchiectasis, *Arch Otolaryngol Head Neck Surg* 10:152, 1929.
40. Rachelefsky GS, Katz RM, Siegel SC: Chronic sinusitis in children

with respiratory allergy: the role of antimicrobials, *J Allergy Clin Immunol* 69:382, 1982.
41. Racehelefsky GS, Katz RM, Siegel SC: Chronic sinusitis in the allergic child, *Pediatr Clin North Am* 35:1091, 1988.
42. Reichler MR and others: The spread of multiply resistant streptococcus pneumoniae at a day care center in Ohio, *J Infect Dis* 166:1346, 1992.
43. Riegle EV and others: Comparison of vasoconstrictors for functional endoscopic sinus surgery in children, *Laryngoscope* 102:820, 1992.
44. Shapiro GG: Role of allergy in sinusitis, *Pediatr Infect Dis J* 4:S55, 1985.
45. Shapiro GG: Sinusitis in children, *J Allergy Clin Immunol* 81:1025, 1988.
46. Shapiro ED and others: Bacteriology of the maxillary sinuses in patients with cystic fibrosis, *J Infect Dis* 146:589, 1982.
47. St Clair T, Negus VE: *Diseases of the nose and throat*, London, 1937.
48. Stammberger H: Endoscopic endonasal surgery: concepts in treatment of recurring rhinosinusitis. I: anatomic and pathophysiologic considerations, *Otolaryngol Head Neck Surg* 94:143, 1986.
49. Stammberger H: Endoscopic endonasal surgery: concepts in treatment of recurring rhinosinusitis. II: surgical technique, *Otolaryngol Head Neck Surg* 94:147, 1986.
50. Stammberger H: Nasal and paranasal sinus endoscopy: a diagnostic and surgical approach to recurrent sinusitis, *Endoscopy* 18:213, 1986.
51. Stammberger H: *Functional endoscopic sinus surgery*, Philadelphia, 1991, Mosby.
52. Stammberger H, Posawetz W: Functional endoscopic sinus surgery: concept, indications and results of the Messerklinger technique, *Eur Arch Otorhinolaryngol* 247:63, 1990.
53. Stevenson RS: The treatment of subacute maxillary sinusitis especially in children, *Proc R Soc Med* 40:854, 1947.
54. Tan TQ, Mason EO, Kaplan SL: Systemic infections due to streptococcus pneumoniae relatively resistant to penicillin in a children's hospital: clinical management and outcome, *Pediatrics* 90:928, 1993.
55. Wald ER: The diagnosis and management of sinusitis in children: diagnostic considerations, *Pediatr Infect Dis J* 4:S61, 1985.
56. Wald ER: Diagnosis and management of acute sinusitis, *Pediatr Ann* 17:629, 1988.
57. Wald ER: Management of sinusitis in infants and children, *Pediatr Infect Dis J* 7:449, 1988.
58. Wald ER and others: Sinusitis and its complications in the pediatric patient, *Pediatr Clin North Am* 28:777, 1981.
59. Wald ER and others: Treatment of acute maxillary sinusitis in childhood: a comparative study of amoxicillin and cefaclor, *J Pediatr* 104:297, 1984.
60. Walker FM: Tonsillectomy and adenoidectomy: unsatisfactory results due to chronic maxillary sinusitis, *BMJ* 908, 1947.
61. Williams WW and others: Immunization policies and vaccine coverage among adults, *Ann Intern Med* 108:616, 1988.
62. Wilson R: Beat frequency of cilia from sites of purulent infection, *Thorax* 41:453, 1986.

Chapter 9

Salivary Gland Disease

David L. Walner
Charles M. Myer, III

Salivary gland disease in the pediatric population is uncommon. Several pathologic processes cause salivary gland disease; thoughtful history and thorough physical examination are necessary for accurate diagnosis and to formulate an appropriate management plan. The physician should consider that similar disease entities differ in incidence between adults and children. In children, inflammatory disease is more common than neoplastic disease. Inflammatory diseases include acute conditions, which are generally infectious (bacterial or viral), and chronic conditions caused by an obstruction, a granulomatous process, or necrotizing sialometaplasia. However, neoplastic disease should be considered. When a solid salivary gland tumor is identified, the chance of malignancy is greater in a child than in an adult. It is also important to be aware of congenital conditions.

A study of parotid masses in children found that nearly 60% were caused by inflammatory processes rather than neoplasms. The most common inflammatory processes were cat-scratch disease, atypical mycobacterial infections, and reactive hyperplasia of peri- or intraparotid lymph nodes.[18] However, a complete differential diagnosis should be considered in any child with salivary gland disease. The differential diagnosis should include inflammatory disease, neoplastic disease, congenital problems, traumatic injuries, autoimmune disease, and numerous less common processes (Box 9-1).

Anatomy and physiology

The salivary system is made up of the major paired parotid, submandibular, and sublingual glands and the minor salivary glands. The major and minor salivary glands are derivatives of ectoderm. During their development, they pierce the surrounding mesenchyme and arborize before terminating as multiple acini.

It is important to recognize salient differences in the anatomy and physiology of the salivary system in children and adults. The overall proportion weight of the salivary glands to total body weight is nearly the same in newborns and adults. However, in infants, the parotid gland is lighter, and the submandibular and sublingual glands proportionally heavier. Each gland increases in weight by three times in the first 6 months of life and by five times in the first 2 years of life. Histologic characteristics are the same as in adults by the age of 2 years.[20]

The infant parotid gland is rounder than that in the adult. It lies wedged between the masseter muscle and the ear. The gland gradually grows during childhood over the surface of the parotid duct. With regard to the submandibular gland in the infant, it is usually continuous with the sublingual gland.

The facial nerve in newborns and children younger than 2 years of age exits the skull base just deep to the subcutaneous tissue underlying the skin. After 2 years of age, the tympanic ring and mastoid tip start to form, allowing the facial nerve to take a deeper position in relation to the skin. After exiting the stylomastoid foramen, the nerve takes a more abrupt lateral course than in the adult. The marginal mandibular branch of the facial nerve frequently courses over the mandible in a superficial position and can be injured easily if not definitively identified.[48] Parotid surgery is one of the most common causes of facial paralysis in children.[2] Experience with pediatric salivary gland surgery is helpful before undertaking pediatric facial nerve dissection.

Flow in the glands is controlled by the autonomic nervous system. Although almost no saliva is secreted during the

Box 9-1. Differential diagnosis of pediatric salivary gland diseases

- Inflammatory
  - Acute
    - Bacterial
      - Suppurative
      - Lymphadenitis
    - Viral
      - Mumps
      - Human immunodeficiency virus
      - Other
  - Chronic
    - Obstructive
      - Sialectasis
      - Sialolithiasis
      - Mucocele or cyst
    - Granulomatous
      - Mycobacterial
      - Actinomycosis
      - Cat-scratch disease
      - Sarcoid
      - Toxoplasmosis
    - Necrotizing sialometaplasia
- Neoplastic
  - Benign
    - Vasoformative tumor
      - Hemangioma
      - Lymphangioma
      - Vascular malformation
    - Pleomorphic adenoma
    - Other
  - Malignant
    - Mucoepidermoid carcinoma
    - Acinic cell carcinoma
    - Other
- Congenital
  - Dermoid cyst
  - Branchial cleft cyst
  - Branchial pouch cyst
  - Congenital ductal cyst
  - Agenesis of the salivary gland
- Traumatic
  - Penetrating cheek trauma
  - Blunt trauma
  - Radiation injury
- Autoimmune
  - Benign lymphoepithelial disease
  - Sjögren's syndrome
- Other
  - Allergy
  - Chronic sialorrhea
  - Cystic fibrosis
  - Drug induced
  - Pneumoparotitis
  - Systemic conditions

night, resting salivary flow increases during the day and peaks in the late afternoon. An average of 50 ml of saliva is secreted during the day; at mealtime, the flow may be as high as 4 ml/min. About 90% of flow is produced by the parotid and submandibular glands. At rest, the submandibular glands produce the bulk of the secretions. The saliva produced is important for protection of the underlying mucosa from trauma and drying and for maintenance of normal deglutition and dental hygiene.

History and physical examination

The history is important in the evaluation of children with salivary gland disease. The family and primary care physician can help obtain this information, which should include the onset, duration, and severity of symptoms. Swelling may be unilateral or bilateral and may be accompanied by pain. It is important to determine if the complaint is a diffuse swelling or a discrete mass and if it is progressive or associated with intermittent postprandial gland enlargement. The character, quality, and quantity of the salivary secretions are also important. The presence of fevers, chills, or a recent upper respiratory infection should be ascertained. Questioning should elicit any history of trauma, including injury from blunt or sharp objects, animal scratches, or recent dental procedures. The presence of congenital anomalies or cysts should be identified. Awareness of underlying systemic disease, which may include immune deficiency, allergy, or autoimmune disease, can be helpful.

The physical examination should include bimanual palpation of all major salivary glands. This consists of simultaneous palpation of the salivary gland structures intraorally and extraorally. Bimanual examination will help distinguish salivary gland enlargement from cervical lymphadenopathy. It is important to identify if the mass is cystic or solid, tender or nontender, mobile or fixed. Facial movement (cranial nerve [CN] VII) should be assessed for subtle asymmetry or weakness. Symmetry and mobility of the tongue (CN XII) and sensation of the tongue (CN V) should be checked. Careful inspection of the salivary gland orifices should be performed routinely and attention focused to the quantity (minimal, adequate, or excessive) and consistency (serous or suppurative) of the salivary content while palpating or "milking" the gland. Repeat examination may be helpful and necessary to follow the natural history of the disease.

Laboratory studies

Laboratory studies are helpful in some instances. If an infectous etiology is present, following the leukocyte count can help determine if appropriate and adequate therapy is being used. Patients with risk factors or suspicion for human immunodeficiency virus (HIV) need to be tested appropriately. A purified protein derivative skin test and chest radiograph would be appropriate if tuberculosis or atypical tuberculosis are being considered in the differential diagnosis. Aerobic and anaerobic cultures of purulent material draining from duct orifices help direct appropriate antibiotic coverage.

Fine-needle aspiration (FNA) has become a commonly used diagnostic tool to evaluate masses within the head and neck. It is an easy and relatively safe technique for the diagnosis of many palpable or deep lying masses. In adults, as high as 93% of benign and malignant lesions of the salivary glands can be differentiated. Cytologic reports agreed with the final histopathologic diagnosis in 74% of cases.[36] Although Batsakis, Sneige, and El-Nagger[11] stated that FNA of major salivary gland tumors is not clinically useful, other authors use FNA routinely and find it helpful. Cytologic evaluation of sialadenitis shows many polymorphonuclear leukocytes in a background of necrotic cellular debris. In cases due to infection, a culture may be obtained at the time of FNA. FNA is helpful to rule out benign disease and allows preoperative planning in cases that require surgery. Pleomorphic adenoma and Warthin's tumor are relatively easy to diagnose by FNA, whereas cystic lesions and poorly differentiated carcinomas are more difficult to diagnose. The usefulness of FNA often depends on the institution. At an institution with a well-trained cytopathologist, FNA can be a useful diagnostic tool. However, at an institution at which FNA is infrequently performed or the pathologist is not well versed in cytology, the test is not helpful except for differentiating abscesses, cysts, and noninfectious, noncystic lesions.

Radiology

Radiology helps confirm a diagnosis suspected from the history and physical examination. Radiology is unnecessary in most salivary gland diseases. The benefit of the study should be considered, including what additional information it will provide to the diagnosis and management plan versus the cost and potential radiation exposure.

The imaging techniques most commonly used to evaluate the salivary glands include plain-film radiography, sialography, radionucleotide scanning, ultrasonography, computed tomography (CT), and magnetic resonance imaging (MRI).

Plain-film radiography is performed easily and can detect the presence of radiopaque ductal stones. Twenty percent of submandibular calculi and 80% of parotid calculi are radiolucent and thus not visualized.

Sialography involves the injection of contrast medium into the salivary duct, thus outlining the salivary ductal system. Sialography can be used to evaluate calculi, obstructive disease, inflammatory lesions, penetrating trauma, and mass lesions. If calculi are present, a filling defect and possible dilation of the main duct or intraglandular ducts will be seen. Chronic sialadenitis may show sialectasis or ductal ectasia. A salivary fistula or sialocele may be seen following trauma. Malignant lesions often show ductal destruction, irregular borders, ductal encasement, and cystic cavities.[45] Examination should not be performed in the face of acute sialadenitis.

Radioisotope scanning uses technetium to study parenchymal function and mass lesions. This study is best used for detecting Warthin's tumor, which is rare in children.

Ultrasonography can be used alone to detect intrinsic versus extrinsic masses, calculi, and inflammatory lesions. This study also can be used to direct a fine-needle biopsy. Lesions can be measured and easily followed with repeat examinations. Advantages include low cost, avoidance of radiation, and avoidance of anesthesia.

CT is an excellent tool to study intrinsic and extrinsic masses of the parotid gland. A CT sialographic study can differentiate benign from malignant masses, show the relationship of the mass to the facial nerve, and differentiate superficial from deep lobe parotid tumors.[47]

MRI is superior to CT for delineating soft tissues. In addition, contrast-enhanced MRI allows visualization of the course of the facial nerve. Sedation or general anesthesia usually is required to image infants and young children.

Biopsy

Open biopsy is necessary in certain instances, e.g., a solid, firm mass that persists for greater than 6 weeks. An incisional biopsy is inappropriate unless a known malignancy is present and the cell type needs to be determined to direct management. An excisional biopsy is appropriate and should be performed when FNA is nondiagnostic or has a high index of suspicion for a malignancy or when cytopathology is not available.

Appropriate steps in evaluating salivary gland masses are shown in Figures 9-1 through 9-4.

INFLAMMATORY

Acute

Acute inflammatory disease of the parotid gland is generally infectious. It most commonly presents as suppurative bacterial sialadenitis and less frequently as viral sialadenitis.

Bacterial

Acute suppurative sialadenitis. Acute suppurative sialadenitis more commonly occurs in the parotid glands than in the submandibular glands. The more serous saliva of the parotid glands contains less bacteriostatic activity compared with the more mucinous saliva of the submandibular glands.[56] Children commonly incur recurrent and severe acute sialadenitis.[42] Some children may have occurrences only once per year, whereas others may have episodes every few months. The primary cause appears to be salivary stasis and is thought to result from ductal obstruction or decreased production of saliva. Predisposing factors may include calculi, duct stricture, dehydration, autoimmune disorders, and

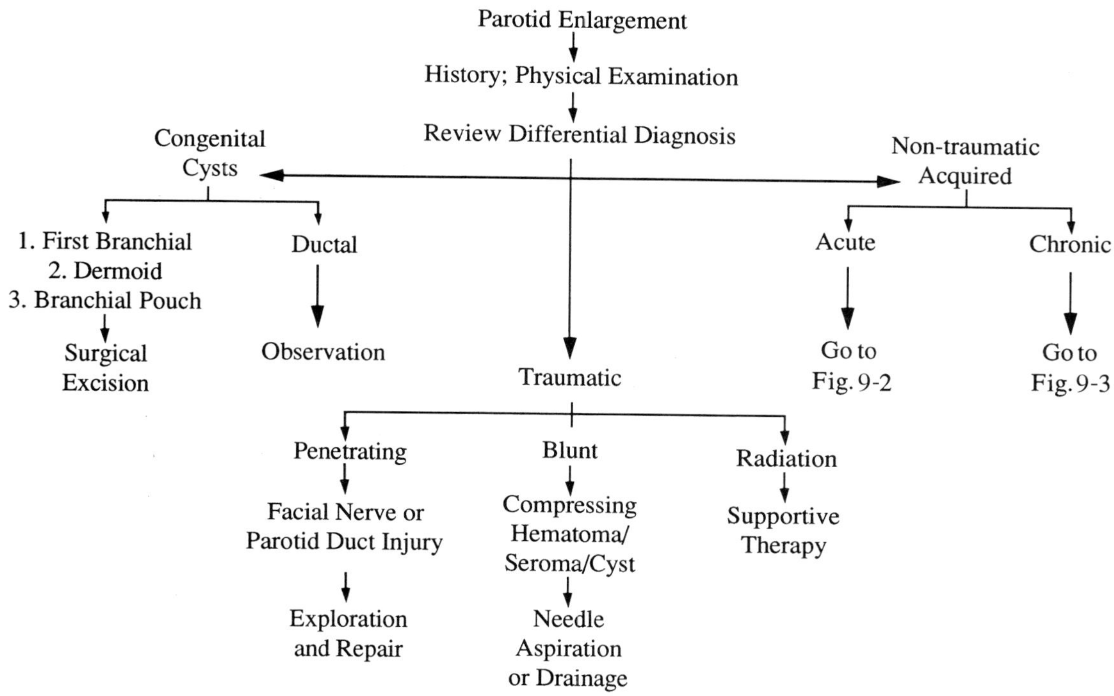

Fig. 9-1. Parotid enlargement.

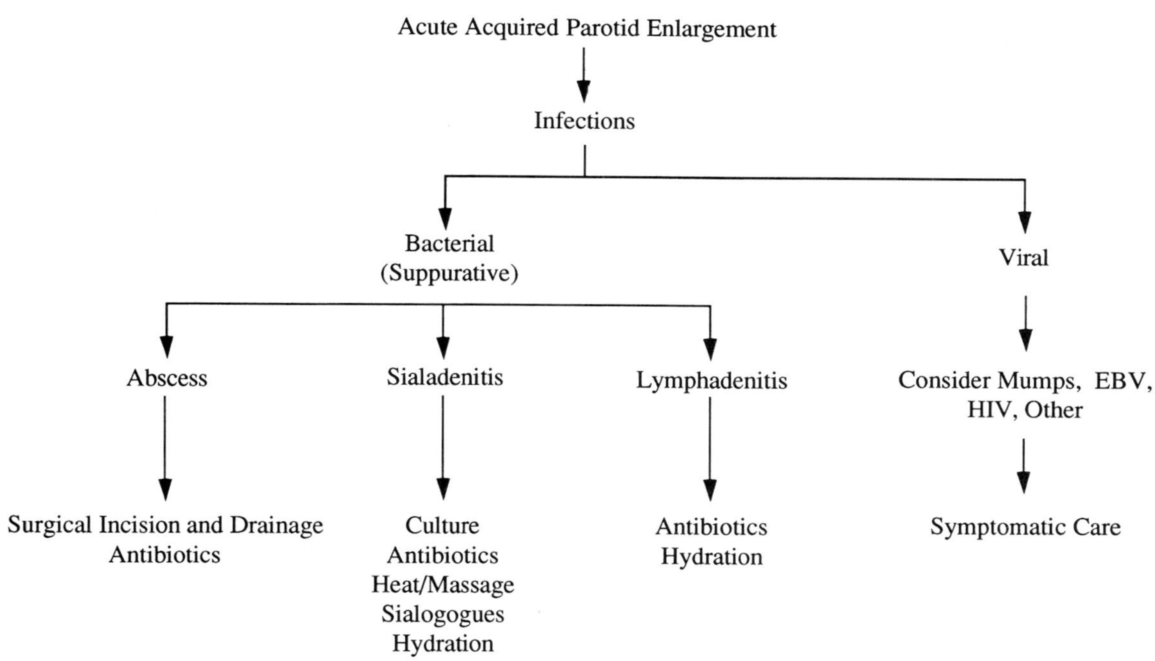

Fig. 9-2. Acute acquired parotid enlargement. EBV—Epstein-Barr virus; HIV—Human immunodeficiency virus.

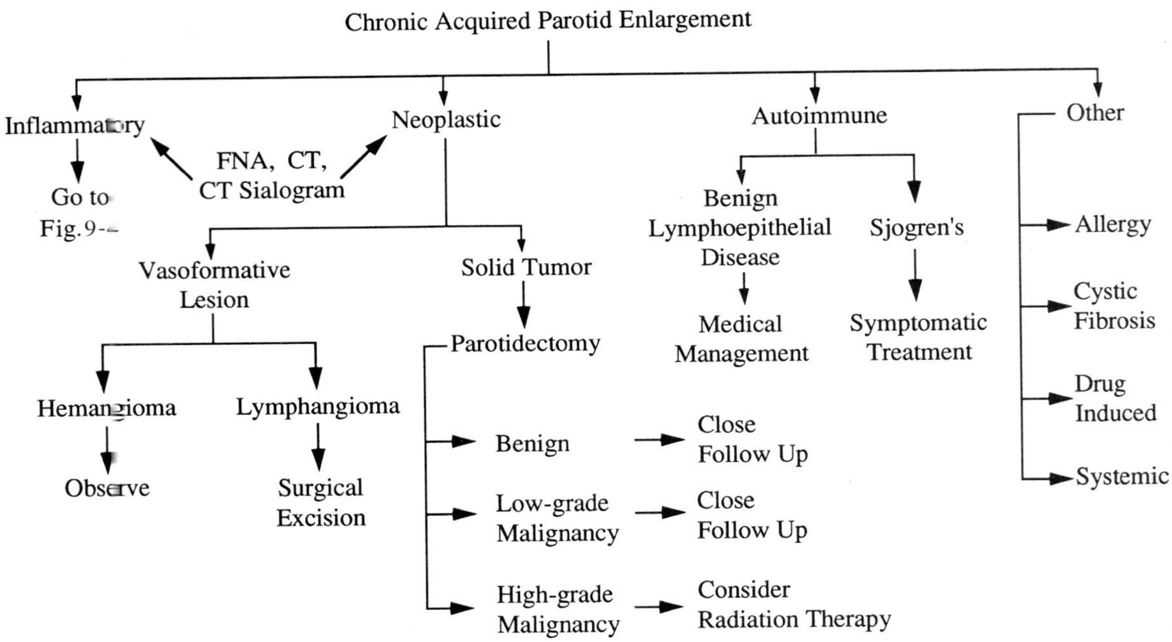

Fig. 9-3. Chronic acquired parotid enlargement.

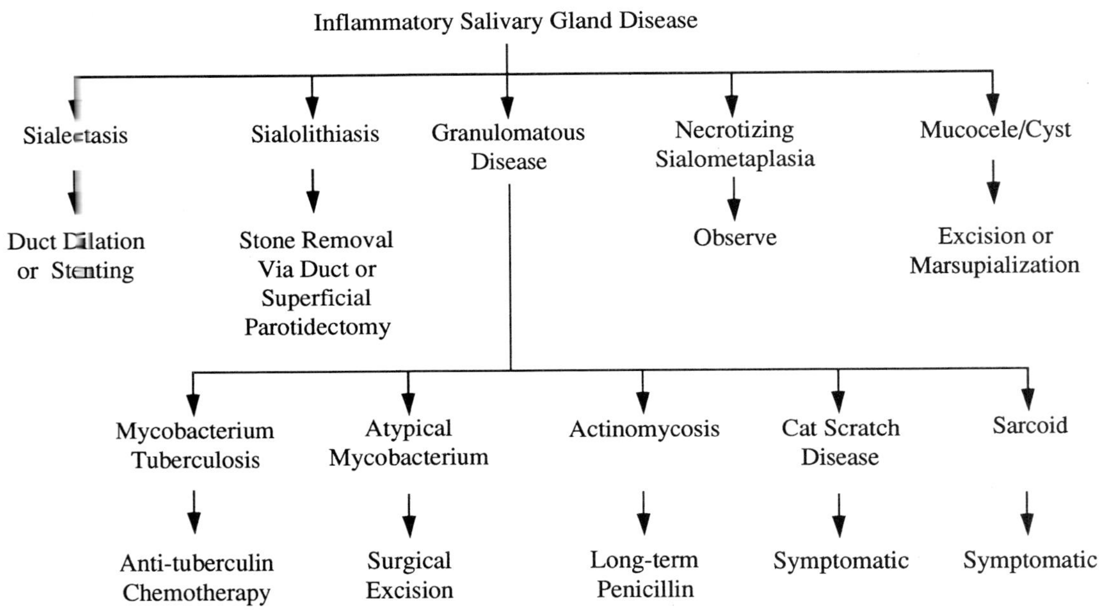

Fig. 9-4. Inflammatory salivary gland disease.

congenital sialectasis. Infrequently, repeated episodes of sialadenitis may include trauma from repetitive biting of the orifice of the parotid duct, dental appliances, and tooth eruption.[65]

Signs and symptoms are characteristic and usually sudden. Local pain and tenderness are observed with edema of the soft tissues overlying the affected gland. Purulent discharge may be seen draining from the involved gland's duct. Most children are otherwise healthy and often remain nontoxic during acute episodes. As the acute phase passes, residual induration and enlargement of the gland may persist for several months. The most common organisms are coagulase-positive *Staphylococcus aureus* and *Streptococcus viridans*. Less commonly identified bacteria include *Streptococcus*

Table 9-1. Acute suppurative sialadenitis

Most common organisms	*Staphylococcus aureus* (coagulase-positive) *Streptococcus viridans*
Less common organisms	*Streptococcus pneumoniae* *Esherichia coli* *Bacteroides melaninogenicus* *Streptococcus micros*

pneumoniae, *Esherichia coli*, *Bacteroides melaninogenicus*, and *Streptococcus micros*[40] (Table 9-1).

Management is similar in adults and children and includes the use of systemic antibiotics, local heat and massage, fluids, and sialogogues (lemon juice, sour candy).[68] A penicillinase-resistant antistaphylococcal antibiotic is recommended for initial therapy and may be adjusted based on culture results or management failure. Rarely, patients not responding to initial therapy may require intravenous antibiotics and hospitalization. Persistent inflammation, progressive edema of the soft tissues overlying the gland, and hyperpyrexia suggest the possibility of an abscess. However, the gland is not fluctuant until very late in the course of the disease because of the multiple fascial investments within the gland. Appropriate workup to rule out an abscess includes FNA with ultrasonography or CT if necessary. If an abscess is identified, surgical incision and drainage is appropriate. Drainage is accomplished through a standard parotidectomy incision with opening of the glandular fascia parallel to the branches of the facial nerve. Multiple drains are placed, and the wound is closed loosely and allowed to heal secondarily. It is necessary to observe for spread of disease into the contiguous fascial spaces of the neck.

Recurrent infections lead to ductal metaplasia with an increased number of mucous glands and saliva that is more viscous and liable for stasis. Once the glandular architecture is altered by several acute infections, the opportunistic oral flora is more likely to cause recurrent acute sialadenitis.[46]

Children often have recurrent acute sialadenitis involving the parotid gland. Each episode should be managed with appropriate antimicrobial therapy. A conservative approach is usually advised because spontaneous resolution generally occurs by puberty. Until that time, gentle probing of the duct during remission may be done to ensure ductal patency.[69] If the patient does not improve spontaneously and sialography shows an alteration in glandular architecture, surgical intervention is necessary. When the submandibular gland is involved, excision of the gland is the management of choice. The procedure is relatively simple to perform and is associated with minimal morbidity.

Historically, recurrent parotitis has been managed by radiotherapy, repeated dilation of the parotid duct, injection of iodized oil into the gland, drugs to decrease the viscosity of the saliva (potassium iodide, pilocarpine), massage, removal of septic foci (teeth, tonsils), oral hygiene, autogenous vaccines, long-term antibiotics, duct ligation, tympanic neurectomy and chorda tympani nerve section, and parotidectomy. Although the most effective and reliable mode of therapy is parotidectomy, many surgeons delay definitive surgery for fear of injuring the facial nerve during surgical dissection. A total parotidectomy with preservation of the facial nerve is the management of choice for recurrent parotitis because superficial parotidectomy alone appears to increase the risk of recurrent disease.[1]

Neonatal sialadenitis. Sialadenitis involving the neonate is a distinct entity. Neonatal sialadenitis is more common in the parotid gland than in the submandibular gland. Because secretions from the submandibular gland have a higher mucous content than parotid secretions, the submandibular gland is rendered relatively immune from infection by the bacteriostatic effects of the mucous. This benefit is diminished, however, when calculi obstruct the duct and retained secretions predispose the gland to infection. Other possible causes of neonatal sialadenititis are anatomic deformities of the oral cavity, dehydration, and prematurity. Approximately 40% of neonates with parotitis are premature for no well-defined reason.

The most common causative organism in neonatal sialadenitis is *S. aureus*. Other organisms that have been identified are various streptococci, *E. coli, Pseudomonas aeruginosa*, and *Branhamella catarrhalis*. The salivary secretions should be cultured and a Gram's stain obtained. The disease is usually limited to a single gland, and signs and symptoms of systemic disease may not be seen. Diagnosis is confirmed by physical examination when a warm, tender, erythematous mass is palpated and pus is expressed from the accompanying salivary duct. Appropriate antimicrobial therapy and adequate hydration result in resolution of the disease in less than 1 week. Recurrence is uncommon.[6]

Lymphadenitis. Lymphadenitis of nodes surrounding the parotid or submandibular gland, or both, can mimic sialadenitis. This may be difficult to determine on physical examination; radiography is helpful in cases not responding to conservative medical management (hydration, antibiotics). Infections involving the scalp, face, or nasopharynx need to be considered.

Viral

For many years, the mumps virus has been considered as the most common cause of viral sialadenitis. Because of the extensive use of the mumps vaccine and the many states that have enacted mumps immunization laws, the number of reported mumps cases continues to decline. According to the National Notifiable Disease Surveillance System, the 1692 cases of mumps reported in 1993 in the United States represent the fewest number of cases ever reported. This was

A
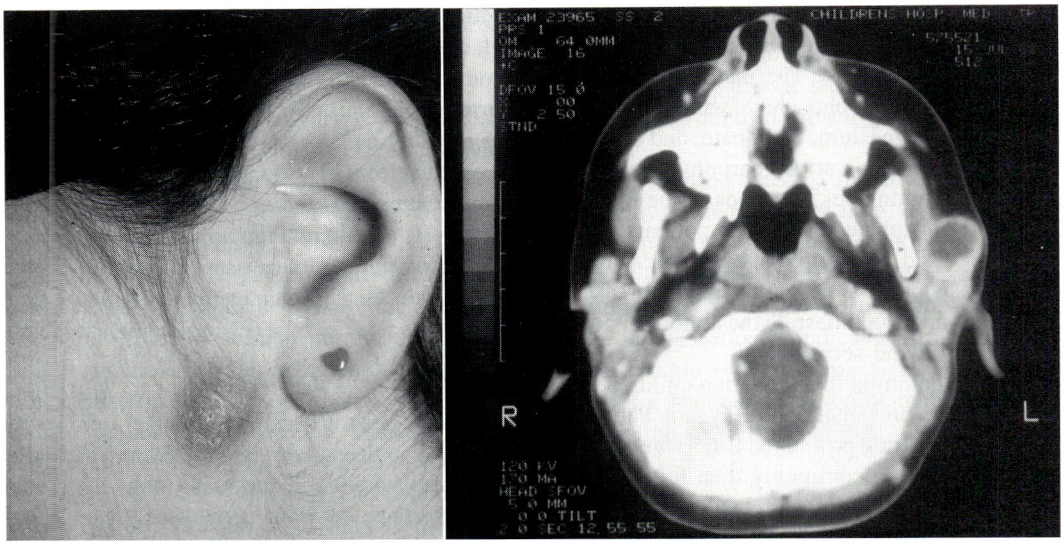

B

Fig. 9-5. A, A patient with an atypical mycobacterium infection involving the parotid gland. **B,** Computed tomography with contrast of the same patient. Notice the rim-enhancing parotid lesion.

and exclusion of other diseases. FNA may help to rule out an abscess; however, culture results can take 6 weeks until an organism is seen. Management of nontuberculous mycobacterial infection usually requires surgical removal of the disease process. If the parotid gland is affected, a superficial parotidectomy with facial nerve preservation is necessary. Antituberculous drugs have not been effective in managing this condition. Use of a macrolide (e.g., clarithromycin) as an adjunct to surgery, especially in cases of incomplete excision, appears to be effective.[61]

Mycobacterial cervical lymphadenitis is known as scrofula. This may be caused by *M. tuberculosis* or an atypical mycobacterium. An excisional biopsy sample of a neck mass should be examined for acid-fast bacilli (AFB). Cultures should be examined for the causative agent. Scrofula caused by *M. tuberculosis* will have a positive chest radiograph in 20% to 50% and a positive PPD. Scrofula caused by atypical tuberculosis will generally have a negative chest radiograph and a weakly positive or negative skin test.[37] Smears or stains for AFB are positive 20% to 50% of the time. Cultures have a 6-week incubation time and in 20% to 50% of cases help differentiate *M. tuberculosis* from atypical mycobacteria. Excisional biopsy is the recommended surgical approach and will reveal caseating granulomas.[3]

Actinomycosis. Actinomycosis is an infectious disease caused by a gram-positive anaerobic organism. Occurrence is usually in the cervicofacial region and frequently involves the salivary glands. Infections often follow dental extraction or oral trauma. The precipitating event allows mucosal invasion of the organism and a slowly progressive inflammatory reaction. Typically, patients have a painless, indurated enlargement of the gland that mimics a neoplasm. Lymph node necrosis characteristically leads to multiple draining cutaneous fistulas.

FNA or fistulous tract drainage culture will reveal the characteristic sulfur granules along with the gram-positive rods. Biopsy specimens are often multiloculated abscesses with whitish-yellow pus. Anaerobic cultures are positive.

Management is with penicillin and consists of a 6-week parenteral course followed by 6 months of oral administration.[27] Cure rates approach 90%.

Cat-scratch disease. Cat-scratch disease is a granulomatous lymphadenitis. Cutaneous inoculation occurs through scratch trauma from a domestic cat. The organism is thought to be a pleomorphic non–acid-fast gram-negative bacillus. Most cases involve the head and neck. The lymph nodes and skin surrounding the parotid and submandibular glands show reticular cell hyperplasia, granuloma formation, and microabscesses.[30]

Patients present with low-grade fever, malaise, adenopathy, and a history of exposure to a cat. A biopsy specimen should be stained with Warthin-Starry silver stain to identify the intracellular bacilli.

Management is conservative and symptomatic. Analgesics, local heat, and aspiration of suppurative nodes can be helpful. Adenopathy generally resolves in a few months.

Sarcoid. Sarcoidosis is an idiopathic granulomatous disease. Sarcoidosis clinically affects the salivary glands in 6% of adults and histologically in 30%.[25] Sarcoidosis is less common in children but, when present, occurs in the second decade of life. It presents with bilateral diffuse enlargement of the parotid glands. Uveoparotid fever (Heerfordt's syndrome) is a form of sarcoidosis characterized by uveitis, parotid enlargement, and facial paralysis. Symptoms may include fever, malaise, weakness, nausea, and night sweats.

Chest radiography looking for hilar adenopathy and an acetylcholinesterase level will assist with the diagnosis. A biopsy from the lip or tail of the parotid will confirm the diagnosis. The disease is self-limited, so no specific management is necessary with regard to salivary gland disease. Systemic involvement or complications may necessitate corticosteroid use.

Toxoplasmosis. The responsible organism is *Toxoplasmosis gondii*, generally in a domestic cat. When this disease involves the parotid gland, it is usually through single or multiple intra- or periparotid lymph nodes. The lymphadenopathy may wax and wane for months and finally resolve spontaneously. The disease is most commonly limited to the lymph nodes but may become disseminated. When dissemination occurs, the patient can develop myocarditis, pericarditis, and hepatosplenomegaly. Serologic testing is the only way to make a definitive diagnosis. Management is supportive unless disseminated disease has occurred.

Tularemia. The rabbit has been implicated as the host of this gram-negative organism called *Francisella tularensis*. A papule is found at the entry site of the disease and may involve the parotid gland with associated lymphadenopathy. Aminoglycoside therapy is used with persisting disease managed by surgical excision.

Necrotizing sialometaplasia

Necrotizing sialometaplasia is a benign, self-healing (reactive) inflammatory process of salivary gland tissue that clinically and histologically mimics a malignant neoplasm.[63] It most commonly affects adults but has been reported in adolescents. It arises in mucus-secreting cells and can be found in the maxillary sinus, nasal cavity, parotid gland, sublingual gland, hard and soft palate, retromolar trigone, lower lip, and tongue. Its clinical appearance ranges from minor submucosal edema with overlying erythema to an erosive ulcer. It usually presents as a painless ulcerated lesion or a nodular swelling. Most cases involving the extrapalatal minor salivary glands and major salivary glands are iatrogenically induced after surgery, trauma, or radiotherapy, with a mean duration of 18 days from the insult to the development of the lesion. In the major salivary glands, necrotizing sialometaplasia occurs secondary to focal lobular sialadenitis and prior surgical manipulation.[10] Typically, the process appears as a 1- to 3-cm crater-like ulcerative lesion. Histologically, lobular necrosis is present with pools of mucin that elicit a granulation tissue reaction with associated acute and chronic inflammation. In addition, extensive squamous cell metaplasia is present.

The lesion heals spontaneously in 6 to 12 weeks. Although total excision of the lesion may be carried out as definitive therapy, it is not necessary or indicated.[24]

Table 9-2. Salivary gland neoplasms in children

Benign*		Malignant†	
Hemangioma	111	Mucoepidermoid carcinoma	122
Mixed tumor	94	Acinic cell carcinoma	30
Vascular proliferative tumor	40	Undifferentiated carcinoma	22
Lymphangioma	18	Adenocarcinoma	19
Lymphoepithelial tumor	3	Adenoid cystic carcinoma	16
Cystadenoma	3	Malignant mixed tumor	10
Warthin's tumor	3	Rhabdomyosarcoma	6
Plexiform neurofibroma	2	Undifferentiated sarcoma	5
Xanthoma	2	Mesenchymal sarcoma	5
Neurolemmoma	1	Unclassified carcinoma	4
Adenoma	1	Squamous cell carcinoma	3
Lipoma	1	Lymphoma	3
TOTAL	279	Ganglioneuroblastoma	1
		TOTAL	246

* Adapted from Schuller DE, McCabe BF: Salivary gland neoplasms in children, *Otolaryngol Clin North Am* 10:399, 1977.

† Adapted from Shikhani AH, Johns ME: Tumors of the major salivary glands in children, *Head Neck Surg* 10:257, 1988.

NEOPLASTIC

Salivary gland neoplasms in children are uncommon. In most large reviews, less than 5% of salivary gland neoplasms occur in patients 16 years of age or younger.[43] Salivary gland tumors account for 8% of all pediatric head and neck tumors.[53] In children and adults, the parotid is the most common location for salivary gland tumors. Several features are important when comparing salivary gland neoplasms in children and adults. Children have more vasoformative tumors, whereas adults have more solid tumors. A solid salivary gland neoplasm is more likely to be malignant in a child than in an adult. Low-dose radiotherapy has been implicated in the development of salivary gland neoplasms.[33] The most common salivary gland neoplasm in neonates and infants is the vasoformative tumor. The most common epithelial tumor in children is the pleomorphic adenoma (Table 9-2). The most common malignant salivary gland neoplasms in children are mucoepidermoid and acinic cell carcinomas.[38] If vasoformative tumors are excluded, approximately 50% of salivary gland tumors in children are malignant.[34]

Benign

Vasoformative tumors

Vasoformative tumors include hemangiomas, lymphangiomas, and vascular malformations. Vasoformative tumors are nonepithelial and comprise the greatest percentage of salivary gland neoplasms in neonates and infants.

Hemangiomas. Hemangiomas of the parotid gland are the most frequent tumor of any type in the first year of life and occur most often in girls and on the left side. Most are

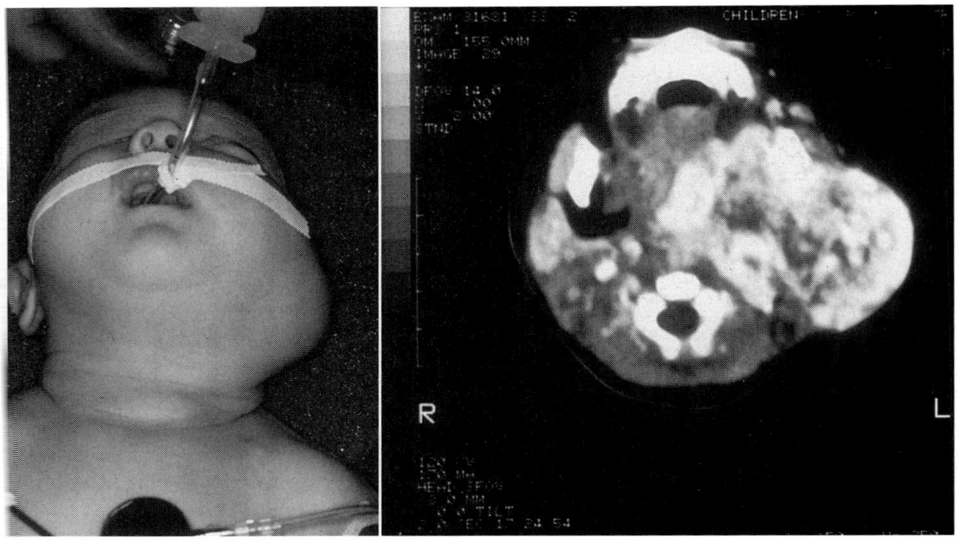

A B

Fig. 9-6. **A,** A patient with a hemangioma of the parotid gland. **B,** Computed tomography with contrast shows a parotid gland mass consistent with a hemangioma and extension into the retropharyngeal space.

identified within 1 month of birth, and 90% are identified within the first year of life. Eighty percent are single lesions, whereas 20% are multiple lesions. Of salivary gland hemangiomas, 80% occur in the parotid gland, 18% in the submandibular gland, and 2% in the minor salivary glands.[51] Hemangiomas can cause the parotid gland to increase up to five times its normal size.[7] The tumor generally is contained within the intracapsular portion of the gland and rarely extends into the submucosal tissues or skin (Fig. 9-6). Histologically, the number of lobules of the gland increases, but the general lobular architecture is preserved. The parenchyma is replaced by vasoformative elements, specifically endothelial proliferation with vascular differentiation. The acini and ductal structures are unaffected. A lymphangiomatous component can also be present.[49] Several types of hemangiomas have been identified histologically, including capillary, cavernous, mixed, and hypertrophic. Separation of these types is relatively arbitrary, and the lesions are most likely part of a broad continuum.[12]

Hemangiomas usually are discovered at or shortly after birth. The patients have facial asymmetry and a fluctuant mass. The tumor is soft to rubbery and usually asymptomatic. In 50% of cases, a parotid hemangioma is associated with other cutaneous hemangiomas.[64] After it appears, the hemangioma grows rapidly over months and plateaus for a period of time prior to its slow but progressive involution. Of affected children, 50% have complete involution of the lesion by age 5 years, 70% have involution by 7 years of age, and 90% by 9 years of age. The earlier the involution, the more complete.[28]

Diagnosis is usually by history and physical examination. If necessary, CT or MRI will confirm the diagnosis. Biopsy is unnecessary, however, if the mass is firm, painful, or rapidly grows, histologic sampling may be necessary to rule out a malignancy.

Most of these tumors undergo spontaneous involution, which requires the use of observation to follow up most of these lesions. Potential complications of hemangiomas may include a localized consumptive coagulopathy known as the Kasabach-Merritt syndrome. Excision of a salivary gland hemangioma is indicated when there is excessively rapid growth of the mass, functional impairment, infection, hemorrhage, or ulceration or complete involution has not occurred and residual disease is causing a functional or cosmetic problem. Surgery, if necessary, would include a subtotal parotidectomy with facial nerve preservation or total submandibular gland excision. Other possible methods of management are systemic corticosteroids and the application of pressure.[41]

Lymphangiomas. The second type of vasoformative tumor found in the salivary glands is the lymphangioma (cystic hygroma). These tumors are soft, painless, compressible benign masses that represent areas of regional lymphatic dilation. Lymphangiomas have been divided into three histologic groupings (simple or capillary, cavernous, cystic) depending on the size of the lymph channels present. All the histologic patterns may coexist in the same lesion.[15] Unlike hemangiomas, salivary gland lymphangiomas do not replace the normal glandular parenchyma. Rather, islands of normal salivary tissue are next to thin-walled lymph-containing vessels.

Lymphangiomas are commonly seen shortly after birth. Approximately 50% to 60% of patients present with these tumors before age 1 and about 90% of the tumors occur prior to the end of the second year of life. The growths may be located in any of the major or minor salivary glands and

A

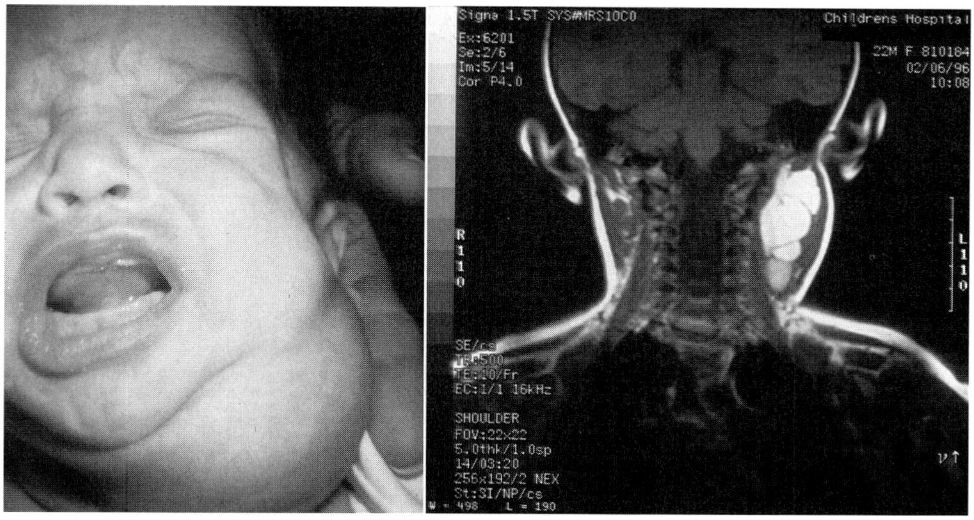

B

Fig. 9-7. **A,** Lymphangioma with involvement of the submandibular and parotid glands. **B,** Magnetic resonance imaging (T1-weighted) shows multiple loculated spaces consistent with a lymphangioma.

usually present as an asymptomatic fluctuant mass (Fig. 9-7). Gradual enlargement can be associated with extension into the neck or mediastinum, with hemorrhage or infection complicating the situation.

The diagnosis can be confirmed when cystic areas are seen with septations on imaging with ultrasound, CT, or MRI.

Unlike hemangiomas, lymphangiomas infrequently undergo spontaneous resolution. Because of this, surgical excision is the only acceptable therapy. Complete surgical excision is the goal; however, healthy structures should not be sacrificed. Definitive therapy usually can be delayed until the child is several years old to make surgical dissection less difficult. Prompt removal of lymphangiomas is necessary when the potential for airway obstruction exists. This potential is highest in tumors of the sublingual glands, submandibular glands, or minor salivary glands. A tracheotomy may be necessary if lymphangioma cannot be removed completely. Recurrence of lymphangioma is uncommon when all evidence of gross tumor is removed. If residual disease remains, recurrence is estimated to occur in approximately 15% of cases.[32]

Vascular malformation. Vascular malformations are the third type of vasoformative lesion. Most are noted at birth and tend to grow with the child. These lesions are divided into low- and high-flow lesions. CT and MRI play a part in workup and therapy and can include embolization, sclerosing agents, and surgery.

Pleomorphic adenoma (benign mixed tumor)

The most common nonvascular or epithelial salivary gland tumor in children is the pleomorphic adenoma.[52] In the pediatric age group, the peak incidence is at 10 years of age. The terms *pleomorphic adenoma* and *benign mixed tumor* are used interchangeably. The original terminology of benign mixed tumor was used to incorporate the two components of the tumor, mesenchymal and epithelial.

The tumor most often presents as a slow-growing, firm, discrete, nodule that is freely mobile and about 1 cm in diameter. Facial paralysis is unusual. Although the tumors appear encapsulated, they have a highly lobular architecture that prohibits enucleation as a therapeutic alternative. Multiglandular involvement in children would be very unusual. Most of these tumors are 1 to 3 cm when diagnosed, which is often greater than 1 year from the time they were first recognized.

The diagnosis can be made by FNA. If FNA is inadequate or unavailable, biopsy consisting of a lateral parotid lobectomy with facial nerve preservation or a submandibular gland excision is appropriate.

Management of pleomorphic adenoma consists of a superficial parotidectomy with facial nerve preservation if the parotid gland is involved or submandibular gland excision if the submandibular gland is involved. Rarely, a mixed tumor abutting the parotid gland but not infiltrating it can be removed with a completely intact capsule sparing parotid tissue and facial nerve dissection. Recurrence after superficial parotidectomy for pleomorphic adenoma in the pediatric population is reported by Shikhani and Johns to be as high as 19.5%.[53]

Other benign neoplasms

Several rare benign neoplasms have been described in the pediatric population. These include basal cell adenoma plexiform neurofibroma, teratoma, papillary cystadenolymphomatosum (Warthin's tumor), xanthoma, neurolemmoma, and lipoma.

Malignant

A child who presents with a firm salivary gland mass should be suspected of harboring a malignancy. As mentioned, if vasoformative lesions are excluded, 50% of pediatric salivary gland tumors are malignant, whereas in adults, only about 25% of salivary gland neoplasms are malignant.[13]

Malignant salivary gland neoplasms are more frequently symptomatic than benign lesions. Local pain and facial paralysis suggest malignancy. When tumors grow rapidly, a high grade malignancy is suggested. In addition, neoplasms in the submandibular glands and the minor salivary glands are much more likely to be malignant than parotid neoplasms. Metastatic disease can be present in the regional lymph nodes or distantly.

FNA may be performed as an initial diagnostic test. When this is not available or inconclusive, a parotidectomy is necessary for diagnosis. Incisional biopsy of a salivary gland neoplasm should never be performed. CT, MRI, or both can help delineate the tumor and help preoperative planning.

Mucoepidermoid carcinoma and acinic cell carcinoma account for 60% of the malignant epithelial salivary neoplasms in children.

Mucoepidermoid carcinoma

Mucoepidermoid carcinoma is the most common malignant epithelial salivary gland neoplasm in children, accounting for approximately 50% of salivary gland malignancies. Most are low-grade lesions that tend to have a good prognosis.[17] Mucoepidermoid carcinomas are composed of cells with squamous differentiation and cells with mucinous differentiation. Lower grade neoplasms are commonly cystic, showing predominant mucinous differentiation. Higher grade neoplasms show greater squamous differentiation and resemble squamous cell carcinoma.[23]

Management is essentially the same in children and adults. Low-grade malignancies of the parotid gland are managed by an appropriate parotidectomy sufficient to remove the tumor with a generous cuff of normal parotid, preserving the facial nerve. The lymph nodes around the digastric triangle should be evaluated at the time of surgery and, if involved, a neck dissection should be done. High-grade malignancies are managed with total parotidectomy. The facial nerve is preserved in all cases unless gross tumor invasion into the nerve is present. If tumor is invading the nerve, resection of the nerve should be performed until frozen sections reveal no further disease. In this scenario, immediate facial nerve grafting is performed. Postoperative radiotherapy is often given to patients with high-grade malignancies.[31]

Submandibular gland malignancies are managed with submandibular gland excision and submandibular triangle nodal dissection. High-grade tumors are often given postoperative radiotherapy. Ten-year survival rates for low-grade mucoepidermoid carcinoma have approached 95%.[19]

Acinic cell carcinoma

Acinic cell carcinoma counts for approximately 12% of the total number of epithelial malignancies of the salivary gland in children.[35] Most acinic cell carcinomas are low-grade malignancies. They are characterized by cells with bland nuclei and an abundant basophilic cytoplasm.

Patients present with a slow-growing solitary mass with or without associated pain. Management is the same as low-grade mucoepidermoid carcinoma: an appropriate parotidectomy sufficient to remove the tumor with a generous cuff of normal parotid tissue, preserving the facial nerve.

Other malignant neoplasms

Adenocarcinoma and undifferentiated carcinoma, adenoid cystic carcinoma, and malignant mixed tumors are rare but can occur in the pediatric population.[29] Primary sarcomas of the salivary glands in children also are uncommon. When present, rhabdomyosarcoma is the most common.

An epithelial salivary gland tumor identified in the first month of life is termed an *embryoma* or *sialoblastoma* and is malignant in 25% of cases. These tumors are usually classified as adenocarcinomas or adenoid cystic carcinomas.[9]

CONGENITAL

Congenital salivary gland cysts are most frequently found in the parotid gland. They can be classified as dermoid cysts, branchial cleft cysts, branchial pouch cysts, and congenital ductal cysts.

Dermoid cysts

Dermoid cysts consist of keratinizing squamous epithelium with associated skin appendages (e.g., hair follicles, sweat glands, sebaceous glands). They are composed of elements from all three germinal layers. Dermoid cysts usually appear as isolated masses within the substance of the parotid gland. Total removal is necessary to prevent recurrence; this is best accomplished by a subtotal parotidectomy with facial nerve preservation.

Branchial cleft cysts

Patients with first branchial abnormalities usually present with unilateral painless swelling of the parotid gland (Fig. 9-8). Bilateral swelling is rare. The first arch branchial cysts account for less than 1% of all branchial anomalies.[4] These cysts have been classified by Work[67] as types I and II.

Type I branchial defects are duplication anomalies of the membranous external auditory canal. These defects are composed only of ectoderm. Located within the periauricular soft tissues and the parotid gland, they commonly present as sinus tracts or areas of localized swelling near the postauricular sulcus, concha, or anterior tragus. The tympanic membrane and middle ear space are rarely involved. Complete surgical removal is curative. Histologic examination

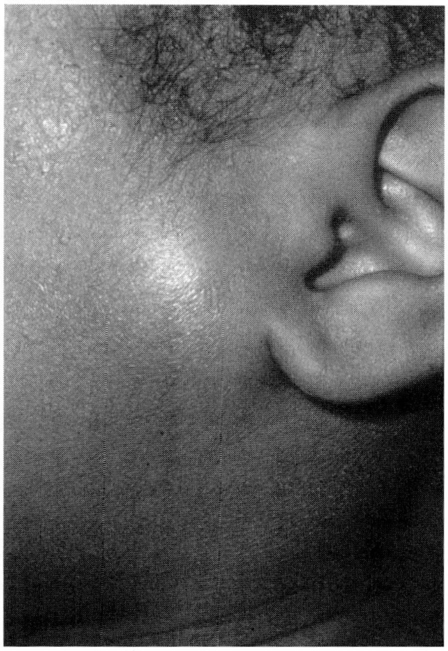

Fig. 9-8. A first branchial cleft anomaly that has become an infected cyst.

reveals a squamous epithelial lining without skin appendages. When the lesion extends into the parotid gland, the facial nerve should be identified and preserved.

Type II first branchial anomalies are less common. The defect is a duplication anomaly consisting of an anomalous membranous and cartilaginous external auditory canal. Unlike type I cysts, type II cysts are composed of ectoderm (squamous epithelium, hair follicles, sweat glands, sebaceous glands) and mesoderm (cartilage). They commonly present in the upper neck immediately posterior or inferior to the angle of the mandible and can extend into the external auditory canal or middle ear cavity. Abscess formation is common, and a fistula or sinus tract also may be present. Complete surgical excision during an asymptomatic period is the management of choice. The cyst is frequently near the facial nerve and may lie medial, lateral, or between branches of the nerve. Careful identification of the facial nerve during the surgical dissection is essential.

Branchial pouch cysts

Branchial pouch cysts are associated with first branchial pouch anomalies and usually occur in the retromandibular portion of the parotid gland. Management is similar to that of other congenital cysts, with complete surgical excision being diagnostic and therapeutic.

Congenital ductal cysts

Congenital ductal cysts generally manifest in infancy. Children with these congenital retention cysts of the parotid gland present with enlargement of the gland. The diagnosis is confirmed with sialography. Observation is advised unless there are multiple episodes of infection.

Agenesis of the salivary glands

Agenesis of the major salivary glands has been reported.[60] Diagnosis can be confirmed with pertechnetate nuclear medicine imaging. The scan may be diagnostic in a child with idiopathic xerostomia. Early identification is important so that proper oral hygiene can be started.

TRAUMATIC

Injury to the major salivary glands is often a component of multiple trauma. When this occurs, major systemic injuries should be managed before dealing with the salivary gland injury. When evaluating trauma to the parotid gland, a physician should be concerned primarily with injuries to the facial nerve and the parotid duct. Injuries may be external, intraoral, or combined. The traumatic event may be caused by penetration of the cheek, blunt trauma to the parotid, radiation, or a foreign body.

Penetrating cheek trauma

Most salivary gland injuries are seen in association with penetrating wounds of the cheek; few cause serious injury to the facial nerve or salivary duct system.[5] Any penetrating wound deep to the parotideomasseteric fascia can injure these structures. If the laceration extends anterior to a line dropped from the lateral canthus of the eye, the facial nerve does not need to be explored. Satisfactory reinnervation will occur through peripheral nerve branches. When a laceration is posterior to this line and the facial nerve is paralyzed, exploration of the wound and reapproximation of the proximal and distal segments of the nerve are obligatory.

Exploration of the facial nerve should occur within 72 hours of the injury so that electrical stimulation of the distal segment is possible. Epineural repair of the severed branches can be accomplished with the aid of an operating microscope. A 6-0 to 8-0 nylon suture is ideal for this purpose. If tension exists on the suture line, a cable graft is preferable. The best results are obtained when the anastomosis is accomplished with fresh, sharp nerve ends. Recovery of facial nerve function after transection and repair requires 6 to 12 months.

The parotid duct (Stensen's duct) is located on a line drawn from the tragus to the midpoint between the upper lip margin and the columella. The parotid duct is likely to be injured if a laceration courses through the masseter muscle. Pooling of saliva in the wound is a frequent finding. Lacerations involving Stensen's duct should be repaired when they are detected because the resultant inflammatory response leads to a high probability of a salivary fistula, sinus tract, or an obstructive cyst. This repair should occur as early as the patient is medically stable and staff is available. The preferable method is to perform the ductal repair using 6-0 or 7-0 nylon suture over a small stent (polyethylene tubing).

The tubing remains in place approximately 10 days. When the orifice of Stensen's or Wharton's duct has undergone significant injury, surgical rerouting of the remaining duct through the buccal mucosa may be necessary.

Blunt trauma

Blunt trauma to the salivary glands may cause less obvious injury than penetrating trauma. Injury to the parotid duct can result in a salivary pseudocyst with associated swelling and recurrence after FNA. Repeat aspiration and a pressure dressing may be necessary. Children who require dental appliances can develop chronic irritation of the salivary ducts resulting in stasis. Salivary gland swelling has been described in neonates resulting from a compression-type birth injury from a forceps delivery.

Radiation

Radiotherapy can injure tissue and compromise function of the salivary glands. Xerostomia is a common finding in patients who have undergone radiotherapy as a result of a loss of secretory activity and damaged salivary cells. External radiation has been implicated as a carcinogen. The incidence of salivary tumors is higher in children who had been irradiated for nonmalignant conditions.[39]

AUTOIMMUNE

Benign lymphoepithelial disease

Benign lymphoepithelial disease typically is seen in children older than 5 years. Although the cause is unknown, an autoimmune mechanism is suspected. It is characterized by unilateral or bilateral enlargement of the major or minor salivary glands or lacrimal glands.[8] Its presentation is different in children as compared with adults.

Salivary gland enlargement in children with benign lymphoepithelial disease is usually sudden and is characterized by a tender gland accompanied by a fever. It persists for a variable length of time. In some cases, episodes of swelling are recurrent and the gland can remain enlarged. The condition usually spontaneously resolves during adolescence.

Benign lymphoepithelial disease is managed in an identical fashion to acute sialadenitis when purulent secretions are present. With recurrent disease, sialectasis and, rarely, cavitary changes can be shown on sialography. Medical therapy is appropriate unless cavitary changes occur. When this occurs, the gland should be removed. If an affected gland develops nodularity, distinction from a neoplasm is necessary. If FNA cannot differentiate the two, surgical excision is required.

Sjögren's syndrome

Primary Sjögren's syndrome in children is uncommon. Sjögren's syndrome is characterized by lymphocyte-mediated destruction of the exocrine glands leading to xerostomia and keratoconjunctivitis sicca. Symptoms include burning oral discomfort and a sandy sensation in the eye. Patients with Sjögren's syndrome have a greater incidence of recurrent parotitis. If a child has recurrent parotitis and a history of dry eyes or xerostomia, further evaluation is indicated. Immunologic tests for antinuclear antibodies and antibodies to Sjögren's syndrome antigens A and B (SS-A and SS-B) are present in 50% to 80%.[26] The sialographic abnormalities show varying degrees of sialectasis. This entity involves the minor salivary glands in 70% of patients and a diagnosis can be obtained with a labial, palatal, or tail of parotid biopsy. Management is symptomatic. In adults, this lesion is associated with an increased incidence of lymphoma.

OTHER DISORDERS

Metabolic and endocrine disorders are associated with salivary gland swelling in children. The parotid swelling is usually bilateral, diffuse, and asymptomatic. This is known as *diffuse parotid swelling* and histologically shows disruption of the normal glandular architecture by a fatty infiltrate, with ductal elements remaining normal.

Allergy

Allergic reactions can cause bilateral parotid enlargement. The enlargement is usually of rapid onset and transient nature. Resolution is usually spontaneous when the offending allergen is eliminated. Certain foods (seafood, strawberries) may precipitate this reaction.[50] Investigation of the saliva or leukocyte differential may reveal a relative eosinophilia.

Chronic sialorrhea

Children who present with drooling or sialorrhea pose an unusual problem for the clinician. Most patients have cerebral palsy or some other debilitating neurologic condition, although otherwise healthy children also may experience sialorrhea. In healthy children who drool, nasal obstruction should be carefully assessed because management may be directed at this problem, including adenoidectomy, turbinectomy, allergic desensitization, or nasal septal reconstruction. Constantly wet clothing and frequent bib changes complicate care of the impaired child and may lead to healthy children being perceived as impaired.

An initial attempt at speech therapy or physical therapy is appropriate prior to beginning extensive medical or surgical management. This method provides a physiologic approach to the problem because drooling is usually secondary to an inability to swallow secretions as opposed to hypersecretion. Even with months of therapy, only a few patients are successfully managed in this manner. Medical regimens involve the use of oral drugs (e.g., antihistamines) or topical patches containing scopolamine. Generally, they have been unsuccessful because of side effects, including blurred vision and urinary retention.

Surgical management of sialorrhea has undergone an evolution. Bilateral submandibular gland excision with parotid duct ligation has most consistently controlled drooling. It has supplanted other surgical options, including submandibular duct rerouting, submandibular duct rerouting with bilateral tympanic neurectomies and chorda tympani nerve sections, and tympanic neurectomies with chorda tympani nerve sections alone. The current procedure is safe and reliable and results in few complications.[54]

Cystic fibrosis

Patients with cystic fibrosis can develop salivary gland enlargement. The submandibular gland is involved more frequently than the parotid gland. When a child younger than 2 years of age presents with diffuse parotid enlargement without an associated infection, a sweat chloride test should be performed to rule out cystic fibrosis. The mechanism of the swelling is unknown, but increased concentrations of calcium and phosphorus are found in the saliva.

Drugs

Salivary gland enlargement has been associated with several drugs, including phenytoin, thiourea, isoproterenol, methimazole, phenothiazine, thiocyanate, iodine compounds, and heavy metals.

Pneumoparotitis

Pneumoparotitis may result from any factor that increases intrabuccal pressure. This entity has been described in glass blowers or musicians who play wind instruments and has followed intubation in reported cases. This problem also can surface in association with malingering.

Systemic conditions

Systemic conditions in which bilateral diffuse salivary enlargement can occur include obesity, alcoholism, portal cirrhosis, malnutrition (kwashiorkor, hypovitaminosis A), gastrointestinal absorption disease (celiac disease, Chagas' disease), chronic pancreatitis, uremia, thyroid disease (hypothyroidism), diabetes, and abnormalities of the pituitary-adrenal axis.

REFERENCES

1. Afzelius LE, Walter CG: The surgical treatment of chronic parotitis, *J Laryngol Otol* 96:1131, 1982.
2. Alberti PE, Biagioni E: Facial paralysis in children-review of 150 cases, *Laryngoscope* 82:1013, 1972.
3. Alleva M and others: Mycobacterial cervical lymphadenitis: a persistent diagnostic problem, *Laryngoscope* 98:855, 1988.
4. Aronsohn RS and others: Anomalies of the first branchial cleft, *Arch Otolaryngol Head Neck Surg* 102:737, 1976.
5. Bailey BJ: *Trauma.* In Cummings CW and others, editors: *Otolaryngology–head and neck surgery*, St Louis, 1993, Mosby.
6. Banks WW and others: Neonatal submandibular sialadenitis, *Am J Otolaryngol* 1:261, 1980.
7. Batsakis JG: *Non-neoplastic diseases of the salivary glands.* In Batsakis JG, editor: *Tumors of the head and neck: clinical and pathological considerations*, Baltimore, 1979, Williams & Wilkins.
8. Batsakis JG: Lymphoepithelial lesion and Sjögren's syndrome, *Ann Otol Rhinol Laryngol* 96:354, 1987.
9. Batsakis JG, Frankenthaler R: Embryoma (sialoblastoma) of salivary glands, *Ann Otol Rhinol Laryngol* 101:958, 1992.
10. Batsakis JG, Regezi JA: Selected controversial lesions of salivary tissues, *Otolaryngol Clin North Am* 10:309, 1977.
11. Batsakis JG, Sneige N, El-Nagger AK: Fine needle aspiration of salivary glands: its utility and tissue effects, *Ann Otol Rhinol Laryngol* 101:185, 1992.
12. Biachi A, Cudmore RE: Salivary gland tumors in children, *J Pediatr Surg* 13:519, 1978.
13. Biorkland A, Eneroth CM: Management of parotid gland neoplasms *Am J Otolaryngol* 1:155, 1980.
14. Bodner L, Azaz B: Submandibular sialolithiasis in children, *J Oral Maxillofac Surg* 40:551, 1982.
15. Brock ME, Smith RJ, Parey SE: Lymphangioma: an otolaryngologic perspective, *Int J Pediatr Otorhinolaryngol* 14:133, 1987.

15a. Brown NA: *The Epstein-Barr virus.* In Feigin RD, Cherry JD, editors: *Textbook of pediatric infectious diseases*, Philadelphia, 1987, WB Saunders.

16. Bullock KN: Salivary duct calculi presenting as trismus in a child, *BMJ* 280:1357, 1980.
17. Callender DL and others: Salivary gland neoplasms in children, *Arch Otolaryngol Head Neck Surg* 118:472, 1992.
18. Camacho AE, Goodman ML, Eavey RD: Pathologic correlation of the unknown solid parotid mass in children, *Otolaryngol Head Neck Surg* 101:566, 1989.
19. Conley J, Tinsley PP Jr: Treatment and prognosis of mucoepidermoid carcinoma in the pediatric age group, *Arch Otolaryngol Head Neck Surg* 111:322, 1985.
20. Crelin ES: *Functional anatomy of the newborn*, New Haven, 1973, Yale University Press.
21. Du Moulin GC and others: Concentration of *Mycobacterium avium* by hospital hot water systems, *JAMA* 260:1599, 1988.
22. Falloon J and others: Human immunodeficiency virus infection in children, *J Pediatr* 114:1, 1989.
23. Reference deleted in pages.
24. Grillon GL, Lally ET: Necrotizing sialometaplasia literature review and presentation of five cases, *J Oral Maxillofac Surg* 39:747, 1981.
25. Reference deleted in pages.
26. Hearth-Holmes M and others: Autoimmune exocrinopathy presenting as recurrent parotitis of childhood, *Arch Otolaryngol Head Neck Surg* 119:347, 1993.
27. Hensher R, Bowereman J: Actinomycosis of the parotid gland, *Br J Oral Maxillofac Surg* 23:128, 1985.
28. Jackson IT and others: Hemangiomas, vascular malformations, and lymphovenous malformations: classification and method of treatment, *Plast Reconstr Surg* 91:1216, 1993.
29. Jaques DA, Krolls SO, Chambers RG: Parotid tumors in children, *Am J Surg* 132:469, 1976.
30. Kane WJ, McCaffrey TV: *Infections.* In Cummings CW and others, editors: *Otolaryngology–head and neck surgery*, St Louis, 1993, Mosby.
31. Kaplan MJ, Johns ME: *Malignant neoplasms.* In Cummings CW and others, editors: *Otolaryngology–head and neck surgery*, St Louis, 1993, Mosby.
32. Karmody CS, Fortson JK, Calcaterrs VE: Lymphangiomas of the head and neck in adults, *Otolaryngol Head Neck Surg* 90:283, 1982.
33. Katz AD, Preston-Martin S: Salivary gland tumors and previous radiotherapy to the head and neck, *Am J Surg* 147:345, 1984.
34. Kessler A, Handler SD: Salivary gland neoplasms in children: a 10-year survey at The Children's Hospital of Philadelphia, *Int J Pediatr Otorhinolaryngol* 29:195, 1994.
35. Lack EE, Upton MP: Histopathologic review of salivary gland tumors in childhood, *Arch Otolaryngol Head Neck Surg* 114:898, 1988.
36. Layfield LJ, Tan P, Glasgow BJ: Fine-needle aspiration of salivary

gland lesions: comparison with frozen sections and histologic findings, *Arch Pathol Lab Med* 111:346, 1987.

37. Levin-Epstein AA, Lucente FE: Scrofula: the dangerous masquerader, *Laryngoscope* 92:938, 1982.
38. Luna MA, Batsakis JG, El-Naggar AK: Pathologic consultations: salivary gland tumors in children, *Ann Otol Rhinol Laryngol* 100:869, 1991.
39. Modan B and others: Radiation induced head and neck tumors, *Lancet* 1:277, 1974.
40. Myer CM: *Salivary gland disease in children.* In Gates GA, editor: *Current therapy in otolaryngology—head and neck surgery* Philadelphia, 1990, Mosby
41. Myer CM III: *Salivary gland disease in children.* In Johnson JT and others, editors: *Instructional courses*, vol 2, St Louis, 1989, Mosby.
42. Myer C, Cotton R: Salivary gland disease in children: a review. Part 1: acquired non-neoplastic disease, *Clinical Pediatr (Phila)* 23:314, 1986.
43. Myer C, Cotton RT Salivary gland disease in children: a review. Part 2: congenital lesions and neoplastic diseases, *Clinical Pediatr (Phila)* 25:353, 1986.
44. Myer CM III, Holmes DK, Cotton RT: *Salivary gland disease in children.* In Granick MS, Hanna DC III, editors: *Management of salivary gland lesions*, Baltimore, 1992, Williams & Wilkins.

44a. Nascimento AG and others: Mucoepidermoid carcinoma of salivary glands, *Head Neck Surg* 8:409, 1986.

45. Rice DH: *Diagnostic imaging.* In Cummings CW and others, editors: *Otolaryngology—head neck surgery*, St Louis, 1993, Mosby.

45a. Rice DH: *Diseases of the salivary glands-non neoplastic.* In Bailey B, editor: *Head and neck surgery—otolaryngology*, Philadelphia, 1993, JB Lippincott

46. Rice DH: *Non-neoplastic salivary gland disorders.* In Gates GA, editor: *Current therapy in otolaryngology—Head and Neck Surgery.* Trenton, 1983, Mosby.
47. Rice DH, Mancuso AA, Hanafee WN: Computerized tomography with simultaneous sialography in evaluating parotid tumors, *Arch Otolaryngol Head Neck Surg* 106:472, 1980.
48. Sammarco JG, Ryan RF, Longnecker CG: Anatomy of the facial nerve in fetuses and stillborn infants, *Plast Reconstr Surg* 37:566, 1966.
49. Schuller DE, McCabe BF: Salivary gland neoplasms in children, *Otolaryngol Clin North Am* 10:399, 1977.
50. Seibert RW: *Diseases of the salivary glands.* In Bluestone CD, Stool SE, Kenna MA, editors: *Pediatric otolaryngology*, Philadelphia, 1996, WB Saunders.
51. Seifert G and others: *Salivary disease in children.* In Seifert G and others, editors: *Diseases of the salivary glands*, Stuttgart, 1986, Thieme.
52. Seifert G, Okabe H, Caselitz J: Epithelial salivary gland tumors in children and adolescents: analysis of 80 cases, *ORL J Otorhinolaryngol Relat Spec* 48:137, 1986.
53. Shikhani AH, Johns ME: Tumors of the major salivary glands in children, *Head Neck Surg* 10:257, 1988.
54. Shott SR, Myer CM III, Cotton RT: Surgical management of sialorrhea, *Otolaryngol Head Neck Surg* 101:47, 1989.
55. Soberman N and others: Parotid enlargement in children seropositive for human immunodeficiency virus, *Am J Roentgenol* 157:553, 1991.
56. Spatt J: Etiology and therapy of acute pyogenic parotitis, *Surg Gynecol Obstet* 112:391, 1961.
57. Reference deleted in pages.
58. Starke JR: Childhood tuberculosis in the 1990's, *Pediatr Ann* 22:550, 1993.
59. Starke JR, Jacobs RF, Jereb J: Resurgence of tuberculosis in children, *J Pediatr* 120:839, 1992.
60. Sucupira MS and others: Salivary gland imaging and radionuclide dacrocystography in agenesis of salivary glands, *Arch Otolaryngol Head Neck Surg* 109:197, 1983.
61. Tessier MH and others: Clarithromycin for atypical mycobacterial lymphadenitis in non-immunocompromised children, *Lancet* 344:1778, 1994 (letter).
62. van Loon FP and others: Mumps surveillance: United States, 1988–1993, *MMWR CDC Surveill Summ* 44:1, 1995.
63. Wenig BM: *Non-neoplastic lesions of the oral cavity, nasopharynx, tonsils, and neck.* In Wenig BM, editor: *Atlas of head and neck pathology.* Philadelphia, 1993, WB Saunders.
64. White AK: Salivary gland disease in infancy and childhood: non-malignant lesions, *J Otolaryngol* 21:422, 1992.
65. Wilson WR, Eavey RD, Lang DW: Recurrent parotitis during childhood, *Clin Pediatr (Phila)* 19:235, 1980.
66. Wolinsky E: Mycobacterial lymphadenitis in children: a prospective study of 105 nontuberculous cases with long-term follow-up, *Clin Infect Dis* 20:954, 1995.
67. Work WP: Cysts and congenital lesions of the parotid gland, *Otolaryngol Clin North Am* 10:339, 1977.
68. Work WP: Non-neoplastic disorders of the parotid gland, *J Otolaryngol* 10:35, 1981.
69. Work WP, Hecht DW: *Inflammatory diseases of the major salivary glands.* In Paparella MM, Shumrick DA, editors: *Otolaryngology*, Philadelphia, 1980, WB Saunders.
70. Work WP, Hecht DW: Non-neoplastic lesion of the parotid gland, *Ann Otol Rhinol Laryngol* 77:462, 1968.

Chapter 10

Cleft Lip and Palate

Robert W. Seibert
Gregory J. Wiet
Robert M. Bumsted

Cleft lip and palate deformities are common congenital disorders. Patients with a cleft lip or palate have numerous associated problems, including basic anatomic deformity, deficient facial growth, dental problems (e.g., missing, malformed, or supernumerary teeth, malocclusion) speech problems (e.g., velopharyngeal incompetence, secondary articulation disorders), otologic problems (e.g., eustachian tube dysfunction, chronic ear disease, hearing loss), psychologic disorders, and additional congenital anomalies. These problems are discussed in detail, with special emphasis on the timing and various therapeutic approaches necessary for management.

An overall program of care should be developed to maximize the benefits of each therapeutic approach for the patient.

CLASSIFICATION

Although numerous systems for classification of cleft lip and palate exist, no standard classification is universally accepted. The following is a basic classification:

I. Cleft lip
   A. Unilateral or bilateral
   B. Complete or incomplete
II. Cleft palate
   A. Location in reference to incisive foramen
      1. Primary—anterior
      2. Secondary—posterior
   B. Unilateral or bilateral
   C. Complete or incomplete
III. Submucous cleft palate

Figure 10-1 shows one functional classification.

Clefts of the lip can be unilateral or bilateral; the extent of the cleft is classified as complete or incomplete. A complete cleft involves the entire lip and is usually associated with involvement of the underlying alveolar arch (premaxilla). An incomplete cleft involves a portion of the lip and may vary from a muscular diastasis with intact overlying skin to wider clefts with only a small band or residual tissue connecting the two sides of the lip. The most severe deformities consist of wide complete clefts of the lip and alveolar ridge, with 15 mm or more of separation between the maxillary components. The small amount of residual tissue frequently called Simonart's bar or band is shown in Figure 10-2.

Clefts of the palate can be classified according to the side (unilateral or bilateral) and the degree of involvement (complete or incomplete). Congenital clefts can be classified by the area of involvement, which is based on the embryologic development. The incisive foramen is the dividing line. The primary palate, formed initially, consists of the portion of the palate located anterior to this foramen, including the alveolar arch, and bears the incisor teeth. The secondary palate, which forms later in embryonic development, is located posterior to the incisive foramen. A unilateral cleft of the secondary palate occurs in those clefts in which the palatal process of the maxilla of one side is fused with the nasal septum. A bilateral complete cleft of the secondary palate has no connection between either palatal process and the nasal septum. Figures 10-3 and 10-4 show clefts of the palate. A complete cleft of the entire palate involves all of the palate and one or both sides of the premaxilla (alveolar arch). This type of cleft is usually associated with a cleft of the lip. An incomplete cleft of the palate usually involves only the secondary palate. The degree of abnormality may vary from submucous cleft palate to a cleft ex-

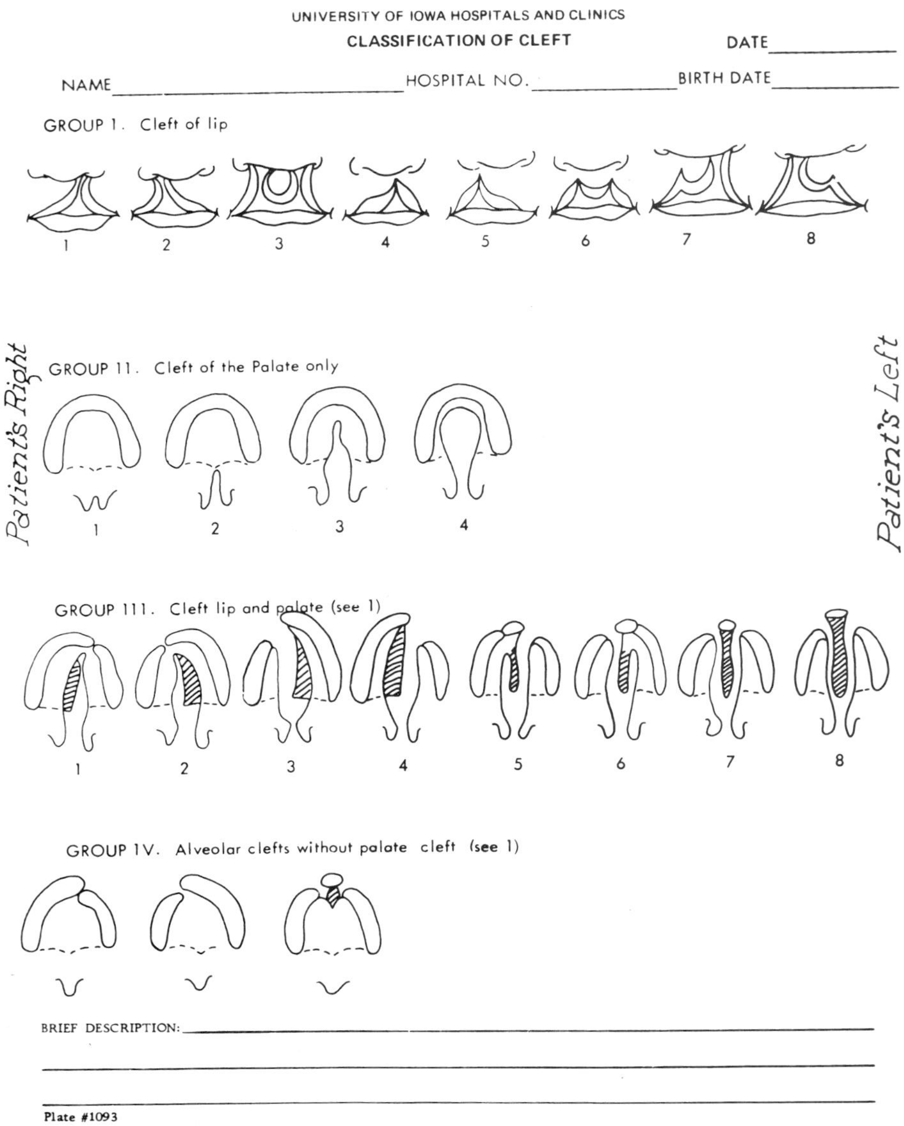

Fig. 10-1. Classification system used by the University of Iowa Cleft Palate Team.

tending to the incisive foramen. A submucous cleft palate, which is caused by a mesodermal deficiency of the muscles of the palate with intact overlying oral and nasal mucous membranes, is characterized clinically by the presence of a bifid uvula; muscular diastasis of the muscles of the soft palate, resulting in a bluish midline streak (zona pellucida); and loss of the posterior nasal spine or frank notching of the posterior hard palate (Fig. 10-5).

EMBRYOLOGY

Development of the upper lip

The critical period for craniofacial development is 4 to 8 weeks postconception. The upper lip is composed of three facial primordia that appear in the fourth week. First, the frontonasal prominence develops from mesenchymal proliferation ventral to the forebrain, forming the cranial boundary of the lip. During the fourth week, rapid proliferation of ectomesenchyme within the frontonasal prominence results in nasal swellings lateral and medial to the nasal placodes, producing the medial and lateral nasal prominences.[46,88] By selective death and proliferation of tissue, the nasal pits are formed and extend into the primitive mouth.[46] The medial nasal prominences merge in the midline, forming the intermaxillary segment, which gives rise to the philtrum of the lip (part of the primary palate).[88]

The lateral upper lip components derive from the two maxillary prominences.[3] During the fifth and sixth weeks, the maxillary swellings enlarge through proliferation of ectomesenchyme of the first pharyngeal arch. The complete

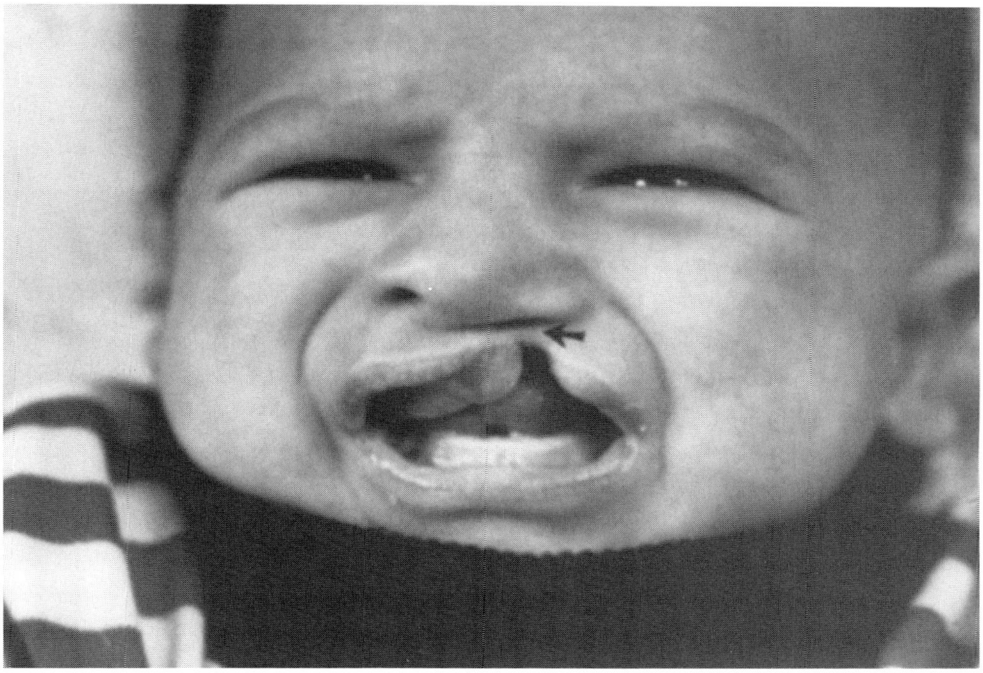

Fig. 10-2. *Arrow* indicates Simonart's band connecting two sides in a patient with incomplete unilateral cleft lip.

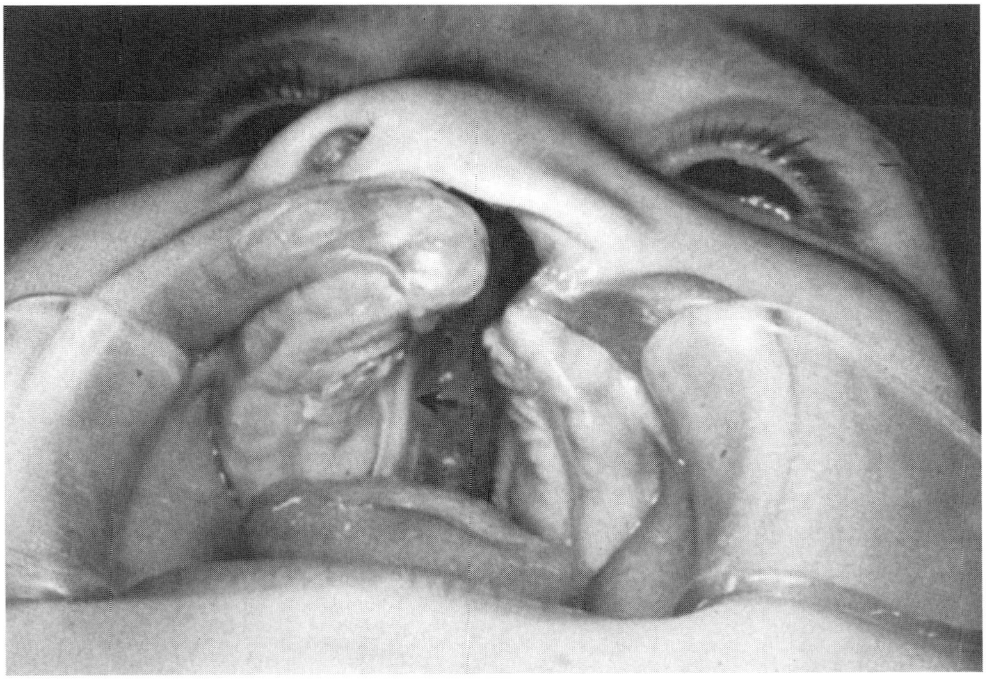

Fig. 10-3. A patient with complete unilateral cleft of lip and palate. *Arrow* marks the junction of the nasal septum with the noncleft side of the palate.

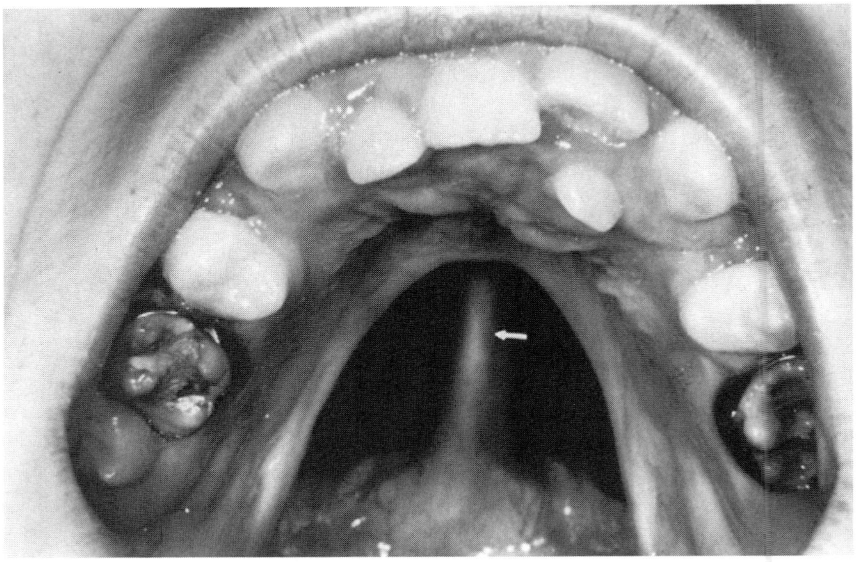

Fig. 10-4. A patient with bilateral incomplete cleft of palate. *Arrow* marks the nasal septum, which is not connected to either palatal shelf.

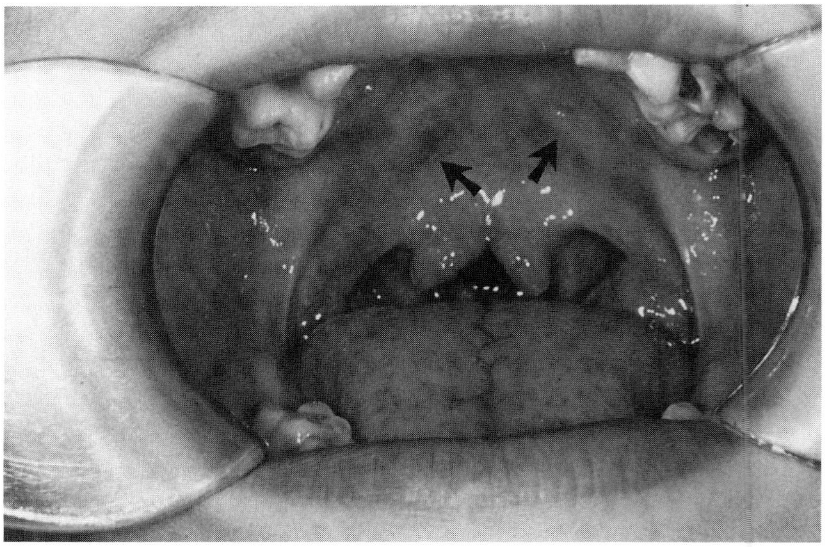

Fig. 10-5. Submucous cleft palate with bifid uvula and muscular diastasis *(arrows)*.

merging of the proliferating medial nasal prominences and the lateral maxillary prominences in the sixth and seventh weeks constitute the smooth and uninterrupted form of the upper lip. The lateral nasal prominences do not contribute to the formation of the upper lip but rather to the lateral nasal alae.[46] Mesenchyme from the second branchial arch invades the lips and cheeks to form the facial muscles and the facial nerve, both of which derive from the second arch.[88]

Development of the palate

Palatogenesis starts at the end of the fifth week, with complete palatal fusion occurring by the twelfth week.[88] The palate arises from the primary (anterior) and secondary (posterior) primordia. The embryologic distinction between these primordia is the basis for the most common classification scheme of palatal clefting, as described. The primary palate derives from the intermaxillary segment, which, as noted, is formed by the merged medial nasal prominences. This includes the bony segment of the anterior palate, which extends to the incisive foramen, the segment of the dental arch that holds the incisor teeth, and the philtrum of the upper lip.[46]

The secondary palate includes bony and muscular components (hard and soft palate) extending posteriorly from the primary palate. The posterior or deep portions of the maxillary prominences form two horizontal, mesodermal shelf-like structures—the lateral palatine processes—that appear at about the sixth week. These structures initially project downward on each side of the tongue. During the seventh week, as the head expands, the tongue moves downward, leaving the lateral processes to grow medially and over the tongue. Mechanisms of palatal processes elevation and horizontal positioning include contractile proteins, located perhaps in the fibroblast; swelling due to hydration of mucopolysaccharides; and differential cell proliferation on lateral and medial surfaces.[2] Fusion of the hard palate, beginning anteriorly and continuing posteriorly, occurs during the eighth week. It appears that a combination of processes, including programmed cell death and the production of a sticky coat, occurs during palatal fusion. Programmed cell death of the medial edge of the horizontal processes allows the exposure of mesenchyme, which, when in contact with its partner, allows an epithelial free fusion.[46] Before fusion, the free edges of the palatal processes produce a sticky coat of cell surface glycoprotein and desmosomes, which, when contact is made, provide an adherent substrate for palato-palato and palato-septo fusion. Production of this sticky coat apparently is directed by the underlying mesenchyme through a cyclic adenosine monophosphate (AMP) second messenger pathway. This pathway theoretically directs cell differentiation including synthesis of glycosaminoglycans, production of sticky glycoconjugates, and autolysis of the epithelial cells at sites of fusion.[2] The nasal septum grows inferiorly and joins the cephalic portion of the newly formed palate, probably through the same mechanisms. From the ninth to twelfth weeks, palato-septo fusion is completed. Bone develops in the primary palate first, with eventual extension posteriorly into the lateral processes to form the complete hard palate.

The posterior portion of the palate remains without underlying bone, forming the soft palate and uvula.[88] During the eighth week, the soft palate and uvula are formed by progressive posterior displacement of epithelium by growth, migration, and coalescence (merging) of two growth centers at the caudal end of the hard palate. Cohen and others[24,25] have hypothesized that the structures within a particular developmental field originate from a common field of primordial cells in the embryo. In their study, the palatal muscles and related bony structures appeared sequentially as densely staining mesenchymal subfields within the larger soft palate field during the first 6 to 9 weeks. The tensor veli palatini appeared first, and the musculus uvulae last. Morphogenesis of the surrounding masticator and soft palate muscles followed a definite timeline, with the masticatory muscles emerging and maturing before the soft palate musculature. By 16 to 17 weeks, the postnatal soft palate morphology was in place. Their analysis showed that muscular morphogenesis of the soft palate field appeared to be independent of maxillary shelf position.

Abnormal development

Gorlin, Cohen, and Levin and Cohen and others[24,25] agree that any factor that interrupts the critically timed nature of fusion and merging can result in abnormal morphogenesis of the lip and palate. Examples include but are not limited to disrupted flow or decreased number of neural crest cells and altered programmed cell death. Environmental influences and genetic aberrations appear to account for such disruptions in the case of formation of the lip and palate.[46]

Failure of merging of the upper lip varies from a mild notch of the vermilion to complete separation of the lip, floor of the nose, alveolar ridge, and palate. This involves abnormal or a lack of merging of the medial nasal prominences with the maxillary prominences.[153] Minor defects of upper lip development (e.g., vermilion notching, cutaneous philtral defects) are frequently referred to as *minimal clefts* and represent the most mild visible indication of aberrant maxillary process development. However, Martin, Jones, and Benirschke[77] found the mildest defect in maxillary process development and, hence, lip formation as a subepithelial cleft of the orbicularis muscle with a normal appearing lip. This results from a deficiency in mesodermal proliferation beneath an intact and fused ectoderm.

A complete cleft palate consists of a bony defect between the right and left halves of the hard palate and an associated defect of the tissues comprising the soft palate. The right and left levator veli palatini muscles, which normally interdigitate with insertion into the midline of the soft palate, are separated by the cleft and thus cannot function properly to elevate the soft palate and provide a seal between the nasopharynx and oropharynx during swallowing and speech. Disturbances during the integration of many structures within the developmental or morphologic fields (4 to 10 weeks) may alter the normal course of morphogenesis of the structures that arise from these fields.[25,26] Soft palate muscles in cleft specimens show delayed development in 10- to 12.5-week fetuses. The delay affects all bony and muscle structures in the masticatory and soft palate fields, with the most striking delay in the soft palate field. Older cleft specimens show distinctly disorganized muscle architecture, which is worse closer to the medial epithelial edge of the palatal shelf. These findings suggest that there is an abnormality in the muscles that persists throughout prenatal life, is apparent in the early development of soft palate mesenchymal fields, and is present at the time of cleft soft palate repair. These abnormalities may explain why some palates, despite adequate anatomic approximation, maintain abnormal function. The most important (and abnormal) muscle of the soft palate as far as speech is concerned is the tensor veli palatini.

Deficient mesenchymal proliferation of the lip and palatal shelves leading to a breakdown in epithelial covering, which ultimately stretches and breaks down, also may be the mechanism by which clefting occurs.[153] The timing and integration of embryologic processes may occur independently of each other and may therefore be affected independently. Abbott and others[1] studied the effects of fluorouracil on the developing rat and found that progressive inhibition of proliferation and growth in cell culture results in two morphologic outcomes: cleft palate resulting from narrowed oral cavity and an increased incidence of anterior palatal fusion under conditions of strong growth reduction. This study shows that elevation and fusion can occur in the absence of growth and proliferation. Based on these observations, severe inhibition of growth or proliferation is not necessarily sufficient to induce cleft palate formation. Johnston and Bronsky[59] provided an up-to-date and complete review of normal and abnormal craniofacial development.

ETIOLOGY

Cleft lip and palate are considered intrinsic disorders of morphogenesis rather than a disruption caused by extrinsic or mechanical constraints *in utero*.[88] This disordered morphogenesis is not completely elucidated. Most researchers believe that a combination of factors, acting at the right time and under the right circumstances, result in the phenotype of the cleft lip or palate. These factors include major genes, minor genes, environmental influences, and random or chance occurrence.[80]

Two entities can be classified within facial and palatal clefting: cleft lip with or without a cleft palate (CL/P) and cleft palate alone. Differences in the epidemiology and etiology of these entities are distinct.* When possible, a distinction between etiology and genetics will be made. Furthermore, facial clefts can be divided into syndromic and nonsyndromic forms. Syndromic clefts include cognitive deficits or structural abnormalities outside of the region of the cleft.[91] It is reported that 30% to 65% of all clefts are associated with a syndrome.[46,51,119] Jones,[60] in a prospective study of 428 patients, found the incident to be 14% with CL/P and 55% with cleft palate alone for associated multiple malformation syndromes, further illustrating the separation of these two entities. Reportedly, more than 300 associated syndromes appear within the CL/P and cleft palate only.†

Early in the study of the inheritance of CL/P and cleft palate only, it became evident that the recurrence risk of clefting did not correspond to mendelian inheritance patterns and that environmental factors acted in concert with some genetic aberration to produce the cleft phenotype. Environmental factors exerting their teratogenic effects on the morphogenesis of the lip and palate have been numerous in animal models.[46] Those with proven clefting potential in humans include phenytoin, retinoic acid (vitamin A) derivatives,[47] and folic acid antagonists.[43,59,91] Additionally, cigarette smoking creating fetal hypoxia (preventing morphogenetic movements of the lateral or medial nasal prominences and fusion of the maxillary prominences[59]) and alcohol use in the first trimester of pregnancy increase the risk of clefting.[91] Vitamin supplements may be capable of reducing the risk of CL/P. Notably, several researchers[141,181] found up to a 65% reduction in the risk of all nonsyndromic orofacial clefting in women at risk who used multivitamins with folic acid.

To explain the etiology of orofacial clefting, the multifactorial/threshold model was established in the late 1960s.[80,86] Its basic tenet was that CL/P depended on a backdrop of several minor mutant genes. Accumulation of these genetic aberrations coupled with environmental insults were compensated for by the developing embryo up to a certain point. Beyond that point or threshold, the embryo's ability to compensate is overwhelmed and the phenotype is expressed. However, recent evidence centered on the hypothesis that a major gene effect (recessive, dominant with reduced penetrance, or codominant) influences the expression of the cleft phenotype.

Conclusions from twins studies are based on the premise that monozygotic (MZ) twins are genetically identical.[20,21,32] In MZ twins who exhibit phenotypic differences, environmental influences are the primary determinant of the condition because the genotypes are identical. Any exclusive, genetically determined condition would show a concordance rate between the MZ twins of 100%. In contrast, dizygotic (DZ) twins share as few as 50% of their genes but are affected by similar environmental influences during intrauterine development. The concordance rates of any genetically determined phenotype in DZ twins are lower than those of MZ twins.[32] The largest studies involve twin pairs in Denmark.[20,21] For nonsyndromic cleft palate only, the overall concordance rates were 50% for MZ twins and 0% for DZ twins.[20] Earlier reports did not show as dramatic a difference with CL/P (MZ, 36%; DZ, 4.7%), and with cleft palate only (MZ, 22%; DZ, 4.6%).[46] These results indicate that CL/P and cleft palate only have major genetic influences and that there is a stronger genetic basis for CL/P than cleft palate only (results consistent with these being two entities). Additionally, these studies point out that clefting is heterogeneous and probably results from several of the above-mentioned processes, including major genes, minor genes, environmental insults, and a developmental threshold.[46]

Researchers believe that they may identify the gene or collection of major genes responsible for clefting in the near future. Other epidemiologic evidence has shown that a major gene component to CL/P etiology (most probably recessive) is likely, that genetic heterogeneneity within and between populations exists, and that there are many sporadic cases (1/2 to 2/3).[68,80] Genetic heterogeneity and many sporadic cases make the powerful technique of linkage analysis (findings in the human genome showing for genetic linkages between the affected genotype and nearby known markers) much more complicated to use. Despite of this, research continues to use more complex linkage models, association, studies, and epidemiologic and animal studies.* Orofacial clefting has been linked to several gene loci. Ardinger and others[3] were the first to observe a significant association between nonsyndromic CL/P and the major gene locus for

* Refs. 20–22, 46, 63, 91, 111.

† Refs. 23, 44-46, 51, 91, 99, 119.

* Refs. 3, 19, 34, 35, 37, 80, 86, 91.

transforming growth factor alpha (*TGFA*). Others confirmed this association[19,35] and showed an association of this gene with cleft palate only.[117] *TGFA* and glucocorticoids are believed to regulate the proliferation and differentiation of palatal epithelial cells and possibly inhibit palatal fusion.[3] Mutations of this gene may affect its timing and tissue specific expression. Another gene showing linkage with CL/P is the retinoic acid receptor alpha (*RARA*) gene,[19] which is especially interesting given the teratogenic effects of retinoic acid in inducing CL/P. Variation at the *RARA* gene locus may increase susceptibility to retinoic acid.[19] Lastly, a gene involved in B-cell leukemias and lymphomas (*BLC3*) has been linked to nonsyndromic CL/P.[134] The strongest evidence implicates a primary gene on 6p and a role for *TGFA* as a modifier of clefting status with involvement or *RARA*, *BCL3*, and genes on 4q.[91] Other contributory factors may include genes that code for variant of a reduced form of nicotinamide-adenine dinucleotide dehydrogenase and cytochrome P-450.[59]

In summary, recent scientific evidence from epidemiologic and genetic studies suggests that genetic factors play a major role in the etiology of CL/P and cleft palate only. Strong evidence exists for a recessive single major polygenic influence and for environmental or stochastic (chance) influences. The concensus is unclear as to the exact etiology of orofacial clefting.

Epidemiology

The incidence and morphology of CL/P vary considerably according to race. The incidence in whites is about 1:1000 live births. The highest incidence is in American Indians: more than 3.6:1000 live births; Japanese: 2.1:1000 live births; and Chinese: 1.7:1000 live births. Blacks have the lowest incidence: 0.3:1000 live births. The more severe the defect, the more males affected (CL/P, 2:1, cleft lip, 1.5:1; bilateral greater than unilateral). Defects are unilateral in 80% of cleft patients and bilateral in 20%. An associated cleft palate is present in about 85% of bilateral and 70% of unilateral clefts. Incomplete cleft lips occurs in about 10% and may present with a Simonart's bar or band.

The incidence of cleft palate only is generally thought to be about half the incidence of CL/P (more than 1:2000 live births). There is usually little difference between racial groups. The incidence is much higher (about 4:1) in females than in males. About 20% to 30% of human cleft palate only are syndromic.[59] Submucous clefts occur in about 1:1200 to 1:2000 live births; more than 50% occur in males. A notch in the posterior edge of the hard palate and bifid uvula is evident in most patients.

GENERAL MANAGEMENT

The multidisciplinary cleft team approach

The basis of a team approach to cleft management is a recognition that (1) no discipline possesses all the necessary expertise for the many problems faced by the cleft patient, and (2) the best approach is patient- rather than specialty-oriented. The comprehensive multidisciplinary team often is incorporated into a craniofacial team and consists of a surgeon (plastic, pediatric surgery, oromaxillofacial surgery, or otolaryngology) otolaryngologist/otologist, dentist (pedodontist, orthodontist, prosthodontist, oral surgeon), speech language pathologist, audiologist, geneticist, social worker, nurse, nutritionist, and psychiatrist/psychologist. The minimally staffed team should consist of a surgeon, dentist, speech pathologist, and audiologist. Experienced members should meet frequently and have a sufficient case load to maintain expertise. Continuing education (e.g., courses sponsored by the American Cleft Palate Craniofacial Association and the American Academy of Facial Plastic and Reconstructive Surgery) should be undertaken frequently. Long- and short-term management plans and outcome results are important responsibilities of the team. Patient assessment begins as soon as possible after birth with general examination, nutrition and feeding instruction, airway support (infants with Robin's sequence), genetic and hearing screening, and psychologic support. Parents are given written and verbal information, and the general plan of management for the first year of life is discussed. Patients are subsequently evaluated by the entire team as needed or at least every 2 to 3 years. Basic surgical, otologic, dental, and speech and hearing assessments are carried out at least annually.

Table 10-1 presents the usual age at which various procedures are performed. However, the timing and sequence of these procedures may vary significantly in individual patients.

Psychologic issues

The birth of a child with a cleft deformity is often devastating for parents, who may react with disappointment, guilt, resentment, grief, and feelings of inadequacy.[140] These feel-

Table 10-1. Usual age of cleft patient for various therapeutic procedures

Procedure	Age at initial procedure	Age at second procedure
Lip adhesion	2-4 wk	3 mo
Lip repair		
Primary	2-3 mo	4-5 mo
After adhesion	5-7 mo	7-10 mo
Palate repair	12-30 mo	
Correction of velopharyngeal incompetence	≥4 yr	
Orthodontic therapy	≥4 yr	
Lip revision	≥4 yr	
Premaxillary recession	5 yr	
Nasal reconstruction		
Tip	6-10 yr	
Dorsum and septum	15-17 yr	

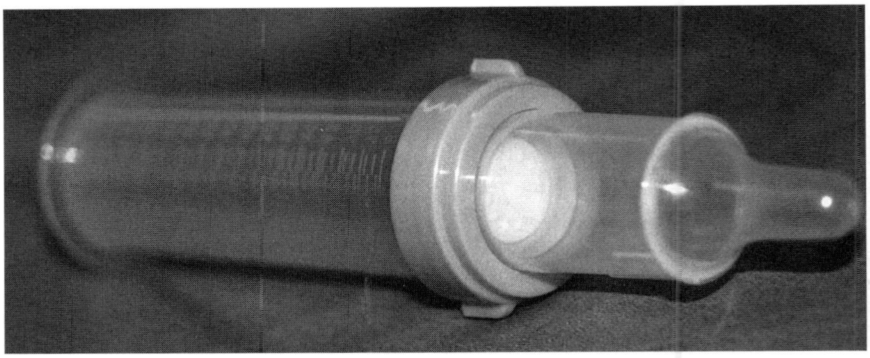

Fig. 10-6. Haberman feeder (Mandela, Inc., McHenry, Ill).

ings may have an adverse effect on the parent's relationship with the child, which in turn complicates the child's character and personality development.[105] During counseling, it is vital that parents verbalize these feelings and be reassured they are not to blame for the cleft deformity. A general outline for the child's long-term care should be presented to increase the parents' understanding of the deformity and methods available for correcting it.

Numerous conditions in cleft patients may adversely affect intellectual, social, and personal development. These factors include care and feeding problems in infancy, the parental reaction to the cleft deformity, the frequent surgical procedures that may be required during early childhood, and possible defective speech, hearing loss, and facial disfigurement associated with the cleft. However, the frequent occurrence of these factors in cleft patients has not been clinically found to produce a typical "cleft palate personality" (i.e., a personality significantly different from that of noncleft children).[151]

Speech problems are found in most cleft palate patients; in 25%, these problems are so severe that speech is difficult to understand.[73] Hearing loss of varying severity also is more common in cleft palate patients. Although the incidence decreases with increasing age, hearing loss may affect speech, learning, and psychologic development in cleft palate patients.[42] Other congenital malformations are present in 14% to 55% of patients with cleft lip and palate.[60] In addition, intelligence tests have shown that cleft palate children have a greater incidence of less-than-average intelligence or retardation.[3,109] Usually, the deficit is greater in verbal than in nonverbal intelligence. This may be related to the delayed speech development of cleft patients rather than to a basic underlying neurologic problem.

Nursing care

Special problems in the nursing care of cleft patients include feeding difficulties, prevention of airway and bleeding complications associated with frequent surgical procedures, and special diets. In addition, parents often initially verbalize guilt feelings to the nursing staff; for this reason, the staff's knowledge and education in the management of psychologic problems associated with cleft disorders is extremely beneficial. The staff frequently provides instructions to parents on daily care of the cleft child.

Neonates with cleft palate frequently have feeding problems, and devices such as an Asepto syringe (Grahm Field, Hauppauge, NY) with rubber tubing or bulb syringe may initially be required. A compressible feeder (e.g., Mead-Johnson, Evansville, Ind. feeder) is successful in most infants. The Haberman cleft feeder in Figure 10-6 may be used in more difficult feeding problems. Trial and error is required until the best feeding device and technique are found. In infants with wide complete clefts, a palatal feeding prosthesis may be of benefit. This device is constructed by a prosthodontist or an orthodontist and is well tolerated when placed in the first few days to weeks of life. Parents are instructed how to remove and clean the prosthesis once each day. A nutritionist evaluates the patient's feeding regimen for optimal growth (ideally 5 to 8 oz/wk as determined by weekly weight checks.) Often concentrating the formula from 20 to 24 Kcal/oz is necessary. During the feeding, the infant should be placed in a slightly upright position, with the nipple or bulb placed in the buccal area of the cheek opposite the cleft. Aerophagia is likely to occur, requiring more frequent burping than noncleft children need. Breastfeeding is rarely successful for children with cleft palates but may be attempted for children with clefts involving only the lip. Feeding difficulties do not seem to be correlated with the severity of the cleft palate. Larger birth weight infants (4 kg and greater) have a definite advantage in achieving desired weight gain.

Experienced, well-trained nurses providing care after primary and secondary surgical procedures on cleft patients are invaluable. Postoperative airway obstruction and bleeding may be life-threatening, and early detection and proper management including inpatient pulse oximetry monitoring are essential. Lip suture lines should be cleaned as necessary with hydrogen peroxide to remove crusts, and an antibiotic ointment is applied two to three times each day. The nursing staff performs this task initially and show the parents how to perform this care after discharge.

ANATOMY

Cleft lip deformity

The anatomic deformity associated with a cleft lip usually involves the bony skeleton and the soft tissue of the lip and nose. The degree of deformity often depends on the severity of the cleft lip.

In healthy patients, the orbicularis oris muscle forms a complete sphincter around the oral cavity. Patients with an incomplete unilateral cleft lip that involves less than two thirds of the height of the lip have intact upper fibers of this muscle, which pass over the top of the cleft and connect the medial and lateral lip segments to form a partial oral sphincter. In these patients, the lower muscle fibers are directed upward and usually attach to the subcutaneous tissue of the cleft margins or to the underlying bone (Fig. 10-7). In a complete unilateral cleft lip, the muscle fibers are directed upward, parallel to the margins of the cleft, and terminate beneath the ala nasi (laterally) and the base of the columella (medially). Frequently, a contracted muscle bulge exists in the lateral segment. This may be detected visually or by palpation. In addition, the musculature of the medial segment is often underdeveloped, and muscle fibers may be disorganized and fail to extend to the cleft margin.[71] Figure 10-8 shows the muscle deformity of the complete unilateral cleft lip.

The muscle deformity of the bilateral incomplete cleft lip is similar to that of the incomplete unilateral cleft lip. In the complete bilateral cleft lip, the lateral segments are similar to those of the unilateral cleft. However, muscle fibers are absent in the prolabial (medial) segment, which is composed of collagenous connective tissue (Fig. 10-9).

The arterial supply of various cleft lip deformities is shown in Figures 10-8 and 10-9. Frequently, the arterial supply is less than normal on the medial portion of the unilateral cleft defect and markedly reduced in the prolabium with a bilateral cleft lip.

Cleft palate deformity

Clefts of the secondary palate have varying deficiencies of bone (hard palate) and muscle (soft palate). Mucosal deficiency is always present except in a submucous cleft palate. Normal structure and function of the soft palate involve numerous muscles, including the tensor veli palatini, palatopharyngeal, palatoglossus, and uvular muscles. The attachments of these palatal muscles occur in a midline raphe normally, forming the so-called levator sling in the middle third of the soft palate; the anterior third is an aponeurotic segment. In cleft patients, these muscles are directed anteriorly, have an abnormal insertion into the posterior margin of the bony palate, and are usually hypoplastic (Fig. 10-10). This abnormal muscle insertion often prevents adequate palatal function, which leads to additional retardation of palatal muscular development. In general, the levator and tensor veli palatini and uvular muscles are more hypoplastic and

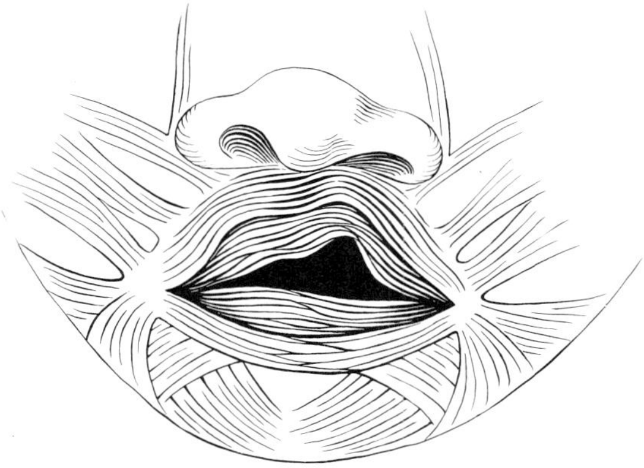

Fig. 10-7. Muscle abnormality in an incomplete cleft lip that involves less than two thirds of the lip. Lower muscle fibers insert into tissue at the cleft margins; upper muscle fibers in the medial and lateral segment connect over the top of the incomplete cleft, forming a partial oral sphincter.

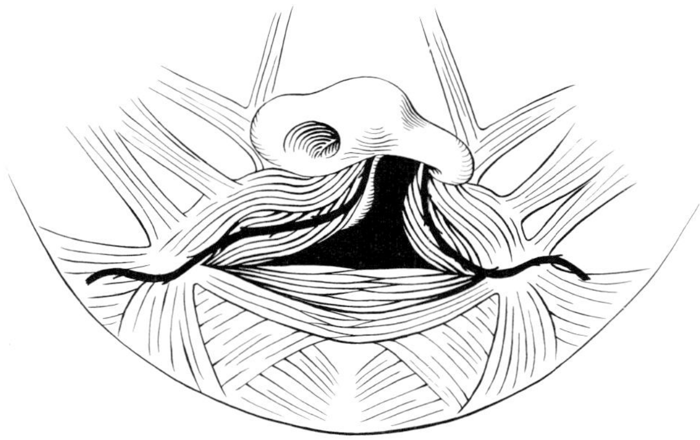

Fig. 10-8. Abnormal direction and insertion of muscle fibers of medial and lateral segments of the cleft into the cleft margin, the area of the ala nasi (laterally), and the base of the columella (medially). *Dark line* indicates arterial supply.

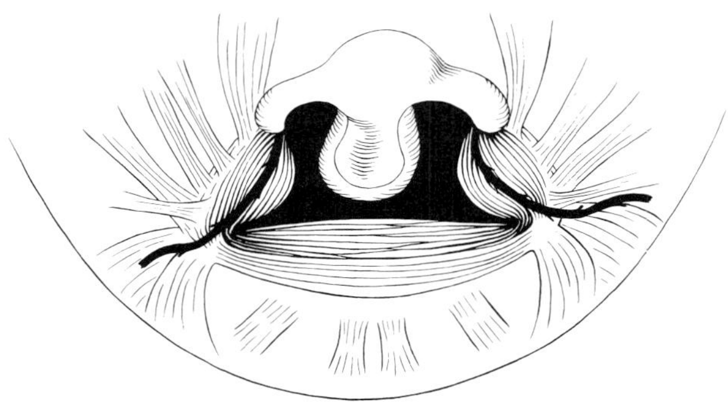

Fig. 10-9. Abnormal muscle anatomy of a complete bilateral cleft. Both lateral muscle segments insert into the ala nasi with the prolabium completely devoid of muscle tissue. Arterial supply is indicated by a *dark line*.

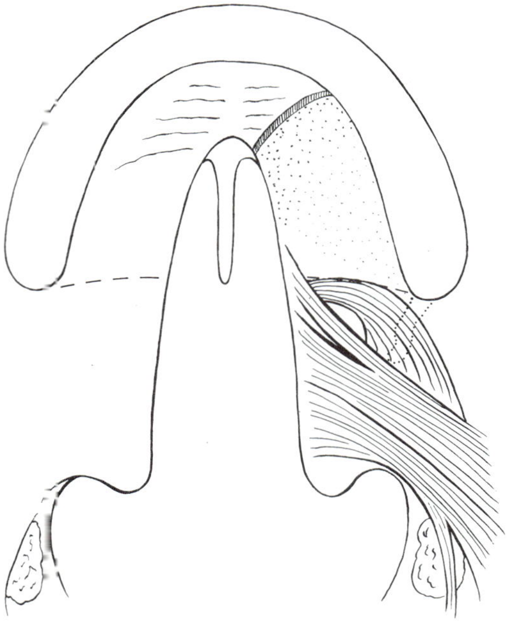

Fig. 10-10 Abnormal muscle insertion into the posterior margin of the hard palate in a cleft patient. Muscles are directed along the margins of the cleft rather than across the soft palate, as occurs normally.

show greater functional abnormalities than the other palatal muscles.[109]

Facial skeleton

The facial skeleton is frequently deformed in patients with CL/P.[33] The severity of the skeletal deformity is often directly related to the severity (unilateral or bilateral, incomplete or complete) of the cleft.

Common deformities of the unilateral cleft include lateral displacement of the premaxilla to the noncleft side, frequent upward tilting of the premaxilla into the cleft defect, malformation of the lower nose, distortion of the nasal septum, and frequent underdevelopment of the maxilla on the side of the cleft. Malalignment of the alveolar arches may be marked.

In patients with a bilateral CL/P, the premaxilla is frequently protruding (located anterior to the maxillary alveolar arches) and often grossly deficient in bone. The overlying midportion of the lip commonly attaches directly to the nasal tip with a nearly total absence of the columella. The maxillary alveolar arches are often underdeveloped and are frequently collapsed in an upward and inward direction. Figure 10-11 shows these deformities. The deformities of both unilateral and bilateral clefts result from a disturbance in the balance between soft tissue and skeletal elements.

Facial growth

Causes of the cleft, the cleft itself, and the surgical procedures used to correct the deformity appear to influence the ultimate form of the face. The cleft itself can produce deformation and growth disorders of the facial skeleton by influencing the interplay between primary and secondary growth centers.[71] The primary growth centers are formed of cranial base cartilage at about the fifth week of gestation. The anterior portions of this cartilage are important for forward facial growth, which occurs by endochondral proliferation under the influence of endogenous factors.[61] Secondary growth centers are suture lines within the facial skeleton that are governed exclusively by functional or exogenous factors, such as muscle pull and the interaction of the two bones at the suture line. A functional connection is thought to exist between the primary and secondary growth centers by way of the mimetic muscles of the face, which act as mediators between the two growth centers.[71] Formation of a cleft lip, alveolus, or palate prevents the perioral and perinasal muscle rings from closing, thus preventing the anatomic connection between the growth centers, which can no longer develop normally. Some recent reports documented cases that illustrate the effect of the cleft itself on general craniofacial growth. Capelozza, Taniguchi, and da Silva[18] showed significant changes in the mandible and the maxilla in unoperated adult cleft patients. Molsted, Kjaer, and Dahl[87] found increased cranial base width and angulation of the sphenoid in 3-month-old children with complete cleft lip and palate. Harris[50] showed a significant difference in the flexure in the cranial base but not in the size. These studies point to the cleft itself or the cause of the cleft as affecting overall facial formation and growth.

Others contend that surgery to correct the cleft defect is responsible for facial growth abnormalities. Previously reported studies[9,10,66,97] showed that most clefts can develop essentially normal facial skeleton except in the area immediately adjacent to the cleft defect. Patients with repaired CL/P may show impaired maxillary growth with collapse of the maxillary arches, producing midface retrusion (Fig. 10-12).[107]

In general, facial growth appears to be adversely influenced by the age at which the palate is repaired (greater inhibition of growth with earlier palate repair), the type of repair used (better growth with less traumatic procedures), and the tension of the closure (increased tension produces greater inhibition of growth).*

The timing and the age at which palatal cleft repair is undertaken impact future facial growth. Some authors advocate repair of the soft palate at 3 months of age followed by lip and hard palate closure at 6 months. In theory, lip closure exerts a posterior pressure on the maxillary segments, increasing the risk of maxillary collapse, and early soft palate closure results in a more anterior tongue position, exerting counterpressure to the future lip repair.[76,106] Others advocate delaying primary repair until 6 months of age, at which time the lip and soft palate are closed along with a mucoperiosteal closure of the alveolar defect followed by hard palate closure at a later date.[129]

* Refs. 38-40, 53, 76, 79, 93, 100, 106-108.

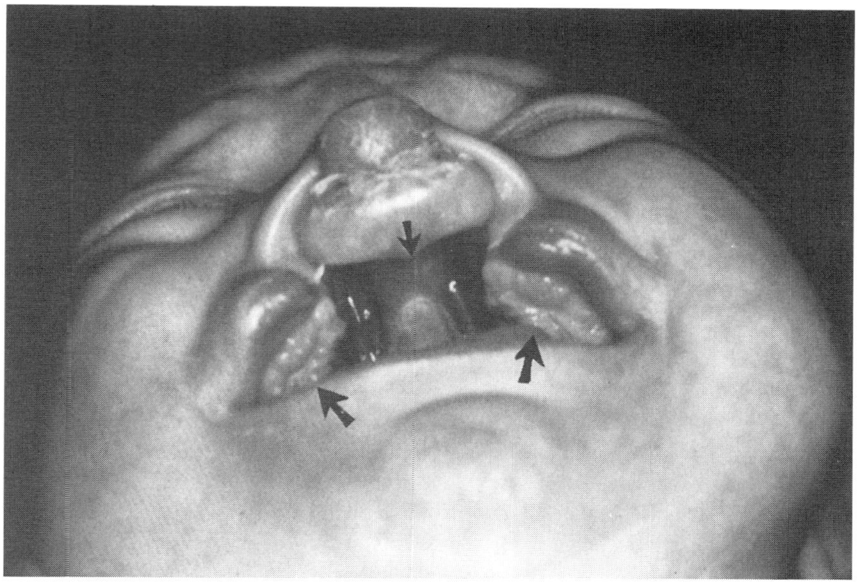

Fig. 10-11. A patient with complete bilateral cleft lip and palate: *Top arrow*, protruding premaxilla; *bottom arrows*, collapse of alveolar arches.

A

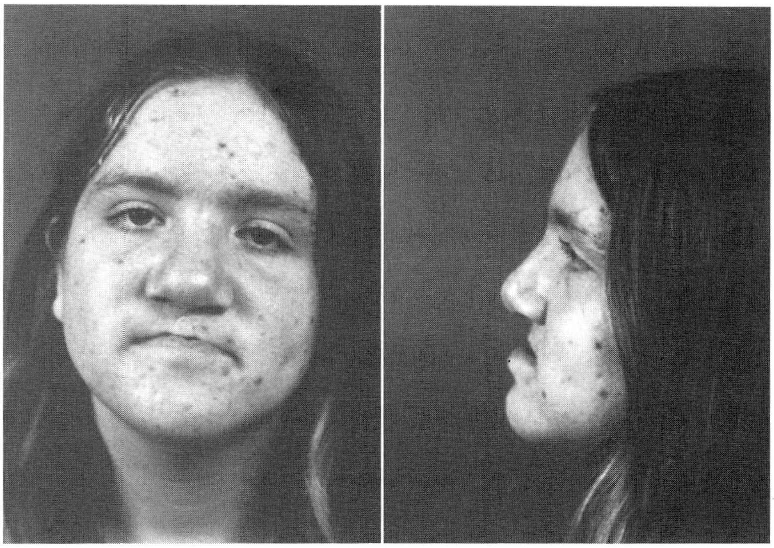

B

Fig. 10-12. A patient with a previously repaired cleft lip and palate; note the reduced midface growth, with retrusion of the midface. **A,** Frontal view. **B,** Side view. (From Bumsted RM: *The management of cleft lip and palate*, Iowa City, Iowa, 1980, American Academy of Otolaryngology-Head and Neck Surgery.)

Traditionally, palates repaired at an earlier age result in more profound maxillary growth deficiencies, including a decreased anterior or posterior dimension, a more narrow dental arch, and abnormal height.[82,93] Maxillary growth retardation appears to be secondary to the production of scar tissue at mucoperiosteal flap donor sites and beneath elevated mucoperiosteum near the dental alveolus[39,40,76,82,100] and pressure exerted by an early lip repair.[53,65] Some authors advocate very limited mucoperiosteal dissection and elevation.[39,76,100,106]

Bardach and others[5-7] recently published several installments in their series of reports on the effects of CL/P surgery on facial development in beagles. Using an established, well-controlled experimental model that allows statistical analysis, the authors commented on the effects of repair sequence (lip first versus palate first versus simultaneous repair immediately versus delayed) on facial growth. Their conclusion was that palate repair performed in the traditional sequence (lip first followed by delayed closure of the palate) is less detrimental to maxillofacial growth and shape than is simultaneous repair or the palate-first, lip-second sequence. Also, these authors showed that wide lip supraperiosteal undermining resulted in a more significant deviation in maxillary size and shape than control animals. Although these results cannot be transferred readily to the clinical setting, they may suggest a direction for a clinical approach and focus attention on specific technical or biologic problems.[7] Bardach and others[5-7] advocate a multidisciplinary and multistage approach to the management of CL/P patients using early lip repair followed by delayed palate repair.

The true cause, however, remains elusive; recent prospective randomized trials on humans verify the timing and technique of any surgical approach. Most reports are anecdotal, use historical controls, or compare normal cephalometric radiographs with those of cleft children without controls for cleft subtype, orthopedics, or other factors affecting overall growth in cleft patients. A series of longitudinal growth studies[121-128] offer little more than simply documenting the deformities. It is difficult to sort out which factors (i.e., lip repair, palate repair, primary pharyngeal flap, timing, orthopedics, effects of the cleft itself) are responsible. These factors shed little light on the specific causes of facial growth disturbances in the cleft patient.

The recent cephalometric study of Kapucu and others[62] of a few unilateral CL/P patients who underwent cleft lip repair only in childhood supports the view that closure of the lip alone is responsible for anterior maxillary growth retardation. Tissue deficiency, however, was the critical factor in degree of maxillary retrusion. Another confounding variable was the older age at surgical repair of these patients.

In summary, although the cleft itself or causes of the cleft cannot be ruled out, much of the abnormal facial growth observed in cleft patients appears to be related to surgical procedures performed to correct the cleft deformity. Careful consideration should therefore be given to the possible effect on the future facial growth of all procedures performed on cleft patients, especially surgical procedures performed on a young patient.

CLEFT LIP REPAIR

Basic goals of primary lip repair include lip reconstruction with correct alignment of the orbicularis oris muscle and Cupid's bow, symmetric reconstruction of the vermilion, creation of a nasal floor and sill, and symmetric placement of the base of the ala and columella.

The timing of lip repair has marked variation in previously reported series. In some countries, the lip is repaired within 48 hours of birth.[16,74] In the United States, some surgeons still use the "rule of 10s," in which surgical repair is performed when the infant is at least 10 weeks old, weighs 10 pounds, and has a hemoglobin level of 10 g. The advantages of immediate repair are that the possibility of maximal healing exists, the surgical procedure prevents a separate hospitalization and is thus less traumatic, and parents leave the hospital with a relatively healthy-appearing child. Advantages of the delayed lip repair include more tissue for the repair, ample time to allow complete pediatric evaluation of the patient, and increased understanding by the parents of the congenital defect, often increasing parental tolerance of any residual deformity after surgical reconstruction. Recently, repair of the lip at 4 to 6 weeks was highly satisfactory in healthy infants. A surgical procedure in such small infants may require special pediatric anesthesia expertise, the use of magnification during the operation, and the absence of other significant congenital problems.

Lip adhesion

Lip adhesion may be used as a preliminary procedure in the therapy of cleft lip. This procedure is usually performed within the first month of life, with definitive lip repair performed 4 to 6 months later. It may be performed with laterally based flaps obtained from the lip itself[101] or inferiorly based flaps of vermilion[147] to convert a complete cleft of the lip into an incomplete cleft. After a lip adhesion, the approximated lip can act as an orthodontic appliance improving the alignment of the maxillary arches and narrowing the alveolar defect. Figure 10-13 shows one technique of unilateral lip adhesion.[114]

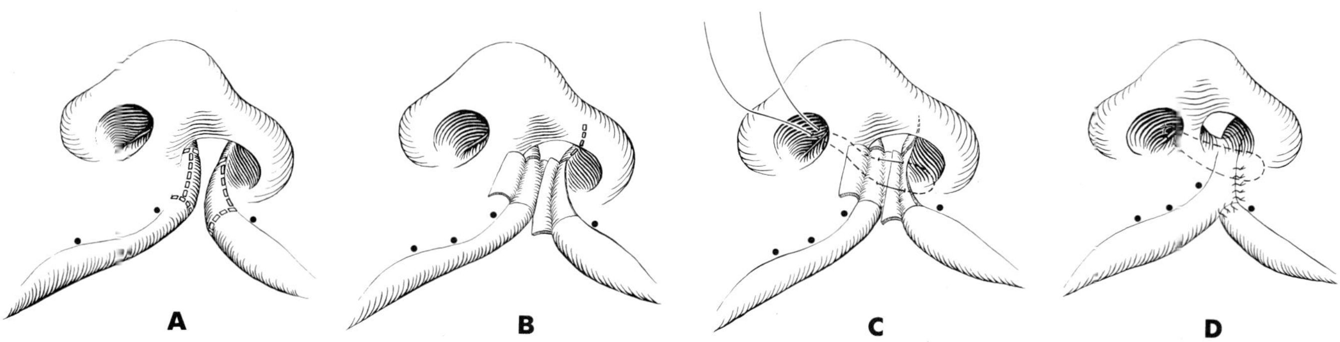

Fig. 10-13. The technique of lip adhesion uses medially and laterally based rectangular flaps from the margin of the cleft. Note the tension-bearing suture through the membranous septum. Unilateral lip adhesion: **A,** landmarks and incisions; **B,** flaps elevated and undermined; **C,** placement of 3-0 nylon retention suture; **D,** final suturing.

The primary advantages of lip adhesion are conversion of a wide complete cleft into an incomplete cleft, improvement of the alignment of the maxillary arches, and occasional occurrence of considerable growth of the prolabium in patients with bilateral clefts.[104] Disadvantages of lip adhesion include the additional operation of the unilateral cleft or symmetric bilateral cleft, possibly increased formation of scar tissue produced by the adhesion, and risk of dehiscence of the adhesion. Staged adhesions may be indicated in a bilateral cleft with a deviated premaxilla as an orthopedic maneuver.

No universally accepted indications currently exist for the use of lip adhesion. Some surgeons never use this technique, whereas others use it in all complete clefts. In general, it appears to be most beneficial in wide clefts with marked malalignment of the alveolar arches that may prevent obtaining a satisfactory result in primary lip repair (Fig. 10-14).

Definitive cleft lip repair procedures

Although numerous methods of definitive lip repair have been described in the literature, three basic types of procedures are available: straight-line closure, rotation advancement flaps, and interdigitation of triangular or rectangular flaps. Straight-line closure is rarely used and is not discussed in this chapter.

Rotation advancement

Millard[83] originally described the rotation advancement method, commonly known as Millard's repair (Fig. 10-15). This technique uses a downward rotation of the superiorly displaced medial lip segment with advancement of the lateral lip segment medially into the defect created below the nose. Advantages of the rotation advancement method include minimal discarding of tissue, creation of a suture line that simulates the philtral column, construction of a nasal sill, repositioning of the base of the ala nasi to a more normal position, and adjustability of the repair. Disadvantages of this technique include difficulty in closing wide clefts without extensive undermining of soft tissue overlying the face of the maxilla, especially without a lip adhesion; occasional sacrifice of excessive mucosa and lip tissue when the height of the lateral lip segment is inadequate; and excessive medial placement of the alar base, which results in an abnormally small nostril. Surgical judgment and experience with this repair may be necessary to obtain excellent results. Although this lip repair technique does not lend itself to the use of exacting measurements to reconstruct the lip, it is probably the most frequently used repair in the United States and appears to be the method of choice for the repair of most clefts of the lip.[92]

Triangular flaps

The second most common method of lip repair is the interdigitation of triangular flaps (basically a Z-plasty technique) for reconstruction of the lip. The Tennison-Randall technique[103,139] uses a single inferiorly based triangular flap on the lateral side of the cleft, which is inserted into an incision on the medial side of the lower portion of the lip (Fig. 10-16). Other surgeons used two triangular flaps, superior and inferior, to obtain sufficient lip length and break up the scar line. These techniques are based on exact, careful measurements and definitive landmarks; they can be more easily used on wide clefts, require minimal discarding of tissue, and preserve the Cupid's bow (Fig. 10-17). Disadvan-

A
B
C
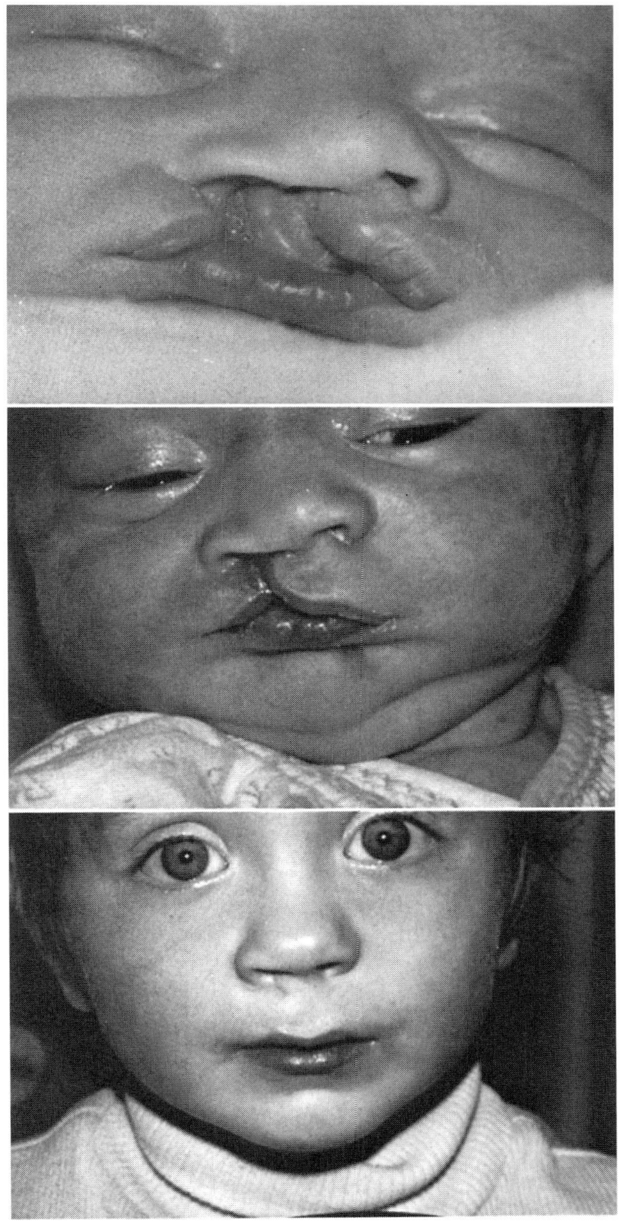

Fig. 10-14. A, A 3-week-old male with right complete cleft lip and palate. **B,** One week after lip adhesion at 4 weeks of age. **C,** The patient at 2 years after rotation advancement cleft closure at 4 months of age.

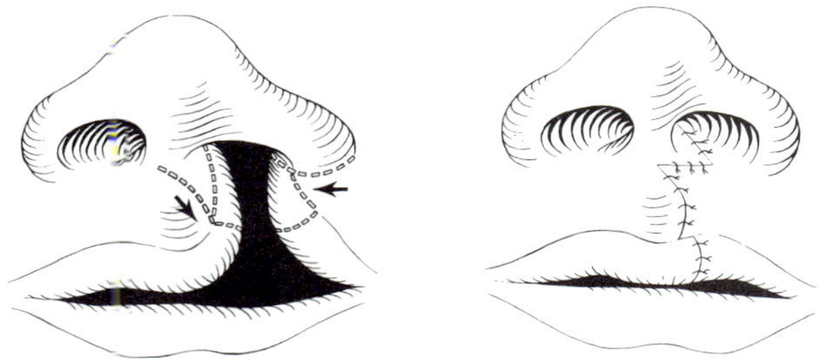

Fig. 10-15. Millard's rotation advancement technique. The medial segment is rotated downward, and the lateral segment is advanced medially for repair of cleft.

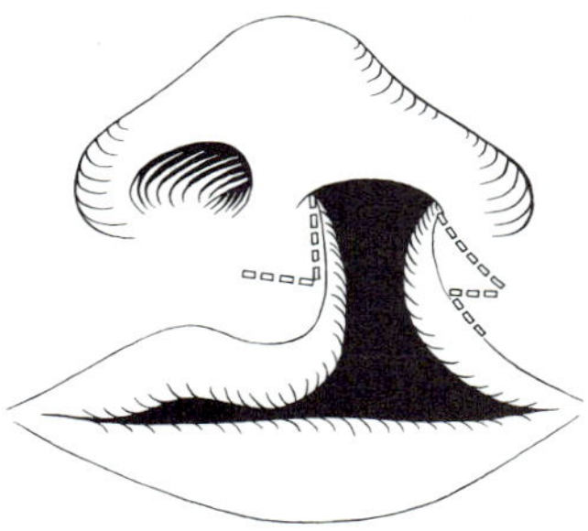

Fig. 10-16. Interdigitation of triangular flaps for lip repair. A single laterally based triangular flap (Tennison-Randall technique) is used.

tages of the transposition flaps include (1) a zigzag scar of the lip rather than a scar following the line of the philtrum and (2) difficulty in modifying the repair significantly once it is designed and incisions are performed.

Repair of bilateral cleft lip

Repair of a bilateral cleft lip is frequently more complex and challenging than repair of a unilateral cleft lip because of the prolabium and premaxilla.

The prolabium is frequently extremely small, deficient in muscle and vermilion, and attached to the nasal tip or based on an extremely short nasal columella. This markedly deficient prolabial segment is used to reconstruct the entire central portion of the lip. Growth of this segment before the definitive cleft procedure can sometimes be obtained with daily massage by the parents or by performing a preliminary lip adhesion. If the lip repairs are staged (two procedures), significant growth of this segment frequently follows reconstruction of one side of the cleft due to improved blood supply to the area created by the initial reconstruction.

The premaxilla frequently shows marked variation in size and position. It usually protrudes forward from the maxillary arch and is often deviated. In addition, the cleft maxillary arches may be collapsed, with insufficient space between them for the premaxillary segment. The abnormal position of the premaxilla and maxillary arches combined with the

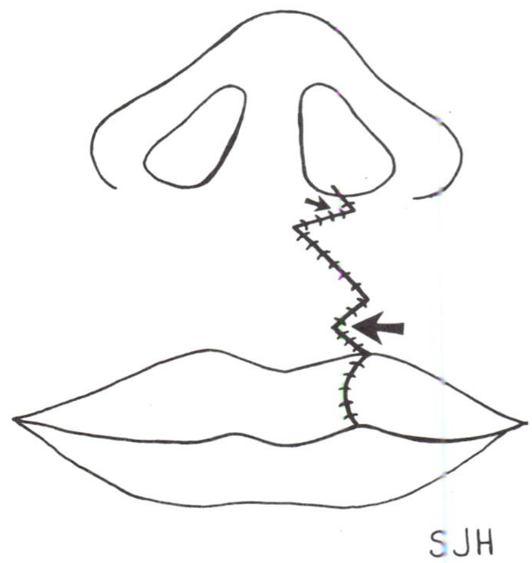

Fig. 10-17. Interdigitation of triangular flaps for lip repair. Two triangular flaps are used. A laterally based flap is placed inferiorly *(large arrow)*, and a medially based flap is located superiorly *(small arrow)*.

markedly deficient prolabium frequently results in extremely difficult surgical reconstruction of the bilateral cleft lip.

Bilateral clefts of the lip may be repaired in one or two stages. The two-stage method allows closure of the cleft with reduced tension, converts a bilateral into a unilateral cleft, and may promote significant growth of the prolabium between the two stages of repair. The initial repair is usually performed at 3 months of age, and the second repair is performed 2 to 3 months later. Although staged repair of a bilateral cleft lip requires additional surgery and hospitalization, it may be the most prudent course for the relatively inexperienced cleft surgeon. Any basic surgical repair of the unilateral cleft lip may be used in staged bilateral cleft repair.

By maintaining or creating bilateral symmetry in these severe deformities, excellent results may be obtained by a single-stage definitive repair of the bilateral cleft lip. This technique is best performed by an experienced cleft surgeon when the bilateral deformity is relatively mild or after a bilateral adhesion.[113] It provides lip reconstruction in a single procedure, eliminating the need for an additional operation and hospitalization.

Surgery

Rotation advancement technique

After a preliminary lip adhesion has been performed, the Millard rotation advancement technique is indicated for unilateral lip deformities, from the microform or minimal clefts to wide complete clefts. Although a few measurements are made, this technique is basically ''cut as you go.'' Fine adjustments depend on skills that can be gained only from experience. The goal to create a lip that is functionally and cosmetically symmetric is one of the most difficult challenges in reconstructive surgery.

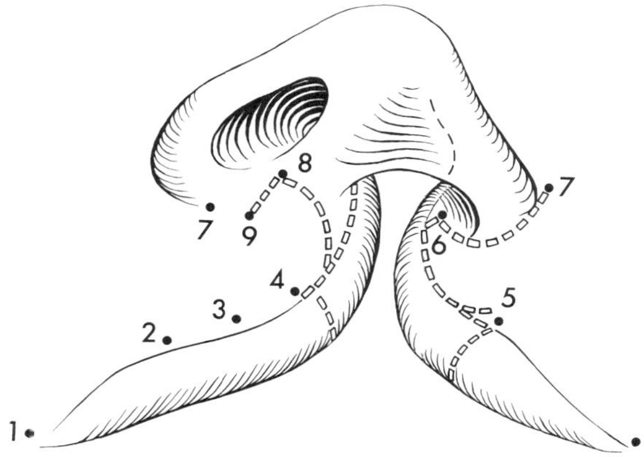

Fig. 10-18. Rotation advancement technique: landmarks and incisions.

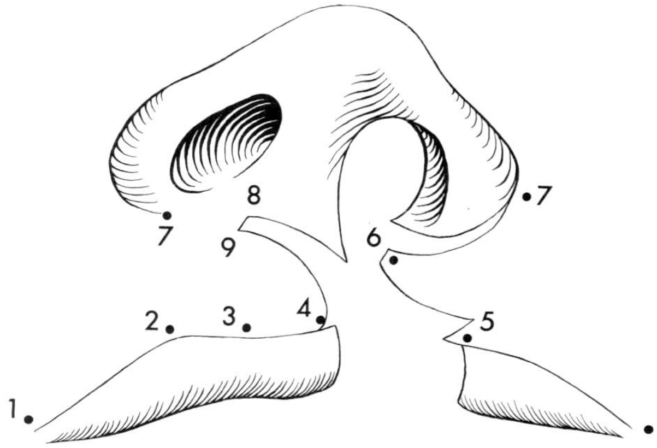

Fig. 10-19. Rotation advancement technique: flaps incised and elevated.

As for the lip adhesion, definitive cheiloplasty is performed with the patient under general inhalation anesthesia through an endotracheal tube secured to the midline of the lower lip and chin without distorting the lip. The surgeon sits at the patient's head, and loupe magnification is used. Lip landmarks are marked out with gentian violet (Fig. 10-18). Point *1* represents the foot of the ala nasi at the lip on the normal side. Point *2* is the high point of Cupid's bow on the normal side. Point *3* is the lowest point of Cupid's bow. Point *4* is the high point of Cupid's bow on the medial side of the cleft. This point may be determined by marking off a distance equal to the distance between points *2* and *3*. Point *5* represents the peak of Cupid's bow on the lateral side of the cleft, usually at the point where the white roll begins to attenuate on the lateral lip. Point *6* is the upper end of the advancement flap and is not determined until the rotation incision from points *4* to *8* has been placed. Point *7* is located along the alar crease so that the distance between points *5* and *7* equals the distance between points *1* and *2*. This determines the height of the lip on the cleft side. Point *8* is the lateral limit of the rotation incision, which ascends the vermilion cutaneous junction to swing across the lip where columella meets lip. It should not extend into the normal philtral column. Point *9* is at the end of the back cut of the rotation incision. In most cases, the back cut is necessary to achieve sufficient downward rotation of the medial flap

Incisions. Skin incisions are made with a 6300 Beaver blade (Becton Dickinson, Franklin Lakes, NJ). The incisions are scored first, and the cleft edge mucosa flaps are elevated. The major flaps may be cut through-and-through with the Beaver blade or with a No. 11 Bard-Parker blade (Becton Dickinson, Franklin Lakes, NJ). Next, the rotation incision is made and carried across the base of the columella far enough to allow point *4* to drop down to a position symmetric with point *2*, the normal Cupid's bow peak. This usually requires a short back cut through skin and muscle. A small, triangular-shaped piece of tissue that remains attached to the columella (Millard's C flap) may be used in lengthening the short side of the columella or may provide the medial portion of the nasal sill.

Length of the advancement flap medial edge (points *5* to *6*) is not determined until adequate downward rotation of point *4* is achieved; i.e., when both cleft edges (points *4* to *9* and points *5* and *6*) are of equal length. Point *6* can be placed slightly higher into the nasal vestibule, or point *5* can be placed 1 to 2 mm more laterally to gain additional length.

Along with the circumalar incision, an incision in the intercartilaginous area of the nasal vestibule down to the pyriform aperture frees the ala nasi to advance medially, independently of the lip. A triangular white roll flap is cut to match the height of the white roll on the normal side. Incision for the interdigitation of this flap medially just above the vermilion cutaneous junction is not made until approximation of the major flaps is satisfactory. The lateral and medial lip segments are freed by sharp dissection from the underlying maxilla in a supraperiosteal plane. Only enough dissection to allow approximation of the lip segments without undue tension is performed (Fig. 10-19).

Suturing. Cleft edge mucosal flaps may be excised when the alveolar ridge is intact; however, in patients with wider clefts, these flaps may be rotated upward to help with closure of the alveolar cleft and anterior floor of nose. The lateral mucosal flap may be rotated into the intercartilaginous incision in the nose to avoid a raw surface at this point. The first suture is a 3-0 or 4-0 polyglactin 910 that grasps the lip muscle back along the upper edge of the advancement flap and along the depths of the back cut of the rotation incision (Fig. 10-20). This suture bears a great deal of tension and creates a more normal convex lip contour. It helps lengthen an often deficient vertical lip dimension (points *5* to *7*), a difficult problem in patients with more severe unilateral

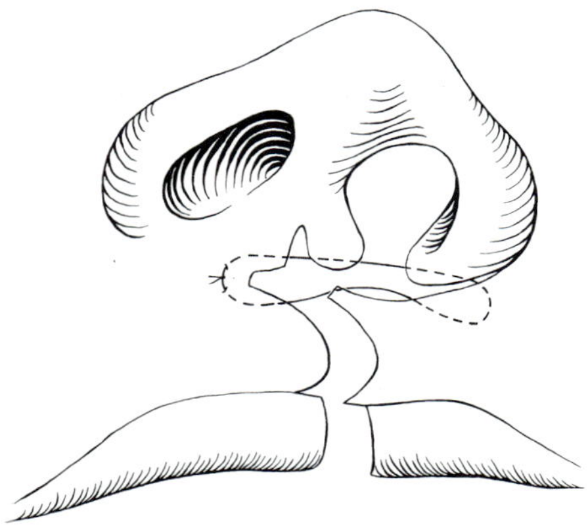

Fig. 10-20. Placement of key suture advances the lateral lip medially.

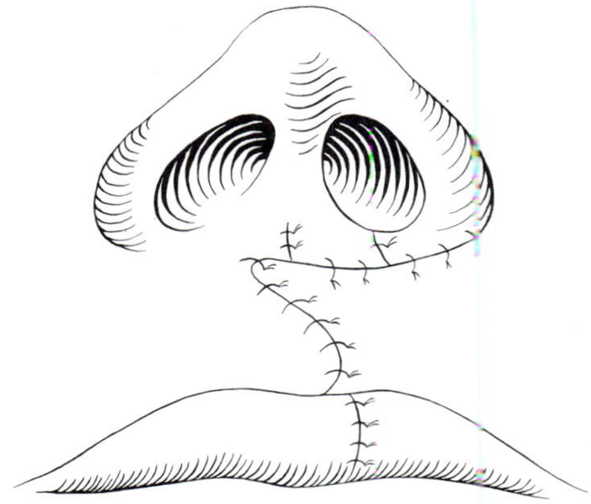

Fig. 10-21. Rotation-advancement technique: final suturing.

clefts, by facilitating lip advancement medially. The orbicularis oris muscles are then approximated with 4-0 polyglactin 910 sutures, with care taken not to shorten the lip. The C flap may be advanced on itself to lengthen the columella by placing a single-prong skin hook in the midline of the columella and retracting the C flap superiorly so it folds on itself. Sutures of 7-0 nylon on a P-6 needle are placed. The C flap is not trimmed until it is ascertained that this tissue will not be needed for nasal sill reconstruction. The ala nasi is then sutured medially with a deep 3-0 or 4-0 polyglactin 910 suture. Little or no trimming of the alar foot should be done to avoid nostril stenosis. At this point, the rotation advancement flaps should be snugly together, with the white roll flap overlapping the medial side of the cleft. If there is a tendency toward peaking of the cleft side of Cupid's bow because of inadequate rotation or inadequate length of the edge of the advancement flap, the repair is taken down and adjusted. Finally, skin edges are trimmed and slightly undermined. The skin is approximated with interrupted 7-0 nylon sutures, and the skin edges are slightly everted. The white roll flap is inserted along the medial side of the cleft in an incision, which creates slightly more rotation, or after excision of an area of skin of the same size and dimensions as the white roll flap. At the vermilion, the lip should be snugly together with deep sutures of 4-0 or 5-0 polyglactin 910. Cutaneous sutures of 7-0 nylon are placed, beginning at the vermilion cutaneous junction and advancing toward the mucosa (Fig. 10-21). Any tendency toward a notch or whistle deformity along the free border of the lip can be corrected by careful suturing or transposition of a mucosal flap from the fuller side to the deficient side to balance the lip. A Z-plasty of mucosa may be performed posteriorly to break up a straight-line closure and to minimize any tendency for contracture of the lip with healing.

The primary goal of cheiloplasty is to create symmetric lip contour in all three dimensions. The form achieved on the operating table will be the final result after healing and scar maturation. Slight discrepancies will not improve with time. In some patients who are hypertrophic scar formers, contracture and shortening may occur at the time of initial healing. With scar maturation, the lip assumes the configurement achieved during the operation.

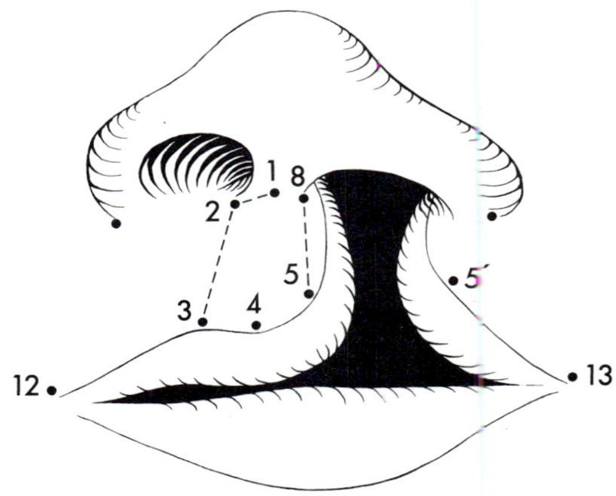

Fig. 10-22. Anatomic landmarks used for repair of the unilateral cleft lip: *12* and *13*, lateral commissures; *3*, high point of Cupid's bow on noncleft side; *4*, midpoint or low point of central portion of lip; *2* and *8*, at base of columella on noncleft and cleft sides; and *5*, high point of Cupid's bow on side of cleft. Point 5 can be located by placing it so that distance from *3* to *4* equals that of *4* to *5*. *5′* is the high point of Cupid's bow on the lateral segment of the cleft and is determined by marking the distance from *3* to *12* equal to that of *5′* to *13*.

Triangular flaps

Once the infant has been prepared and draped, important anatomic landmarks can be determined and marked with gentian violet, which is applied with a cotton-tipped applicator stick broken to create a fine point. These landmarks (Fig. 10-22) include the high point of the Cupid's bow on the noncleft side, the base of the columella on the cleft and

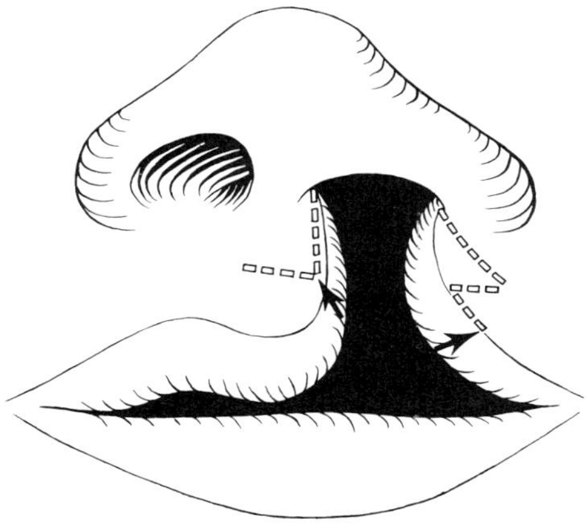

Fig. 10-23. Incisions for the single triangular flap method of lip repair. *Arrows* mark location of points 5 and 5′ (Fig. 10-22).

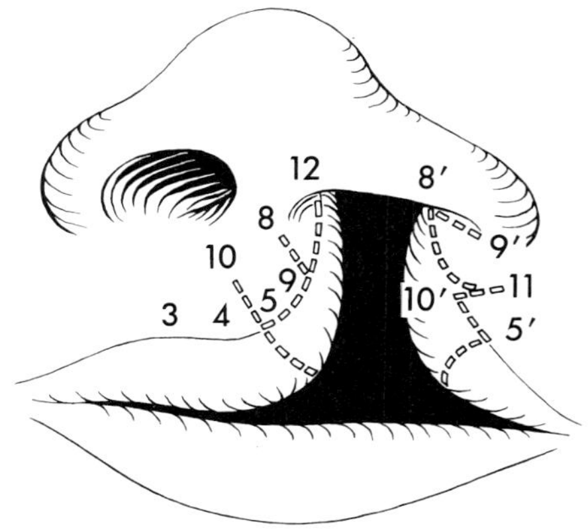

Fig. 10-24. Outline of incisions for the two triangular flap (Bardach) method of lip repair (Fig. 10-17). (Modified from Bumstead RM: *The management of cleft lip and palate*, Iowa City, Iowa, 1980, American Academy of Otolaryngology-Head and Neck Surgery.)

noncleft sides, and the low or middle point of the central portion of the lip.

If the single triangular flap technique is used, an equilateral triangular flap is created on the lateral cleft segment, with the sides of the triangle equal to the previously measured difference in lip length plus 2 mm (Fig. 10-23). The initial portion of this triangle is drawn, starting at the high point of the Cupid's bow on the lateral segment and continuing the predetermined distance upward on the vermilion cutaneous junction. After this, an equilateral triangle is constructed (see Fig. 10-23). The triangle is inserted into a defect created by an equally long incision drawn perpendicular to the vermilion cutaneous junction from the high point of the Cupid's bow on the medial segment of the cleft.

If the two triangular, or Bardach, technique is used, the previously measured difference in lip length of the cleft and noncleft sides plus 2 mm is halved, and an equilateral triangle is constructed in the lower portion of the lip, similar to that described. The upper equilateral triangular flap is based on the medial cleft segment. This incision is started at the base of the columella and meets the vermilion cutaneous junction at the previously determined length necessary for construction of a side for the triangle. A superiorly based equilateral triangle is constructed based on this line and is inserted into a defect created by an incision of equal length located in the crease of the nasal sill on the lateral segment (Fig. 10-24). When the cleft lip is associated with a cleft palate, the incision along the vermilion cutaneous junction is extended into the nose to create flaps used to reconstruct the nasal floor. On the medial segment, this incision is carried along the base of the septum, so that a flap can be created by upward elevation. The lateral incision is also carried posteriorly beneath the inferior turbinate so that a similar flap may be developed. These flaps are sutured together to close the floor of the nose.

Once the drawing of the repair is complete, the incisions are performed. Incisions along the vermilion cutaneous junction of the lateral segment extend completely through the lip tissue at a right angle to the surface incised, creating a laterally based vermilion flap, which may be used to augment the vermilion of the medial segment of the lip. On the medial segment of the lip, the vermilion cutaneous junction incision extends to (but not through) the mucosal layer. This creates a medially based flap of vermilion on the mucosal surface of the lip to provide additional mucosal lining for lip reconstruction.

The triangular skin flaps are created by incisions through the skin, leaving the underlying muscle intact. Similar flaps are created in the mucosa opposite the skin incisions. Following this, a blunt and sharp dissection is made to elevate the overlying skin and underlying mucosa from the abnormally directed cleft musculature for approximately 1 cm from the cleft margin along the entire length of the lip (Fig. 10-25). The upper portion of the abnormally directed muscle fibers is transected from the base of the columella medially and the ala nasi laterally (Fig. 10-26). This creates two flaps of muscle, which may be rotated downward to reconstruct the orbicularis oris muscle completely.

When a cleft of the alveolus and palate is associated with a cleft lip, the previously described flaps from the septum and lateral nasal wall are elevated and closed with interrupted 4-0 chromic sutures. After this, the muscular flaps from the margins of the cleft are rotated downward, and the orbicularis oris muscle is reconstructed by suturing the ends of the muscular flaps together with two or three 4-0 Polyglactin 910 or chromic sutures. These muscular flaps should be adequately separated from the underlying and overlying mucosa and skin to allow adequate length of the reconstructed lip (Fig. 10-27). The skin flaps are then transposed and sutured in place with 7-0 synthetic sutures. The vermilion cutaneous junction of both segments is accurately approximated. These high points of the Cupid's bow—which

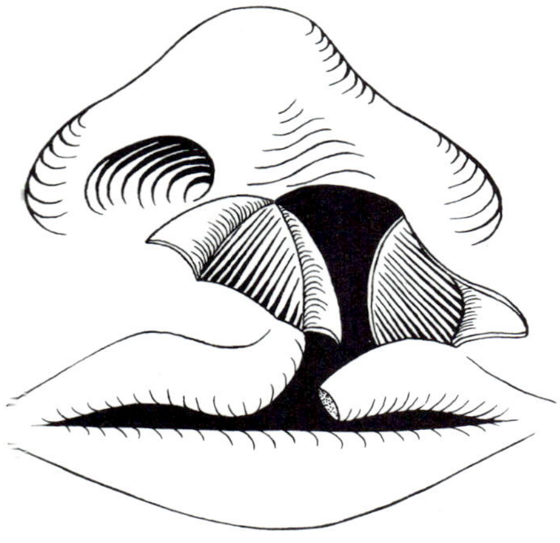

Fig. 10-25. Skin elevation from underlying muscle. Following this elevation, the mucosa is elevated in a similar manner from the undersurface of the muscle tissue.

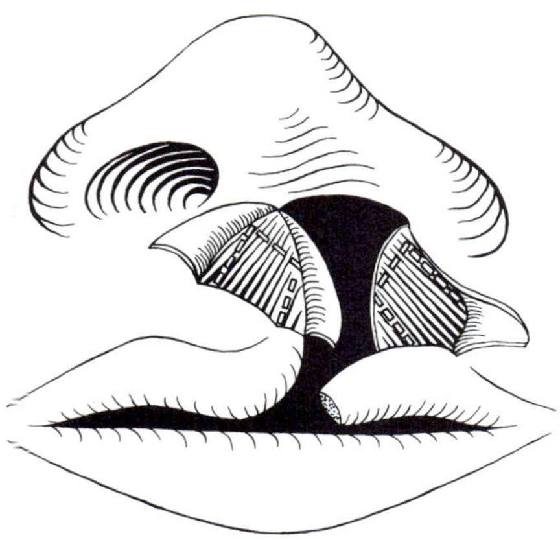

Fig. 10-26. *Heavy line* shows muscle incisions made to create muscle flaps of abnormally directed cleft musculature to reconstruct the orbicularis oris muscle.

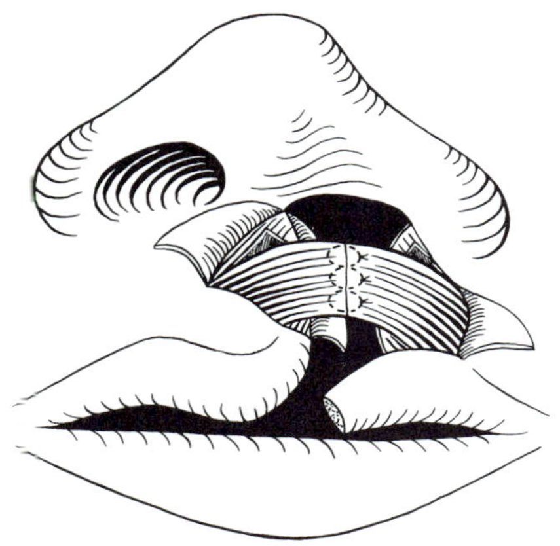

Fig. 10-27. Muscle flaps are sutured together to reconstruct the orbicularis oris muscle. Skin and mucosal layers are closed according to basic techniques of lip repair.

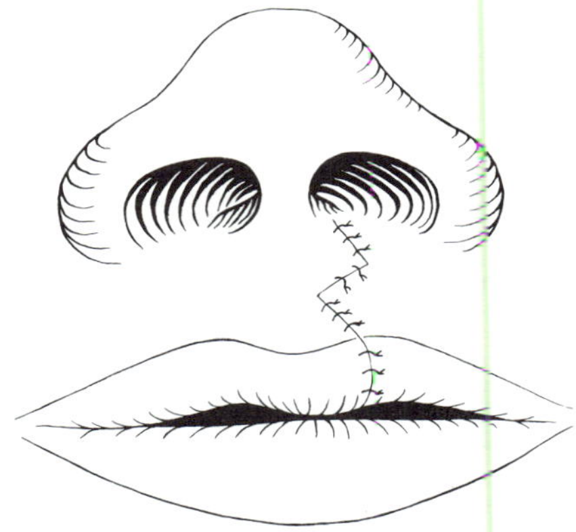

Fig. 10-28. Completed closure after the single triangular flap (Tennison-Randall) repair.

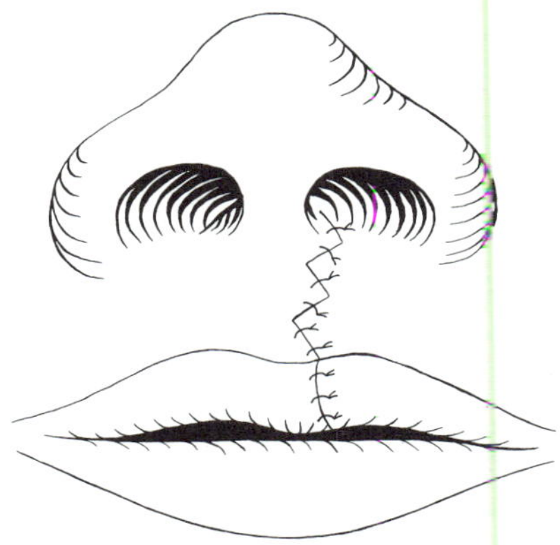

Fig. 10-29. Completed closure after the two triangular flap (Bardach) repair.

were permanently marked with a 25-gauge needle, dipped in gentian violet, and inserted before the initiation of any incision for surgical repair—provide accurate approximation. This repair is shown in Figures 10-28 and 10-29.

Once the lip length is determined to be satisfactory, the underlying mucosa is closed with interrupted 5-0 chromic sutures. After any necessary modification, the inner layer of the vermilion is also reconstructed with the same suture; 6-0 synthetic sutures are used on the external surface.

The rotation advancement and triangular flap methods of lip repair may produce satisfactory results. The specific surgical method is selected based on the experience and ability of the surgeon.

One-stage bilateral cleft lip repair

Figures 10-30 through 10-35 show one-stage bilateral cleft lip repair. This technique,[82] has several advantages: symmetric lip and nasal reconstruction with orbicularis oris

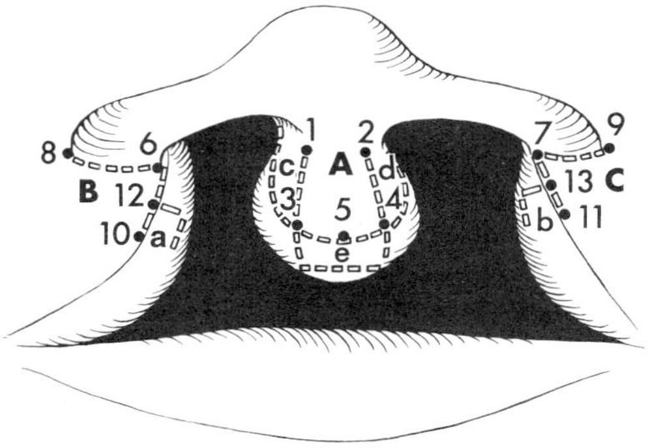

Fig. 10-30. Bilateral cleft lip repair: landmarks and incisions. Prolabium provides philtral flap; *A* forked flaps, *c* and *d* tubercle reinforcing flap, *e*. Lateral lip provides flaps *B* and *C* and midline vermillion flaps, *a* and *b*.

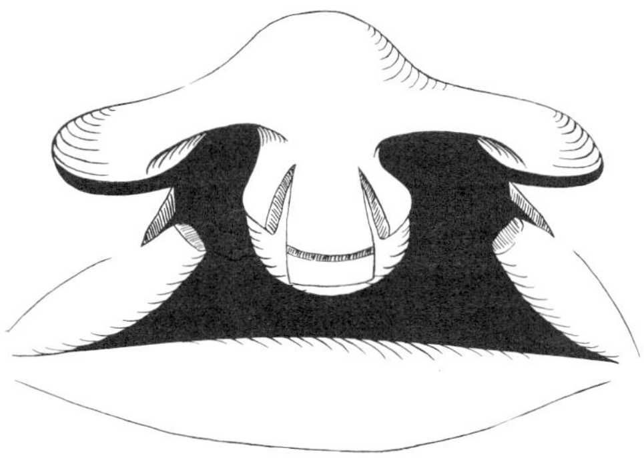

Fig. 10-31. Bilateral cleft lip repair: flaps incised and elevated.

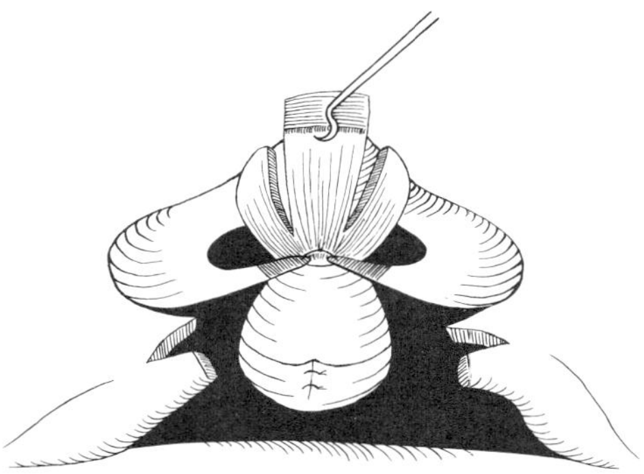

Fig. 10-32. Tips of the ala nasi de-epithelized and sutured medially at the base of the prolabium. Excess prolabial mucosa provides the medial lining of the labial sulcus.

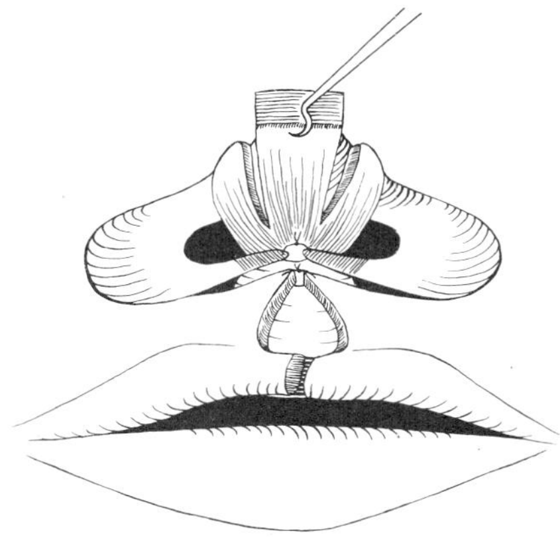

Fig. 10-33. Tips of the flaps sutured medially beneath the prolabium.

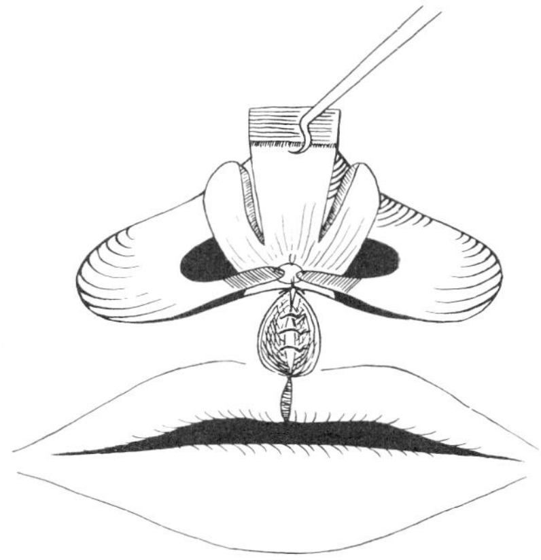

Fig. 10-34. Bilateral cleft lip repair: orbicularis oris muscle and mucosal approximation.

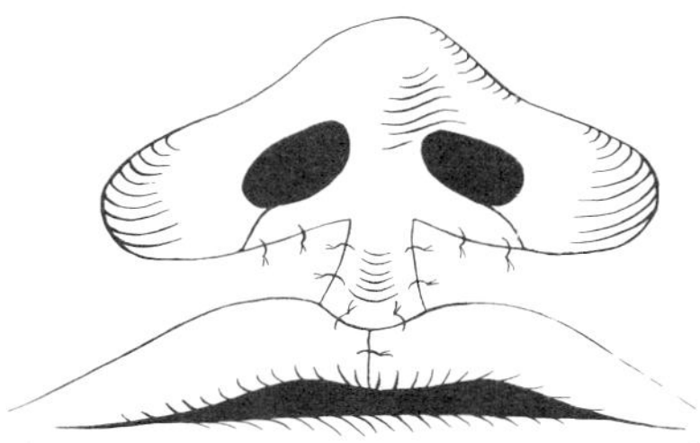

Fig. 10-35. Placement of forked flaps in the nasal sill and final suturing. Flap *e* may be used to reinforce tubercle from behind.

muscle continuity, mucosal-lined labial sulcus, symmetric Cupid's bow, midline lip tubercle, occasionally a philtral dimple, and flaps saved for a columella lengthening at a second stage. Figure 10-30 shows a typical bilateral complete symmetric cleft lip with landmarks and incisions indicated. The height of the lip is determined by the vertical height of the prolabium as indicated by incisions *1* to *3* and *2* to *4*. The philtral flap should be made as narrow as feasible because of its tendency to stretch and widen with healing, especially when the premaxilla protrudes markedly. The small quadrilateral shaded flap just below the vermilion cutaneous junction is used to reinforce a midline vermilion tubercle. Both lateral lip elements are handled in the same way with the cleft edge incisions *6* to *10* and *7* to *11* matching the prolabial height. The small flaps of lengths *10* and *12* to *13* consist of vermilion/mucosa and submucosa and are brought beneath the prolabial flap to reconstruct the midline vermilion. The lip and nose are freed by circumalar incisions (*6* to *8* and *7* to *9*), and the lip is freed from the maxilla to allow medial advancement without tension. The ala nasi may be freed by an incision in the intercartilaginous area of the nose for medial advancement. The forked flaps are full-thickness flaps, which will be saved and banked later in the nasal sill. Figure 10-31 shows that all incisions have been made. The vermilion flap remains attached to the infero/posterior aspect of the prolabial flap, which has been thinned posteriorly. Incisions *10* to *12* and *11* to *13* are placed at the vermilion cutaneous junction. Including white skin in the flap often results in a conspicuous scar across the philtrum above the vermilion cutaneous junction, especially with the growth of the lip. Figure 10-32 shows the prolabial flap retracted superiorly. The tips of the ala nasi have been brought medially and sutured to the periosteum in the region of the anterior nasal spine. To achieve the best asymmetry, each flap may be sutured separately. Excess vermilion from the prolabium is trimmed and sutured onto the anterior surface of the premaxilla to provide medial labial sulcus lining. Figure 10-33 shows that the superior portions of the lateral lip flaps have been secured medially in the same fashion as the alar flaps. Again, separate suturing may be required for the best symmetry. Orbicularis oris muscles are approximated (Fig.10-34), skin edges are trimmed and adjusted as necessary, and a philtral dimpling stitch is placed from the undersurface of the prolabial flap to the reconstructed muscle. Final suturing with subcutaneous and skin stitches is applied (Fig. 10-35). When there is a tendency for vermilion deficiency (whistle deformity) in the midline, the flap attached to the prolabium may be tucked behind the vermilion flaps to help create a midline tubercle.

Postoperative care

A tongue stitch is applied to help control the airway until the patient is fully awake. The patient is kept in arm restraints, and feedings through an Asepto syringe are begun the day after surgery. The patient is discharged when taking feedings well and when the parents are comfortable with feeding technique and care of the incision. Antibiotic ointment is applied to the sutures twice per day. Sutures are removed at 7 days in an outpatient procedure with sedation. Arm restraints and specialized feedings are continued for 10 days after operation.

CLEFT PALATE REPAIR

The basic goals of palate repair include separation of the nasal and oral cavities, construction of a watertight and airtight velopharyngeal valve, preservation of facial growth, and development of aesthetic dentition and functional occlusion.

The timing of surgical closure of the palate is controversial; the optimal age for this procedure has not been settled. The desirability of creating adequate mechanism for normal speech is balanced with the possible effect of the surgical procedure on facial growth and dental occlusion. An adequate velopharyngeal valve is necessary for normal speech. Studies indicate that the earlier the palate is repaired and velopharyngeal competence established, the better the resultant speech will be.[31,48] Early surgical repair, however, may increase abnormalities in facial growth, increase maxillary arch collapse, and exacerbate orthodontic problems.

In the 1960s, the tendency was to wait until after the deciduous molars had erupted[9] to minimize facial growth retardation. However, by the early 1980s, increasing emphasis was placed on palatal closure by 12 months of age to minimize speech problems.[31] Most centers complete palate closure by 18 months of age if not by 12 months. Some perform a soft palate repair concurrently with cheiloplasty at 3 to 6 months of age, with hard palate closure by a vomer flap at 12 months.[69] Nearly all cleft palates are successfully repaired by surgery, including massive clefts, in which the size of the cleft is larger than the size of the remaining palatal tissue.[15] However, equally effective results may be obtained by dental obturation of the palatal defect without the associated trauma and morbidity of surgery and its possible subsequent secondary effects on facial growth. Dental obturation of palatal clefts cannot be performed as early in life as palatoplasty because of the necessity for patient cooperation and adequate dentition to secure the appliance. In patients age 3 to 4 years, obturation is usually highly successful.

Palatoplasty techniques

The basic surgical techniques of palate repair include Schweckendiek's procedure or primary veloplasty, Von Langenbeck's palatoplasty, V-Y push-back,[64,148] double reversing Z-plasty[41] (Furlow's palatoplasty), and two-flap palatoplasty. A combination of palatoplasty and pharyngeal flap may be used for the repair of extremely large clefts[15] and occasionally for primary palate repair.[133]

Basic considerations in the repair of any cleft palate should include the described pathologic anatomy (see Fig. 10-30). Although methods of palate repair do not emphasize

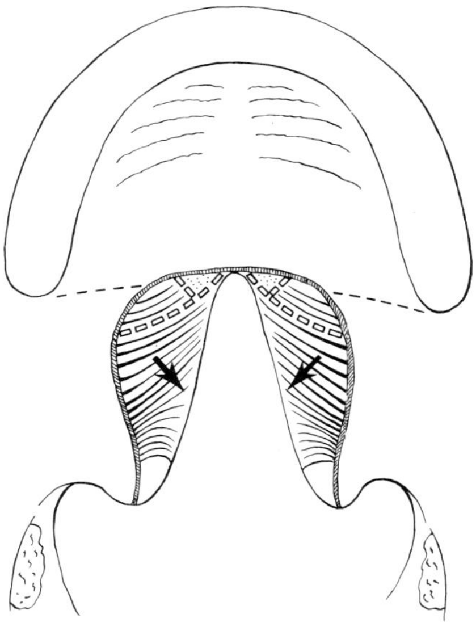

Fig. 10-36. The mucosa overlying the abnormally directed and inserted palatal musculature has been dissected from muscles. *Dark lines* mark incisions to be made along margins of the muscle bundles. These muscle bundles are rotated in direction of *arrows* for reconstruction of a levator sling.

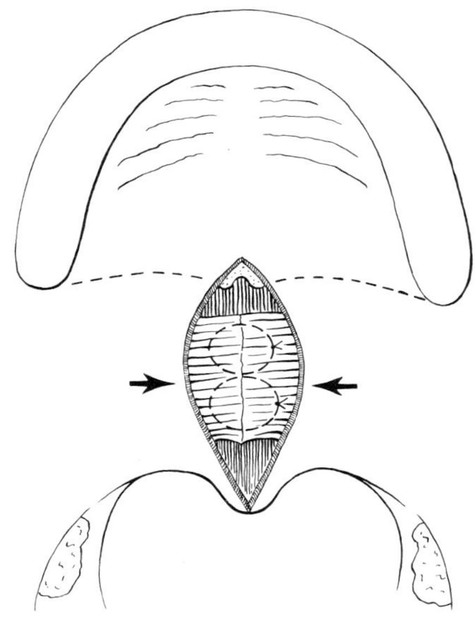

Fig. 10-37. Muscle bundles are sutured together *(arrows)* to reconstruct a levator sling.

reconstruction of the muscular sling of the palate, such reconstruction appears to be significant in subsequent palatal and eustachian tube function. Reconstruction of the muscular sling (Fig. 10-36) requires dissection of the oral and nasal mucosa from the muscular bundle inserting into the posterior portion of the remaining hard palate. This muscular insertion is transected, and each muscle bundle is rotated to the midline and sutured together, thereby reconstructing the muscular sling (Fig. 10-37).

Schweckendiek's technique

Schweckendiek's procedure (primary veloplasty) consists of closure of only the soft palate cleft (Fig. 10-38). This initial repair is usually performed at age 3 to 12 months, with delayed closure of the hard palate at a later date. A dental prosthesis is usually necessary to close the remaining defect in the hard palate until the secondary procedure is performed (usually at 4 to 5 years of age). Advantages of this technique include construction of a velopharyngeal valve at an early age, minimal disturbance in future facial growth, and the narrowing of the width of the remaining palatal cleft with increasing age. Disadvantages include the necessity of an additional operative procedure and hospitalization, a required dental prosthesis that should be changed frequently (time and expense), and significant speech disorders that are hard to manage with speech therapy.[144] In addition, eustachian tube function did not clinically improve in patients with primary veloplasty compared with those without surgical closure of the soft palate defect.[14] This technique is rarely indicated.

Von Langenbeck's palatoplasty

Von Langenbeck's palatoplasty[146] used bipedicle mucoperiosteal flaps of the hard and soft palate for repair of the defect (Fig. 10-39). These anteriorly and posteriorly based bipedicle flaps are advanced medially to close the palatal cleft. This method is simple to perform, requires less dissections, and results in decreased denuded palatal bone. Disadvantages include failure to provide any additional palatal length, inability to close complete clefts of the primary and secondary palate, and poorer speech resulting in more extensive palatal clefts.[66] This technique is used frequently, primarily for clefts involving only the soft palate.

V-Y *push-back*

The V-Y push-back (Oxford method) involves the creation of two posteriorly based unipedicle flaps with single or double (depending on the extent of the cleft), anteriorly based, unipedicle, palatal flaps (Fig. 10-40). The anterior flaps, if present, are advanced or rotated medially, and the posterior flaps are retrodisplaced with a V to Y technique, increasing the length of the reconstructed palate. Advantages include lengthening of the reconstructed palate, avoidance of a straight-line closure (presumably decreasing subsequent scar contracture and shortening of the reconstructed palate), and improved speech resulting in more extensive palatal clefts than those obtained by Von Langenbeck's method. Disadvantages include failure to provide mucosal coverage of the retrodisplaced palate's nasal surface, which reduces the palatal lengthening obtained in the final result secondary to scar contracture of the raw nasal surface, and the difficulty of closing the cleft's alveolar portion. Also, fistulas tend to occur in the thin mucoperiosteal membrane near the

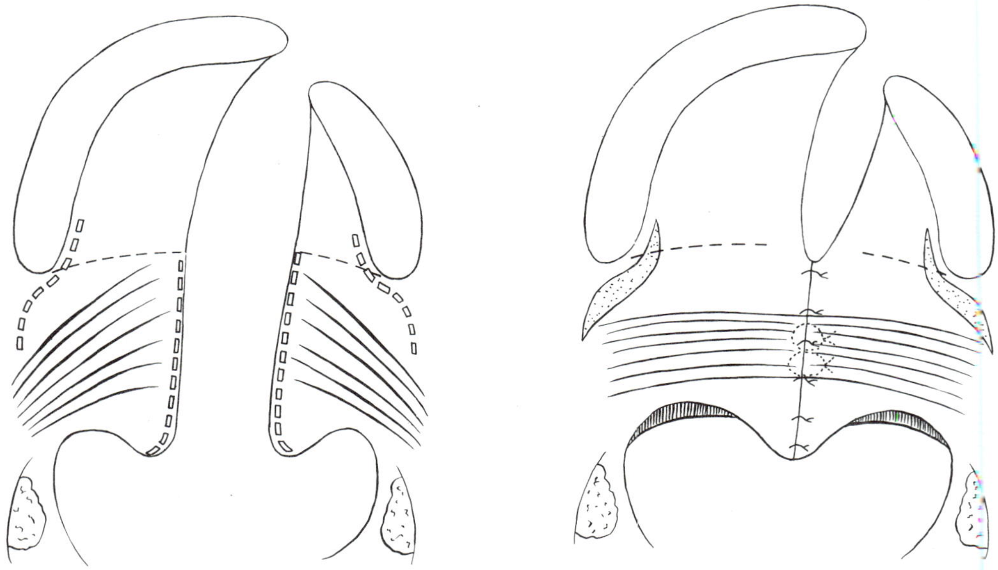

Fig. 10-38. Schweckendiek's procedure (primary veloplasty). Incisions are made in the soft palate, muscle bundles are dissected, a levator sling is reconstructed (as previously described), and the soft palate is closed.

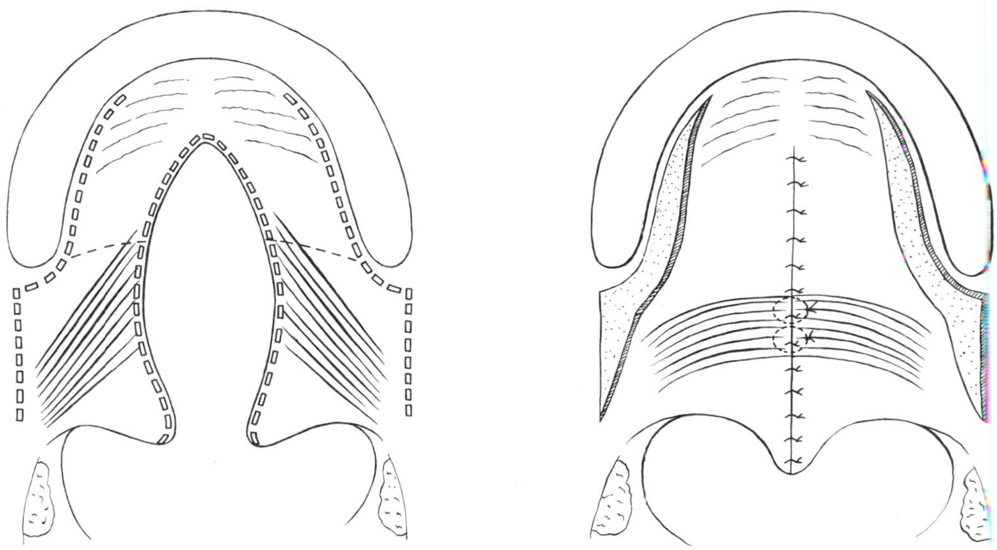

Fig. 10-39. Von Langenbeck's palatoplasty. Incisions are indicated by *dark lines*. A levator sling is reconstructed by dissecting and repositioning the palatal musculature; palatal closure is obtained by use of bipedicle mucoperiosteal palatal flaps.

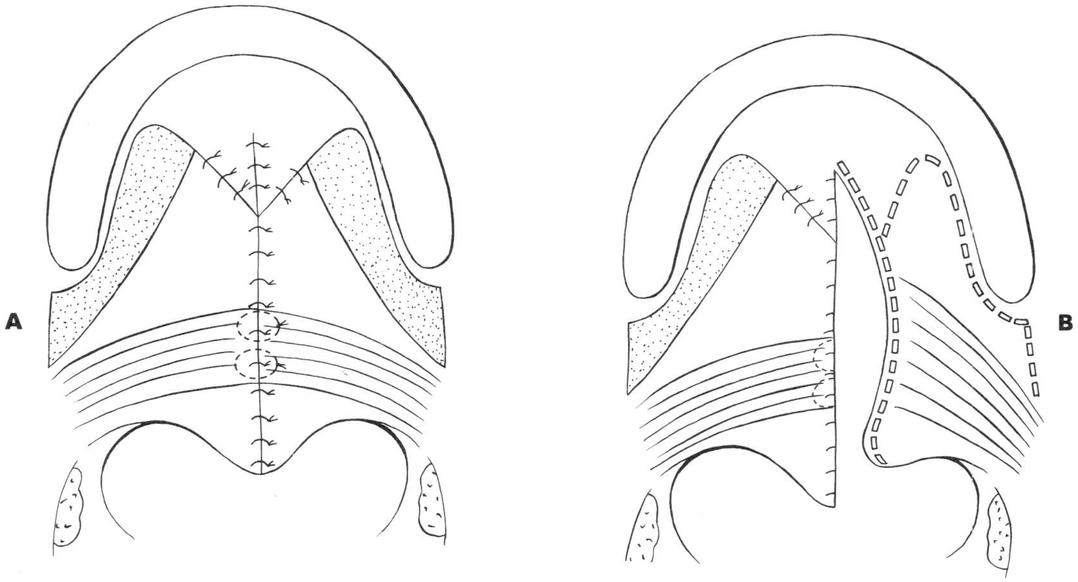

Fig. 10-40. A, V-Y push-back palatoplasty after completion of the procedure. A levator muscular sling is reconstructed, and palate lengthening is obtained by V-Y push-back.

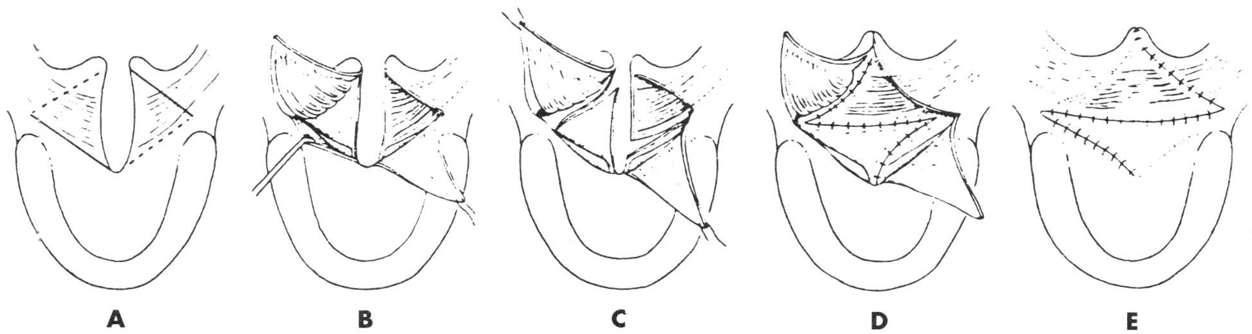

Fig. 10-41. A to **E,** Furlow palatoplasty. **A,** Two mirror-image Z-plasties are drawn with the cleft as their central limbs. **B,** The oral-side Z-plasty flaps are elevated with the levator-palatopharyngeus muscle in the posteriorly based flap. Only the mucosa is elevated in the anteriorly based flap. **C,** The nasal flaps are elevated with the remaining muscle in the posteriorly based flap. **D** and **E,** Transposing the two sets of flaps overlaps the palatal muscles and lengthens the soft palate. (From Furlow L Jr: Cleft palate repair by double reversing Z-plasty, *Plast Reconstr Surg*, 78:725, 1978. Used by permission.)

hard/soft palate junction. This technique appears to be the best procedure for most incomplete clefts extending into the maxillary alveolus.

Furlow's palatoplasty

Furlow's double reversing Z-plasty operation[41] lengthens the velum and creates a functional levator muscle sling. Technically difficult to perform in wide clefts, it is ideal for narrow or submucous clefts for which Von Langenbeck's procedure might otherwise be considered. Four triangular flaps are created. The two muscle-bearing flaps transpose posteriorly, and the two thin nonmuscular flaps reconstruct the anterior soft palate (Fig. 10-41). Speech appears to be good, and the results in 2- to 3-year-old submucous cleft palate children with velopharyngeal insufficiency are encouraging.

Two-flap palatoplasty

Two-flap palatoplasty involves the creation of two posteriorly unipedicle-based flaps that extend to the alveolar portion of the cleft (Fig. 10-42). These flaps are rotated and advanced medially to reconstruct the defect. This method does not allow closure of the alveolar cleft or lengthen the palate unless a Z-plasty is used in the soft palate. It is used primarily in complete clefts of the palate and alveolus. The levator muscles are easily dissected and approximated, and posterior fistulas are extremely uncommon.

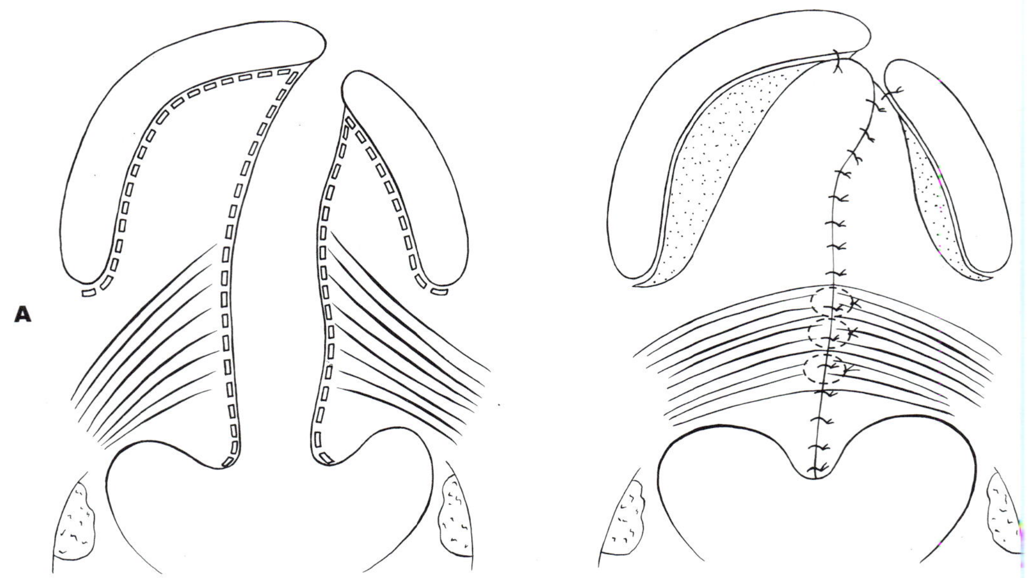

Fig. 10-42. Two-flap palatoplasty. **A,** *Dark lines* indicate incisions used to create palatal flaps. **B,** A muscular levator sling has been reconstructed, and closure has been completed.

Palatoplasty and pharyngeal flap combination

The combination of a palatoplasty and pharyngeal flap is rarely used for primary palate closure. This technique may be indicated in patients with extremely wide palatal clefts; however, it should be performed at an older age rather than at the time of customary palate repair. The main disadvantage is an inability to identify patients who fail to develop adequate velopharyngeal closure after palatoplasty and who would therefore require a pharyngeal flap as a secondary procedure. Use of this technique thus subjects most patients to an unnecessary additional procedure at the time of palatoplasty with a resultant increase in morbidity, especially postoperative upper airway obstruction, and blood loss. In the repair of extremely wide palatal clefts at an older age, this combined technique appears to offer an advantage by providing a complete two-layer closure of the defect.

Surgical technique

At the time of palatoplasty, the patient is positioned with the head in the seated surgeon's lap, with exposure of the palate obtained by a self retaining mouth gag. A hypopharyngeal pack is placed to prevent aspiration of blood during the procedure. Decreased blood loss and easier elevation of the mucoperiosteal flaps overlying the remaining hard palate can be obtained by the injection of 1% lidocaine with 1:100,000 epinephrine before creation of the palatal flaps.

Two-flap palatoplasty. In two-flap palatoplasty, a single mucoperiosteal flap is elevated from each palatal shelf. The flap is based posteriorly on the descending palatine artery. This technique allows excellent exposure for dissection and levator sling reconstruction. The incidence of fistulization is extremely low. A disadvantage is that part of the distal flap may be lost if a neurovascular bundle is transected.

The procedure is performed with the patient under general inhalation anesthesia via an endotracheal tube taped to the midline. A towel roll is placed under the patient's shoulders. The Dingman (Storz, St Louis, Mo) self-retaining mouth gag is used for exposing the oral cavity and pharynx and for holding the endotracheal tube in place. The mouth gag is not suspended from a Mayo (Wilson DIV Affiliated Hospital Products, Columbus, Ga) stand; however, a folded towel is often placed beneath the handle of the gag.

Incisions. The cleft margins, adjacent hard palate, and retromolar areas are infiltrated with 1% lidocaine and 1:100,000 epinephrine. The cleft margins are incised with a 6300 Beaver or No. 11 Bard-Parker blade, and the relaxing incisions are made laterally with a No. 15 Bard-Parker blade (Fig. 10-43). At the hard palate cleft, the incision is made 2 to 3 mm lateral to the cleft edge. To avoid injury to a developing tooth, care is taken not to bring the relaxing incisions too far laterally over the alveolar ridge. The relaxing incisions are carried posteriorly just into the medial retromolar area and just through the mucosa at this point.

Mucoperiosteal flaps are then elevated from the hard palate using a Freer elevator (Baxter, Deerfield, Ill) (Fig. 10-44). This elevation is easy to accomplish once the subperiosteal plane is entered against bare bone. The neurovascular bundle coming from the greater palatine foramen is identified and preserved. On the noncleft side, mucoperiosteum also is elevated from the vomer. This vomer flap is kept

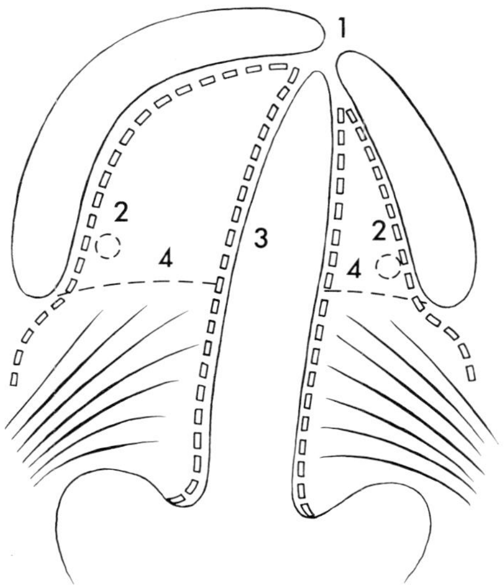

Fig. 10-43. Two-flap palatoplasty. Landmarks and incisions: *1,* alveolar cleft; *2,* neurovascular bundle; *3,* vomer; *4,* posterior edge of hard palate.

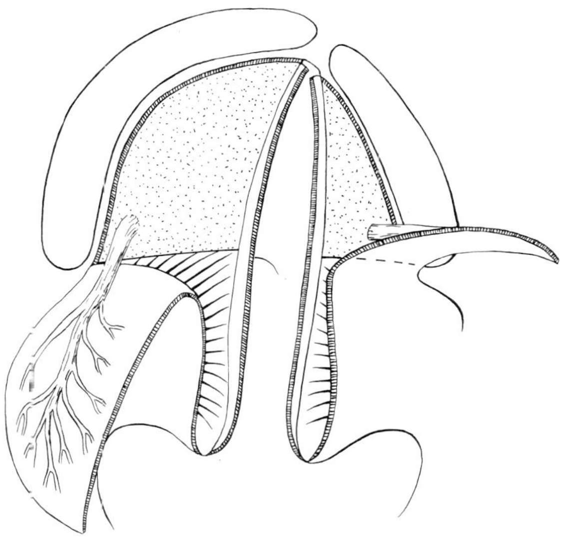

Fig. 10-44. Two-flap palatoplasty: flaps incised and elevated.

continuous posteriorly with the nasal mucosa layer of the soft palate. Care is taken in dissecting around the vomer premaxillary suture. Velar muscle fibers turn anteriorly and insert along the medial and posterior edge of the hard palate (Veau's muscle). It is necessary to dissect these fibers sharply from bone using a dental type of elevator. Muscle fibers are dissected from the soft palate nasal mucosa for 1 to 2 cm. The medial edges of the soft palate are prepared for suturing by freeing mucosa around muscle for 2 mm.

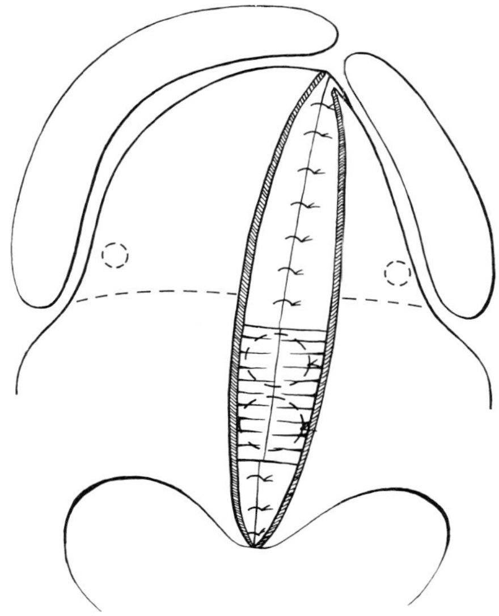

Fig. 10-45. Two-flap palatoplasty: nasal mucosa and mucoperiosteal closure and levator reconstruction.

Medial mobility of the soft palate is enhanced by blunt dissection through posterior extension of the relaxing incision in the plane between the pterygoid and superior constrictor muscles. This plane is almost avascular, and blunt dissection is performed with little bleeding. In patients with wider clefts, it may be necessary to infracture the hamulus process medially and sometimes to strip the levator veli palatini muscle tendon from the hamulus. Mucoperiosteum is tightly bound to the maxillary palatine suture and should be freed from the suture to provide sufficient medial mobility of the flaps in most clefts. Finally, nasal mucoperiosteum is elevated from the nasal surface of the hard palate on the cleft side using right-angle dental type of elevators.

Suturing. The palate is closed in three layers. Figure 10-45 shows the closure of the nasal layer by a vomer mucoperiosteal flap to a palatal mucoperiosteal flap and velar mucosa posteriorly. This closure is performed with a 4-0 or 5-0 polyglactin 910 suture with the knots placed on the nasal side. In patients with wide clefts, approximating the nasal layer at the hard/soft palate junction may be impossible. This closure may be facilitated by performing a Z-plasty of the nasal mucosa or by leaving a small gap for secondary healing. Next, the palatal muscles are carefully approximated with multiple buried horizontal sutures of 3-0 or 4-0 polyglactin 910 so that the levator muscle sling can be reconstructed. This closure brings oral mucosa into close approximation. The mucoperiosteal flaps are sutured anteriorly with buried 4-0 polyglactin 910 through the periosteum, which tends to evert the edges. The oral layer may be tacked down to the nasal layer to decrease dead space. The oral mucosa is ap-

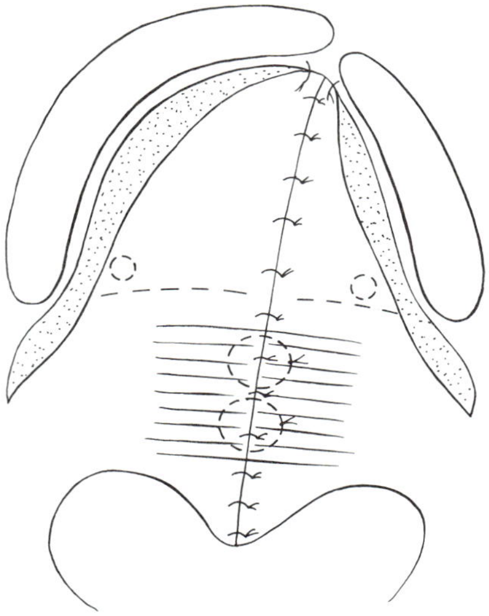

Fig. 10-46. Two-flap palatoplasty: oral layer closure.

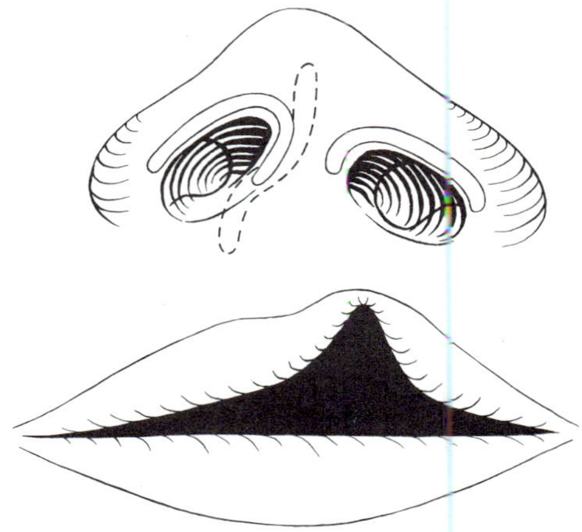

Fig. 10-47. Nasal deformities that occur in unilateral cleft lip. The anterior nasal spine and inferior nasal septum are deviated to the noncleft side. The columella and medial crus are shortened on the side of the cleft. The lateral crus is elongated and has an abnormal configuration; its angle of junction with the medial crus is less acute than normal. The alar base is displaced laterally and posteriorly. Hypertrophy of the inferior turbinate on the cleft side occurs frequently.

proximated with simple everting sutures of 4-0 or 5-0 chronic catgut. Vertical mattress sutures may be placed if there is any gaping of the muscle. Two or three sutures also are placed from the tips of the flaps anteriorly to the alveolar ridge mucosa (Fig. 10-46). The relaxing incisions are packed with microfibrillar collagen. Hemostasis is ensured by electrocautery and pressure.

Complications

The most common complication of palatoplasty is hypernasal speech; this has been described in up to 30% to 40% of cleft patients, especially with later repairs (greater than 2 years).[48] The incidence of hypernasal speech varies with the severity of the cleft, the type of repair performed, the patient's age at repair, and variation in the definition of adequate speech or velopharyngeal competence in reports of various cleft palate procedures. However, in general, the more severe the cleft defect, the poorer the speech result.

Fistula formation reportedly occurred in up to 21% of patients after palatoplasty, but this incidence should be 10%. These fistulas are most commonly located anteriorly on the lingual surface of the maxillary alveolus and posteriorly at the hard/soft palate junction. Hemorrhage and excessive blood loss are uncommon, averaging 60 to 140 ml.[30,138]

Airway impairment may occur intraoperatively and postoperatively. Bleeding and oral secretions are the most common intraoperative causes, and edema is the most common postoperative cause. An endotracheal tube and a hypopharyngeal pack protect against airway obstruction during the operation. Allowing the patient to awaken with the endotracheal tube in place prevents obstruction in the immediate postoperative period. A heavy silk suture is routinely placed through the tongue tip before the patient is extubated. This aids in control of the upper airway and is invaluable in Robin's sequence patients with glossoptosis. The suture is usually removed in the postanesthetic recovery room after the patient is completely awake but may be left in place overnight or longer if required. Mortality in palatoplasties is less than 0.5% and is usually associated with inadvertent extubation, aspiration pneumonia, and congenital heart disease.

CLEFT NOSE REPAIR

Most patients with a cleft lip have an associated nasal deformity of variable severity. In general, cleft nose deformity becomes more apparent with increasing age. The unilateral cleft lip nose has abnormalities of the columella, tip, ala, and internal nose[55] (Figs. 10-47 and 10-48). The columella is shortened on the side of the cleft, with its base and underlying anterior nasal spine directed into the noncleft side. The nasal tip is deflected toward the side of the cleft by displacement of the medial crus of the lower lateral cartilage in an inferior or downward direction. In addition, the angle between the medial crus and the lateral crus of the lower nasal cartilage on the side of the cleft is less acute than normal, with the lateral crus displaced downward, causing the nostril to hood and buckle in on itself (producing an S-shaped fold on the lateral crus). This angle is frequently longer than the noncleft side.

Frequent underdevelopment of the maxilla on the cleft side displaces the alar base laterally, posteriorly, and downward, producing a widened naris on the cleft side with its usual orientation horizontally rather than vertically. A bowstring contracture of the nostril from its apex continues along the upper border of the lateral crus to the piriform aperture on the side of the cleft, producing a relative stenosis

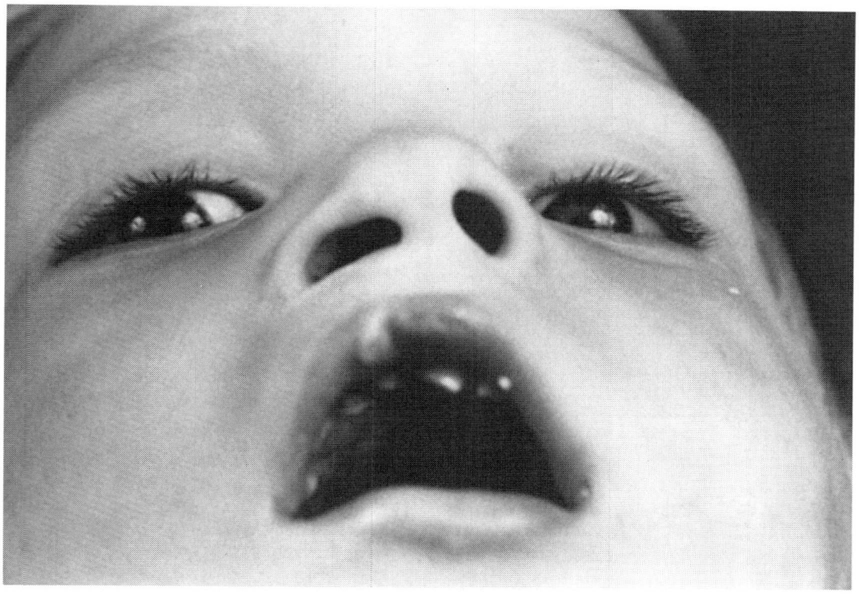

Fig. 10-48. Classic nasal deformity associated with the unilateral cleft lip (Fig. 10-45).

of the internal nares. Interruption of the circumnasal superficial musculo-aponeurotic system (SMAS) may significantly contribute to this deformity[54,137,145] because of the disrupted insertion of the upper nasolabial muscular periosteum. The most important constituent of the deformity is the transverse head of the nasal muscle complex. Precise repair of the perinasal SMAS allows for a more normal, natural form of the nasal sill, alar base, columella, and lower lateral cartilage orientation.[137] Internally, the caudal or anterior end of the cartilaginous septum is frequently deviated into the noncleft side, with an associated inferior septal deviation into the same side and the upper portion of the septum deviated into the cleft side. In addition, the inferior turbinate is often hypertrophied on the side of the cleft, and many patients have an inadequate nasal airway.[14] Approximately 60% of CL/P patients have an airway that is inadequate for normal nasal breathing and average a 30% smaller nasal airway than noncleft patients.[149]

The bilateral cleft lip nose has deformities of the columella, ala, alar base, and internal nares similar to those described for the unilateral cleft, but they present bilaterally. This frequently results in an extremely short columella; a broad, flattened nasal tip; and horizontal orientation of the nares. The columella, caudal septum, and anterior nasal spine are frequently displaced forward or downward (Fig. 10-49).

The goals of surgery for the cleft nasal deformity include reconstruction of the nasal floor and sill, columellar lengthening, correction of the deformed ala, repositioning of the alar base, provision of adequate nasal tip support and symmetry, straightening of the nasal dorsum (if necessary), and achievement of an adequate intranasal airway. Often, obtaining these goals requires one or more operations at different ages.

The described techniques of lip repair reconstruct the nasal floor and sill at the time of the primary lip repair. In addition, the base of the ala may be placed in a more symmetric position and the columella lengthened (in the Millard repair). Some surgeons also perform a partial correction of the nasal tip and alar cartilage during primary lip repair. These can range from simple suturing techniques to perialar incisions and advancements[135] to complete open rhinoplasty with large areas of undermining over the nasal cartilages, over the nasal dorsum, and extending over the maxilla to the infraorbital rim.[27,54,70,142,143] This provides immediate results; however, long-term studies on the effects on nasal and facial growth have not been done. Repair at preschool age may result in difficulties in growth and appearance, which do not show up until adolescence.[136]

Reconstruction of moderate to severe deformities of the nasal tip is frequently performed at 6 to 10 years of age, using tip rhinoplasty with insertion of an implant or graft under the alar base on the side of the cleft (if there is maxillary deficiency). A deficient maxillary platform may be improved when an alveolar ridge bone graft is performed. Other indications are to provide bony support for erupting permanent teeth and to close fistulas. Minor deformities of the nasal tip, intranasal septum, and nasal bones are usually repaired at 14 to 18 years of age. This delay may allow for the use of local anesthesia and minimizes possible disturbance of facial growth.

Surgical techniques

Many surgical techniques are available to correct the cleft nasal deformity. Standard intranasal rhinoplasty approaches for correction of the cleft nasal deformity are usually inadequate, often producing a less-than-desired result. An external approach appears to provide the best results. Basic external

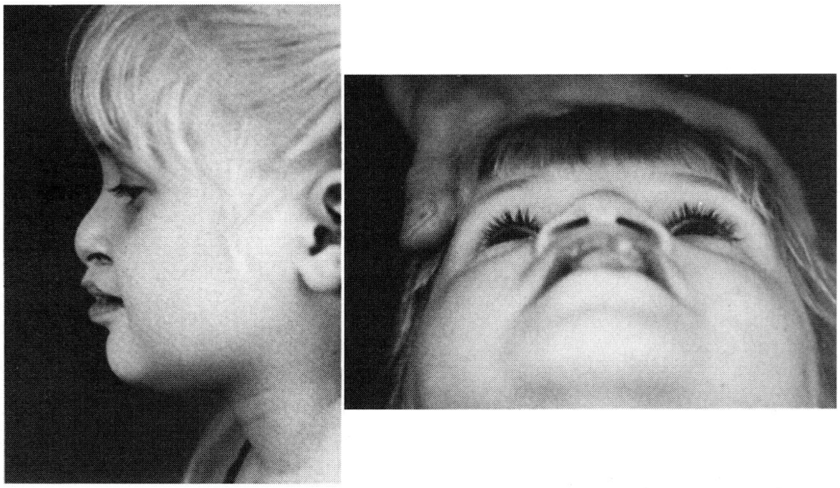

Fig. 10-49. A patient with typical nasal deformity associated with a bilateral cleft lip. The columella is extremely short, the nasal tip is broad and flattened with horizontal orientation of the external nares, and the alae are displaced laterally and posteriorly. **A,** Side view. **B,** View from below.

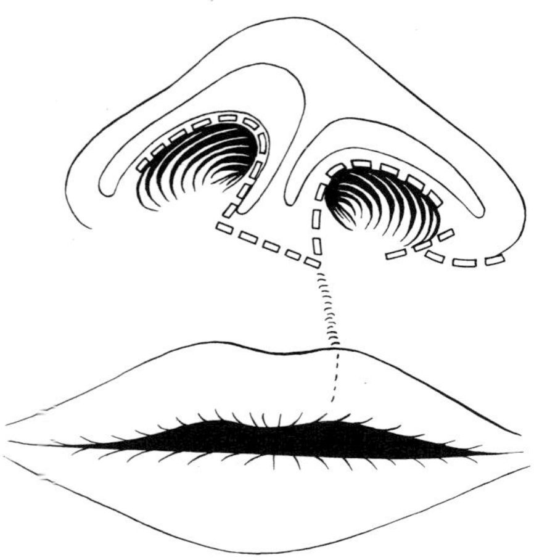

Fig. 10-50. Repair of the unilateral cleft nose: incisions for the external (Bardach) approach. The columella is lengthened by asymmetric V-Y advancement, using skin from the midportion of the lip. In bilateral clefts, columellar lengthening is obtained by using tissue from the same area; however, incisions of upper lip use symmetric V-Y advancement rather than asymmetric advancement.

techniques for correcting the cleft nasal deformity include the approach described by Dibbell[29] and Bardach[8] (Fig. 10-50).

Dibbell technique

The surgical technique developed by Dibbell[29] involves extensive surgical incisions of the ala nasi, the lateral alar margin, and the lip. The horizontally directed cleft ala and nares are rotated into a vertical orientation, excessive skin at the margin of the cleft ala is excised, the alar base is rotated and advanced into a correct anatomic location (requiring advancement of the lateral portion of the lip to correct the resultant deformity), and the misplaced and deformed lateral crus of the alar cartilage is inserted into proper position and maintained with sutures. This technique can correct most cleft nose deformities, achieving excellent cosmetic results. However, this technique involves extensive surgery, and obtaining these results requires advanced surgical ability and judgment.

Bardach technique

The external approach described by Bardach[8] is shown in Figures 10-51 through 10-53. This method of correction lengthens the columella by the use of a triangular skin flap from the middle portion of the upper lip in bilateral and unilateral cleft nasal deformities. A V-Y advancement technique is used, with the apex of the V-shaped skin flap located beneath the middle of the columella in the bilateral cleft and at the lateral margin of the shortened side of the columella in the unilateral cleft. This incision in the upper lip skin is extended superiorly at the base of the columella just caudal to the caudal margin of the medial crus. Superiorly, the incision continues laterally as a marginal incision along the caudal margin of the lower lateral cartilage. Subcutaneous dissection and elevation of the lip and columellar skin as a superiorly based flap provide excellent exposure of the nasal tip. The lateral crura of the lower cartilages are dissected from the underlying vestibular skin and trimmed so that they are symmetric, and the lateral crus of the cleft side is advanced medially and partially incorporated into the shortened medial crus on this side. This lengthens the medial crus. The tip is supported by suturing the apices of the medial crura together to create appropriate tip projection. If hooding of the alar margin on the side of the cleft is still present,

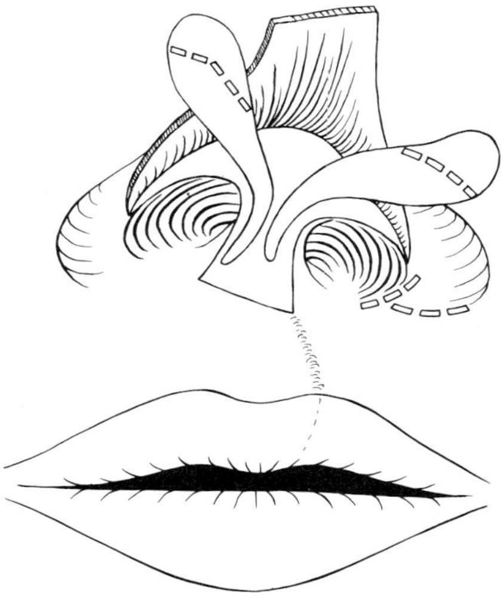

Fig. 10-51. A superiorly based flap of the columellar and lip skin has been elevated, exposing lower lateral cartilages. These cartilages are dissected totally free from underlying nasal mucosa and trimmed to be asymmetric *(dotted lines)*.

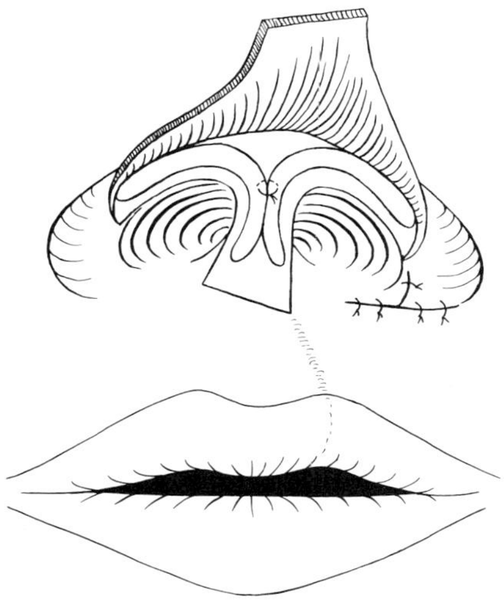

Fig. 10-52. A deformed lateral crus on the cleft side has been scored and advanced medially, lengthening the shortened medial crus on the cleft. To maintain a symmetric tip with adequate projection, permanent suture is placed between reconstructed medial crura at their junction with lateral crura.

further elevation of the lateral crus may be obtained by suturing it to the upper lateral cartilage. A V-Y closure of the skin of the upper lip elongates the columellar skin and narrows the base of the ala. The malpositioned ala may also be corrected at this time by a V-Y advancement technique. If the maxilla on the side of the cleft is deficient, the alar base may be elevated by implanting irradiated cartilage or an iliac crest bone graft beneath the repositioned base. This procedure is often performed in a patient aged 6 to 10 years. A

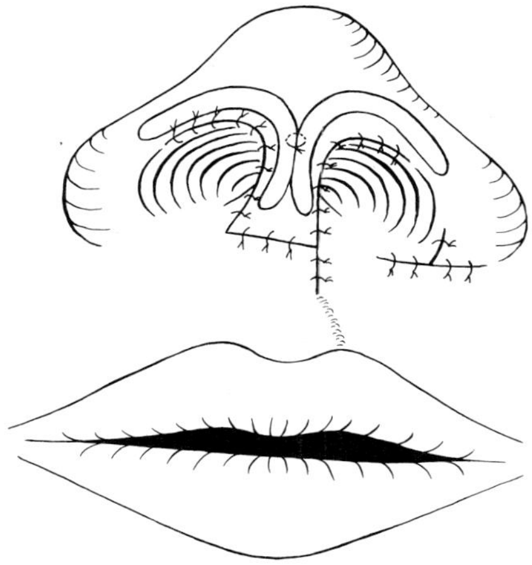

Fig. 10-53. Completed skin closure.

result obtained with this technique is shown in Figure 10-54.

Correction of the septum, inferior turbinate, and bony external nose is usually performed in a patient aged 14 to 18 years using conventional septorhinoplasty techniques.

SPEECH DISORDERS IN CLEFT PALATE

The goal of cleft palate repair is an intact, normal physiologically functioning mechanism that allows development of normal speech. The reported incidence of speech disorders in cleft patients varies widely. Some speech abnormality exists in many cleft palate patients. Such marked variation may be related to the definition of acceptable and normal speech that is used in evaluating these patients. Although success rates of 60% to 70% with primary surgery were acceptable in the past,[89] current techniques should result in at least a 90% incidence of a functionally adequate velopharyngeal mechanism for speech.

Failure to achieve this results in primary and secondary effects on speech. Primary effects include altered nasal resonance (hypernasality); audible nasal emission of air through the nose or nasal turbulence; and articulation disorders, including the absence or distortion of certain sounds, especially those requiring a buildup and sudden release of oral pressure (plosives). Secondary effects include abnormal articulation due to glottic stops, pharyngeal fricatives, and nasal grimace produced by attempts to interrupt or constrict the flow of air in the vocal tract. In addition, there may be omissions or substitutions of speech elements (phonemes). Although there is no such thing as typical cleft palate speech, these patients do tend to make certain types of articulation errors more frequently than noncleft patients with speech disorders[131] (e.g., most commonly, affricative and fricative errors stops; glides; nasal semivowels).[132]

Adequate velopharyngeal function is the most important determinant of articulation and listener understanding in cleft palate patients.[89] Other factors influencing speech in

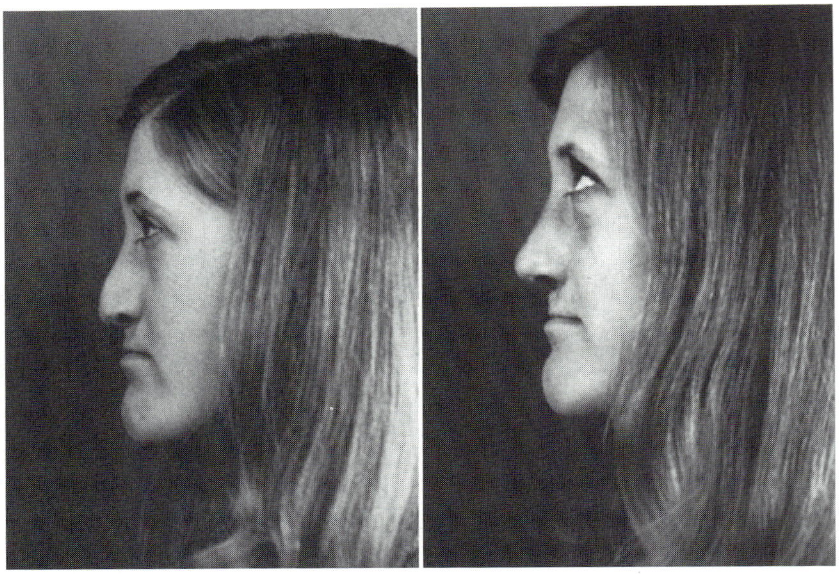

Fig. 10-54. A, Preoperative and **B,** postoperative views after external tip rhinoplasty using an external (Bardach) approach. (From Bumsted RM: *The management of cleft lip and palate*, Iowa City, Iowa, 1980, American Academy of Otolaryngology-Head and Neck Surgery.)

cleft patients include dentition, the presence and severity of associated hearing loss, and muscular and neurologic defects. In addition, the abnormal compensatory patterns of speech production learned by cleft patients before closure of the palate defect and velopharyngeal competence are also significant for speech results after secondary surgical procedures. Previously learned incorrect speech patterns usually continue, and speech therapy is needed to obtain normal speech.

The role of experienced speech pathologists in the diagnosis and therapy of speech disorders in cleft patients cannot be overemphasized. Speech pathologists perform articulation tests in isolated and connected speech and evaluations of the patient's response to standard speech therapy. Speech production is an easier task using isolated words rather than running conversation. This fact may result in a marked difference in articulation proficiency between isolated responses and connected speech. In addition to the results of the specific articulation tests, observation of the patient's articulation in conversational speech provides an evaluation of the speaker's intelligibility level and the degree of the communication handicap. Additional clinical features of velopharyngeal incompetence include facial grimaces associated with the production of pressure sounds, audible nasal emission of air, and improved articulation when the nostrils are manually occluded. In some patients, the response to speech therapy may provide valuable diagnostic information.

Radiographic evaluation of patients with speech disorders may include videofluoroscopy and lateral radiography. Multiview videofluoroscopy is best used to evaluate the degree of palatal movement and velopharyngeal closure during conversational speech. Lateral radiography of the head can determine palatal position and motion during the production of a speech sound, such as a sustained /s/, which requires an essentially complete velopharyngeal closure. Lateral radiography provides information on the degree of palatal elevation and posterior wall movement and the degree of closure obtained in an anteroposterior direction during the production of isolated words rather than the degree of closure actually obtained during conversational speech. The degree of lateral pharyngeal wall motion cannot be determined by this technique; it requires a basilar view, which is more difficult to obtain and evaluate clinically.

Clinical examination of the depth of the nasopharynx and palatal length and estimation of the degree of palatal mobility may be obtained during phonation. However, there may be a marked difference between palatal mobility in connected speech and in phonation of a single sound. Additional information regarding palatal and pharyngeal wall motion may be obtained by nasopharyngoscopy performed with a flexible fiberoptic endoscope. This technique allows direct visualization of palatal motion, pharyngeal wall motion (including the lateral and posterior pharyngeal walls), and the extent and pattern of any velopharyngeal gap during speech.[26] Disadvantages of nasoendoscopy includes its invasiveness, the skill required to properly use and interpret the resulting image, and the difficulty to obtain cooperation in children younger than 4 years. It also provides no quantitative data. In patients who have undergone operations such as a pharyngeal flap with residual velopharyngeal insufficiency, it is the only diagnostic method currently available. Manometry also may be used to compare the maximal pressures obtained with rapid, forced expirations in the open and manually occluded nares. The ratio of open to occluded pressures allows a gross quantitative measurement of velopharyngeal competence; a value of 0.5 or less usually indicates significant velopharyngeal incompetence. The greater the degree of incompetence, the lower the ratio. The nasometer is a microcomputer that measures the difference between nasal and oral acoustic energy output during speech. A ratio of the two energy sources is computed as a ''nasalance'' score, which provides a quantitative assessment of nasality. Drawbacks of the nasometer are its dependence on accurate normative data and calibration and its expense.

These tests provide useful measurements of different aspects of velopharyngeal function. Fundamentally, however, the trained ear plays an important role in determining velopharyngeal adequacy. Studies by Morris and Van Demark show a greater than 90% correlation between a trained speech pathologist's assessment, articulation tests, and radiography that still applies today.

Speech therapy

Speech therapy is the initial method of choice in all patients with speech disorders. The speech therapist conducts initial parental counseling, preferably before the child is 6 months old. The importance of talking and playing with the child is reinforced to the parents who frequently assume that speech stimulation is unnecessary because the infant has an abnormal mechanism for speech production. Formal speech therapy is usually not initiated until 3 to 4 years of age and is used only after the speech pathologist can determine which aspects of the speech abnormality can be improved by therapy. Biofeedback using a device such as a nasometer to allow a visual correlation of velopharyngeal function has been successful in some patients.[36,67] Failure to respond to speech therapy may be important in selecting patients who need secondary surgical procedures to correct velopharyngeal incompetence.

In addition to the diagnostic role of the speech therapist, additional speech therapy is frequently needed after correction of the anatomic defect by dental or surgical techniques. Prior speech therapy familiarizes patient and parents with this approach, which is more readily accepted and effective after the secondary procedure. Once therapy has been established by an experienced speech pathologist, further therapy may often be obtained in the local community or school system.

Failure to obtain significant improvement in velopharyngeal competence after 6 to 12 months of programmed speech therapy usually indicates a need for secondary methods of management. Articulation errors may require correction of dental abnormalities; however, once dental problems are corrected, the only available method of correction of articulation errors is speech therapy.

The basic goal of secondary procedures for the correction of velopharyngeal incompetence is the development of a clinically competent velopharyngeal sphincter to produce normal speech. This need not be a completely airtight velopharyngeal port because, as Bjork[12] showed, speech is usually not affected if the size of the velopharyngeal port during speech production is less than 20 mm^2; ''however, the non-trained listener cannot detect this.''[12]

Dental prostheses

Dental prostheses that may be used for the correction of velopharyngeal incompetence include palatal lifts and obturators. A palatal lift is rarely used in patients with cleft palate and velopharyngeal incompetence and is indicated only for patients with a poorly mobile palate and with adequate palatal length to close the velopharyngeal port on elevation of the palate. In most cleft palate patients, a dental obturator is necessary. These prosthetic devices occlude the nasopharynx so that the patient may obtain velopharyngeal competence during speech. These obturators are best used as a primary method of management in an unoperated cleft palate because it is difficult to obtain satisfactory results in patients with prior attempts at surgical repair of the palatal defect.

Use of a dental prosthesis constructed by an experienced and qualified prosthodontist is a highly effective method of obtaining velopharyngeal competence. A dental prosthesis is indicated in patients who refuse surgery, certain patients for whom surgery has been a failure, and high-risk patients for whom surgery is contraindicated. Advantages of this method are avoidance of surgery with its associated morbidity and mortality and a success rate approximating that obtained by surgery. Disadvantages of a prosthesis include the need for modification as the patient grows; the need for repairs as it wears out; and the frequent failure of insurance plans to reimburse the patient for the cost of constructing, modifying, and repairing the prosthesis. In addition, compliance in younger children is difficult, assuming a prosthesis can be constructed for them at all. Such devices have been used successfully in selected patients with neurologic deficits such as hypesthesia of the palate.

Patients who successfully use a dental prosthesis for speech production should be persuaded to continue its use because their speech production after surgical correction may be less satisfactory than presurgical speech. In addition, construction and successful use of a dental prosthesis may be extremely difficult or impossible after a failed surgical procedure, which could result in permanent poorer speech. This situation should be repeatedly stressed to the patient and relatives before undertaking any attempt at surgical correction.

Surgical correction

The best type of surgical correction for velopharyngeal insufficiency depends on correct assessment of the problem. The importance of determining the pattern, the location, and the degree of participation of the velum and the lateral and posterior pharyngeal walls cannot be overemphasized. At times, a combination of techniques such as palatal push-back and pharyngeal flap may be indicated.

Palatal elongation. Small deficiencies in velar elevation (<0.5 cm) as seen on lateral radiography or endoscopy may be corrected by palatal push-back techniques similar to those described for primary palatoplasty.[41] However, it is uncommon to use this technique alone. In older children and adults undergoing primary palatoplasty, a push-back technique is often used with a primary pharyngeal flap because of the reduced likelihood of achieving velopharyngeal competency with palatoplasty alone.

Pharyngeal implants and rolls. Posterior pharyngeal wall implants and pharyngeal wall procedures are considered together because both involve projecting the posterior pharyngeal wall anteriorly, in effect creating a permanent Passavant's ridge. They may be effective in patients with midline defects of 1 cm or less and a mobile soft palate on endoscopy. Implant materials include cartilage, both autograph and cadaveric irradiated, and synthetic materials such as polymeric silicone or alloplastic, which risk infection and extrusion. Polytef paste injections, although highly effective, are no longer federally approved for this area.

The pharyngeal roll operation consists of raising a small superiorly based flap from the posterior pharyngeal wall, rolling it like a jelly roll, and suturing it to the prevertebral fascia at the correct level.

Pharyngoplasty techniques. Pharyngoplasty is the use of various flaps of pharyngeal tissue to narrow the pharynx or produce a forward projection of the posterior pharyngeal wall. Pharyngoplasty basically involves the transposition of local flaps of posterolateral pharyngeal wall tissue, which are sutured into an incision in the posterior pharyngeal wall. Hynes[57] created superiorly based flaps consisting of a salpingopharyngeal muscle and a significant portion of the lateral pharyngeal wall musculature. These flaps were transposed and sutured together into a horizontal incision across the posterior pharynx; closure of the flap donor sites narrows the entire velopharyngeal port. Orticochea[96] described a technique that attempts to produce a dynamic sphincter in the velopharyngeal port area by use of bilateral superiorly based flaps of the posterior tonsillar pillars (palatopharyngeal muscles), which are sutured into an inferiorly based pharyngeal flap. Orticochea believed that, after a healing period, this procedure would create a diaphragm-like sphincter, which would produce a circular, contractible hole in the center of the velopharyngeal port. This hole could be closed during speech production and swallowing, thereby providing velopharyngeal competence. The incidence of postoperative airway obstruction appears to be greater with this technique.

Recently, pharyngoplasty techniques without the posterior pharyngeal flap have become popular over the past decade.[57a,120a] These may be the procedures of choice when lateral pharyngeal wall mobility is absent or poor and velar elevation is good (coronal pattern of closure). The palatopharyngeal flaps require rotation and placement high into the nasopharynx (Fig. 10-55). They may be sutured end to end or overlap to further narrow the velopharyngeal port. The advantages of this technique include rapid recovery due to decreased pain and dysphasia and, usually, less airway obstruction than with a posterior pharyngeal flap.

Pharyngeal flap. A pharyngeal flap is created by elevating mucosa and its underlying constrictor muscle from the posterior pharyngeal wall; it is then sutured into the palate. This produces tissue obturation of most of the velopharyngeal valve with the only remaining openings located between the lateral margin of the flap and the lateral pharyngeal wall. Thus, during speech, only these lateral port areas should be occluded to obtain velopharyngeal competence (Fig. 10-56). A pharyngeal flap is the most common surgical technique for correcting velopharyngeal incompetence. It is indicated when there is poor velar elevation with good medial mobility of the lateral pharyngeal walls (sagittal pattern of closure) as determined by videofluoroscopy and endoscopy.

Significant improvements in the surgical construction of pharyngeal flaps include the creation of as wide a based flap as possible,[150] mucosal coverage of the raw surface of the flap to minimize flap contracture during healing,[13] control of the surgically constructed lateral pharyngeal port's size,[52] and variable lateral port size based on the degree of lateral pharyngeal wall motion.[58] Hogan[52] designed an operation (lateral port control) to limit the combined size of lateral ports to less than 20 mm^2, which is reported by Bjork[12] to be the maximal velopharyngeal port opening during clinically normal speech. This was accomplished by suturing the lateral margin of a superiorly based pharyngeal flap to an incision in the lateral pharyngeal wall so that it was snug around a 14 French catheter. This provided 97% success in obtaining velopharyngeal competence. However, this high rate of success also is associated with a high incidence of significant nasal airway obstruction.

Use of a variable approach to lateral port size produces a high rate of velopharyngeal competence and reduces the incidence of nasal airway obstruction in patients in whom a larger port can be used. Patients with little or no lateral pharyngeal wall motion require lateral ports of less than 20 mm^2 to obtain satisfactory velopharyngeal competence. A high incidence of nasal airway obstruction results; patients should be informed of this before the procedure. Patients with moderate or large degrees of lateral pharyngeal wall motion can maintain velopharyngeal competence with larger port size and have a low incidence of postoperative nasal airway obstruction.

Most surgeons prefer a superiorly rather than an inferiorly based pharyngeal flap; however, studies have failed to show any significant difference in speech using these flaps.[152] The superiorly based flap allows a flap of any length to be constructed, a more normal situation because the flap tends to

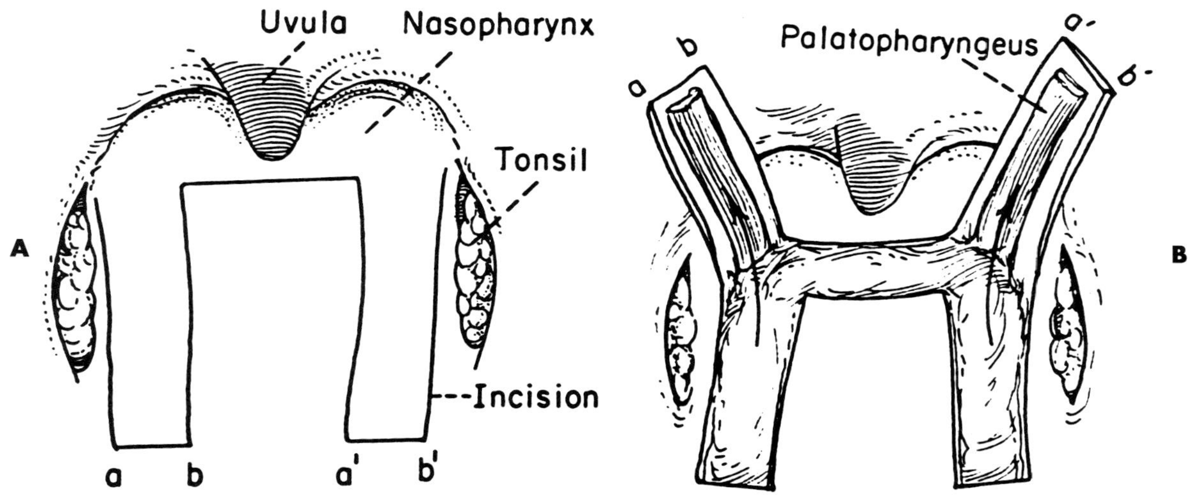

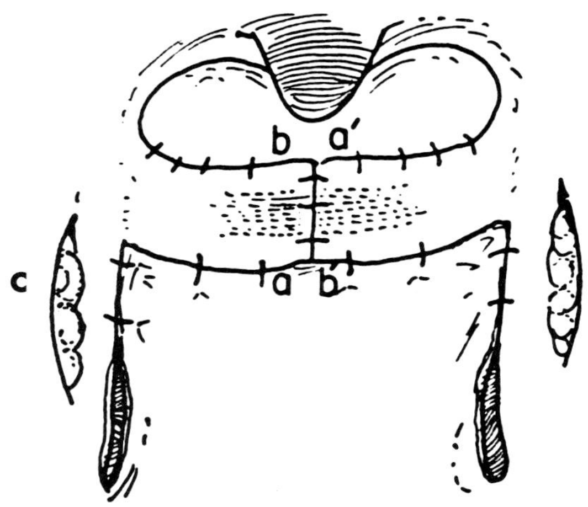

Fig. 10-55. **A,** Posterior tonsillar pillar flaps outlined with a transverse incision across the posterior pharyngeal wall. **B,** Tonsillar pillar flaps elevated with the palatopharyngeal muscles. **C,** Pillar flaps rotated 90° and sutured across the transverse defect and posterior pharyngeal wall end to end. The lateral defects are closed. (From Jackson IT: Clinics in plastic surgery, *Plast Reconstr Surg* 12:714, 1985. Used by permission.)

elevate rather than depress the soft palate; postoperatively, the raw surface is accessible if bleeding occurs, unlike an inferiorly based flap, which is inacesssible.

The indications for a prepharyngeal flap adenoidectomy include an extremely large adenoid mass that may partially occlude the lateral ports or make creation of the pharyngeal flap difficult, chronic eustachian tube dysfunction that has not responded to prior insertion of ventilating tubes, recurrent respiratory infections or chronic nasal drainage associated with clinical evidence or recurrent adenoiditis, and chronic sinus disease in a child who needs a pharyngeal flap. The pharyngeal flap prevents access to the nasopharynx for adenoidectomy, which is usually performed 6 weeks before the flap procedure. Staging of these operations is necessary because postoperative bleeding from the nasopharynx is inaccessible after the flap is created, and the adenoidectomy may result in diminished vascularity at the base of a superiorly based flap.

Surgical technique. A pharyngeal flap is performed on a patient under general anesthesia and in a position similar to that assumed for a palatoplasty, with endotracheal intubation and hypopharyngeal pack insertion. Injection of 0.5% lidocaine with 1:1,000,000 epinephrine into the posterior pharyngeal wall and palate decreases operative bleeding. Vertical incisions in the posterior pharyngeal wall should be made just medial to the junction of the lateral and posterior pharyngeal walls superiorly with a gentle curve medially toward the inferior extent of the flap (Fig. 10-57). These incisions extend through the superior constrictor muscle to the prevertebral fascia, on which blunt and sharp dissection is used to elevate a superiorly based flap. Flap elevation begins at the apex and extends superiorly to the level of the hard palate. Electrocautery is used to control bleeding.

The opening in the palate may be created by a midline incision that transects the soft palate (lateral port control technique) or by a horizontal incision on the nasal surface of the soft palate that extends into the midportion of the palate (sandwich technique) (Fig. 10-58). Both techniques use the mucosa of the nasal surface of the palate as a flap based on the posterior margin of the palate to provide mucosal coverage of the raw surface of the superiorly based pharyngeal flap. In the sandwich technique, a pocket is cre-

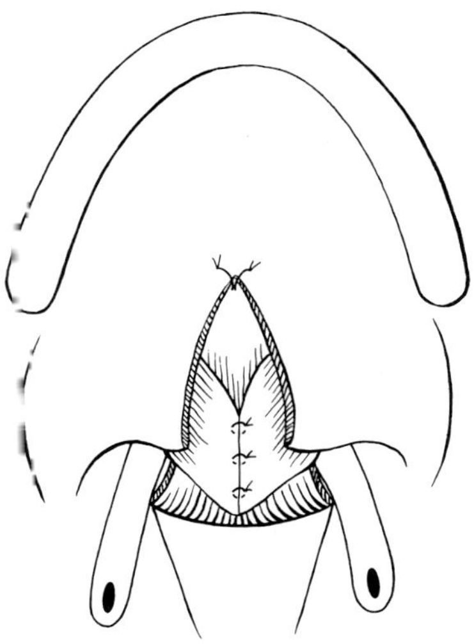

Fig. 10-61. Lateral port control method. Palatal lining flaps are sutured over the raw surface of the pharyngeal flap.

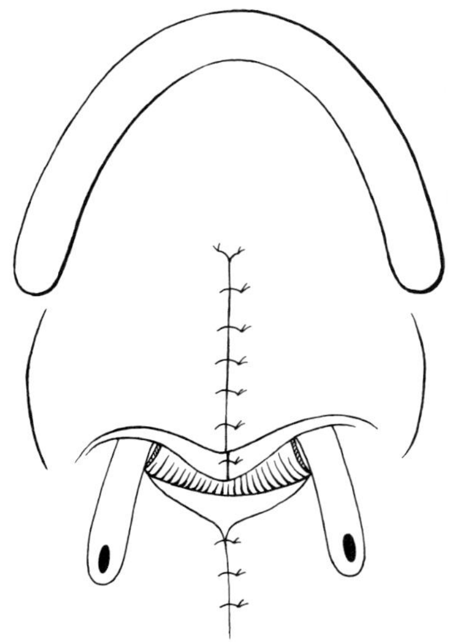

Fig. 10-62. Lateral port control method. The soft palate is repaired in layers, and the flap donor site is closed.

occurs, resulting in total nasal obstruction and denasal voice. A polysomnogram may be indicated to document obstructive sleep apnea. The lateral ports may be enlarged with a Z-plasty technique or by laser excision of the port margin followed by prolonged (4 to 6 weeks) endotracheal tube stenting of the enlarged ports. Occasionally, entire release of the flap pedicle should be done to relieve airway obstructive symptoms. Deterioration in velopharyngeal function for speech is rare.[17]

DENTAL MANAGEMENT

Adequate dental care is necessary and desirable in all patients; however, cleft patients have more severe dental problems than the normal population has. A dentist or pedodontist can often deliver routine dental care. All teeth should be preserved if possible because future occlusion and the ability to retain a dental prosthesis may depend on the presence of an adequate number of teeth. In addition to basic dental problems, cleft children frequently have congenitally missing teeth (50%) and an abnormally formed tooth (27%) in the area of the cleft.[95] Supernumerary teeth occur in 21% of cleft patients compared with 1% of the normal population. Frequently, cleft patients require additional specialized dental care by an experienced prosthodontist and orthodontist.

A maxillofacial prosthodontist is frequently involved in the lifelong management of cleft patients. Prosthodontic cleft care includes the use of presurgical orthopedics, fixed prosthodontics (crown and bridge), and removable prostheses.

Presurgical orthopedics involve the use of a prosthetic to obtain a more favorable relationship of the maxillary arches before lip repair in unilateral cleft lip and palate. Improved alignment of the maxillary arches often facilitates lip repair by improving the relationship of the underlying bony structures in patients who have wide clefts or severe malalignment of the maxillary arches. The appliance is usually constructed during the second week of life and is designed so that pressure is applied to specific areas of the maxillary arch to move segments into a more favorable anatomic position. This appliance is usually fitted to the bottle nipple and pacifier and functions when the child sucks. It should be modified every week because the segments change position and growth occurs in this area. This appliance is usually used for 3 to 6 months before closure of the lip, and most patients undergo lip surgery after 4 months of use.[72]

A bridge is a fixed dental prosthesis permanently placed in the mouth by using two or more remaining teeth as abutments and restoring a segment of missing teeth or an individual tooth. A crown is a fixed dental prosthesis that restores the normal contour and function of a damaged or malformed tooth; however, it uses the remaining tooth and root structure rather than adjacent teeth for retention. Cleft patients frequently require these types of fixed prostheses for maintenance of teeth and for replacement of teeth lost secondary to disease or to the congenital defect.

Removable prosthetic appliances include dentures (partial or complete) and dental appliances (e.g., palatal lifts, obturators). Removable partial dentures may be used instead of fixed bridges to restore missing or malformed anterior teeth in cleft patients. A dental obturator may provide velopharyngeal competence or be used to close a defect in the palate by physically occluding the opening between the oral cavity and nose, thereby improving speech and swallowing. Basic indications for the use of a dental prosthesis to occlude palatal defects include replacement of missing teeth, medical problems contraindicating surgery, patient refusal of surgery, extensive defects difficult to close surgically, and prior failure of surgical closure in patients who do not desire additional surgery. The primary disadvantages of prostheses are the problems associated with wearing them and the necessity for their intermittent replacement.

The main goals of orthodontic care in cleft patients are to establish a functional dental occlusion, create an acceptable facial appearance, facilitate facial growth, and assist in speech production and development. Olin[94] divided orthodontic care of the cleft patient into phase I—therapy delivered during primary dentition, which consists mainly of expansion of the maxillary arches; phase II—therapy during mixed dentition; and phase III—final corrections performed after the eruption of all permanent teeth.

The most common orthodontic deformity in patients with cleft palates is an anterior or posterior crossbite, which usually occurs on the side of the cleft. With this condition, there is an abnormal occlusion, with the teeth of the maxillary arch contacting the mandibular teeth medial to the normal anatomic position. These occlusion abnormalities may be corrected by orthodontic expansion of the maxillary arch to an appropriate anatomic position. Repair of an oronasal fistula in a patient with a crossbite should be delayed until the maxillary expansion is complete to prevent dehiscence or recurrence of the fistula secondary to this expansion. Rotated, malaligned, or missing teeth adjacent to the cleft defect may frequently be corrected by basic orthodontic techniques. If a significant bony defect exists in addition to the abnormal occlusion, surgery may be necessary for correction. This procedure can involve a maxillary or mandibular osteotomy, depending on the patient's appearance, the occlusion, and cephalometric analysis. With proper orthodontic care, most patients can eventually be provided with functional and aesthetically normal dental occlusion.

This description of the dental care in cleft patients shows the vital role of dental specialists in multidisciplinary management. The interaction of these specialists with other team members in regard to the method and timing of various secondary surgical procedures is also very important. Without this input into overall patient management, surgical correction of various deformities can complicate orthodontic therapy or result in recurrence of the original problem once the orthodontic therapy is completed. Dental specialists are thus necessary in the management of CL/P patients.

EAR DISEASE

Patients who have clefts involving only the lip have an incidence of middle ear disease similar to that in the general population. However, many authors have reported a greater incidence of hearing loss in patients with cleft palate.* Although these studies have shown an increased incidence of hearing loss, there is disagreement regarding the type and degree of hearing loss. This variation appears to be related to the definition of hearing loss used in the studies and to the age of the cleft patient evaluated for hearing loss.

Abnormal insertion of the levator and tensor veli palatini muscles into the posterior margin of the hard palate and the muscular hypoplasia appears to be the primary cause of eustachain tube dysfunction in cleft patients. However, there is recent evidence that the nature of middle ear effusions in cleft patients is different from that in noncleft patients. Hutton and others[56] recently published a study on the characterization of mucin from the effusions of cleft patients. When compared with mucoid and serous effusions from noncleft patients, the mucin in the middle ears of cleft patients, contained larger glycopeptides with a larger hydrodynamic size. This suggests that infections in cleft patients may be different from those in noncleft patients.

Severeid[115] found evidence of eustachian tube dysfunction resulting in conductive hearing loss or middle ear effusion in 84% of patients with cleft palate. The only significant variable that correlated with the incidence of eustachian tube dysfunction was the age of the patient. With increasing patient age, the incidence of eustachian tube function decreased; in most cases, normal eustachian tube function eventually developed with increasing patient age. During long-term follow-up of these patients, 7% developed cholesteatomas despite regular otolaryngologic examinations every 3 to 6 months from birth.[116] At Washington University, 96.2% of 132 children with cleft palate developed middle ear disease significant enough to require tympanostomy tube placement before or at palatoplasty.[90] Nearly 50% of these children required repeat tube placement. The incidence of middle ear complications included persistent perforation in 13%, cholesteatoma in about 1%, and chronic otorrhea in 6%. A trend was noted toward decreasing rate of tube insertion with increasing age because less than 50% of the population required tubes after age 3. Management of cleft palate patients with respect to ear disease should be aggressive because the already delayed speech development related to the cleft itself will be only compounded by significant hearing loss during the critical ages for speech development. Paradise, Elster, and Tan[98] showed that artificially fed breast milk provided some protection against the development of otitis media in infants with cleft palate.

Currently, the goal of the management of ear disease in cleft palate patients is to provide adequate hearing, maintain ossicular continuity, maintain adequate middle ear space, and prevent deterioration of the tympanic membrane until the patient develops adequate eustachian tube function. All patients are carefully examined at least every 3 to 6 months until they develop adequate eustachian tube function. After this they are evaluated at maximal intervals of 1 year. Any patient with recurrence of eustachian tube dysfunction is evaluated at least every 3 to 6 months until the problem resolves and is adequate on two consecutive examinations.

Indications for myringotomy and insertion of ventilating tubes include those which are widely accepted (persistent

* Refs. 49, 75, 78, 84, 85, 110, 120, 130.

middle ear effusion with a conductive hearing loss despite adequate medical management, recurrent acute otitis media failing prophylaxis, a combination of both, or presence of a retraction pocket). Borderline cases should be managed aggressively in this population given the high incidence of middle ear complications and persistent eustachian tube dysfunction. Ventilation tubes should improve the patient's hearing and may improve speech. In addition, this aggressive management and frequent evaluation may provide early detection of complications, allowing for management at an earlier stage.

REFERENCES

1. Abbott BD, and others: Effects of 5-fluorouracil on embryonic rat palate in vitro: fusion in the absence of proliferation, *Teratology* 47: 541, 1993.
2. Amwayi F: The development of the secondary palate: update on concepts and mechanisms, *East Afr Med J* 70:588, 1993.
3. Ardinger HH, and others: Association of genetic variation of the transforming growth factor-alpha gene with cleft lip and palate, *Am J Hum Genet* 45:348, 1989.
4. Bardach J: *Cleft lip and palate*, Warsaw, 1967, Polish Institute of Medical Publications (in Polish).
5. Bardach J, Kelly KM, Salyer KE: A comparative study of facial growth following lip repair performed in sequence and simultaneously: an experimental study in beagles, *Plast Reconstr Surg* 91:1008, 1993.
6. Bardach J, Kelly KM, Salyer KE: The effects of lip repair with and without soft-tissue undermining and delayed palate repair on maxillary growth: an experimental study in beagles, *Plast Reconstr Surg* 94:343, 1994.
7. Bardach J, Kelly KM, Salyer KE: Relationship between the sequence of lip and palate repair and maxillary growth: an experimental study in beagles, *Plast Reconstr Surg* 94:343, 1994.
8. Reference deleted in pages.
9. Bernstein L: The effect of timing of cleft palate operations on subsequent growth of the maxilla, *Laryngoscope* 78:1510, 1968.
10. Bishara SE and others: Facial and dental relationships of individuals with unoperated clefts of the lip and/or palate, *Cleft Palate Craniofac J* 13:238, 1976.
11. Bishara SE, Krause CJ, Olin WH: Cephalometric findings in two cases with unrepaired bilateral cleft lip and palate, *Cleft Palate Craniofac J* 15:232, 1978.
12. Bjork L: Velopharyngeal function in connected speech, *Acta Radiol Suppl* 202:1, 1961.
13. Blackfield HM and others: Cinefluorographic analysis of the surgical treatment of cleft palate speech, *Plast Reconstructr Surg* 31:542, 1963.
14. Bumsted RM: A study of intranasal anatomy and function in mature patients with complete unilateral cleft lip and palate. Paper presented at the International Meeting on Cleft Lip and Palate, Acapulco, May 7, 1981.
15. Bumsted RM: A new method for achieving complete two-layer closure of a massive palatal cleft, *Arch Otolaryngol Head Neck Surg* 108:147, 1982.
16. Cannon RH: Unilateral cleft lip, *N Engl J Med* 227:583, 1967.
17. Caouette-Laberge L, Egerszegi EP, De Remont A: Long-term follow-up after division of a pharyngeal flap for severe nasal obstruction, *Cleft Palate Craniofac J* 29:27, 1992.
18. Capelozza L Jr, Taniguchi SM, da Silva OG Jr: Craniofacial morphology of adult unoperated complete unilateral cleft lip and palate patients, *Cleft Palate Craniofac J* 30:376, 1993.
19. Chenevix-Trench G and others: Cleft lip with or without cleft palate: associations with transforming growth factor alpha and retinoic acid receptor loci, *Am J Hum Genet* 51:1377, 1992.
20. Christensen K, Fogh-Anderson P: Cleft lip (+/− cleft palate) in Danish twins, 1970–1990, *Am J Med Genet* 47:910, 1993.
21. Christensen K, Fogh-Anderson P: Isolated cleft palate in Danish multiple births, 1970–1990, *Cleft Palate Craniofac J* 30:469, 1993.
22. Christensen K, Fogh-Anderson P: Etiological subgroups in non-syndromic isolated cleft palate: a genetic-epidemiological study of 52 Danish birth cohorts, *Clin Genet* 46:329, 1994.
23. Cohen MM: Syndromes with cleft lip and palate, *Cleft Palate Craniofac J* 15:306, 1978.
24. Cohen SR and others: Soft palate myogenesis: a developmental field paradigm, *Cleft Palate Craniofac J* 31:345, 1994.
25. Cohen M, Polley JW, Figueroa AA: Secondary (intermediate) alveolar bone grafting, *Clin Plast Surg* 20:691, 1993.
26. Cohen SR and others: Patterns of abnormal myogenesis in human cleft palates, *Cleft Palate Craniofac J* 31:345, 1994.
27. Cook TA, Davis RE, Israel JM: The extended Skoog technique for repair of the unilateral cleft lip and nose deformity, *Facial Plast Surg* 9:195, 1993.
28. Croft CB and others: The occult submucous cleft palate and the musculus uvulae, *Cleft Palate Craniofac J* 15:150, 1978.
29. Dibbell DG: Cleft lip nasal reconstruction correction of the classic unilateral defect, *Plast Reconstructr Surg* 69:264, 1982.
30. Dingman RO, Ricker OL, Lob V: Blood loss in infant cleft lip and palate surgery, *Plast Reconstructr Surg* 4:333, 1949.
31. Dorf DF, Curtin JW: The early cleft palate repair and speech outcome, *Plast Reconstr Surg* 70:74, 1982.
32. Eufinger H and others: Clefts of the lip and palate in twins: use of DNA fingerprinting for zygosity determination, *Cleft Palate Craniofac J* 30:564, 1993.
33. Fara M: *The musculature of cleft lip and palate.* In Converse TM, editor: *Reconstructive plastic surgery*, vol 4, Philadelphia, 1977, WB Saunders.
34. Farrall M, Holder S: Familial recurrence-pattern analysis of cleft lip with or without cleft palate, *Am J Hum Genet* 50:270, 1992.
35. Feng H and others: Evidence from family studies for linkage disequilibrium between TGFA and a gene for nonsyndromic cleft lip with or without cleft palate, *Am J Hum Genet* 55:932, 1994.
36. Fletcher S: *Diagnosing speech disorders: cleft palate*, New York, 1978, Grune & Stratton.
37. Fraser FC: Invited editorial: mapping the cleft-lip genes: the first fix, *Am J Hum Genet* 45:345, 1989.
38. Friede H, Lilja J: Dentofacial morphology in adolescent or early adult patients with cleft lip and palate after a treatment regimen that included vomer flap surgery and pushback palatal repair, *Scand J Plast Reconstr Surg Hand Surg* 28:113, 1994.
39. Friede H: Abnormal craniofacial growth, *Acta Odontol Scand* 53:203, 1995.
40. Friede FH and others: Maxillary dental arch and occlusion in patients with repaired clefts of the secondary palate: influence of push back palatal surgery, *Scand J Plast Reconstr Surg Hand Surg* 27:297, 1993.
41. Furlow LT Jr: Cleft palate repair by double opposing Z-plasty, *Plast Reconstr Surg* 78:724, 1986.
42. Goldstein L: Intellectual impairment in children with cleft palate, *J Speech Hear Disord* 4:287, 1961.
43. Gorlin RJ, Cohen MM, Levin LS: *Orofacial clefting syndromes: other syndromes.* In Motulsky AG and others, editors: *Syndromes of the head and neck*, vol 19, ch 2, ed 3, New York, 1990, Oxford Press.
44. Gorlin RJ, Cohen MM, Levin LS: *Orofacial clefting syndromes: associations.* In Motulsky AG and others, editors: *Syndromes of the head and neck*, vol 19, ch 23, ed 3, New York, 1990, Oxford Press.
45. Gorlin RJ, Cohen MM, Levin LS: *Orofacial clefting syndromes: other syndromes.* In Motulsky AG and others, editors: *Syndromes of the head and neck*, vol 19, ch 22, ed 3, New York, 1990, Oxford Press.
46. Gorlin RJ, Cohen MM, Levin LS: *Orofacial clefting syndromes: gen-*

eral aspects. In Motulsky AG and others, editors: *Syndromes of the head and neck*, vol 19, ed 3, New York, 1990, Oxford Press.

47. Goulding EH, Pratt RM: Isotretinoin teratogenicity in mouse whole embryo culture, *J Craniofac Genet Dev Biol* 6:99, 1986.
48. Grabb WC: *General aspects of cleft palate surgery.* In Grabb WC, Rosenstein SW, Bzoch KR, editors: *Cleft lip and palate*, Boston, 1971, Little, Brown.
49. Graham MD: A longitudinal study of ear disease and hearing loss in patients with cleft lips and palates, *Trans Am Acad Ophthalmol Otolaryngol* 67:213, 1963.
50. Harris EF: Size and form of the cranial base in isolated cleft lip and palate, *Cleft Palate Craniofac J* 30:170, 1993.
51. Hofstee Y, Kors N, Hennekam RC: Genetic survey of a group of children with clefting: implications for genetic counseling, *Cleft Palate Craniofac J* 30:447, 1993.
52. Hogan VM: A clarification of the surgical goals in cleft palate speech and the introduction of the lateral port control (LPC) pharyngeal flap, *Cleft Palate Craniofac J* 10:331, 1973.
53. Honda Y and others: Longitudinal study on the changes of maxillary arch dimensions in Japanese children with cleft lip and/or palate: infancy to 4 years of age, *Cleft Palate Craniofac J* 32:149, 1995.
54. Horswell BB, Pospisil OA: Nasal symmetry after primary cleft lip repair: comparison between Delaire cheilorhinoplasty and modified rotation-advancement, *J Oral Maxillofac Surg* 53:1025, 1995.
55. Huffman WC, Lierle DM: Studies on the pathologic anatomy of the unilateral harelip nose, *Plast Reconstr Surg* 4:225, 1949.
56. Hutton DA and others: Preliminary characterization of mucin from effusions of cleft palate patients, *Otolaryngol Head Neck Surg* 109: 1000, 1993.
57. Hynes W: Observations in pharyngoplasty, *Br J Plast Surg* 20:224, 1967.

57a. Jackson I: Sphincter pharyngoplasty, *Clin Plast Surg* 12:711, 1985.

58. Johns DF, Salyer KE: A method of correcting difficult problems of velopharyngeal incompetency. Paper presented at the Third International congress on Cleft Palate and Related Craniofacial Anomalies, Toronto, June 1977.
59. Johnston MC, Bronsky PT: Prenatal craniofacial development: new insights on normal and abnormal mechanisms, *Crit Rev Oral Biol Med* 6:25, 1995.
60. Jones MC: Etiology of facial clefts: prospective evaluation of 428 patients, *Cleft Palate Craniofac J* 25:16, 1988.
61. Joos U: Skeletal growth after muscular reconstruction for cleft lip, alveolus and palate, *Br J Oral Maxillofac Surg* 33:139, 1995.
62. Kapucu RM and others: The effect of cleft lip repair on maxillary morphology in patients with unilateral complete cleft lip and palate, *Plast Reconstr Surg* 97:1371, 1996.
63. Khoury MJ, Erickson JD, James LM: Maternal factors in cleft lip with or without cleft palate: evidence from interracial crosses in the United States, *Teratology* 27:351, 1983.
64. Kilner TP: Cleft lip and palate repair technique, *St Thomas Hosp Rep* 2:127, 1937.
65. Kramer GJ, Hoeksma JB, Prahl-Anderson B: Palatal changes after lip surgery in different types of cleft lip and palate, *Cleft Palate Craniofac J* 31:376, 1994.
66. Krause CJ, Van Demark D, Tharp R: Palatoplasty: a comparative study, *Trans Am Acad Ophthalmol Otolaryngol* 80:551, 1975.
67. Kunzel HJ: First applications of a feedback device for the therapy of velopharyngeal competence in vocation, *Folia Phoniatr (Basel)* 34: 92, 1982.
68. Kurnit DM: Genetics, chance and morphogenesis, *Am J Hum Genet* 41:979, 1987.
69. Larosa and others: *The furlow double reversing Z-plasty for cleft palate: the first 10 years of experience.* In Bardach J, Morris HL, editors: *Multidisciplinary management of cleft lip and palate*, Philadelphia, 1990, WB Saunders.
70. LaRossa D, Donath G: Primary nasoplasty in unilateral and bilateral cleft nasal deformity, *Clin Plast Surg* 20:781, 1993.
71. Latham RA: *The anatomy of the facial skeleton in cleft lip and palate.* In Converse JM, editor: *Reconstructive plastic surgery*, vol 4, Philadelphia, 1977, WB Saunders.
72. Lavelle WE, Bardach J: When is presurgical orthopaedic treatment indicated in the unilateral cleft lip and palate patient? Paper presented at the Tenth Annual Meeting of the American Academy of Facial Plastic Reconstructive Surgery, Palm Beach, Fla April 22, 1974.
73. Levine ES: *Auditory disability.* In Garrett JF, Levine ES, editors: *Psychological practices with the physically disabled*, New York, 1962, Columbia University Press.
74. Lewin ML: Management of cleft lip and palate in the United States and Canada: report of a summary, *Plast Reconstr Surg* 33:383, 1964.
75. Linthicum FH, Body H, Keaster J: incidence of middle ear disease in children with cleft palate, *Cleft Palate Bull* 9:23, 1959.
76. Markus AF, Delaire J: Functional primary closure of cleft lip, *Br J Oral Maxillofac Surg* 31:281, 1993.
77. Martin RA, Jones KL, Benirschke K: Extension of the cleft lip phenotype: the subepithelial cleft, *Am J Med Genet* 47:744, 1993.
78. Masters FW, Bingham HG, Robinson DW: The prevention and treatment of hearing loss in the cleft palate child, *Plast Reconstr Surg* 25: 203, 1960.
79. Mazaheri M and others: Evaluation of maxillary dental arch form in unilateral clefts of lip, alveolus, and palate from one month to four years, *Cleft Palate Craniofac J* 30:90, 1993.
80. Melnick M: Cleft lip (± cleft palate) etiology: a search for solutions, *Am J Med Genet* 42:10, 1992.
81. Millard DR Jr: *Cleft craft: the evolution of its surgery, the unilateral deformity*, vol 1, Boston, 1976, Little, Brown.
82. Millard D: *Cleft craft: the evolution of its surgery-alveolar and palatal deformities*, vol 3, Boston, 1980, Little, Brown.
83. Millard DR: A radical rotation in single harelip, *Am J Surg* 95:318, 1958.
84. Miller MH: Hearing problems associated with cleft palate, *Ann Otol Rhinol Laryngol* 68:90, 1959.
85. Miller MH: Hearing losses in cleft palate cases, *Laryngoscope* 66A: 1491, 1959.
86. Mitchell LE, Risch N: Mode of inheritance of nonsyndromic cleft lip with or without cleft palate: a reanalysis, *Am J Hum Genet* 51:323, 1992.
87. Molsted K, Kjaer I, Dahl E: Cranial base in newborns with complete cleft lip and palate: radiographic study, *Cleft Palate Craniofac J* 32: 199, 1995.
88. Moore GE: Molecular genetic approaches to the study of human craniofacial dysmorphologies, *Int Rev Cytol* 77:158, 1995.
89. Morris HL: Velopharyngeal competence and primary cleft palate surgery, 1960–1971: a critical review, *Cleft Palate Craniofac J* 10:62, 1973.
90. Muntz HR: An overview of middle ear disease in cleft palate children, *Facial Plast Surg* 9:177, 1993.
91. Murray JC: Face facts: genes, environment, and clefts, *Am J Hum Genet* 57:227, 1995 (editorial).
92. Musgrave RH, Garrett WS: *The unilateral cleft lip.* In Converse JM, editor: *Reconstructive plastic surgery*, vol 4, Philadelphia, 1977, WB Saunders.
93. Nystrom M, Ranta R: Effect of timing and method of closure of isolated cleft palate on development of dental arches from 3 to 6 years of age, *Eur J Orthod* 16:377, 1994.
94. Olin WH: *Orthodontics.* In Grabb WC, Rosenstein SW, Bzoch KR, editors: *Cleft lip and palate*, Boston, 1971, Little, Brown.
95. Olsen NH: *Pediatric dentistry.* In Grabb WC, Rosenstein SW, Bzoch KR, editors: *Cleft lip and palate*, Boston, 1971, Little, Brown.
96. Orticochea M: Results of the dynamic muscle sphincter operation in cleft palates, *Br J Plast Surg* 23:108, 1970.

97. Ortiz-Monasterio F and others: A study of untreated adult cleft palate patients, *Plast Reconstr Surg* 38:36, 1966.
98. Paradise JL, Elster BA, Tan L: Evidence in infants with cleft palate that breast milk protects against otitis media, *Pediatrics* 94:853, 1994.
99. Pashayan HM: What else to look for in a child born with a cleft lip and/or palate, *Cleft Palate Craniofac J* 20:54, 1983.
100. Precious DS, Delaire J: Clinical observations of cleft lip and palate, *Oral Surg Oral Med Oral Pathol* 75:141, 1993.
101. Randall P: A lip adhesion operation in cleft lip surgery, *Plast Reconstr Surg* 35:371, 1965.
102. Randall P: A triangular flap operation for the primary repair of unilateral clefts of the lip, *Plast Reconstr Surg* 23:331, 1959.
103. Randall P: A triangular flap operation for the primary repair of unilateral clefts of the lip, *Plast Reconstr Surg* 23:331, 1959.
104. Randall P, Graham UP III: *Lip adhesion in the repair of bilateral cleft lip.* In Grabb WC, Rosenstein SW, Bzoch KR, editors: *Cleft lip and palate*, Boston, 1971, Little, Brown.
105. Ross A: *The exceptional child in the family.* In Wirls C, editor: *Psychological aspects of cleft lip and palate*, Boston, 1971, Little, Brown.
106. Ross RB: Growth of the facial skeleton following the Malek repair for unilateral cleft lip and palate. *Cleft Palate Craniofac J* 32:194-98, 1995.
107. Ross RB: *Facial growth in cleft lip and palate.* In Converse JM, editor: *Reconstructive plastic surgery*, vol 4, Philadelphia, 1977, WB Saunders.
108. Ross RB: Treatment variables affecting facial growth in complete unilateral cleft lip and palate, *Cleft Palate Craniofac J* 24:5, 1987.
109. Ruess A: A comparative study of cleft palate children and their siblings, *J Clin Psychol* 21:354, 1965.
110. Sataloff J, Fraser M: Hearing loss in children with cleft palates, *Arch Otolaryngol Head Neck Surg* 55:61, 1952.
111. Schendel SA, Cholonb A, Delaire J: Histochemical analysis of cleft palate muscle, *Plast Reconstr Surg* 94:919, 1994.
112. Schweckendiek W: Primary veloplasty: long-term results without maxillary deformity, a 25 year report, *Cleft Palate Craniofac J* 15: 268, 1978.
113. Seibert RW: Lip adhesion in bilateral cleft lip, *Arch Otolaryngol Head Neck Surg* 109:434, 1983.
114. Seibert RW: *Unilateral cleft lip and palate*, vol 4, Philadelphia, 1990, Mosby.
115. Severeid LR: *A longitudinal study of eustachian tube function and middle ear disease in cleft palate children*, Iowa City, 1971, University of Iowa (Master's thesis).
116. Severeid LR: *Development of cholesteatoma in children with cleft palate: a longitudinal study.* In McCabe BF, Sade J, Abrahamson M, editors: *Cholesteatoma: first international conference*, Birmingham, Ala, 1977, Aesculapius Publishing.
117. Shaing R and others: Association of transforming growth-factor alpha gene polymorphisms with nonsyndromic cleft palate only (CPO), *Am J Hum Genet* 53:836, 1993.
118. Shaw GM and others: Risks of orofacial clefts in children born to women using multivitamins containing folic acid periconceptionally, *Lancet* 346:393, 1995.
119. Shprintzen RJ and others: Anomalies associated with cleft lip, cleft palate or both, *Am J Med Genet* 20:585, 1985.
120. Skolnik WM: Otologic evaluation in cleft palate cases, *Laryngoscope* 68:1908, 1958.
120a. Sloan GM, Reinisch JR, Nichter LS: Surgical treatment of velopharyngeal insufficiency: pharyngoplasty vs. pharyngeal flap, *Plast Surg Forum* 13:123, 1990.
121. Smahel Z, Mullerova Z: Effects of mandibular growth patterns on the development and configuration of the face in patients with unilateral cleft lip and palate, *Scand J Plast Reconstr Surg Hand Surg* 28:207, 1994.
122. Smahel Z, Mullerova Z: Facial growth and development during puberty in unilateral cleft lip and palate: a longitudinal study, *J Craniofac Genet Dev Biol* 14:57, 1994.
123. Smahel Z: Treatment effects on facial development in patients with unilateral cleft lip and palate, *Cleft Palate Craniofac J* 31:437, 1994.
124. Smahel Z, Mullerova Z: Facial growth and development in unilateral cleft lip and palate during the period of puberty: comparison of the development after periosteoplasty and after primary bone grafting, *Cleft Palate Craniofac J* 31:106, 1994.
125. Smahel Z: The prediction of restoration of a positive overjet in unilateral cleft lip and palate, *Acta Chir Plast* 36:42, 1994.
126. Smahel Z and others: Facial growth and development in unilateral complete cleft lip and palate from palate surgery to adulthood, *J Craniofac Genet Dev Biol* 13:57, 1993.
127. Smahel Z, Mullerova Z: Craniofacial growth and development in unilateral cleft lip and palate: clinical implications, *Acta Chir Plast* 37: 29, 1995 (review).
128. Smahel Z, Mullerova Z: Facial growth and development in unilateral cleft lip and palate from the time of palatoplasty to the onset of puberty: a longitudinal study, *J Craniofac Genet Dev Biol* 15:72, 1995.
129. Smith WP, Markus AF, Delaire J: Primary closure of the cleft alveolus: a functional approach, *Br J Oral Maxillofac Surg* 33:156, 1995.
130. Spriesterbach D: Hearing loss in children with cleft palates, *Plast Reconstr Surg* 30:336, 1962.
131. Spriesterbach DC, Morris HL: *Speech problems in patients with cleft lip and palate.* In Converse JM, editor: *Reconstructive plastic surgery*, Philadelphia, 1977, WB Saunders.
132. Spriesterbach DC and others: Hearing loss in children with cleft palates, *Plast Reconstr Surg* 30:336, 1962.
133. Stark RB, DeHann CR: The addition of a pharyngeal flap to primary palatoplasty, *Plast Reconstr Surg* 26:378, 1960.
134. Stein J and others: Nonsyndromic cleft lip with or without cleft palate: evidence of linkage to BCL3 in 17 multigenerational families, *Am J Hum Genet* 57:257, 1995.
135. Sugihara T and others: Primary correction of the unilateral cleft nose, *Cleft Palate Craniofac J* 30:231, 1993.
136. Takato T, Yoneharra Y, Susami T: Early correction of the nose in unilateral cleft lip patients using an open method: a 10-year review, *J Oral Maxillofac Surg* 27:183, 1995.
137. Talmant JC: Nasal malformations associated with unilateral cleft lip: accurate diagnosis and management, *Scand Hand Surg* 27:183, 1993.
138. Tempest MN: Some observations on blood loss in harelip and cleft palate surgery, *Br J Plast Surg* 11:34, 1958
139. Tennison CW: The repair of the unilateral cleft lip by the stencil method, *Plast Reconstr Surg* 23:331, 1959.
140. Tiza V, Gumpertz E: The parents' reaction to the birth and early care of children with cleft palate, *Pediatrics* 30:86, 1962.
141. Tolarova M, Harris J: Reduced recurrence of orofacial clefts after periconceptional supplementation with high-dose folic acid and multivitamins, *Teratology* 51:71, 1995.
142. Trott JA, Mohan N: A preliminary report on one stage open tip rhinoplasty at the time of lip repair in bilateral cleft lip and palate: the Alor Setar experience, *Br J Plast Surg* 46:215, 1993.
143. Trott JA, Mohan N: A preliminary report on open tip rhinoplasty at the time of lip repair in unilateral cleft lip and palate: the Alor Setar experience, *Br J Plast Surg* 46:363, 1993.
144. University of Iowa Cleft Palate Team: Unpublished data, 1962.
145. Verwoerd CD and others: The nose in children with unilateral cleft lip and palate, *Int J Pediatr Otorhinolaryngol* 32(suppl) S45, 1995.
146. Von Langenbeck B: Die uranoplastik Mittels ablosung der mukosperistalen Gaumenuberzuges, *Arch Klin Chir* 2:205, 1861.
147. Walker J Jr and others: Physiologic consideration in cleft lip closure: the C-W technique, *Plast Reconstr Surg* 37:552, 1966.
148. Wardill WEM: The technique of operation for cleft palate, *Br J Surg* 25:117, 1937.

149. Warren DW, Dalston RM, Mayo R: Hypernasality in the presence of adequate velopharyngeal closure, *Cleft Palate Craniofac J* 30:150, 1993.
150 Webster RC and others: Methods of surgical correction of velopharyngeal sphincter incompetence using palatal and posterior pharyngeal tissue: proposed system of classification, *Plast Reconstr Surg* 18:474, 1956.
151. Westlake H, Rutherford D: *Cleft palate*, Englewood Cliffs, NJ, 1966, Prentice-Hall.
152. Whitaker LA and others: A prospective and randomized series comparing superiorly and inferiorly based posterior pharyngeal flaps, *Cleft Palate Craniofac J* 9:304, 1972.
153. Wilroy RS: Embryology and genetics of cleft lip and palate, *Continuing Education* 73, 1979.

Table 11-1. Muscles of the velopharyngeal mechanism

Muscle	Origination	Attachment	Function	Innervation
Tensor veli palatini	Vertical portion arises from the scaphoid fossa at the base of the internal pterygoid plate, from the spine of the sphenoid, and from outer side of the cartilaginous portion of the eustachian tube	Terminates in a tendon that winds around the hamular process	Tenses the soft palate; opens the auditory tube during swallowing	Mandibular branch of the trigeminal nerve
Levator veli palatini	Arises from the undersurface of the apex of the petrous portion of the temporal bone and from the inner surface of the cartilaginous portion of the eustachian tube; found to occupy the intermediate 40% of the length of the soft palate[6]	Fibers spread out in the soft palate where they blend with those of the opposite side	Acts as a sling when contracted to pull the velum in a posterosuperior direction;[65] major elevator of the velum;[41] positions the velum[17]	Pharyngeal plexus derived from the glossopharyngeal and vagus nerves and the facial nerve;[50] course of the facial nerve is through the greater petrosal nerve[34]
Musculus uvulae	Palatal aponeurosis in a circumscribed area posterior to the hard palate[2]	Inserts into the uvula	Adds bulk to the dorsal surface of the soft palate	Pharyngeal plexus; pharyngeal plexus derived from the glossopharyngeal and vagus nerves and the facial nerve[50]
Palatoglossus	Has a fan-shaped attachment from the anterior surface of the soft palate[40]	Courses through loose connective tissue within the anterior faucial pillar and has a tapering termination in the side of tongue[40]	Elevates the tongue upward and backward to constrict the pillars and probably lowers the velum;[44] positions the velum[17]	Pharyngeal plexus composed of branches from the glossopharyngeus and vagus cranial nerves and from the sympathetic trunk
Palatopharyngeal	Arises from the soft palate	Inserts with the stylopharyngeus into the posterior border of the thyroid cartilage	Adducts the posterior pillars, constricts the pharyngeal isthmus, narrows the velopharyngeal orifice, raises the larynx, and lowers the pharynx;[46] positions the velum[17]	Pharyngeal plexus
Superior constrictor	Arises from the lower third of the posterior margin of the internal pterygoid plate and its hamular process	Inserts into the median raphe	Medial movement of the lateral aspect of the pharyngeal walls;[65] high levels of activity are related to laughter;[41] may function to draw the velum posteriorly;[41] pulls the posterior wall and posterolateral angle anteriorly[17]	Pharyngeal plexus derived from the glossopharyngeal and vagus nerves and the facial nerve[50]

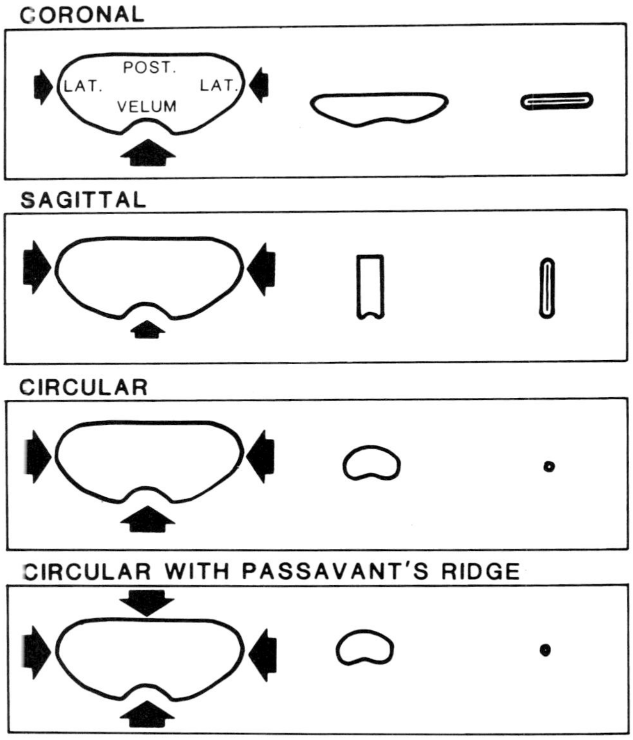

Fig. 11-2. Velopharyngeal closure patterns. These descriptive patterns are based on the shape of the gap as it closes.

common closure pattern, found in only 10% to 15% of the population.

Circular

A circular closure pattern occurs when both the lateral pharyngeal walls and the velum (soft palate) provide significant contributions to closure. In this pattern, not only is the soft palate making contact with the posterior surface of the pharyngeal wall, but there is also significant medial motion of the lateral pharyngeal walls so that the result of closure looks like a circle getting smaller. This pattern is present in about 10% to 20% of the population.

Circular with Passavant's ridge

Circular closure with Passavant's ridge is recognized when a circular closure pattern is present and the posterior pharyngeal wall moves anteriorly. This anterior movement or sphincteric action across the posterior pharyngeal wall is described as *Passavant's ridge*. Therefore, this closure pattern occurs when all four pharyngeal walls are involved in closure of the velopharyngeal port. It is found in about 15% to 20% of the population.

Describing velopharyngeal closure patterns is clinically useful and in some cases may help in deciding the type of therapy required. When the velopharyngeal mechanism is dysfunctional, an additional descriptive method is employed.

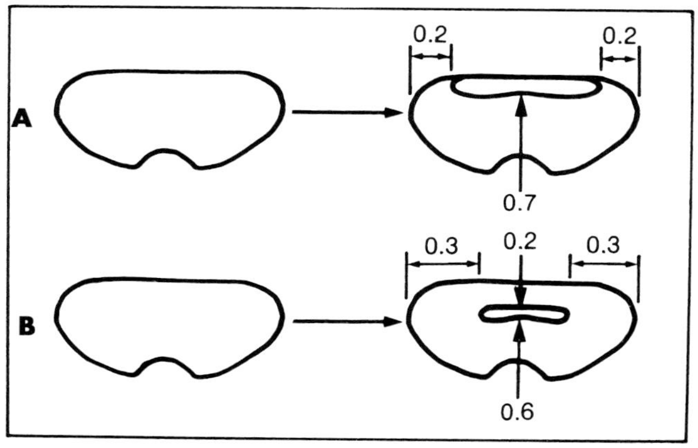

Fig. 11-3. Describing velopharyngeal closure patterns is performed first by naming the type of closure pattern involved and then showing with arrows the amount of motion present in each particular wall. A ratio of movement for the wall being described to the opposite wall is performed. **A,** A coronal closure pattern with the velum showing 0.7 motion and the two lateral pharyngeal walls showing motion rated at 0.2. **B,** A circular closure pattern with posterior wall motion. This could also be considered a coronal closure. This would be a very unusual closure pattern but is used here for descriptive purposes. In this case, the anterior wall shows 0.6 motion, both lateral pharyngeal walls show 0.3, and the posterior wall shows 0.2 with a resultant small coronal-shaped gap.

Aside from describing the velopharyngeal closure patterns, the relative contributions of the pharyngeal walls are rated. Although absolute measurements of the velopharyngeal gap or pharyngeal wall motion have been performed, these are difficult in a clinical setting. In 1988 an international working group proposed rating pharyngeal wall contribution to closure as a ratio of motion from one wall to the other.[22] Therefore, pharyngeal wall motion is graded by the degree of movement of that wall to the opposite wall. If complete closure to the opposite wall occurs, then a ratio of 1 is given. If motion toward the opposite wall is only halfway, then the ratio is 0.5. In this way pharyngeal wall dysfunction and resultant gaps in closure can be described (Fig. 11-3).

The vertical level of closure is an equally important anatomic location. In performing reconstructive velopharyngeal surgery, it is preferable to take advantage of existing velopharyngeal motion. Videofluoroscopy or nasopharyngoscopy can be used to identify the point of maximal pharyngeal wall motion. This level of closure should be ascertained for each individual; this has generally been done using multivideofluoroscopy. Using multivideofluoroscopy, Finkelstein and others[18] found that Passavant's ridge exists in about 40% of individuals and is formed by fibers of the superior constrictor muscle. Using the torus tubarius as a landmark, they found that the upper limit of lateral pharyngeal wall motion was approximately 1 cm below the torus. Vertical length of closure can be variable. It can be fairly short, making it necessary to be precise about the vertical level of any reconstructive sphincter, or it can be longer, in which case precise placement may be less critical.[9]

CAUSES OF VELOPHARYNGEAL INSUFFICIENCY

The causes of VPI are diverse, ranging from paralytic conditions (e.g., following strokes or base-of-skull surgery) to anatomic congenital abnormalities of the palate. Any interference with the velopharyngeal sphincter may result in dysfunction.

Congenital anatomic conditions affecting velopharyngeal function are most commonly caused by clefting of the palate and associated anomalies. Cleft palates occur in approximately 1 of every 750 live births.[23] The incidence of VPI following cleft palate repair varies, partly depending on how a particular research group is defining VPI. However, it appears that about 50% of children with cleft palates have some VPI. Many of these patients can be managed successfully with speech therapy; others require surgical intervention. Palatal clefting can be considered on a continuum ranging from frank, overt clefting of the palate to submucous clefting; an entity known as *occult submucous cleft* also exists. In 10,836 school-age children, Weatherley-White and others[76] determined the incidence of submucous clefting to be 1 in 1200. Most of these children were asymptomatic for VPI.

A submucous cleft is defined by a bifid uvula, muscular diastasis of the soft palate, and notching of the posterior border of the hard palate (loss of the posterior nasal spine). The bifid uvula and muscular diastasis are generally identifiable by visual inspection; the notch in the hard palate requires palpation for identification. The presence of a bifid uvula alone does not constitute a submucous cleft palate but rather serves as a harbinger warranting further inspection. Bifid uvulas have an incidence of 1 in 80 whites.[23] An occult submucous cleft suggests that the usual triad of submucous cleft signs is not present. In the occult submucous cleft palate, there is no musculus uvulae or diastasis of the levator palatini muscle. This finding is recognized on nasoendoscopy as an absence of the bulge from the contraction of the musculus uvulae that is typically present on the nasal surface of the soft palate during speech (Fig. 11-4). Many children with VPI who have no obvious cleft are identified as having occult submucous clefts.

Occult submucous clefts or submucous clefts predispose children to VPI because of the abnormal musculature of their velopharyngeal sphincter. Consequently, these children may acquire VPI when changes occur to the anatomy of the velopharynx, such as an adenoidectomy or even involution of the adenoid pad.[20,43,58] For this reason, a preoperative evaluation for adenoidectomy should include a careful inspection of the palate, both visually and with palpation.[49]

VPI may occur following adenoidectomy even in children without a submucous cleft palate, but its occurrence in relatively healthy children can be hard to predict.[81] Huge adenoids may assist in easy velopharyngeal closure. When these adenoids are removed, considerable palatal motion may be required to obtain closure. Shorter palates, a relatively deep nasopharynx, or palatal hypotonia may all be factors in the development of VPI following adenoidectomy. Ren, Isberg, and Henningsson[58] showed that VPI following adenoidectomy is often associated with enlarged tonsils or remaining prominent adenoid tissue.

Incomplete removal of adenoid tissue can cause VPI. If there is concern that the child's palate may not be able to make the complete excursion back to the new position of the posterior pharyngeal wall, then a partial adenoidectomy can be performed. This has been described in various ways, but generally a superior-half adenoidectomy is performed either with suction electrocautery or using a Thompson-Sinclair adenoid forceps or adenoid curette. If VPI exists after adenoidectomy, the current recommendations are for a 3- to 6-month trial of speech therapy. Useful adjuncts to this therapy are biofeedback using nasometry and occasionally continuous positive airway pressure (CPAP) therapy for those with touch-closure VPI findings.[39,55,82] The authors have found both posterior-wall augmentation and sphincter pharyngoplasty to be useful surgically.

Many conditions or syndromes can result in or predispose children to VPI. Furthermore, any condition that can affect the timing of the palate with speech, such as developmental delays or mental retardation, will also result in VPI. Velocardiofacial (VCF) syndrome and Down syndrome warrant special comment.

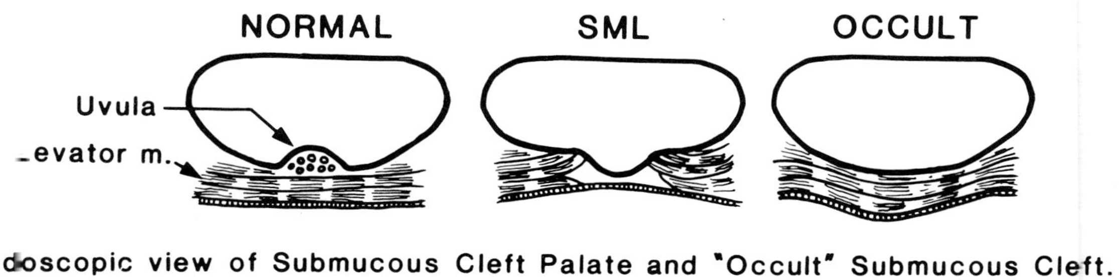

Fig. 11-4. Nasal endoscopic view of the soft palate.

Velocardiofacial syndrome

Velocardiofacial syndrome is being diagnosed with increasing frequency as a result of better awareness about the syndrome as well as the availability of chromosome testing for diagnosis. This condition has rather typical facies: prominent nose, retruded mandible, cardiovascular anomalies, possibly cleft palate, and often learning disabilities. Inheritance is autosomal dominant with variable expressivity. Failure to thrive in infancy is present in about 25% of patients, and about 35% have short stature. Obstructive sleep apnea may also occur. Mental disability is experienced by nearly all individuals with VCF syndrome.

Facial appearance in VCF syndrome is fairly characteristic: a long face with vertical maxillary excess, malar flatness, and mandibular retrusion. Pierre Robin syndrome may be present. The nose is usually prominent with a square nasal root and narrow nasal passages.

Over 80% of patients have cardiac anomalies. Ventricular septal defect is the most common, but other cardiac anomalies such as a right-sided aortic arch, tetralogy of Fallot, and aortic valve disease are also found. Of significant importance to the otolaryngologist is that the internal carotid arteries can be displaced medially along the posterior pharyngeal wall.[13] When considering velopharyngeal surgery in patients with VCF syndrome, it is critical to consider internal carotid location. This is often visible with nasoendoscopy. The authors have used radiographic techniques rarely to precisely map the location related to the proposed surgery.

Diagnosis of VCF syndrome can be difficult. Reporting on 21 patients with VCF syndrome, Finklestein and others[17,18] found that only 11 (52%) had typical manifestations. Fortunately, genetic testing is now possible for these patients. Microdeletions of the q11 region of chromosome 22 have been found in patients with VCF syndrome. This is the same area in which microdeletions occur in DiGeorge syndrome. The microdeletions in some patients with VCF syndrome have encompassed the DiGeorge chromosome locus.[62] Thus patients with VCF syndrome have been found to have DiGeorge syndrome and vice versa. The possibility of these syndromes occurring together should be recognized by the otolaryngologist caring for these patients.

Down syndrome

Down syndrome (trisomy 21) occurs in 1.5 of 1000 live births and is associated with mental handicaps, hearing loss, and muscular hypotonia,[16,71] all of which can be risk factors for the development of VPI. A review of 74 tonsillectomies and adenoidectomies in children with Down syndrome identified two children with postoperative VPI.[37] Kavanagh and Kahane[37] point out the possible risk of developing VPI in children with known hypotonia and articulation problems. Considering their predisposing factors it is somewhat surprising that postadenoidectomy VPI does not occur more often. The predisposing factors may be offset by the narrow oropharynx and velopharynx as well as the shallow skull base at the adenoid site that are found in present in patients with Down syndrome.

NASOPHARYNGOSCOPY

Flexible nasopharyngoscopy is effective for viewing the velopharyngeal orifice. Nasopharyngoscopy allows for visualization of the contribution of the pharyngeal walls and fairly accurate analysis of the closure patterns and deficiencies of velopharyngeal motion. Drawbacks of nasopharyngoscopy are that endoscopic images are prone to distortion and vertical-level assessments may be more difficult.[22] Nasopharyngoscopy is usually performed so that both the video and audio can be recorded.

When properly prepared, most children can tolerate nasopharyngoscopy. Topical anesthesia is used for the nose; systemic sedation is generally not advisable. A speech pathologist is generally in attendance and helps perform the speech examination. Both nasal chambers can be examined, and then the nasopharyngeal area is examined during speech. Despite the shortcomings of nasoendoscopy, this method has been reliable in assessing VPI and is the standard method for viewing the nasopharyngeal area.[12]

NONSURGICAL MANAGEMENT

Successful management of velopharyngeal dysfunction depends on careful evaluation of both velopharyngeal function and speech. It is also influenced by the type and severity of defect, client age, cognitive ability, motivation, availability of services, and expertise of service providers.[19,47] Integration of services provided by an interdisciplinary team of specialists is usually required to develop and implement effective treatment plans. Management decisions must be based not only on subjective practitioner impressions but should also include data provided by objective procedures such as nasopharyngoscopy, videofluoroscopy, aerodynamic and/or nasometric studies, and in-depth articulation analysis.[53]

For individuals who do not have the basic anatomy or function necessary to obtain adequate velopharyngeal closure for speech, surgical management is generally recommended.[5] These patients often present with a consistent lack of velopharyngeal closure with varied speech demands and have hypernasality measurements in the moderate to severe range.

Nonsurgical management options may be used prior to, in conjunction with, or instead of surgery. These options include, but are not limited to, prosthetic dental management, speech therapy, biofeedback management using nasometry, and resistance exercises performed while CPAP is introduced into the nasal cavities. To date, however, research data on the efficacy of these management options and factors affecting outcome are limited.

Prosthetic devices have been used successfully over the past 30 years to assist with inadequate velopharyngeal closure.[3,83] These devices are particularly helpful when there are contraindications to surgery for significant velopharyngeal dysfunction, when dysfunction is secondary to neuromuscular involvement, or when velopharyngeal movements are poorly timed.[45,78] There are two basic types of prosthetic devices: obturators and palatal lifts.

An obturator is a device designed and constructed by a prosthetic dentist to substitute for missing or incomplete tissue; it is attached to the teeth by dental wires or bands.[1] The obturator usually used to improve velopharyngeal function is a thin acrylic plate that extends back into the pharyngeal area.

Customized fabrication and fitting of the obturator use data provided by nasopharyngoscopy, aerodynamic measurements, videofluoroscopy, and/or nasometric studies.[36,55,57,72] A gradual reduction in obturator size has been advocated for some patients; this usually involves adjusting the size of the original obturator. It is postulated that as the size of the obturator is gradually reduced, velopharyngeal function may improve and, in some cases, eliminate the need for either the obturator or surgical intervention.[3,45]

Unlike obturators, palatal lifts are designed to elevate the soft palate when its length is adequate. Lifts are particularly useful in patients who have limited or no dynamic palatal movement. It is unclear at this time whether palatal lifts improve the neuromuscular ability of the velopharynx.[78] Use of obturators or palatal lifts can be difficult in young children, particularly if cooperation or cognitive ability is compromised.

Hypernasality, nasal emissions, and articulatory/phonologic deficits can be the result of mislearning rather than VPI. These problems respond well to speech treatment, particularly phoneme-specific nasal emissions occurring with a select group of sounds. *Surgical intervention is contraindicated in these cases.* For children, diagnostic speech therapy is often recommended prior to physical management, particularly in cases of borderline, mild, or inconsistent hypernasality.[25,26]

Speech or language management is strongly recommended for children with severe articulatory/phonologic deficiencies or a limited ability for expressive language. Compensatory articulation error patterns such as glottal stops restrict airflow below the velopharyngeal valve.[7,29] Radiographic or nasopharyngoscopic observation of the velopharyngeal mechanism is appropriate for children who are able to demonstrate correct articulatory placement for some oral consonant sounds and who have enough language ability to provide a varied speech sample.

Diagnostic speech therapy frequently uses a microcomputer-based instrument called a Nasometer (Kay Elemetrics Corporation, Lincoln Park, NJ), which measures sound energy and has proven to be an effective biofeedback device to reduce nasality levels in some patients.[5,19] Nasometers graphically calculate and display the ratio of oral versus nasal sound energy or nasalance. Elevated nasalance scores on passages containing only oral sounds are significantly correlated with listener judgment ratings of hypernasality.[11] Reduced nasalance scores on passages containing primarily nasal sounds are correlated with listener judgment ratings of hyponasality.[10] Nasometric scores in children with hypernasality are also significantly correlated with aerodynamic estimates of velopharyngeal area and to nasoendoscopic findings.[11,56]

Management using a Nasometer encourages such strategies as ear training, promoting lower posterior tongue placement, increasing loudness, speaking at a lower pitch, using a more open-mouth posture, controlling the type of consonants and vowels used in speech training, and slowing speech rate.[5,57] The duration of any speech therapy to reduce hypernasality should be carefully monitored. If continued improvement in hypernasality is not demonstrated within 3 to 6 months, speech therapy to reduce hypernasality should be discontinued and other treatment options explored.[26]

Video-recorded nasopharyngoscopy has been used successfully in biofeedback therapy for adults with VPI.[82,84] A case study of an older child showed correction of phoneme-specific nasal emissions using nasopharyngoscopy.[82] Nasopharyngoscopy biofeedback therapy may prove to be a useful tool in training some children to achieve better velopharyngeal function, but further research is necessary.

A new therapy for hypernasality uses CPAP, which is introduced into the nasal cavities during speech production.[39] It is theorized that when hypernasality is related to physiologic limitations, resistance training might strengthen the muscles involved in velopharyngeal closure. As positive air pressure is delivered to the nasal cavities, levator veli palatini muscle activity increases.[42] Therapy can occur in the patient's home—a major management advantage. Preliminary case reports suggest that CPAP therapy is useful for patients with mild to moderate hypernasality, regardless of the underlying cause.

SURGICAL MANAGEMENT

Pharyngoplasty

To improve velopharyngeal competence surgically, procedures that obturate the middle of the velopharyngeal area or the lateral portion of the velopharynx can be used. Hynes[33] was the first to conceive of a procedure that obturated the lateral part of the velopharynx. His goal in designing this operation was to construct a dynamic sphincter. He believed that raising lateral flaps of superior origin would lead to a neuromuscular flap that would contract. Nearly two decades later, Orticochea[52] reported using lateral-based flaps for the management of VPI. In his description of the Orticochea pharyngoplasty, he used the posterior tonsillar pillars as donor flaps and created a recipient site by raising a small inferior pharyngeal flap.

Nearly a decade later, Jackson[35] modified the Orticochea technique, and it is essentially this later description of pharyngoplasty that has gained so much popularity. The posterior tonsillar pillars are still used as the donor flaps to be sutured across the nasopharynx. However, an inferior pharyngeal flap is not created. Instead the transverse incision is made higher in the nasopharynx, and a small superior pharyngeal flap can be created if needed.

Further modifications of this technique have occurred, most of which have centered on getting an adequate superior placement and covering raw tissue areas. Several studies have assessed the success of a sphincter pharyngoplasty to improve VPI. In 1984 Riski and others[60] reported a correction of hypernasality in 78% of patients. In 1992 a more complete evaluation of the sphincter pharyngoplasty had similar success rates, although the surgical technique changed during the study.[59] An objective study was performed by Witt and others,[80] who found that nasal resonance improved in 79% of the patients. In their study, the sphincter pharyngoplasty was employed to correct hypernasality in patients exhibiting all velopharyngeal closure patterns, instead of selecting out certain patients for other techniques.[80] This study also appropriately documented potential problems with all types of velopharyngeal obturating surgery. They found that 30% of their patients were judged to be hyponasal postoperatively.[80] Sloan and others[69] compared a modified Hynes pharyngoplasty with inferiorly and superiorly based pharyngeal flaps. They concluded that sphincter pharyngoplasty was a better technique for management of VPI.[69]

Indications

Sphincter pharyngoplasty is a good choice when one of the following criteria are present: closure of the persistent velopharyngeal gap in which there is poor lateral-wall motion and good velar motion or significant augmentation of the posterior pharyngeal wall. A sphincter pharyngoplasty may also be indicated for those with poor motion of any of the pharyngeal walls, including the velum. These patients have a relatively adynamic sphincter, and typically their velopharyngeal port is described as a black hole because there is no light reflection of the sphincter during nasoendoscopy.[79] Because the sphincter pharyngoplasty pulls the lateral pharyngeal walls medially and because the flaps are sewn across the back wall, both the lateral and posterior portions of the velopharyngeal port are obturated. The degree of obturation can be varied by the thickness of the flaps, the snugness (tightness) with which the flaps are sutured together, and the extension of the flaps toward the uvula.

Technique

Proper patient preparation includes having recently reviewed the nasoendoscopy tape and videofluoroscopy results, if performed. If possible, a recording of the nasoendoscopy should be present in the surgical suite so it can be reviewed during surgery. The need for a possible tonsillectomy or adenoidectomy should also have been previously determined. If proper positioning and placement of the sphincter will be through the adenoid pad, an adenoidectomy should have been performed. Placing a sphincter pharyngoplasty through the adenoid can increase the difficulty of the procedure. We prefer to perform adenoidectomy or tonsillectomy (if the tonsils are so large that they preclude obtaining a healthy palatopharyngeal muscular flap) approximately 8 weeks prior to placement of the sphincter pharyngoplasty. Care should be taken during tonsillectomy not to injure the posterior tonsillar pillars and to induce minimal scarring of the palatopharyngeal muscle.

Following intubation with an oral Ray tube, a Dingman or Davis mouth gag may be used to obtain adequate exposure of the posterior tonsillar pillars. Exposure to the nasopharynx is obtained by using a uvula retractor. With the soft palate retracted superiorly, the proper vertical level for sphincter pharyngoplasty is determined by comparing the anatomic landmarks found either by videofluoroscopy or nasoendoscopy with those present by viewing or palpating the nasopharynx directly during surgery. After this site is determined it is injected with a vasoconstrictive agent such as 1% lidocaine 1 : 100,000 epinephrine. The posterior tonsillar pillars are likewise mildly injected to improve hemostasis. A No. 15 blade is used to make an incision along the anterior surface of the posterior tonsillar pillar. The posterior tonsillar pillar is detached inferiorly just above the inferior pole of the tonsil. A combination of a No. 15 blade and lower lateral crural right-angle scissors is used to elevate the palatopharyngeal muscle superiorly. The posterior incision, which is close to the junction of the lateral and posterior pharyngeal walls, is carried superiorly to the level of the desired vertical placement across the nasopharynx. The palatopharyngeal flaps are then elevated up to nearly this level. The anterior incision should not extend as superiorly as the posterior incision. In fact, the anterior incision of the palatopharyngeal muscle usually does not extend even as high as the superior pole of the tonsil, because in so doing the reconstructed velopharyngeal port can become quite narrow (Fig. 11-5).

The further superiorly and toward the uvula the anterior incision extends, the more narrow the reconstructive port will become. If the surgeon's intent is to keep the velopharyngeal port fairly open while creating significant obturation of the lateral and posterior portion of the nasopharynx, then the anterior incision can be extended across the back of the tonsillar pillars and curved up along the posterior and superior (nasal) surface of the soft palate or pharynx. This type of extension allows the palatopharyngeal flap to be elevated more superiorly without necessarily constricting the velopharyngeal port.

The two palatopharyngeal muscles can also be elevated superiorly with some blunt dissection (using a Herd dissector) or finger dissection. With the two palatopharyngeal muscles elevated, an incision is made across the nasopharynx at the desired level of sphincter placement. This usually requires palatal retraction with the uvula retractor. The palato-

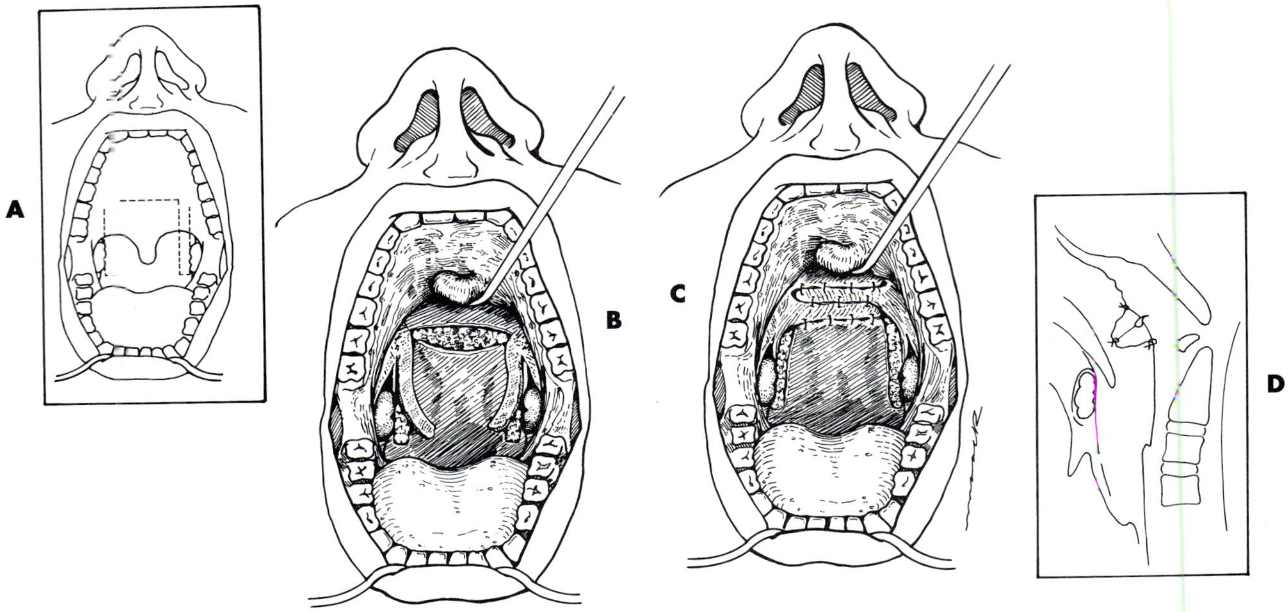

Fig. 11-5. Sphincter pharyngoplasty technique. **A,** The height or vertical level the sphincter usually needs to be placed in relation to the pharynx. The soft palate is retracted. The *broken dashed lines* represent an approximation of the surgical incisions, although this is difficult to represent two-dimensionally. **B,** The soft palate is retracted superiorly, and the posterior tonsillar pillars (palatopharyngeal muscle) have been elevated. Note that the anterior incision stops at the superior pole but may extend further vertically and medially along the nasal surface of the soft palate toward the uvula if the surgeon desires a narrow, tight port. Note also that the medial or posterior incision for the flaps extends up to the horizontal incision so that the flap can be easily rotated. **C,** The flaps have been sutured into the sphincter position overlapped. The flaps may also be sutured end to end. This illustration better demonstrates that the sphincter could be adjusted closed by pulling the flaps in more tightly, by creating a larger posterior wall ridge (harvesting larger and thicker flaps), and by extending the anterior incision medially along the nasal side of the soft palate (this step is usually not needed and can lead to severe narrowing of the port). **D,** Lateral view following pharyngoplasty. Note that the sphincter is in the nasopharynx, above the soft palate. (Permission granted by the copyright owner: *Facial Plastic Clinics of North America*, Philadelphia, 1996, WB Saunders.)

pharyngeal flaps are sutured transversely across the nasopharynx. These flaps can be sutured either end to end or in an overlapping fashion. Vicryl 4-0 is generally used to suture these flaps together and to the nasopharynx. If a very snug sphincter is created, then an obstructive breathing pattern may occur immediately after surgery. In this case the authors place a soft nasal trumpet through the sphincter until the following morning.

Pharyngeal flaps

An operation designed to obturate the midline of the velopharyngeal port is termed a *pharyngeal flap*. In this procedure, a flap of tissue is pedicled superiorly or inferiorly to the posterior pharyngeal wall and then sutured to the palate. Success has been reported using both the inferiorly and superiorly based pharyngeal flaps. Placement in the midline divides the velopharyngeal port into two smaller lateral ports. Mobile lateral pharyngeal walls are needed for ports to be open during breathing and closed during speech. Posterior-wall and velar motion are relatively unimportant when choosing this procedure.

In the last decade preoperative nasopharyngoscopy has facilitated better preoperative planning. More attention has been focused on proper vertical placement of flaps. One of the criticisms of inferiorly based pharyngeal flaps is that the pharyngeal flap is tethered inferiorly and that with additional scar contracture the flap will be pulled out of optimal position.[77] For this reason, the trend in the United States has been toward superiorly based pharyngeal flaps.

Pharyngeal flaps have been effective in reducing hypernasality. Morris and others[48] studied 65 subjects, more than half of whom underwent pharyngeal flap surgery more than 10 years previously. Eighty-three percent showed normal velopharyngeal function, and 66% showed normal or near-normal speech production. Eight of the sixty-five patients had surgical revision of the flap: one required reduction in the size of the lateral ports; the other seven required either flap takedowns or lateral port enlargements. Likewise,

Hirschberg[31] reported a series of 500 pharyngeal flaps in which 90% of the patients demonstrated improvement in hypernasality and 74% showed improved speech. The best speech results were obtained when the width of the flap was appropriately matched with relative motion of the lateral pharyngeal walls. Matching the width of the flap to obturate the remaining gap area, which is determined by maximal medial motion of the lateral pharyngeal walls, is termed *tailoring* of the pharyngeal flap.[64] In theory, tailor-made flaps are a good concept. In practice, however, achieving precise millimeter dimensions in the lateral ports can be difficult because of the many forces of scar contracture. Inconsistency of scar contracture between individuals leads to some of the reported complications.

Many good long-term studies have thoroughly documented the drawbacks and benefits of this procedure.[73] Sleep apnea is a reported complication from pharyngeal flaps.[38,85] Sleep apnea is more likely to occur early in the postoperative period, and within 3 months obstructed sleep problems should be much resolved.[51,67] In a long-term follow-up study, Morris and others[48] examined the electrocardiograms of 33 of the 65 subjects in the pharyngeal flap study. Those chosen for electrocardiographic monitoring had either complained of sleep difficulty or had a history of snoring. There were no clear findings of right ventricular hypertrophy, which can be a pathologic response to obstructive sleep apnea. Their conclusion was that although symptoms of nasal airway obstruction may be present, they are rarely serious enough to cause pathology.

Indications

Patients with relatively good lateral wall motion but a central persisting gap are good candidates for pharyngeal flap surgery. A sagittal closure pattern is also an indication for this procedure.

Technique

The pharyngeal flap is performed by placing a Dingman mouth gag and injecting the posterior pharyngeal wall and the palate with 1% lidocaine 1:100,000 epinephrine. Two different procedures can be used for performing the pharyngeal flap. The fish-mouth technique essentially requires bivalving the soft palate (separating nasal mucosa from oral tissue) to create a pocket into which the pharyngeal flap is pulled and sutured.[61] The pocket is usually placed just superior and anterior to the edge of the soft palate on the nasal side. The other technique, which involves splitting the palate, has been well described by Croft, Shprintzen, and Rakoff[9] and Hogan.[32] Both of these reports describe adjustments to the lateral ports.

The width of the flap is decided by previous nasoendoscopy or videofluoroscopy. The superiorly based flap is elevated a little higher than the level ascertained to be appropriate for maximum medial motion of the lateral pharyngeal walls. With scar contracture, the flap usually descends a couple millimeters. The fish-mouth or palatal splitting technique is used to sew the flap into position. Prior to suturing the flap, small endotracheal tubes are placed in both ports to assist in postoperative breathing and to provide some guidance on lateral port size.

After the small endotracheal tubes have been removed postoperatively, the patient should be monitored for obstructive apnea. The tubes are usually left in place the first night, and the patient should not be discharged from the hospital until indications are clear that serious obstructive apnea is not present. Parents need to be cautioned that if obstruction seems to be getting worse, the patient should be brought back to the hospital for monitoring and reevaluation.

Augmentation of the Posterior Pharyngeal Wall

The concept of augmenting the posterior pharyngeal wall in an effort to improve velopharyngeal competence has received and will continue to receive attention for a number of reasons: (1) the risk of inducing hyponasality and nasal obstruction is theoretically lower; (2) it is relatively easy to perform most of the procedures; (3) the majority of persistent velopharyngeal gaps are continuous with the posterior pharyngeal wall; and (4) in many VPI patients the velum or soft palate has relatively good motion. The concept of simply bringing the posterior pharyngeal wall forward to correct the gap in many patients with VPI is appealing. In practice, many posterior pharyngeal wall augmentation techniques have failed to meet expectations. One of the best techniques currently used to augment the posterior pharyngeal wall is a sphincter pharyngoplasty, in which a large shelf of tissue is placed across the posterior pharyngeal wall. However, this section focuses on those techniques that augment the posterior wall.

Various materials have been used to augment the posterior wall, either by injection or implantation.[4,14,24] Tissue implants such as cartilage and fascia have been used.[27,30,54,74] The most common injectable material over the last few decades has been Teflon (Mentor Medical Systems, Oshawa, Ontario).[75] To treat marginal VPI, Smith and McCabe[70] injected Teflon into the posterior pharyngeal wall to create a transverse ridge. They also discuss the possible necessity of repeated Teflon injections. Disadvantages of using Teflon are that migration may occur and that the material is not approved by the Food and Drug Administration for such use. One inadvertent carotid artery injection has occurred with Teflon. Obviously, it is important to palpate the posterior wall for the great vessels prior to any sort of posterior pharyngeal wall procedure. Conversely, an anecdotal advantage of Teflon injection is that as the Teflon migrates and the posterior wall bulges less, the velopharyngeal sphincter may slowly make adjustments to maintain competence, much like sphincter improvement in obturator reduction.

Because of the continuing theoretic advantages of poste-

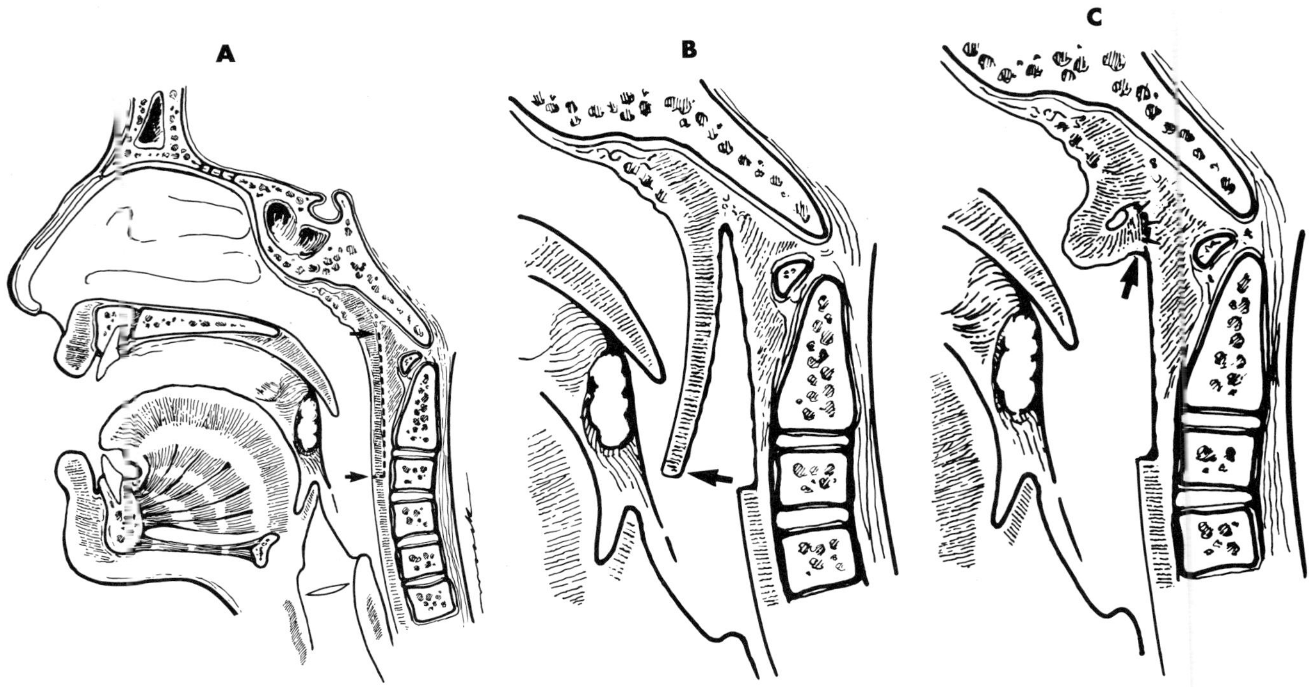

Fig. 11-6. Augmentation of the posterior pharyngeal wall. **A,** The section of the posterior pharyngeal wall to be elevated; the inferior level is at about the inferior pole of the tonsil. **B,** The constrictor muscle is raised with the flap and is elevated quite superiorly. **C,** The flap has been folded and sutured into place. Even though the flap was elevated higher, the fold and maximum area of augmentation occur a little lower. Although not shown in **C,** sutures are often placed on the folded flap laterally to close some of the dead space, sometimes creating a bit more stability. (Permission granted by the copyright owner: *Facial Plastic Clinics of North America*, Philadelphia, 1996, WB Saunders.)

rior wall augmentation, there has been renewed interest in using posterior wall tissue to create a shelf or ledge along the posterior wall. In this procedure a superiorly based pharyngeal flap is lifted up and buckled to create a ridge across the posterior wall.

Indications

Posterior wall augmentation is selected when there is a small central midline gap and velopharyngeal closure can be completed by simply bringing the posterior wall forward. Because patients may achieve velopharyngeal closure but the closure may not be tight enough, pressure occasionally causes leakage of the air through the velopharyngeal port. This condition is referred to as a *touch-closure* problem because the pharyngeal walls touch together but do not achieve competent closure. Under these conditions slight augmentation of the posterior pharyngeal wall is enough to provide a competent seal. Another indication for posterior wall augmentation can be VPI following adenoidectomy. If significant augmentation of the posterior pharyngeal wall is required, then a sphincter pharyngoplasty is usually a better technique. Posterior wall augmentation works best for 1- to 3-mm gaps or for touch-closure problems.

Technique

Posterior wall augmentation using a buckled or folded pharyngeal flap is relatively easy to perform. A superiorly based pharyngeal flap is raised and then folded on itself at the level of maximum pharyngeal wall motion in the area of the velopharyngeal port. This procedure is performed by placing a Davis mouth gag and injecting the posterior pharyngeal wall with a vasoconstrictive solution. A superiorly based pharyngeal flap is then elevated such that the constrictor muscle is present within the flap. The width of the flap is decided by ascertaining the width of the gap to be obturated and making the flap slightly larger. Because the flap shrinks once it is elevated a wider flap than anticipated is usually required (Fig. 11-6).

The lateral incisions are made first and carried through the constrictor muscle until the white fascia is encountered posteriorly. At this point, a right-angle elevator can be used to elevate the remaining muscle off the fascia. The flap is detached inferiorly at about the level of the inferior pole of the tonsil. The flap is elevated superiorly to slightly above the level of the desired augmentation. Once the flap has been elevated above the level of augmentation, the buckle of the flap will be correctly positioned. The flap can then be sutured

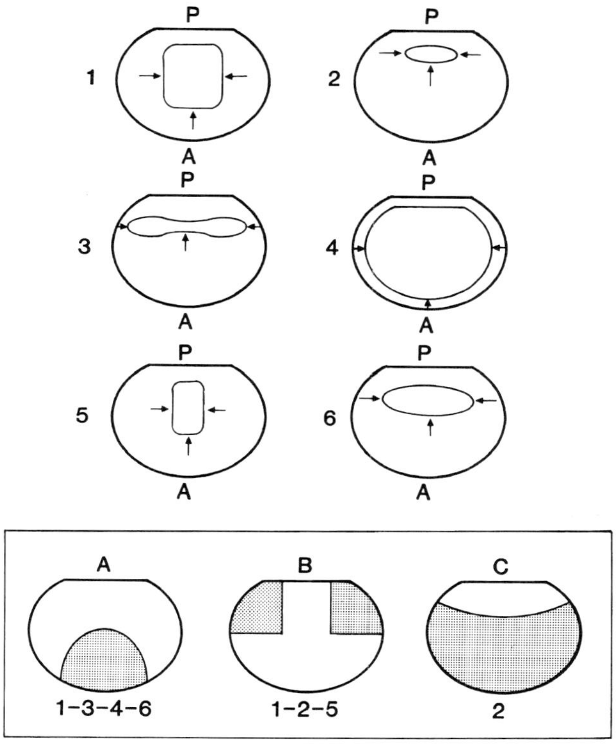

Fig. 11-7. The types of obturation that can be expected with the three surgical methods described. The *shaded areas* represent parts of the velopharyngeal area left open following the surgery; the *white areas* show what is obturated with tissue during the surgery. Remember that in all of these examples there are variations; with surgery more or less can be obturated than is demonstrated. **A,** The type of obturation obtained with a sphincter pharyngoplasty. Significant augmentation and closure of the posterior and lateral pharyngeal walls occurs. The area left open is midline and located just behind the uvula. This helps demonstrate why someone with good soft palatal motion will generally do well with a sphincter pharyngoplasty. A sphincter pharyngoplasty would work well in treating the patients in *1* (this sphincter would need to be a little bit snug), *3*, *4* (black hole patterns are usually best treated with a very snug or tight sphincter or with a prosthetic obturator), and *6*. **B,** Obturation following a pharyngeal flap attachment to the soft palate. Because the lateral areas (ports) are left open, it is apparent why this surgery works best in people with good lateral wall motion. Matching the obturated pattern over *1* to *6*, it can be seen that a good match could be made in the patients in *1* (wider pharyngeal flap would be needed), *2*, and *5*. **C,** The folded or rolled pharyngeal flap mildly augments the posterior wall. The best match for this procedure is the patient in *2*. Although this patient could be treated by any of the surgical methods, described augmentation of the posterior wall is the least aggressive and leaves the most unobturated area. Therefore, it is less likely to cause airway obstruction. (Permission granted by the copyright owner: *Facial Plastic Clinics of North America*, Philadelphia, 1996, WB Saunders.)

on itself or to the posterior wall so that the fold is in the desired location vertically. Usually three to four sutures are placed across the inferior edge of the flap to hold it in proper position, and then one or two sutures are placed on the lateral aspects of the folded flap for stability and to close any dead space between the two flap layers.

One of the drawbacks to this procedure is some variability in flap atrophy. Another drawback is that even though large buckles can be created, they are functionally not very useful because large buckles have a tendency to flap (move up and down) depending on the amount of pressurized air present. For this reason, small gaps of 1 to 3 mm can be closed successfully but large gaps are inconsistently closed because a large folded flap is not vertically stable in its position.

SUMMARY

Management of VPI requires careful evaluation by a team of professionals, including a speech/language pathologist and a surgeon who have expertise in speech disorders. Care needs to be individualized. Surgical care requires preoperative assessment of the velopharynx by nasoendoscopy, videofluroscopy, or both. Selection of the surgical procedure depends on the pattern of velopharyngeal closure, the degree of closure, and associated medical conditions. A sample of common nasopharyngoscopic findings and selected surgical procedures is provided in Figure 11-7.

REFERENCES

1. Adisman IK: *Cleft palate prosthetics.* In Grabb WC, Rosenstein SW, Bzoch KR, editors: *Cleft lip and palate*, Boston, 1971, Little, Brown.
2. Azzam NA, Kuehn DP: The morphology of musculus uvulae, *Cleft Palate J* 14:78, 1977.
3. Blakely RW: Temporary speech prosthesis as an aid in speech training, *Cleft Palate Bull* 10:63, 1960.
4. Blocksma R: Correction of velopharyngeal insufficiency by silastic pharyngeal implant, *Plast Reconstr Surg* 31:268, 1963.
5. Boone DR, McFarlane SC: *The voice and voice therapy*, Englewood Cliffs, NJ, 1994, Prentice Hall.
6. Boorman JG, Sommerlad BC: Levator palatini and palatal dimples: their anatomy, relationship and clinical significance, *Br J Plast Surg* 38:326, 1985.
7. Broen PA, Doyle SS, Bacon CK: The velopharyngeally inadequate child: phonologic change with intervention, *Cleft Palate Craniofac J* 30:500, 1993.
8. Crockett DM, Bumstead RM, Van Demark DR: Experience with surgical management of velopharyngeal incompetence, *Otolaryngol Head Neck Surg* 99:1, 1988.
9. Croft CB, Shprintzen RJ, Rakoff SJ: Patterns of velopharyngeal valving in normal and cleft palate subjects: a multiview videofluoroscopic and nasoendoscopic study, *Laryngoscope* 91:265, 1981.
10. Dalston RM, Warren DW, Dalston ET: A preliminary investigation concerning the use of nasometry in identifying patients with hyponasality and/or nasal airway impairment, *J Speech Hear Res* 34:11, 1991.
11. Dalston RM, Warren DW, Dalston ET: Use of nasometry as a diagnostic tool identifying patients with velopharyngeal impairment, *Cleft Palate Craniofac J* 28:184, 1991.
12. D'Antonio L and others: Reliability of flexible fiberoptic nasopharyngoscopy for evaluation of velopharyngeal function in a clinical population, *Cleft Palate J* 26:217, 1989.
13. D'Antonio LL, Marsh JL: Abnormal carotid arteries in velocardiofacial syndrome, *Plast Reconstr Surg* 80:471, 1987.

14. Eckstein H: Paraffin for facial and palatal defects. *Dermatol Ztschr*

42. Kuehn DP, Moon JB, Folkins JW: Levator veli palatini muscle activity

Chapter 12

Pharyngitis and Adenotonsillar Disease

Brian J. Wiatrak
Audie L. Woolley

Infectious and inflammatory diseases involving the pharynx, tonsils, and adenoids account for a significant proportion of childhood illnesses and pediatric healthcare expenditures and often result in two of the most common surgical procedures of childhood, tonsillectomy and adenoidectomy (Fig. 12-1). Recent clinical research has helped to illuminate this vast area of pediatric otolaryngology, including the effects of adenotonsillar hypertrophy on obstructive sleep apnea, the microbiologic flora of the tonsils and adenoids and their role in chronic adenotonsillar hypertrophy, the relationship between adenotonsillar hypertrophy and craniofacial growth, and new techniques for adenotonsillectomy with improved management of perioperative morbidity. This chapter reviews our current understanding of pharyngitis and adenotonsillar disease processes.

HISTORY

Celsus was the first to report removal of the tonsils.[38] Describing his surgical technique, Celsus indicated that "the tonsils are loosened by scrapping around them and then torn out."[36] Hemostasis was obtained using a vinegar mouthwash and painting the tonsillar fossa with a medication to reduce bleeding.[26] Aëtius of Amida on the Tigris described a technique for tonsillectomy in the first half of the sixth century in which a hook was used to snare the tonsil and a knife was used for amputation; he warned of the severe dangers of hemorrhage when excising too deeply.[179] Subsequent surgical techniques were described by Paul of Aegina in 625, and Physick described a forcep to facilitate extirpation of the tonsil, which became the forerunner for the modern tonsil guillotine.[36,122] Mackenzie[89a] improved on the Physick tonsillotome and popularized its use for surgery of the tonsils in the late nineteenth century.

The adenoids were first described by the Danish physician Meyer. In his 1868 paper "Adenoid vegetations in the nasopharyngeal cavity," Meyer described in detail his technique of posterior rhinoscopy to diagnose adenoid hypertrophy and recommended removal of adenoid tissue with the aid of a ring knife.[165] In 1885, Gottstein described the first adenoid curette.[165]

Crowe reviewed 1000 consecutive tonsillectomies performed between 1911 and 1917. In his paper "Relation of tonsillar and nasopharyngeal infection to general systemic disorders," Crowe provided a detailed description of a meticulous surgical technique by sharp dissection and described using the Crowe-Davis mouth gag.[33] The low complication rate he described compares favorably to modern reports of tonsillectomy.

ANATOMY

Waldeyer's ring

Together, the lingual tonsils anteriorly, the palatine tonsils laterally, and the pharyngeal tonsils (adenoids) posterosuperiorly form a ring of lymphoid or adenoid tissue about the upper end of the pharynx known as *Waldeyer's tonsillar ring*. All the structures of Waldeyer's ring have a similar histology and presumably similar functions.

Palatine tonsil

The palatine tonsil represents the largest accumulation of lymphoid tissue in Waldeyer's ring and, in contrast to the lingual and pharyngeal tonsils, constitutes a compact body with a definite thin capsule on its deep surface.[72] Tonsillar crypts, blind tubules from the epithelium on the surface of the tonsil that are lined with stratified squamous epithelium, extend deeply into this tissue.

The tonsillar capsule is a specialized portion of the pharyngobasilar fascia that covers the surface of the tonsil and extends into it to form septa that conduct the nerves and vessels.[72] The tonsil is not, therefore, easily separated from its capsule, but the capsule is united largely by loose connective tissue to the pharyngeal muscles. The tonsil can be easily dissected from its normal position by separating the capsule from the muscle through this loose connective tissue.

The tonsillar fossa is composed of three muscles: the palatoglossus muscle, which forms the anterior pillar; the palatopharyngeal muscle, which is the posterior pillar, and the superior constrictor muscle of the pharynx, which forms the larger part of the tonsillar bed.[72] The muscular wall is thin, and immediately against it on the outer wall of the pharynx is the glossopharyngeal nerve. This nerve can be easily injured if the tonsillar bed is violated, and not uncommonly the nerve is temporarily affected by edema following tonsillectomy that produces both a transitory loss of taste over the posterior third of the tongue and referred otalgia.

The arterial blood supply of the tonsil enters primarily at the lower pole, with branches also at the upper pole. There are typically three arteries at the lower pole: the tonsillar branch of the dorsal lingual artery anteriorly, the ascending palatine artery (a branch of the facial artery) posteriorly, and the tonsillar branch of the facial artery between these entering the lower aspect of the tonsillar bed.[72] At the upper pole of the tonsil the ascending pharyngeal artery enters posteriorly, and the lesser palatine artery enters on the anterior surface. The tonsillar branch of the facial artery is the largest. Venous blood drains through a peritonsillar plexus about the capsule.[72] The plexus drains into the lingual and pharyngeal veins, which in turn drain into the internal jugular vein.

The nerve supply of the tonsillar region is through the tonsillar branches of the glossopharyngeal nerve about the lower pole of the tonsil and through the descending branches of the lesser palatine nerves, which course through the pterygopalatine ganglion.[72] The cause of referred otalgia with tonsillitis is through the tympanic branch of the glossopharyngeal nerve. Efferent lymphatic drainage courses through the upper deep cervical lymph nodes, especially the jugulodigastric or tonsillar node located behind the angle of the mandible.[72]

Adenoids

The adenoid or pharyngeal tonsils form the central part of the ring of lymphoid tissue surrounding the oropharyngeal isthmus. The adenoid is composed of lymphoid tissue, with its apex pointed toward the nasal septum and its base toward the roof and posterior wall of the nasopharynx. The adenoid is covered by a pseudostratified ciliated columnar epithelium that is plicated to form numerous surface folds. The adenoid develops as a midline structure by the fusion of two lateral primordia that become visible during early fetal life, are fully developed during the seventh month of gestation, and continue to grow until the fifth year of life, often causing some degree of airway obstruction.[153] Thereafter the adenoid gradually atrophies, the nasopharynx grows, and the airway improves.[76]

The blood supply and drainage are from the ascending pharyngeal artery, the ascending palatine artery, the pharyngeal branch of the maxillary artery, the artery of the pterygoid canal, and contributing branches from the tonsillar branch of the facial artery.[60] Venous drainage is to the pharyngeal plexus, which communicates with the pterygoid plexus and then drains into the internal jugular and facial veins. The nerve supply is from the pharyngeal plexus. The efferent lymphatic drainage of the adenoids is to the retropharyngeal and pharyngomaxillary space lymph nodes.[60]

IMMUNOLOGY OF THE ADENOIDS AND TONSILS

The adenoids and tonsils are predominately B-cell organs: B lymphocytes comprise 50% to 65% of all adenoid and tonsillar lymphocytes.[134] T-cell lymphocytes comprise approximately 40% of adenoid and tonsillar lymphocytes, and 3% are mature plasma cells. Conversely, 70% of the lymphocytes in peripheral blood are T cells.[65] The immunoreactive lymphoid cells of the adenoids and tonsils are found in four distinct areas: the reticular cell epithelium, the extrafollicular area, the mantle zone of the lymphoid follicle, and the germinal center of the lymphoid follicle.[134]

There is ample evidence that the adenoids and tonsils are involved in inducing secretory immunity and regulating secretory immunoglobulin production. They contain a system of channels covered by specialized endothelium that can mediate antigen uptake in a fashion similar to Peyer's patches of epithelium in the bowel.[74,113] Both the adenoids and tonsils are favorably located to mediate immunologic protection of the upper aerodigestive tract as they are exposed to airborne antigens. Both organs, specifically the tonsils, are particularly designed for direct transport of foreign material from the exterior to the lymphoid cells.[134] This is in contrast to lymph nodes, which depend on antigenic delivery through afferent lymphatics. The tonsillar crypts are covered by stratified squamous epithelium. There are 10 to 30 of these crypts in the tonsils, and they are ideally suited to trapping foreign material and transporting it to the lymphoid follicles.[134]

The tonsils and adenoids rank among the secondary lymphatic organs. Intratonsillar defense mechanisms eliminate weak antigenic signals. Only when additional higher antigenic concentrations are presented does proliferation of anti-

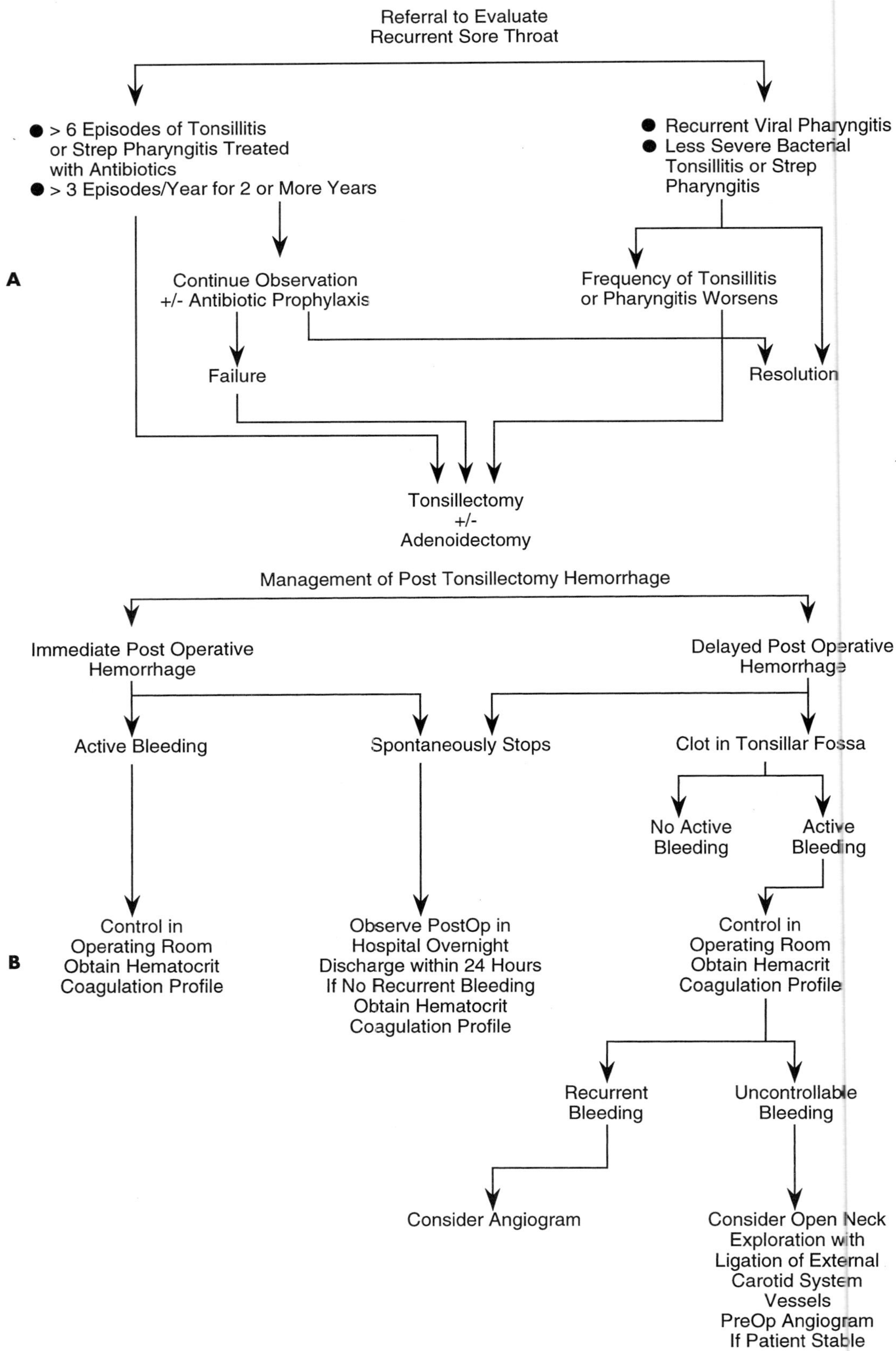

Fig. 12-1. Management algorithms of pediatric pharyngitis and adenotonsillar disease.

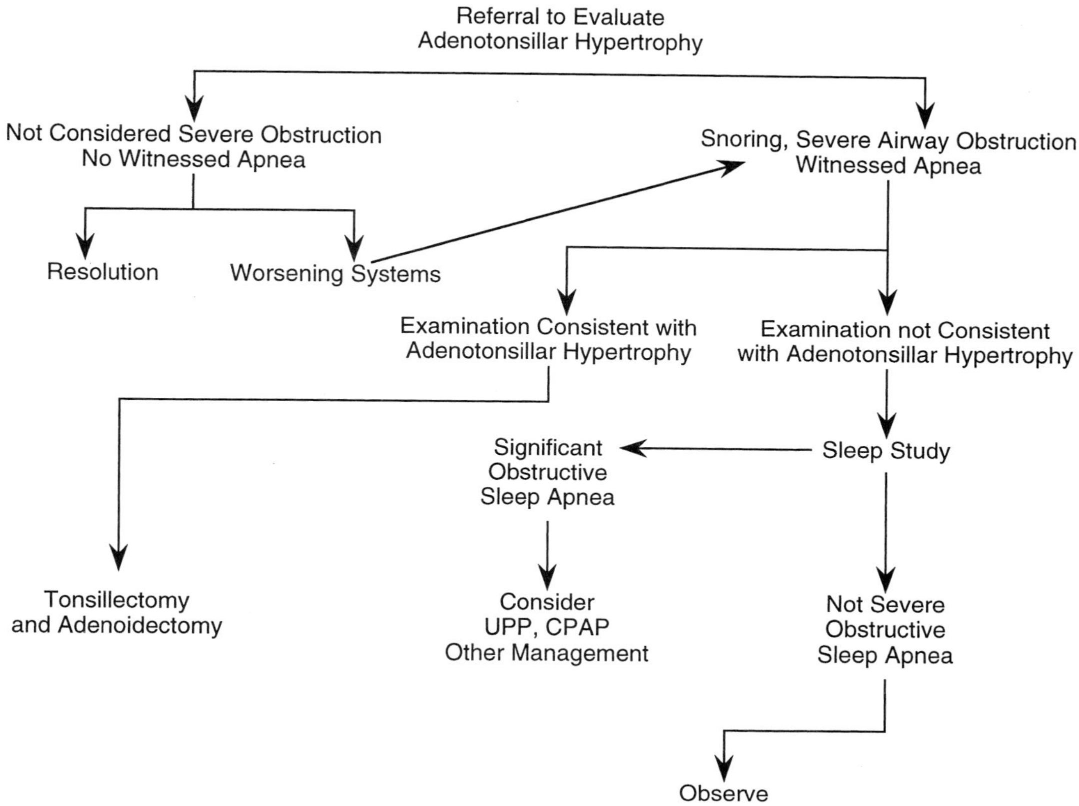

C

Fig. 12-1, cont'd. For legend see opposite page.

gen-sensitive B cells occur in the germinal centers.[134] Low antigen doses effect the differentiation of lymphocytes to plasma cells, whereas high doses produce B-cell proliferation. The generation of B cells in the germinal centers of the tonsils is considered by Siegel to be one of the most essential tonsillar functions.[152]

Immunoglobulins (Igs) produced by the adenoid include IgG, IgA, IgM, and IgD.[134] IgG appears to pass into the nasopharyngeal lumen by passive diffusion.[134] The tonsil produces antibodies locally as well as B cells that migrate to other sites around the pharynx and periglandular lymphoid tissues to produce antibodies.

T-cell functions such as interferon-γ production and presumably production of other important lymphokines have been shown to be present in tonsils and adenoids.[133] The role played by tonsillar and adenoid T cells in tumor response is still unknown.

The human tonsils are immunologically most active between the ages of 4 and 10 years. Involution of the tonsils begins after puberty, resulting in a decrease of the B-cell population and a relative increase in the ratio of T to B cells.[134] Although the overall Ig-producing function is affected, considerable B-cell activity is still seen in clinically healthy tonsils even at 80 years of age.[11] The situation is different in disease-associated changes, such as when recurrent tonsillitis and adenoid hyperplasia are observed. Inflammation of the reticular crypt epithelium results in shedding of immunologically active cells and decreasing antigen transport function with subsequent replacement by stratified squamous epithelium.[92,158] These changes lead to reduced activation of the local B-cell system, decreased antibody production, and an overall reduction in density of the B-cell and germinal centers in extrafollicular areas.[159] In contrast to recurrent tonsillitis, the changes are less pronounced in adenoid hyperplasia, where the immunoregulatory conditions necessary for maintenance of the B-cell population are well preserved. The reason for this is most likely that the reticular epithelium is less affected in inflammation of adenoids than in tonsils.

There are conflicting reports regarding the immunologic consequences of tonsillectomy and adenoidectomy, yet it is clear that no major immunologic deficiencies result from these procedures.[151] Ogra[109] showed a three- to fourfold drop in titers in children previously immunized with live poliovirus vaccine. Serum IgA levels in posttonsillectomy patients were lower than in age-matched controls, but this immunologic change did not appear to be clinically significant.[37,41] Children who were previously immunized orally with live poliovirus vaccine dropped their titers three- to fourfold after tonsillectomy and adenoidectomy.[109] Attempts to vaccinate seronegative children subjected to tonsillectomy and adenoidectomy have resulted in delayed and lowered nasopharyngeal secretory immune responses as measured by IgA antibodies to the poliovirus.[134] Fortunately, poliovirus epidemics are no longer an annual threat.

It is clear that the adenoids and tonsils are active immunologic organs that generally reinforce the mucosal immunity of the entire upper aerodigestive tract. The immunologic role of these organs should be considered before a patient undergoes adenoidectomy or tonsillectomy; nonetheless, clinical consideration still forms the actual basis of surgery.

BACTERIOLOGY

Establishment of normal flora in the upper respiratory tract begins at birth. *Actinomyces, Fusobacterium,* and *Nocardia* are acquired by 6 to 8 months of age.[19] Subsequently, *Bacteroides, Leptotrichia, Propionibacterium,* and *Candida* are also established as part of the oral flora.[37,154] *Fusobacterium* populations reach high numbers after dentition and reach maximal numbers at 1 year of age.[37] The ratio of anaerobic to aerobic bacterium in saliva is approximately 10:1.[37] This is due to variations in oxygen concentration throughout the oral cavity.

Healthy children up to 5 years of age can harbor known aerobic pathogens. Ingvarsson, Lundgren, and Irving[75] revealed that *Streptococcus pneumoniae* was recovered in 19% of healthy children, *Haemophilus influenzae* in 13%, group A *Streptococcus* in 5%, and *Moraxella (Branhamella) catarrhalis* in 36%. The frequency of pathogens decreases with age, possibly due to increased immunity. Changes in the pharyngeal bacteria flora noted during viral illnesses are thought to be due to the increased adherence of *Staphylococcus aureus* as well as gram-negative enteric organisms.[147] Oral pharyngeal colonization during illness-free periods was found to vary from 12% to 18% for gram-negative enterics and from 5% to 14% for *S. aureus.*[128] During an episode of viral upper respiratory tract infection, the colonization of gram-negative organisms and *S. aureus* increased to 60% and 43%, respectively.

Brodsky and Koch[15] found substantive differences in the type and number of aerobic bacteria found in nondiseased and diseased adenoids. The core samples of normal adenoids revealed that 75% of children who were relatively free of upper respiratory disease, otitis media, and symptoms of adenoid obstruction had either no bacterial growth on culture or bacteria that are considered to be part of the normal flora and not pathogenic. This compares with only 45% of children who had chronic adenoid infection and 39% who had obstructive adenoid hypertrophy; the bacteria found in these children were more likely to be β-lactamase producers.

INFECTIONS OF WALDEYER'S RING

Many organisms can induce inflammation of Waldeyer's ring. These include aerobic as well as anaerobic bacteria, viruses, yeasts, and parasites. Some of the infectious organisms are part of the normal oral pharyngeal flora whereas others are external pathogens. Because the oropharynx is colonized by many organisms, most infections of Waldeyer's ring are polymicrobial. These organisms work synergistically and can be demonstrated in mixed aerobic and anaerobic infections.[20]

Another feature of mixed infections is the ability of organisms resistant to an antimicrobial agent to protect an organism susceptible to that agent by the production of an antibiotic degrading enzyme that is secreted into the tissues.[22] Because of the polymicrobial nature of most infections around Waldeyer's ring, it is often difficult to interpret data derived from clinical samples obtained from mucosal surfaces and to differentiate between organisms that are colonized and those that are invaders.

VIRUSES

The classic ''common cold'' is the most frequent cause of otolaryngologic infection in children. A multitude of offending viral pathogens have been implicated in causing pharyngitis, including rhinovirus, influenzavirus, parainfluenzavirus, adenovirus, coxsackievirus, echovirus, reovirus and respiratory syncytial virus. Viral pharyngitis is usually mild in presentation with patients complaining of a sore throat and dysphagia. Most patients will have a fever with erythema of the pharyngeal mucosa. The tonsils may be enlarged but frequently there is no associated exudate.

Herpangina caused by coxsackievirus is characterized by small vesicles with erythematous bases that become ulcers and are spread over the anterior pillar tonsils, palate, and posterior pharynx (Fig. 12-2). Herpes simplex commonly causes the well known ''cold sore.'' This virus can also cause exudative or nonexudative pharyngitis mainly in older children and young adults. In younger children, the herpesvirus may induce gingivostomatitis.

Management of viral infections is nonspecific and symp-

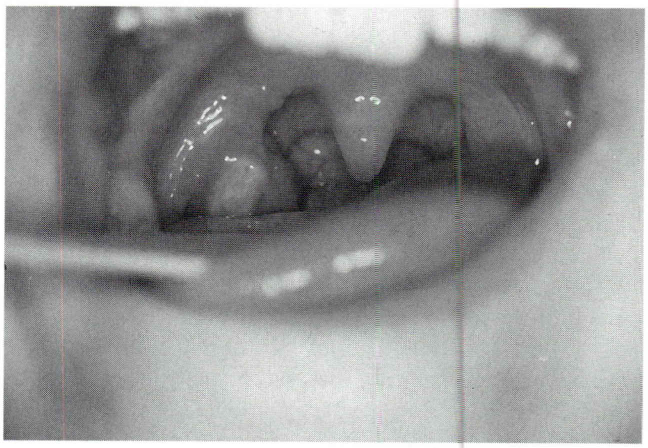

Fig. 12-2. Viral ulcer on the right tonsil, consistent with coxsackievirus infection.

tomatic. Antibiotics are helpful in cases of secondary bacterial infection.

Epstein-Barr virus

One particular type of viral infection that deserves special attention is the Epstein-Barr virus (EBV). EBV induces the mononucleosis syndrome, which consists of high fever; general malaise; large, swollen, dirty-gray tonsils (Fig. 12-3); sore throat; dysphagia; and odynophagia. Petechiae located at the junction of the hard and soft palate are highly suggestive of EBV although not pathognomonic. Often these patients have hepatosplenomegaly with resultant liver damage. The method of transmission most likely is oral contact.

Diagnosis of EBV is confirmed by laboratory studies. A differential blood count showing 50% lymphocytosis with 10% atypical lymphocytes is characteristic of EBV infection. Serologic studies include monospot and serum heterophil antibody titers. These tests may be negative initially, and repeat testing in 1 to 2 weeks is warranted if the results are clinically suspicious. The heterophil antibody titers are detected by the Paul-Bunnell-Davidsohn or Ox-cell hemolysis test. If the heterophil antibody agglutination test is negative the disease may still be present. Only 60% of patients with infectious mononucleosis have a positive test within the first 2 weeks after onset of the illness; 90% have a positive test 1 month after onset.[121] Management of this condition is symptomatic. Recovery may take weeks, and antibiotics are used to treat secondary bacterial infections. Ampicillin should be avoided because a rash may occur despite previous intake without similar reactions. Upper-airway obstruction from severely enlarged tonsils can be life-threatening and should be managed promply with the insertion of a nasopharyngeal airway and short-term high-dose steroid therapy. If the obstruction is severe and unrelieved by these measures, a tonsillectomy or tracheotomy may need to be performed.

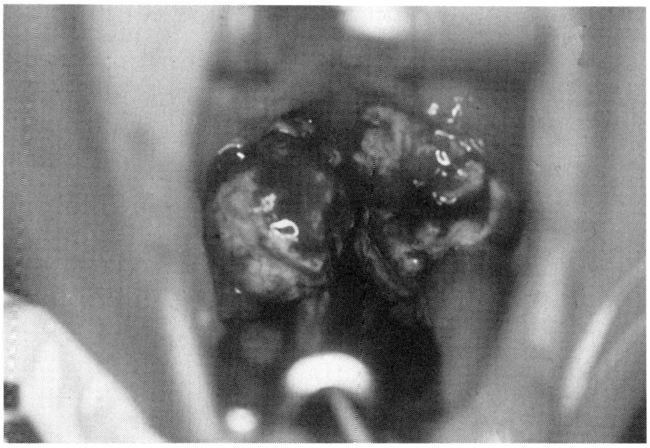

Fig. 12-3. Tonsillar hypertrophy and mononucleosis with significant airway obstruction.

CANDIDA

Candidiasis can result in severe pharyngitis, particularly in patients who are immunocompromised or who have been undergoing treatment with antimicrobial agents. It is a fairly unmistakable syndrome consisting of coherent white plaques on the oral pharyngeal mucosa. Removal of these plaques may reveal a raw, bleeding surface. Management is with nystatin (Bausch & Lomb) or, in refractory cases, fluconazole (Pfizer).

NEISSERIA

Pharyngitis due to *Neisseria gonorrhoeae* is common in homosexual males. It has been detected in 6% of adolescents with acute pharyngitis.[182] Although the infection is often asymptomatic, it can result and persist after treatment. Acute exudative tonsillitis is a manifestation of gonococcal pharyngitis. The clinical syndrome may range from an asymptomatic to an exudative pharyngitis, but most cases tend to fall toward the exudative pharyngitis end of the spectrum. Nonetheless, disseminated gonococcemia can result even from mild or asymptomatic infection. Penicillin or tetracycline are the most effective therapeutic agents.

VINCENT'S ANGINA

Vincent's angina is secondary to *Spirochaeta denticolata* and Vincent's fusiform bacillus Borrelia vincentii (*Treponema vincentii*). This condition arises slowly, manifesting both mild local and systemic symptoms. The infection arises most commonly in overcrowded conditions. Patients present with complaints of high fever, headache, sore throat, and physical findings of cervical lymphadenopathy and a membrane on the tonsil that, when removed, reveals an ulcer that remains confined to the surrounding tissue and usually heals in 7 to 10 days.[187] Management is with penicillin. Local treatment in the form of oral hygiene is helpful. This condition may be confused with trench mouth, which is caused by the same organisms but the oral cavity ulcers in trench month include the gums and oral mucous membranes.[187]

SYPHILIS

Treponema pallidum infections in both the primary and secondary stages of syphilis can be associated with oral pharyngeal lesions. In primary syphilis, the appearance of oral chancres is about 3 weeks after exposure. Grayish superficial mucous membrane patches surrounded by an erythematous border are generally found in patients with secondary syphilis.

CORYNEBACTERIUM DIPHTHERIAE

The incidence of *Corynebacterium diphtheriae* (Klebs-Löffler bacillus) infection has declined markedly since the introduction of vaccination. This organism causes an early exudative pharyngotonsillitis with a thick pharyngeal membrane. Infection can then spread to the throat, tonsils, palate, and larynx.[40] *C. diphtheriae* organisms can also produce a lethal exotoxin that can damage cells in distant organs. Today only 200 to 300 cases of diphtheria occur in the United States each year, usually but not exclusively in people who have not been immunized.[161] The organism is a gram-positive pleomorphic aerobic bacillus that can be identified in a routine throat culture, particularly when the microbiologist is made aware of a clinical suspicion of this diagnosis. Only toxigenic strains infected with a bacteriophage can produce diphtheria.[162] Laryngeal inflammation combined with an exudative, necrotic, gray, pharyngeal membrane may result in airway obstruction. Removal of this membrane causes bleeding. Early diagnosis is critical, and the goal of therapy is neutralization of unbound toxin with antitoxin. Myocarditis and neurologic sequelae resembling Guillain-Barré syndrome or poliomyelitis may result.[162] Identification of this disease is by fluorescent antibody studies. The presence of Klebs-Löffler bacillus in the membrane can be diagnosed by Gram's staining.[187] Because diphtheria is an emergency condition, antitoxin should be given in the first 48 hours of onset to be effective. Airway obstruction should be managed by tracheotomy. Penicillin in high doses should be administered.

STREPTOCOCCAL TONSILLITIS–PHARYNGITIS

Group A streptococcus is the most common bacterial cause of acute pharyngitis.[7] Its public health importance lies not only in its frequency but also on the fact that it is a percursor of two serious sequelae: acute rheumatic fever and poststreptococcal glomerulonephritis. Although the incidence of rheumatic fever has decreased, all groups of β-hemolytic streptococcus have been associated with rheumatic fever.[19]

Acute streptococcal tonsillitis is a disease of childhood, with a peak incidence at about 5 to 6 years of age but can occur in children younger than 3 years of age and in adults over age 50.[187] Outbreaks may arise in epidemic forms in institutional settings such as recruit camps and daycare facilities. Acute tonsillitis is manifested by a dry throat, malaise, fever, fullness of the throat, odynophagia, dysphagia, otalgia, headache, limb and back pain, cervical adenopathy, and shivering. Examination will reveal a dry tongue, erythematous enlarged tonsils, and yellowish-white spots; in severe cases, a tonsillar or pharyngeal membrane or purulent exudate may exist along with jugulodigastric lymph node enlargement.[137]

The diagnosis of acute tonsillitis depends mainly on clinical grounds. The clinical manifestations of streptococcal and nonstreptococcal pharyngitis overlap so broadly that it is often impossible to make the diagnosis with certainty. For this reason, most authorities recommend that the diagnosis of group A β-hemolytic streptococcal (GABHS) pharyngitis be verified or ruled out by microbiologic tests in patients who appear likely, on the basis of clinical and epidemiologic considerations, to have this illness.[7,31] The time-honored method of diagnostic confirmation is the throat culture. This is a simple and extremely useful test but must be skillfully performed by swabbing the posterior pharynx and tonsillar areas.[7] The test must also be appropriately processed and read. Such selective use of throat cultures represents good medical practice.

One of the major problems in the use of throat cultures in everyday medical practice has been the delay in obtaining results. These can range from 18 to 48 hours, delaying appropriate management; however, a delay of this length will not increase the development of rheumatic fever. Nevertheless, it can be difficult for physicians to convince parents of the wisdom of withholding antibiotics, especially if their children are cranky and febrile. If group A streptococcal pharyngitis is treated early in the clinical course, the period of communicability is reduced.[129] Management is thus initiated before culture results are available and unfortunately may not be terminated even when negative results are obtained. Development of rapid tests for the detection of the group A streptococcal antigen has therefore presented a useful advance.

Several rapid tests to detect group A streptococcal antigen in the pharynx have been developed and employ either latex agglutination or enzyme-linked immunosorbent assay (ELISA) methods to extract the antigen from a swab. The streptococcal group A carbohydrate may be detected within a matter of minutes. These kits are suitable for use in a physician's office. Although the rapid detection tests are highly specific, they are unfortunately not as sensitive as routine throat culture.[7,43,54] A negative rapid detection test may instigate the practitioner to withhold antibiotic therapy while awaiting culture results. Most guidelines suggest that throat cultures should be performed when the body temperature is greater than 38.3° C or when the illness is characterized exclusively by a sore throat.[73] The most accurate and cost-effective method to diagnose acute GABHS infection is the use of the rapid strep test; this is followed by standard throat culture in patients with a negative rapid strep test result and a strong suspicion of streptococcal tonsillitis.

Even if optimally obtained and processed, throat cultures are not without flaws. Throat culture cannot reliably differentiate acute from chronic infection. Managing all patients who have positive cultures results in overmanagement. There are occasional false-negative results (approximately 10% of cases), but a recent report has stated that these patients are most likely carriers who do not require treatment.[7] Studies have reported that a single throat culture is 90% to 97% sensitive and 90% specific for GABHS growth.[144] The carrier state can be elucidated by serologic testing. A true infection is demonstrated by a positive throat culture and at least a two-dilutional rise in the antistreptolysin-O titer.[148] A GABHS carrier without acute infection will have a positive culture with no change in dilution titer.[1] Excluding the diagnosis of group A streptococcal pharyngitis is quite important

with a history of adenotonsillar hypertrophy, and adenotonsillar hypertrophy is the most common cause of sleep apnea in children.[46] It is important to elicit the severity of symptomatology by obtaining a thorough history from the patient's primary caregiver. Findings that suggest significant sleep disturbance include witnessed apneic episodes, excessively loud snoring, chronic mouth-breathing, frequent awakening during the night, hypersomnolence, enuresis, nightmares, poor school performance, dysphasia, hyponasal speech (rhinolalia clausa) or, rarely, hypernasal speech (rhinolalia aperta) caused by enlarged tonsils impinging on normal palatal movement.[132] Children with chronic adenotonsillar hypertrophy and airway obstruction may also present with failure to thrive.[23,83,143] In adults, obstructive sleep apnea is often associated with the classic obesity-related pickwickian syndrome. Describing polysomnographic findings, Leach and others[83] noted that obesity was not a factor in children with obstructive sleep apnea caused by adenotonsillar hypertrophy.

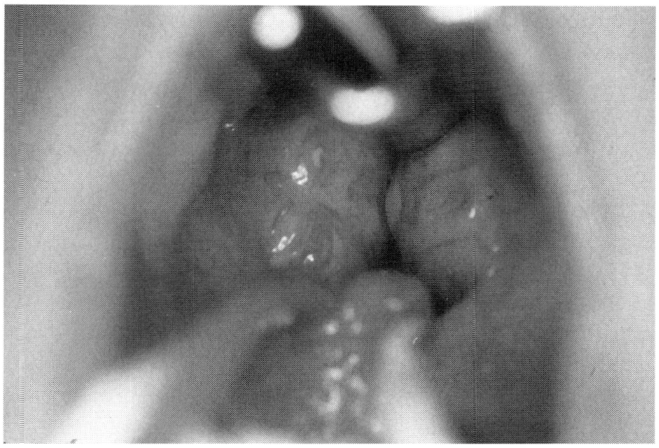

Fig. 12-7. Tonsillar hypertrophy with significant pharyngeal obstruction.

Most children with airway obstruction related to adenotonsillar hypertrophy have a history of significant snoring at night.[59,83,112,132,188] Excessive snoring in itself may be a significant indicator of obstructive sleep apnea, even without a history of witnessed apnea, as indicated by polysomnography.[25,188] Descriptions parents may use in cases of significant obstruction include the child snoring like an adult or that they can hear the child snoring outside of the child's bedroom. Enuresis is another indicator of severe underlying airway obstruction in children. Weider and others[175,176] described enuresis related to chronic adenotonsillar hypertrophy and significant airway obstruction that was relieved by adenotonsillectomy. In their study, all patients with secondary enuresis (developed later during childhood) responded to adenotonsillectomy, whereas 24 patients with primary enuresis (congenitally present) did not respond to surgery, possibly as a result of other neurologic factors. A proposed cause of enuresis is poor nocturnal regulation of antidiuretic hormone release that is related to disorders of rapid eye movement (REM) sleep. Patients with chronic adenotonsillar hypertrophy and airway obstruction may also develop failure to thrive, possibly related to abnormal regulation of growth hormone release. During REM sleep, growth hormone may be severely disrupted in children with obstructive sleep apnea.[83]

A

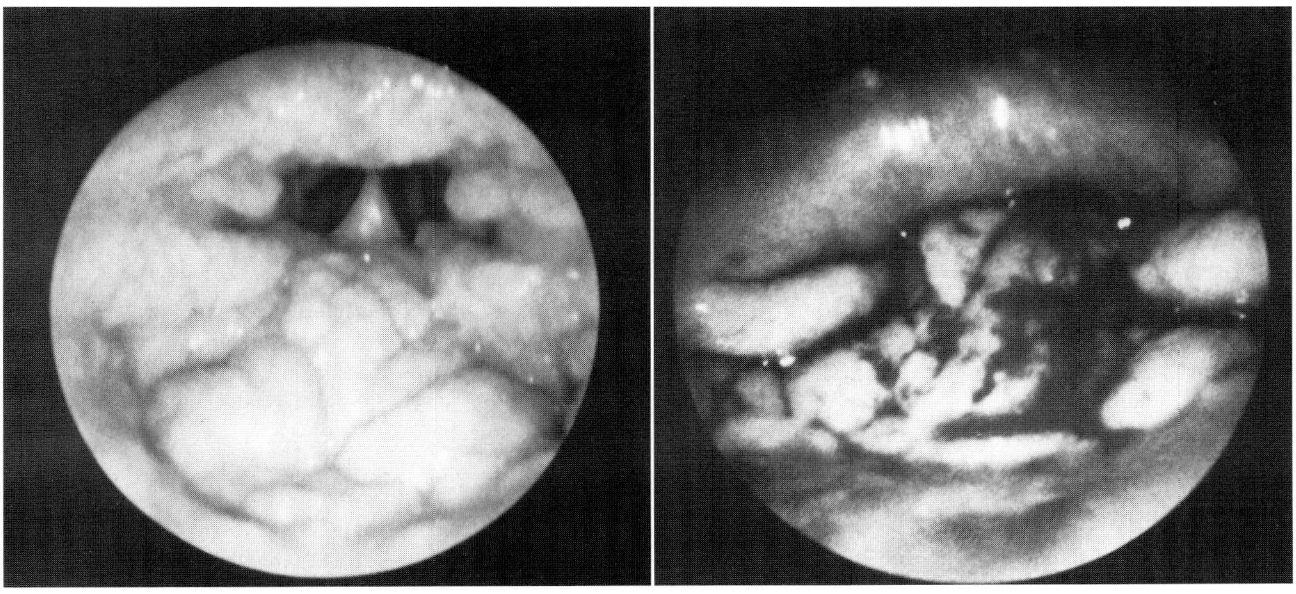

B

Fig. 12-8. A, Endoscopic view of mild adenoid hypertrophy. **B,** Severe adenoid hypertrophy with total choanal obstruction.

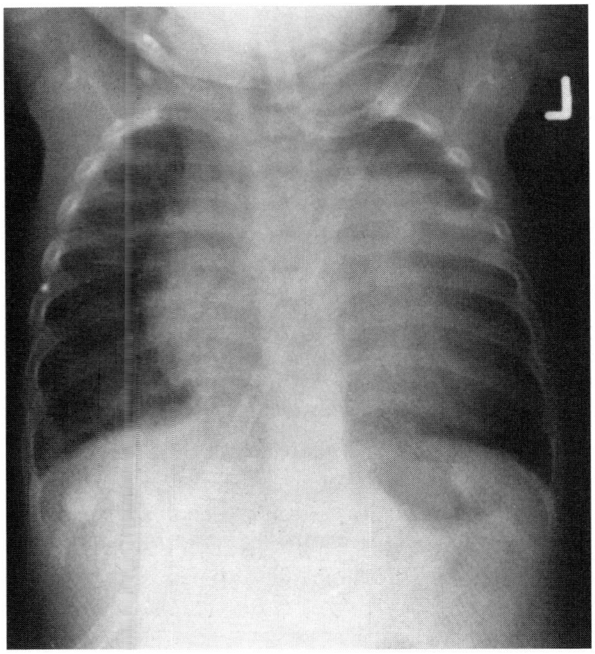

Fig. 12-9. Posteroanterior chest radiograph of a patient with adenotonsillar hypertrophy, severe airway obstruction, pulmonary vascular hypertension, and cor pulmonale.

The role of polysomnographic testing in children has been previously reported.[23,83,132] Sleep sonography is another reliable method to detect evidence of obstructive sleep apnea in children and may be performed in the child's home, thereby potentially saving the costs of expensive polysomnographic studies. Sleep sonography entails analysis of a tape-recording of the patient's nocturnal sleeping pattern. Excellent correlation between sleep sonography and polysomnography has been reported.[123] Because of the high cost of polysomnography, it is important for the otolaryngologist to be selective in referring patients for this diagnostic modality. Patients with obvious symptoms related to adenotonsillar hypertrophy confirmed by physical examination most likely will not require polysomnographic testing. Patients with significant symptomatology suggesting sleep apnea or a significant sleep disturbance without evidence of significant adenotonsillar hypertrophy on examination should undergo polysomnographic testing to determine the severity of the sleep disturbance. Screening chest radiography and electrocardiography are also recommended in the preoperative assessment of severe cases.

Craniofacial growth and adenotonsillar hypertrophy

Chronic mouth-breathing secondary to adenotonsillar hypertrophy and upper-airway obstruction has been shown to affect craniofacial growth patterns in children. As early as 1872, Tomes[168] reported that children who were chronic mouth-breathers secondary to adenoid hypertrophy displayed evidence of malocclusion and maxillofacial growth abnormalities. Mouth-breathing leads to displacement of the mandible and tongue downward and backward and potential postural changes of the head and neck that may secondarily affect dental occlusion and jaw growth.[111] Numerous animal and human studies have demonstrated the effect of chronic nasal obstruction on maxillofacial growth patterns. Harvold[67] demonstrated that chronic nasal obstruction may lead to narrow maxillary dental arches in rhesus monkeys. Linder-Aronson, Woodside, and Lundstrom[87] demonstrated the classic stigmata of adenoid facies in children with chronic nasopharyngeal obstruction from adenoid hypertrophy; these consisted of longer total anterior face height with a tendency toward a retrognathic mandible compared with controls.

The postural changes of chronic mouth-breathing disturb the normal equilibrium of forces exerted on the teeth and oral facial soft tissues by the tongue and lip, resulting in an open bite, a protrusive maxilla, and a buccal posterior crossbite. The severity of adenotonsillar hypertrophy and resulting airway obstruction as measured by surgical findings and lateral cephalometric radiographs is directly related to the degree of maxillofacial growth disturbance and malocclusion.[111] Adenotonsillectomy has been shown to reverse some of these findings.[61,87] Other investigators have confirmed the relationship between chronic nasal obstruction, adenotonsillar hypertrophy, and increased facial height.[42,169] Although there is significant support in the literature for the effect of upper-airway obstruction and adenotonsillar hypertrophy on craniofacial growth, other studies have been less conclusive about this relationship.[66,101,180] Maxillofacial growth disturbances in children who are mouth-breathers also may be multifactorial in etiology.[174] As a result of this apparent relationship between upper-airway obstruction, adenotonsillar hypertrophy, and craniofacial growth disturbance, an otolaryngologic evaluation may be warranted in children undergoing orthodontic procedures for malocclusion who show evidence of adenotonsillar hypertrophy and mouth-breathing.

Diagnostic assessment of the tonsils and adenoids

The physical examination of patients with suspected adenotonsillar disease should include a thorough head and neck examination to rule out manifestations of chronic adenotonsillar hypertrophy (i.e., the craniofacial stigmata of chronic nasal obstruction, which includes open-mouth breathing, an elongated face, dark circles under the eyes, and evidence of dental malocclusion). Other causes of nasal obstruction that may also result in these findings (e.g., turbinate hypertrophy secondary to allergic rhinitis) should also be evaluated. It is important to listen to the patient's speech to assess the presence of hyponasality. Having the child repeat words such as *Mickey Mouse*, which emphasize nasal emission, and *baseball*, which does not, will better illuminate the presence of hyponasality.[14]

A

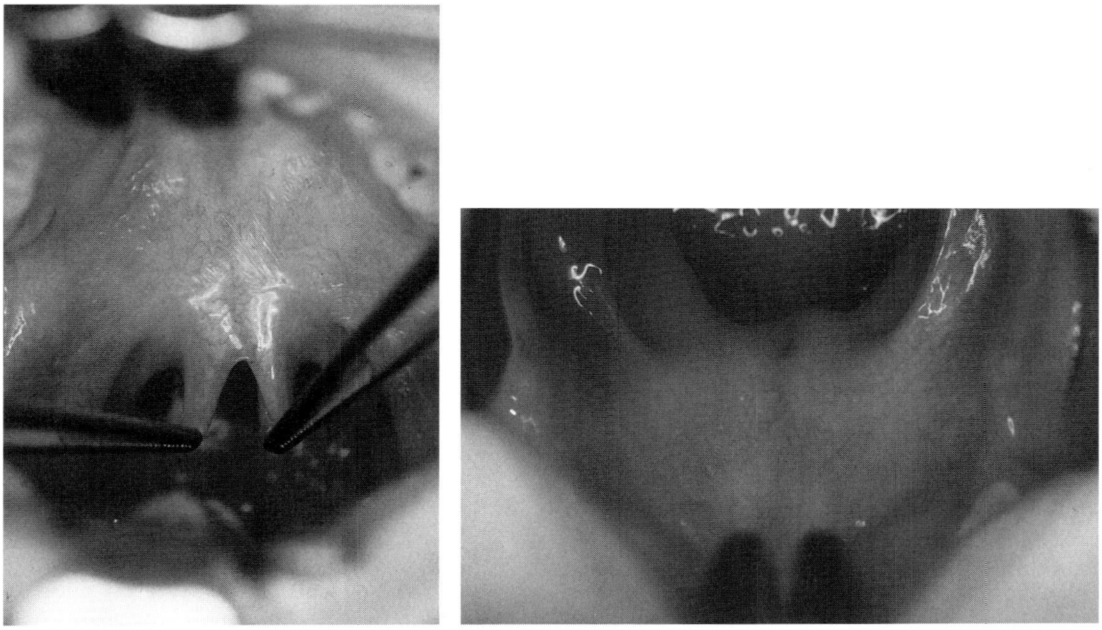

B

Fig. 12-10. **A,** Bifid uvula in a patient with a submucous cleft palate. **B,** Submucous cleft palate.

Brodsky, Moore, and Stanievich[16] described an assessment scale for tonsillar hypertrophy. In their scale, 0 indicates that the tonsils do not impinge on the airway; 1+ indicates less than 25% airway obstruction; 2+ indicates 25% to 50% airway obstruction; 3+ indicates 50% to 75% airway obstruction; and 4+ indicates more than 75% airway obstruction. It is also important to assess the palate on oral examination. Patients with evidence of overt or submucous cleft palate are at increased risk for the development of velopharyngeal insufficiency (VPI) after adenoidectomy. Submucous cleft palate may manifest only as a bifid uvula. However, notching of the posterior hard palate may be palpable and an obvious translucent line through the mid-soft palate may be evident (Fig. 12-10). Although diagnostic assessment of the tonsils is apparent on oral examination, evaluation of adenoid tissue is much more difficult because it is not easily accessible on physical examination.

Lateral neck radiography may be helpful in assessing adenoid hypertrophy (Fig. 12-11). Fujioka, Young, and Girdany[47] determined that the adenoid : nasopharyngeal ratio, measured by lateral neck radiography, closely correlated with clinical symptomatology related to adenoid hypertrophy; this has been confirmed by other reports.[30] However, physiologic variations during nasal and oral breathing may affect these nasopharyngeal dimensions as measured by lateral neck radiography.[12]

Lateral neck radiography is not necessary for the evaluation of all patients with suspected adenoid hypertrophy. Patients with significant obstructive symptomatology and obvious tonsillar hypertrophy most likely require surgical intervention, and lateral neck radiography would not alter the decision to proceed with surgery. Patients with significant nasal obstruction and insignificant tonsillar hypertrophy should undergo radiologic assessment of the nasopharynx. Patients with significant nasal obstruction and evidence of allergic rhinitis may have concurrent underlying adenoid hypertrophy and would benefit from lateral neck radiography.

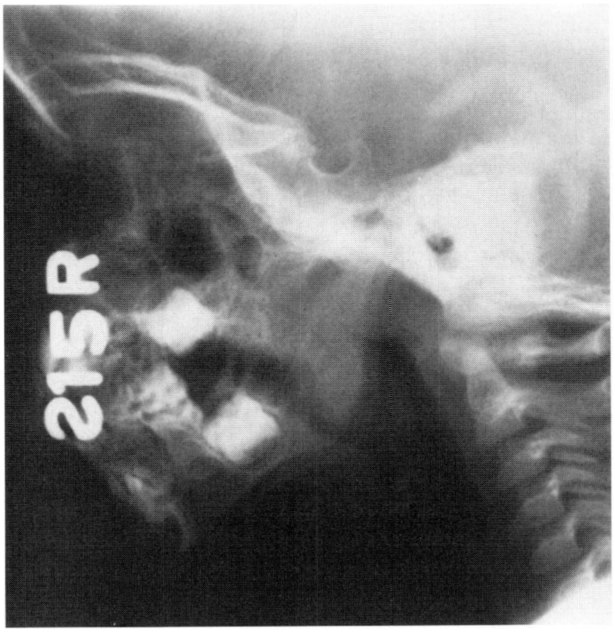

Fig. 12-11. Lateral neck radiograph demonstrating significant adenoid hypertrophy and nasal pharyngeal obstruction.

Flexible endoscopic nasopharyngoscopy may also be valuable in the assessment of adenotonsillar disease. With appropriate topical anesthesia, pediatric endoscopes, and reassurance from the physician, this procedure is generally tolerated well by children. The presence of adenoid tissue obstructing the posterior nasal choana will be apparent by this technique; the degree of hypopharyngeal extension of tonsillar hypertrophy may also be apparent. VPI secondary to tonsillar hypertrophy impinging on palatal movement will be apparent by nasopharyngoscopy. The presence of adenoiditis may also be diagnosed by the presence of purulent secretions covering the adenoid pad. Wormald and Prescott[184] and Wang and others[173] demonstrated the efficacy of flexible nasopharyngoscopy compared with lateral neck radiography and clinical symptomatology in the assessment of adenoid hypertrophy in children. Rhinomanometry has also been demonstrated to correlate with the presence of nasal obstruction secondary to adenoid hypertrophy. However, this test is not well tolerated by children, is difficult and time-consuming to administer, and is probably not of clinical benefit in its current form.[119]

Preoperative assessment

Preoperative assessment in patients undergoing adenotonsillectomy is crucial and may reveal potential problems that may complicate either surgery or the patient's postoperative course. It is crucial to elicit the existence of any coagulation abnormalities. A family history of coagulation disorders or easy bruising may be a warning sign of an underlying bleeding disorder warranting further hematologic evaluation. Routine evaluation of coagulation studies before surgery in patients undergoing adenotonsillectomy is controversial. Manning and others[95] examined the records of 994 of 1050 consecutive patients undergoing tonsillectomy, adenoidectomy, or adenotonsillectomy and determined that evidence of coagulation disorders in patients with no clinical history of or examination consistent with a hematologic disorder was extremely low, thereby not justifying routine preoperative coagulation studies. This was confirmed by Close and others,[29] who suggested that excessive bleeding associated with tonsillectomy was usually not the result of an identifiable coagulation disorder.

Conversely, Kang and others[78] studied the risk of postoperative hemorrhage in 1061 children undergoing adenotonsillectomy. In their study, 2.5% of the children had at least one abnormality on preoperative coagulation screening, which consisted of prothrombin time, partial thromboplastin time, bleeding time, and platelet count. The authors suggested that although hematologic disorders were diagnosed infrequently by preoperative coagulation screening, the coagulation profile may detect patients who are more likely to bleed postoperatively.[78] This is consistent with the findings of Bolger, Parsons, and Potempa,[10] who demonstrated abnormal initial coagulation screening results in 11.5% of patients undergoing adenotonsillectomy. It is apparent that patients who have an obvious family or clinical history of excessive bleeding or an underlying hematologic disorder require close monitoring of their coagulation profiles and consultation with a hematologist. Use of preoperative coagulation screening should be left to the discretion of the surgeon until its role is better clarified by further study.

Patients with obvious severe airway obstruction secondary to adenotonsillar hypertrophy may require polysomnography, chest radiography, electrocardiography, and possibly cardiology consultation. Patients with cor pulmonale and hypercapnia may require postoperative intensive care monitoring with mechanical ventilation to avoid postobstructive pulmonary edema. If the severity of airway obstruction is not clear by parental history, then polysomnography may be warranted.

Patients with other medical conditions may require further testing or preoperative consultation. Patients with a history of significant bronchospasm may require pulmonary medicine evaluation and management in the perioperative period. Black patients should be screened for sickle-cell disease preoperatively, and female patients of reproductive age should undergo a preoperative β-human chorionic gonadotropin to rule out pregnancy. Velocardiofacial syndrome may require preoperative angiography to determine the presence of abnormally medially displaced carotid arteries, which may be at risk during tonsillectomy.[45]

ADENOTONSILLECTOMY

The technique of adenotonsillectomy has evolved significantly over the past 2000 years, and various techniques are used today for extirpation of the tonsils and adenoids. Multiple tonsillectomy techniques exist, including the sharp dissection initially described by Crowe, Watkins, and Rottholz[33]; various electrocauterization techniques; lasers (including potassium-titanyl—phosphate [KTP] and CO_2); and the tonsil guillotine. The number of adenotonsillectomies performed in the United States appears to have peaked in the 1940s and 1950s.[136] In 1959, 1.4 million tonsillectomies were performed; this number decreased to 500,000 in 1979 and fell even further to 340,000 in 1985.[105a,136] In the past 30 years there has been a significant decrease in the number of adenotonsillectomies performed in the United States as well as a change in the preoperative indications for surgery. Whereas chronic infection was the primary surgical indication for adenotonsillectomy in the 1950s and 1960s, airway obstruction and obstructive sleep apnea have now become important preoperative indications for surgery.[136] Apparent decreases in the number of adenotonsillectomies performed in the United States reflect a higher degree of selectivity by otolaryngologists and referring primary care physicians and have become important in the new era of managed healthcare.

Indications

The current indications for tonsillectomy and adenoidectomy are shown in Boxes 12-1 and 12-2. Generally, the indications for adenotonsillectomy can be related primarily to

Box 12-1. Surgical indications for tonsillectomy

Infection

Recurrent, acute tonsillitis (more than six episodes per year or three episodes per year for ≥ 2 years)
Recurrent acute tonsillitis associated with other conditions:
- Cardiac valvular disease associated with recurrent streptococcal tonsillitis
- Recurrent febrile seizures

Chronic tonsillitis that is unresponsive to medical therapy associated with:
- Halitosis
- Persistent sore throat
- Tender cervical adenitis

Streptococcal carrier state unresponsive to medical therapy
Peritonsillar abscess
Tonsillitis associated with abscessed cervical nodes
Mononucleosis with severely obstructing tonsils that is unresponsive to medical therapy.

Obstruction

Excessive snoring and chronic mouth-breathing
Obstructive sleep apnea or sleep disturbances
Adenotonsillar hypertrophy associated with:
- Cor pulmonale
- Failure to thrive
- Dysphagia
- Speech abnormalities

Craniofacial growth abnormalities
Occlusion abnormalities

Other

Suspected neoplasia–asymmetric tonsillar hypertrophy

chronic upper-airway obstruction in conjunction with adenotonsillar hypertrophy, which is manifesting as snoring, obstructive sleep apnea, or chronic infectious conditions such as chronic recurrent tonsillitis.

Upper-airway obstruction

Patients with airway obstruction related to adenotonsillar hypertrophy typically manifest excessive snoring and possibly obstructive sleep apnea. The severity of the condition can often be elicited by a parental history. However, there may often be no indications of airway obstruction other than loud snoring. It has been demonstrated that patients who snore excessively loudly at night may manifest significant sleep apnea by polysomnographic testing when no significant parental history of obstructive sleep apnea has been noted.[25,188] Signs of severe airway obstruction related to adenotonsillar hypertrophy, in addition to loud snoring, include daytime somnolence, failure to thrive, and possibly enuresis.

Patients who have obvious adenotonsillar hypertrophy on physical examination, a significant history of loud snoring, and witnessed episodes of obstructive sleep apnea do not

Box 12-2. Surgical indications for adenodoidectomy

Infection

Purulent adenoiditis
Adenoid hypertrophy associated with:
- Chronic otitis media with effusion
- Chronic recurrent acute otitis media
- Chronic otitis media with perforation
- Otorrhea or chronic tube otorrhea

Obstruction

Adenoid hypertrophy associated with excessive snoring and chronic mouth-breathing
Sleep apnea or sleep disturbances
Adenoid hypertrophy associated with:
- Cor pulmonale
- Failure to thrive
- Dysphagia
- Speech abnormalities

Craniofacial growth abnormalities
Occlusion abnormalities
Speech abnormalities

Other

Suspected neoplasia
Adenoid hypertrophy associated with chronic sinusitis

necessarily need preoperative polysomnographic testing. If the parental history is unclear regarding the severity of airway obstruction or if the physical examination and history are not consistent then preoperative polysomnographic testing is warranted to demonstrate the severity of airway obstruction. Patients whose polysomnographic tests demonstrate a significant number of events (>10/hour) or significant oxygen desaturation (<90%) are candidates for surgical intervention.

Chronic infections

Patients with chronic recurrent tonsillitis or chronic tonsillitis may benefit from tonsillectomy and possibly adenoidectomy. In 1995, the American Academy of Otolaryngology–Head and Neck Surgery *Clinical Indicators Compendium* stated that patients with three or more infections of the tonsils and/or adenoids per year, despite adequate medical therapy, are candidates for tonsillectomy and adenoidectomy.[3] Other indications include chronic tonsillitis unresponsive to medical therapy that results in a persistent foul taste or halitosis or recurrent tonsillitis associated with the streptococcal state and has not responded to β-lactamase–resistant antimicrobial therapy.[3] The efficacy of elective tonsillectomy for recurrent sore throats has been demonstrated by numerous investigators.[98,116] The efficacy of elective tonsillectomy has also been demonstrated in children with recurrent throat infections, including GABHS.[116]

In a study by Paradise and others,[116] 187 children participated in a randomized clinical trial. Inclusion criteria for the study included patients with seven or more sore throat episodes in the preceeding year who were treated with antibiotics; five or more sore throat episodes in the 2 preceding years; or three or more episodes in each of the 3 preceding years. These patients benefited from elective tonsillectomy and/or adenoidectomy compared with a control group of children who were managed nonsurgically. Factors that should be taken into account when considering surgery for recurrent throat infections in children include (1) the severity of each episode, (2) how well the children have responded to medical therapy, and (3) quality-of-life issues (e.g., missed days at school.)

Tonsillectomy and adenoidectomy should be considered in patients with recurrent tonsillitis as well as other medical conditions such as cardiac valvular disease with recurrent streptococcal tonsillitis, a history of febrile seizures, poorly controlled diabetes, and possibly ventricular peritoneal shunts. Systemic infections in these situations could become life-threatening.

Tonsillectomy is the management of choice for peritonsillar abscess in children who will not tolerate needle aspiration. Peritonsillar abscesses that have been successfully drained by needle aspiration are not necessarily an absolute indication for tonsillectomy. However, tonsillectomy is definitely indicated in cases of recurrent peritonsillar abscess.[8,28,70,-8]

Although diphtheria is currently unusual, tonsillectomy may be warranted in patients who are diphtheria carriers and have not responded to antibiotic therapy. Finally, patients with chronic halitosis related to debris in the tonsillar crypts or secondary to chronic tonsillitis are candidates for tonsillectomy.

ADENOIDECTOMY

Indications

Adenoid hypertrophy or chronic adenoiditis may cause significant problems requiring adenoidectomy in situations in which the tonsils themselves are not diseased and are not contributing to symptomatology. Patients with chronic adenoid hypertrophy causing craniofacial morphology problems, excessive snoring, or possibly quality-of-life issues (e.g., poor olfaction) are candidates for adenoidectomy.[57] Adenoid hypertrophy may be confirmed by flexible nasopharyngoscopy or lateral cervical radiography.

Patients with a history of chronic recurrent sinusitis may also benefit from adenoidectomy. Patients with chronic sinusitis and significant adenoid hypertrophy may initially benefit from adenoidectomy rather than undergoing more extensive sinus surgery.[135] In addition, patients with chronic purulent rhinitis secondary to chronic adenoiditis may also respond to adenoidectomy if they have not responded well to appropriate medical therapy. Patients with hyponasal speech (rhinolalia clausa) are also candidates for adenoidectomy. Hypernasal speech (rhinolalia aperta) is not an indication. However, in unusual cases, excessive tonsillar hypertrophy may impede palatal movement, and this may improve after tonsillectomy.[91]

Although surgical intervention should be considered in cases of severe nasal obstruction related to adenoid hypertrophy, there is evidence that alternative medical therapy exists to manage adenoid hypertrophy. Demain and Goetz[38] demonstrated that aqueous nasal beclomethasone therapy led to significant improvement of nasal obstruction secondary to adenoid hypertrophy, which was confirmed by pre- and post-management flexible nasopharyngoscopy. In addition, patients with underlying inhalant allergies may benefit from antihistamine therapy and possibly from allergic immunologic desensitization therapy.

Conservative adenoidectomy should be performed in patients with a cleft palate or submucous cleft palate, leaving the lower portion of the adenoid pad intact to decrease the risk of postoperative VPI.

ADENOIDECTOMY AND OTITIS MEDIA

The role of the adenoids in the etiology of otitis media has been controversial. However, recent investigations have demonstrated that appropriate management of the adenoids plays an important role in the diagnosis and management of chronic otitis media in children. Bluestone and others[9] and McKee[100] indicated that surgical manipulation of the eustachian tube during adenoidectomy may predispose children to eustachian tube malfunction and the subsequent development of otitis media with effusion. In addition, numerous reports have demonstrated that adenoidectomy alone or in conjunction with myringotomy tube placement may reduce the incidence of future episodes of otitis media and possibly reduce the necessity for future ventilation tubes.[53,117] Gates and others[53] randomly assigned 578 children between the ages of 4 and 8 years into four management groups: group 1 received bilateral myringotomy and no ventilation tube placement; group 2 received placement of ventilation tubes; group 3 underwent adenoidectomy alone; and group 4 underwent adenoidectomy and placement of ventilation tubes. It was demonstrated with statistical significance that patients who underwent adenoidectomy in conjunction with bilateral myringotomy had significantly lower postmanagement morbidity, as measured by hearing loss secondary to middle-ear effusion and the number of subsequent placements of ventilation tubes. Paradise and others[117] randomly studied 213 children who had previously received ventilation tubes that had since extruded. These patients were randomized into two groups—adenoidectomy and no adenoidectomy (control group). The adenoidectomy group had statistically significant less otitis media as compared with control subjects.

The actual mechanism by which adenoidectomy affects the course of otitis media in children is unclear. Surgical extirpation of the adenoids may remove a nasopharyngeal

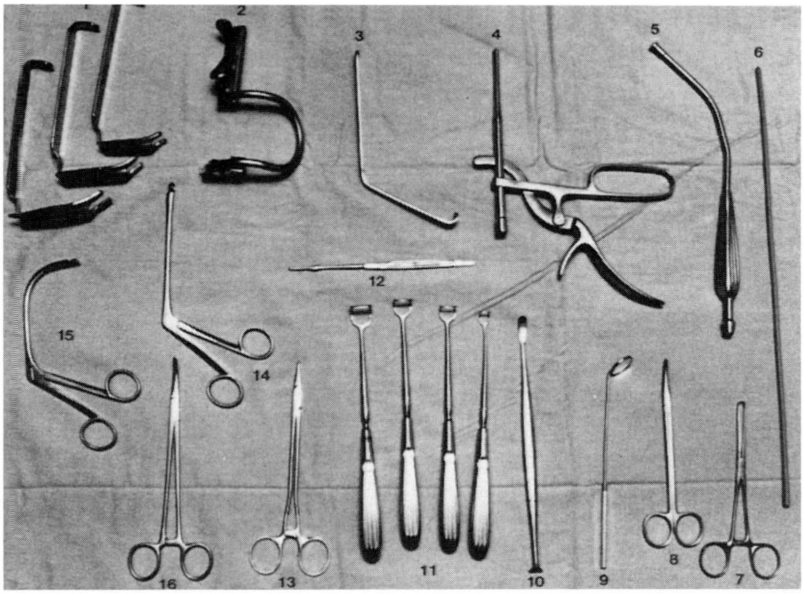

Fig. 12-12. Instrumentation used in tonsillectomy and adenoidectomy procedures.

nidus of contaminated tissue that secondarily acts as a source of infection in the middle ear, or adenoidectomy may simply remove an anatomic obstruction of the eustachian tube. The actual size of the adenoid pad has not necessarily been implicated in the etiology of chronic otitis media with effusion; many authors have failed to determine the relationship between adenoid size and chronic otitis media with effusion.[51,52,93,139]

Based on current evidence, adenoidectomy should be considered in children undergoing ventilation tube placement who have symptomatology suggestive of chronic nasal obstruction or adenoid hypertrophy that is confirmed by nasopharyngoscopy or nasopharyngeal radiography. Patients who require subsequent sets of ventilation tubes also may be candidates for adenoidectomy, regardless of adenoid size or symptomatology.

ADENOTONSILLECTOMY

Surgical technique

Many surgical techniques have been described for extirpation of the tonsils and adenoids. Crowe, Watkins, and Rothholz[33] described the first meticulous surgical dissection technique using sharp instrumentation. More recently, however, dissection using electrocautery has become popular. Current techniques include CO_2 or KTP laser tonsillectomy and tonsillectomy using various electrocautery devices (e.g., standard Bovie electrocautery and bipolar electrocautery.* Evidence suggests that sharp dissection may lead to slightly less postoperative pain. However, there may be less intraoperative blood loss with electrocautery techniques.[84,86,142]

* Refs. 2, 86, 90, 97, 107, 115, 155, 177.

Guillotine tonsillectomy techniques are still used and have been shown to have a low complication rate.[99,170,172] In China, the technique of guillotine tonsillectomy in children without anesthesia has been described.[186]

We believe that electrocautery tonsillectomy using a meticulous dissection technique and low electrocautery wattage results in very minimal intraoperative blood loss and acceptable postoperative discomfort. This technique will be described in detail; instrumentation is shown in Figure 12-12.

Patients should not eat solid foods for 8 hours before surgery. If the patient is closely supervised, he or she may drink clear liquids until 3 hours before surgery. Preoperative sedation with midazolam hydrochloride (0.5 to 1 mg/kg) approximately 30 minutes before surgery may be necessary for patients with excessive preoperative anxiety. Anesthesia is typically induced by mask ventilation, with subsequent intravenous access after the anesthetic has taken effect. Patients usually receive intravenous antibiotics such as ampicillin (20 mg/kg; maximum dose, 1 g). Telian and others[163] demonstrated that intravenous antibiotics followed by a 1-week course of postoperative oral antibiotics significantly decreased morbidity after tonsillectomy.

Patients who have a significant history of obstructive sleep apnea or are younger than 3 years of age receive intraoperative corticosteroids, most commonly dexamethasone (0.5 mg/kg). Catlin and Grimes[27] reported that one dose of intraoperative intravenous corticosteroids improved recovery time in children following tonsillectomy. However, Ohlms, Wilder, and Weston[110] and Volk and others[171] demonstrated no significant effects on recovery time from a single dose of intravenous steroids. The authors use corticosteroids to potentially reduce airway edema in patients who are

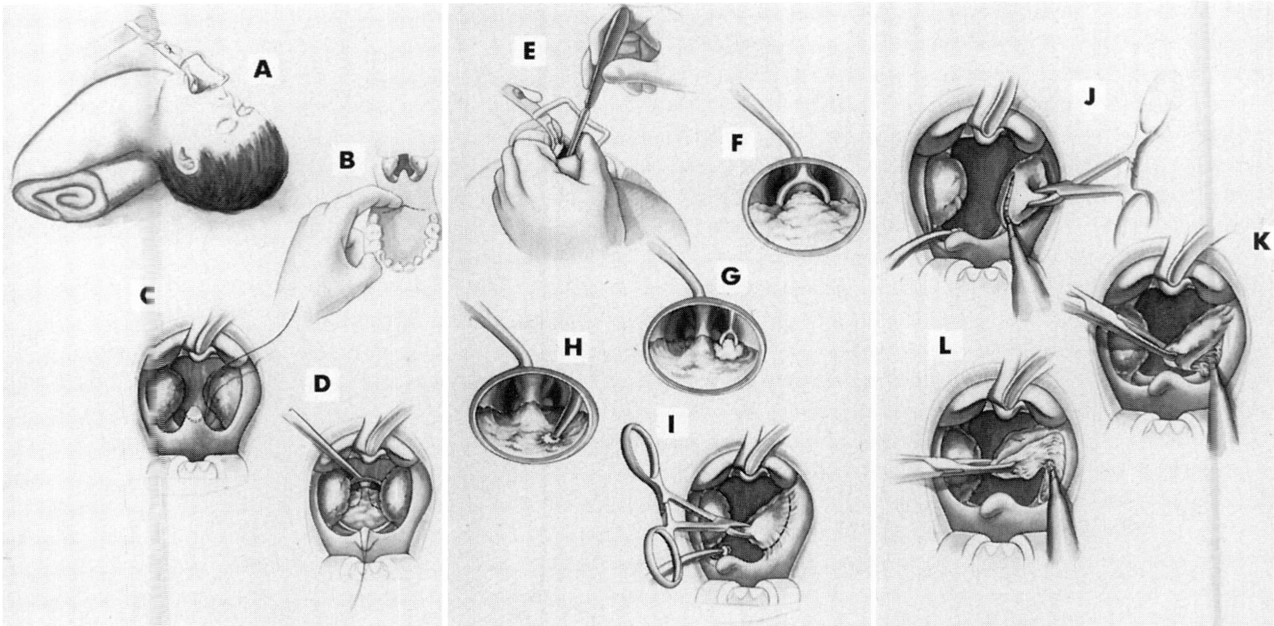

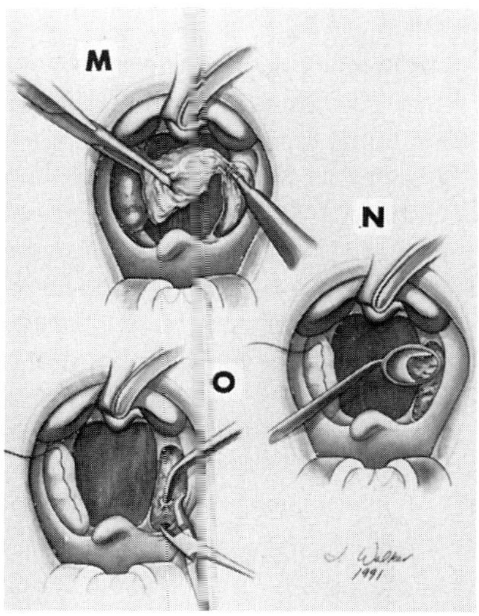

Fig. 12-13. Adenotonsillectomy technique. **A,** Patient placed in Rose's position. **B,** Palate inspected for presence of submucous cleft. **C,** Nylon suture placed through uvula for retraction. **D,** Nasopharynx inspected with mirror. **E** and **F,** Positioning of curette for adenoid removal. **G,** Removal of adenoid remnants with small curette. **H,** Removal of adenoid remnants and control of bleeding using suction cautery. **I** and **J,** Grasping of right tonsil and incision of mucosa using cautery. **K** to **M,** Dissection of tonsil with cautery. **N,** Inspection of superior pole with mirror. **O,** Control of bleeding using suction cautery.

more susceptible to airway complications after tonsillectomy. Although we do not use routine peritonsillar infiltration with local anesthetic agents, numerous reports have described short-term benefit with regard to postoperative pain in the immediate recovery period after tonsillectomy.[13,77,156] Peritonsillar infiltration with local anesthesia may also decrease intraoperative blood loss in patients undergoing sharp-dissection tonsillectomy.[13]

After induction of general anesthesia and placement of an endotracheal tube, the patient is placed in Rose's position (Fig. 12-13) and a Crowe-Davis mouth gag is placed for exposure of the oropharynx. A red rubber catheter is placed through the right nares and brought back out through the oral cavity and clamped with a Kelly clamp to retract the soft palate for better visualization of the nasopharynx. At this point the hard and soft palate is examined by visual inspection and palpation for evidence of a submucous cleft palate. Adenoidectomy should not be performed in the presence of an occult submucous cleft palate unless absolutely necessary. Conservative adenoidectomy should be considered in these situations.

Adenoidectomy is typically performed using adenoid curettes, which have either straight or curved handles. The LaForce adenotome also has been described as an instrument for adenoid extirpation.[80] The nasopharynx is inspected with a nasopharyngeal mirror to assess the size of the adenoid pad and guide placement of the curette. The curette is placed high in the nasopharynx so it abuts the posterior aspect of the nasal septum. The adenoid pad is then carefully curetted, with care taken not to penetrate deeply into the prevertebral region. Care must also be taken when using the curette not to extend too far laterally, thus potentially risking damage to the torus tubarius and eustachian tube orifice. Small curettes may be used to remove residual adenoid tissue in the posterior choanal region. This entails removal of the superior portion of the adenoid pad and preservation of the inferior aspect using cautery or curettes. Packs are placed into the nasopharynx to obtain hemostasis.

After tonsillectomy has been performed, the nasopharynx is reexamined and hemostasis is obtained using suction electrocautery. It is important to remember that the mouth-gag tongue blade places pressure on the base of tongue and should be released intermittently to allow blood circulation in the tongue and possibly aid in reducing postoperative pain. A throat pack may be used to prevent blood and secretions, which may be swallowed and lead to postoperative nausea and vomiting, from entering the esophagus. In addition, blood oozing around the endotracheal tube may form a laryngeal clot, which may lead to postextubation airway obstruction. Children undergoing adenotonsillectomy typically have an uncuffed endotracheal tube, which may allow leakage of air around the tube with positive pressure ventilation. Fires and endotracheal tube explosions have been reported during tonsillectomy, presumably related to oxygen leaking around uncuffed endotracheal tubes.[79]

At this point, the tonsillectomy is performed with electrocautery. The tonsil is grasped with an Allis clamp or tenaculum. It is then retracted medially, and the superior pole is incised with the electrocautery identifying the tonsillar capsule and carefully dissecting the avascular plain between the capsule and the tonsillar bed. When sharp dissection is used, the superior mucosal incision may be made with a knife, and blunt dissection may be used to separate the tonsil from the tonsillar bed using a Thompson dissector or a Fischer knife. Using the electrocautery, the tonsil is carefully dissected down to its inferior extent where it is amputated. With sharp dissection, a tonsil snare can be used to amputate the tonsil at the inferior pole. If bleeding is noted at this point, a pack may be placed in the tonsillar fossa and the opposite tonsil is then excised in the same manner. Care must be taken to preserve the mucosa and muscle in the posterior pillar, especially superiorly. Extensive cauterization and tissue loss of the posterior pillar may predispose the patient to postoperative nasopharyngeal stenosis. If electrocautery is being used, great care must be taken so that other metal instrumentation in the oropharynx (e.g., the mouth gag or Yankauer suction) is not touched, which could lead to burns of the oropharynx or lips. In addition, the electrocautery blade should be guarded with a nonconducting material. After removal of the tonsillar fossa packs, residual bleeding may be controlled using electrocautery on a low wattage setting. Significant bleeders may need to be clamped and ligated. Great care should be taken when using suture ligatures in the tonsillar fossa. The external maxillary and lingual arteries may inadvertently be ligated in the region of the inferior tonsillar pole, thus leading to sloughing and severe hemorrhage. In addition, the internal carotid artery, which is in close proximity to the tonsillar fossa, may be damaged inadvertently, resulting in complications such as pseudoaneurysm formation and excessive hemorrhage.[105] After hemostasis has been obtained in the oropharynx and nasopharynx, the oral and nasal cavities should be thoroughly irrigated. The hypopharynx is suctioned, evacuating all secretions and potential blood clots, and the stomach should also be suctioned at this point. The patient is then awakened and extubated.

Patients who have a significant history of obstructive sleep apnea, those younger than 3 years of age, or those with other medical problems or extenuating circumstances are admitted to the hospital after surgery for overnight observation. If they are taking oral fluids adequately, all other patients are discharged after an observation period of approximately 4 to 6 hours. Intravenous fluids are administered based on deficit replacement and maintenance until oral intake resumes satisfactorily; lactated Ringer's solution or ½ normal saline is used. Acetaminophen with or without codeine is given for analgesia. A 1-week course of oral antibiotics is also prescribed. The patient's diet advances from clear liquids on the day of surgery to a soft diet the following day and then solid foods subsequently as tolerated. Soft foods are generally well tolerated. However, patients with unrestricted diets have not been shown to have significant complication rates postoperatively.[18,64,164] Patients are instructed to return immediately to the emergency room if there is any evidence of bright red bleeding from the nose or oral cavity.

Inpatient versus outpatient procedures

It has been clearly demonstrated in the literature that adenotonsillectomy in appropriately selected children may be performed on an outpatient basis.* It is important that patients are observed postoperatively and that they obtain significant postoperative intravenous rehydration. Postoperative observation times discussed in the literature vary from 136 minutes to 6 to 8 hours.[69,106] Although short-stay outpatient tonsillectomy has been demonstrated as a safe and cost-effective procedure, it is important preoperatively to select outpatients who are at risk for postoperative complications and who may benefit from longer observation periods following surgery.

Numerous authors believe that children younger than 3 years of age should be admitted for observation after surgery because they are at increased risk for postoperative complications, most of which are airway-related.† The ultimate decision for postoperative admission lies with the surgeon. Other situations that may warrant admission after adenotonsillectomy include (1) patients with a history of an abnormal bleeding disorder or abnormal coagulation profile preopera-

* Refs. 48, 63, 106, 131, 146, 150, 167.

† Refs. 6, 56, 68, 137, 167, 181.

tively; (2) patients with evidence of obstructive sleep apnea; (3) patients with underlying craniofacial abnormalities such as Down syndrome; and (4) patients with systemic disorders such as cardiopulmonary disease or asthma. Postoperative admission also should be considered for patients undergoing tonsillectomy for peritonsillar abscess, for patients who live a long distance from the hospital (>60 miles or 1 hour driving time), or for patients whose home situation is not consistent with close postoperative observation.[70,88,178]

Complications

Serious postoperative complications secondary to surgery of the tonsils and adenoids are primarily related to pain, hemorrhage, airway obstruction, postoperative pulmonary edema, VPI, nasopharyngeal stenosis, and death. Meticulous attention to surgical technique and technical advances in modern anesthesiology have significantly reduced the number of complication related to adenotonsillectomy. Paradise and others[116] reported an overall complication rate of 14%; all of these complications were self-limiting. Richmond and others reported a series of 794 adenotonsillectomy patients, of whom 4.2% had variable degrees of postoperative bleeding and 1.3% had self-limiting postoperative airway obstruction. In 9409 pediatric patients undergoing adenotonsillectomy, Crysdale and Russel[34] reported an overall hemorrhage rate of 2.15%, with only 0.06% of the patients requiring a second general anesthetic for hemostasis. For reasons other than the hemorrhage, (including fever, airway distress, pneumonia, inadequate oral intake, vomiting, and pain), 0.6% of the patients required delayed hospitalization. The incidence of serious surgical complications has been reported to be approximately 15 cases per 1000.[58] Pulmonary abscess, although dreaded in the past, is now extremely rare. However, this complication may still be encountered, as well as other rare complications, including Horner's syndrome, optic neuritis, meningitis, brain abscess, paralysis of the glossopharyngeal and recurrent laryngeal nerves, salivary fistulae from the submandibular gland to the tonsillar fossa, and mediastinal emphysema.[125,126,166]

Chronic postoperative pain related to fibrosis and calcification of the stylohyoid ligament (Eagle's syndrome) may be encountered occasionally. Pain referred to the ipsilateral ear may be diagnosed by palpating the tonsillar fossa and obtaining radiographic studies that may demonstrate an elongated styloid process. Aspiration of foreign bodies (e.g., dislodged teeth, sponges, and lymphoid tissue) also may be encountered. If a tooth aspiration is suspected, a radiographic study should be obtained immediately; if a permanent tooth has been dislodged, a dental consultation should be obtained. A thorough investigation, including endoscopy, must be performed when a suspected foreign body has been aspirated.

Postoperative hemorrhage

Postoperative hemorrhage is the most common serious complication related to adenotonsillectomy. Reported postoperative hemorrhage rates range from 0.5% to 10%, although variable rates have been reported with different surgical techniques.[34,81,94,138,160] Meticulous attention to surgical technique and intraoperative hemostasis, regardless of which technique is used, will lead to acceptable postoperative hemorrhage rates. Patients with underlying coagulation disorders that have been determined either by history and physical examination or by preoperative screening in appropriately selected patients will help avert significant intraoperative blood loss. Appropriate preoperative and intraoperative measures are taken in conjunction with a hematology consult. Certain analgesics (e.g., ketorolac tromethamine) have been associated with increased hemorrhage rates when given in the perioperative period and should be avoided in patients undergoing adenotonsillectomy.[49,141]

The extensive blood supply of the tonsillar fossa is comprised of a complex network of anastomosing arteries, primarily arising from the ipsilateral external carotid artery system. However, contributions from the internal carotid and vertebral arteries exist, and contralateral vessels circulate through the circle of Willis.[149] Therefore, extensive intraoperative or postoperative hemorrhage may not always cease after ligation of the external carotid artery. In rare, severe cases, ligation of other branches (e.g., the maxillary, facial, lingual, or superior thyroid artery) may be necessary.[81]

The arterial blood supply of the nasopharynx and adenoids arises from both the internal and external carotid arterial system. However, bleeding in this region can be controlled most commonly with compression and electrocautery. In severe cases, application of caustic agents (e.g., tannic acid, bismuth subgallate) or hemostatic agents (e.g., avitene) may be beneficial. Aberrant arterial vessels in the oropharynx and nasopharynx may be damaged intraoperatively (Fig. 12-14). McKenzie and Wolfe[102] reported an aberrant carotid artery arising in Rosenmüller's fossa that was injured during adenoidectomy, necessitating subsequent ligation of the common carotid artery with resultant transient hemiplegia.[102]

Bleeding can occur intraoperatively, immediate postoperatively (within 24 hours), or delayed (after 24 hours). Intraoperative hemorrhage may be related to an underlying coagulopathy or possibly to major arterial damage in severe cases. Steps to control major intraoperative hemorrhage include using suction cautery or ligation or possibly placing a pack in the tonsillar fossa and oversuturing the tonsillar pillars to provide constant compression of the fossa. Suture ligatures may cause damage to underlying arterial vessels, thereby worsening the bleeding or possibly leading to delayed postoperative hemorrhage and also should be placed with extreme care if they are used.[50,105] In severe cases, ligation of larger arteries through an open-neck exploration may be necessary. However, this should be an extremely uncommon step. Persistent hemorrhage from the nasopharynx after adenoidectomy is often related to residual remnants of adenoid tissue that should be completely removed to best obtain hemostasis.

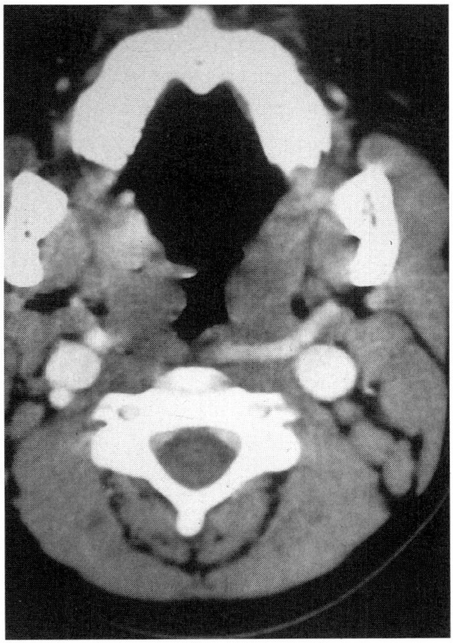

Fig. 12-14. Computed tomogram with contrast enhancement demonstrating an aberrant artery in the left retropharyngeal region.

Immediate postoperative bleeding after adenoidectomy may be controlled initially with topical decongestant nose drops. However, patients with severe bleeding should be taken back to the operating room for examination of the nasopharynx and definitive hemostasis in which the clots are suctioned, adenoid remnants are removed, and the nasopharyngeal pad is definitively cauterized.

Delayed postoperative bleeding, although typically not as dangerous as intraoperative or immediate bleeding, may be fatal if not managed appropriately. Patients should be well informed before discharge about the possibility of delayed postoperative hemorrhage and should be told to return for immediate evaluation if there is any evidence of bright red bleeding from the nose or mouth. The most common time for delayed postoperative bleeding is between the fifth and seventh postoperative days. When hemorrhage occurs, patients should be returned to the operating room for immediate hemostasis if active bleeding is confirmed on physical examination. If no active bleeding is apparent and a blood clot is evident in the tonsillar fossa, it should not be disturbed. However, if it cannot be determined whether active bleeding is taking place, the clot should be suctioned to allow better examination. Blood clots often hide bleeding vessels and may prevent appropriate coagulation as a result of fibrinolysis.[130] Patients with delayed hemorrhage who are not actively bleeding and have a blood clot present in the tonsillar fossa should be admitted for overnight observation; a coagulation profile and hematocrit should be obtained.

Airway obstruction and pulmonary edema

Postoperative airway obstruction may occur after adenotonsillectomy, especially in children under 3 years of age.[6,18] Edema of the tongue, nasopharynx, and palate may necessitate replacement of a nasal trumpet temporarily and also may require intravenous corticosteroid therapy. Dislodging of pharyngeal clots may obstruct the larynx postoperatively, resulting in death.[35] Therefore, all clots should be evacuated from the pharynx before termination of the procedure.

Postoperative pulmonary edema may arise in patients with long-term upper-airway obstruction related to adenotonsillar hypertrophy, often necessitating prolonged mechanical ventilation. Patients with a prolonged history of obstructive sleep apnea as documented by polysomnography and evidence of cor pulmonale should be observed closely after surgery with pulse oximetry in a monitored setting. Patients with persistent hypercapnia, may require planned postoperative mechanical ventilation until P_{CO_2} levels return to normal.

Velopharyngeal insufficiency

Velopharyngeal insufficiency, or hypernasality, is a relatively unusual complication primarily related to adenoidectomy. In patients with excessively large tonsils and preoperative VPI, the VPI may actually improve after the obstructive tonsils have been removed. Patients with a history of cleft palate or evidence of an occult submucous cleft palate on physical examination (see Fig. 12-10) should not undergo adenoidectomy unless it is absolutely necessary, and in these situations conservative or partial adenoidectomy should be performed. The actual incidence of VPI after adenoidectomy in otherwise healthy children has been estimated to be between 1 in 750 and 1 in 1459.[58,183] It is important to determine preoperatively whether there is a family history of VPI or if the patient had a prior history of hypernasal speech or nasal regurgitation as an infant. These signs may herald the development of postoperative VPI. If an underlying speech abnormality exists preoperatively, speech therapy evaluation should be performed. It also is important to determine whether reported hyponasal speech is truly related to a nasal obstruction or is actually related to hypernasal speech, which could be misinterpreted by the parents.

Patients who develop postoperative VPI should be evaluated and managed initially by a speech pathologist. Most cases are transient and will resolve with time. However, severe cases may require surgical intervention such as a pharyngeal flap, sphincteroplasty, or possibly posterior pharyngeal wall augmentation. Reconstructive surgery should be considered in patients with persistent VPI who have not responded to speech therapy for at least 1 year. Habit palsy is transient postoperative VPI that develops secondary to pain when the patient has altered pharyngeal muscle control during speech and swallowing. If not resolved shortly after surgery, speech therapy is usually successful.

Nasopharyngeal stenosis

Nasopharyngeal stenosis is an extremely difficult management problem that requires surgical intervention for satisfactory resolution. This situation may arise from excessive cauterization with extensive mucosal destruction involving the nasopharynx, lateral nasopharyngeal wall, and superior tonsillar pillar along with excessive resection of posterior tonsillar pillar tissue. Other predisposing factors include performing surgery during an acute episode of pharyngitis or purulent sinusitis, revision adenoid surgery with removal of lateral pharyngeal bands, and keloid formation.[85] Figi[44] described 37 cases of nasopharyngeal stenosis, 22 of which were secondary to adenotonsillectomy.[45] Guggenheim[62] reported 18 cases of nasopharyngeal stenosis secondary to adenoidectomy caused by stripping of the lymphoid tissue from the torus tubarius, Rosenmüller's fossa, and the lateral nasopharynx.[63]

Numerous techniques have been described for surgical repair using a combination of skin flaps, local mucosal flaps, stents, skin grafts, and scar incisions.[37] Cotton[32] described a technique using incision of the stenosis with rotation of a lateral and inferior-based pharyngeal flap to reline the naso-

A

B

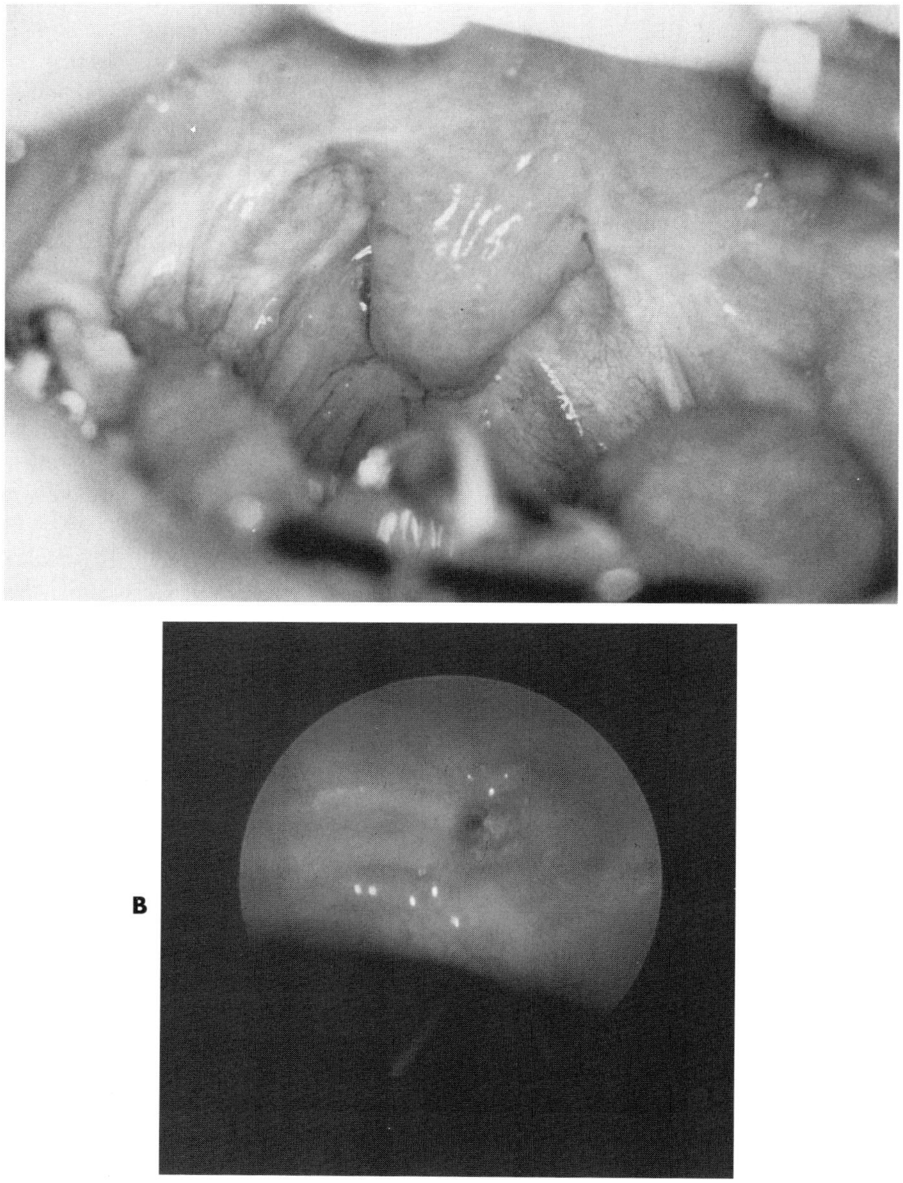

Fig. 12-15. A, Orpharyngeal view of postadenotonsillectomy nasopharyngeal stenosis. **B,** Endoscopic view of nasopharyngeal stenosis using a 120° rod-lens telescope.

pharynx. Occasionally, second-stage repair is necessary. On physical examination, patients with nasopharyngeal stenosis typically demonstrate the uvula scarred down to the posterior pharyngeal wall with possibly a small opening visible by mirror examination or flexible nasopharyngoscopy (Fig. 12-15). The majority of the scarring is based laterally in the region of the posterior tonsillar pillars. This results in partial or complete obstruction of the nasopharyngeal airway and can be extremely debilitating.

Cervical spine complications

A rare complication of adenoidectomy or tonsillectomy is atlantoaxial subluxation (Grisel's syndrome). Although up to 10% of patients may report neck pain after adenoidectomy, patients with Grisel's syndrome will have deep calcification of the anterior arch of the atlas and laxity of the anterior transverse ligament between the atlas and axis.[39,140] This leads to complaints of stiff neck with spasm of the sternocleidomastoid or deep cervical muscle. The patient will hold his or her head to one side with slight rotation toward the opposite side. Radiographic evaluation in suspected cases should include anteroposterior and lateral cervical spine radiography in addition to flexion-extension radiographs, which may detect mild subluxation. CT and possibly magnetic resonance imaging may demonstrate evidence of decalcification in severe cases; this may be associated with cervical spine osteomyelitis. Most cases of atlantoaxial subluxation are related to infection or trauma and only rarely are secondary to adenotonsillectomy.[5] Patients with Down syndrome are more prone to traumatic atlantoaxial subluxation following adenotonsillectomy and should undergo preoperative cervical spine radiographic screening. Great care should be taken in cervical spine manipulation during surgery in patients with Down syndrome.[118]

Management of atlantoaxial subluxation after adenoidectomy or adenotonsillectomy should be individualized based on the duration and the symptoms present. Intravenous antimicrobial therapy and possibly cervical traction may be necessary. In the presence of cervical osteomyelitis, long-term (4 to 8 weeks) intravenous antimicrobial therapy, coupled with cervical stabilization, will be necessary.[5] Retropharyngeal abscess has also been reported following adenoidectomy.[124]

REFERENCES

1. Amir and others: Group A beta-hemolytic streptococcal pharyngitis in children younger than 9 years, *Isr J Med Sci* 30:619, 1994.
2. Andrea M: Microsurgical bipolar cautery tonsillectomy, *Laryngoscope* 103:1177, 1993.
3. Anonymous: *1995 Clinical indicators compendium*, Alexandria, Va, 1995, American Academy of Otolaryngology-Head and Neck Surgery.
4. Reference deleted in pages.
5. Baker LL, Bower CM, Glasier CM: Atlanto-axial subluxation and cervical osteomyelitis: two unusual complications of adenoidectomy, *Ann Otol Rhinol Laryngol* 105:295, 1996.
6. Berkowitz RG, Zalzal GH: Tonsillectomy in children under 3 years of age, *Arch Otolaryngol Head Neck Surg* 116:685, 1990.
7. Bisno AL: Acute pharyngitis: etiology and diagnosis, *Pediatrics* 97: 949, 1996.
8. Bluestone CD: Current indications for tonsillectomy and adenoidectomy, *Ann Otol Rhinol Laryngol Suppl* 155:58, 1992.
9. Bluestone CD and others: Eustachian tube function as related to adenoidectomy for otitis media, *Trans Am Acad Ophthalmol Otolaryngol* 76:1325, 1972.
10. Bolger WE, Parsons DS, Potempa L: Preoperative hemostatic assessment of the adenotonsillectomy patient, *Otolaryngol Head Neck Surg* 103:396, 1990.
11. Brandtzaeg P and others: Immunoglobulin systems of human tonsils: I. Control subjects of various ages: quantification of Ig-producing cells, tonsillar morphonometry and serum Ig concentration, *Clin Exp Immunol* 31:367, 1978.
12. Britton PD: Effect of respiration on nasopharyngeal radiographs when assessing adenoidal enlargement, *J Laryngol Otol* 103:71, 1989.
13. Broadman LM and others: The effects of peritonsillar infiltration on the reduction of intraoperative blood loss and post-tonsillectomy pain in children, *Laryngoscope* 99:578, 1989.
14. Brodsky L: Modern assessment of tonsils and adenoids, *Pediatr Clin North Am* 36:1551, 1989.
15. Brodsky L, Koch RJ: Bacteriology and immunology of normal and diseased adenoids in children, *Arch Otolaryngol Head Neck Surg* 119: 821, 1993.
16. Brodsky L, Moore L, Stanievich JF: A comparison of tonsillar size and oropharyngeal dimensions in children with obstructive adenotonsillar hypertrophy, *Int J Pediatr Otorhinolaryngol* 13:149, 1987.
17. Brodsky L, Moore L, Stanievich J: The role of *Haemophilus influenzae* in the pathogenesis of tonsillar hypertrophy in children, *Laryngoscope* 98:1055, 1988.
18. Brodsky L, Radomski K, Gendler J: The effect of post-operative instructions on recovery after tonsillectomy and adenoidectomy, *Int J Pediatr Otorhinolaryngol* 25:133, 1993.
19. Brook I: The clinical microbiology of Waldeyer's ring, *Otolaryngol Clin North Am* 20:259, 1987.
20. Brook I, Walker RI: Pathogenicity of anaerobic gram-positive cocci, *Infect Immun* 45:320, 1984.
21. Brook I, Yocum P: Bacteriology of chronic tonsillitis in young adults, *Arch Otolaryngol Head Neck Surg* 110:803, 1984.
22. Brook I, Yocum P: In vitro protection of group A beta hemolytic streptococci from penicillin and cephalothin by *Bacteroides fragilis*, *Chemotherapy* 29:18, 1983.
23. Brouillette RT, Fernbach SK, Hunt CE: Obstructive sleep apnea in infants and children, *J Pediatr* 100:31, 1982.
24. Brown OE, Manning SC, Ridenour B: Cor pulmonale secondary to tonsillar and adenoidal hypertrophy: management considerations, *Int J Pediatr Otorhinolaryngol* (review), 6:131, 1988.
25. Carroll JL and others: Inability of clinical history to distinguish primary snoring from obstructive sleep apnea syndrome in children, *Chest* 108:610, 1995.
26. Catlin FI: Pulmonary complications of tonsillectomy as originally described by Samuel J. Crowe, M.D., *Laryngoscope* 91:52, 1981.
27. Catlin FI, Grimes WJ: The effect of steroid therapy on recovery from tonsillectomy in children, *Arch Otolaryngol Head Neck Surg* 117: 649, 1991.
28. Christensen PH, Schonsted-Madsen U: Unilateral immediate tonsillectomy as the treatment of peritonsillar abscesses: results with special attention to pharyngitis, *J Laryngol Otol* 97:1105, 1983.
29. Close HL and others: Hemostatic assessment of patients before tonsillectomy: a prospective study, *Otolaryngol Head Neck Surg* 111:733, 1994.

30. Cohen LM, Koltai PJ, Scott JR: Lateral cervical radiographs and adenoid size: do they correlate? *Ear Nose Throat J* 71:638, 1992.
31. Committee on Infectious Diseases of the American Academy of Pediatrics: *1994 red book: report of the Committee on Infectious Diseases,* 1994, The American Academy of Pediatrics (abstract).
32. Cotton RT: Nasopharyngeal stenosis, *Arch Otolaryngol Head Neck Surg* 3:145, 1985.
33. Crowe SJ, Watkins SS, Rothholz AS: Relation of tonsillar and nasopharyngeal infections to general systemic disorders, *Bull Johns Hopkins Hosp* 28:1, 1917.
34. Crysdale WS, Russel D: Complications of tonsillectomy and adenoidectomy in 9409 children observed overnight, *Can Med Assoc J* 135: 1139, 1986.
35. Cummings GO: Morbidities and mortalities following 20,000 tonsillectomies and adenoidectomies, *Laryngoscope* 64:647, 1954.
36. Curtin JM: The history of tonsil and adenoid surgery, *Otol Clin North Am* 20:415, 1987.
37. D'Amelio R and others: Serum IgA in salivary levels in normal subjects: comparison between tonsillectomized and non-tonsillectomized subjects, *Int Arch Allergy Appl Immunol* 68:256, 1982.
38. Demain JG, Goetz DW: Pediatric adenoidal hypertrophy and nasal airway obstruction: reduction with aqueous nasal beclomethasone, *Pediatrics* 95:355, 1995.
39. Derkay CS, Kenna MA, Pang D: Refractory torticollis: an uncommon complication of adenotonsillectomy, *Int J Pediatr Otorhinolaryngol* 14:87, 1987.
40. Dobie RA, Tobey DN: Clinical features of diphtheria in the respiratory tract, *JAMA* 242:2197, 1979.
41. Donovan R, Soothill JF: Immunological studies in children undergoing tonsillectomy, *Clin Exp Immunol* 14:347, 1973.
42. Dunn GF and others: Relationships between variation of mandibular morphology and variation of nasopharyngeal airway size in monozygote twins, *Angle Orthod* 43:129, 1973.
43. Facklam RR: Specificity study of kits for detection of group A streptococci directly from throat swabs, *J Clin Microbiol* 25:504, 1987.
44. Figi FA: Cicatricial stenosis of the nasopharynx: correction by means of skin graft, *Plast Reconstr Surg* 2:97, 1947.
45. Finkelstein Y and others: The otolaryngologist and the patient with velocardiofacial syndrome, *Arch Otolaryngol Head Neck Surg* 119: 563, 1993.
46. Frank Y, Kravath RE, Pollak CP: Obstructive sleep apnea and its therapy: clinical and polysomnographic manifestations, *Pediatrics* 71: 737, 1983.
47. Fujioka M, Young LW, Girdany BR: Radiographic evaluation of adenoid size in children: adenoid-nasopharyngeal ratio, *Am J Radiol* 133: 401, 1979.
48. Gabalski EC and others: Ambulatory tonsillectomy and adenoidectomy, *Laryngoscope* 106:77, 1996.
49. Gallagher JE, Blauth J, Fornadley JA: Perioperative ketorolac tromethamine and postoperative hemorrhage in cases of tonsillectomy and adenoidectomy, *Laryngoscope* 105:606, 1995.
50. Gardner JF: Sutures and disasters in tonsillectomy, *Arch Otolaryngol Head Neck Surg* 88:551, 1968.
51. Gates GA and others: Chronic secretory otitis media: effects of surgical management, *Ann Otol Rhinol Laryngol Suppl* 138:2, 1989.
52. Gates GA, Avery CA, Prihoda TJ: Effect of adenoidectomy upon children with chronic otitis media with effusion, *Laryngoscope* 98: 58, 1988.
53. Gates GA and others: Effectiveness of adenoidectomy and tympanostomy tubes in the treatment of chronic otitis media with effusion, *N Engl J Med* 317:1444, 1987.
54. Gerber MA: Comparison of throat cultures and rapid strep tests for diagnosis of streptococcal pharyngitis, *Pediatr Infect Dis J* 8:820, 1989.
55. Gerber MA, Markowitz M: Management of streptococcal pharyngitis reconsidered, *Pediatr Infect Dis J* 4:518, 1985.
56. Gerber ME and others: Selected risk factors in pediatric tonsillectomy, *Arch Otolaryngol Head Neck Surg* 122:811, 1996.
57. Ghorganian SN, Paradise JL, Doty RL: Odor perception in children in relation to nasal obstruction, *Pediatrics* 72:510, 1983.
58. Gibb AG: Unusual complications of tonsil and adenoid removal, *J Laryngol Otol* 83:1159, 1969.
59. Gislason T, Benediktsdottir B: Snoring, apneic episodes, and nocturnal hypoxemia among children 6 months to 6 years old: an epidemiologic study of lower limit of prevalence, *Chest* 107:963, 1995.
60. Goeringer GC, Vidic B: The embryogenesis and anatomy of Waldeyer's ring, *Otolaryngol Clin North Am* 20:207, 1987.
61. Gryczynska D, Powajbo K, Zakrzewska A: The influence of tonsillectomy on obstructive sleep apnea children with malocclusion, *Int J Pediatr Otorhinolaryngol* 32(suppl):S225, 1995.
62. Guggenheim P: Cicatricial stenosis of the nasopharyngeal isthmus: result of lateral adenoidectomy, *Arch Otolaryngol Head Neck Surg* 77:13, 1963.
63. Guida RA, Mattucci KF: Tonsillectomy and adenoidectomy: an inpatient or outpatient procedure? *Laryngoscope* 100:491, 1990.
64. Hall MD, Brodsky L: The effect of post-operative diet on recovery in the first twelve hours after tonsillectomy and adenoidectomy, *Int J Pediatr Otorhinolaryngol* 31:215, 1995.
65. Hanson LA: Comparative immunological studies of the immune globulins of human milk and of blood serum, *Int Arch Allergy Appl Immunol* 18:241, 1961.
66. Hartsook JT: Mouthbreathing as a primary etiologic factor in the production of malocclusion, *J Dent Child* 13:91, 1946.
67. Harvold EP: *Neuromuscular and morphological adaptations in experimentally induced oral respiration.* In McNamara JMJ, editor: *Nasorespiratory function and craniofacial growth, monograph 9. Craniofacial growth series,* Ann Arbor, Mich, 1979, Center for Human Growth and Development.
68. Helmus C: Tonsillectomy and adenoidectomy in the one and two-year old child, *Laryngoscope* 89:1764, 1979.
69. Helmus C, Grin M, Westfall R: Same-day-stay adenotonsillectomy, *Laryngoscope* 100:593, 1990.
70. Herzon FS: Peritonsillar abscess: incidence, current management practices and a proposal for treatment guidelines, *Laryngoscope* 74(suppl):1, 1995.
71. Hinton AE and others: Parental cigarette smoking and tonsillectomy in children, *Clin Otolaryngol* 18:178, 1993.
72. Hollinshead WH: *The pharynx and larynx.* In Hollinshead WH, editor: *Anatomy for surgeons: the head and neck.* Philadelphia, 1982, JB Lippincott.
73. Honikman LH, Massel BF: Guidelines for the selective use of throat cultures in the diagnosis of streptococcal respiratory infections, *Pediatrics* 48:573, 1971.
74. Howie AJ: Scanning and transmission electron microscopy on the epithelium of human palatine tonsils, *J Pathol* 130:191, 1980.
75. Ingvarsson L, Lundgren K, Irving J: The bacterial flora in the nasopharynx in healthy children, *Acta Otolaryngol Suppl (Stockh)* 386: 94, 1982.
76. Jeans WD and others: A longitudinal study of the growth of the nasopharynx and its contents in normal children, *Br J Radiol* 54:117, 1981.
77. Jebeles JA and others: Tonsillectomy and adenoidectomy pain reduction by local bupivacaine infiltration in children, *Int J Pediatr Otorhinolaryngol* 25:149, 1993.
78. Kang J and others: Coagulation profile as a predictor for post-tonsillectomy and adenoidectomy (T + A) hemorrhage (see comments), *Int J Pediatr Otorhinolaryngol* 28:157, 1994.
79. Keller C, Elliott W, Hubbell RN: Endotracheal tube safety during

electrodissection tonsillectomy (see comments), *Arch Otolaryngology Head Neck Surg* 118:643, 1992.

80. Kornblut AD: A traditional approach to surgery of the tonsils and adenoids, *Otol Clin North Am* 20:349, 1987.

81. Kornmesser HJ: Blutunger und blutsillung im bereich des gesichtsschaedels, des halses und des mittelohres, *Arch Otorhinolaryngol Head Neck Surg* 219:209, 1978.

82. Krober MS, Bass JW, Michels GN: Streptococcal pharyngitis: placebo-controlled double-blind evaluation of clinical response to penicillin therapy, *JAMA* 253:1271, 1985.

83. Leach J and others: Polysomnographic and clinical findings in children with obstructive sleep apnea, *Arch Otolaryngol Head Neck Surg* 118:741, 1992.

84. Leach JL, Manning S, Schaefer SD: Comparison of two methods of tonsillectomy, *Laryngoscope* 103:619, 1993.

85. Lehman WB, Pope TH, Hudson WR: Nasopharyngeal stenosis, *Laryngoscope* 78:371, 1968.

86. Linden BE and others: Morbidity in pediatric tonsillectomy, *Laryngoscope* 100:120, 1990.

87. Linder-Aronson S, Woodside DG, Lundstrom A: Mandibular growth direction following adenoidectomy, *Am J Orthod Dentofacial Orthop* 89:273, 1986.

88. Lockhart R, Parker GS, Tami TA: Role of Quinsy tonsillectomy in the management of peritonsillar abscess, *Ann Otol Rhinol Laryngol* 100:569, 1991.

89. Luke MJ and others: Chronic nasopharyngeal obstruction as a cause of cardiomegaly, cor pulmonale, and pulmonary edema, *Pediatrics* 37:762, 1966.

89a. Mackenzie M: *The pharynx.* In Anonymous: *Diseases of the pharynx,* New York, 1880, William Wood and Co.

90. MacGregor FB, Albert DM, Bhattacharyya AK: Post-operative morbidity following paediatric tonsillectomy: a comparison of bipolar diathermy dissection and blunt dissection, *Int J Pediatr Otorhinolaryngol* 31:1, 1995.

91. MacKenzie-Stepner K and others: Velopharyngeal insufficiency due to hypertrophic tonsils: a report of 2 cases, *Int J Pediatr Otorhinolaryngol* 14:57, 1987.

92. Maeda S, Mogi G, Oh M: Microcrypt extensions of tonsillar crypts, *Ann Otol Rhinol Laryngol* 91:1, 1982.

93. Mandel EM and others: Effect of adenoidectomy on eustachian tube function: preliminary results of a randomized clinical trial, *Adv Otorhinolaryngol* 47:227, 1992.

94. Maniglia AJ, Kushner H, Cozzi L: Adenotonsillectomy: a safe outpatient procedure [see comments], *Arch Otolaryngol Head Neck Surg* 115:92, 1989.

95. Manning SC and others: An assessment of preoperative coagulation screening for tonsillectomy and adenoidectomy, *Int J Pediatr Otorhinolaryngol* 13:237, 1987.

96. Mantanoski GM, Price WH, Ferencz C: Epidemiology of streptococcal infections in rheumatic and nonrheumatic families. IV. The effect of tonsillectomy on streptococcal infections, *Am J Epidemiol* 87:226, 1968.

97. Martinez SA, Akin DP: Laser tonsillectomy and adenoidectomy, *Otolaryngol Clin North Am* 20:371, 1987.

98. Mawson SR, Adlington P, Evans M: A controlled study evaluation of adenotonsillectomy in children, *J Laryngol Otol* 81:777, 1967.

99. McGuire NG: A method of guillotine tonsillectomy with an historical review, *J Laryngol Otol* 81:187, 1967.

100. McKee WJE: A controlled study of the effects of tonsillectomy and adenoidectomy in children, *Br J Prev Soc Med* 17:49, 1963.

101. McKenzie AM: Adenoids, deformities of the palate and artificial infant feeding: an analysis of 222 cases, *Br Dent J* 30:159, 1909.

102. McKenzie W, Wolfe CI: Carotid abnormalities and adenoid surgery, *J Laryngol Otol* 73:596, 1959.

103. Menashe VD, Farrehi C, Miller MS: Hypoventillation and cor pulmonale due to chronic upper airway obstruction, *J Pediatr* 67:198, 1965.

104. Mullens PD, Nagaraj HS, McMurray GT: Upper airway obstruction resulting in cor pulmonale, *J Ky Med Assoc* 76:223, 1978.

105. Myer CM III: Tonsillectomy, *Patient of the Month Program* 18:11, 1988.

105a. Anonymous: National Center for Health Statistics. 1984 summary: National hospital discharge survey. Advance data from vital and health statistics. 112, 1985 (abstract).

106. Nicklaus PJ, Herzon FS, Steinle IV EW: Short-stay outpatient tonsillectomy, *Arch Otolaryngol Head Neck Surg* 121:521, 1995.

107. Nishimura T and others: Laser tonsillectomy, *Acta Otolaryngol Suppl (Stockh)* 454:313, 1988.

108. Noonan JA: Reversible cor pulmonale due to hypertrophied tonsils and adenoids: studies in two cases, *Circulation* 32:164, 1965.

109. Ogra PL: Effect of tonsillectomy and adenoidectomy on nasopharyngeal antibody responses to poliovirus, *N Engl J Med* 284:59, 1971.

110. Ohlms LA, Wilder RT, Weston B: Use of intraoperative corticosteroids in pediatric tonsillectomy, *Arch Otolaryngol Head Neck Surg* 121:737, 1995.

111. Oulis CJ and others: The effect of hypertrophic adenoids and tonsils on the development of posterior crossbite and oral habits, *J Clin Pediatr Dent* 18:197, 1994.

112. Owen GO, Canter RJ, Robinson A: Overnight pulse oximetry in snoring and non-snoring children, *Clin Otolaryngol* 20:402, 1995.

113. Owen RL, Nemanic S: Antigen processing structures of the mammalian intestinal tract: a SEM study of lymphoepithelial organs, *Scanning Microsc* 2:269, 1978.

114. Palumbo FM: Pediatric considerations of infections and inflammations of Waldeyer's ring, *Otolaryngol Clin North Am* 20:311, 1987.

115. Pang YT: Paediatric tonsillectomy: bipolar electrodissection and dissection/snare compared, *J Laryngol Otol* 109:733, 1995.

116. Paradise JL and others: Efficacy of tonsillectomy for recurrent throat infection in severely affected children: results of parallel randomized and nonrandomized clinical trials, *N Engl J Med* 310:674, 1984.

117. Paradise JL and others: Efficacy of adenoidectomy for recurrent otitis media in children previously treated with tympanostomy-tube placement: results of parallel randomized and nonrandomized trials. *JAMA* 263:2066, 1990.

118. Parfenchuk TA and others: Posterior occipitoatlantal hypermobility in Down syndrome: an analysis of 199 patients, *J Pediatr Orthop* 14: 304, 1994.

119. Parker AJ, Maw AR, Powell JE: Rhinomanometry in the selection for adenoidectomy and its relation to preoperative radiology, *Int J Pediatr Otorhinolaryngol* 17:155, 1989.

120. Perkin RM, Anas NG: Pulmonary hypertension in pediatric patients, *J Pediatr* 105:511, 1984.

121. Petersdorf RG and others, editors: *Harrison's principles of internal medicine*, New York, 1983, McGraw-Hill.

122. Physick PS: Description of a forceps, employed to facilitate the extirpation of the tonsil, *Am J Med Sci* 2:116, 1828.

123. Potsic WP: Comparison of polysomnography and sonography for assessing regularity of respiration during sleep in adenotonsillar hypertrophy, *Laryngoscope* 97:1430, 1987.

124. Prado VM and others: Retropharyngeal abscess after adenoidectomy, *Ear Nose Throat J* 74:54, 1995.

125. Pratt LW: Tonsillectomy and adenoidectomy: mortality and morbidity, *Trans Am Acad Ophthalmol Otolaryngol* 74:1146, 1970.

126. Pratt LW, Hornberger HR, Moore VJ: Mediastinal emphysema complicating tonsillectomy and adenoidectomy, *Ann Otol Rhinol Laryngol* 71:158, 1962.

127. Pruet CW, Duplan DA: Tonsil concretions and tonsilloliths, *Otolaryngol Clin North Am* 20:305, 1987.

128. Ramirez-Ronda CH, Fuxench-Lopea Z, Nevarez M: Increased pha-

ryngeal bacterial colonization during viral illness, *Arch Intern Med* 141:1599, 1981.
129. Randolf MF and others: Effect of antibiotic therapy on the clinical course of streptococcal pharyngitis, *J Pediatr* 106:870, 1985.
130. Rasmussen N: Complications of tonsillectomy and adenoidectomy, *Otolaryngol Clin North Am* 20:383, 1987.
131. Reiner SA and others: Safety of outpatient tonsillectomy and adenoidectomy, *Otolaryngol Head Neck Surg* 102:161, 1990.
132. Richardson MA and others: Evaluation of tonsils and adenoids in sleep apnea syndrome, *Laryngoscope* 90:1106, 1980.
133. Richtsmeier WJ: Human interferon production in tonsil and adenoid tissue cultures, *Am J Otolaryngol* 4:325, 1983.
134. Richtsmeier WJ, Shikhari AM: *The physiology and immunology of the pharyngeal lymphoid tissue.* In *Otolaryngology Clinics North Am* Philadelphia, 1987, WB Saunders.
135. Rosenfeld RM: Pilot study of outcomes in pediatric rhinosinusitis, *Arch Otolaryngol Head Neck Surg* 121:729, 1995.
136. Rosenfeld RM, Green RP: Tonsillectomy and adenoidectomy: changing trends, *Ann Otol Rhinol Laryngol* 99:187, 1990.
137. Rothschild MA, Catalano P, Biller HF: Ambulatory pediatric tonsillectomy and the identification of high-risk subgroups (see comments), *Otolaryngol Head Neck Surg* 110:203, 1994.
138. Roy A, De la Rosa C, Vecchio YA: Bleeding following tonsillectomy, *Arch Otolaryngol Head Neck Surg* 102:9, 1976.
139. Roydhouse N: Adenoidectomy for otitis media with mucoid effusion, *Ann Otol Rhinol Laryngol* 89:312, 1980.
140. Rundle FW: Post tonsillectomy morbidity: a clinical trial of a local penicillin-steroid-anesthetic mixture, *Ann Otol Rhinol Laryngol* 76:1060, 1967.
141. Rusy LM and others: A double-blind evaluation of ketorolac tromethamine versus acetaminophen in pediatric tonsillectomy: analgesia and bleeding, *Anesth Analg* 80:226, 1995.
142. Salam MA, Cable HR: Post-tonsillectomy pain with diathermy and ligation techniques: a prospective randomized study in children and adults, *Clin Otolaryngol* 17:517, 1992.
143. Schiffmann R, Faber J, Eidelman AI: Obstructive hypertrophic adenoids and tonsils as a cause of infantile failure to thrive: reversed by tonsillectomy and adenoidectomy, *Int J Pediatr Otorhinolaryngol* 9:183, 1985.
144. Schulman ST: Streptocococcal pharyngitis: diagnostic considerations, *Pediatr Infect Dis J* 13:567, 1994.
145. Schwartz RH, Weintzen RW, Pedreira F: Penicillin V therapy for group A streptococcal pharyngitis, *JAMA* 246:1790, 1981.
146. Segal C, Berger G, Basker MB: Adenotonsillectomies on a surgical day clinic basis, *Laryngoscope* 93:1205, 1983.
147. Selinger DS, Reed WP, McLaren LC: Model for studying bacterial adherence to epithelial cells infected with viruses, *Infect Immun* 32:941, 1981
148. Shapiro NL, Cunningham MJ: Streptococcal pharyngitis in children, *Curr Opin Otolaryngol Head Neck Surg* 3:369, 1995.
149. Sholehvar J, Hunsicker RC, Stool SE: Arteriography in posttonsillectomy hemorrhage, *Arch Otolaryngol Head Neck Surg* 95:581, 1972.
150. Shott SR, Myer CM III, Cotton RT: Efficacy of tonsillectomy and adenoidectomy as an outpatient procedure: a preliminary report, *Int J Pediatr Otorhinolaryngol* 13:157, 1987.
151. Siegel G: The influence of tonsillectomy on cell mediated immune response, *Arch Otolaryngol Head Neck Surg* 239:205, 1984.
152. Siegel G: Theoretical and clinical aspects of the tonsillar function, *Int J Pediatr Otorhinolaryngol* 6:61, 1983.
153. Snook T: The development of the human pharyngeal tonsil, *Am J Anat* 55:323, 1934.
154. Socransky SS, Maniganiello SD: The oral microbiota of man from birth to senility, *J Periodontol* 42:485, 1971.
155. Strunk CL, Nichols ML: A comparison of the KTP/532-laser tonsillectomy vs. traditional dissection/snare tonsillectomy, *Otolaryngol Head Neck Surg* 103:966, 1990.
156. Stuart JC and others: Peritonsillar infiltration with bupivacaine for paediatric tonsillectomy, *Anaesth Intensive Care* 22:679, 1994.
157. Sugita R and others: Microorganisms isolated from peritonsillar abscess and indicated chemotherapy, *Arch Otolaryngol Head Neck Surg* 108:655, 1982.
158. Surjan L: Reduced lymphocyte activation in repeatedly inflammed human tonsils, *Acta Otolaryngol (Stockh)* 89:187, 1980.
159. Surjan L, Brantzaeg P, Berdal P: Immunoglobulin system of human tonsils: II. Patients with chronic tonsillitis or tonsillar hyperplasia: quantification of Ig-producing cells, tonsillar morphometry and serum Ig concentrations, *Clin Exp Immunol* 31:382, 1978.
160. Szeremeta W, Novelly NJ, Benninger M: Postoperative bleeding in tonsillectomy patients, *Ear Nose Throat J* 75:373, 1996.
161. Teele DW: *Inflammatory diseases of the mouth and pharynx.* In Bluestone CD, Stool SE, editors: *Pediatric otolaryngology*, Philadelphia, 1983, WB Saunders.
162. Telian SA: Sore throat and antibiotics, *Otolaryngol Clin North Am* 19:103, 1986.
163. Telian SA and others: The effect of antibiotic therapy on recovery after tonsillectomy in children: a controlled study, *Arch Otolaryngol Head Neck Surg* 112:610, 1986.
164. Thomas PC, Moore P, Reilly JS: Child preferences for post-tonsillectomy diet, *Int J Pediatr Otorhinolaryngol* 31:29, 1995.
165. Thornval A: Wilhelm Meyer and the adenoids, *Arch Otolaryngol Head Neck Surg* 90:383, 1969.
166. Tolczynski B: Tonsillectomy, its hazards and their prevention, *Eye Ear Nose Throat Mo* 48:378, 1969.
167. Tom LW and others: Is outpatient tonsillectomy appropriate for young children? *Laryngoscope* 102:277, 1992.
168. Tomes C: On the developmental origin of the V-shaped contracted maxilla, *Monthly Rev Dent Surg* 1:2, 1872.
169. Trask G and others: The effects of perennial allergic rhinitis on dental and skeletal development: A comparison of siblings. *Am J Orthod* 92:286, 1987.
170. Unlu Y and others: Guillotine and dissection tonsillectomy in children, *J Laryngol Otol* 106:817, 1992.
171. Volk MS and others: The effects of preoperative steroids in tonsillectomy patients, *Otolaryngol Head Neck Surg* 109:726, 1993.
172. Wake M, Glossop P: Guillotine and dissection tonsillectomy compared, *J Laryngol Otol* 403:588, 1989.
173. Wang DY and others: Fiberoptic examination of the nasal cavity and nasopharynx in children, *Acta Otorhinolaryngol Belg* 45:323, 1991.
174. Watson WG: Open bite: a multifactorial event, *Am J Orthod* 80:443, 1981.
175. Weider DJ, Hauri PJ: Nocturnal enuresis in children with upper airway obstruction, *Int J Pediatr Otorhinolaryngol* 9:173, 1985.
176. Weider DJ, Sateia MJ, West RP: Nocturnal enuresis in children with upper airway obstruction, *Otolaryngol Head Neck Surg* 105:427, 1991.
177. Weimert TA, Babyak JW, Richter HJ: Electrodissection tonsillectomy, *Arch Otolaryngol Head Neck Surg* 116:186, 1990.
178. Weinberg E and others: Needle aspiration of peritonsillar abscess in children [review], *Arch Otolaryngol Head Neck Surg* 119:169, 1993.
179. Weir N: *Otolaryngology: an illustrated history*, London, 1990, Butterworth & Co.
180. Whitaker RHR: The relationship of nasal obstruction to contracted arches and dental irregularities, *Dent Rec* 31:425, 1911.
181. Wiatrak BJ, Myer CM III, Andrews TM: Complications of adenoton-

sillectomy in children under 3 years of age, *Am J Otolaryngol* 12: 170, 1991.

182. Wiesner PJ: Gonococcal pharyngeal tonsillar infections, *Clin Obstet Gynecol* 18:121, 1981.
183. Witzel MA and others: Velopharyngeal insufficiency after adenoidectomy: an 8-year review, *Int J Pediatr Otorhinolaryngol* 11:15, 1986.
184. Wormald PJ, Prescott CAJ: Adenoids: comparison of radiological assessment methods with clinical and endoscopic findings, *J Laryngol Otol* 106:342, 1992.
185. Yellon RF, Bluestone CD: *Head and neck space infections in children.* In Bluestone CD, Stool SE, Kenna MA, editors: *Pediatric otolaryngology*, Philadelphia, 1996, WB Saunders.
186. Yuan HC, Tang SJ, Cheng RQ: Clinical observation on guillotine tonsillectomy without anesthesia, *Acta Otolaryngol (Stockh)* 454:273, 1988.
187. Zalzal GH, Cotton RT: *Pharyngitis and adenotonsillar disease.* In Cummings C and others, editors: Otolaryngology—Head and Neck Surgery, St Louis, 1986, Mosby.
188. Zucconi M, and others: Habitual snoring and obstructive sleep apnea syndrome in children: effects of early tonsil surgery, *Int J Pediatr Otorhinolaryngol* 26:235, 1993.

Chapter 13

Obstructive Sleep Apnea

Laura M. Sterni
David E. Tunkel

The stupid-lazy child who frequently suffers from headaches at school, breathes through his mouth instead of his nose, snores and is restless at night, and wakes up with a dry mouth in the morning, is well worthy of the solicitous attention of the school medical officer.

—W. Hill, 1889[34]

Over 100 years ago clinicians began to recognize the manifestations of sleep-related breathing obstruction in children. In 1976, Guilleminault and others[29] published the first description of the obstructive sleep apnea syndrome (OSAS) in children. Numerous subsequent reports have resulted in the recognition of OSAS as a common cause of significant morbidity in children. Sleep-related upper-airway obstruction in children can lead to a variety of nighttime and daytime symptoms. Serious complications of OSAS such as cor pulmonale and hypertension were common in the early reports of affected children.[10,29,30] Today, increased awareness and understanding of childhood OSAS have led to earlier diagnosis and therapy with improved outcomes.

CLASSIFICATION OF SLEEP-RELATED UPPER-AIRWAY OBSTRUCTION

Snoring is the common feature of three clinical syndromes of sleep-related upper-airway obstruction in children. The diagnoses of primary snoring (PS), upper-airway resistance syndrome (UARS), and OSAS separate patients according to the severity of their sleep-related upper-airway obstruction and resulting clinical complications.

Primary snoring

Approximately 10% of children snore during sleep on most or all nights,[1,3,18] and most are considered to have PS. PS has been defined as snoring during sleep without associated apnea, hypoventilation, or hypoxemia. Children with PS have no associated sleep disturbance and no daytime symptoms referable to nighttime breathing difficulties.[16] PS can be extremely loud and disturbing, even frightening, to others in the home. The factors that predispose children to PS are similar to those described for OSAS and are discussed below. Adenotonsillar hypertrophy is a frequent cause of snoring in children.[81] Snoring in 6- to 13-year-old children has been strongly associated with parental cigarette smoking.[18]

The natural history of PS in healthy children is unknown. Ali, Pitson, and Stradling[4] found that 50% of children who were described by their parents as habitual snorers at 4 years of age had stopped snoring without treatment at 2-year follow-up. While the authors of this chapter currently do not recommend therapy for children with PS, the natural history of this entity is unknown and long-term consequences may exist.

Upper-airway resistance syndrome

Children with UARS have snoring and partial upper-airway obstruction during sleep that are sufficient to cause sleep disruption and/or daytime symptoms in the absence of gas-exchange abnormalities. Guilleminault and others[31] first described this syndrome in adult patients in 1993. In their study, individuals with UARS presented with snoring and excessive daytime sleepiness but did not meet the diagnostic criteria for OSAS as measured by overnight polysomnography. These patients did have numerous arousals in response to increased upper-airway resistance that led to sleep fragmentation. Continuous positive airway pressure (CPAP) eliminated the snoring, sleep fragmentation, and daytime sleepiness in these patients.[31]

Downey, Perkin, and MacQuarrie[21] retrospectively analyzed the overnight polysomnographic recordings of children who were referred for suspected OSAS, were clinically symptomatic (symptoms were not specified), and had presumably negative sleep studies. Their analysis revealed that these patients did have more arousals and awakenings than children with snoring and no other reported symptoms.[21] Several other studies have demonstrated normal sleep efficiency and architecture in children with OSAS,[17,22] so the presence of UARS in children is still debated. We consider offering therapy to children who snore but have normal polysomnographic recordings when there are significant daytime symptoms that may be caused by nocturnal upper-airway obstruction.

Obstructive sleep apnea syndrome

Approximately 3% of children will have OSAS.[25] As many as 40% of snoring children referred to a sleep clinic or otolaryngologist may have OSAS.[17,26] OSAS describes sleep-related upper-airway obstruction that may result in significant physiologic abnormalities or associated daytime symptoms. Childhood OSAS has been defined as episodes of upper-airway obstruction during sleep that are usually associated with a reduction in oxyhemoglobin saturation or hypercarbia. In its most severe form, OSAS can lead to cor pulmonale, developmental delay, failure to thrive, or even death.[15] Sleep-related upper-airway obstruction in children may manifest as obstructive apnea or obstructive hypoventilation.[70] Obstructive hypoventilation results from continuous partial airway obstruction, which leads to paradoxical respiratory efforts, hypercarbia, and often hypoxemia. Diagnosis of obstructive hypoventilation in children requires end-tidal CO_2 monitoring during polysomnography. Despite the absence of complete airway obstruction during sleep, children with obstructive hypoventilation are at risk for all of the reported complications of nighttime breathing obstruction.

Obstructive hypoventilation is generally not seen in adults with OSAS. There are other differences in OSAS in children versus adults; some of the important characteristics of OSAS in the two populations are compared in Table 13-1.

SYMPTOMS AND SIGNS OF CHILDHOOD OBSTRUCTIVE SLEEP APNEA SYNDROME

Children with OSAS almost always present with a history of snoring and difficulty breathing during sleep.[10,30,68] Parents often report nighttime sweating, restlessness, and unusual sleeping positions in their affected children. Patients will manifest increased respiratory effort during sleep. Chest retraction, use of accessory muscles, and paradoxical rib cage motion during inspiration occur during episodes of upper-airway obstruction. Paradoxical breathing (inward movement of the thorax during inspiration) can be normal during sleep in infants and toddlers. During rapid eye movement (REM) sleep, the tonic and phasic activity of the intercostal muscles disappears and the infant chest wall becomes more compliant. The negative intrathoracic pressures generated during inspiration result in the paradoxical inward movement of the thorax. Paradoxical breathing decreases with age and is rare in healthy children over 3 years of age.[24] Paradoxical respirations in older children are almost always the result of upper-airway obstruction.

Enuresis has been associated with OSAS in children but is not a consistent finding.[11,22,29,30] Enuresis associated with OSAS may be related to disrupted, restless sleep patterns that affect arousal. Several studies have reported resolution of nocturnal enuresis following adenotonsillectomy in children with symptoms of nocturnal upper-airway obstruction or polysomnography that is diagnostic for OSAS.[29,87,88]

Daytime symptoms of OSAS include those of adenotonsillar hypertrophy. Mouth-breathing, hyponasal speech, and

Table 13-1. Childhood versus adult obstructive sleep apnea syndrome

	Adults	Children
Presentation		
Excessive daytime sleepiness	Main presenting complaint	Infrequent complaint
Associated obesity	Majority of patients	Minority of patients
Underweight/failure to thrive	Not seen	Frequent finding
Daytime mouth-breathing	Not seen	Frequent finding
Gender	Males:female = 2:1	Male:female = 1:1
Enlarged tonsils and adenoids	Not seen	Frequent finding
Sleep pattern		
Obstructive	Obstructive apnea	Obstructive apnea or obstructive hypoventilation
Arousal with obstruction	Common	Not often seen
Disrupted	Common	Not often seen
Management		
Surgical	Minority of patients	Definitive therapy in most patients
Medical (positive airway pressure)	Most common management	Only in selected patients

Adapted from Carroll JL, Loughlin GM: Diagnostic criteria for obstructive sleep apnea syndrome in children, *Pediatr Pulmonol* 14:71, 1992.

an increased frequency of upper respiratory infections have been reported.[11,17] Morning headaches have been associated with nighttime breathing obstruction,[30] but controlled studies comparing children with OSAS with children with normal polysomnography results have found no significant difference in the frequency of this complaint.[11,43] Adults with OSAS often present with excessive daytime sleepiness, but this is rarely seen in children with OSAS.[11,17] Children are less likely than adults to terminate an obstructive episode with arousal.[55] Furthermore, in contrast to adult OSAS patients, children with OSAS generally have normal sleep architecture and efficiency.[17,22] The preservation of sleep quality in children with OSAS may explain the lack of excessive daytime sleepiness.

Daytime behavioral disturbances have been reported in children with sleep-related upper-airway obstruction. In 1982, Brouillette, Fernbach, and Hunt[10] reported that 5 of 22 children with OSAS presented with "behavioral disturbances" and developmental delay, both of which improved following therapy for upper-airway obstruction. Two other children in this study had hypoxic brain damage from severe OSAS.[10] Hyperactivity, aggressiveness, social withdrawal, and learning problems have also been described in children with OSAS.[11,22,30] Obese children with OSAS have more deficits in memory, vocabulary, and learning as assessed by standardized neurocognitive tests than do obese children without OSAS.[67]

Failure to thrive[10,30,43] was reported as a common sequela of OSAS in children. Although overt failure to thrive now occurs less frequently as a result of early diagnosis and management of OSAS, children with OSAS often grow poorly. Improved growth has been reported in childhood OSAS after treatment with adenotonsillectomy.[46,78,90] Marcus and others[46] reported decreased growth in children with even mild OSAS, and this appeared to be related to the increased work of breathing during sleep. Following adenotonsillectomy the patients had improved growth and decreased energy expenditure during sleep.[46] OSAS should be considered in the differential diagnosis of failure to thrive or impaired growth that is unexplained by other conditions.

Severe untreated OSAS can lead to pulmonary hypertension and cor pulmonale.[10,30] Pulmonary hypertension results from the recurrent, severe, nocturnal hypoxemia, hypercarbia, and acidosis. Systemic hypertension, a frequent complication of adult OSAS, has also been reported in children with OSAS.[29,30,68,74] Chest radiography, electrocardiography, and echocardiography should be considered for any child with symptoms or signs of congestive heart failure or hypertension. Children with multiple, lengthy, or extreme episodes of hypoxemia on polysomnography may require cardiopulmonary evaluation as well. Children with cardiovascular complications of OSAS should have repeat polysomnography after therapy to confirm resolution of OSAS.

PATHOPHYSIOLOGY

The upper airway is a collapsible muscular tube that includes the nasopharynx, oropharynx, and hypopharynx. Patency of the upper airway is determined by the tonic activity of the pharyngeal dilating muscles as well as phasic contraction of these muscles in response to negative upper-airway pressure (inspiration). Skeletal and soft-tissue structures such as the tonsils and adenoids affect upper-airway diameter and resistance and are important in determining airway patency. During sleep, reduced upper-airway inspiratory muscle tone and diminished reflex dilation lead to airway narrowing. These effects are most pronounced in REM sleep, leading to increased obstructive events in predisposed patients.

In otherwise healthy children, adenotonsillar hypertrophy is a significant risk factor for OSAS.[43] However, there is no strict correlation between size of the lymphoid tissues and the presence of severity of sleep-related breathing obstruction.[2,19] One child with significantly enlarged tonsils and adenoids may be asymptomatic, whereas another with only moderate adenotonsillar hypertrophy will have severe OSAS. Furthermore, only a small percentage of children with adenotonsillar hypertrophy develop OSAS.

Marcus and others[51] demonstrated that the pediatric upper airway behaves as a Starling resistor. In the Starling resistor model, maximum inspiratory flow through the collapsible upper airway is determined by upstream (nasal) pressure and the pressure surrounding the collapsible segment. When airway collapse occurs, flow is independent of the downstream (tracheal) pressure. Airway collapse occurs when the pressure surrounding the airway becomes greater than the pressure within the collapsible segment. The pressure outside the airway is dictated by structural factors as well as activity of the airway dilator muscles. Marcus and others[51] demonstrated that children with OSAS had greater airway collapsibility than those with PS. Although airway collapsibility was reduced following adenotonsillectomy in children with OSAS, it remained greater than in the patients with PS. It appears that children with OSAS have subtle abnormalities in upper-airway structure or neuromuscular control in addition to adenotonsillar hypertrophy.

HIGH-RISK GROUPS

Adenotonsillar hypertrophy is the leading cause of childhood OSAS. There are, however, a number of other medical conditions that are strongly associated with OSAS. Children in these high-risk groups should be followed closely for the development of signs and symptoms that may suggest sleep-related airway obstruction.

Obesity

Obese children are at risk for sleep-related breathing obstruction.[48,76] Deposition of adipose tissue within the muscles and soft tissues surrounding the upper airway[36] and external compression from the neck and jowls lead to upper-airway narrowing in these patients. Upward displacement of the diaphragm by the obese abdomen when the individual is supine and decreased chest wall compliance lead to lower lung volumes during sleep, decreased oxygen stores, and increased risk of desaturation with obstructive events.

Craniofacial abnormalities

Children with craniofacial anomalies usually have a multifactorial etiology for OSAS. Evaluation is directed toward examination of craniofacial issues such as skull base shape, maxillary size and shape, tongue size and support, and mandibular size and shape. Concomitant central nervous system abnormalities affecting pharyngeal tone as well as coexisting laryngotracheal anomalies should be evaluated. OSAS in such children may persist after adenotonsillectomy, and additional surgical and nonsurgical therapy may be necessary. Infants with craniofacial anomalies can be difficult to treat and may require tracheotomy.

Children with skeletal dysplasias such as achondroplasia may have mixed apnea syndromes. Compression of the brainstem at the craniocervical junction may cause abnormalities of ventilatory drive and central apnea. Cervicomedullary compression can also affect upper-airway control, leading to airway obstruction during sleep. Adenotonsillar enlargement and the craniofacial features seen in these patients may also cause OSAS.[66] Adenotonsillectomy may be helpful, but additional therapy with CPAP or tracheotomy may be needed in such complicated patients. Craniocervical decompression has been used in some patients with achondroplasia but the effects in OSAS remain controversial.[60]

Neuromuscular disease

Cerebral palsy in children is associated with decreased pharyngeal tone, resulting in OSAS. These children are at high risk for respiratory complications after adenotonsillectomy.[27,54,71] When pharyngeal hypotonia is marked, tracheotomy is necessary to relieve OSAS. Children with primary muscular diseases such as Duchenne muscular dystrophy can also develop OSAS secondary to loss of upper-airway muscle tone.[40]

Patients with Down syndrome have a high incidence of OSAS. A study of OSAS in these patients found that adenotonsillectomy alone was not adequate therapy for over 60% of the patients studied.[50] It was concluded that the generalized hypotonia and anatomic abnormalities such as obesity, macroglossia, and midfacial and mandibular hypoplasia all contribute to nocturnal airway obstruction in these patients.

Mucopolysaccharidoses

Mucopolysaccharidoses such as Hunter's and Hurler syndromes are associated with severe progressive OSAS in affected children. The head and neck manifestations in these syndromes include short neck, depressed nasal dorsum, macroglossia, adenotonsillar enlargement, and craniofacial abnormalities.[75] Bredenkamp and others[7] reported upper-airway obstruction in 17 of 45 patients (38%) with mucopolysaccharidoses, 7 (16%) of whom required tracheotomy. Laryngeal tissues can be infiltrated and tracheal size decreased from mucopolysaccharide deposition, leading to airway obstruction at multiple levels.[62] Adenotonsillectomy and tracheotomy may be part of the surgical treatment of OSAS in such complicated cases.[72]

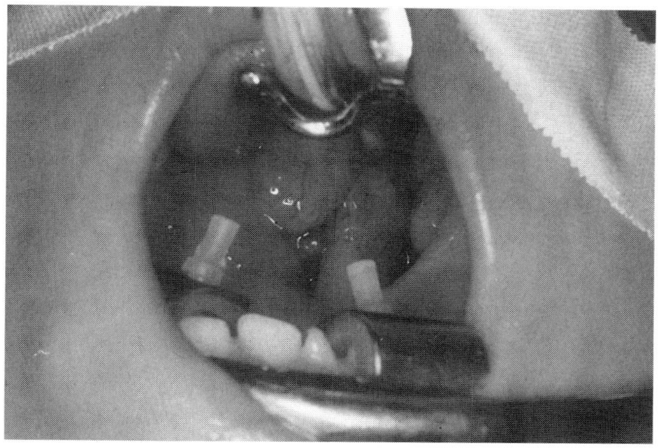

Fig. 13-1. Unilateral enlargement of a tonsil in a child who developed obstructive sleep apnea syndrome over a 2-week period. Pathology revealed Burkitt's lymphoma.

Acute-onset/rapidly progressive obstructive sleep apnea syndrome

Abrupt onset or rapid progression of OSAS in children suggests rapid enlargement of lymphoid tissue in the pharynx or other lesions rapidly growing near the airway. Viral syndromes can be associated with marked lymphoid hyperplasia and severe OSAS in children, with the most classic example being infectious mononucleosis secondary to Epstein-Barr virus infection. Acute OSAS associated with Epstein-Barr virus infection is treated with a nasopharyngeal airway and steroids.[77]

Malignant disease of the head and neck may cause sleep-related upper-airway obstruction, as discussed later in this chapter. A full head and neck examination should be directed at intrinsic and extrinsic masses causing airway compromise. Biopsy should be performed to direct additional therapy (Fig. 13-1).

DIAGNOSIS

History

Several studies have demonstrated that OSAS cannot be distinguished from PS in children based on clinical history and physical examination alone.[17,26,43,80] In one report, 89% of parents of children with OSAS observed their child struggling to breath during sleep, as did 58% of parents of children with PS. The majority of parents of children with both disorders were frightened by their child's nighttime breathing, often staying up nights to watch the child breathe.[17] Goldstein and others[26] evaluated 30 snoring children referred to a pediatric otolaryngology clinic using a focused history and physical examination in addition to a review of audiotaped breathing of the children during sleep. In only half of the 18 children believed to have definite OSAS clinically was polysomnography diagnostic for OSAS.[26] Although the clinical history may not be diagnostic, a thorough evaluation of daytime and nighttime symptoms is helpful in planning and interpreting subsequent studies.

Physical examination

The diagnosis of childhood OSAS is suggested by the patient's history and confirmed by polysomnography. The physical examination should note height and weight because growth may be impaired by OSAS. Cardiopulmonary abnormalities associated with OSAS should be identified. A full otolaryngologic examination of the head and neck should establish the likely site or sites of dynamic or static airway obstruction.

Tonsil and adenoid size should be assessed in children with symptoms of nocturnal airway obstruction. Signs of adenoidal hypertrophy include decreased nasal airflow with an adequate nasal airway on rhinoscopy, a hyponasal speech pattern, and an open-mouth breathing posture. Nasal examination should be focused to exclude obstructive septal deformity, intranasal masses, and mucosal or turbinate swelling within the nose. The oral examination should center around tonsil size and symmetry, pharyngeal dimensions, palate shape and size, and tongue size and motion.

Routine oral and nasal examination can be supplemented with fiberoptic nasal endoscopy to assess nasal patency, adenoid size, and effect of tonsil size and anatomy on awake respiration.[85] Croft and others[19] used fiberoptic endoscopy to evaluate the site of obstruction in children with polysomnogram-proven OSAS. The authors identified distinct adenoidal, adenotonsillar, tongue base, and laryngeal sites of obstruction based on fiberoptic endoscopy and planned successful surgical therapy based on these findings.[19]

The physical examination of children with craniofacial anomalies is directed at craniofacial structure, jaw size and position, and tongue size and position. Assessment of pharyngeal and laryngeal tone is necessary in children with neuromotor diseases such as cerebral palsy or muscular dystrophy. When sleep-disordered breathing is accompanied by awake airway symptoms such as stridor or hoarseness, laryngotracheal examination with flexible or rigid endoscopy should be performed.

Polysomnography

Overnight polysomnography in a sleep laboratory is the gold standard for diagnosing childhood OSAS. Pediatric sleep laboratories should involve clinicians with expertise in pediatric respiratory disorders and/or sleep medicine to ensure that the studies are performed and interpreted appropriately for this age group. The presence of the child's caregiver during the study provides comfort and reassurance to the patient. Caregivers can also provide an assessment of the child's sleep patterns in the laboratory; it is important to know whether the study captured a typical night's sleep and if the nighttime breathing abnormalities witnessed at home were seen during the study.

Overnight polysomnography is recommended. Although a nap study that is positive for obstructive sleep apnea correlates well with the presence of obstructive apnea on an overnight study, negative nap studies do not exclude OSAS during full polysomnographic studies.[49] Nap studies are limited by the short recording time and the possible absence of REM sleep periods. The use of sedatives and sleep deprivation are not recommended because both may increase upper-airway obstruction artifactually.[14,33]

In children, end-tidal CO_2 should be monitored to detect obstructive hypoventilation. The consensus statement adopted by the American Thoracic Society, *Standards and Indications for Cardiopulmonary Sleep Studies in Children*, also recommends measurement of (1) respiratory effort, as assessed by movement of the chest wall and abdomen; (2) airflow at the nose and/or mouth; (3) measurement of arterial oxygen saturation (Sao_2) by pulse oximetry (Spo_2); (4) electrocardiographic recording to monitor cardiac rate and rhythm; (5) electromyography in the anterior tibial region to monitor arousals; and (6) appropriate electroencephalography, electro-oculography, and electromyography measurements for sleep staging (Table 13-2).[5]

Sleep-related upper-airway obstruction is diagnosed in children who have more than one obstructive apneic episode per hour or evidence of significant obstructive hypoventilation. In adults, obstructive apneas are considered abnormal only if they last more than 10 seconds. Significant obstructive apneas in children are often shorter than 10 seconds. Due to the higher oxygen consumption in children and the

Table 13-2. Polysomnography for obstructive sleep apnea syndrome in children

Sleep state
Electroencephalogram
Electro-oculogram (right and left)
Electromyogram (submental)
Respiratory variables
Abdominal and chest wall movement (strain gauges, inductive plethysmography)
Oronasal airflow (thermistor)
End-tidal CO_2
Arterial oxygen saturation with pulse oximetry
Nonrespiratory variables
Electrocardiogram
Electromyogram (tibial) to document movements and arousals
Recommended but not required
Audiovideo recording

fall in functional residual capacity during sleep, an infant or toddler may have falls in Sao_2 after only a few seconds of upper-airway obstruction. Obstructive apneas lasting two or more consecutive breaths are generally considered abnormal in children. Obstructive hypoventilation is diagnosed when peak end-tidal CO_2 ($Petco_2$) is greater than 53 mm Hg or when $Petco_2$ is greater than 50 mm Hg for 8% or more of total sleep time in the presence of paradoxical respirations or snoring and in the absence of lung disease.[52] Hypoxemia is defined as an Spo_2 of less than 92% and is correlated with the child's baseline readings and respiratory events. Sleep architecture is examined because an adequate study should contain at least one REM period. Sleep efficiency and frequency of arousal from sleep in association with a respiratory events are also analyzed.

No standard guidelines exist for classifying the severity of OSAS. In our laboratory we classify children as having either mild, moderate, or severe OSAS based on clinical picture, number of obstructive events per hour, $Petco_2$ or duration of elevated end-tidal CO_2 measurements, and frequency and severity of oxygen desaturation. Representative polysomnographic tracings from pediatric patients are shown in Figure 13-2.

Other studies

Airway radiography, cephalometric studies, and computed tomography have limited use in the diagnosis of OSAS because they provide no functional information. These studies may assist in the management plan for children with OSAS who have unusual anatomic abnormalities. Preliminary studies suggest that evaluation of nighttime breathing difficulties may be accomplished in the home using video and cardiorespiratory recordings with extended oximetry [38,59] Additional validation of unattended home studies is needed before they can be recommended.

INDICATIONS FOR POLYSOMNOGRAPHY

The diagnosis of OSAS in children is problematic because children with the syndrome may have symptoms and signs that are indistinguishable from those of children with PS. Polysomnography remains the gold standard for diagnosing sleep apnea in children because clinical assessment alone is sensitive but not specific for OSAS.

Children who undergo adenotonsillectomy for recurrent pharyngeal infection may have obstructive symptoms as well. These children do not require polysomnography on a routine basis. Polysomnography is recommended for patients with non–sleep-related indications for adenotonsillectomy if there is concern that the patient may also have severe OSAS and thus require intensive postoperative monitoring. The use of preoperative polysomnography is most controversial in healthy children with obstructive adenotonsillar hypertrophy and no other surgical indication. Historically, adenotonsillectomy has been used to manage obstructive symptoms in healthy children without preoperative polysomnography. We should recognize that this practice may allow children without OSAS to undergo adenotonsillectomy.

Trained observers have occasionally diagnosed OSAS by direct observation of a sleeping child or by review of a videotape. Such observations may allow the polysomnogram to be deferred when the examination, history, and direct observations are consistent.

Ideally, polysomnography would be inexpensive, accessible, and have no effects on routine sleep patterns. However, the sleep study may be costly and may not be available to all patients. Sleep in the pediatric laboratory may not be representative of the patient's usual sleep pattern, and obtaining a sleep study may significantly delay treatment of OSAS in some cases.

Additional study of the natural history of OSAS and other nocturnal breathing disorders of childhood is necessary in order to use polysomnography most appropriately. We suggest the use of polysomnography when possible both to diagnose OSAS and to assess perioperative risk. We urge that polysomnography be performed in high-risk patients, including those with craniofacial anomalies, neuromotor disease, or associated medical conditions that may complicate surgical management of OSAS. Baseline preoperative polysomnography is useful to assess postoperative improvement in such high-risk patients. Polysomnography is also useful in the evaluation of children for whom information from the history or physical examination may be inconsistent.

Repeat polysomnography is recommended for children who exhibit persistent snoring or other symptoms of sleep-related upper-airway obstruction 4 to 6 weeks after surgery. A follow-up sleep study should also be considered for patients with significant complications from OSAS (e.g., cor pulmonale, failure to thrive), patients with severe OSAS on initial sleep study, or very young (younger than 1 year) patients to ensure resolution of nighttime breathing abnormalities.[5] Figure 13-3 presents an algorithm for the diagnosis and management of OSAS in both healthy and high-risk children.

SURGICAL MANAGEMENT

Tonsillectomy and/or adenoidectomy

Tonsillectomy, adenoidectomy, or adenotonsillectomy is the most common surgical treatment of childhood OSAS. Adenoid and tonsillar hyperplasia appears to be a key element in the compromise of airway patency during sleep in otherwise healthy children with OSAS.[28,44] Brodsky, Moore, and Stanievich[8] demonstrated that children undergoing adenotonsillectomy for obstruction had decreased lateral oropharyngeal dimensions compared with children undergoing adenotonsillectomy for chronic infection. They suggest that decreased oropharyngeal size, in addition to adenotonsillar hyperplasia, may contribute to OSAS in children. Removal of enlarged lymphoid tissues in Waldeyer's ring is curative for most of these children.[9,63,78]

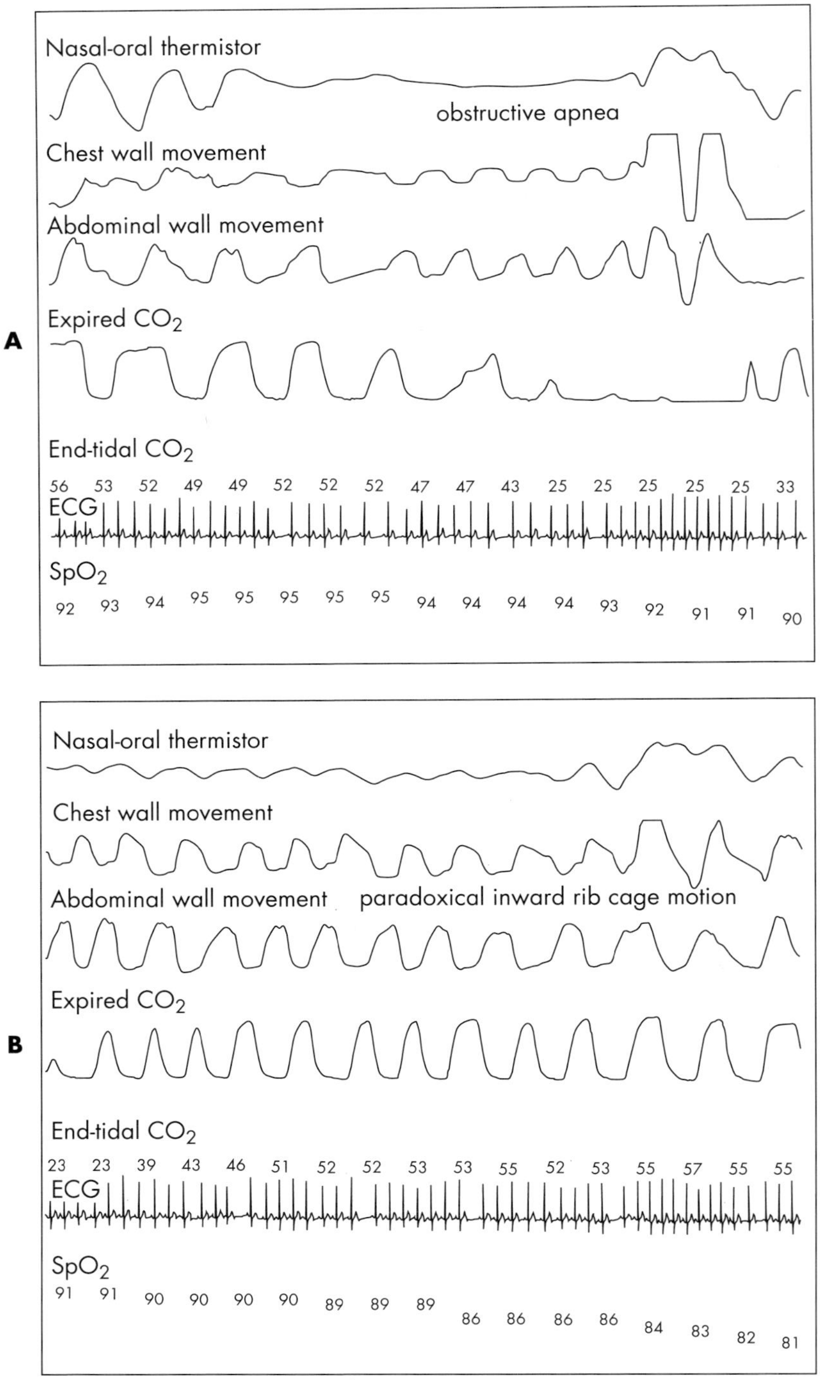

Fig. 13-2. Typical polysomnographic recordings. **A,** Obstructive apnea. **B,** Obstructive hypoventilation. Note the paradoxical inward rib cage motion seen in both tracings. In **A,** nasal–oral thermistor and expired CO_2 tracings flatten during the obstructive apnea while respiratory efforts continue. Note the fall in arterial oxygen saturation measured by pulse oximetry (Spo_2) that occurs shortly after the approximately 10-second event. In **B,** continuous partial airway obstruction results in elevated end-tidal CO_2 readings and a fall in Spo_2.

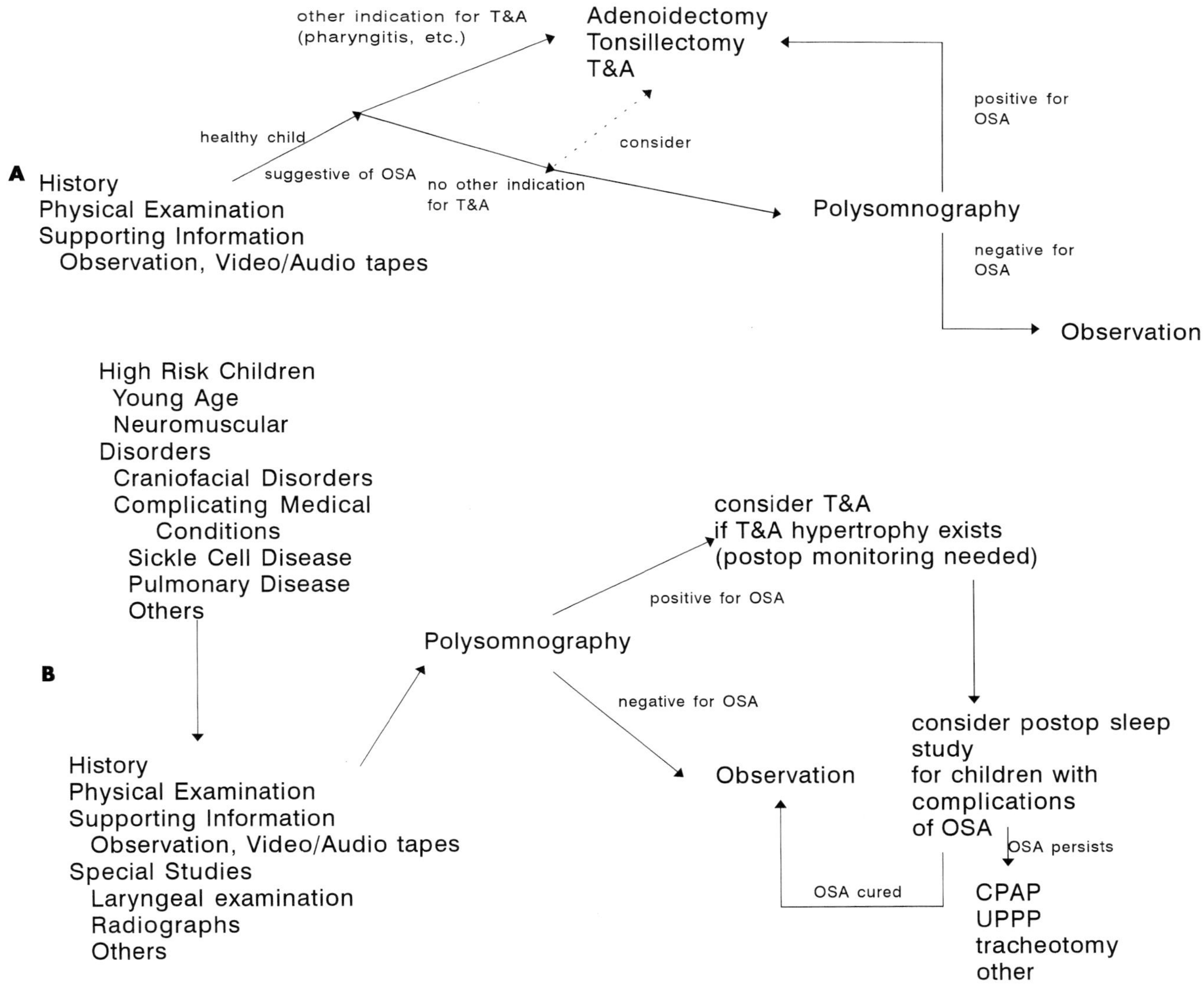

Fig. 13-3. Evaluation and management of obstructive sleep apnea syndrome in **A**, healthy children and **B**, high-risk children.

Perioperative management of children undergoing adenotonsillectomy for OSAS should be individualized, recognizing that these children have more frequent postoperative complications and the potential for serious respiratory compromise.[54,71] Children younger than 3 years of age, children with severe OSAS documented by polysomnography, and children with craniofacial anomalies or neuromotor impairment are at greatest risk for perioperative respiratory compromise.[27,54,73,89] Suen, Arnold, and Brooks[80] reported that children with severe OSAS on polysomnography were more likely to have persistent OSAS after adenotonsillectomy, and those with a preoperative respiratory event index less than 19.1 were likely to be cured after adenotonsillectomy.[80]

Preoperative risk assessment centers around the severity of sleep disturbance as documented by polysomnography. Chest radiography and electrocardiography can document the cardiopulmonary sequelae of OSAS (e.g., right ventricular hypertrophy).[12] Patients with severe OSAS may be treated with CPAP prior to adenotonsillectomy if surgery is to be delayed of if significant cardiovascular complications are present. Children with OSAS should undergo routine assessment of hemostatic factors[37] and anesthetic risk for adenotonsillectomy.[57]

Adenotonsillectomy is performed using standard techniques, with attention to minimizing edema in children at risk for postoperative obstruction. The majority of children who undergo adenotonsillectomy for mild OSAS have immediate improvement as shown by sleep studies performed on the first postoperative night.[32] However, children with severe OSAS or complicating anatomic or neuromotor disorders often have prolonged recovery or incomplete relief of OSAS.[27,54,71] Inpatient postoperative management, along with cardiorespiratory monitoring and pulse oximetry, is necessary for high-risk children who have moderate to severe OSAS.[54,65,79] Recovery should occur in an area where signs of respiratory depression and airway swelling can be recognized and prompt intervention can occur.

Narcotics should be used judiciously, and postoperative oxygen supplementation should be carefully monitored for signs of depression of ventilatory drive. Steroids are often administered perioperatively, and nasopharyngeal airways are used in high-risk patients to support the airway after surgery. Brown, Manning, and Ridenour[12] suggested endotracheal intubation and mechanical ventilation for several days after adenotonsillectomy in children with severe OSAS resulting in cor pulmonale.[12] CPAP or bilevel positive airway pressure (BiPAP) can be used for postoperative airway support in children with obstructive symptoms after adenotonsillectomy.[53,85]

Other Pharyngeal Surgery

Resection of palatal and pharyngeal tissue in children as management of OSAS is almost always performed in combination with or subsequent to adenotonsillectomy. Uvulopalatopharyngoplasty (UPPP) is not widely used for the management of children with OSAS[1]; it is used primarily for children at high risk for persistent obstruction due to neuromuscular dysfunction after adenotonsillectomy. Seid and others[73] reported on the use of UPPP in combination with adenotonsillectomy in 10 children with obstructive apnea and mental retardation with neuromotor disease of diverse etiologies. Only two patients required additional surgery to relieve OSAS, and one 15-month-old patient with cerebral palsy required subsequent tracheotomy. Tracheotomy was avoided in nine patients, but postoperative sleep studies were not performed. Kosko and Derkay[41] noted similar favorable results with UPPP combined with adenotonsillectomy in neurologically impaired children with OSAS, with 12 of 15 children showing improvement on pulse oximetry or formal polysomnography Donaldson and Redmond[20] and Strome[79] have successfully used UPPP as part of the surgical management of OSAS in children with Down syndrome.

Potential postoperative velar dysfunction and voice alteration should be considered in the decision-making process for such high-risk children with OSAS. Fiberoptic endoscopy of velopharyngeal anatomy may be useful before considering UPPP, especially in children with poor pharyngeal tone secondary to neuromotor disease.

Tongue reduction surgery has been proposed for the management of macroglossia in conjunction with OSAS, such as is seen in Beckwith-Wiedemann and Down syndromes.[58] Anterior tongue reduction probably improves cosmesis more than airway function, because central and posterior tongue size may be more critical to airway patency. Rimell and others[69] noted that children with Beckwith-Wiedemann syndrome often required tracheotomy when airway obstruction occurred during the neonatal period. They also found that adenotonsillectomy was probably more beneficial than tongue reduction for managing OSAS in these children with macroglossia. Central tongue reduction has been reported to improve OSAS in children with Down syndrome and other craniofacial disorders.[13,56]

Obstructive sleep apnea has been described in children who have undergone pharyngeal flap surgery for correction of velopharyngeal incompetence.[42,61] Sleep-associated airway obstruction is usually most pronounced in the immediate postoperative period, and obstructive symptoms improve as the flap atrophies over several months. A subset of these children may develop chronic OSAS that may require flap revision or takedown. Predisposing anatomic factors may include tonsillar or adenoidal hypertrophy, micrognathia, or abnormalities of pharyngeal tone.

Craniofacial surgery

A variety of surgical procedures have been proposed to manage OSAS in children with complex craniofacial disorders or neuromotor disease. Burstein and others[13] successfully used mandibular advancement, tongue reduction, tongue–hyoid suspension, and other nasal and pharyngeal procedures to manage children with OSAS with abnormal craniofacial anatomy with or without neuromuscular disease. Tracheotomy was avoided in 89% of this heterogeneous group of children with complex OSAS, including children with hemifacial microsomia, Down syndrome, and cerebral palsy.

Children with micrognathia often have severe OSAS that may benefit from techniques such as mandibular advancement and tongue suspension. Tracheotomy is often required in neonates and infants with these conditions to secure the airway until craniofacial growth and neuromotor maturation relieve the sleep-disordered breathing. Tomaski, Zulzal, and Saal[82] have noted that children with isolated Pierre-Robin sequence can usually be managed conservatively with nasopharyngeal tubes and positioning, whereas syndromic children with associated anomalies often require tracheotomy for relief of airway obstruction (Fig. 13-4).

Midfacial hypoplasia, as seen in Crouzon's disease and Apert's syndrome, is associated with childhood OSAS. Craniofacial corrective surgery with maxillary advancement often results in improvement of obstructive symptoms.[64]

Tracheotomy

Tracheotomy is indicated for the management of severe OSAS in children with complicated anatomic or neuromotor issues. Recent reviews of pediatric tracheotomy indicate that tracheotomy is now performed more often for dynamic airway issues such as severe OSAS than for fixed airway lesions.[83] Tracheotomy bypasses the area(s) of airway obstruction during sleep.

Tracheotomy should be considered for patients with severe OSAS associated with neuromotor disease. Tracheotomy can be avoided in some cases by UPPP, pharyngeal

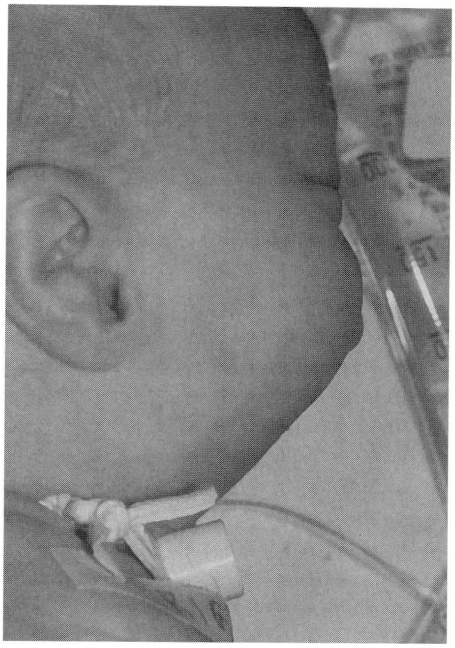

Fig. 13-4. A child with severe micrognathia who required tracheotomy as a neonate for obstructive sleep apnea syndrome.

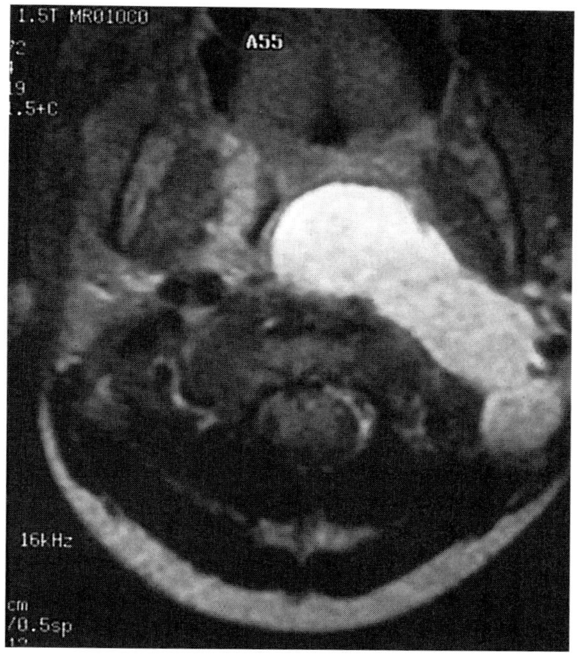

Fig. 13-5. Axial T2-weighted magnetic resonance image of a child with obstructive sleep apnea syndrome. This mass was a parapharyngeal and cervical cystic hygroma. Excision relieved obstructive symptoms.

surgery (including mandibular advancement or tongue–hyoid suspension), and CPAP.[13,41,53]

Laryngeal surgery

Children with acquired or congenital laryngeal abnormalities may have OSAS. Laryngeal anomalies usually present with awake airway symptoms such as hoarseness, stridor, aspiration, and cough. Flexible and rigid endoscopy combined with radiographic studies can define abnormal laryngeal anatomy.[84]

Laryngomalacia is the most common cause of neonatal stridor, with inspiratory collapse of supraglottic tissues seen on fiberoptic endoscopy. Belmont and Grundfast[6] found symptoms of OSAS in 23% of infants with laryngomalacia. Laryngomalacia is almost always self-limited, and symptoms usually resolve before the second year of life. Supraglottoplasty (resection of obstructive supraglottic tissues) can be attempted in cases of severe obstruction or failure to thrive.[35,39,91] Marcus, Crockett, and Ward[47] documented improvement of OSAS from laryngomalacia on polysomnography after supraglottoplasty.

Other surgical management

Some children with OSAS may have compressing anatomic lesions extrinsic to the airway. We have seen several children with head and neck masses that encroach on the airway who presented initially with nocturnal upper-airway obstruction. Lymphangiomas (cystic hygroma) in the parapharyngeal space can cause symptoms of obstructive sleep apnea (Fig. 13-5). Excision of such masses can relieve airway symptoms.

OSAS may be caused or worsened by nasal abnormalities or nasopharyngeal masses. Choanal atresia or stenosis can cause OSAS in neonates, and transnasal and transpalatal approaches for repair have been described. Nasal septal deviation as an isolated finding rarely causes childhood OSAS. Septoplasty and turbinate reduction have been used to relieve nasal obstruction and improve nocturnal breathing in adults.

Intranasal masses can cause snoring and/or OSAS in young infants, and removal is usually curative. Obstructive intranasal masses in children include foreign bodies, inflammatory polyps, mucoceles, and congenital masses such as nasolacrimal duct cysts.

Malignancies of the head and neck can present with symptoms of OSAS. Nasopharyngeal carcinoma, juvenile nasopharyngeal angiofibroma, lymphoma, and rhabdomyosarcoma can present with obstructive symptoms when nasal or pharyngeal patency is affected (Fig. 13-6). Appropriate oncologic treatment using combinations of surgery, chemotherapy, and radiotherapy can relieve airway symptoms, but airway support may be necessary until tumor regression occurs.

NONSURGICAL MANAGEMENT

Children who fail to respond to or are not candidates for surgical intervention are now being managed successfully with CPAP or BiPAP. Recent reports demonstrate that

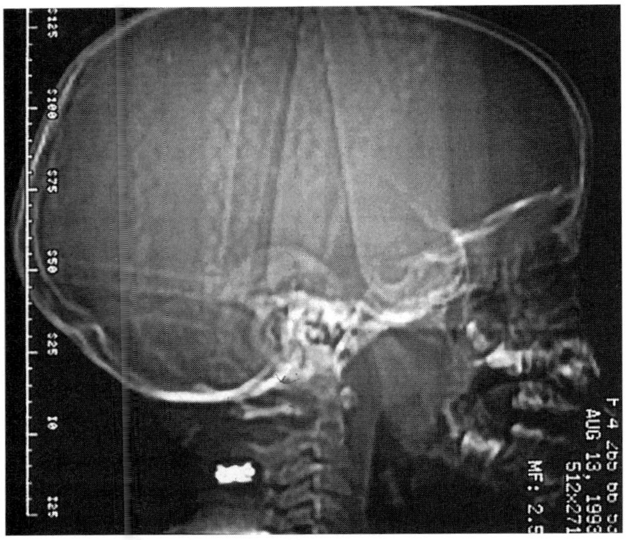

Fig. 13-6. Lateral radiograph of a 3-year-old with rapidly progressive obstructive sleep apnea syndrome. The nasopharynx is obliterated with soft tissue. Biopsy revealed rhabdomyosarcoma.

CPAP is safe, efficacious, and well tolerated by children.[53,86] In our experience, BiPAP has also been used safely and effectively to manage childhood OSAS and may be better tolerated by patients. BiPAP allows independent adjustment of delivered positive pressure during inspiration and expiration. The pressure delivered during expiration can be reduced, usually without compromising airway patency. Patients may find exhaling against a lower applied pressure to be more comfortable, thus improving compliance and acceptance. The level of positive pressure required to eliminate obstructive apneas and normalize ventilation and nighttime oxygen saturation must be determined in the sleep laboratory. The positive pressure requirements of growing children must be reevaluated intermittently with polysomnography.[53] Complications of CPAP or BiPAP include noncompliance, local discomfort or irritation from poor mask fit, and nasal congestion. One review also reported hypoventilation and increased central apneas in 8 of 32 children,[86] again stressing the importance of assessing pressure requirements in the sleep laboratory. Poor compliance is the greatest limitation to the use of CPAP and BiPAP in the management of OSAS.

Oxygen supplementation is not generally considered a management option for OSAS. In patients with severe OSAS, supplemental oxygen may worsen obstructive apnea due to suppression of the hypoxic respiratory drive and depression of upper-airway motor tone.[23] A recent study has demonstrated that supplemental oxygen can be used safely in some children with mild to moderate OSAS but should be considered palliative until definitive therapy occurs.[45] Initial oxygen supplementation in patients with OSAS should be delivered under monitored conditions.

As in adults, weight loss is an important component in management of OSAS in obese children. Nutritional counseling with aggressive follow-up is necessary for these patients.

REFERENCES

1. Abdu MH, Feghali JG: Uvulopalatopharyngoplasty in a child with obstructive sleep apnea: a case report, *J Laryngol Otol* 102:546, 1988.
2. Ahlqvist-Rastad J, Hultcrantz E, Svanholm H: Children with tonsillar obstruction: indications for and efficacy of tonsillectomy, *Acta Paediatr Scand* 77:831, 1988.
3. Ali NJ, Pitson DJ, Stradling JR: Snoring, sleep disturbance, and behaviour in 4-5 year olds, *Arch Dis Child* 68:360, 1993.
4. Ali NJ, Pitson D, Stradling JR: Natural history of snoring and related behaviour problems between the ages of 4 and 7 years, *Arch Dis Child* 71:74, 1994.
5. American Thoracic Society: Standards and indications for cardiopulmonary sleep studies in children, *Am J Respir Crit Care Med* 153:866, 1996.
6. Belmont JR, Grundfast K: Congenital laryngeal stridor (laryngomalacia): etiologic factors and associated disorders, *Ann Otol Rhinol Laryngol* 93:430, 1984.
7. Bredenkamp JK and others: Otolaryngologic manifestations of the mucopolysaccharidoses, *Ann Otol Rhinol Laryngol* 101 472, 1992.
8. Brodsky L, Moore L, Stanievich JF: A comparison of tonsillar size and oropharyngeal dimensions in children with obstructive adenotonsillar hypertrophy, *Int J Pediatr Otorhinolaryingol* 13:149, 1987.
9. Brooks LJ: Treatment of otherwise normal children with obstructive sleep apnea, *Ear Nose Throat J* 72:77, 1993.
10. Brouillette RT, Fernbach SK, Hunt CE: Obstructive sleep apnea in infants and children, *J Pediatr* 100:31, 1982.
11. Brouillette R and others: A diagnostic approach to suspected obstructive sleep apnea in children, *J Pediatr* 105:10, 1984.
12. Brown OE, Manning SC, Ridenour B: Cor pulmonale secondary to tonsillar and adenoidal hypertrophy: management considerations, *Int J Pediatr Otorhinolaryngol* 16:131, 1988.
13. Burstein FD and others: Surgical therapy for severe refractory sleep apnea in infants and children: application of the airway zone concept, *Plast Reconstr Surg* 96:34, 1995.
14. Canet E and others: Effects of sleep deprivation on respiratory events during sleep in healthy infants, *J Appl Physiol* 66:1158, 1989.
15. Carroll JL, Loughlin GM: *Obstructive sleep apnea syndrome in infants and children: clinical features and pathophysiology.* In Ferber R, Kryger MH, editors: *Principles and practice of sleep medicine in the child*, Philadelphia, 1995, WB Saunders.
16. Carroll JL, Loughlin GM: *Primary snoring in infants and children.* In Ferber R, Kryger MH, editors: *Principles and practice of sleep medicine in the child*, Philadelphia, 1995, WB Saunders.
17. Carroll JL and others: Inability of clinical history to distinguish primary snoring from obstructive sleep apnea syndrome in children, *Chest* 108: 610, 1995.
18. Corbo GM and others: Snoring in children: association with respiratory symptoms and passive smoking [published erratum appears in *BMJ* 300:226, 1990, *BMJ* 299:1491, 1989.
19. Croft CB and others: Endoscopic evaluation and treatment of sleep-associated upper airway obstruction in infants and young children, *Clin Otolaryngol* 15:209, 1990.
20. Donaldson JD, Redmond WM: Surgical management of obstructive sleep apnea in children with Down syndrome, *J Otolaryngol* 17:398, 1988.
21. Downey R, Perkin RM, MacQuarrie J: Upper airway resistance syndrome: sick, symptomatic but underrecognized, *Sleep* 16:620, 1993.
22. Frank Y and others: Obstructive sleep apnea and its therapy: clinical and polysomnographic manifestations, *Pediatrics* 71:737, 1983.
23. Gauda EB and others: Effect of oxygenation on breath-by-breath re-

sponse of the genioglossus muscle during occlusion, *J Appl Physiol* 71:1231, 1991.

24. Gaultier C: *Respiratory adaptation during sleep from the neonatal period to adolescence*. In Guilleminault C, editor: *Sleep and its disorders in children*, New York, 1987, Raven Press.
25. Gislason T, Benediktsdottir B: Snoring, apneic episodes, and nocturnal hypoxemia among children 6 months to 6 years old: an epidemiologic study of lower limit of prevalence, *Chest* 107:963, 1995.
26. Goldstein NA and others: Clinical diagnosis of pediatric obstructive sleep apnea validated by polysomnography, *Otolaryngol Head Neck Surg* 111:611, 1994.
27. Grundfast K, Berkowitz R, Fox L: Outcome and complications following surgery for obstructive adenotonsillar hypertrophy in children with neuromuscular disorders, *Ear Nose Throat J* 69:756, 1990.
28. Grundfast KM, Wittich DJJ: Adenotonsillar hypertrophy and upper airway obstruction in evolutionary perspective, *Laryngoscope* 92:650, 1982.
29. Guilleminault C and others: Sleep apnea in eight children, *Pediatrics* 58:23, 1976.
30. Guilleminault C, Korobkin R, Winkle R: A review of 50 children with obstructive sleep apnea syndrome, *Lung* 159:275, 1981.
31. Guilleminault C and others: A cause of excessive daytime sleepiness: the upper airway resistance syndrome, *Chest* 104:781, 1993.
32. Helfaer MA and others: Polysomnography after adenotonsillectomy in mild pediatric obstructive sleep apnea, *Crit Care Med* 24:1323, 1996.
33. Hershenson M and others: The effect of chloral hydrate on genioglossus and diaphragmatic activity, *Pediatr Res* 18:516, 1984.
34. Hill W: On some causes of backwardness and stupidity in children, *BMJ* 2:711, 1889.
35. Holinger LD, Konior RJ: Surgical management of severe laryngomalacia, *Laryngoscope* 99:136, 1989.
36. Horner RL, Mohiaddin RH, Lowell DG: Sites and sizes of fat deposits around the pharynx in obese patients with obstructive sleep apnoea and weight matched controls, *Eur Respir J* 2:613, 1989.
37. Hutchinson RE, Davey FR, Henry JB: Evaluation of coagulation disorders in patients with diseases of Waldeyer's ring, *Otolaryngol Clin North Am* 20:317, 1987.
38. Jacob SV and others: Home testing may be preferable to conventional polysomnography for the diagnosis of pediatric obstructive sleep apnea, *Am Rev Respir Dis* 147:762, 1993 (abstract).
39. Kelly SM, Gray SD: Unilateral endoscopic supraglottoplasty for severe laryngomalacia, *Arch Otolaryngol Head Neck Surg* 121:1351, 1995.
40. Khan Y, Heckmatt JZ: Obstructive apnoeas in Duchenne muscular dystrophy, *Thorax* 49:157, 1994.
41. Kosko JR, Derkay CS: Uvulopalatopharyngoplasty: treatment of obstructive sleep apnea in neurologically impaired pediatric patients, *Int J Pediatr Otorhinolaryngol* 32:241, 1995.
42. Kravath RE and others: Obstructive sleep apnea and death associated with surgical correction of velopharyngeal incompetence, *J Pediatr* 96:645, 1980.
43. Leach J and others: Polysomnographic and clinical findings in children with obstructive sleep apnea, *Arch Otolaryngol Head Neck Surg* 118:741, 1992.
44. Mangat D, Orr WC, Smith RO: Sleep apnea, hypersomnolence, and upper airway obstruction secondary to adenotonsillar enlargement, *Arch Otolaryngol* 103:383, 1977.
45. Marcus CL and others: Supplemental oxygen during sleep in children with sleep-disordered breathing, *Am J Respir Crit Care Med* 152:1297, 1995.
46. Marcus CL and others: Determinants of growth in children with the obstructive sleep apnea syndrome, *J Pediatr* 125:556, 1994.
47. Marcus CL, Crockett DM, Ward SL: Evaluation of epiglottoplasty as treatment for severe laryngomalacia [published erratum appears in *J Pediatr* 118:168, 1991, *J Pediatr* 117:706, 1990.
48. Marcus CL and others: Evaluation of pulmonary function and polysomnography in obese children and adolescents, *Pediatr Pulmonol* 21:176, 1996.
49. Marcus CL, Keens TG, Ward SL: Comparison of nap and overnight polysomnography in children, *Pediatr Pulmonol* 13:16, 1992.
50. Marcus CL and others: Obstructive sleep apnea in children with Down syndrome, *Pediatrics* 88:132, 1991.
51. Marcus CL and others: Upper airway collapsibility in children with obstructive sleep apnea syndrome, *J Appl Physiol* 77:918, 1994.
52. Marcus CL and others: Normal polysomnographic values for children and adolescents, *Am Rev Respir Dis* 146:1235, 1992.
53. Marcus CL and others: Use of nasal continuous positive airway pressure as treatment of childhood obstructive sleep apnea, *J Pediatr* 127:88, 1995.
54. McColley SA and others: Respiratory compromise after adenotonsillectomy in children with obstructive sleep apnea, *Arch Otolaryngol Head Neck Surg* 118:940, 1992.
55. McGrath-Morrow SA and others: Termination of obstructive apnea in children is not associated with arousal, *Am Rev Respir Dis* 141:195, 1990.
56. Mixter RC, Ewanowski SJ, Carson LV: Central tongue reduction for macroglossia, *Plast Reconstr Surg* 91:1159, 1993.
57. Montgomery JN, Watson CB, Mackie AM: Anesthesia for tonsillectomy and adenoidectomy, *Otolaryngol Clin North Am* 20:331, 1987.
58. Morgan WE and others: Surgical management of macroglossia in children, *Arch Otolaryngol Head Neck Surg* 122:326, 1996.
59. Morielli A and others: Can sleep and wakefulness be distinguished in children by cardiorespiratory and videotape recordings? *Chest* 109:680, 1996.
60. Nelson WF and others: Neurological basis of respiratory complications in achondroplasia, *Ann Neurol* 24:89, 1988.
61. Orr WC, Levine NS, Buchanan RT: Effect of cleft palate repair and pharyngeal flap surgery on upper airway obstruction during sleep, *Plast Reconstr Surg* 80:226, 1987.
62. Peters ME and others: Narrow trachea in mucopolysaccharidoses, *Pediatr Radiol* 94:225, 1985.
63. Potsic WP and others: Relief of upper airway obstruction by adenotonsillectomy, *Otolaryngol Head Neck Surg* 94:476, 1986.
64. Potsic WP, Wetmore RF: Sleep disorders and airway obstruction in children, *Otolaryngol Clin North Am* 23:651, 1990.
65. Price SD, Hawkins DB, Kahlstrom EJ: Tonsil and adenoid surgery for airway obstruction: perioperative respiratory morbidity, *Ear Nose Throat J* 72:526, 1993.
66. Reid CS and others: Cervicomedullary compression in young patients with achondroplasia, *J Pediatr* 110:522, 1987.
67. Rhodes SK and others: Neurocognitive deficits in morbidly obese children with obstructive sleep apnea, *J Pediatr* 127:741, 1995.
68. Richardson MA and others: Evaluation of tonsils and adenoids in sleep apnea syndrome, *Laryngoscope* 90:1106, 1980.
69. Rimell FL and others: Head and neck manifestations of Beckwith-Weidemann syndrome, *Otolaryngol Head Neck Surg* 113:262, 1995.
70. Rosen CL, D'Andrea L, Haddad GG. Adult criteria for obstructive sleep apnea do not identify children with serious obstruction, *Am Rev Respir Dis* 146:1231, 1992.
71. Rosen GM and others: Postoperative respiratory compromise in children with obstructive sleep apnea syndrome: can it be anticipated? *Pediatrics* 93:784, 1994.
72. Ruckenstein RJ and others: The management of otolaryngological problems in the mucopolysaccharidoses: a retrospective review, *J Otolaryngol* 20:177, 1991.
73. Seid AB and others: Surgical therapy of obstructive sleep apnea in children with severe mental insufficiency, *Laryngoscope* 100:507, 1990.
74. Serratto M, Harris VJ, Carr I: Upper airway obstruction: presentation with systemic hypertension, *Arch Dis Child* 56:153, 1981.
75. Shapiro J, Strome M, Crocker AC: Airway obstruction and sleep apnea

in Hurler and Hunter syndromes, *Ann Otol Rhinol Laryngol* 94:458, 1985.

76. Silvestri JM and others: Polysomnography in obese children with a history of sleep-associated breathing disorders, *Pediatr Pulmonol* 16: 124, 1993.
77. Snyderman NL: Otorhinolaryngologic presentations of infectious mononucleosis, *Pediatr Clin North Am* 28:1011, 1981.
78. Stradling JR and others: Effect of adenotonsillectomy on nocturnal hypoxaemia, sleep disturbance, and symptoms in snoring children, *Lancet* 335:249, 1990.
79. Strome M: Obstructive sleep apnea in Down syndrome children: a surgical approach, *Laryngoscope* 96:1340, 1986.
80. Suen JS, Arnold JE, Brooks LJ: Adenotonsillectomy for treatment of obstructive sleep apnea in children, *Arch Otolaryngol Head Neck Surg* 121:525, 1995.
81. Teculescu DB and others: Snoring in French preschool children, *Pediatr Pulmonol* 13:239, 1992.
82. Tomaski SM, Zulzal GH, Saal HM: Airway obstruction in the Pierre-Robin sequence, *Laryngoscope* 105:111, 1995.
83. Tunkel DE and others: Polysomnography in the evaluation of readiness for decannulation in children, *Arch Otolaryngol Head Neck Surg* 122: 721, 1996.
84. Tunkel DE, Zalzal G: Stridor in infants and children: ambulatory evaluation and operative diagnosis, *Clin Pediatr* 31:48, 1992.
85. Wang D and others: Fiberoptic evaluation of the nasal and nasopharyngeal anatomy in children with snoring, *J Otolaryngol* 23:57, 1994.
86. Waters KA and others: Obstructive sleep apnea: the use of nasal CPAP in 80 children, *Am J Respir Crit Care Med* 152:780, 1995.
87. Weider DJ, Hauri PJ: Nocturnal enuresis in children with upper airway obstruction, *Int J Pediatr Otorhinolaryngol* 9:173, 1985.
88. Weider DJ, Sateia MJ, West RP: Nocturnal enuresis in children with upper airway obstruction, *Otolaryngol Head Neck Surg* 105:427, 1991.
89. Wiatrak BJ, Myer CM, Andrews TM: Complications of adenotonsillectomy in children under 3 years of age, *Am J Otolaryngol* 12:170, 1991.
90. Williams EF and others: The effects of adenotonsillectomy on growth in young children, *Otolaryngol Head Neck Surg* 104:509, 1991.
91. Zalzal GH, Anon JB, Cotton RT: Epiglottoplasty for the treatment of laryngomalacia, *Ann Otol Rhinol Laryngol* 96:72, 1987.

Chapter 14

Head and Neck Malignancies

Richard J.H. Smith
Robert A. Robinson

Each year in the United States, cancer is diagnosed in 1 of every 333 persons under 20 years of age. It affects 7500 children before their fifteenth birthday and 3500 young adults between 15 and 20 years of age.[76] Data collected by the Surveillance, Epidemiology, and End Results Program of the National Cancer Institute (NCI) suggest that these numbers are on the rise. In 1972, 12 cancers were diagnosed per 100,000 children under the age of 15 years; by 1990, that number had climbed to nearly 14 per 100,000.[76,121] During this same period, cancer-related mortality decreased, although malignancies remain the most common cause of death from disease in late infancy to early adulthood. Childhood cancers are exceeded only by accidents as the leading cause of death in children older than 1 year of age. More than 100,000 person-years of life are lost annually due to cancer.[64]

The types and relative frequencies of childhood cancers are vastly different than those of adults. Nearly one third of pediatric malignancies are leukemias, most commonly acute lymphocytic leukemia, and an additional 12% are either Hodgkin's lymphoma (HL) or non-Hodgkin's lymphoma (NHL). Nonhematologic solid tumors comprise the remaining 55%. Of all solid tumors in children younger than 15 years of age, brain tumors are most common, followed in frequency by neuroblastoma and rhabdomyosarcoma (RMS).

Impressive gains have been made in survival rates for some childhood cancers. Overall, survival in children under 15 years of age who are diagnosed with solid tumors has more than doubled, from 28% in 1960 to 70% in 1990.[76] Particularly impressive survival gains have been achieved with Wilms' tumor and HL, both of which now have cure rates exceeding 90%.[76] Outcome data over this 30-year period show that the slopes of curves describing survival over time have remained fairly constant for all types of tumors. Upswings or jumps that would reflect the discovery of "magic bullets" or major technologic breakthroughs are lacking. Advances in treatment and gains in survival have been achieved in a slow, incremental manner.

This progress largely reflects the impact of clinical trials. Initiated first in 1948 to enable Farber, Diamond, and Mercer[37] to document the efficacy of methotrexate in inducing remission in some children with acute lymphocytic leukemia, most clinical trials today are conducted by the Children's Cancer Group or the Pediatric Oncology Group. In these trials, standard therapy is compared with a modification of that therapy, and if the modified protocol is superior it then becomes the new standard. Progress is tedious, but from the perspective of time it has been tremendously rewarding.

The possibility of more rapid advances in diagnosis and management is becoming increasingly real as studies in the molecular biology of childhood malignancies elucidate several requisite steps for tumorigenesis. Two important cytogenetic events, translocation and amplification, are important in tumor development and can act synergistically to generate potent oncogenic activity.[6] Nonrandom chromosomal translocations typically activate oncogenes by one of two mechanisms.[90] The first mechanism, frequently found in lymphoid malignancies, places the coding sequence of one gene under the regulatory control of a second gene. This juxtaposition results in increased or inappropriate expression of the first gene. The second mechanism generates a new gene, which is a chimera of two other genes that is formed by joining their coding regions. For amplification events, additional

Table 14-1. Age-incidence ranking for head and neck tumors in children

Age (years)			
0–1	**1–5**	**6–10**	**11–20**
Neuroblastoma	Rhabdomyosarcoma	Lymphoma	Lymphoma
Rhabdomyosarcoma	Lymphoma	Rhabdomyosarcoma	Thyroid malignancies
Lymphoma	Neuroblastoma	Nonrhabdomyosarcoma soft-tissue sarcoma	Nasopharyngeal malignancies
Nonrhabdomyosarcoma soft-tissue sarcoma	Nonrhabdomyosarcoma soft-tissue sarcoma	Thyroid malignancies	Salivary gland neoplasms

copies of a cellular gene are generated in the form of double-minute chromosomes or homogeneously staining regions.[102]

Head and neck tumors of childhood are reviewed in this chapter. This subset of malignancies represents less than 5% of all childhood cancers, and by order of relative prevalence includes lymphomas (59%), RMSs (13%), thyroid carcinomas (10%), nasopharyngeal carcinomas (5%), neuroblastomas (5%), nonrhabdomyosarcoma soft-tissue sarcomas (NRSTS; 4.5%), salivary gland malignancies (2.5%), and malignant teratomas (1%).[23] Age has a marked effect on tumor type and modifies this order of prevalence considerably; this factor is obviously pertinent to a directed evaluation and diagnostic workup (Table 14-1). Discussion is limited to lymphomas, RMSs, neuroblastomas, NRSTSs, salivary gland malignancies, and malignant teratomas; thyroid and nasopharyngeal carcinomas are adequately covered elsewhere.

LYMPHOMAS

Non-Hodgkin's lymphomas

Lymphomas are the third most common cancers in children in the United States,[94] and NHLs represent 60% of these diagnoses. The annual incidence in children younger than 15 years of age is 7 to 8 per 1,000,000, with peak ages between 7 and 11 years. Boys are preferentially affected by a 3:1 margin,[78,120] and the disease is twice as common in whites as in blacks.[98] Since 1973, the annual incidence of NHL has risen by approximately 30%. Although the reasons for this increase remain unclear, specific populations of children who are at greater risk for NHL have been identified. These groups include children with congenital immunodeficiency syndrome (Wiskott-Aldrich syndrome), children with acquired immunodeficiency syndrome (AIDS), and children who have received immunosuppressive therapy for organ or bone marrow transplants. Common to all patients is deficient or impaired T-cell function.

Geographic differences in the incidence rates and subtypes of NHL are striking. For example, NHL is rare in Japan, whereas in equatorial Africa and northeastern Brazil, Burkitt's lymphoma (BL) is endemic and accounts for approximately 50% of all cancers.[94] An association with Epstein-Barr virus (EBV) and BL has been demonstrated in these areas[42]; and even in cases of sporadic BL in the United States that are negative by standard screening,[93] EBV genomic DNA can be detected with molecular biology.

Presentation and evaluation

Non-Hodgkin's lymphomas are classified as low-, intermediate-, or high-grade lesions based on their clinical aggressiveness. More than 90% of children have high-grade disease, probably reflecting the cellular composition and function of an immature immune system. Characterized by an acute onset with rapid progression, prompt diagnosis and initiation of therapy are important to reduce morbidity and ensure long-term survival.[117] In 23% to 46% of affected children, primary disease occurs within the abdominal cavity and involves, in decreasing order of frequency, the distal ileum, cecum, and appendix.[79,103] Mediastinal primary tumors are slightly less common and are diagnosed in 15% to 45% of cases.[118] Primary head and neck involvement occurs in 5% to 10% of children and originates in the salivary glands, larynx, paranasal sinuses, orbit, scalp, and Waldeyer's ring.[103] Proximity to the central nervous system makes direct extension possible.

The rapid progression of disease mandates prompt referral to a specialized management center prior to biopsy so that a pediatric oncologist can expedite the diagnostic and staging evaluation (Table 14-2) and determine the site and procedure to obtain tissue for histologic, cytologic, immunophenotyping, and genotyping analyses, with consultation from the surgeon and pathologist if necessary. Definitive diagnosis requires biopsy, sometimes by excision of a cervical node. Disseminated disease is the rule, however, and not infrequently adequate numbers of malignant cells are found in the bone marrow, spinal fluid, or pleural or ascites fluid, obviating surgical intervention entirely. The presence of pancytopenia suggests bone marrow involvement, and when more than 25% of the marrow is replaced with tumor, children are assigned a diagnosis of acute lymphoblastic leukemia.

Management

Dramatic improvement in overall cure rates among children with NHL reflects the incremental development of effective multimodal chemotherapeutic regimens through

Table 14-2. Diagnostic and staging evaluation for non-Hodgkin's lymphoma

Essential	Useful	Occasionally indicated
History	Intravenous urography	Contrast studies of the gastrointestinal tract
Physical examination	Special radiologic views (airway)	CT, MRI of brain
Specimens for histology, cytology, immunophenotyping, genotyping	CT, MRI of primary site	Myelography, CT, MRI of spinal cord
Complete blood count	Radionuclide, radiologic skeletal survey	Lymphangiography
Serum chemistries	Radionuclide liver–spleen scan	Creatinine clearance
Bone marrow aspiration	Coagulation profile	Urinary uric acid
Cerebrospinal fluid analysis	Epstein-Barr virus studies	Serum lactic acid
Urinalysis	Protein electrophoresis	Bone marrow biopsy
Chest radiography	Acid–base studies	Liver biopsy
Gallium-67 scanning		
Abdominal imaging		

CT—Computed tomography; MRI—Magnetic resonance imaging.

well-planned clinical trials. Systemic therapy is imperative because occult micrometastases affect more than 80% of children with NHL and cure rates are less than 20% when only local therapy is used.[117] Management protocols are based on the extent of disease as determined by the staging workup and the histologic subtype.

Although several different staging systems have been applied to NHL (Table 14-3), each shares the essential purpose of identifying relatively homogeneous subcategories of disease to ensure that therapeutic trials address increasingly specific questions and are comparable to each other.[116] Chemotherapy is the backbone of management, traditionally with agents used for acute lymphoblastic leukemia (i.e., cyclophosphamide, doxorubicin, vincristine, prednisone). Radiotherapy is reserved for massive disease, and surgery is only used occasionally in children with life-threatening tracheal compression. Response to therapy is monitored by following tumor size and activity using a variety of imaging modalities or invasive techniques.

Histopathology and molecular biology

The histopathology of NHL is extremely variable and has been categorized in various ways. The traditional and widely adopted Rappaport classification uses histologic pattern, cell type, and degree of differentiation to categorize tumors. In children, only three categories are seen with any frequency: small, noncleaved-cell; lymphoblastic; and large-cell lymphomas. The diffuse histologic pattern is almost universal within these categories.[117] The first category can also be further subdivided as Burkitt's (homogeneous) or non-Burkitt's (pleomorphic) types, but this distinction lacks clinical relevance.

The development of immunologic markers has added refinement to categorization and contributed to the identification of molecular mechanisms in pathogenesis. Best studied are the small, noncleaved-cell lymphomas, particularly BL (Fig. 14-1). The role of EBV, a B-cell mitogen, in BL probably fosters the establishment of a premalignant state by expanding the pool of lymphocytes in which chromosomal transformations can occur. Classic to BL is the translocation of the *myc* gene from chromosome 8 to a position juxtaposed to an immunoglobulin receptor subunit gene on chromosomes 2, 14, or 22 (t[8;2], t[8;14], t[8;22], respectively).[30,110] Unregulated expression of the *myc* gene disrupts regulation of the expression of target genes that are required for the normal progression of the cell cycle.[14,84,88]

Most theories about the pathogenesis of lymphoblastic lymphomas are based on the unproven, although reasonable, assumption that lymphoblastic lymphomas and T-cell leukemias are different manifestations of a single disease entity.[98] In both cancers, the translocation of transcription factor genes to either chromosomes 7 or 14 places the former chromosome under shared regulatory control with the latter. The result is the activation of developmental processes that are not usually operative in T cells.[119] The precise mechanism of malignant transformation following translocation has not been determined.

Approximately 50% of large-cell lymphomas have a t(2;5) chromosomal rearrangement.[99] Consequently, the catalytic domain of the anaplastic lymphoma kinase gene (*ALK*) on chromosome 2 is fused to the amino-terminal portion of nucleophosmin gene (*NPM*) on chromosome 5.[77] The chimeric protein product that is produced engages in activities foreign to both derivative genes and probably inappropriately phosphorylates substrates in the cytoplasm. The precursor RNA can be detected by a reverse-transcriptase–polymerase chain reaction assay, which has become an important diagnostic tool.[33] It has been found in some nonanaplastic lymphomas, some CD30+ anaplastic lymphomas, and some lymphomas that lack cytogenetic evidence of the translocation. Although the impact of molecular biology has yet to revolutionize clinical practice, it will inevitably refine our diagnostic capabilities and permit the development of target tumor-specific therapy.

Table 14-3. Staging systems for non-Hodgkin's lymphoma

Stage	System: Ann Arbor	St Jude Children's Research Hospital	Memorial Sloan-Kettering Cancer Center	Prince of Wales Children's Hospital, Autralia
I	Involvement of a single lymph node region (I) or of a single extralymphatic organ or site (I_E)	Single tumor (extranodal) or single anatomic area (nodal) excluding the mediastinum or abdomen	A single site	A single site
II	Involvement of two or more lymph node regions on the same side of the diaphragm or localized involvement of extralymphatic organ or site and of one or more lymph node regions on the same side of the diaphragm	Single extranodal site with regional lymph node involvement; two or more nodal areas on the same side of the diaphragm; two single extranodal tumors ± regional node disease on the same side of the diaphragm; primary gastrointestinal tract tumor, usually in the ileocecal area ± involvement of associated mesenteric nodes	Two or more sites above or below the diaphragm	Two or more sites above or below the diaphragm
III	Involvement of lymph node regions on both sides of the diaphragm ± extranodal involvement ± splenic involvement	Two single extranodal tumors ± regional node disease on opposite sides of the diaphragm; two or more nodal areas on opposite sides of the diaphragm; all extensive primary intraabdominal disease; all primary intrathoracic tumors	Two or more sites above and below the diaphragm; extensive intrathoracic and extensive intraabdominal involvement	Above and below the diaphragm (III-O) All primary intrathoracic (III-T) Extensive intraabdominal (III-Ab)
IV	Diffuse involvement of one or more extralymphatic organs or tissues ± associated lymph node enlargement	Any of the above + initial CNS ± bone marrow involvement	Any of the above + bone marrow ± CNS involvement	Marrow infiltration by <25% tumor cells (IV-M) Marrow infiltration by >25% tumor cells (IV-M) CNS infiltration (IV-N)

CNS—Central nervous system.

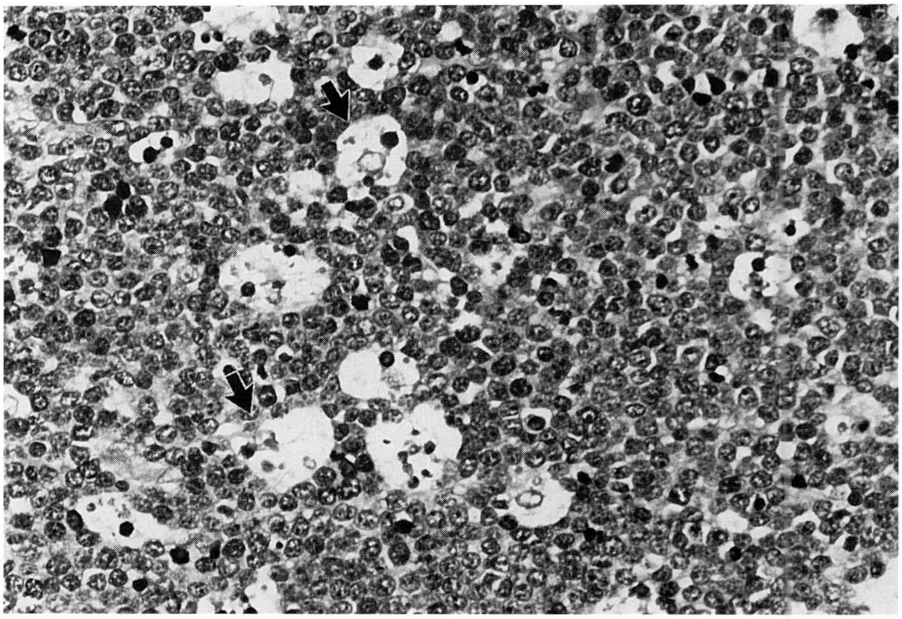

Fig. 14-1. Non-Hodgkin's lymphoma categorized as malignant lymphoma with diffuse, small, noncleaved cells (Burkitt's lymphoma EBL⁻). Small noncleaved lymphocytes diffusely replace this lymph node. The size is monotonous, differentiating it from non-BL, which has more variation in of nuclei size and shape. Histiocytes *(arrows)* with their abundant pale cytoplasm and engulfed cellular material are scattered among the malignant lymphocytes giving a "starry-sky" appearance. (Original magnification, ×400.)

Hodgkin's lymphoma

In 1832, Thomas Hodgkin described the disease that now bears his name. Although characterized by the presence of mononuclear cells (Hodgkin's cells) and binucleated or multinucleated tumor cells (Reed-Sternberg [RS] cells) in a background of variable and often abundant reactive cells, a single unifying principle of the biologic nature of HL and of the origin of the RS cell has remained elusive.[50] Current data suggest that HL represents a group of diseases with an uncertain relationship to each other.[18] Age at diagnosis follows a bimodal distribution, with the first peak occurring between 15 and 40 years of age and the second peak occurring after age 50. Approximately 4% of cases occur in children younger than 10 years of age, and 11% are found in children between the ages of 10 and 16 years.[25]

Presentation and evaluation

In more than 90% of childhood and adult cases, HL arises in the lymph nodes, typically causing an asymmetric adenopathy that is firm, rubbery, and nontender. Particularly common is the combination of mediastinal and right supraclavicular nodal disease. The spleen is the most common extranodal site of involvement. Constitutional symptoms may be present and include fever of 38° C or higher, drenching night sweats, or unexplained loss of 10% or more of body weight. Diagnosis is made by lymph node biopsy, and the disease then is staged using the classification developed in 1971 by the Ann Arbor workshop[19] and modified 18 years later to incorporate newer procedures like computed tomography (CT).[63] This system is based on the premise that HL spreads through the lymphatics to contiguous nodal groups and through the circulation to extranodal sites, although these modes of spread have not been clearly established and multifocal involvement may represent multicentric disease.[18]

Clinical staging procedures include history, physical examination, radiologic procedures, and laboratory tests (excluding biopsies). Chest radiography and abdominal studies are most important, although CT has limited sensitivity in detecting abdominal adenopathy in children.[4] Pathologic staging procedures include bone marrow biopsy, splenectomy, liver biopsy, and lymph node biopsy. Surgical findings result in a change in stage in approximately one third of children, most frequently because the disease burden is greater than expected.[25]

Stage I designates disease in a single node group; stage II indicates involvement of two or more nodal groups on one side of the diaphragm, the number of which is noted by a subscript; stage III signifies disease in nodal groups and/or the spleen on both sides of the diaphragm (III_1 = splenic, hilar, celiac axis, and/or portal nodes; III_2 = periaortic, iliac, inguinal/femoral, and/or mesenteric nodes); and stage IV denotes disease at other sites as indicated by a subscript (M = bone marrow; H = liver; L = lung; O = bone; P = pleura; D = skin). Other modifiers include the following subscripts: X for bulky disease (maximum dimension > 10 cm or, in the case of mediastinal disease, one third of the thoracic diameter at T5-6 on a 6-foot posteroanterior chest radiograph); E for extension from a lymph node to an adjacent extranodal site; A for asymptomatic disease; and B for the constitutional symptoms listed previously.[107]

Stage at presentation is similar among children and adults, with about 60% of patients presenting with stage I or II disease and 40% presenting with stage II or IV disease regardless of age.[25] In children under 10 years of age, however, stage I disease is more common (18%) and stage IV disease is less common (3%) than in adolescents (8% and 15%, respectively) and adults (11% and 11%, respectively). Systemic "B" symptoms are also less likely in younger patients (19%) than in adolescents (30%) and adults (32%).

Management

Management of HL varies according to stage. In most centers, radiation therapy is recommended for stage IA and IIA disease. For cervical disease, most protocols include the involved nodal groups with margins of 7 cm. Because of the high relapse rate in children with stage IIA disease of the mediastinum, chemotherapy may also be given.[70] For more advanced disease, chemotherapy either alone or as part of combined regimen including radiotherapy is used.[3]

Long-term results of pediatric patients with early-stage HL suggest a prognosis similar to that of adults, with cure rates of approximately 90%.[62] Using combined-modality therapy for stage IV disease, overall survival rates are slightly lower (about 80%).[3] When patients who have received only chemotherapy relapse at nodal sites, salvage radiotherapy should be considered.[12]

Histopathology and molecular biology

The major histologic types of HL recognized by the Lukes/Bulter and Rye classifications include lymphocytic predominance, nodular and diffuse, classical nodular sclerosis, lymphocytic depletion, reticular, and diffuse types[18] (Fig. 14-2). There is probably no need for further subclassification because current management protocols have eliminated differences in survival rates between the most common types (mixed cellularity and nodular sclerosis).

Micromanipulation of histologic sections to isolate and analyze individual Hodgkin's and RS cells has verified an origin from B-lineage cells at various stages of development.[60] Ig heavy chain rearrangements have also been detected by polymerase chain reaction amplification in approximately 25% of cases.[68] These studies suggest that HL represents a clonal lymphocyte population and that different chromosomal rearrangements may be associated with different subclasses of disease.

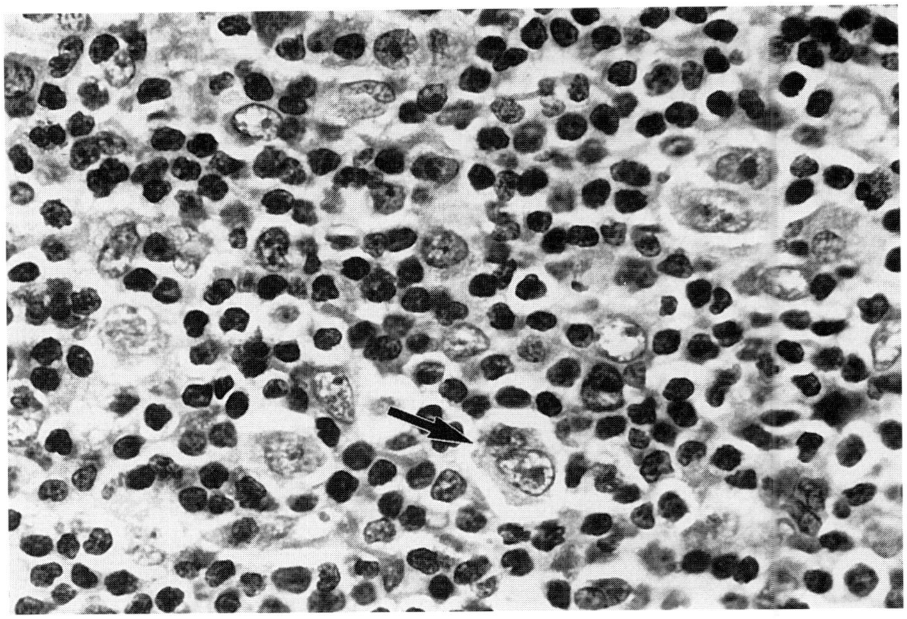

Fig. 14-2. Hodgkin's lymphoma of the nodular sclerosing subtype. A mixed population of lymphocytes, histiocytes, and plasma cells along with binucleated Reed-Sternberg cells (*arrows*) are present. (Original magnification, ×480.)

SARCOMAS

Rhabdomyosarcoma

Rhabdomyosarcoma is the most common soft-tissue sarcoma of childhood, representing 13% of all pediatric malignancies and affecting 250 children in the United States each year.[26,85] Forty percent of these children present with disease in the head and neck. Sites of involvement include the orbit, nose and paranasal sinuses, oropharynx, soft tissues, nasopharynx, and external ear or mastoid. Because of the high possibility of contiguous spread to the central nervous system, the paranasal sinuses, infratemporal fossa, middle ear, and nasopharynx are classified as parameningeal sites.

In the 1960s, fewer than one third of children with RMS survived, but cure rates now approximate 70%, largely reflecting advances made by the Intergroup Rhabdomyosarcoma Study Committee (IRSC).[38,85] Prior to formation of the IRSC in 1972, the relatively small numbers of patients, short follow-up times, and the confounding effects of varied treatments limited univariate and multivariate analyses, especially for small subgroups of patients. However, when three pediatric centers agreed to pool patients and investigate resources, it became possible to identify prognostic variables of crucial importance for stratifying patients in clinical trials. Valid comparisons of alternative therapies were developed, and therapies were tailored according to the risk of relapse.

Presentation and evaluation

The majority of affected children are younger than 5 years of age when the diagnosis of RMS is made.[113] The spectrum of presenting signs and symptoms varies greatly depending on the site of the primary tumor, the age of the child, and the presence or absence of metastatic disease. Presentation in the head and neck is most frequently heralded by a local swelling. Less than half of these children have pain. Nasal discharge or obstruction, signs of cranial nerve involvement, otorrhea, hearing loss, fetor, and proptosis are even less frequent.[46]

The orbit is involved in nearly one third of RMSs of the head and neck,[46] with the typical presentation being a rapidly developing, unexplained proptosis. In decreasing order of frequency, RMS also affects the oral cavity and pharynx (29%), the face and neck region (24%), and the ears and sinuses (9%). Nasopharyngeal and paranasal sinus involvement can cause nasal obstruction or epistaxis, and otitis media is often the presenting symptom of temporal bone disease.[8]

The diagnostic workup of children with suspected RMS must address two complementary issues: the nature and extent of the primary disease and the presence or absence of locoregional or metastatic disease. To assess the former, CT and magnetic resonance imaging (MRI) are essential; to assess the latter, common sites for metastases must be evaluated, including the lungs, bone, and bone marrow. A minimal test battery mandates a CT of the chest, a ^{99m}Tc-diphosphonate bone scan, and bilateral aspiration and biopsy of iliac bone marrow.

Surgery is a necessary part of the diagnostic and staging evaluation and is an essential component in the Intergroup Rhabdomyosarcoma Study clinical grouping classification (IRSCGC; Table 14-4). Although this staging system is widely used, it has recently come under criticism.[113] Radical surgery for RMS in the head and neck is often feasible,[46] although tumor extirpation may be limited only to partial removal or excision biopsy to establish the diagnosis. As a

Table 14-4. Intergroup Rhabdomyosarcoma Study clinical grouping classification

Group	Definition
I	Localized disease, completely resected
II	Compromised or regional resections with microscopic residual disease
III	Incomplete resection or biopsy with gross residual disease
IV	Distant metastatic disease present at onset

result, children in group III represent a heterogeneous collection of patients who have resectable and unresectable tumors. Additional important variables that are not considered in the IRSCGC are the degree of local extension and the status of the primary echelon nodes. To address these shortcomings, in 1991 the IRSC adopted a TNM classification (primary tumor, regional lymph nodes, and distant metastasis) that is similar to one used to characterize disease extent in adults with solid tumors (Table 14-5). Current IRSC studies rely on both staging systems.

Management

Multimodal, multiagent therapy is the mainstay of management of RMS. Several different chemotherapeutic agents are used, with appropriate selections based on the initial extent of disease and its site of origin. Some children, like those with orbital RMS, require less intensive, two- or three-drug therapy and do well. In contrast, children with metastatic disease require extremely intensive therapy and still do poorly: Although they respond to initial chemotherapy, 75% relapse within 18 to 24 months.[57] To improve this outcome, efforts are ongoing to develop new active chemotherapeutic agents and to use dose-intensifying regimens with hematopoietic growth factors and/or autologous hematopoietic progenitor cells.

Radiotherapy is required to eradicate residual tumor cells at the primary site or to treat gross persistent disease. Guidelines for dosage and radiation fields evolved during the Intergroup Rhabdomyosarcoma Studies I, II, and III. Local control is achieved in 80% to 90% of children using 4000 to 4500 cGy for microscopic residual disease and 4500 to 5000 cGy for tumors larger than 5 cm.[71] Prophylactic irradiation of clinically uninvolved regional nodes is unnecessary. With parameningeal tumors, 4500 to 5500 cGy is required; if there is overt parenchymal, meningeal, or cerebrospinal fluid involvement, whole-brain irradiation and intrathecal chemotherapy are indicated.[39,71] Hyperfractionation is currently under evaluation as an approach to maintain local control rates and to reduce late side effects. Intergroup Rhabdomyosarcoma Study IV is also assessing whether doses less than 4000 cGy can eradicate microscopic residual disease and whether alternative radiation delivery methods (e.g., brachytherapy) can achieve local control in infants and young children without unacceptable damage to the surrounding normal tissue.[80]

With the refinement of aggressive craniofacial and intracranial surgical techniques that minimize postoperative morbidity, surgery is playing a more important role in selected patients with head and neck RMS. For most children in group III, intensification of therapy using a risk-based study design has significantly improved management outcome. The largest gains have been realized in children with gross residual tumor after biopsy. In selected patient subsets, it has also been possible to decrease therapy.[28]

Histopathology and molecular biology

The histologic classification of RMS is based on the resemblance of these tumors to normal fetal skeletal muscle before innervation. The first formal classification was proposed by Horn and Enterline[49] in 1958 and was subsequently adopted by the IRSC and the World Health Organization. Embryonal RMS of the botryoid subtype is the most common variant, accounting for 60% of tumors. It is characterized by variable amounts of spindle and primitive cells that are either tightly packed or loosely dispersed in a myxoid background. Rhabdomyoblasts are present in a variety of shapes, leading to unusual designations like tadpole, racquet, or strap cells (Fig. 14-3). The botryoid subtype accounts for 5% of cases and tends to arise in the mucosal-lined organs of the nasopharynx, external auditory canal, and genital urinary tracts. It is characterized grossly by the presence of polypoid masses and microscopically by the presence of subepithelial aggregates of tumor cells known as the *cambium layer.* Metastases are rare and the prognosis is excellent. Alveolar RMSs are diagnosed in 20% of affected children and are characterized by the presence of fibrovascular septa that form alveolar-like spaces that contain freely floating monomorphous round malignant cells with abundant eosinophilic cytoplasm. Pleomorphic RMSs show features of both embryonal and alveolar RMS but are uncommon in children.[85]

Cytogenetic studies of alveolar RMS have identified frequent chromosomal rearrangements and amplification. The most commonly recognized translocation events, t(2;13) and t(1;13), are found in 64% and 18% of cases, respectively.[114] The result is fusion of the *PAX3* gene on chromosome 2 or the *PAX7* gene on chromosome 1 with the *FKHR* gene on chromosome 13. In the case of *PAX3*, the new chimeric transcription factor excessively activates transcription from binding targets of wild-type *PAX3*. Molecular assays for *PAX3* and *PAX7* fusion genes have identified additional cases that do not have cytogenetically detectable rearrangements. Based on these more sensitive studies, the overall frequency of *PAX3/PAX7-FKHR* chimera appears to be higher than 90%.[6] The prevalence and presumed importance of these fusion genes in tumorigenesis suggest that drugs designed to block their intracellular activity may be effective chemotherapeutic agents.

Table 14-5. TMN* classification (as modified by the Intergroup Rhabdomyosarcoma Study Committee)

Stage	Sites	T	Size	N	M
1	Orbit Head and neck (excluding parameningeal area)	T1 or T2	a or b	Any N	M0
2	Bladder/prostate Extremity Cranial parameningeal sites Other (includes trunk, retroperitoneum)	T1 or T2	a	N0 or NX	M0
3	Bladder/prostate Extremity Cranial parameningeal sites Other (includes trunk, retroperitoneum)	T1 or T2	a b	N1 Any N	M0 M0
4	All	T1 or T2	a or b	N0 or N1	M1

* Tumor: T1—confined to anatomic site of origin, (a ≤ 5 cm in diameter; b > 5 cm in diameter); T2—Extension or infiltration into surrounding tissue (a ≤ 5 cm in diameter; b > 5 cm in diameter).
Nodes: N0—No evidence of regional lymph node involvement; NX—The minimum requirements to assess regional lymph node involvement cannot be met; N1—Evidence of regional lymph node involvement.
Metastases: M0—No evidence of distant metastases; M1—Evidence of distant metastases.

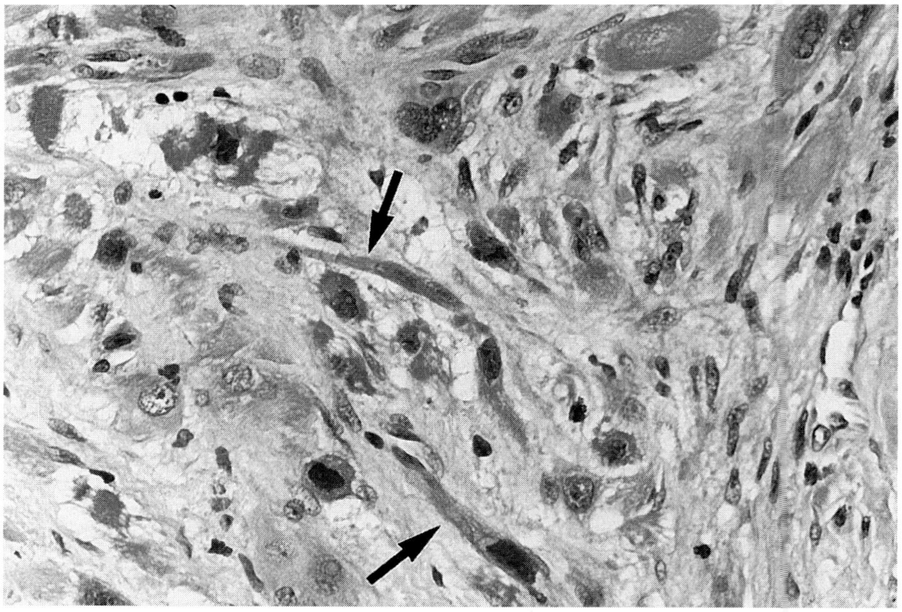

Fig. 14-3. Embryonal rhabdomyosarcoma. The cells show a mixture of shapes but a spindled or elongated morphology is evident overall. Strap cells *(arrows)*, which resemble primitive muscle cells and are classically described in rhabdomyosarcomas, are easily seen in this example but may be difficult to identify in some cases. Immunohistochemical staining for muscle-specific markers can be useful in these instances. (Original magnification, ×350.)

Nonrhabdomyosarcoma soft-tissue sarcomas

Nonrhabdomyosarcoma soft-tissue sarcomas of childhood have a combined annual incidence of about 2 to 3 cases per 1,000,000 and comprise a large number of uncommon tumors, including fibrosarcoma, dermatofibrosarcoma protuberans (DFSP), epitheloid sarcoma, synovial sarcoma, malignant fibrous histiocytoma, hemangiopericytoma, chondrosarcoma, osteosarcoma, leiomyosarcoma, liposarcoma, and soft-tissue clear-cell sarcoma.[113] The diagnostic evaluation for a child with a suspected NRSTS is identical to that for a child with RMS because tumor distinction is impossible on clinical grounds alone. This limitation makes it imperative to obtain enough tissue to establish a diagnosis without compromising the possibility of future surgical extirpation.

The rarity of these tumors has made the IRSCGC the most commonly used staging system (see Table 14-5), although the TNM system for soft-tissue sarcomas in adults has also been applied by modifying the histologic grading classification (Table 14-6).[87,91] The pathologic evaluation of these tumors typically takes into consideration factors such as necrosis, mitotic activity, cellularity, matrix formation, and pleomorphism. Measures of ploidy and the demonstration of certain molecular genetic abnormalities will undoubtedly prove valuable in guiding prognostically based management protocols in the future.

Table 14-6. American Joint Committee on Cancer Staging protocol of soft-tissue sarcomas

Stage	Grade	Tumor	Nodes	Metastases
IA	1	1	0	0
IB	1	2	0	0
IIA	2	1	0	0
IIB	2	2	0	0
IIIA	3	1	0	0
IIIB	3	2	0	0
IVA	1–3	1–2	1	1
IVB	1–3	1–2	0–1	1

Histologic Grading System:

Grade 1	Grade 2	Grade 3
Myxoid and well-differentiated liposarcomas	Sarcomas not specifically included in grades 1 or 3	Pleomorphic round-cell liposarcoma
Deep-seated dermatofibrosarcoma protuberans		Mesenchymal chondrosarcoma
Well-differentiated fibrosarcoma		Extraskeletal osteosarcoma
Well-differentiated and infantile hemangiopericytoma		Malignant Triton tumors
Well-differentiated peripheral nerve sheath tumor		Alveolar soft-part sarcoma
Extraskeletal myxoid chondrosarcoma		Sarcomas not in grade 1 with >15% necrosis or with >4 mitoses/10 high-power fields (40×)
Angiomatous malignant fibrous histiocytoma		Marked atypia or cellularity

Tumor: 1 = ≤5 cm; 2 = >5 cm.
Nodes: 0—No regional node involvement; 1—Regional nodes involved with tumor.
Metastases: 0—None; 1—Distant disease.

Currently, the most important factors determining the likelihood of cure are histologic grade and tumor resectability.[45] The latter is particularly important for high-grade malignancies. Unfortunately, tumor size and invasiveness preclude complete resection in 30% to 50% of cases, and long-term locoregional control with adjuvant chemoradiotherapy is usually unsuccessful in the presence of either gross residual or metastatic disease (1 of 26 survivors with gross residual or metastatic disease versus 29 of 36 survivors with completely resected tumors or microscopic residual disease). Although the roles of radiotherapy and chemotherapy have not yet been standardized, data from the NCI Pediatric Branch indicate that a substantial number of children may benefit from appropriate intense multimodal therapy. Management of these children should be based on select clinical protocols designed to assess responsiveness and long-term outcome.

Fibrosarcoma

Fibrosarcoma is a rare malignancy of the head and neck, with only 7 of 53 cases (13%) reported by the Armed Forces Institute of Pathology and 22 of 110 cases (20%) reported by Soule and Pritchard.[106] Neck disease occurs most commonly, followed in descending order of frequency by involvement of the oral cavity, scalp, auriculoparotid region, and face.[111] Hematogenous and lymphatic spread are extremely rare.[40]

Children of all ages are affected and typically present with an asymptomatic, slowly enlarging mass.[108] In infants a unique form of congenital fibrosarcoma occurs that is considered a histologically low-grade fibrosarcoma.[101] Although these tumors can be large, the long-term outlook is quite good, perhaps reflecting an enhanced sensitivity to chemotherapeutic agents; some unresectable congenital fibrosarcomas respond to preoperative chemotherapy, permitting a later, less mutilating surgical procedure with clear margins.[15,82] In contrast, fibrosarcoma is more aggressive in older children, survival is lower, and the impact of multimodal therapy is not obvious. Management requires wide local excision to optimize the chances of survival. The absence of a true capsule makes intraoperative assessment of the degree of tumor spread difficult.

The excised mass is typically gray-tan with hemorrhagic and necrotic areas.[27] Comprised mostly of spindle-shaped fibroblasts or myofibroblasts with scanty cytoplasm, histologic grading is possible based on degree of cellularity, cellular maturity, and amount of collagen production (Fig. 14-4). Cytogenetic studies have shown an association with trisomies of chromosomes 8, 11, 17, and 20.[1,67]

Dermatofibrosarcoma protuberans

Dermatofibrosarcoma protuberans is a nodular cutaneous tumor with a high propensity for local recurrence after simple excision. It usually appears as a firm, solitary, flesh-

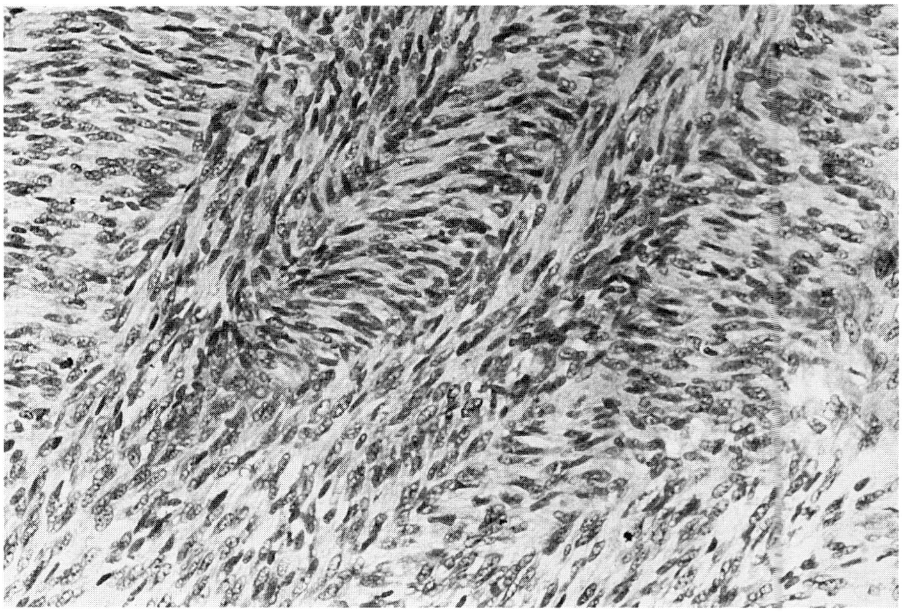

Fig. 14-4. Fibrosarcoma. Discrete fascicles of spindle cells form intersecting patterns, sometimes producing a herringbone effect. (Original magnification, ×200.)

colored nodule although multiple masses or an area of induration can occur. The trunk is the favored site of involvement, followed by the extremities and the head and neck, especially the scalp and supraclavicular fossa.[69]

Approximately 12% of affected persons are older children,[69] but DFSP has been diagnosed in patients under 10 years of age. Time to diagnosis may exceed 2 years, with size at diagnosis up to 2 cm. Management requires wide excision for a successful long-term outcome, reflecting the "pseudocapsule" and finger-like extensions of DFSP. With surgical margins less than 2 cm, recurrence rates approximate 40%; with margins larger than 2 cm, recurrence rates drop to 25%; and with margins larger than 3 cm, few recurrences are reported.[11,96] However, given the regional anatomy of the head and neck, achieving a 2.5- to 3-cm margin can be difficult; even with the Mohs' technique, extensive surgery may be required.[72] Although local recurrence rates of 50% to 70% are reported, with repeated procedures, 90% of affected patients can be rendered free of disease.[5,69]

There is no consensus regarding the cell of origin of DFSP. The primary mass is usually grossly encapsulated and well-circumscribed, although it can send multiple pseudopod-like projections laterally and deeply (3 cm or more).[48] These extensions are easily missed on histologic sectioning. Histologic examination shows elongated cells with a storiform organization (Fig. 14-5).

Epithelioid sarcoma

Epithelioid sarcoma can easily be confused with a variety of benign and malignant conditions such as necrobiotic granuloma, rhabdoid tumor, RMS, and Ki-1 lymphoma.[23,34,47,86] It occurs throughout infancy and early childhood, although most individuals are not diagnosed until the second to fourth decades of life.[56] Approximately 10% of cases involve the head and neck, produce nontender, nonulcerated swelling, and follow a protracted course of repeated local recurrences with eventual distant metastases. More aggressive tumors that metastasize early are uncommon. Once the diagnosis has been made, complete surgical resection should always be attempted because the role and efficacy of chemotherapy and radiotherapy have not been clearly established.

The characteristic histologic pattern is one of nodules separated by fibrous septa (Fig. 14-6). The cells inside the nodules are polygonal, variable in size, and may cluster, suggesting squamous differentiation. Areas of necrosis and an inflammatory infiltrate are common. The molecular biology of epithelioid sarcoma has shown multiple structural changes, most frequently the deletion of 1p21-22.[56]

NEUROBLASTOMAS

Neuroblastomas are the most common extracerebral solid tumors of infancy and childhood.[2] Their annual incidences in white and nonwhite children under 15 years of age are 9 and 4.5 per 1,000,000, respectively.[59,74] Arising from primitive neuroectodermal cells of neural crest origin as embryonal tumors of the sympathetic nervous system, neuroblastomas can develop anywhere sympathetic nervous tissue is found. Primary tumors occur paravertebrally along the sympathetic chain from the neck to the pelvis and from paraganglia from the adrenal medulla, the organ of Zuckerkandl, or the retroperitoneal, inguinal, paratesticular, testicular, oviductal, or ovarian paraganglia. The most unusual aspect of this tumor is the frequent occurrence of spontaneous regression, typically in infants with a small primary tumor, liver involvement, subcutaneous nodules, and patchy bone mar-

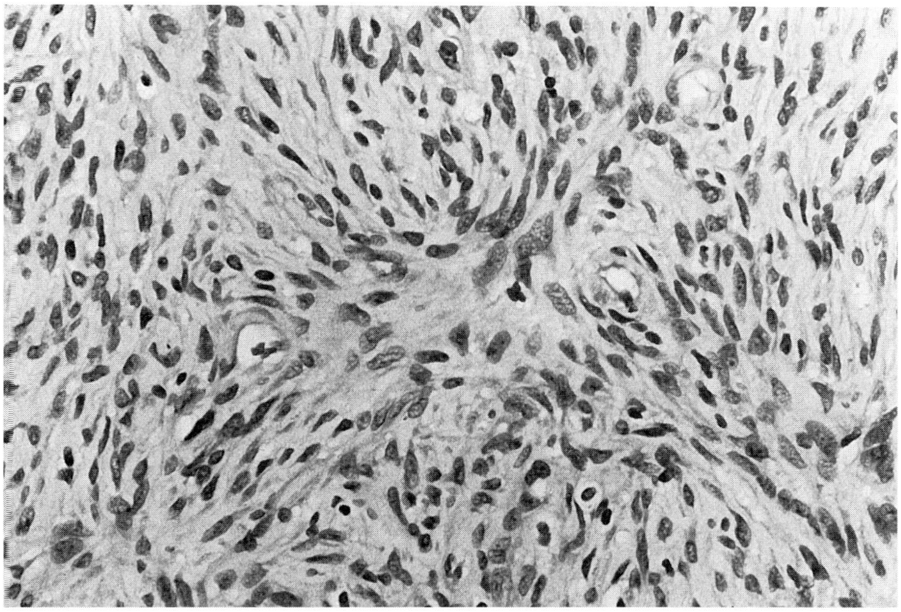

Fig. 14-5. Dermatofibrosarcoma protuberans. This intermediate-grade malignancy is in the group of fibrohistiocytic tumors. Many of the tumors in this group have plump spindle cells arranged in patterns frequently described as cartwheel, whorling or storiform (from the Latin ''storea''—a rush mat'') because of its woven appearance. (Original magnification, ×275.)

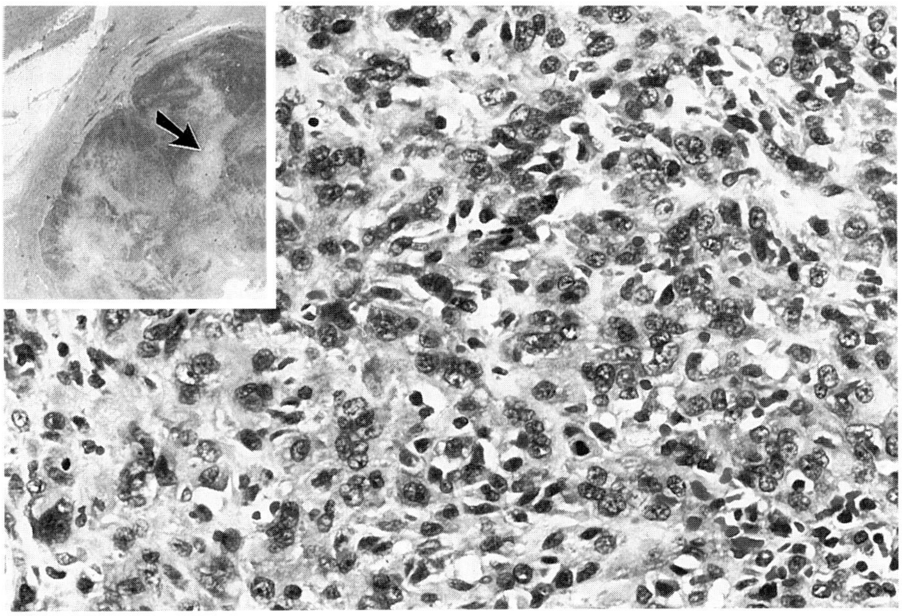

Fig. 14-6. Epithelioid sarcoma. This unusual tumor is composed of epithelial-like cells that have polygonal shaped cytoplasm. Necrosis *(arrow)* in the center of the nodules is characteristic. The lower-power view *(inset)* reveals a distinct nodular appearance. (Original magnification, ×400; low-power inset, original magnification, ×5.)

row infiltration without major replacement of hematopoietic cells.[13]

Presentation and evaluation

Primarily a tumor of infancy and early childhood, as many as 50% of cases are diagnosed in infants under 1 year of age and 80% are detected in children younger than 5.[104] Presenting signs and symptoms depend on the site of the primary lesion, the presence and site of metastases, and the secretion of hormones and vasoactive substances. The most common site of origin is the adrenal medulla or adjacent retroperitoneum, but 2% to 5% of neuroblastomas develop in the head and neck region.

Primary cervical tumors are generally detected at an earlier age and at a lower stage than tumors detected elsewhere, reflecting the greater facility with which abnormalities in the neck are recognized. Laryngotracheal or pharyngeal compression can lead to airway obstruction, dysphagia, or aspiration. Ipsilateral ptosis occurs if the superior cervical ganglion is involved. Primary neuroblastoma of the orbit may cause proptosis, periorbital ecchymoses (panda eyes), and ocular muscle paresis, although more subtle findings

Table 14-7. Clinical criteria for staging of neuroblastoma

Stage	Evans	Stage	Pinkel/St. Jude
I	Confined to the organ or structure of origin	I	Localized, completely resected tumor
II	Extension in continuity beyond the organ or structure of origin but not crossing the midline	IIA	Localized, resected tumor with residual microscopic disease
		IIB	Localized tumor partially or not resected
III	Extension in continuity beyond the midline	IIIA	Regional or systemic spread of disease without involvement of bone or bone marrow
IV	Remote disease (skeleton, organs, soft tissue, distant lymph node groups)	IIIB	Same as IIIA with single, localized destructive lesion of bone
IV-S	Otherwise class I or II except for remote disease confined to the liver, skin, and/or bone marrow	IIIC	Generalized tumor in bone, bone marrow, or both

such as edema of the conjunctivae or eyelids, papilledema, and retinal hemorrhage may occur. Because the sympathetic nervous system is intimately associated with the development and maintenance of eye color, heterochromia irides is possible.[51] Another finding peculiar to the head and neck is the cardiofacial syndrome or ''asymmetric crying face.'' This type of congenital facial weakness becomes most apparent with crying and reflects disease involvement of the motor cortex, the nucleus or peripheral root cranial nerve VII, or the muscles of facial expression.[61]

Paraspinal neuroblastoma may extend through adjacent intervertebral foramina into the spinal cord (''en sablier'' tumors) to produce paraplegia. Although this finding is most commonly associated with mediastinal and retroperitoneal tumors, it also occurs with cervical disease.[89,109] Neuroblastoma is also a noteworthy cause of congenital paraparesis, although clinical features of neurologic dysfunction in neonates are difficult to recognize and diagnosis may be delayed.

The diagnostic and metastatic evaluation of children with neuroblastoma of the head and neck requires multiple imaging studies, immunocytochemistry studies, routine histology, and cytogenetic analysis. For suspected cervical disease, CT and MRI to evaluate the neck should be complemented by abdominal CT and MRI, intravenous pyelography, bone scans, and liver–spleen scans to appropriately stage the tumor. The staging system created by Evans is most widely used,[35,36] although a TNM staging system was proposed in 1982.[44] Both systems are based on clinical experience with neuroblastoma and reflect the degree of tumor burden, surgical resectability, and the pattern of metastatic spread (Tables 14-7 and 14-8).

Tumor markers such as catecholamine metabolites, ferritin, neuron-specific enolase, and the ganglioside GM_2 are helpful in diagnosis and disease monitoring.[13] The frequency of abnormal elevations depends on disease burden and therefore hampers detection of neuroblastoma at an early stage. Certain cutoff levels of ferritin and neuron-specific enolase can be used, but both of these markers are quite nonspecific. Catecholamines and their metabolites (vanillylmandelic acid, homovanillic acid, and dopamine) are elevated in 80% to 85% of children with neuroblastoma and have been very successfully developed by the Japanese for use in urine screening programs despite high false-negative rates.[100] Tests on 115,000 infants suggest that the majority of neuroblastomas can be discovered before the age of 1 year, when prognosis is most favorable.[100]

Table 14-8. TMN clinical criteria for staging of neuroblastoma

Stage	Criteria
I	Primary tumor ≤5 cm; no evidence of regional node disease; no evidence of distant disease
II	Primary tumor >5 but ≤10 cm; no evidence of regional node disease; no evidence of distant disease
III	Stage I or II with evidence of regional node disease or primary tumor >10 cm ± regional node disease; no evidence of distant disease
IV	Primary single tumor ± regional node disease; evidence of distant metastases
V	Multicentric tumors ± regional node disease ± distant metastases

TMN Postsurgical clinical criteria for staging of neuroblastoma

Stage	Criteria
I	Complete excision, margins free; lymph nodes negative or not assessed; no evidence of distant disease
II	Complete excision, margins free; lymph nodes positive, involved nodes resected or extent of involvement not assessed; no evidence of distant disease
IIIA	Microscopic residual disease
IIIB	Macroscopic residual disease or complete resection with evidence of lymph node disease and incomplete resection of involved nodes
IV	Evidence of distant metastases
V	Multicentric tumor

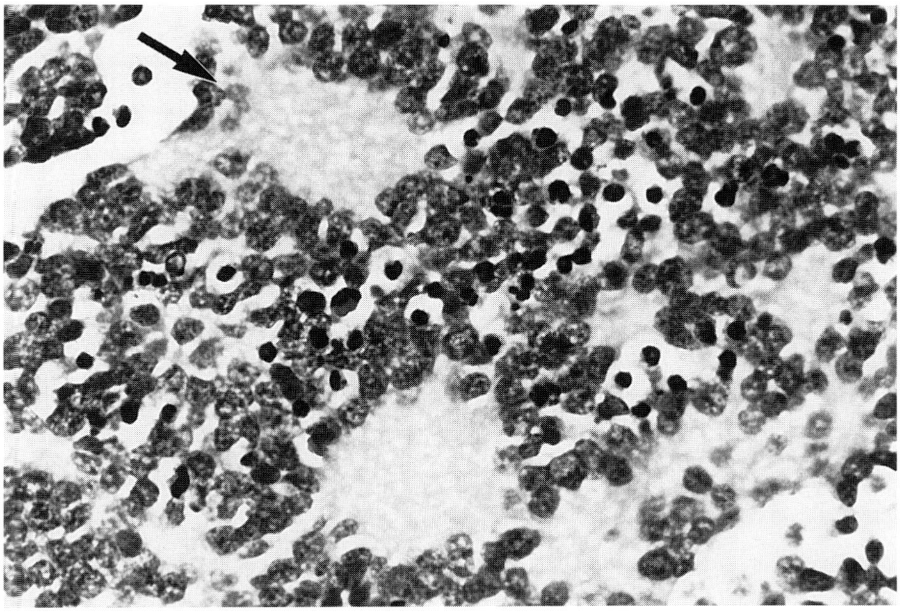

Fig. 14-7. Neuroblastoma. Small blue cells characterize this neoplasm. The differential diagnosis of ''small blue-cell'' tumors in children also includes lymphoma and peripheral neuroectodermal/tumor Ewing's sarcoma. Other tumors can also be considered in this group. Neuroblastoma can be differentiated by its relatively uniform cell appearance and neurofibrillary material between the cells. Pseudorosettes (Homer-Wright) are illustrated *(arrow)*, but are often not seen. Immunohistochemical marking and electron microscopy can be useful to demonstrate neural-associated proteins or neural-associated structures (e.g., neurosecretory granules). (Original magnification, ×425.)

Management

Management of neuroblastoma is determined by the stage of disease and sites of involvement. In the head and neck, surgical intervention most commonly implies excisional biopsy. A cervical sympathetic ganglion is usually involved and is resected. Adjacent, enlarged nodes should also be removed, although a formal radical neck dissection is not required.[81] In cases in which complete resection would cause unacceptable morbidity, a second surgical procedure can be planned 12 to 24 weeks following completion of chemotherapy.[105] Unfortunately, despite the large number of chemotherapeutic agents that are active in newly diagnosed patients, long-term remission remains elusive for children over 1 year of age with International Neuroblastoma Staging System stage IV disease (approximately 45% of all children with neuroblastoma).

Histopathology and molecular biology

Grossly, neuroblastoma is a discrete solid mass with well-circumscribed contours. Coagulative necrosis may develop in nonviable areas, sometimes with dystrophic calcification. Microscopically, the tumor represents one of the ''small blue-cell'' neoplasms of childhood that is exquisitely susceptible to smear or crush artifact. Iatrogenic damage may obscure cytologic details, making it difficult to make an unequivocal histologic diagnosis.[31] The prototype neuroblastoma is composed of small uniform cells that are 7 to 10 μm in diameter and have dense hyperchromatic nuclei with minimal perinuclear cytoplasm. Immunohistochemistry has revolutionized diagnostic histopathology, and a battery of selected antibodies is used to evaluate specific cellular and subcellular aspects of these neoplasms (Fig. 14-7).

Molecular biology has also impacted diagnosis and management protocols. Deletions in the short arm of chromosome 1 (1p36) are the most common structural aberration and identify children with a poor prognosis.[2] A less frequent abnormality is amplification of the *N-myc* oncogene.[16,17] This event is associated with advanced stages of disease and rapid tumor progression, perhaps because amplification usually accompanies 1p deletions. The effect of ploidy is more controversial. Diploid and tetraploid neuroblastomas tend to be associated with unfavorable structural aberrations (like 1p36 deletions) and gene amplification (like *N-myc*) more often than do triploid neuroblastomas.[13,20]

Many of the favorable genetic findings, (e.g., triploidy, lack of *N-myc* amplification, and presence of 1p heterozygosity) correlate with favorable histologic findings as indicated by the presence of ganglionic cells and abundant Schwann-cell stroma. The converse also is true. Diploid or tetraploid tumors with 1p deletions do not show spontaneous development of Schwann-cell stroma.[2]

The clinical implication of these studies is that infants with stage I, II, or IV-S disease in addition to 1p deletions, *N-myc* amplification, and diploidy or tetraploidy are at high risk for recurrence and require aggressive therapy at diagnosis. Management failures appear to be due to the development of multidrug resistance associated with overexpression of *MRP* (multidrug-resistance–associated protein), even when a diverse range of structurally and functionally unrelated chemotherapeutic agents is used.[83]

Based on advances in the molecular biology of neuroblastoma, priorities for future trials will include defining subsets of children who do not require therapy, improving durability of remissions for disseminated disease by exploiting cytokines for dose intensification, defining the place of autologous bone marrow transplantation, exploring means for reversing drug resistance, evaluating tumor-targeted radiotherapy, and identifying new active chemotherapeutic agents. By evaluating biologic response modifiers, it may be possible to impact the biologic determinants of tumor initiation, progression, and spontaneous regression.

SALIVARY GLAND MALIGNANCIES

Childhood malignancies of the salivary glands are rare. In a review of 2135 children under 16 years of age who developed salivary gland tumors, only 17 (0.79%) malignancies were recorded (15 [0.7%] mucoepidermoid and 2 [0.09%] acinar cell carcinomas).[21] Most of these malignancies involved the parotid gland. Other authors have confirmed this bias, and from an overview of nine different studies, Rasp and Permanetter[92] concluded that the parotid gland is the favored site (88.5%), followed by the submandibular gland (7.7%), the minor salivary glands (3.3%), and the sublingual gland (0.5%). A unique feature of these tumors is that most appear to be induced by radiation.[55]

Presentation and evaluation

Children with salivary gland malignancies are usually in their second decade of life at diagnosis. The majority also are survivors of another malignancy, most frequently acute lymphoblastic leukemia diagnosed 10 years earlier for which cranial radiotherapy was required.[95] Chemotherapy, age at the time of therapy, and genetic susceptibility are additional risk factors that may contribute to the development of secondary salivary gland malignancies.[55]

Regardless of location, the most common presentation is as an asymptomatic mass, although facial nerve involvement occasionally accompanies parotid gland disease.[95] The presence of cervical adenopathy does not imply metastatic disease; it more likely reflects common childhood reactive hyperplasia seen as a sequela of repeated upper-respiratory infections. Evaluation by CT and MRI is helpful to delineate tumor boundaries and for planning surgical resection.

Management

Salivary gland malignancies in children should be excised. Although the primary principle of surgical excision is accepted, however, the extent of the procedure and the value of multimodal therapy are not as clearly defined. For parotid gland disease, subtotal parotidectomy is required, and unless tumor invasion dictates otherwise, the facial nerve should be spared. Complete excision should also be the goal for tumors of the submandibular, sublingual, and minor salivary glands. Radiotherapy is reserved for children with high- or intermediate-grade malignancies of the major salivary glands and high-grade malignancies of the minor salivary glands. Its value as adjuvant therapy in intermediate-grade tumors of the soft palate is debatable.

Histopathology and molecular biology

Mucoepidermoid and acinic cell carcinomas account for 60% of childhood salivary gland malignancies (45% and 15%, respectively),[65] although the former is the only type that has been diagnosed in the intraoral salivary glands.[41,112] Mucoepidermoid carcinomas are usually low-grade and are seldom fatal (Fig. 14-8), whereas acinic cell carcinomas behave like their adult counterparts (Fig. 14-9). Probably the only epithelial salivary gland tumor unique to children is the embryoma.[10] Recognized only in newborns or during the first year of life, this malignancy is morphologically similar to stages in the development of the embryonic anlage of salivary gland tissue. Fewer than one quarter show either biologic or histologic signs of malignancy, and complete surgical excision is curative.[10]

TERATOMAS

Teratomas are the most common extragonadal germ-cell tumors of childhood. They arise most commonly in a midline or paraaxial location from the brain to the sacral area and involve the head and neck once in every 40,000 births.[58] In this region, sites of involvement include the soft tissues of the neck (cervical teratomas), superficial facial structures in and about the temporal fossa and zygomatic area, oral cavity, oronasopharynx, and orbit.[7]

Presentation and evaluation

Over 75% of cervical teratomas are diagnosed in neonates, two thirds of whom have respiratory distress significant enough to cause stridor.[53] Hydramnios, stillbirth, and premature labor are other frequent accompaniments.[7] This information, in addition to age at diagnosis and respiratory ability, was used by Jordan and Gauderer[53] to define five different disease types (Table 14-9). The high mortality rate in the adult group (type V) reflects the correspondingly high rate of malignant transformation. In contrast, death in neonates usually results from respiratory obstruction due to lesion bulk and location. Malignant degeneration is much less common, although it does occur.

Rothschild and others[97] described seven neonates with teratomas that metastasized to the cervical nodes, lungs, and liver. The metastatic deposits were composed of either mature glial tissue or a mixture of mature and immature elements. Differentiation suggests that the presence of metastases does not necessarily portend a bleak prognosis[9]—an impression also supported by Rothschild and others,[97] who found that in only one patient with metastases was death secondary to metastatic disease. Benign teratomas arising in the paranasal sinuses are extremely rare, and all of the malignant lesions of the sinonasal tract have occurred in adults.[7]

Management

The recommended management for head and neck teratomas is surgical excision. When a neonate is experiencing respiratory difficulty, the first priority should be stabilization of the airway.

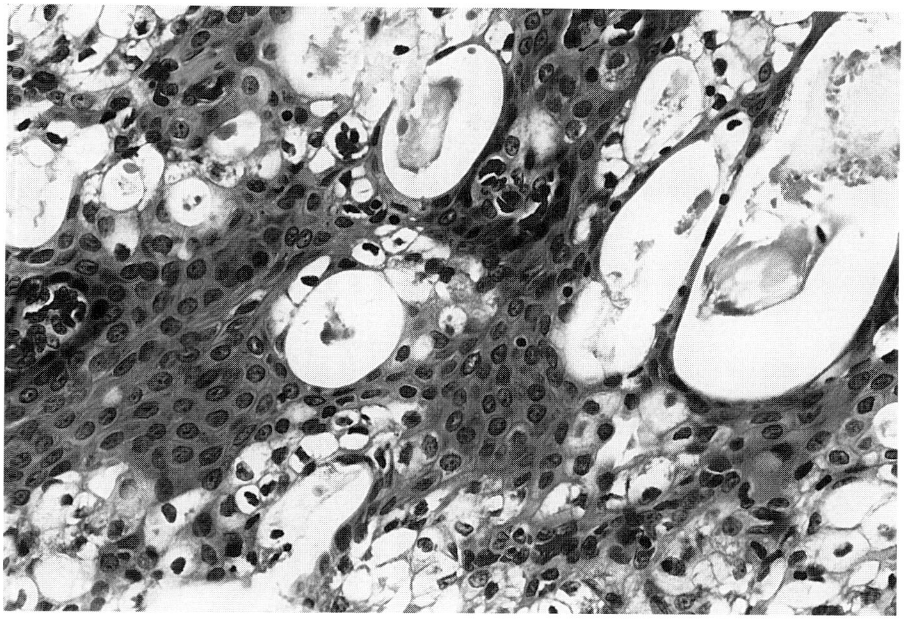

Fig. 14-8. Mucoepidermoid carcinoma. Mucus-producing and squamous tumor cells are the prime histologic components of mucoepidermoid carcinomas. Mucus cells containing rounded intracytoplasmic mucus droplets are evident along with pavement-like squamous cells with distinct cellular boundaries. Larger cysts containing mucus are also present. (Original magnification, ×320.)

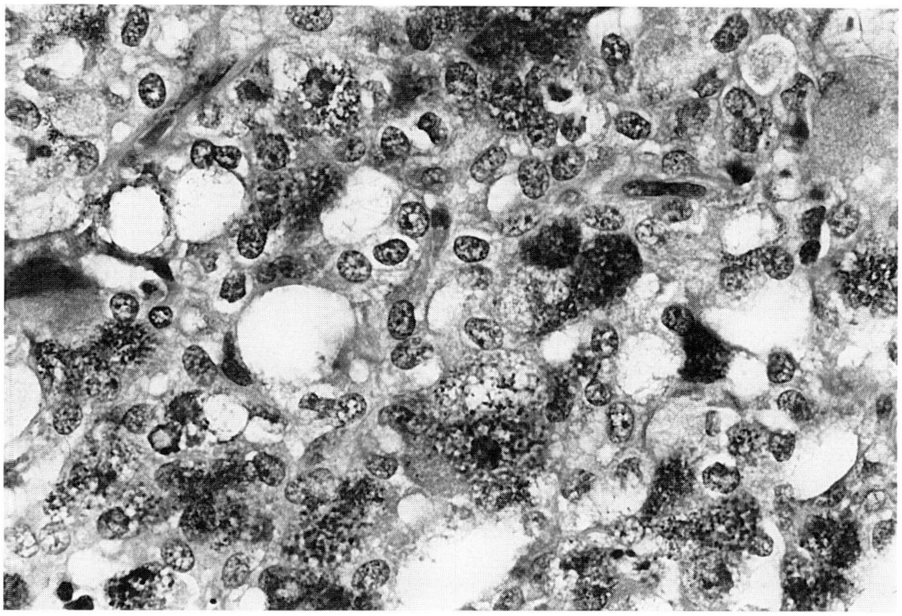

Fig. 14-9. Acinic cell carcinoma. Tumor cells appear similar histologically to normal acinar unit cells, but their lack of arrangement of organization into functional units helps in differentiation. These cells have a granular appearance, and some show large basophilic granules. Microcystic changes are seen in this case. (Original magnification, ×420.)

Histopathology and molecular biology

Teratomas in neonates and infants contain tridermic tissue elements. Although the preponderant tissue is most often neuroepithelium, other tissues that can be involved include fetal cartilage, myogenic tissue, and epithelium (squamous, ciliated, columnar, enteric, and endocrine). In type II and III teratomas, malignancy is not equated with the degree of immaturity of the tissue elements and instead reflects immaturity of the host[7] (Fig. 14-10).

SEQUELAE OF MANAGEMENT

The morbidity of managing head and neck cancers in children must be measured not over a 5- to 10-year interval but over a lifetime of 70+ years. As cure rates improve, therapy must be refined to optimize growth potential and fertility and minimize the risk of second malignancies without sacrificing the primary goal of tumor eradication. The immediate sequelae of radiotherapy to the head and neck are similar in both children and adults. Acutely, mucositis,

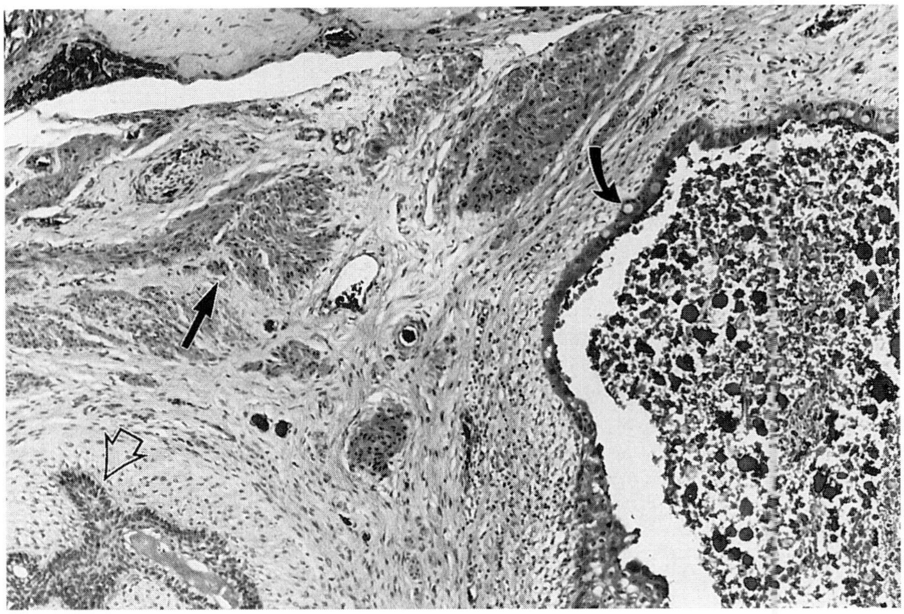

Fig. 14-10. Teratoma. Multiple cell types in a haphazard arrangement are evident in this low-power view showing squamous cells *(open arrow)*, mucus-containing goblet cells *(curved arrow)* lining a cyst, and smooth muscle cells *(solid straight arrow)*. (Original magnification, ×50.)

Table 14-9. Teratoma types

Type*	Cases (%)	Hydramnios (%)	Mortality (%)
I	12.4	56	100
II	45.6	23	43.4
III	17.1	8.1	2.7
IV	14.3	—	3.2
V	10.6	—	43.5

* I—Moribund neonate or stillborn infant; II—Neonate with respiratory distress; III—Neonate without respiratory distress; IV—Child 1 month to 18 years of age; V—Adult.

otitis externa, and alopecia are common; subacutely, somnolence develops in about one third of children who receive whole-brain radiation. Transient demyelination can also occur and lead to a sensation of electric shocks at various levels below the neck that are elicited by flexion of the head or torso (Lhermitte's syndrome). Late effects include problems with transverse myelopathy, sensorineural hearing loss, endocrinopathies, and normal development of irradiated structures.[54]

Most disheartening of all is the possibility of another malignancy. This risk is not insubstantial: Children who have survived one malignancy are 10 to 20 times more likely to develop another cancer than is the general population.[75] Contributing factors include radiotherapy, chemotherapy, age at treatment, and genetic susceptibility. Especially vulnerable are children previously treated for retinoblastoma and survivors of HL who receive mantle irradiation. Reported tumors include acute leukemias, bone and soft-tissue sarcomas, and carcinomas of the skin, breast, thyroid, and salivary glands.[55]

Most radiation-induced second neoplasms occur more than 15 years after management of the first. Unfortunately, as length of follow-up increases, so too does risk.[66] Among chemotherapeutic agents, cyclophosphamide has been implicated in the development of solid tumors, and etoposide, an epipodophyllotoxin that acts by inhibiting the enzyme topoisomerase II, has been implicated in the development of second leukemias. The sobering reality is that the management of primary malignancies of the head and neck in children is extremely toxic, and the burden of a successful outcome can be immense. Addressing these issues remains the challenge for the twenty-first century.

REFERENCES

1. Adam LR and others: Cytogenetic analysis of a congenital fibrosarcoma, *Cancer Genet Cytogenet* 52:37, 1991.
2. Ambros IM and others: Role of ploidy, chromosome 1p, and Schwann cells in the maturation of neuroblastoma, *N Engl J Med* 334:1505, 1996.
3. Bader SB and others: Pediatric stage IV Hodgkin disease, *Cancer* 72: 249, 1993.
4. Baker LL and others: Staging of Hodgkin's disease in children: comparison of CT and lymphography with laparotomy, *Am J Roentgenol* 154:1251, 1990.
5. Barnes L, Coleman J, Johnson J: Dermatofibrosarcoma protuberans of the head and neck, *Arch Otolaryngol Head Neck Surg* 10:398, 1984.
6. Barr FG and others: In vivo amplification of the PAX3-FKHR and PAX7-FKHR fusion genes in alveolar rhabdomyosarcoma, *Hum Mol Genet* 5:15, 1996.
7. Batsakis JG: Teratomas of the head and neck with emphasis on malignancy, *Ann Otol Rhinol Laryngol* 104:496, 1995.
8. Batsakis JG: *Tumors of the head and neck: clinical and pathological considerations*, Baltimore, 1974, Williams & Wilkins
9. Batsakis JG, Littler ER, Oberman HA: Teratomas of the neck: a clinicopathologic appraisal, *Arch Otolaryngol Head Neck Surg* 79:619, 1964.

10. Batsakis JG and others: Perinatal salivary gland tumors (embryomas), *J Laryngol Otol* 102:1007, 1988.
11. Bendix-Hansen K, Myhre-Jensen O, Kaae S: Dermatofibrosarcoma protuberans: a clinicopathological study of nineteen cases and a review of the world literature, *Scand J Plast Reconstr Surg* 17:247, 1983.
12. Bennett JM and others: Age and Hodgkin's disease: the impact of competing risks and possibly salvage therapy on long term survival: an E.C.O.G. study, *Leukemia Research* 17:825, 1993.
13. Berthold F: *Incidence and overview*. In Pochedly C, editor: *Neuroblastoma: tumor biology and therapy*, Boca Raton, 1990, CRC Press.
14. Blackwood EM, Eisenman RN: Max: a helix-loop-helix zipper protein the forms a sequence-specific DNA-ginding complex with Myc, *Science* 251:1211, 1991.
15. Brock P and others: Infantile fibrosarcoma, *Med Pediatr Oncol* 19: 210, 1991 (letter).
16. Brodeur GM and others: Molecular analysis and clinical significance of N-myc amplification and chromosome 1p monosomy in human neuroblastomas, *Prog Clin Biol Res* 271:3, 1988.
17. Brodeur GM, Seeger RC: Gene amplification in human neuroblastomas: basic mechanism and clinical implications, *Cancer Genet Cytogenet* 19:101, 1986.
18. Butler JJ, Pugh WC: Review of Hodgkin's disease, *Hematol Pathol* 7:59, 1993.
19. Carbone PP and others: Report of the committee on Hodgkin's disease staging classification, *Cancer Res* 31:1860, 1971.
20. Caron H and others: Allelic loss of chromosome 1p as a predictor of unfavorable outcome in patients with neuroblastoma, *N Engl J Med* 334:225, 1996.
21. Castro EB and others: Tumors of the major salivary glands in children, *Cancer* 29:312, 1972.
22. Charache H: Hodgkin's disease in children. *N Y State J Med* 46:507, 1946.
23. Chase DR and others: Keratin in epithelioid sarcomas: an immunohistochemical study, *Am J Surg Pathol* 8:435, 1984.
24. Chilcote RR, Brown E, Rowley JD: Lymphoblastic leukemia with lymphomatous features associated with abnormalities of the short arm of chromosome 9, *N Engl J Med* 313:286, 1985.
25. Cleary SF, Link MP, Donaldson SS: Hodgkin's disease in the very young, *Int J Radiat Oncol Biol Phys* 28:77.
26. Coene MJH and others: Rhabdomyosarcoma of the head and neck in children, *Clin Otolaryngol* 17:291, 1992.
27. Coffin CM, Dehner LP: Fibroblastic-myofibroblastic tumors in children and adolescents: a clinicopathologic study of 108 examples in 103 patients, *Pediatr Pathol* 11:559, 1991.
28. Crist W and others: The third intergroup rhabdomyosarcoma study, *J Clin Oncol* 13:610, 1995.
29. Crist WM, Kelly DR, Radab AH: Predictive ability of Lukes-Collins classification for immunologic phenotypes of childhood non-Hodgkin's lymphoma: an institutional series and literature review, *Cancer* 48:2070, 1981.
30. Dalla-Favera R and others: Human c-myc onc gene is located on the region of chromosome 8 that is translocated in Burkitt lymphoma cells, *Proc Natl Acad Sci U S A* 79:7824, 1982.
31. Dehner LP: *Histiogenesis and histopathology of neuroblastoma*. In Pochedly C, editor: *Neuroblastoma: tumor biology and therapy*, Boca Raton, 1990, CRC Press.
32. Donaldson SS, Link MP: *Childhood lymphomas: Hodgkin's disease and non-Hodgkin's lymphoma*. In Mossa AR, Robson MC, Schimpff SC, editors: *Comprehensive textbook of oncology*, ed 2, Baltimore, 1991, William & Wilkins.
33. Downing JR and others: Molecular detection of (2;5) translocation of non-Hodgkin's lymphoma by reverse transcriptase-polymerase chain reaction, *Blood* 85:3416, 1995.
34. Enzinger FM: Epithelioid sarcoma: a sarcoma simulating a granuloma or a carcinoma, *Cancer* 26:1029, 1970.
35. Evans AE and others: Factors influencing survival of children with nonmetastatic neuroblastoma, *Cancer* 38:661, 1976.
36. Evans AE, D'Angio GJ, Randolph J: A proposed staging for children with neuroblastoma, *Cancer* 27:374, 1971.
37. Farber S, Diamond LK, Mercer RD: Temporary remissions in acute leukemia in children produced by folic acid antagonist 4-aminopteroylglutamic acid (aminopterin), *N Engl J Med* 238:787, 1948.
38. Flamant F, Hill H: The improvement in survival associated with combined chemotherapy in childhood rhabdomyosarcoma: a historical comparison of 345 patients in the same center, *Cancer* 53:2417, 1984.
39. Gasparini M and others: Questionable role of CNS radioprophylaxis in the therapeutic management of childhood rhabdomyosarcoma with meningeal extension, *J Clin Oncol* 8:1854, 1990.
40. Greager JA and others: Fibrosarcoma of the head and neck, *Am J Surg* 167:437, 1994.
41. Gustafsson H and others: Mucoepidermoid carcinoma in minor salivary glands in childhood, *J Laryngol Otol* 101:1320, 1987.
42. Gutierrez ME and others: Molecular epidemiology of Burkitt's lymphoma from South America: differences in breakpont location and Epstein-Barr virus association from tumors in other world regions, *Blood* 79:3261, 1992.
43. Halperin EC and others: *Hodgkin's disease*. In *Pediatric radiation concology*, New York, 1989, Raven Press.
44. Harmer MH, editor: *International union against cancer: TNM classification of malignant tumors*, ed 3, Geneva, 1982, International Union Against Cancer.
45. Hayani A and others: Soft-tissue sarcomas other than rhabdomyosarcoma in children, *Med Pediatr Oncol* 20:114, 1992.
46. Healy GB and others: The role of surgery in rhabdomyosarcoma of the head and neck in children, *Arch Otolaryngol Head Neck Surg* 117:1185, 1991.
47. Hedley DW and others: Method for analysis of cellular DNA content of paraffin-embedded pathological material using flow cytometry, *J Histochem Cytochem* 31:1333, 1983.
48. Hobbs ER and others: Treatment of dermatofibrosarcoma protuberans with Mohs micrographis surgery, *Ann Surg* 207:102, 1988.
49. Horn RC, Enterline HT: Rhabdomyosarcoma: a clinicopathological study and classification of 39 cases, *Cancer* 11:181, 1958.
50. Hsu S and others: Cytokines in malignant lymphomas: a review and prospective evaluation, *Hum Pathol* 24:1040, 1993.
51. Jaffe N and others: Heterochromia and Horner syndrome associated with cervical and mediastinal neuroblastoma, *J Pediatr* 87:75, 1975.
52. Jenkin RDT, Peters MV, Darte JMM: Hodgkin's disease in children, *Am J Roentgenol* 100:222, 1967.
53. Jordan RB, Gauderer MWL: Cervical teratomas: an analysis. Literature review and proposed classification, *J Pediatr Surg* 23:583, 1988.
54. Kao GD, Willi SM, Goldwein J. The sequelae of chemo-radiation therapy for head and neck cancer in children: managing impaired growth, development, and other side effects, *Med Pediatr Oncol* 21: 60, 1993.
55. Kaste SC, Hedlund G, Pratt CB: Malignant parotid tumors in patients previously treated for childhood cancer: clinical and imaging findings in eight cases, *Am J Roentgenol* 162:655, 1994.
56. Kodet R and others: Epithelioid sarcoma in childhood: an immunohistochemical, electron microscopic, and clinicopathologic study of 11 cases under 15 years of age and review of the literature, *Pediatr Pathol* 14:433, 1994.
57. Koscielniak E and others: Metastatic rhabdomyosarcoma and histiologically similar tumors in childhood: a retrospective European multicenter analysis, *Med Pediatr Oncol* 20:209, 1992.
58. Kountakis SE and others: Teratomas of the head and neck, *Am J Otolaryngol* 15:292, 1994.
59. Kramer S and others: Incidence of childhood cancer: experience of a decade in a population-based registry, *J Natl Cancer Inst* 70:49, 1983.
60. Kuppers R and others: Hodgkin disease: Hodgkin and Reed-Sternberg

cells picked from histological sections show clonal immunoglobulin gene rearrangements and appear to be derived from B cells at various stages of development, *Proc Natl Acad Sci U S A* 91:10962, 1994.
61. Lenarsky C and others: Occurrence of neuroblastoma and asymmetric crying facies: case report and review of the literature, *J Pediatr* 107: 268, 1985.
62. Leventhal BG, Donaldson SS: *Hodgkin's disease.* In Pizzo PA, Poplack, DG editors: *Principles and practice of pediatric oncology*, ed 2, Philadelphia, 1993, JB Lippincott.
63. Lister TA and others: Report of a committee convened to discuss the evaluation and staging of patients with Hodgkin's disease: Cotswold Meeting, *J Clin Oncol* 7:1630, 1989.
64. Lukens JN: Progress resulting from clinical trials solid tumors in childhood cancer, *Cancer* 74:2710, 1994.
65. Luna MA, Batsakis JG, El-Naggar AK: Pathology consultation salivary gland tumors in children, *Ann Otol Rhinol Laryngol* 100:869, 1991.
66. Maisel RH, Case M: Squamous cell carcinoma after childhood radiation to the nasopharynx, *Otolaryngol Head Neck Surg* 107:783, 1992.
67. Mandahl N and others: Nonrandom numerical chromosome aberrations (+8, −11, +17, +20) in infantile fibrosarcoma, *Cancer Genet Cytogenet* 40:137, 1989.
68. Manzanal A and others: Evaluation of clonal heavy chain rearrangements in Hodgkin's disease using the polymerase chain reaction (PCR), *Histopathology* 27:21, 1995.
69. Mark RJ and others: Dermatofibrosarcoma protuberans of the head and neck, *Arch Otolaryngol Head Neck Surg* 119:891, 1993.
70. Mauch P, Goodman R, Hellman S: The significance of mediastinal involvement in early stage Hodgkin's disease, *Cancer* 42:1039, 1978.
71. Maurer HM and others: The Intergroup Rhabdomyosarcoma Study-II, *Cancer* 71:1904, 1993.
72. McPeak CJ, Cruz T, Nicastri AD: Dermatofibrosarcoma protuberans: an analysis of 86 cases, five with metastasis, *Ann Surg* 166:803, 1967.
73. Mecucci C, Van Den Berghe H: OKT8-Positive T-cell lymphoma associated with a chromosome rearrangement t(2;17) possibly involving the T8 locus, *N Engl J Med* 313:185, 1985.
74. Michaelis J, Kaatsch P: Cooperative documentation of childhood malignancies in the FRG: system design and five-year resuls, *Mongr Paediatr* 18:56, 1986.
75. Mike V, Meadows AT, D'Angio GJ: Incidence of second malignant neoplasms in children: results of an international study, *Lancet* 2: 1326, 1982.
76. Miller BA and others: Cancer statistics review: 1973-1988, NIH Report No 92-2789, 1992, National Cancer Institute.
77. Morris SW and others: Fusion of a kinase gene, ALK, to a nucleolar protein gene NPM in non-Hodgkin's lymphoma, *Science* 267:316, 1995.
78. Murphy SB: Classification, staging and end results of treatment of childhood non-Hodgkin's lymphomas: similarities and differences from lymphomas in adults, *Semin Oncol* 7:332, 1980.
79. Murphy SB and others: Non-Hodgkin's lymphomas of childhood: an analysis of the histology, staging and response to treatment of 338 cases at a single institution, *J Clin Oncol* 7:186, 1989.
80. Nag S, Grecula J, Ruymann FB: Aggresive chemotherapy, organ-preserving surgery, and high-dose-rate remote brachytherapy in the treatment of rhabdomyosarcoma in infants and young children, *Cancer* 72:2769, 1993.
81. Ninane J and others: Stage II neuroblastoma: adverse prognostic significance of lymph node involvement, *Arch Dis Child* 57:438, 1982.
82. Ninane J, Rombouts JJ, Cornu G: Chemotherapy for infantile fibrosarcoma, *Med Pediatr Oncol* 19:209, 1991 (letter).
83. Norris MD and others: Expression of the gene for multidrug-resistance-associated protein and outcome in patients with neuroblastoma, *N Engl J Med* 334:231, 1996.
84. Packham G, Cleveland JL: Ornithine decarboxylase is a mediator of c-Myc-induced apoptosis, *Mol Cell Biol* 14:5741, 1994.
85. Pappo AS and others: Biology and therapy of pediatric rhabdomyosarcoma, *J Clin Oncol* 13:2123, 1995.
86. Patterson JW: Rheumatoid nodule and subcutaneous granuloma annulare: a comparative histologic study, *Am J Dermatopathol* 10:1, 1988.
87. Peabody TD, Simon MA: Principles of staging of soft-tissue sarcomas, *Clin Orthop* 289:19, 1993.
88. Prendergast GC, Lawe D, Ziff EB: Association of Myn, the murine homolog of Max, with c-Myc stimulates methylation-sensitive DNA binding and ras co-transformation, *Cell* 65:395, 1991
89. Punt J and others: Neuroblastoma: a review of 21 cases presenting with spinal cord compression, *Cancer* 42:3095, 1980.
90. Rabbitts TH: Chromosomal translocations in human cancer, *Nature* 372:143, 1994.
91. Rao BN and others: Pediatric nonrhabdomyosarcomas of the extremities: influence of size, invasiveness, and grade on outcome, *Arch Surg* 126:1490, 1991.
92. Rasp G, Permanetter W: Malignant salivary gland tumors: squamous cell carcinoma of the submandibular gland in a child, *Am J Otolaryngol* 13:109, 1992.
93. Razzouk BI and others: Epstein-Barr virus DNA recombination and loss in sporadic Burkitt's lymphoma, *J Infect Dis* 173:529, 1996.
94. Robison LL: *General principle of the epidemiology of childhood cancer.* In Pizzo PA, Poplack DG, editors: *Principles and practice of pediatric oncology*, ed 2, Philadelphia, 1993, JB Lippincott.
95. Rogers D and others: Primary malignancy of the salivary gland in children, *J Pediatr Surg* 29:44, 1994.
96. Roses DR and others: Surgical treatment of dermatofibrosarcoma protuberans, *Surg Gynecol Obstet* 162:449, 1986.
97. Rothschild MA and others: Evaluation of management of congenital cervical teratoma: case report and review, *Arch Otolaryngol Head Neck Surg* 120:444, 1994.
98. Sandlund JT, Downing JR, Crist WM: Non-Hodgkin's lymphoma in childhood, *N Engl J Med* 334:1238, 1996.
99. Sandlund JT and others: Clinicopathologic features and treatment outcome of children with large-cell lymphoma and the t(2;5) (p23;q35), *Blood* 84:2467, 1994.
100. Sawada T and others: Number and cure rate of neuroblastoma cases detected by the mass screening program in Japan: future aspects, *Med Pediatr Oncol* 15:14, 1987.
101. Schofield DE and others: Fibrosarcoma in infants and children: application of new techniques, *Am J Surg Pathol* 18:14, 1994.
102. Schwab M, Amler LC: Amplification of cellular oncogenes: a predictor of clinical outcome in human cancer, *Genes Chromosom Cancer* 1:181, 1990.
103. Siegel SE, Jenkin D, Wilson J: *Long-term survival in childhood non-Hodgkin's lymphoma.* In Burchenal JH, Oettgen HF, editors: *Cancer: achievements, challenges and prospects for the 1980s*, vol 2, New York, 1981, Grune & Stratton.
104. Smith RJH, Katz CD: *Neuroblastoma of the head and neck.* In Pochedly C, editor: *Neuroblastoma: tumor biology and therapy*, Boca Raton, 1990, CRC Press.
105. Smith EI and others: The impact of chemotherapy and radiation therapy on secondary operations for neuroblastoma, *Ann Surg* 191:561, 1980.
106. Soule EH, Pritchard DJ: Fibrosarcoma in infants and children, *Cancer* 40:1711, 1977.
107. Straus DJ: Treatment of early stage Hodgkin's disease, *Blood Rev* 7: 34, 1993.
108. Swain RE, Sessions DG, Ogura JH: Fibrosarcoma of the head and neck: a clinical analysis of forty cases, *Ann Otol* 83:439, 1974.
109. Traggis DG and others: Prognosis for children with neuroblastoma presenting with paralysis, *J Pediatr Surg* 12:419, 1977.
110. Tsujimoto Y, Yunis J, Onorato-Show L: Molecular cloning of the chromosomal breakpoint of B-cell lymphomas and leukemias with the t(11;14) chromosome translocation, *Science* 224:1403, 1984.

111. Unmat S, Nasser JG: Fibrosarcoma of the infratemporal fossa in childhood: a challenging problem, *J Otolaryngol* 21:441, 1992.
112. Waldron CA, El-Mofty SK, Gnepp DR: Tumors of the intraoral minor salivary glands: a demographic and histologic study of 426 cases, *Oral Surg Oral Med Oral Pathol* 66:323, 1988.
113. Wexler LH, Helman LJ: Pediatric soft tissue sarcomas, *CA Cancer J Clin* 44:211, 1994.
114. Whang-Peng J and others: Cytogenetic studies in subgroups of rhabdomyosarcoma, *Genes Chromosom Cancer* 5:299, 1992.
115. White L, Meyer PR, Benedict WF: Establishment and characterization of human T-cell leukemia line (LALW-2) in nude mice, *J Natl Cancer Inst* 72:1029, 1984.
116. White L, Siegel SE: *Non-Hodgkins lymphoma in childhood.* In Sutow WW, Fernbach DF, Vietti TJ, editors: *Clinical pediatric oncology*, St Louis, 1984, Mosby.
117. White L, Siegel SE, Quah TC: Non-Hodgkin's lymphomas in children: I. Patterns of disease and classification, *Crit Rev Oncol Hematol* 13:55, 1992.
118. Wollner H: Non-Hodgkin's lymphoma in children, *Pediatr Clin North Am* 23:371, 1976.
119. Xia Y and others: TAL2, a helix-hoop-helix gene activated by the (7; 9)(p34;q32) translocation in human T-cell leukemia, *Proc Natl Acad Sci U S A* 88:11416, 1991.
120. Young Jr JL, Miller RE: Incidence of malignant tumours in US children, *J Pediatr* 86:254, 1975.
121. Young JL and others: Cancer incidence, survival, and mortality for children younger than age 15 years, *Cancer* 58:598, 1986.

Chapter 15

Differential Diagnosis of Neck Masses

Ralph F. Wetmore
William P. Potsic

The presentation of a neck mass in a pediatric patient has many diagnostic possibilities not normally encountered in an adult (Fig. 15-1). Neoplastic disease, especially malignant, is the primary consideration in the evaluation of a neck mass in an adult. In contrast, diagnosis of a pediatric neck mass can be categorized, depending on the location, growth factors, and the child's age. The possibility of malignancy should always be considered in the differential diagnosis in pediatric patients; however, it is not as overriding a concern as in adults.

The two major categories of pediatric neck masses include congenital and acquired lesions. Congenital masses have a high incidence (>50% in some series[47]), which initially differentiates them from acquired masses. The primary type of acquired masses are inflammatory (acute and chronic), which further narrows the differential diagnosis. Benign and malignant lesions are rare in the pediatric patient.

The approach to the child with a neck mass depends on the history and physical examination. Radiographic and laboratory studies may prove helpful, but some masses require surgical biopsy to establish the diagnosis. Thus, the pediatric neck mass often poses a challenge to the surgeon.

History

In the evaluation of a pediatric patient with a neck mass, a detailed history alone can often exclude many lesions in the differential diagnosis. Consideration of temporal relationships can often prove helpful. A history of infection elsewhere in the patient or recent travel or exposure to farm animals may suggest an infectious origin. Preceding trauma may signal a hematoma, whereas an increase in the size of the mass or pain with eating may point to a salivary gland problem. Exposure to drugs such as phenytoin may also be contributory.

The growth characteristics of the neck mass are important. Slow growth suggests a benign process, whereas rapid enlargement occurs with infectious or malignant lesions. Some masses fluctuate in size (e.g., hemangiomas increase in size with straining and crying). Fever, weight loss, night sweats, or fatigue suggest a malignant process.

Physical examination

In the evaluation of a child with a neck mass, comprehensive head and neck evaluation is essential. Clues to the pathogenesis of the neck mass may be found anywhere in the head. Likewise, a total physical examination should be performed with special attention to other lymph node groups, such as the axillae and groin. Palpation for an enlarged spleen should always be attempted.

Infants frequently have small palpable lymph nodes in the posterior cervical region, whereas older children have palpable nodes in the anterior cervical, posterior cervical, and submandibular regions. Any node larger than 2 cm in diameter falls outside the range of these normal hyperplastic nodes and should be evaluated further.

In examination of abnormal lymph nodes or a neck mass, the location is important for determining the site of the precipitating infection or the primary source of a malignant neoplasm. For example, infection in the nasopharynx tends to drain into the posterior cervical region, whereas tonsillitis

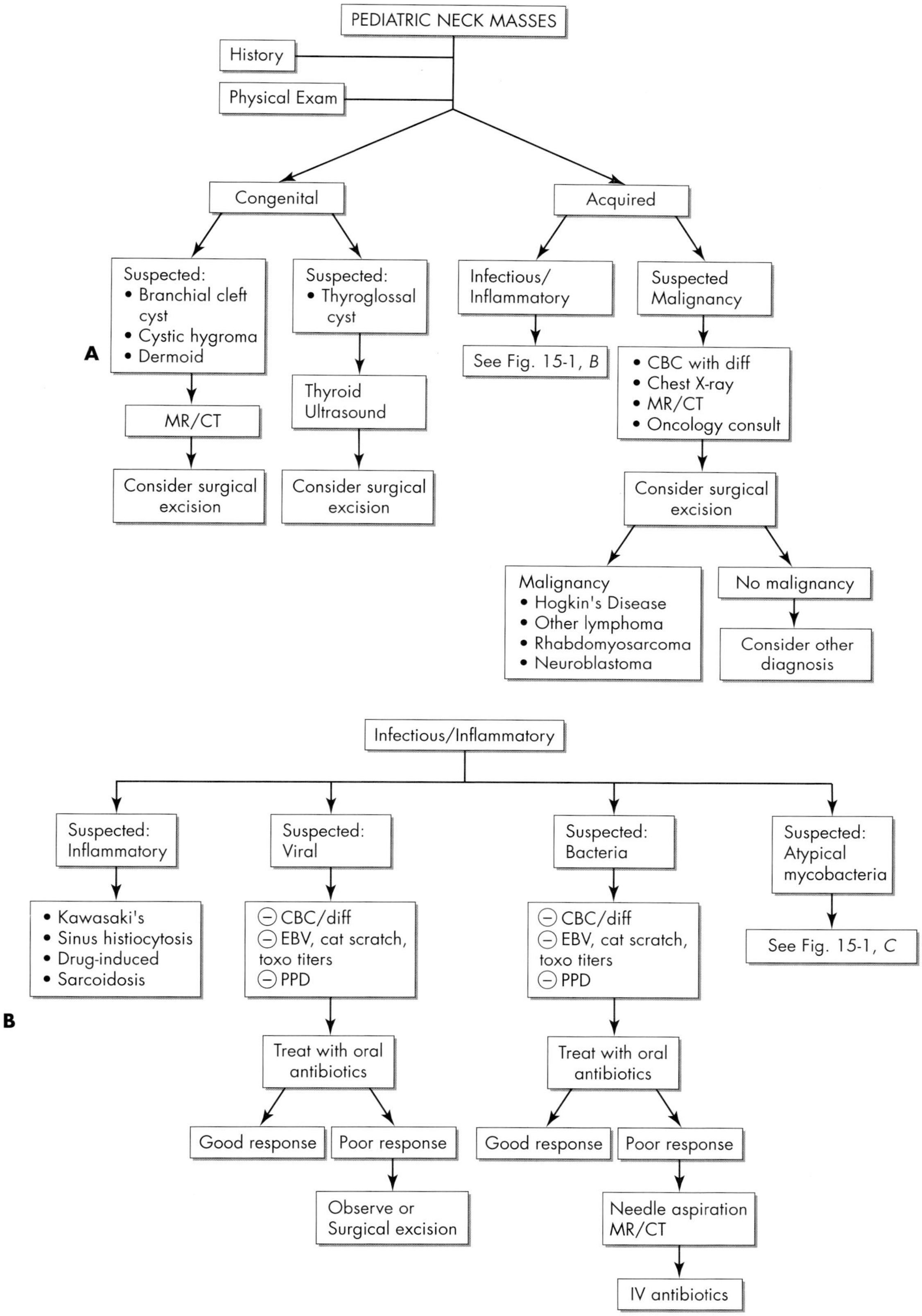

Continued.

Fig. 15-1. A to **C**, Algorithms for the differential diagnosis of neck masses.

may cause enlargement in the anterior cervical region. Moussatos[38a] and Putney[40a] noted an increased incidence of malignancy in the posterior cervical triangle; in contrast, Torsiglieri and others[47] reported an increased incidence in the supraclavicular region.

The consistency of a neck mass is frequently helpful in categorizing the mass. For example, hard masses tend to occur with infection or a malignant process. Fixation of a mass to the skin or deeper structures of the neck suggests a malignancy. A fluctuant mass tends to occur with abscess formation or a cyst.

Radiologic studies

Depending on the clinical impression of a neck mass from the history and physical examination, selected radiographic studies may help narrow the differential diagnosis. Chest radiography is helpful if a malignancy, sarcoidoisis, or pulmonary tuberculosis is suspected. In the evaluation of the nasopharynx, cervical spine, or retropharyngeal region, lateral neck radiography may show an abnormality. Likewise, a sinus series may show evidence of an infection or neoplasm in the paranasal sinuses.

In cases of infection in the neck, computed tomography (CT) with contrast may differentiate cellulitis that may respond solely to antibiotic therapy from an abscess with rim enhancement that may necessitate surgery. CT with contrast also helps identify vascular masses such as hemangiomas. Magnetic resonance imaging (MRI) provides even better detail of soft tissue. When combined with contrast, MRI is also useful in the evaluation of vascular lesions.

Ultrasound of the neck is most helpful in differentiating a cystic structure from a solid mass. It should be included as part of the evaluation of any thyroid mass. Before excision of a thyroglossal duct cyst, ultrasound can confirm the presence of a thyroid gland in its normal position, ruling out the possibility of ectopic thyroid. Use of ultrasound in these cases is easier and more economic. Thyroid scanning remains essential in the evaluation of any thyroid mass.

C

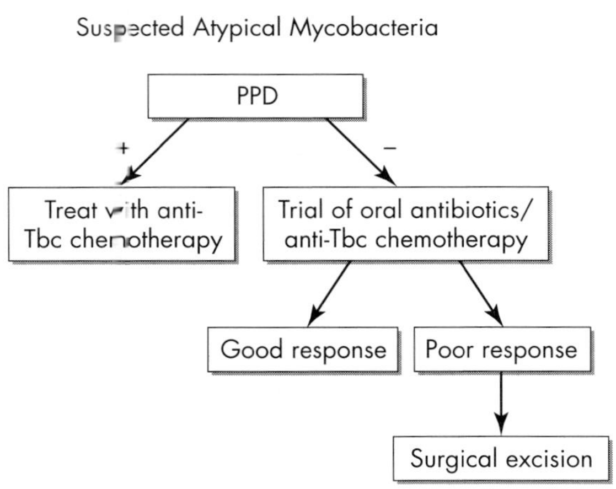

Fig. 15-1, cont'd. For legend see p. 249.

Laboratory studies

As with radiography, selected laboratory studies may be useful in the evaluation of the pediatric neck mass. A complete blood count with differential is indicated if a malignancy or systemic infection is suspected. Serologic testing for Epstein-Barr Virus (EBV), cytomegalovirus, toxoplasmosis, syphilis, or cat-scratch disease may be diagnostic. An elevated serum calcium level is highly suggestive of sarcoidosis, whereas thyroid function studies are necessary in the evaluation of most thyroid masses. Urinary collection for vanillylmandelic acid (VMA) is helpful when neuroblastoma is suspected. Although not as accurate as a culture of infected tissue, skin tests if available remain a reliable indicator of mycobacterial disease.

Surgical diagnosis

Although fine-needle aspiration of a suspected malignancy is not as reliable in children as in adults, fine-needle aspiration of a neck infection decompresses the mass and provides material for culture. In some cases, especially when the diagnosis of malignancy is considered, an incisional or excisional biopsy is indicated. Advantages of a biopsy include inspection of the lesion, providing a cuff of healthy surrounding tissue and tissue for frozen and permanent section, electron microscopy, and tumor markers.

CONGENITAL MASSES

Branchial cleft cysts

Although the definitive mechanism for the development of branchial cleft cysts is unclear, it is suspected that these congenital masses result from the cervical sinus of His be-

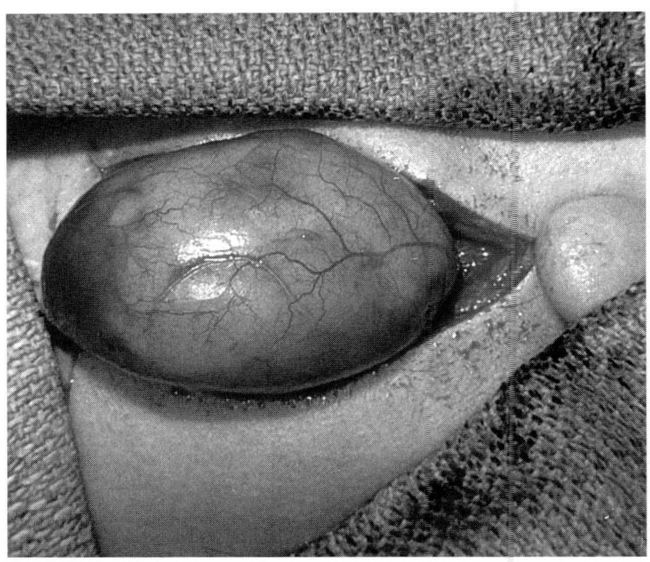

Fig. 15-2. A typical branchial cleft cyst is an epithelium-lined cyst filled with mucoid material. This cyst presents along the anterior border of the sternocleidomastoid muscle.

coming entrapped without an external or internal opening. An epithelium-lined cyst results. Others suggest that these cysts develop from epithelial rests of tissue from Waldeyer's ring.[50] Branchial cleft cysts are relatively common; in one series, they comprise one third of congenital neck masses.[47]

Branchial cleft cysts typically present as nontender, fluctuant masses that may become inflamed and abscess during an upper respiratory infection (Fig. 15-2). First branchial cleft cysts, although rare, typically present near the angle of the mandible (Fig. 15-3). Second branchial cysts are found high in the neck and deep to the anterior border of the sternocleidomastoid muscle. Third branchial cleft cysts, also rare, present near the upper pole of the thyroid gland. Other symptoms, depending on the size of the cyst, include dysphagia, dyspnea, and stridor.

Radiologic evaluation of a branchial cleft cyst may include ultrasound, CT, and MRI. Ultrasound shows a fluid-filled cyst and can differentiate cystic lesions from solid masses. CT or MRI also confirm the cystic characteristics of the mass and, more importantly, delineate the relationship of the cyst with surrounding structures (Fig. 15-4).

Management of branchial cleft cysts is surgical excision. It is advisable, if possible, to manage an infected cyst with antibiotics, allowing the inflammation to resolve before excision is attempted.

Thyroglossal duct cysts

Thyroglossal duct cysts form in a persistent thyroid descent tract that begins as an elongation of the thyroid diverticulum. Beginning at the foramen caecum of the tongue, this tract may extend to the thyroid gland itself, where some tissue may persist in the region of a pyramidal lobe. These remnants are cysts and are not associated with a cutaneous sinus or fistula tract unless surgically drained and inadequately excised. They comprise approximately one third of congenital neck masses in children.[47]

Most thyroglossal duct cysts present in the midline near the level of the hyoid bone because the tract passes just anterior to the hyoid bone (Fig. 15-5). Some cysts may present laterally and are not infrequently found superior to the hyoid or as low as the level of the thyroid gland. Thyroglossal duct cysts that occur off the midline may be difficult to differentiate from branchial cleft cysts, an important factor in their surgical excision. Other unusual presentations of thyroglossal duct cysts include formation on either side of the hyoid bone as dumbbell-shaped lesions and, rarely, as cystic lesions in the larynx. Thyroid tissue is found in surgical specimens in up to 45% of cases.[49]

A thyroglossal duct cyst usually presents as an asymptomatic mass but may be associated with mild dysphagia. Not infrequently, presentation of these cysts may be accom-

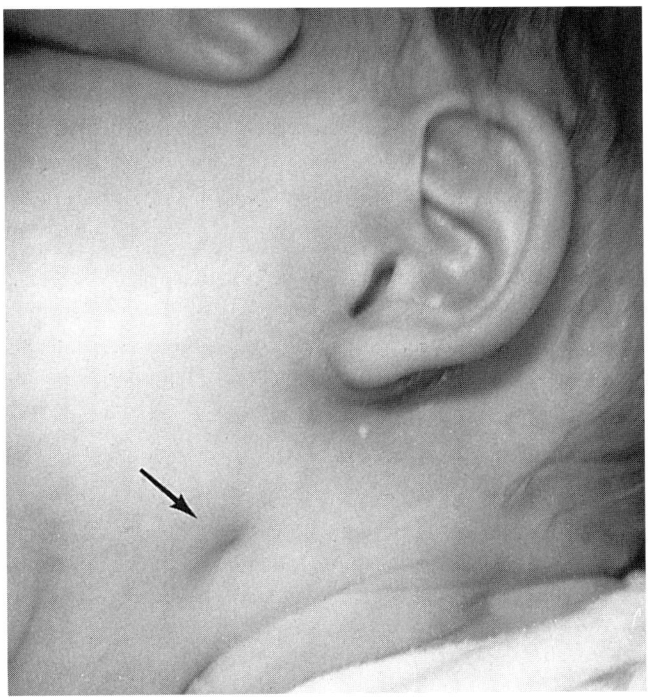

Fig. 15-3. First branchial derivatives present as a pit or a mass near the angle of the mandible *(arrow)*. They frequently originate in or near the external canal and, during their course, involve the facial nerve.

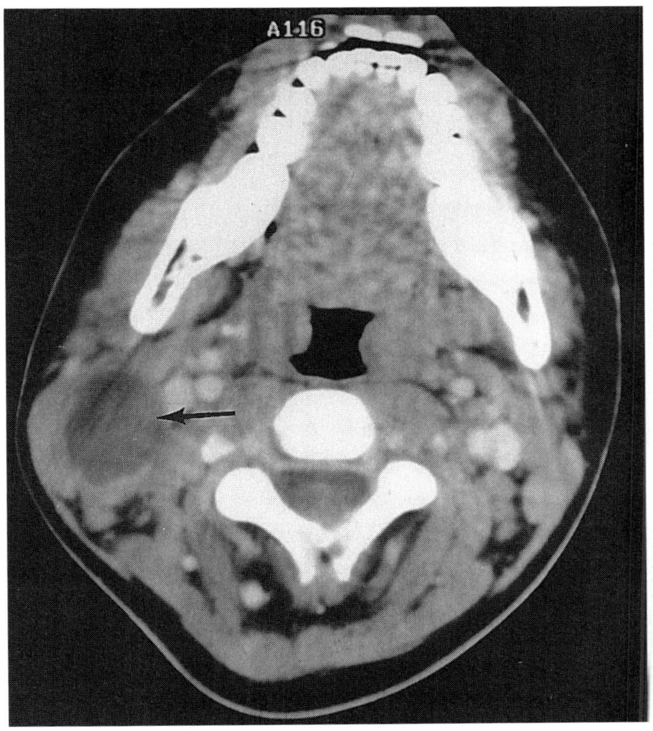

Fig. 15-4. Axial computed tomography of the neck shows a branchial cleft cyst in the hypolucent area *(arrow)*.

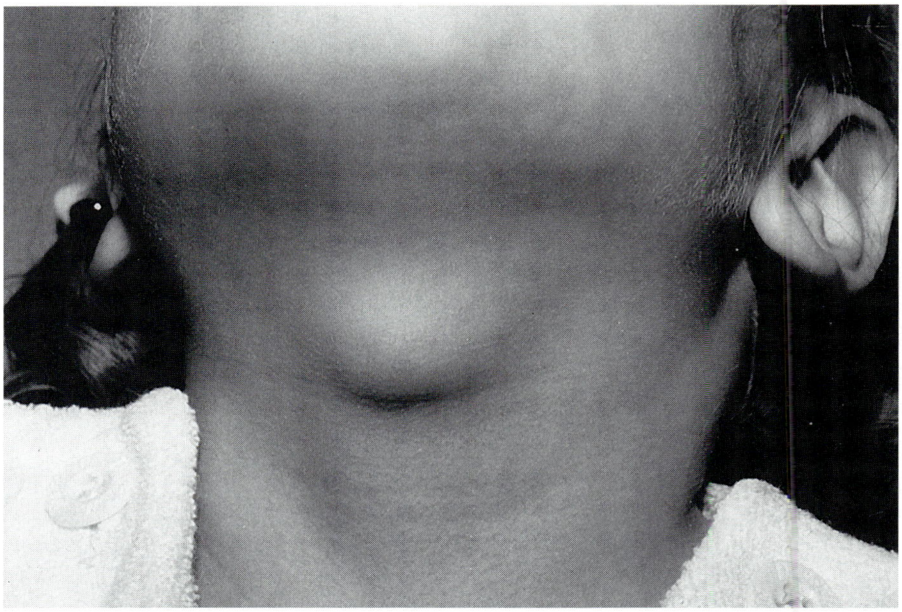

Fig. 15-5. Thyroglossal duct cysts are often found in the midline of the neck at or near the hyoid bone.

panied by infection causing rapid enlargement that may produce significant dysphagia and choking.

In cases in which a thyroglossal duct cyst is suspected, it is important to differentiate ectopic thyroid from a cyst. Although only 10% of ectopic thyroid is found in the neck, it may represent the only thyroid tissue in 75% of patients.[41] Children with ectopic thyroid may be mildly hypothyroid; however, excision of this tissue necessitates hormone replacement for the remainder of the patient's life. Thyroid ultrasound and radionucleotide scanning can differentiate ectopic thyroid from a thyroglossal duct cyst; ultrasound is easier to perform, less expensive, and does not use radioisotopes.

The Sistrunk operation is the standard method of thyroglossal duct cyst excision. The cyst is excised along with a cuff of tissue including the center portion of the hyoid bone. Incision and drainage of an infected cyst should be avoided because violation of the cyst capsule may invite recurrence. Recurrence rates of nearly 10% have been reported in children who have undergone uncomplicated Sistrunk operations.[47]

Lymphangiomas

Lymphangiomas are congenital malformations of lymph tissue that result from the failure of lymph spaces to connect to the rest of the lymphatic system. The resulting neck masses range from lymphangiomas to cystic hygromas. Lymphangioma simplex is composed of small, thin-walled channels. Cavernous lymphagiomas represent larger cystic areas surrounded by fibrous adventitia. Cystic hygromas consist of multiple cystic spaces of varying sizes. Lymphangiomas may be seen in continuity with vascular anomalies forming a lymphangiohemangioma.

A lymphangioma presents as a soft, smooth, nontender mass that is compressible and can be transilluminated (Fig. 15-6). Typically, lymphangiomas fluctuate in size as a result of infection or hemorrhage. They most impact the cosmetic appearance of the child. Depending on the size and location of the mass, there may be respiratory compromise and difficulty in feeding.

Radiographic evaluation with MRI or CT is invaluable for diagnosis and determination of the extent of the lesion. Radiography shows fluid-filled spaces with surrounding connective tissue. Because these malformations lack a capsule and extend along the lymphatic channels, MRI or CT is essential in defining normal anatomic structures that should be preserved when surgical excision is performed.

The goals of surgery are to improve cosmetic appearance and to counter impaired breathing or eating. Because of the infiltrative nature of these malformations, complete surgical excision is often difficult; debulking of the mass often accomplishes these goals. Some experts recommend staging of surgical excision in extensive cases.[22] Management with radiotherapy and sclerosing agents has not been effective.[22]

Hemangiomas

Similar to lymphangiomas, hemangiomas represent malformations of vascular tissue rather than true neoplasms. Histologic classification includes capillary, cavernous, and juvenile types. Hemangiomas present at birth, grow rapidly during the first year of life and begin to slowly involute at 18 to 24 months of age. Hemangiomas occur in up to 10% of children with a female-to-male ratio of 2:1.[26]

Hemangiomas present as a red or bluish soft mass that frequently has a skin component. Typically, these masses are compressible and increase in size with straining or

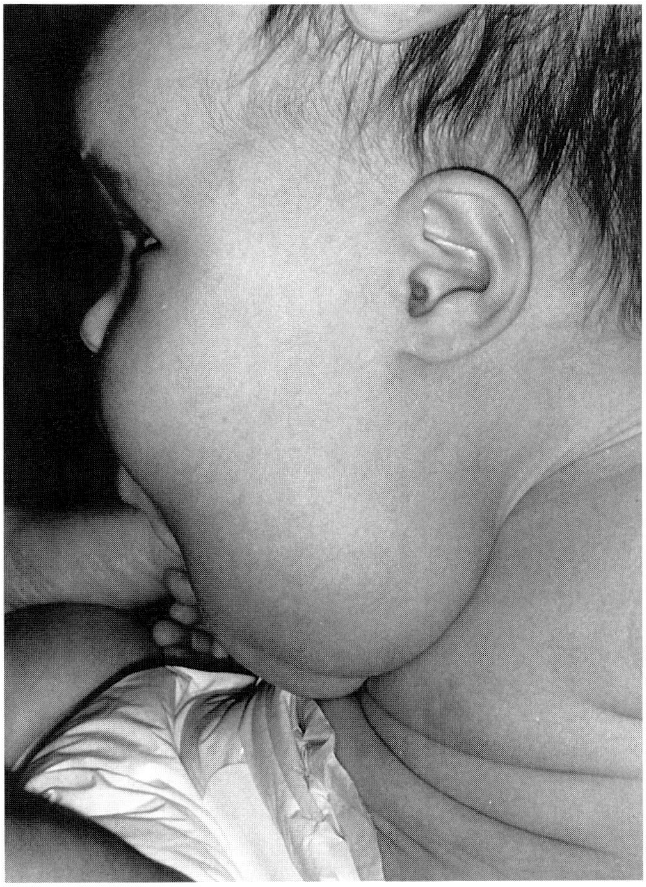

Fig. 15-6. Lymphangiomas of the neck may cause significant cosmetic deformity and may impair respiration or alimentation.

crying. With large hemangiomas, a bruit may be heard over the lesion. CT or MRI with contrast often confirms the diagnosis of a vascular lesion (Fig. 15-7).

Because hemangiomas typically involute after several years, the usual management is observation, unless there is functional impairment, bleeding, skin necrosis, or a coagulopathy caused by thrombocytopenia. Use of systemic corticosteroids may be helpful in the management of complications such as skin ulceration, dysphagia, dyspnea, thrombocytopenia, or cardiac failure.[7,14,17,18] Surgical excision or laser therapy may be helpful in cases of incomplete involution or when mild functional or cosmetic abnormalities remain. Management with radiotherapy may lead to malignant transformation, and the use of sclerosing agents and cryotherapy has produced poor results.[19,22]

Teratomas

Teratomas in the head and neck are rare, comprising only 3.5% of all teratomas in one series.[1] Although there is a female-to-male preponderance of 6:1 in other body regions, the female-to-male ratio is equal in the head and neck.[8] Teratomas arise from pluripotential cells and consist of tissues foreign to the site from which they arise. A history of maternal polyhydramnios has been noted in up to 18% of neonates who have a cervical teratoma (Fig. 15-8).

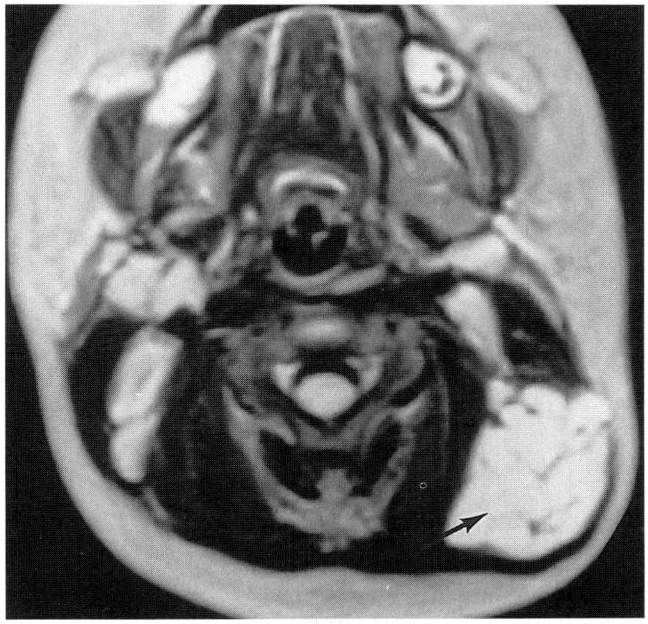

Fig. 15-7. Magnetic resonance imaging with contrast shows an enhancing vascular lesion in the posterior neck, consistent with a hemangioma *(arrow)*.

Most teratomas present as firm neck masses. With large teratomas, there may be symptoms of respiratory compromise caused by tracheal compression. Intrinsic calcifications may be seen on CT or MRI, a finding that may assist diagnosis. Management is by surgical excision; failure of complete excision may result in recurrence.

Dermoid cysts

Similar to teratomas, to which they are pathologically related, dermoid cysts arise from epithelium that has been entrapped in tissue during embryogenesis or by traumatic implantation. Dermoid cysts consist of epithelium-lined cavities filled with skin appendages (e.g., hair, hair follicles, sebaceous glands). They are found at other sites in the head and neck, including the orbit, nose, nasopharynx and oral cavity.

Typically, dermoid cysts present in the midline of the neck, usually in the submental region (Figs. 15-9 and 15-10). They are attached to and move with the overlying skin and are painless unless infected. Management is by complete surgical excision.

Laryngoceles

A laryngocele is an abnormal dilation or herniation of the saccule of the larynx. If this dilation lies within the limits of the thyroid cartilage, the laryngocele is internal. If it ex-

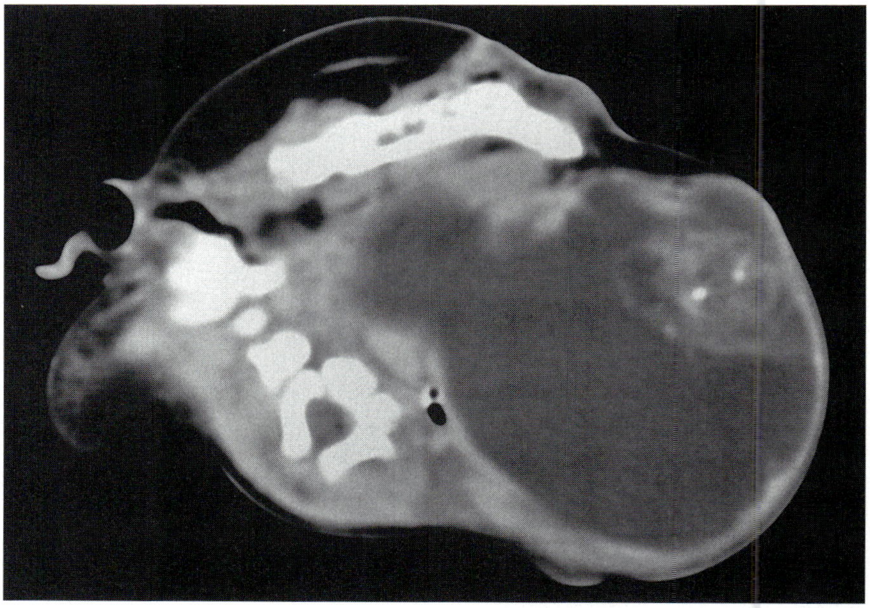

Fig. 15-8. Computed tomography shows a large teratoma cyst in a newborn that severely compromised the respiratory tract and required a tracheostomy.

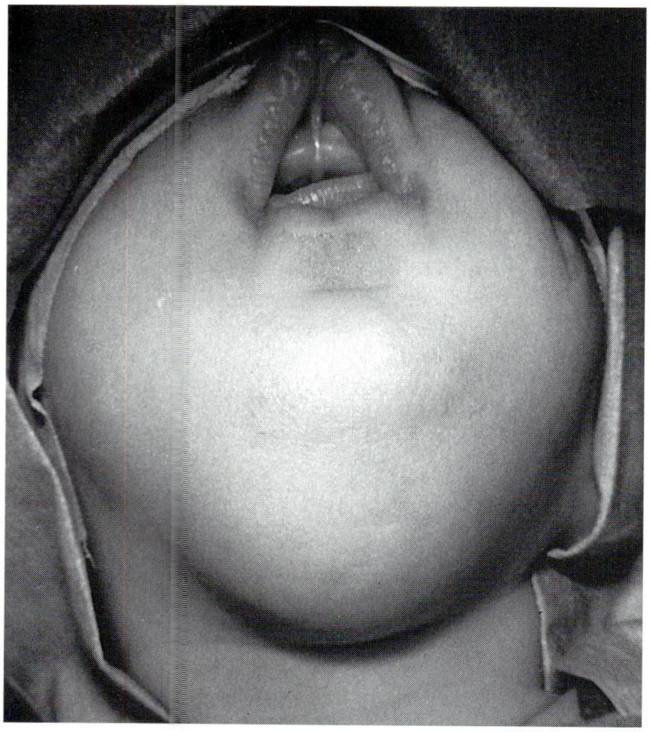

Fig. 15-9. A large dermoid cyst presents in the midline of the submental region.

tends beyond the thyroid cartilage in a cephalad direction to protrude through the thyrohyoid membrane, the laryngocele is external. Some laryngoceles present with internal and external components. Laryngoceles are rare in infants and children but may present congenitally in newborns. Clinical differentiation of air-filled laryngoceles from fluid-filled saccular cysts may be impossible.[12]

Hoarseness, cough, dyspnea, and dysphagia suggest a laryngocele. CT may be helpful in diagnosis, especially in delineating the extent of the lesion and differentiating the laryngocele's air-filled space from the fluid of a saccular cyst. Surgical excision through an external approach is the management of choice.

Thymic cysts

The thymus develops from the third pharyngeal pouch and descends into the chest. An implant of thymic tissue along this descent tract anywhere in the neck may result in a thymic cyst. Thymic cysts may be more common than suggested by several reports in the literature.[38] Almost all are unilateral (most commonly on the left side of the neck), and 90% are cystic.[29]

Typically, a thymic cyst presents as an asymptomatic mass, but it may be painful if infected or if there is a rapid increase in its size. CT or MRI may help differentiate a thymic cyst comprising a single cystic lesion from a cystic hygroma that has multiple large cysts within the mass. The preferred management is surgical excision. Diagnosis is confirmed by histologic identification of Hassall's corpuscles.

Venous malformations

Anomalies of the external jugular vein may occasionally result in a neck mass.[2] Typically, the external jugular vein empties into the subclavian vein, but it may empty into the

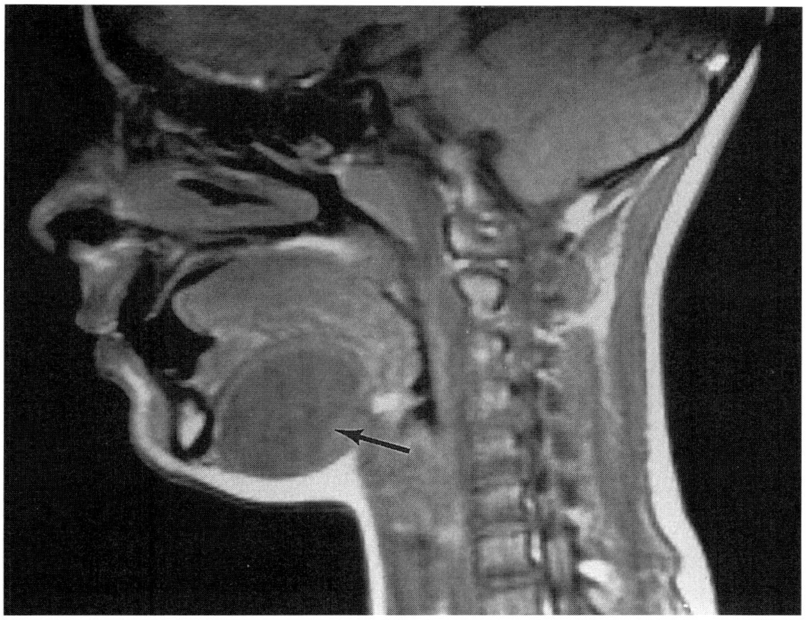

Fig. 15-10. Magnetic resonance imaging (sagittal view) shows a large dermoid cyst in the submental region just deep to the tongue *(arrow)*.

internal jugular vein outside the carotid sheath, forming a venous plexus. Jugular malformations present as soft, compressible masses along the anterior border of the sternocleidomastoid muscle. Management is by ligation or excision of the anomaly.

Sternocleidomastoid tumors of infancy

Neonates with sternocleidomastoid tumors present with neck masses that are usually not apparent at birth but appear at 1 to 8 weeks of age. Pathologically, the mass is characterized by dense fibrous tissue and the absence of normal striated muscle (Fig. 15-11). As the mass resolves, the remaining muscle continues to degenerate into fibrous tissue. The etiology of this disorder, also known as congenital torticollis, is unclear; however, birth trauma, ischemia of the muscle, and intrauterine positioning have been implicated.

Most patients are firstborn;[37] siblings are rarely affected.[46] Congenital torticollis presents as a firm, painless, discrete, fusiform mass within the sternocleidomastoid muscle that slowly increases in size for 2 to 3 months and then slowly regresses for 4 to 8 months (Fig. 15-12). Because the mass disappears in more than 80% of cases,[24] conservative management with physiotherapy (passive and active motion) prevents the development of restrictive torticollis. In resistant cases, surgical section of the sternocleidomastoid muscle may be required.

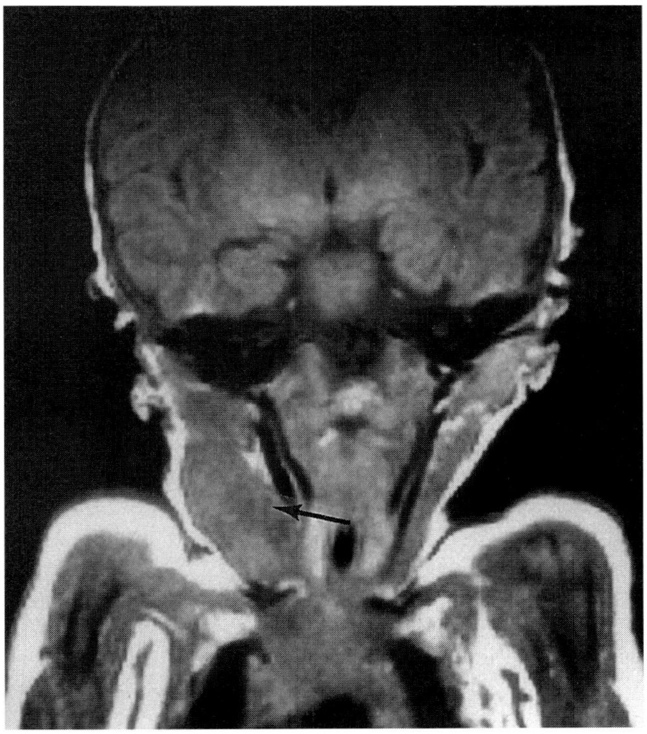

Fig. 15-11. Magnetic resonance imaging of an infant with congenital torticollis shows enlargement of the sternocleidomastoid muscle *(arrow)*.

ACQUIRED MASSES

Viral lymphadenopathy

Reactive lymph nodes result from viral upper respiratory tract infections, such as adenovirus, rhinovirus, or enterovirus (coxsackievirus A and B). EBV often presents with mas-

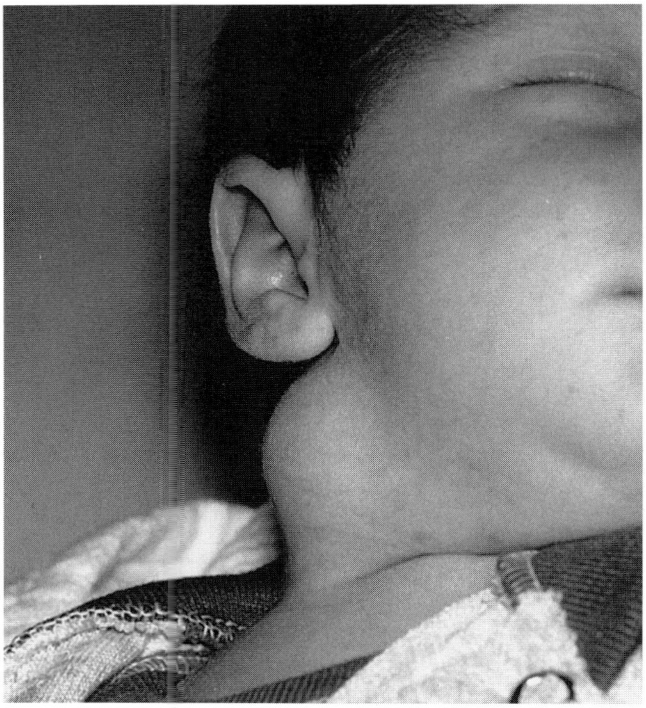

Fig. 15-12. A firm mass in the midportion of the sternocleidomastoid muscle is seen in an infant with congenital torticollis.

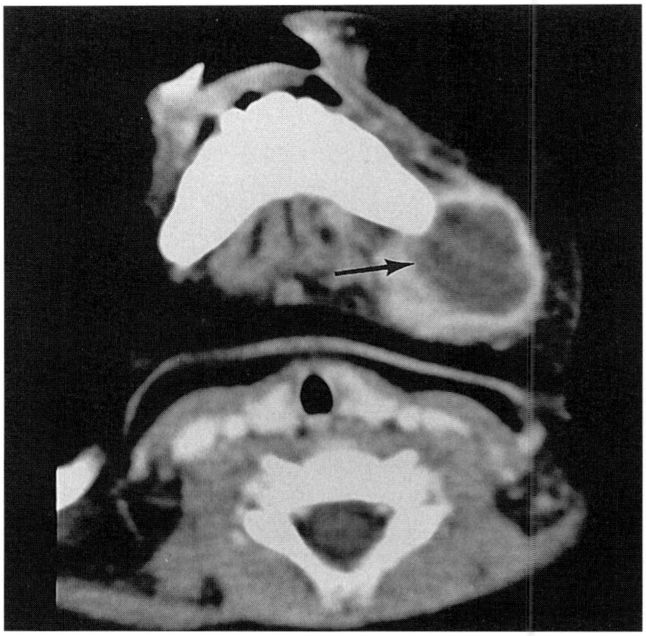

Fig. 15-13. Computed tomography with contrast shows a neck abscess in the submandibular triangle *(arrow)*. Abscess formation is characterized by hypolucency and rim enhancement.

sive lymphadenopathy in addition to enlargement of other lymphoid tissue (e.g., tonsils, spleen). On pathologic examination, there is a proliferation of normal cells; however, in contrast to neoplastic disease, the node architecture is intact.

Reactive lymphadenopathy is frequently bilateral and is associated with symptoms of the underlying respiratory infection. Management is observation, although not infrequently these nodes are biopsied because their consistency mimics lymphoma and their regression in size is often slow.

Unlike most cases of viral lymphadenopathy, human immunodeficiency virus infection may result in the acquired immunodeficiency syndrome whose associated findings, aside from generalized lymphadenopathy, include hepatosplenomegaly; weight loss; susceptibility to viral, bacterial, and fungal infections; and fevers. Pediatric AIDS should be suspected in cases in which multiple neck nodes are involved with bacterial infection and in cases that fail to respond to adequate antibiotic therapy.

Bacterial lymphadenopathy

Suppurative lymphadenopathy

Staphylococcus aureus and group A β-streptococcus are the most common causative organisms of suppuration in the neck, although other bacteria such as *Haemophilus* and *Moraxella* have been implicated. Brodsky and others[9] found a 19% incidence for anaerobic bacteria versus 67% for aerobic bacteria. Brook[10] reported a similar anaerobic incidence and β-lactamase–positive organisms in 34%. In neonates, the offending organisms may be *Staphylococcus* or *Streptococcus*, but *Pseudomonas* and other gram-negative bacteria have also been reported.[4,6]

There appears to be no major differences between the *Staphylococcus* and *Streptococcus* groups when demographic factors and occurrence of symptoms are compared. Frequently, the neck mass develops in the submandibular region, but it may occur in the anterior and posterior cervical triangles (Fig. 15-13).[5] Associated symptoms include a history of upper respiratory infection, sore throat, earache, and skin lesions.[5] Initial management is with antibiotic therapy, given, orally or intravenously depending on the severity of the infection. Failure to respond to medication may indicate the need for fine-needle aspiration or incision and drainage.

Cat-scratch disease

Most cases of cat-scratch disease occur in patients younger than 20 years,[25] and males are affected more frequently than females.[34] More than 90% of patients have a history of feline contact, and there is a fall and winter prevalence. Although the symptom complex of cat-scratch disease has been recognized for almost 50 years, only recently has the bacterium *Rochalimaea henselae* been implicated as the etiologic agent.[51] Serologic testing by indirect fluorescent antibodies to this organism has a high sensitivity and specificity. Typically, affected children present with lymphade-

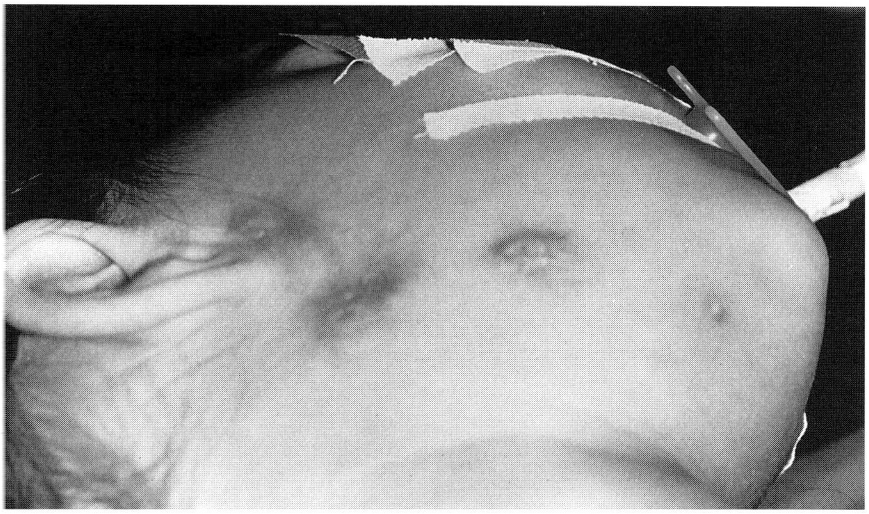

Fig. 15-14. Atypical mycobacterial infection frequently involves the submandibular triangle and preauricular regions.

nopathy associated with mild fever and other symptoms of malaise. There is no effective medical management of this disorder. Rarely is the infection severe enough to require surgery.

Toxoplasmosis

Infection with *Toxoplasma gondii* is usually contracted through the consumption of poorly cooked meat or ingestion of oocytes excreted in cat feces. Symptoms include fever, malaise, sore throat, and myalgias. Cervical adenitis occurs in more than 90% of cases.[36] Complications of toxoplasmosis include myocarditis and pneumonitis. The diagnosis is confirmed by serologic testing, and management is with pyrimethamine or sulfonamides.

Mycobacterial infection

Most atypical mycobacterial infections are caused by a variety of mycobacteria, including *Mycobacterium avium-intracellulare, Mycobacterium scrofulaceum, Mycobacterium kansasii, Mycobacterium fortuitum*, and *Mycobacterium haemophilum*. In the past few years, the reemergence of *Mycobacterium tuberculosis* has been noted; *M. tuberculosis* as a cause of cervical adenopathy is associated with pulmonary tuberculosis in endemic areas of the United States. In a series on the cause of mycobacterial neck infections, Hawkins and others[23] showed a 59% incidence for atypical mycobacteria compared with 29% for *M. tuberculosis*.

Skin tests for *M. tuberculosis* and atypical mycobacteria are available[33] and were positive in 95% of cases in the series by Hawkins and others.[23] Mycobacterial infection is definitively diagnosed by culture, which frequently takes weeks.

The most common site of mycobacterial infection in the neck is the anterior superior cervical region, followed by the posterior cervical, middle cervical, supraclavicular, and submental regions. Atypical mycobacterial infection is not infrequently found in the preauricular region (Fig. 15-14). It tends to occur unilaterally, whereas *M. tuberculosis* is more diffuse and frequently bilateral.[23] A painless, firm, enlarging mass in the face of antibiotic therapy suggests the diagnosis. The overlying skin is frequently discolored with atypical mycobacterial infection. In patients with *M. tuberculosis* infection, weight loss, fever, and anorexia may also be present.

The current management of *M. tuberculosis* infection is with antituberculous chemotheraphy, usually including two drugs. Although lymph nodes infected with atypical mycobacteria are best managed by surgical excision or incision and curettage, Hawkins and others[23] showed resolution of neck masses in 4 of 18 cases of atypical mycobacterial infection with chemotheraphy alone.[23]

Tularemia

Infection of the neck with *Francisella tularensis* is rare. The organism is transmitted to humans by rabbits, ticks, or contaminated drinking water. Symptoms include fever, tonsillitis, painful adenitis, ulcers, chills, fatigue, and headache. Diagnosis is by serology and culture. Intramuscular streptomycin is the management of choice.

Brucellosis

Brucellosis is caused by several species of the genus *Brucella*, which are small gram-negative bacilli. Children acquire brucellosis by the ingestion of unpasteurized milk. This is rare in the United States but not uncommon in undeveloped countries. In addition to generalized lymphadenopathy involving the neck and other body regions, there may be fatigue, malaise, and fever. The diagnosis is confirmed by serology and culture. Management in adults is with tetracycline, whereas children younger than 9 years of age should receive trimethoprim-sulfamethoxazole.

Fungal infections

Fungal infections of the neck typically present in immunocompromised patients with symptoms and signs that suggest viral or bacterial infection. The usual pathogens include *Candida, Histoplasma*, and *Aspergillus*. The diagnosis is made by serology or fungal smear and culture. Management of fungal lymphadenopathy requires intravenous amphotericin B.

Sialadenitis

The salivary glands are susceptible to viral and bacterial infection and, at times, may resemble infection of surrounding lymph nodes. Although rare since the development of a vaccine, mumps is a paramyxoviral infection that may cause orchitis, meningitis, or sensorineural hearing loss. One or both parotid or submandibular glands may be involved. Management includes supportive measures, such as analgesics and hydration.

In addition to viral infection, dehydration and generalized disability of patients often predisposes to bacterial infection of the salivary glands. The causative organisms include *S. aureus, Streptococcus* species, and *Haemophilus influenzae*.

Children with sialadenitis present with the rapid onset of pain and swelling of the affected glands. Fever, chills, and malaise may also occur. Examination of the oral cavity may reveal purulent discharge from the ducts of the involved glands (Stensen's or Wharton's). Management of bacterial sialadenitis is hydration and oral or intravenous broad-spectrum antibiotic therapy.

Noninfectious inflammatory disorders

Kawasaki disease (mucocutaneous lymph node syndrome)

Kawasaki disease is an acute multisystem vasculitis of unknown etiology that tends to affect children younger than 5 years of age.[20] To confirm this diagnosis, the patient should have fever persisting for 5 days and four of the following features: (1) acute, nonpurulent cervical lymphadenopathy that is usually unilateral; (2) erythema, edema, and desquamation of the hands and feet; (3) polymorphous exanthem; (4) bilateral painless conjunctival injection; (5) erythema and injection of the lips and oral cavity.

Associated findings in the acute stage include thrombocytosis and cardiac signs of pericardial effusion.[40] In the subacute stage, coronary artery aneurysms may develop in 15% to 20% of cases.[20] The goal of management is to reduce the inflammatory response with aspirin and γ-globulin therapy.

Sinus histiocytosis (Rosai-Dorfman disease)

Children with sinus histiocytosis present with massive nontender cervical lymphadenopathy that is similar to infectious mononucleosis or lymphoma. The disease is thought to represent an abnormal histiocytic response to some precipitating cause, possibly either a herpes virus or EBV.[28] Biopsy shows dilated sinuses, many plasma cells, and marked proliferation of histiocytes. In addition to massive adenopathy, fever and skin nodules may be present. Management of this disorder is expectant.

Drug-induced lymphadenopathy

Although phenytoin is the most well-known cause of drug-induced lymphadenopathy, pyrimethamine, allopurinol, and phenylbutazone have also been implicated.[48] Typically, the adenopathy resolves when drug therapy is discontinued; however, long-term use of phenytoin has been reported to progress to a premalignant pseudolymphomatous state.

Sarcoidosis

The etiology of sarcoidosis is unknown, but clusters of cases tend to suggest an infectious or toxic origin. It is found most commonly in the second decade of life, and males and females are affected equally. Patients typically present with lymph node enlargement, fatigue, and weight loss. Depending on the sites of involvement, there may also be cough, dyspnea, hoarseness, bone and joint pain, visual symptoms, headaches, fever, and skin rash. Abnormalities on chest radiography help suggest the diagnosis, which is confirmed by finding noncaseating granulomas on biopsy of involved tissue. Management is expectant, although corticosteroids may be helpful in acute settings.

BENIGN NEOPLASMS

Lipomas

Lipomas are benign encapsulated fatty tumors found in subcutaneous tissue. In general, they rarely occur in the head and neck. The usual management is surgical excision.

Thyroid adenomas

A thyroid adenoma presents as an isolated mass that is palpable within the thyroid gland. On ultrasound, an adenoma appears as a solid mass in contrast to a thyroid cyst. On thyroid scanning, an adenoma appears as a cold nodule; however, some adenomas take up radionucleotide and show function, although not as much as that seen with typical hyperfunctioning nodules. Thyroid adenomas usually require excision to differentiate them from thyroid carcinomas.

Neurofibromas

Neurofibromas are circumscribed tumors that arise from small cutaneous nerves and are composed of Schwann cells, nerve fibers, and fibroblasts. They may be solitary or more rarely occur as multiple neurofibromas (e.g., in von Recklinghausen's disease). Management is excision, taking care not to injure nearby anatomic structures.

Pleomorphic adenomas

Pleomorphic adenomas are salivary gland tumors that typically arise in the lateral portion of the parotid gland. They present as slow-growing painless masses that show no evidence of nerve or skin involvement. A superficial parotidectomy is necessary for surgical excision.

MALIGNANT NEOPLASMS

Lymphomas

Lymphomas are the most common neck malignancy in large pediatric series.[15,47] They may be divided into two histologic categories, Hodgkin's and non-Hodgkin's, which have different clinical courses and prognoses.

Rye classified Hodgkin's disease into four histologic types: nodular sclerosing, mixed cellularity, lymphocyte predominant, and lymphocyte depleted. Males of any age are more commonly afflicted with Hodgkin's disease than females, although the incidence is nearly equal during the teenage years.[44] Hodgkin's disease often presents as an asymptomatic cervical or supraclavicular mass (Fig. 15-15). Fever is commonly associated with cough, night sweats, and weight loss. After confirmation of cell type by biopsy, management consits of chemotherapy or radiotherapy depending on histology and staging.

Non-Hodgkin's lymphoma is more likely to be disseminated and extranodal. Histologic types include lymphoblastic, large cell, and undifferentiated. The liver, lung, and bone marrow are the most common sites of extralymphatic involvement. In the neck, non-Hodgkin's lymphoma is less common than Hodgkin's disease.[43] Weight loss, night sweats, and fever are common, especially when disease is more disseminated. Chemotherapy is the mainstay of management of non-Hodgkin's lymphoma.

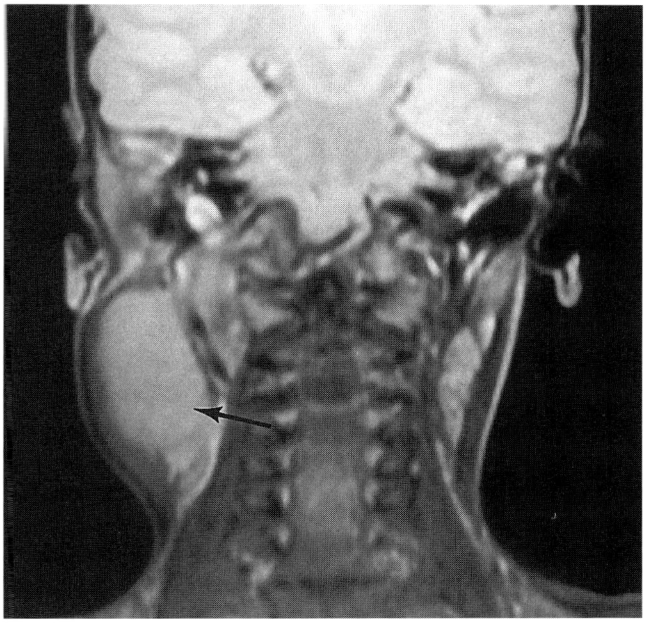

Fig. 15-15. Magnetic resonance imaging of the neck shows Hodgkin's disease presenting in the posterior cervical region *(arrow)*.

Rhabdomyosarcomas

Soft-tissue sarcomas comprise a small percentage of all childhood malignancies. Rhabdomyosarcoma is the most common soft-tissue sarcoma; because it occurs most commonly in the head and neck, it comprises a significant percentage of malignant neck masses in series of pediatric patients.[16] The peak incidence of rhabdomyosarcoma occurs at 2 to 5 years, with another peak between 15 and 19 years of age.[32] White children are affected more often than children of other races, and there is a slight male predominance.[32] Embryonal rhabdomyosarcoma is the most common cell type, followed by alveolar and pleomorphic.[31]

Predominant sites of rhabdomyosarcoma in the head and neck include the orbit, nasopharynx, paranasal sinuses, ears, and oral cavity. Primary involvement of the neck occurred in 89% of cases in one series.[3] Metastatic disease from one area of the head to the neck is rare.[35]

Management of rhabdomyosarcoma includes a combination of surgery, radiotherapy, and chemotherapy. The role of surgery, biopsy, debulking, or radical excision depends on the site, extent, and presence of recurrence. Radiotherapy to the primary site is given at 5000 to 6000 cGy in children older than 3 years at age and lesser doses in younger children.[3] Two thirds of patients experience long-term survival or cure.[16,45]

Thyroid carcinoma

Thyroid carcinoma is uncommon in the pediatric age group but has been associated with exposure to low-dose ionizing radiation.[13] Female children are more commonly affected but less so than female adults. The usual histology is papillary or mixed papillary-follicular. Involved patients present with a solitary mass in the anterior neck. More worrisome signs include rapid growth of the mass, hoarseness, dysphagia, and fixation of the mass to the surrounding structures. Metastases, when present, are found in regional lymph nodes and the lungs or bones. Ultrasound or thyroid scanning are helpful in diagnosis, although frozen section at the time of surgical excision is definitive. Because almost all thyroid carcinoma in children is papillary, management should be subtotal or total thyroidectomy with neck dissection if there is nodal involvement. Thyroid suppression is often used to prevent recurrence, and radioactive iodine helps eliminate unresectable tumor.

Salivary gland malignancies

Mucoepidermoid and acinic cell carcinomas of the salivary glands account for approximately 60% of malignant epithelial neoplasms in children.[30] With mucoepidermoid carcinoma, local invasiveness, regional metastasis, and prognosis depend on histologic differentiation; the behavior of acinic cell carcinoma does not correlate with histology. Mucoepidermoid and acinic cell carcinomas present as solitary firm masses that grow painlessly, usually in the parotid gland. Both tumors tend to be low-grade and are seldom fatal.[30] Depending on which gland is involved, initial management is by superficial parotidectomy or submandibular gland excision. Use of adjuvant therapy, including neck dissection or radiotherapy, depends on cell type and tumor growth characteristics.

Nasopharyngeal carcinoma

Nasopharyngeal carcinoma may present with a mass in the neck associated with a nasopharyngeal mass, unilateral otitis media, rhinorrhea, and nasal obstruction. In advanced cases, there may be one or more cranial nerve palsies. There is an increased incidence of nasopharyngeal carcinoma in black and Asian teenagers.[21,42] Titers of EBV types 2 and 3 have been elevated in patients with nasopharyngeal carcinoma.[39] Although the diagnosis is confirmed by biopsy, CT and MRI may help determine the extent of tumor involvement. Bone or liver metastasis may be identified by the use of bone scan or CT of the abdomen. Management depends on clinical staging and includes radiotherapy with or without chemotherapy.

Neuroblastomas

Neuroblastomas are malignant neoplasms that originate from primitive neuroblasts and neural crest cells. Only 2% to 4% of neuroblastomas originate in the neck.[11] In the neck, these masses may be associated with an ipsilateral Horner's syndrome.[27] Because systemic involvement is common, evaluation of the patient should include MRI and CT of the neck, chest, and abdomen, looking for metastatic spread. Elevated urinary VMA found on 24-hour collection strongly suggests neuroblastoma. Management depends on the extent of involvement and may include surgical excision, radiotherapy, and chemotherapy.

SUMMARY

A neck mass may provide a diagnostic challenge to the clinician and a source of anxiety to the parents. Systematic evaluation, paying particular attention to important details in the history and physical examination, can narrow the differential diagnosis and allow selection of appropriate radiologic and laboratory studies when indicated. In children, congenital and inflammatory masses are most common, but malignancy should be considered, especially if the mass continues to grow after appropriate therapy.

REFERENCES

1. Abemayor E and others: Teratomas of the head and neck in children, *Laryngoscope* 94:1489, 1984.
2. Alonso WA, Chambers RG: Aberrant jugular vein simulating a cervical cyst, *Laryngoscope* 80:244, 1970.
3. Anderson GJ and others: Rhabdomyosarcoma of the head and neck in children, *Arch Otolaryngol Head Neck Surg* 116:428, 1990.
4. Baker CJ: Group B streptococcal cellulitis-adenitis in infants, *Am J Dis Child* 136:631, 1982.
5. Barton LL, Feigin RD: Childhood cervical lymphadenitis: a reappraisal, *J Pediatr* 84:846, 1974.
6. Barton LL, Ramsey RA, Raval DS: Neonatal group B streptococcal cellulitis-adenitis, *Pediatr Dermatol* 1:58, 1993.
7. Bartoshesky LE, Bull M, Feingold M: Corticosteroid treatment of cutaneous hemangiomas: how effective? *Clin Pediatr (Phila)* 17:625, 1978.
8. Berry CL, Keeling J, Hilton C: Teratoma in infancy and childhood: a review of 91 cases, *J Pathol* 98:241, 1969.
9. Brodsky L and others: Needle aspiration of neck abscesses in children, *Clin Pediatr (Phila)* 31:71, 1992.
10. Brook I: Aerobic and anaerobic bacteriology of cervical adenitis in children, *Clin Pediatr (Phila)* 19:693, 1980.
11. Brown R, Syzmula N, Lore J: Neuroblastoma of the head and neck, *Arch Otolaryngol* 104:395, 1978.
12. Civantos FJ, Holinger LD: Laryngoceles and saccular cysts in infants and children, *Arch Otolaryngol Head Neck Surg* 118:296, 1992.
13. Clark DE: Association of irradiation with cancer of the thyroid in children and adolescents, *JAMA* 159:1007, 1955.
14. Cohen SR, Wang C: Steroid treatment of hemangioma of the head and neck in children, *Ann Otol Rhinol Laryngol* 81:584, 1972.
15. Cunningham MJ, Myers EN, Bluestone CD: Malignant tumors of the head and neck in children: a twenty-year review, *Int J Pediatr Otorhinolaryngol* 13:279, 1987.
16. Donaldson SS: Rhabdomyosarcoma: contemporary status and future directions, *Arch Surg* 124:1015, 1989.
17. Edgerton MT: The treatment of hemangiomas: with special reference to the role of steroid therapy, *Ann Surg* 183:517, 1976.
18. Fost NC, Esterly NB: Successful treatment of juvenile hemangiomas with prednisone, *J Pediatr* 72:351, 1968.
19. Garfinkle TJ, Handler SD: Hemangiomas of the head and neck in children: a guide to management, *J Otolaryngol* 9:5, 1980.
20. Gersony WM: Diagnosis and management of Kawasaki disease, *JAMA* 265:2699, 1991.
21. Greene MH, Graumeni JF, Hoover R: Nasopharyngeal cancer among young people in the United States: racial variations by cell type, *J Natl Cancer Inst* 58:1267, 1977.
22. Handler SD, Raney RB: Management of neoplasms of the head and neck in children. I. Benign tumors, *Head Neck Surg* 3:395, 1981.
23. Hawkins DB and others: Mycobacterial cervical adenitis in children: medical and surgical management, *Ear Nose Throat J* 72:733, 1993.
24. Hulbert KF: Congenital torticollis, *J Bone Joint Surg Am* 32:50, 1950.
25. Jackson LA, Perkins BA, Wenger JD: Cat scratch disease in the United States: an analysis of three national databases, *Am J Public Health* 83:1707, 1993.
26. Jacobs AH, Waldon RG: The incidence of birthmarks in the neonate, *Pediatrics* 58:218, 1976.
27. Jaffe N and others: Heterochromia and Horner's syndrome associated with cervical and mediastinal neuroblastoma, *J Pediatr* 87:75, 1975.
28. Levine PH and others: Detection of human herpesvirus 6 in tissues involved by sinus histiocytosis with massive lymphadenopathy (Rosai-Dorfman disease), *J Infect Dis* 166:291, 1992.
29. Lewis CT: Ectoptic thymus of the neck: report of three examples in children, *Postgrad Med J* 51:38, 1975.
30. Luna MA, Batsakis JG, El-Naggar AK: Pathology consultation: salivary gland tumors in children, *Ann Otol Rhinol Laryngol* 100:869, 1991.
31. MacArthur CJ, McGill TJI, Healy GB: Pediatric head and neck rhabdomyosarcoma, *Clin Pediatr (Phila)* 31:66, 1992.
32. Malogolowkin MH, Orega JA: Rhabdomyosarcoma of childhood, *Pediatr Ann* 17:251, 1988.
33. Margileth AM: Cat scratch disease and nontuberculous mycobacterial

disease: diagnostic usefulness of PPD-Battey, PPD-T and cat scratch skin test antigens, *Ann Allergy* 68:149, 1992.
34. Margileth AM: Dermatologic manifestations and update of cat scratch disease, *Pediatr Dermatol* 5:1, 1988.
35. Maurer HM and others: The intergroup rhabdomyosarcoma study: a preliminary report, *Cancer* 40:2015, 1977.
36. McCabe RE and others: Clinical spectrum in 107 cases of toxoplasmic lymphadenopathy, *Rev Infect Dis* 9:754, 1987.
37. McDaniel A and others: Torticollis in infancy and adolescence, *Ear Nose Throat J* 63:478, 1984.
38. Miller MB, DeVito MA: Cervical thymic cyst, *Otolaryngol Head Neck Surg* 112:586, 1995.
38a. Moussatos G, Baffes T: Cervical masses in infants and children, *Pediatrics* 37:251, 1963.
39. Neel HB, Pearson GR, Taylor WF: Antibodies to Epstein-Barr virus in patients with nasopharyngeal carcinoma and in comparison groups, *Ann Otol Rhinol Laryngol* 93:477, 1984.
40. Pontell J, Rosenfeld RM, Kohn B: Kawasaki disease mimicking retropharyngeal abscess, *Otolaryngol Head Neck Surg* 110:428, 1994.
40a. Putney F: The diagnosis of head and neck masses in children, *Otol Clin North Am* 3:277, 1970.
41. Radkowski D and others: Thyroglossal duct remnants: preoperative evaluation and management, *Arch Otolaryngol Head Neck Surg* 117: 1378, 1991.
42. Raney RB, Handler SD: Management of neoplasms of the head and neck in children. II. Malignant tumors, *Head Neck* 3:500, 1981.
43. Sandlund JT, Crist WM: *The non-Hodgkin lymphoma*. In Rudolph AM, Hoffmaln JIE, Rudolph CD, editors: *Rudolph's pediatrics*, ed 20, Stanford, Conn, 1996, Appleton & Lange.
44. Schnitzer B and others: Hodgkin's disease in children, *Cancer* 31:560, 1973.
45. Sercarz JA and others: Pediatric rhabdomyosarcoma of the head and neck, *Int J Pediatr Otorhinolaryngol* 31:15, 1995.
46. Tom LWC and others: The sternocleidomastoid tumor of infancy, *Int J Pediatr Otorhinolaryngol* 13:245, 1987.
47. Torsiglieri AJ and others: Pediatric neck masses: guidelines for evaluation, *Int J Pediatr Otorhinolaryngol* 16:199, 1988.
48. Treyve EL, Duckert LG: Phenytoin-induced lymphadenopathy appearing as a nasopharyngeal malignant neoplasm, *Arch Otolaryngol Head Neck Surg* 107:382, 1981.
49. Ward PH and others: The many faces of cysts of the thyroglossal duct, *Trans Am Acad Ophthal Otolaryngol* 74:310, 1970.
50. Wild G and others: The lateral cyst of the neck: congenital or acquired? *Acta Otolaryngol (Stockh)* 103:546, 1987.
51. Zangwill KM, Hamilton DH, Perkins BA: Cat scratch disease in Connecticut: epidemiology, risk factors, and evaluation of a new diagnostic test, *N Engl J Med* 329:8, 1993.

Chapter 16

Congenital Disorders of the Larynx

Bruce Benjamin

The study of congenital abnormalities of the upper airway in premature babies, neonates, and infants may require consultation among pediatric specialists in the fields of medicine, surgery, neonatology, pulmonology, anesthesiology, and radiology. The pediatric laryngologist is the focal point for definitive endoscopic diagnosis and for determining management of airway obstruction. Although the majority of patients undergoing diagnostic examination are seldom seriously ill, many demanding problems confront the endoscopist and anesthesiologist, sometimes unexpectedly. Mutual understanding and teamwork are essential for the safe sharing of access to the airway. Moreover, when airway obstruction exists, anesthesia and endoscopic instrumentation may precipitate serious or total obstruction, so facilities to overcome this emergency should always be readily at hand.

ANATOMY

Child and adult differences

Structural and functional differences exist between the pediatric and the adult larynx.

The size of the internal larynx at birth is approximately one third of its adult size, and the infant larynx is smaller in proportion to the rest of the body than it is in the adult. The vocal cords are 4 to 4.5 mm long at birth. The laryngeal saccule is variable in size and may be large enough to be seen on a lateral radiograph (Fig. 16-1). The supraglottic airway makes an angle with the subglottic airway at the vocal cords.

The larynx grows until puberty, at which time it is fully developed. Whereas the thyroid cartilage in an infant is short and broad, the adult larynx, especially in the male, develops the laryngeal prominence and thyroid notch.

The thyroid cartilage is closer to the hyoid in the infant. The fetal larynx is positioned high in the neck, usually at the level of the second and third vertebrae, descending to the fourth vertebra at birth, to the fifth at approximately 6 years of age, and to the sixth or seventh at puberty.

The higher larynx of the infant is softer, more easily displaced, and more easily irritated. The epiglottis projects into the oropharynx, and its shape can vary considerably. The so-called infantile epiglottis is longer, narrower, and more tubular. This Ω-shaped structure is seen more often in laryngomalacia but is not a constant finding nor necessarily a diagnostic feature. The aryepiglottic folds are disproportionately large, and the arytenoids vary in shape, being more prominent in the infant than in the adult larynx. The epiglottis is softer and less rigid than in the adult, as is the entire cartilaginous framework of the larynx, which has less resistance to changing pressures. Although this mobility of the musculature and soft tissues of the pharynx and larynx in the newborn is greater, the capacity is also greater for stabilization by the sucking pad in the cheeks and the skeletal muscular action in fixing the mandible and hyoid bones. The normal pharyngeal airway is maintained from the moment of birth, despite variations in head and neck position, opening of the jaw, and various powerful sucking movements. During inspiration there is constriction, and during expiration the upper respiratory chamber of the pharynx normally expands.

The mucous membrane and underlying connective tissue of the immediate subglottic region are loosely attached. Be-

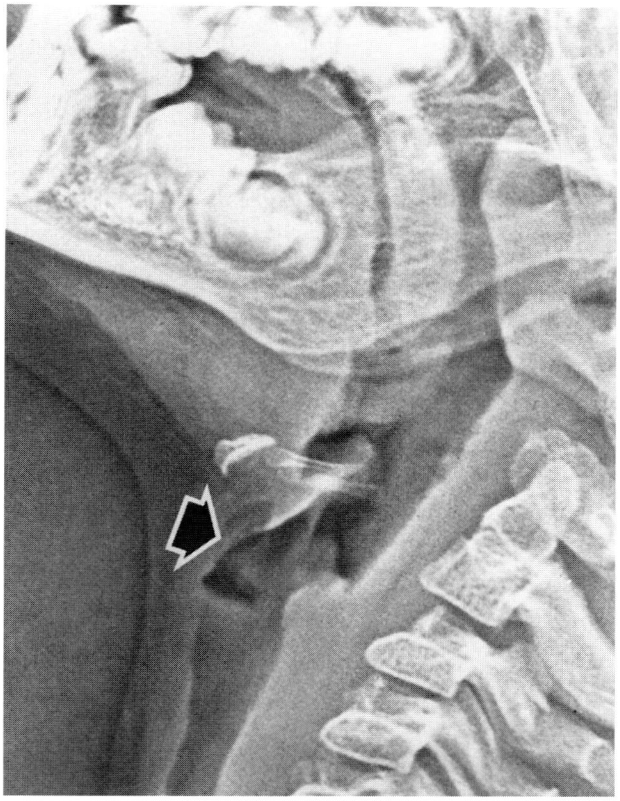

Fig. 16-1. Lateral xerography of the larynx and pharynx. Ventricle of the larynx is clearly seen with the true cords below and the false cords above. *Arrow* points to an air-filled laryngeal saccule, which is sometimes large enough to be seen on radiography under normal circumstances.

cause the subglottic space is bounded by the rigid ring of the cricoid cartilage, the tissues enlarge at the expense of the airway when swelling and edema occur.

Nerve supply

The nerve supply of the larynx, both sensory and motor, is through cranial nerve (CN) X via the superior and inferior laryngeal nerve branches. Laryngeal paralysis is virtually always caused by a peripheral nerve lesion because each side is equally represented in the cerebral cortex. Because the left recurrent laryngeal nerve runs under the arch of the aorta in a longer course than the right nerve does, it is likely to be affected by a greater variety of diseases; thus, motor paralysis is more common on the left side than on the right.

PHYSIOLOGY

Laryngeal reflexes

Several vital laryngeal reflexes exist. Laryngeal spasm, bronchial constriction, slowing of the heart rate, and apnea are life-threatening effects on the cardiovascular and respiratory systems, mediated by well-known laryngeal reflexes. The administration of vagolytic drugs and the application of topical anesthesia reduce the effects of these powerful laryngeal reflexes during endoscopic manipulation.

Protection

The protective function of the larynx prevents contamination of the airway by food and fluid during swallowing as the vocal cords and the laryngeal sphincter mechanism completely close. The shape and backward movement of the epiglottis divert the bolus to each side into the piriform fossae before it enters the esophagus. The cough reflex, activated by receptors in the larynx and upper trachea, triggers an explosive cough against closed vocal cords to remove any foreign substance from the airway before serious aspiration to the lower airways can occur—a vital protective function of the larynx.

Phonation

Phonation is the second primary function of the larynx, and an abnormality of this function in the newborn produces an abnormal or feeble cry or no cry at all.

HISTORY

Significant facts relating to the congenital abnormality are obtained from the parents, the medical attendants (including the obstetrician, pediatrician, or neonatologist), and the nursing staff.

The nature of the mother's pregnancy (hydramnios is associated with tracheoesophageal fistula) and the course of the perinatal period (a traumatic or forceps delivery may cause nasal trauma) are important. Some clinical conditions, such as severe micrognathia, are obvious at birth. Neonatal respiratory distress caused by major airway obstruction may be apparent immediately after birth: bilateral choanal atresia, bilateral vocal cord paralysis, large congenital cyst, or major laryngeal web. Periods of cyanosis can accompany the stridor associated with total nasal obstruction, but if the infant cries and takes a breath through the mouth, the airway obstruction is momentarily relieved.

If both vocal cords are paralyzed, stridor is always present, the cry may be weak, and mucus may be aspirated. A muffled or absent cry suggests supraglottic pharyngeal obstruction caused by a cyst or a mass. A harsh barking cough or biphasic inspiratory and expiratory stridor, especially with retraction of the head and neck, suggests tracheal obstruction caused by stenosis, compression, or collapse.

A history of respiratory distress and aspiration with feeding in the neonatal period signals the possibility of a communication between the respiratory and digestive tracts, such as a tracheoesophageal fistula or a posterior laryngeal cleft.

Some congenital lesions do not present their features at birth and are delayed for days or weeks. Examples include laryngomalacia, in which the stridor may not appear for several days or even 1 week or more after birth; vascular compression of the trachea, which may appear weeks or months after birth; and subglottic hemangioma, the symptoms of which may not appear for several months.

PHYSICAL EXAMINATION

An estimated 10% of all newborns, especially those who are premature, have some form of respiratory difficulty in the first few hours of life, but most recover quickly. Most cases of respiratory distress are caused by hyaline membrane disease; some are caused by respiratory depression from drugs. Probably less than 5% of persistent neonatal respiratory distress is caused by congenital anomalies of the upper respiratory tract but these anomalies are significant. When one anomaly exists, other anomalies may exist in the respiratory tract or in other organ systems.

Examination may show respiratory distress, a rapid or even slow respiratory rate, and signs of hypoxia or cyanosis. The normal respiratory rate is rapid in a newborn and slower in older children. Physical signs on general examination of the baby may lead to suspicion of a specific condition.

Complete nasal obstruction may result in death from asphyxia. For example, bilateral posterior choanal atresia is associated with periods of respiratory obstruction. Vigorous inspiratory efforts produce marked chest retraction and cyanosis, but if the infant cries and takes a breath through the mouth, the airway obstruction is relieved until the crying stops. The mouth closes until the cycle of obstruction is repeated. These features should alert the attending physician to the possibility of serious nasal obstruction and the probability of bilateral choanal atresia.

A baby with obvious signs of Pierre Robin sequence may have serious upper airway problems caused by oropharyngeal obstruction from micrognathia and a retroposed tongue. Similar signs are seen in babies with Treacher Collins syndrome, Crouzon's syndrome, Apert's syndrome, and macroglossia, whether it is idiopathic, caused by lymphangioma or hemangioma or associated with cretinism.

Other obvious conditions on general examination include large neck masses such as a hemangioma or lymphangioma, a large thyroglossal duct cyst, or even a branchial cyst, which may compress the airway in the pharynx or the trachea. Most conditions causing respiratory obstruction in the newborn are congenital, whereas respiratory difficulties in older patients are usually acquired.

In older children, the larynx and hypopharynx can often be inspected by indirect examination with the laryngeal mirror, but this examination is not possible in infants. The larynx and related structures can be adequately inspected only by direct laryngoscopy, which allows accurate visualization of all structures. The laryngologist's clinical examination relies on evaluation of the facies, nasal airways, tongue, oropharynx, and neck and on chest examination and auscultation. The neck and the laryngeal structures are palpated for position and general outline.

Small-diameter pediatric size flexible laryngoscopes are used by otolaryngologists and pulmonologists in infants and children to examine the nasal cavities, pharynx, and larynx in the office, clinic, or ward. Flexible instruments less than 3 mm in diameter or ultrathin fiberoptic bronchoscopes, which have neither a steering mechanism nor a suction channel, can be passed via an endotracheal tube.

The description, duration, and nature of the features described from the history should be correlated with the findings from the physical examination. Although these features or combination of features may suggest the possibility of the underlying pathologic condition, few are diagnostic. Usually the clinician obtains radiologic studies before proceeding to thorough endoscopic examination with the patient under general anesthesia.

Stridor

The cardinal sign of airway obstruction, stridor, is well known to all medical practitioners. The abnormal and distinctive sound is produced by turbulence of the airflow in the upper airways. Stridor is usually inspiratory but occasionally expiratory; it is caused by some degree of respiratory obstruction. It may be accompanied by physical signs of airway obstruction, a weak or absent cry, repeated aspiration, cyanotic or apneic attacks, cough, swallowing difficulty, or lower respiratory tract manifestations such as pneumonia or bronchitis. Stridor is heard by anyone listening beside the patient. A wheeze similar to the expiratory accompaniment of asthma may be heard if it is loud, but it is usually heard by chest auscultation. The vibration set up by severe stridor (e.g., in laryngomalacia) may affect the surrounding tissues in the neck or chest. The parent can often feel it by placing a hand on the child's chest. The parent may state that the child's chest "rattles."

Stridor's cause may be found in the nose or nasal cavities (as in bilateral posterior choanal atresia), in the pharynx (as in micrognathia and glossoptosis), in the larynx (as in laryngomalacia), in the trachea (as in compression of the trachea by a vascular ring), or even in the main bronchi (as in congenital bronchial stenosis). The following are congenital abnormalities of the pharynx and larynx that cause airway obstruction:

Nasopharyngeal obstruction
- Bilateral posterior choanal atresia
- Turbinate hypertrophy (stuffy nose syndrome)
- Deviated septum caused by birth trauma
- Encephalocele, dermoid, chordoma, hamartoma, and others

Facial skeletal abnormalities
- Pierre Robin sequence (micrognathia, glossoptosis, cleft palate)
- Treacher Collins syndrome (mandibulofacial dysostosis)
- Apert's syndrome (acrocephalosyndactyly)
- Crouzon's syndrome (craniofacial dysostosis)

Oropharyngeal obstruction
- Macroglossia

Lingual thyroid or internal thyroglossal duct cyst
Pharyngeal tumors (e.g., cystic hygroma, dermoid, aberrant thyroid tissue)

Laryngeal obstruction

Supraglottic
Laryngomalacia
Ductal retention cyst (epiglottic or vallecula cyst)
Saccular cyst
Cystic hygroma
Bifid epiglottis
Hypoplasia of epiglottis
Pharyngolaryngeal web (probably a variant of normal)

Glottic
Vocal cord paralysis
Web and atresia
Interarytenoid web
Posterior laryngeal cleft
Arthrogryposis multiplex congenita
Cri du chat syndrome
Anterior laryngeal cleft
Congenital neurovascular dysfunction (Plott's syndrome)

Subglottic
Congenital subglottic stenosis
Subglottic hemangioma
Web and atresia
Cysts

Congenital abnormalities of the trachea that cause airway obstruction include tracheoesophageal fistula, tracheomalacia, vascular ring compression, innominate artery compression, stenosis, tracheal compression, hemangioma, webs, atresia, and tracheogenic duplication cyst.

The characteristics of the stridor may be a clue to the location of the obstruction. A harsh, high-pitched, crowing noise during inspiration often indicates an abnormality in the larynx, in the subglottic region, or more often in the supraglottic tissues. Stridor of lower pitch with snoring and excessive secretions may indicate a pharyngeal or nasopharyngeal obstruction. Stridor that is inspiratory and expiratory with a prolonged low-pitched expiratory phase suggests obstruction of the trachea or even main bronchi from compression or collapse.

Stridor and respiratory distress may also be caused by conditions outside the respiratory tract. For instance, a large abdominal mass, a diaphragmatic hernia and eventration, a reduplication cyst, a hemangioma, or a lymphangioma can narrow the major airways.

The clinician should know when the stridor began, how long it has persisted, whether it is constant or intermittent, and what has been its progress and degree. Its relation to inspiration and expiration; the effect of sleeping, eating, crying, or posture; and a possible association with aspiration may all be important. Observation and examination over hours or days may give useful information not detectable at a single examination.

Correlation of the clinical features, physical signs, radiologic abnormalities, and the endoscopic changes is essential to localize the cause and make a correct diagnosis. Endoscopic examination of a patient under general anesthesia always includes the oropharynx, larynx, trachea, and bronchi; often, the esophagus; and when indicated, the nasal cavities and nasopharynx. Laryngoscopy alone is incomplete because pathologic conditions in the tracheobronchial tree may remain undiagnosed. More than 10% of patients have lesions at more than one anatomic site in the upper aerodigestive tract.[15]

Stridor and *congenital laryngeal stridor* are all-inclusive terms but never diagnoses. If possible, the term should refer to the primary cause and anatomic location because not all reasons for stridor in an infant are congenital. Laryngoscopy alone in the investigation of congenital laryngeal stridor without examination of the tracheobronchial tree and, if necessary, the esophagus should be regarded as incomplete.

ENDOSCOPIC EXAMINATION

Diagnostic endoscopic examination to investigate stridor is indicated when one of the following exists:

Severe stridor
Progressive stridor
Stridor associated with unusual features, such as cyanotic attacks, apneic attacks, dysphagia, aspiration, failure to thrive, or a radiologic abnormality
Stridor causing undue parental anxiety

Signs of obstruction

Airway obstruction may be present from birth and persistent, recurring with every breath (e.g., in bilateral vocal cord paralysis). It may also be variable and phasic (e.g., in laryngomalacia) or relentlessly progressive (e.g., with an enlarging cyst.)

Major congenital airway obstruction in a newborn produces stridor, rapid breathing with increased effort indicated by retraction of the chest, epigastric in-drawing, tracheal tug, suprasternal and intercostal retraction, and flaring of the nasal alae during inspiration. As obstruction progresses, even vigorous use of the accessory respiratory muscles and tachypnea might not prevent respiratory failure with impaired pulmonary ventilation, cyanosis, and subsequent bradycardia as the levels of hypoxia and hypercarbia increase.

With chronic airway obstruction, sternal retraction caused by persistent, negative pleural pressure and high compliance of the rib cage may be exaggerated. With a long-standing obstruction, a permanent pectus excavatum may result.

In seriously ill patients with lower airway obstruction and lung parenchymal lesions causing respiratory failure, blood gas and blood pH studies may be required as single or serial examinations to assess the degree of respiratory failure and to assist in the management of respiratory or metabolic acidosis. In patients with obstruction of the upper airways, blood gases may remain normal or near normal even with severe obstruction. Clinical assessment is much more important.

Cry abnormalities

Normal phonation depends on the subglottic air pressure; on the length, tension, and mass of the vibrating vocal cords; and on the ability of the straight free medial margin of the vocal cord to vibrate freely. Any change in these variables produces abnormal vocalization.

When both vocal cords are paralyzed, stridor always exists, and the cry, although usually weak, is clear. With unilateral cord paralysis, the cry may be weak and feeble, but usually no serious airway obstruction exists. Depending on the size of the laryngeal web, complete aphonia or a weak, breathy, and feeble cry may exist; with smaller webs, minimal impairment of phonation may occur. A muffled or absent cry in infants may relate to pharyngeal involvement (e.g., from a cyst or other pharyngeal obstruction). Cysts in or about the larynx affect the voice and obstruct the airway.

Cri du chat syndrome[27] is a rare but interesting cause of a weak and high-pitched abnormal cry resembling the mewing of a cat.

Aspiration

Congenital anomalies and neurologic conditions of the oral cavity, pharynx, larynx, trachea, and esophagus are the most common causes of repeated aspiration and aspiration pneumonia with segmental atelectasis. Recurrent aspiration frequently causes failure to thrive.

Feeding difficulty and incoordinated swallow and aspiration often occur in patients with cleft palate, mandibular hypoplasia and glossoptosis, disorders in the midfacial skeleton, choanal atresia, and esophageal abnormalities (e.g., stenosis, webs, duplication).

The differential diagnosis of repeated aspiration in infants requiring endoscopic investigation includes gastroesophageal reflux with aspiration, neuromuscular incoordination of swallowing in central nervous system disorders, bulbar paralysis, tracheoesophageal fistula, cleft larynx, and vagal paralysis with insensitivity of the superior half of the larynx with ipsilateral recurrent laryngeal nerve paralysis.

Radiologic studies with contrast material used for the esophageal swallow and cineradiography are traditional investigations. Scanning for radioactive-labeled milk may be useful, especially for gastroesophageal reflux. Reflux may occur after swallowing, with return of gastric contents and aspiration into the tracheobronchial tree. Esophagoscopy with biopsy and pH monitoring may give useful information.

In some cases of repeated aspiration, gastric tube feedings are an essential part of the management during investigation and observation to prevent further deterioration and to provide the required nutritional support.

Cough and apnea

Cough is an essential component of the body's defense mechanism and is a primitive reflex that is most reliable in protecting the lower respiratory tract. As a symptom, cough represents a physiologic response to various respiratory tract stimuli. Repeated, persistent cough in a baby is distressing to parents.

Cough is not a common feature of disorders of the respiratory tract in babies. When cough does occur, however, it is an important diagnostic aid. The onset, frequency, and force of the cough and the presence of secretions should be noted. For example, coughing associated with feeding or drinking may be caused by aspiration. A persistent barking cough with or without stridor is a prominent characteristic of tracheal narrowing and is suggestive of tracheomalacia or tracheal compression.

In tracheal compression or collapse, the head and neck may be held in hyperextension, and cyanotic or apneic attacks may occur. Apneic attacks occurring with innominate artery compression of the trachea or with tracheomalacia associated with tracheoesophageal fistula has been termed *reflex apnea* or *dying spells*. Prolonged apneic attack leads to cyanosis, bradycardia, or even cardiac arrest.

RADIOLOGIC EXAMINATION

After correlation of evidence from the history and physical examination, an appropriate radiologic examination should be considered in infants with possible congenital abnormalities of the hypopharynx, larynx, and trachea, especially if stridor and airway obstruction exist.

Anteroposterior chest radiography is a routine requirement. An anteroposterior view of the tracheal air column enhanced by a high-kilovolt technique may be useful (e.g., in subglottic hemangioma or tracheal stenosis). The film should be taken, if possible, during both inspiration and expiration because changes in the mobile soft tissues of the pharynx change the appearance.[2]

Lateral study of the upper airways with radiography or xeroradiography is particularly useful. A well-exposed film with the patient's head and neck in the hyperextended position consistently provides worthwhile information, often of essential diagnostic value. Many variations are seen in normal lateral airway radiography in infants. Experience in interpretation distinguishes the normal from the abnormal. The most reliable landmark in the larynx is the laryngeal ventricle, which is normally distended with air. Apparent abnormalities in an otherwise healthy airway can be produced by poor positioning or exposure technique. When possible, radiography should be undertaken, except in an extreme emergency, before a patient is examined by endoscopy under a general anesthetic.

Xeroradiography has been used for many years in evalu-

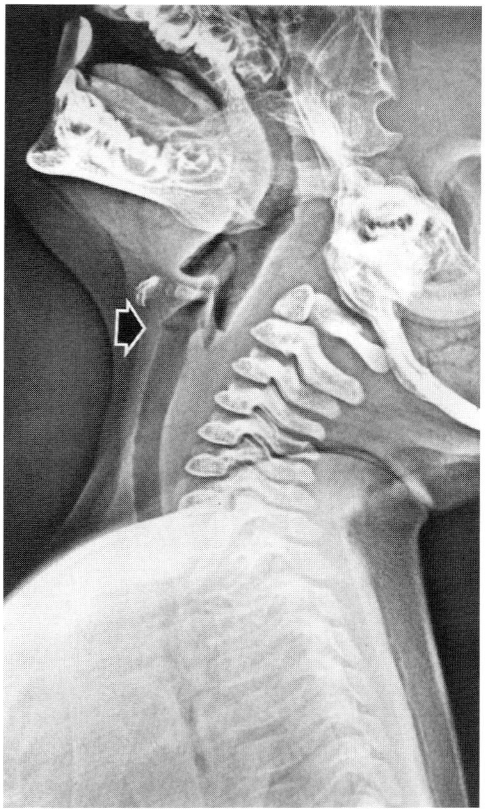

Fig. 16-2. Normal larynx and tracheal air shadow in an infant. The nasopharyngeal airway, soft palate, posterior pharyngeal wall, base of the tongue, and supraglottic structures (including arytenoids and epiglottis) are well outlined. Ventricle of the larynx *(arrow)* is seen with the true cords below and the false cords above. Cervical and intrathoracic parts of the trachea are clearly shown.

ating the upper respiratory tract and has a very useful application in the larynx. Its enhancement of the air–soft tissue edge and wide exposure latitude are distinct advantages over conventional radiologic technique; in many patients, the airway can be seen from the nasal cavities above to the bifurcation of the trachea below. The higher radiation dosage associated with xeroradiography should be carefully considered and balanced against the clinical needs for the particular patient and the possibility of additional useful information (Fig. 16-2). It is now seldom used.

Contrast laryngography has no place in the investigation or documentation of infant laryngeal problems.

The contrast esophagogram is essential in the investigation of some infants and may show gastroesophageal reflux. Although the barium study has traditionally been regarded as a diagnostic radiologic investigation, the unreliability of a single barium swallow examination, even when performed by an experienced radiologist, is well known. However, esophagography may help diagnose a vascular ring, H-type tracheoesophageal fistula, swallowing difficulty caused by neuromuscular incoordination, mediastinal cyst or tumor, and even a posterior laryngeal cleft. There are no studies to show that computed tomography (CT) has additional advantages in assessing the laryngeal airway, but it is of great advantage in investigating a pulmonary or mediastinal mass, whether solid or cystic (e.g., neurogenic tumor, teratoma, lymphosarcoma, bronchogenic or duplication cyst) (Fig. 16-3).

In selected cases, contrast tracheobronchography (as for congenital stenosis of the trachea or bronchi) and occasionally angiocardiography (as for a vascular ring) are helpful. Clearly, investigation of the larynx and pharynx alone without study of the tracheobronchial tree and, if necessary, the esophagus should be regarded as incomplete.

Care should be taken in the interpretation of a single film

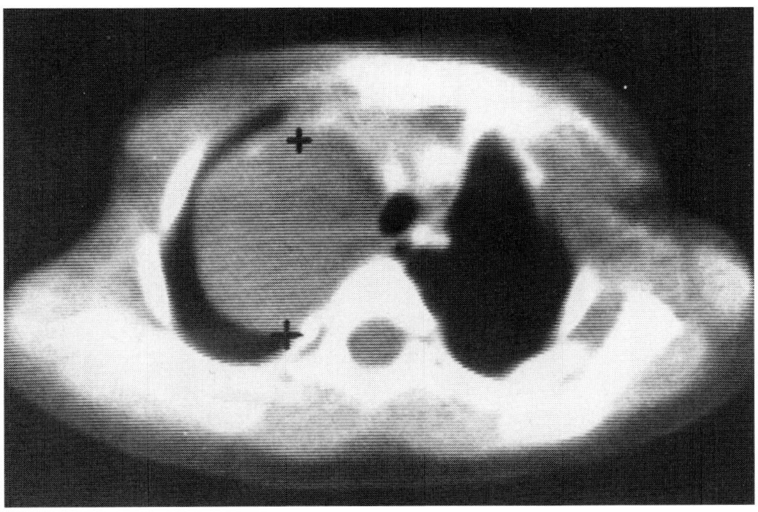

Fig. 16-3. Computed tomography confirms a bronchogenic cyst adjacent to the lower trachea and carina.

because the soft-tissue structures are subject to changes in caliber and appearance. The pharynx, larynx, and trachea may be visualized during any phase of respiration or deglutition. Although two or more films are taken, they may not necessarily represent the phases of respiration because ensuring inspiratory and expiratory film in infants is often difficult.

Symptoms relating to the airway and to the esophagus often coexist in infants who have aspiration caused by gastroesophageal reflux, tracheoesophageal fistula, or a repaired tracheoesophageal fistula. In some cases, secondary lower respiratory tract disease is clinically or radiologically apparent.

ENDOSCOPY

Anesthesia

Cooperation, mutual understanding, and teamwork between the surgeon and the anesthesiologist are imperative for the safety of the baby during endoscopic examination of the upper airways. Patients rarely undergo examination without general anesthesia. Occasionally in sick neonates up to a few weeks of age or in those with suspected vocal cord paralysis, no anesthetic is used, but the anesthesiologist is in attendance. Intubating a baby without general anesthesia may sometimes be preferable in Pierre Robin sequence, in which a difficult airway problem exists.

The most common general anesthetic technique for neonatal endoscopy[4] relies on spontaneous respiration using insufflation of nitrous oxide, oxygen, and halothane. Some anesthesiologists prefer to add methoxyflurane to the gaseous mixture to provide additional analgesia of longer duration, thus ''smoothing out'' the procedure. In the case of an ill child, oxygen only with halothane is used.

Atropine as a single agent is used for premedication in babies. It can be given by intramuscular injection preoperatively or intravenously at or soon after induction of anesthesia. Atropine protects against bradycardia and helps minimize secretions in the respiratory tract. Topical anesthesia using lidocaine (up to 5 mg/kg) in a dilute solution minimizes unwanted reflex activity and is regarded as most important because it usually abolishes laryngeal spasm during endoscopy. However, laryngeal spasm can occasionally be a complication in endoscopy with spontaneous respiration. A venipuncture is always performed with endoscopy, and a muscle relaxant is ready to be given if required.

Instruments

Several sizes and types of pediatric laryngoscopes should be available, including the Holinger anterior commissure infant laryngoscope, the Benjamin-Lindholm laryngoscopes, and the Benjamin subglottiscopes. A complete range of rigid bronchoscopes, starting with the 2.5-mm instrument with adaptations to allow ventilation, is available. Various small-diameter Hopkins fiberoptic rigid telescopes, whose light may be directed straight ahead or at various angles, are necessary. The smallest has an outside diameter of 1.9 mm. Other 2.8- and 4-mm telescopes are used constantly in the larynx, tracheobronchial tree, and esophagus for detailed examination. Telescopes with viewing angles of 0°, 30°, and 70° can be used to examine all parts of the larynx and the tracheobronchial tree with previously unavailable clarity and precision (Fig. 16-4).

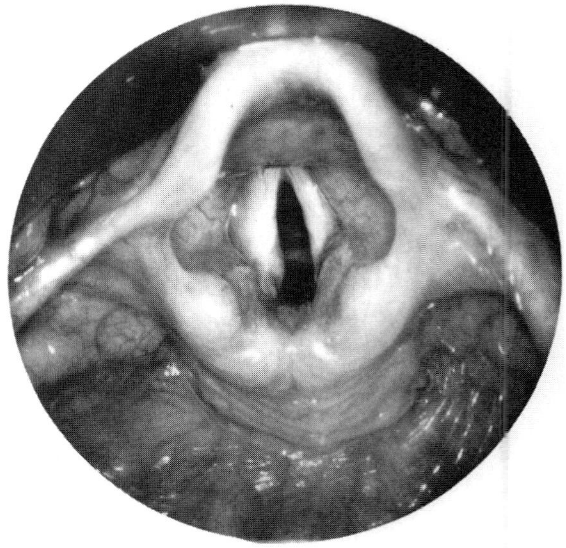

Fig. 16-4. Endoscopy of the normal larynx using a Lindholm laryngoscope. The vocal cords, supraglottic structures, piriform fossae, and epiglottis are shown.

There are few routine uses for the flexible fiberoptic pharyngoscope, laryngoscope, or bronchoscope in the investigation of congenital disorders of the larynx. It may be useful, however, to observe laryngeal dynamics in the infant with laryngomalacia who is awake or under general anesthesia and breathing spontaneously. A flexible neonatalscope, such as that described by Silberman and others,[24] designed for the examination of intubated neonates, should have valuable and interesting applications in placing endotracheal and tracheotomy tubes and in localizing areas of obstruction of the lower respiratory tract.

Technique

A preliminary survey of the larynx and pharynx with the naked eye is accomplished with the hand-held laryngoscope (Fig. 16-5). Hopkins rigid telescopes provide a magnified image for detailed examination of anatomic structure and mucosa. Although direct laryngoscopy is used principally to examine the larynx, other specific anatomic areas are always evaluated, including the oropharynx, the base of the tongue and valleculae, the piriform fossae, the postcricoid region, the epiglottis, the arytenoids, the false cords, the ventricles, the vocal cords (including the anterior and posterior commissure), the subglottic region, and the trachea. External pres-

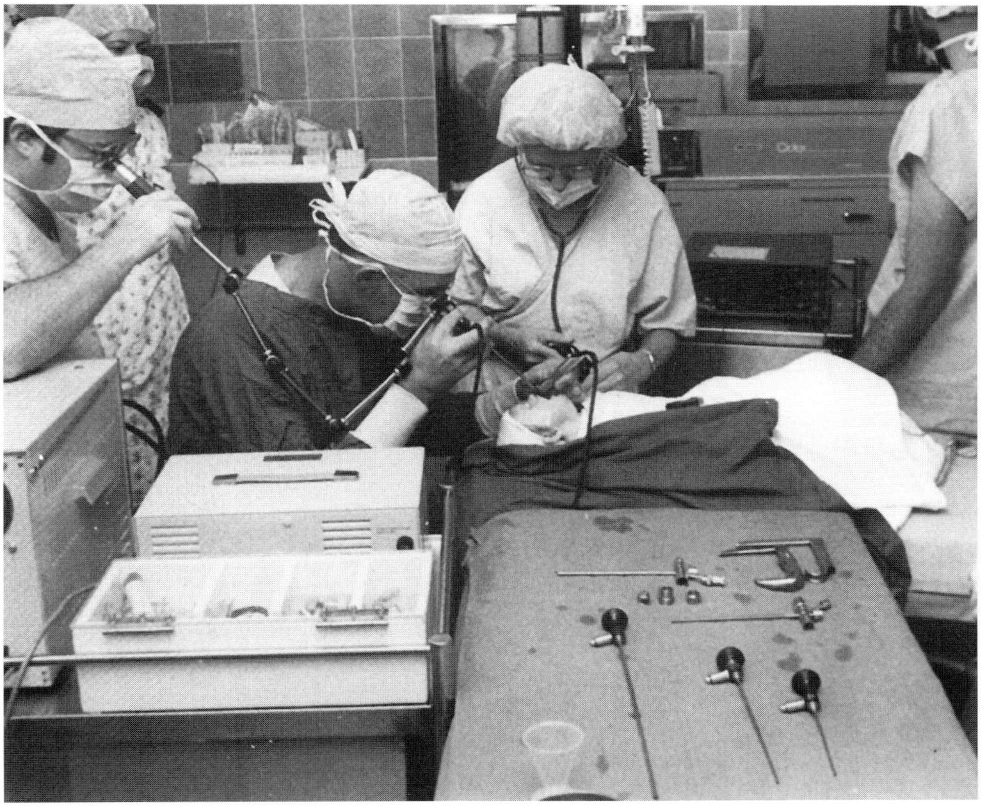

Fig. 16-5. Operating room setup and technique for diagnostic endoscopy. A range of endoscopes suitable for the child's size and age has been selected, suction is readily available, and an anesthesiologist monitors the patient's respiration and heartbeat. Operating room personnel work together as a team.

sure and manipulation of the larynx with a finger or fingers on the neck, with gentle counterpressure from the distal beak of the laryngoscope, rotate or displace the larynx sufficiently to make the other side of the endolarynx or subglottic region more prominent and easier to visualize.

The unique designs of the Lindholm and Benjamin-Lindholm laryngoscopes (Karl Storz, Tuttlingen, Germany) provide a panoramic view of the laryngopharynx by placing the beak of the laryngoscope at the base of the tongue in the vallecula in front of the epiglottis. Although originally designed for adults, the new, small laryngoscope can be used satisfactorily, without trauma, in most infants over 6 to 9 months of age. An infant size instrument is available. These laryngoscopes are especially useful for microlaryngoscopy and laser surgery. The standard slotted Storz pediatric laryngoscopes of 8-, 9.5-, 11-, and 13.5-cm length or the Jackson pediatric laryngoscopes with a slide are used routinely. If the larynx is difficult to expose or examine, a special purpose laryngoscope such as the Holinger pediatric anterior commissure laryngoscope, the Benjamin pediatric operating microlaryngoscope, or the smaller Tucker-Benjamin slotted laryngoscope (Karl Storz, Tuttlingen, Germany) and subglottiscope for newborn and premature infants is useful. These scopes are helpful, for instance, in exposing the larynx in micrognathia or abnormalities of the middle third of the face. The anterior commissures of the posterior glottic space and the interarytenoid region can be seen and displayed by deliberately separating the vocal folds; the subglottic region is more satisfactorily exposed.

Laryngoscopy with telescopes gives a magnified image of the anatomic structures using the standard 0° straight-ahead rigid Hopkins telescope and the 30° or 70° angled telescope for the laryngeal ventricles, the anterior and posterior commissures, and the anterior subglottic region.

Examination of the trachea, main bronchi, and segmental openings is an integral part of endoscopy for congenital airway problems. The patient continues to breathe the anesthetic mixture through the ventilating bronchoscope while the topical analgesic can be applied in measured doses to the tracheal mucosa or to the carina if necessary. The rigid Storz Hopkins telescopes are used alone, passed through a laryngoscope only or through a bronchoscope to examine the contour, caliber, and color of the airways as the dynamics of inspiration and expiration continue. Secretions may be aspirated and collected in a trap bottle for examination and culture. Any abnormal compression, collapse, or pulsation is noted. Biopsy of a lesion is necessary only very occasionally.

It is important that pressure from the tip of the laryngoscope blade or the direction of its introduction does not disturb assessment of vocal cord function and general laryngeal dynamics. Such interference may lead to a false diagnosis of vocal cord paralysis. With the laryngoscope blade in the vallecula and sufficient time for complete evaluation during inspiration and vocalization, the examination will be reliable. Assessment of vocal cord movement and examination of the typical changes of laryngomalacia are best performed when the anesthesia has been discontinued at the end of the procedure and the patient is recovering pharyngeal and laryngeal movements.

Endoscopic examination of the larynx, pharynx, tracheobronchial tree, and esophagus can be successfully and safely performed in a patient at any age, even in premature infants weighing less than 1000 g. The hospital should have the necessary equipment for investigation and experienced anesthetic and endoscopic personnel. A fully staffed postoperative recovery ward and intensive care area with facilities to recognize, diagnose, and manage potential complications immediately are necessary. A multidisciplinary approach with close cooperation between the pediatrician, endoscopist, anesthesiologist, and others involved in the child's care is essential.

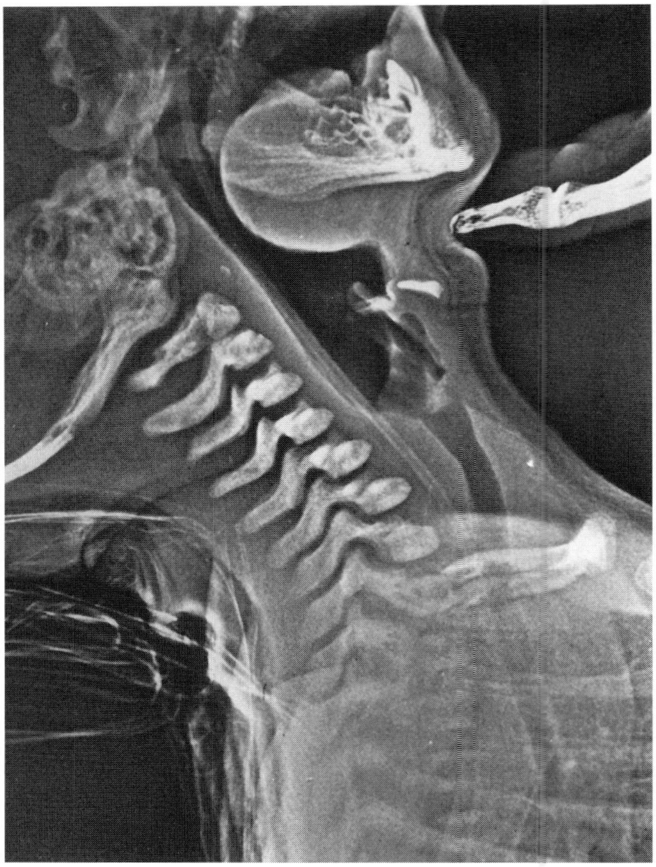

Fig. 16-6. A baby with oropharyngeal obstruction caused by micrognathia and retroposed tongue. Upper airway obstruction is caused by a hypermobile tongue, which has a narrow and unstable origin. The larynx and tracheal air shadow are normal. (From Benjamin B: *Ann Otol Rhinol Laryngol* 90:478, 1981.)

SPECIFIC ABNORMALITIES

Pierre Robin sequence

Pierre Robin sequence consists of mandibular hypoplasia (micrognathia), glossoptosis (retroposed tongue), and an incomplete midline cleft of the palate, although an occasional patient may not have one of these features. The condition usually presents as an isolated anomaly or as part of another syndrome, commonly Stickler's syndrome. Estimates of incidence range from 1:2000 to 1:50,000 births. The cause is unknown, but some patients have a family history of micrognathia or cleft palate.

Upper airway obstruction is common. It is less severe in the prone position as the tongue falls forward, partly relieving pharyngeal obstruction. Severe obstruction may cause cyanotic episodes, cerebral hypoxia, aspiration pneumonia, right-sided heart failure, or fatal asphyxia. In an infant with micrognathia and glossoptosis, the larynx is under the base of the tongue, making direct laryngoscopy and intubation difficult and sometimes impossible (Fig. 16-6).

The onset of obstruction is usually within a few hours of birth, but it is not possible at first to assess the future severity of the airway obstruction. Repeated observation in the neonatal intensive care ward is needed to determine the best method of airway management. Pulse oximetry is performed in every case; a reasonable guide is to have the oxygen saturation in room air greater than 85% at least 90% of the time. Airway management should be individualized until successful control is achieved using the following progressive sequence:

- Posturing in the prone position
- Nasopharyngeal tube
- Endotracheal intubation
- Tracheotomy

The method may partly depend on the severity of associated cardiac and other abnormalities that commonly coexist. Posturing prone is the most important initial part of management; the tongue falls forward, partly clearing the oropharyngeal airway. Posturing can be discontinued when the child can maintain an airway sleeping supine, usually at about 5 or 6 months of age. Nasogastric tube feeding may be needed if aspiration occurs during feeding.

In cases in which posturing is unsuccessful, a nasopharyngeal tube is passed through one nasal cavity and positioned so the tip is below the level of the base of the tongue but just above the larynx to provide an alternate artificial airway. Posturing may still be necessary.

Various operative techniques to secure the tongue forward have been described, but most are no longer used. In an emergency, traction using a toothed forcep or a suture to pull the tongue forward immediately improves the airway.

If posturing prone or a nasopharyngeal tube does not provide a reliable airway, emergency endotracheal intubation or definitive tracheotomy should be considered. Endotracheal intubation under controlled conditions provides an excellent temporary airway, but there are disadvantages. Laryngoscopy for intubation is always difficult and sometimes impossible without special purpose laryngoscopes such as the Holinger pediatric anterior commissure laryngoscope or the smaller Tucker-Benjamin laryngoscope for premature or small babies. The patency of the tube should be carefully maintained. Accidental extubation may occur with failure to reintubate, and laryngeal trauma from prolonged intubation is a distinct possibility. Tracheotomy is the preferred long-term artificial airway.

If other techniques fail, tracheotomy is safe and dependable to successfully bypass the obstruction and should be performed for cyanosis observed clinically and desaturation measured objectively. There should be no reluctance or delay in performing a tracheotomy because of the relatively high chance of hypoxic cerebral damage or death. The tracheotomy can usually be removed between 6 and 18 months of age.

Patients can be divided into three groups according to the airway management found to be necessary for the severity of airway obstruction and the eventual outcome.

Mild	Posture alone
Moderate	Nasopharyngeal tube
Severe	Short-term intubation, tracheotomy, or death

Experience shows that no method of airway management is effective for every patient. Nasotracheal intubation in many cases can secure a certain, safe airway that can be maintained for many weeks with painstaking nursing care, if necessary over a prolonged period. The airway obstruction inevitably improves with time as the anatomic structures assume a more normal anatomic relationship and the tone in the tongue and pharyngeal musculature improves.

The death rate is 10% to 20%. Deaths from respiratory obstruction indicate the prime importance of airway management and the need for tracheotomy in severe cases.

Abnormalities of midfacial skeleton

Infants with Treacher Collins syndrome (mandibulofacial dysostosis), Apert's syndrome (acrocephalosyndactyly), Crouzon's syndrome (craniofacial dysostosis), and other diseases may have nasal airway obstruction, retrognathia, and malocclusion, so that posterior displacement of the midfacial structures causes oropharyngeal upper airway obstruction. In older children with these anomalies, adenoid hypertrophy sometimes exists, worsening the chronic nasopharyngeal obstruction and causing obstructive sleep apnea. In these patients, removal of the adenoids and tonsils may be dramatically effective.

In neonates, however, conservative management of the airway obstruction by vigilant nursing maintenance of a suitable posture and supportive measures is usually sufficient. In severe or refractory cases, a tracheotomy is indicated.

Oropharyngeal obstruction

A cause of oropharyngeal obstruction is macroglossia, which may be primary (cretinism, Beckwith-Weidemann syndrome), secondary (lymphangioma, hemangioma), part of another congenital syndrome, or idiopathic. Reduction of tongue size by surgical excision offers an acceptable functional result with minimal morbidity.[23]

Aberrant thyroid tissue is most commonly seen as lingual thyroid at the foramen cecum in the base of the tongue but has been reported elsewhere in the pharynx as a cause of airway obstruction. Careful consideration is necessary before a lingual thyroid is removed because it may be the only functioning thyroid tissue in the body. A radioactive thyroid scan detects any other functioning thyroid tissue that is present.

Mucous-retention cysts or ductal cysts most frequently occur in the vallecula. Other pharyngeal masses include dermoid cysts, teratomas, and chordomas. Management of these conditions is symptomatic in each case. With a ductal mucous-retention cyst, aspiration, deroofing, or marsupialization may be necessary.

Laryngomalacia

Laryngomalacia is the most common cause of stridor in infants. The term *congenital laryngeal stridor* should never be used as a definitive diagnosis—it is no more a diagnosis than "fever," "pain," or "anemia" in general medicine. Stridor has multiple causes in an infant; not all are congenital, nor is the stridor necessarily generated from the larynx region. The cause of stridor in a particular patient should be properly determined. If *stridor* is used as a diagnostic term and associated with a specific disease, diagnosis of other laryngopharyngeal anomalies may be delayed, forgotten, or inadvertently disregarded.

The cause of laryngomalacia is not known with certainty. The abnormal flaccidity of the laryngeal tissues is probably a temporary physiologic dysfunction that resolves with growth. Most cases resolve spontaneously within 12 to 24 months. Immaturity of tissues or histopathologic abnormality of the cartilage with increased softness has never been proven. The role of cartilaginous rigidity and elasticity is unknown. Some claim that laryngomalacia is a manifestation of delayed development of neuromuscular control or is caused by an anatomic abnormality.[1]

Clinical presentation

The important features of laryngomalacia include variable inspiratory stridor, signs of intermittent upper airway obstruction, a normal cry, and normal general health and development. Although persistent, noisy stridor from laryngomalacia is distressing to anxious parents, the condition seldom affects the baby's general state of health and progress. It is twice as common in boys as in girls.

Stridor very seldom starts at birth but usually begins in the first few days or weeks of life and persists thereafter as a variable inspiratory accompaniment. It is usually described as harsh and crowing, but at times it is low pitched and fluttering. Sometimes vibrations may be felt by a hand on the infant's chest. The stridor is usually worse with crying and feeding, during excitement or activity, or when the child is lying on his back with the head and neck flexed. However, stridor may improve when the child lies prone or when the head and neck are extended. Elevation of the mandible and submental soft tissues with a finger may partly improve the airway obstruction. The stridor is intermittent and variable; the child sleeps quietly at times and seems "mucousy" at other times, but aspiration of mucus from the pharynx does not relieve the symptoms. Observation and reexamination over days or weeks may give useful information that is not apparent at a single examination. If chest retraction is severe and prolonged, pectus excavatum (sternal retraction) may develop.

Laryngomalacia appears to be caused by flaccidity or incoordination of the supralaryngeal structures, including the cartilages and the soft tissue.

Chen and Holinger[8] observed six mechanisms, two or more of which may occur together as the cause of obstruction: inward collapse of the aryepiglottic folds, primarily the cuneiform cartilages; an elongated epiglottis curled on itself; anterior and medial collapsing movements of the arytenoid cartilages; posterior and inferior displacement of the epiglottis; short aryepiglottic folds; and on overly acute angle of the epiglottis. Some patients have an associated micrognathia, but this is not consistently seen. The cry is clear, strong, and normal. Cyanosis is so uncommon that if it occurs, a condition other than laryngomalacia should be suspected. Similarly, feeding is occasionally slow and noisy; if dysphagia exists, especially if associated with aspiration, the clinician should be alerted to some other condition.

Endoscopic examination

The diagnosis of laryngomalacia can be confirmed only by direct endoscopic examination during respiration, which also excludes the possibility of any associated abnormality in the tracheobronchial tree. The clinician completes a careful endoscopic examination of the upper respiratory tract with and without telescopes. As administration of anesthesia is discontinued and the patient regains muscular tone, the examiner reintroduces the laryngoscope to watch for the typical changes, with the blade at the base of the tongue above and in front of the epiglottis. The epiglottis may be abnormal: tall, narrow, and folded in on itself so that its lateral margins lie close together. Traditionally, endoscopists have described the infantile epiglottis with laryngomalacia, but many patients who have neither laryngomalacia nor stridor have an Ω-shaped or tubular epiglottis, indicating that the shape of the epiglottis itself is not as important as the flaccidity and tendency of the supraglottic tissues to collapse. The aryepiglottic folds and arytenoids are tall, thin, pale, and flaccid, appearing lax and redundant. During each inspiration, they are sucked into the larynx. On expiration, they are blown up and out, so that expiration is unimpeded. When the epiglottis and the aryepiglottic folds of the surpaglottic laryngeal introitus are splinted outward by a laryngoscope, the stridor is immediately corrected and the airway is unimpeded. Sometimes the characteristic changes of laryngomalacia are seen during the initial laryngoscopy, but more often they are seen at the end of the procedure as the administration of anesthesia is discontinued (Fig. 16-7).

Flexible fiberoptic laryngoscopy can confirm the abnormality of the supraglottic structures in laryngomalacia, but the examination is inadequate unless the subglottic region and tracheobronchial tree are examined endoscopically because some patients have associated pathologic findings in other areas.

Radiologic examination

Although chest and lateral airway radiography is routine in the investigation of stridor, radiologic examination of laryngomalacia is normal. No diagnostic radiologic features can be seen in single films.

Management

Most infants with laryngomalacia gain weight and mature normally. If general progress is satisfactory, diagnosis by endoscopic examination usually allays the parents' concern. Active management is unnecessary. The parents should be reassured that the symptoms will subside over the following months and with growth and development of the larynx. Only very rarely is surgery required.

A conservative approach for this usually self-correcting condition is appropriate for most infants, but a few with severe obstruction may require surgery. Indications include severe stridor with failure to thrive, obstructive apnea, weight loss, severe chest deformity, cyanotic attacks, pulmonary hypertension, cor pulmonale, and desaturation documented by hospital studies showing hypoxemia and hypercapnia. Coexistent causes of airway obstruction should be excluded.

Surgical procedures, usually done with the laser, that have been advocated include division of the aryepiglottic fold, partial amputation of the epiglottis, epiglottopexy with glossoepiglottic adhesion, removal of redundant supra-arytenoid mucosa and lateral borders of the epiglottis, removal

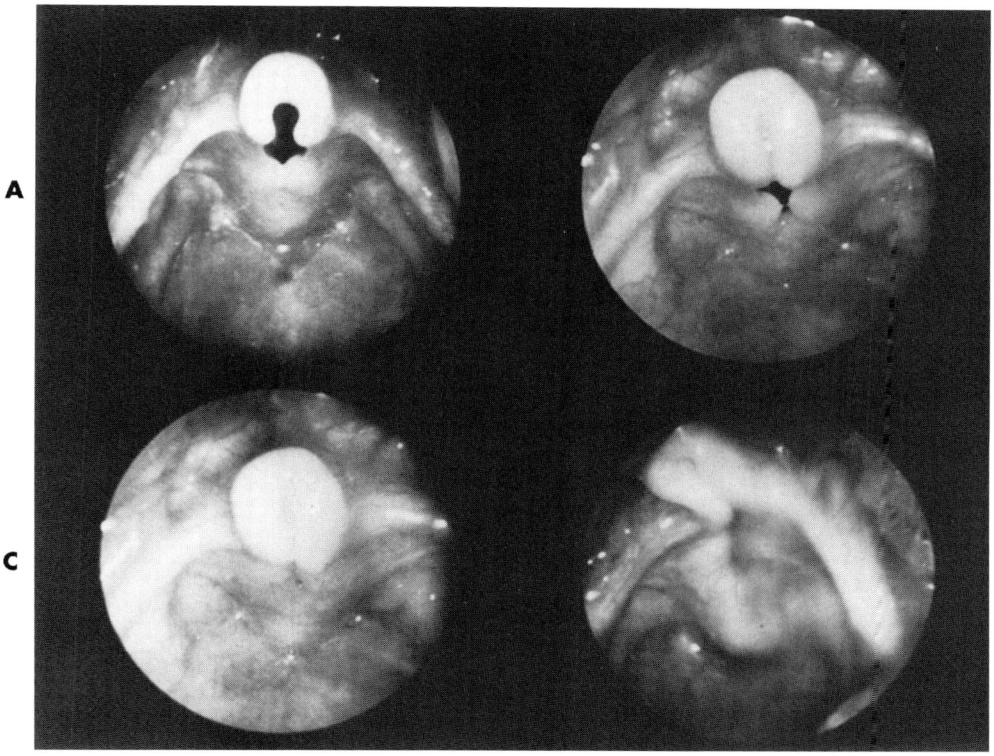

Fig. 16-7. Laryngomalacia. Photographs show changes during the inspiratory cycle. **A,** The epiglottis is small and tightly curled on itself with a well-known Ω shape, so that its lateral margins lie close together, even during expiration. **B** and **C,** As inspiration occurs, tall, floppy, hypermobile arytenoids and aryepiglottic folds are sucked into the supraglottic region, and the posterior edges of epiglottis come together, contributing to inspiratory obstruction. **D,** Violent inspiratory effort causes complete laryngeal obstruction with collapse and gross distortion of the structures.

of the cuneiform and corniculate cartilages and the surrounding mucosa, and in extreme cases, tracheotomy. The most commonly recommended management appears to be endoscopic laser trimming and removal of the prolapsing aryepiglottic fold with the cuneiform cartilage or division of a tight, short aryepiglottic fold. In this way, excessive tissue contributing to obstruction is removed, namely the redundant supra-arytenoid mucosa including the cuneiform cartilage. Most authors believe that identifying and managing gastroesophageal reflux is also important.

Kelly and Gray[21] reviewed the complications of these procedures, including posterior stenosis after bilateral supraglottoplasty. They recommended unilateral endoscopic supraglottoplasty to decrease the likelihood of stenosis in some children who may later require a second procedure on the contralateral side for complete relief of symptoms.

Laryngeal cysts

Cysts of the larynx and pharynx can be classified as follows:

- Ductal cysts, which occur anywhere that a mucous-producing gland exists
- Saccular cysts, either lateral or (less commonly) anterior; the saccule is normally small and contains air
- Thyroglossal duct cysts, which occur at the tongue base at the foramen cecum
- Cystic hygroma or lymphangioma, which is a multilocular cystic developmental abnormality arising from lymph vessels

Ductal cysts

Ductal cysts are also known as *mucous-retention cysts*. They are found in the valleculae within the larynx or the subglottic region. They result from retention of mucus in dilated collecting ducts of the submucosal glands, are usually less than 1 cm in diameter, are superficial, and remain within the mucous membrane. Thus, the common vallecular cyst is merely a ductal cyst in the anatomic region of the vallecula. Similarly, a congenital subglottic cyst is a ductal cyst in the subglottic region of the larynx.

In infants who have undergone prolonged intubation, ductal cysts are not uncommonly seen in the subglottic region (Fig. 16-8) and may be multiple. These cysts are caused by irritation and obstruction of mucous gland ducts. They might

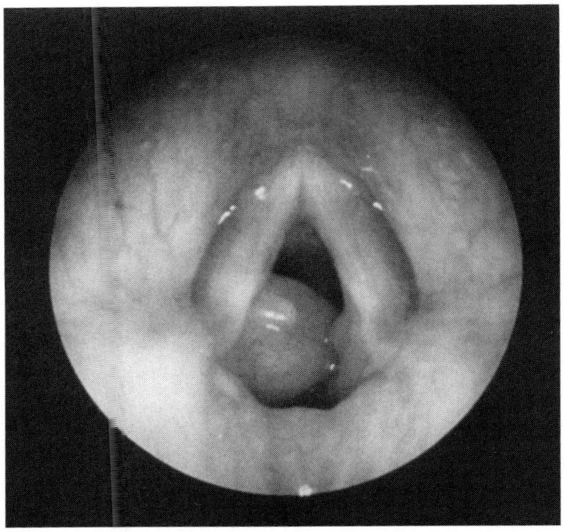

Fig. 16-8. Ductal cysts in the subglottic region of a newborn. The cysts were diagnosed and managed by endoscopy.

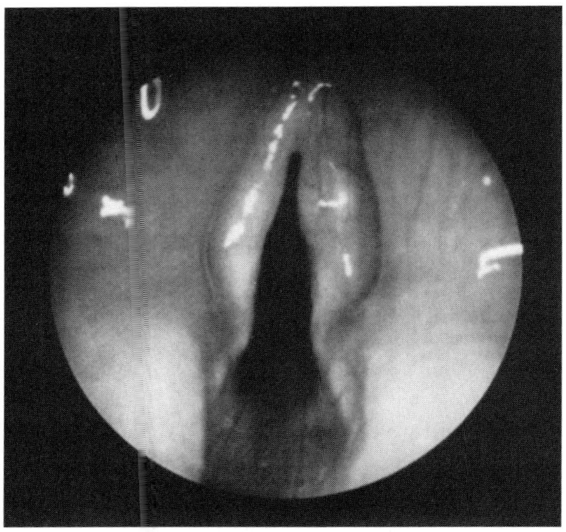

Fig. 16-9. An intracordal cyst in the right vocal cord with some minor reactive changes on the edge of the left vocal cord.

not be clearly seen on lateral airway radiography but are diagnosed on direct endoscopic examination. They are managed by removal by forceps or laser, with care being taken for possible reexamination to manage recurrence. A small intracordal cyst (Fig. 16-9) requires removal by laryngeal microsurgery.

Saccule cysts

The saccule of the laryngeal ventricle (see Fig. 16-1) is a normal structure seen as an outpouching of mucous membrane that contains mucous glands between the false and true vocal cords at the anterior third of the laryngeal ventricle.

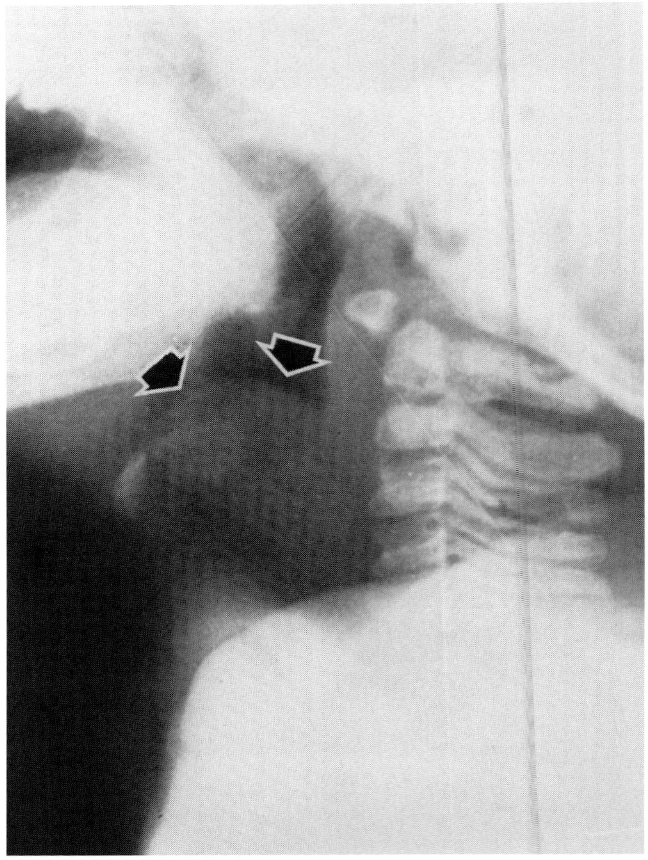

Fig. 16-10. A large congenital saccular cyst *(arrows)* in a newborn causing distortion of the supraglottic structures and severe airway obstruction since birth.

Delicate intrinsic laryngeal muscles lie medial and lateral to the saccule; by compressing the saccule, they are thought to control expression of its secretions onto the vocal cords for lubrication.

A congenital saccular cyst in the newborn (Fig. 16-10) is a dilated saccule filled with mucus that does not communicate with or drain into the laryngeal lumen. Saccular cysts have also been called *congenital cysts of the larynx, laryngeal mucoceles,* and *saccular mucoceles.* Saccular cysts are of two types. Although both are rare, the more common is the lateral saccular cyst that extends up to distend the false vocal cord and the aryepiglottic fold (Fig. 16-11). A lateral saccular cyst is the same as an internal laryngomucocele. The anterior saccular cyst is smaller and extends medially into the laryngeal lumen between the true and false cords (Fig. 16-12).

A laryngocele (most often seen in adults) is an abnormal dilation of a saccule. It is distended with air, which causes it to become pathologic and temporarily symptomatic (Fig. 16-13). Apparently, congenital laryngeal cysts in the region of the ventricle are saccular cysts and are the counterparts of the adult laryngoceles. In the neonate and infant, the sac-

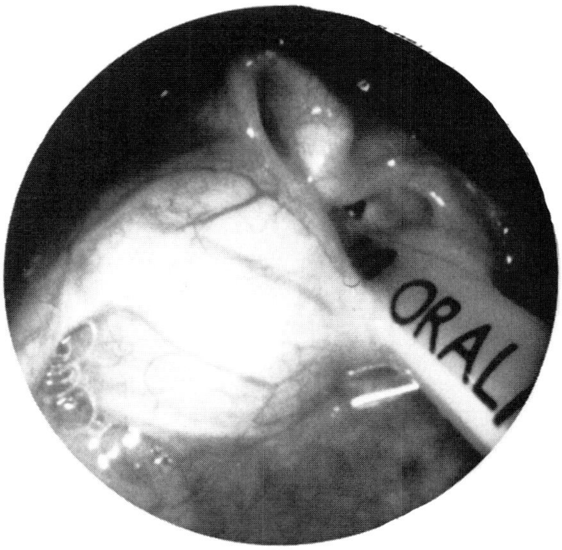

Fig. 16-11. A large lateral saccular cyst in the left hemilarynx of a newborn causing severe obstruction. This lateral saccular cyst is also termed a *mucous-filled internal laryngocele*.

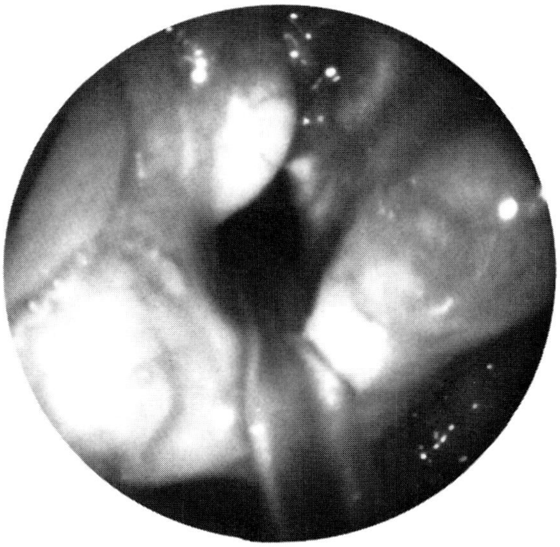

Fig. 16-12. An anterior saccular cyst on the left side of the larynx is filled with mucus. This internal laryngocele arises from the saccule at the anterior aspect of the laryngeal ventricle.

cular cyst is the common pathologic finding. A laryngocele is differentiated from a cyst in that its lumen may be filled with air and, at other times, may be temporarily distended with mucus that discharges into the lumen of the larynx through the normal communication, which has been temporarily obstructed. Holinger and others[19] reported that a developmental spectrum exists among the normal saccule, large saccule, laryngocele, and saccular cyst.

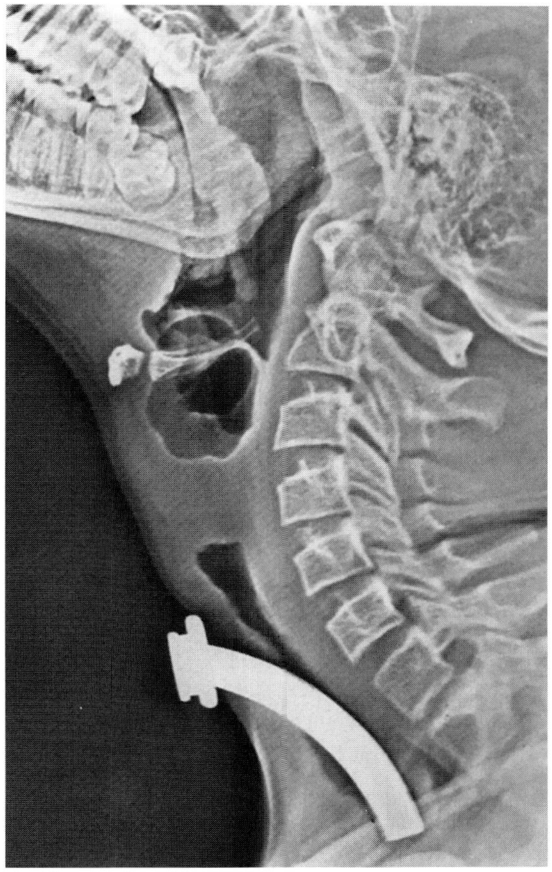

Fig. 16-13. A large, air-containing laryngocele in a teenage boy. A papilloma in the larynx caused partial obstruction of the opening of the laryngeal saccule.

In infants, a saccular cyst may exist at birth and cause severe respiratory distress with inspiratory stridor, episodes of cyanosis, inaudible or muffled cry, and occasionally dysphagia. Although very rare, an external swelling may exist in the neck; if so, investigation is required for an external and an internal laryngocele.

Soft-tissue lateral radiography of the neck and airway shows a cyst in all cases. The diagnosis can be confirmed only at the time of direct laryngoscopy. If radiography reveals the presence of such a problem, the surgeon should be fully prepared (e.g., to decompress a cyst by sucking out its contents or by incising it). Attempts at anesthesia induction can precipitate severe airway obstruction. Endoscopy will reveal a large distended bluish or pink fluid-filled cyst occupying one side of the supraglottic tissues. Consequently, aspiration via a large-bore needle, incision with a sharp instrument, or removal of the dome of the cyst permits drainage of the thick fluid. This procedure may have to be repeated if the cyst reforms. Very rarely, an infant requires an external incision or an excision of the external laryngocele of a persisting

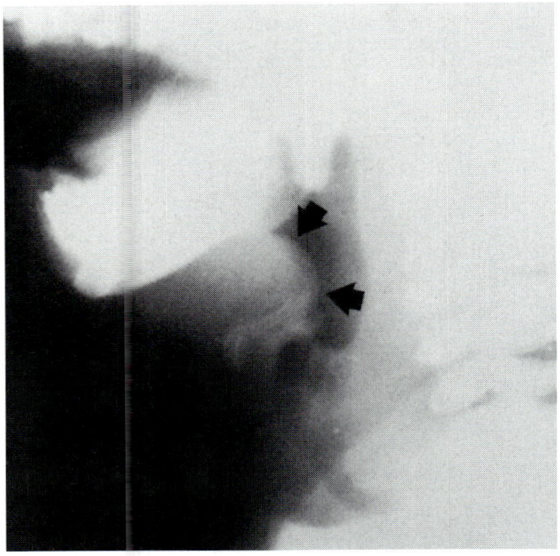

Fig. 16-14. A thyroglossal duct cyst *(arrows)* at the base of the tongue, displacing the epiglottis to a backward position.

cyst. Commonly, recurrence requires repeated aspiration or removal of part of the cyst.

Thyroglossal cyst

Thyroglossal duct cysts (Fig. 16-14) can occur anywhere from the foramen cecum to the thyroid gland and the persisting thyroglossal duct. An internal thyroglossal duct cyst occurs at the base of the tongue in the region of the foramen cecum. Such a cyst, proximal to the hyoid bone, may push the epiglottis backward and down, producing severe obstruction of the supraglottic laryngeal lumen. Management is by incision, drainage, and removal of the roof.

Cystic hygroma

Cystic hygromas (lymphangiomas) are multilocular developmental congenital malformations rather than true neoplasms and are most common in soft tissues of the lateral neck as diffuse, compressible, smooth, nontender masses that transilluminate. They might be obvious at birth or within the first 2 years of life. Histologically they consist of widely dilated lymph vessel spaces. A mass that contains abnormal lymphatics and blood vessels is a lymphangiohemangioma.

Cystic hygromas are usually asymptomatic except for large masses causing cosmetic deformity or masses that stretch or compress tissues of the pharynx and larynx to produce airway obstruction. A cystic hygroma is virtually always a supraglottic mass, whereas a congenital hemangioma causing airway obstruction is usually subglottic.

Management is moderately controversial. Aspiration of the cystic spaces may relieve airway compression if tension within the hygroma is excessive. Management of symptomatic lateral neck lesions is by surgical excision, which may be difficult because of undefined surgical planes. External excision of the bulk by laser or some other modality may be required. For a severe chronic obstruction, a long-term tracheotomy may be necessary.

Vocal cord paralysis

Unilateral or bilateral vocal cord paralysis accounts for about 10% of all congenital laryngeal lesions.[18] Unilateral vocal cord paralysis probably goes undiagnosed in some infants and, with later recovery of laryngeal function, is never documented.

The lesion affecting the motor nerve supply can be located anywhere from the nucleus ambiguus in the brainstem to the neuromuscular junction in the larynx, involving the vagus nerve or its recurrent branch. Consequently, each case should be carefully investigated.[12]

Unilateral vocal cord paralysis is seen more often on the left side than the right. The etiology is often unknown. However, various congenital cardiovascular anomalies can affect the left side, including ventricular septal defect, tetralogy of Fallot, abnormalities of the great vessels, and patent ductus arteriosus. A nerve can be damaged by events such as operation for an H-fistula, cervical esophagostomy, and surgery for a congenital heart defect.

However, bilateral vocal cord paralysis with both vocal cords unable to abduct results in consistent severe stridor and cyanotic attacks. Aspiration is common with recurrent chest infections and scattered small areas of atelectasis on chest radiography. Although bilateral vocal cord paralysis can be seen in an otherwise healthy infant, a strong association exists with central neurologic abnormalities such as meningomyelocele, hydrocephalus, Arnold-Chiari malformation, bulbar palsy, and birth trauma. Bilateral vocal cord paralysis may be associated with birth trauma related to difficult, prolonged second-stage labor with difficult forceps delivery and undue traction on the cervical spine. In these cases, recovery in 6 to 9 months is expected. Hereditary bilateral vocal cord paralysis is extremely rare.[16]

Clinical presentation

The cardinal clinical features of unilateral vocal cord paralysis in a newborn are a weak, breathy cry; often aspiration of pharyngeal secretions; and sometimes cyanotic attacks and choking during feeding. Loss of sensation of the involved hemilarynx contributes to aspiration. Stridor is seldom prominent.

A tracheotomy is almost always necessary in bilateral vocal cord paralysis. However, although a tracheotomy may relieve the airway obstruction when a neurologic abnormality exists, abnormal respiratory function, apnea, and cyanosis may persist. Caudal displacement of the brainstem with the medulla and the cerebellum is thought to stretch CN X and may cause disturbed function of the displaced respiratory center.

Laryngoscopic examination

Clinical suspicion of unilateral or bilateral vocal cord paralysis should be confirmed by indirect flexible laryngoscopy or by direct laryngoscopic examination. Pressure from the laryngoscope blade or the direction of introduction should not distort assessment of vocal cord function and the shape and general dynamics of the larynx. Such interference may cause a false diagnosis of lost vocal cord movement.

The laryngoscope blade should be placed in the vallecula (in front of the epiglottis) at the end of the procedure, when anesthesia has been discontinued. As the patient recovers pharyngeal and laryngeal movement, time is ample for a complete, reliable evaluation during inspiration and vocalization. Vocal cord movement and the mobility of the cricoarytenoid joint are compared with those of the vocal cord on the other side to detect cricoarytenoid joint function. It is generally easy to confirm a diagnosis of unilateral vocal cord paralysis but not to confirm bilateral paralysis. For neonates in whom bilateral vocal cord paralysis is suspected but in whom the diagnosis cannot be confirmed at the first examination, a nasotracheal tube can, be left *in situ* and reexamination performed days or 1 week later. If bilateral vocal cord paralysis is confirmed, a tracheotomy is performed. A tracheotomy is virtually always necessary for bilateral vocal cord paralysis and sometimes necessary in cases of unilateral vocal cord paralysis with stridor and partial airway obstruction or troublesome aspiration.

Vocal cord paralysis can usually be assessed with a flexible fiberoptic laryngoscope in the unanesthetized child or in a patient during spontaneous respiration anesthesia.

Management

Paralysis sometimes resolves spontaneously. In unilateral cases, this results in improved cry. In bilateral cases, airway improvement is usually sufficient for removal of the tracheotomy tube.

Correction of the airway obstruction in unremitting bilateral paralysis is a major problem, and the optimal age for further surgical procedures is conjectural.

No reports have been made of the results of nerve-muscle pedicle reinnervation in the pediatric age group. However, this operation can be considered for patients older than 4 years. The surgery is performed exclusively in the soft tissues of the neck; the integrity of the larynx is not breached. If the operation is unsuccessful, an arytenoidectomy can be performed later at a suitable age. The results of an arytenoidectomy[9] are more predictable in maintaining a good voice and obtaining a good airway so that decannulation is possible. Some patients continue to have stridulous breathing at night and do not obtain normal exercise tolerance.

Recently, transverse cordotomy with or without partial or complete arytenoidectomy has been successfully used in adults and a few older children. A transverse laser incision deeply divides the vocal fold, vocal ligament, and vocalis muscle on one side; after healing, the respiratory glottis is usually sufficiently widened for removal of the tracheotomy tube. The place of these operations in younger children has not been determined.

Laryngeal webs and atresia

Laryngeal webs are uncommon. They are formed during embryogenesis of the laryngotracheal groove. Actively proliferating epithelium temporarily obliterates the developing laryngeal opening, but the lumen is normally reestablished as the vocal cords appear separately on each side. Laryngeal web, subglottic stenosis, and congenital laryngeal atresia result from different degrees of failure of the epithelium's resorption during the seventh and eighth weeks of intrauterine development.

The most common web is at the glottic level and affects the vocal cords (Fig. 16-15). Other types include the posterior glottic web, causing interarytenoid vocal cord fixation[14]; subglottic webs, which may occur with or without cricoid cartilage involvement and subglottic stenosis; and supraglottic webs. Laryngeal atresia, a rare life-threatening anomaly, appears to represent a lack of recanalization of the embryonic larynx. Prompt diagnosis in the delivery room followed by a tracheotomy may prevent death. There is an association with tracheoesophageal fistula.

Clinical presentation

The major presenting clinical features of a laryngeal web are abnormal cry or voice, respiratory distress, and stridor. The cry may be absent or husky. Respiratory distress includes cyanosis at birth or an unexplained airway obstruction, which requires immediate intubation or a tracheotomy to provide an artificial airway before further assessment. Stridor is not often a feature. Recurrent or atypical croup occurs in some patients, especially those whose web is associated with subglottic stenosis. Many patients have major congenital anomalies of other systems, principally of the upper respiratory tract, most often subglottic stenosis. About one chance in three exists of having an associated abnormality of the respiratory tract.[3] Congenital subglottic stenosis is commonly seen when the glottic web is severe.

Endoscopic examination

Most laryngeal webs are located at the level of the glottis. In all cases, definitive diagnosis requires direct endoscopy to assess the web and detect any associated abnormalities of the upper respiratory tract. The larynx is examined with magnification from straight and angled lenses, which allow better evaluation of the site, extent, and thickness of the web than the operating microscope does. Assessing the thickness at and below the anterior commissure is essential. A large, thick web may cause life-threatening obstruction, or there may merely be a small, thin membrane at the anterior commissure. The free posterior edge of the web is thin, round, regular, concave posteriorly, and sharply outlined; the ante-

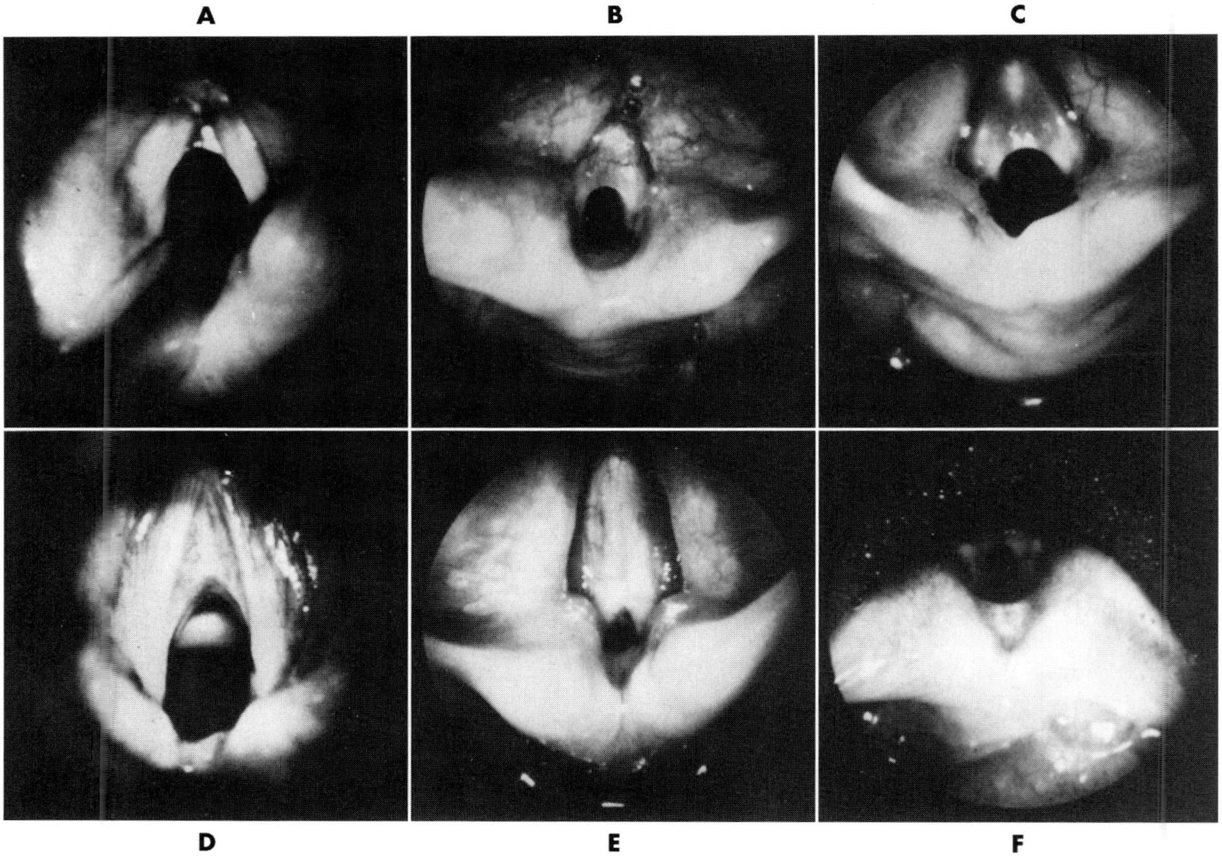

Fig. 16-15. Endoscopy of various congenital laryngeal webs. **A,** Thin web in a newborn. **B,** Thicker web in a newborn. **C,** Medium web. **D,** Thick web with subglottic stenosis. **E,** Severe web with very small glottic opening. **F,** Congenital interarytenoid web. (From Benjamin B: *Ann Otol Rhinol Laryngol* 92:317, 1983.)

rior part is usually thicker, depending on the size of the membranous web itself. The presence and severity of congenital subglottic stenosis can best be assessed by a combination of endoscopic examination and radiography. A lateral radiograph or xeroradiogram may give valuable information about the anterior thickness of the web, the presence or absence of congenital subglottic stenosis, and the site of a subglottic web (Fig. 16-16).

Congenital interarytenoid web is a rare laryngeal anomaly whose distinctive feature is a band of tissue joining the medial surfaces of the arytenoids and restricting abduction of the vocal cords (Fig. 16-17). In addition to the interarytenoid web, which is present to some degree in all patients, associated anomalies may include subglottic stenosis and enlarged bulky arytenoids. Other problems include difficulty exposing the larynx and maintaining the airway during anesthesia and endoscopy. Inspiratory stridor is the cardinal feature; the obstruction may be severe at birth or may worsen over weeks or months. The stridor is episodic and sometimes associated with obstructive cyanotic attacks. Diagnosis depends on direct laryngoscopy, paying particular attention to the posterior larynx without an endotracheal anesthesia tube in place and preferably using a technique of insufflation anesthesia with spontaneous ventilation. Direct inspection of the larynx is difficult to some degree in every case and special purpose hand-held laryngoscopes such as the Holinger pediatric anterior commissure laryngoscope or the Tucker-Benjamin infant laryngoscope and subglottiscope are helpful. They are used with rigid telescopes, both straight and angled, so that the posterior commissure and arytenoids are deliberately separated and palpated to determine the consistency and depth of the web. The arytenoids are often large and bulky, and often a congenital subglottic stenosis is present. Some cases have likely been misdiagnosed as bilateral vocal cord paralysis, cricoarytenoid joint fixation, or posterior glottic stenosis. The association with other congenital anomalies, especially those of the respiratory tract, is high.

Management

Many forms of management for congenital laryngeal webs have been advocated, including (1) dilation, which may be done deliberately (knowing that a web is present) or inad-

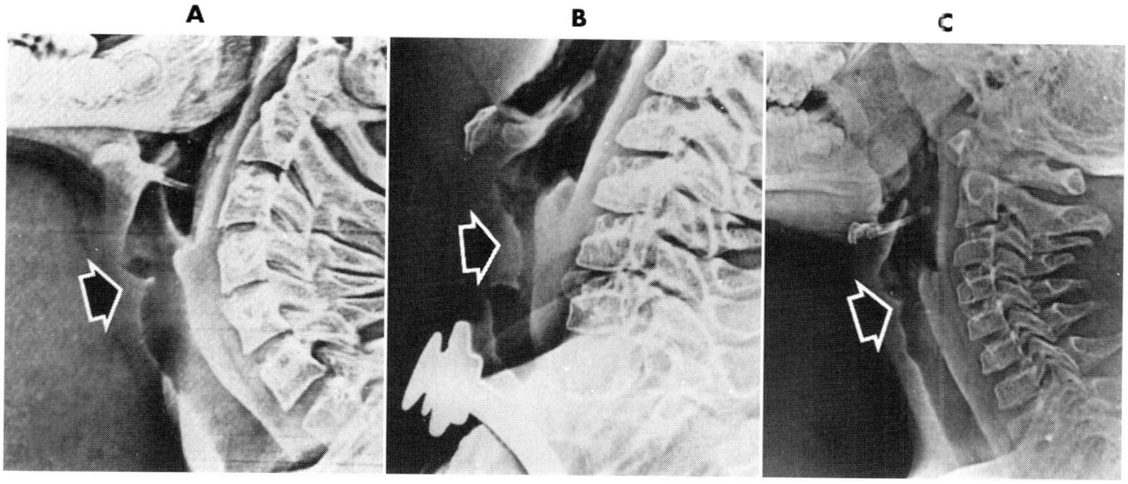

Fig. 16-16. Lateral xerography of congenital laryngeal webs. **A,** The thin posterior edge and the thick edge at the anterior commissure. **B,** A large glottic web with severe subglottic stenosis. **C,** A subglottic web. (From Benjamin B: *Ann Otol Rhinol Laryngol* 92:317, 1983.)

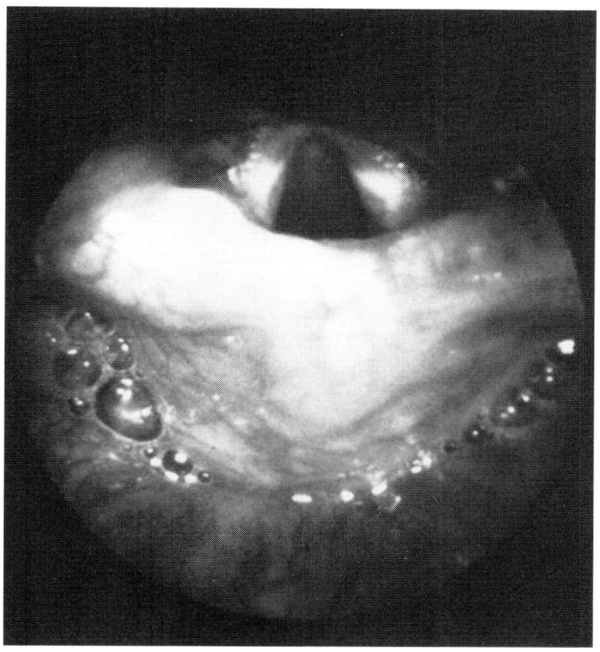

Fig. 16-17. A thick congenital interarytenoid web joining the medial surfaces of the posterior aspect of the arytenoids and causing partial airway obstruction, making laryngoscopy and exposure of the larynx difficult.

vertently (while passing an endotracheal tube or a bronchoscope); (2) simple endoscopic microsurgical division with scissors; (3) endoscopic division with an attempt to prevent recurrence by using sutures through the free cut edge of the web or the repeated use of dilators, (4) endoscopic insertion of a keel; (5) laser management; and (6) laryngofissure to allow removal of redundant soft tissues in the subglottic area with or without the use of a keel.

In general, the simpler the web and the simpler the management, the better the result. Thin glottic webs alone respond well to simple incision or rupture. For the remainder, obtaining a satisfactory result (judged by the voice) is difficult, as is improving the airway to achieve decannulation after a tracheotomy.

Infants with congenital interarytenoid web alone usually do not require an artificial airway. Infants with congenital interarytenoid web and associated congenital subglottic stenosis or other congenital anomaly (involving dysmorphic facies or midface hypoplasia) usually need a tracheotomy, but decannulation is possible after 3 to 5 years with a very good long-term prognosis.

Posterior laryngeal cleft

A posterior cleft of the larynx is difficult to diagnose and is frequently missed.[10] The posterior cleft may be limited to the interarytenoid region, or it may involve the cricoid lamina. A more extensive cleft is termed a *laryngotracheoesophageal cleft.* A classification into four types has recently been proposed (Fig. 16-18).[6]

A posterior cleft of the larynx often has other associated anomalies, such as esophageal atresia, tracheoesophageal fistula, and stenosis of the trachea or bronchi.

Depending on the extent of the cleft, the cardinal presenting feature, especially with oral feedings, is aspiration, which causes choking and cyanosis. Although some change in the cry may occur, there is no specific characteristic. Stridor is unusual; when present, it is usually caused by tracheobronchial obstruction from aspirated secretions. There may be radiographic evidence of aspiration pneumonitis (Fig. 16-19).

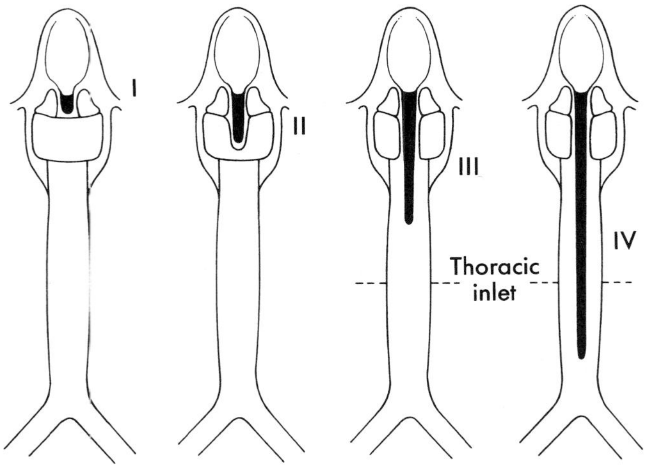

Fig. 16-18. Classification of the cleft larynx. Type 1 is a supraglottic interarytenoid cleft, above the level of the vocal cords. Type 2 is a partial cricoid cleft, extending below the level of the vocal cords and partially through the posterior lamina of the cricoid cartilage. Type 3 is a total cricoid cleft with or without further extension into the cervical tracheoesophageal wall. Type 4 is a laryngotracheoesophageal cleft. (From Benjamin B, Inglis A: *Ann Otol Rhinol Laryngol* 98:4[illegible]9, 1989.)

Final diagnosis depends on endoscopic examination, especially for minor interarytenoid clefts. Failure to diagnose the anomaly may result from inexperience of the endoscopist.

A laryngeal cleft should be sought at endoscopy in any patient with aspiration and stridor. A suitable laryngoscope, such as the Holinger anterior commissure pediatric laryngoscope, can be used to separate the posterior glottis and examine the posterior commissure while the patient is under general anesthesia and breathing spontaneously without an endotracheal tube (Fig. 16-20). Visualizing a small or large cleft can be difficult because of an unstable, collapsing larynx and redundant esophageal mucosa, especially when the cleft has not been suspected clinically. A laryngeal cleft may be found in patients with the VATER (vertebral, anal, tracheal, esophageal, and renal anomalies) association, with tracheoesophageal fistula, and with G syndrome.

Although the clinical features of a minor supraglottic interarytenoid cleft may suggest the presence of laryngomalacia, diagnosis can be confirmed only by careful examination of the larynx with particular attention to the interarytenoid region.

A posterior cleft limited to the larynx might not require surgery. Endogenous secretions are cleared by careful nursing. When feedings are thick, the tendency is to aspirate and choke. With careful medical management and the child's growth and development, symptoms of the condition may completely subside. Some minor clefts with persistent aspiration despite conservative management may require endoscopic microsurgical repair. In larger clefts, surgical repair by the lateral pharyngotomy approach or by the laryngofissure approach has been successful.

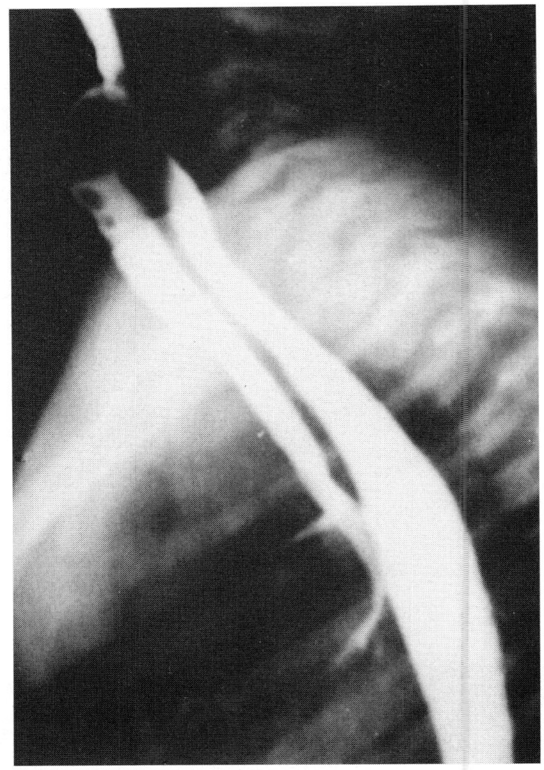

Fig. 16-19. A posterior laryngeal cleft. Barium swallow has outlined the esophagus, trachea, and bronchi. It is preferable to make the diagnosis at endoscopic examination.

Arthrogryposis multiplex congenita

Arthrogryposis multiplex congenita is an uncommon congenital (sometimes familial) disorder characterized by multiple joint deformities and other congenital defects, such as facial diplegia (Möbius' syndrome), difficulty in swallowing, and other central nervous system abnormalities.

Cohen and Isaacs[11] reviewed manifestations of arthrogryposis multiplex congenita. They described Pierre Robin–like features (micrognathia, glossoptosis, cleft palate), severe dysphagia, aspiration pneumonitis, aphonia or changes in the cry, vocal cord paralysis, supraglottic changes similar to those of laryngomalacia, and hypertrophy of the cricopharyngeus and upper third of the esophagus.

Central nervous system dysfunction rather than simple muscle weakness causes the dysphagia and respiratory difficulties. A tracheotomy and feeding gastrostomy are part of management, but the long-term prognosis is poor.

Cri du chat syndrome

Cri du chat syndrome[27] is a chromosomal disorder in which the newborn has a cry similar to the mewing of a cat. Partial deletion of the short arm of chromosome 5 exists.

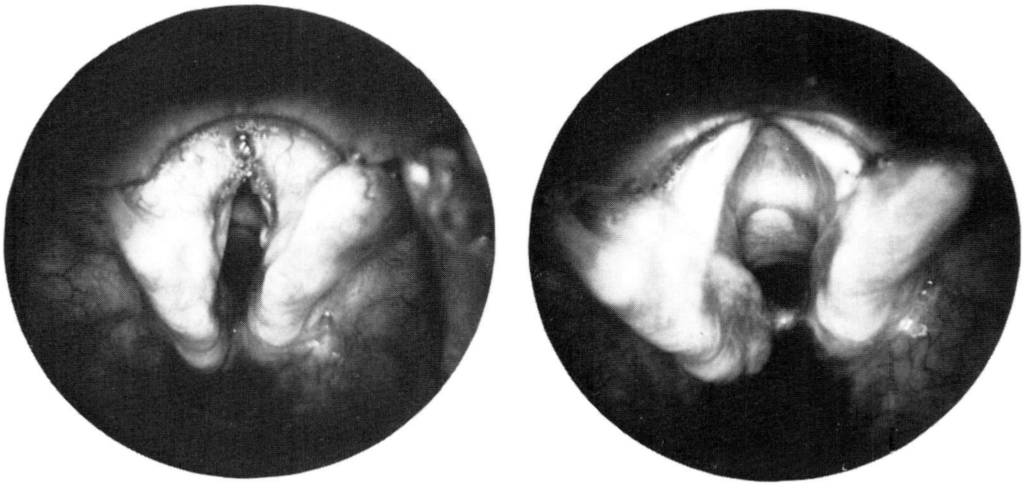

Fig. 16-20. A posterior laryngeal cleft (type 2). The defect is not seen until a laryngoscope is used to open the posterior glottis, showing the cleft extending a few millimeters below the glottic level, constituting a partial cricoid cleft. (From Benjamin B, Inglis A: *Ann Otol Rhinol Laryngol* 98:418, 1989.)

There is a characteristic congenital high-pitched stridor with endoscopic abnormalities seen in the larynx. The endolarynx is said to be elongated and curved with a floppy epiglottis, changes similar to laryngomalacia. On phonation, the posterior part of the larynx shows an open triangle, probably caused by paralysis of the interarytenoid muscle. Sometimes a minor cleft causes recurrent aspiration.

Other associated abnormalities include microcephaly, hypertelorism, generalized hypotonia, severe mental retardation, and low-slung ears with a beak-like profile. In general, the prognosis is poor.

Neuromuscular dysfunction (Plott's syndrome)

Plott[22] described a hereditary disorder with congenital laryngeal adductor paralysis as a feature. Plott's syndrome is X-linked and is associated with mental retardation. The prognosis is poor.

Subglottic stenosis

Congenital subglottic stenosis is the third most common congenital laryngeal anomaly after laryngomalacia and vocal cord paralysis. However, it is the most common congenital laryngeal abnormality causing serious respiratory obstruction and requiring a tracheotomy in infants.

The subglottic larynx is the region extending from the insertion of the conus elasticus into the free edge of the vocal cords above to the inferior margin of the cricoid cartilage below. By definition, congenital subglottic stenosis exists when this anatomic area has a diameter of less than 4 mm in a full-term newborn or less than 3 mm in a premature infant. These diameters are likely to be associated with clinical symptoms. Neoplasms, inflammatory conditions, and acquired strictures after endotracheal intubation are excluded from the definition. Differentiation between congenital and acquired subglottic stenosis should be clear, although the latter can be superimposed on the former. The prognosis is better in purely congenital cases.

Histopathology

Holinger and others[20] emphasized that the more accurate the histopathologic diagnosis of subglottic stenosis, the more precise and appropriate the management. The most common abnormality is generalized circumferential stenosis of the cricoid cartilage, so that the subglottic diameter is small. However, the lumen may be eccentric, and the abnormal shape of the cricoid cartilage may be associated with a large anterior lamina, an oval or elliptic shape, a large posterior lamina, or generalized thickening. A submucosal (occult) cleft or a trapped first tracheal ring[25,26] is a rare deformity. Soft subglottic stenoses of a congenital nature may be caused by submucosal mucinous gland hyperplasia and should be differentiated from a congenital subglottic hemangioma or, less commonly, from ductal cystic disease and acquired soft-tissue subglottic narrowing caused by submucosal fibrosis or granulation tissue. The latter may be acquired and caused by endotracheal intubation, a complication more likely to occur in the patient who has an underlying congenital subglottic stenosis.

Clinical presentation

Manifestations of congenital subglottic stenosis usually occur in the first few weeks or months of life and are not always evident at birth or in the neonatal period. Stridor is the most common feature, followed by respiratory distress, a harsh croupy barking cough, or a hoarse cry. The condition affects males twice as often as females. Associated congenital abnormalities of the upper respiratory tract or other organs are not uncommon.

Clinically, congenital subglottic stenosis may present in the following ways:

1. Subacute, or persistent, croup, in which the stridor lasts 1 to 3 weeks (whereas the usual attack of acute viral laryngotracheitis lasts 1 to 3 days)
2. Recurrent atypical croup, with each attack persisting for longer than usual
3. Difficulty introducing an endotracheal anesthetic tube of average size. Narrowing of the subglottic region is detected when the child is being anesthetized for some unrelated surgical condition.
4. Decannulation difficulty after tracheotomy or extubation after prolonged intubation

A tight endotracheal tube without a leak of gas around the subglottic region may cause reactive mucosal edema after it is removed. Stridor and a croupy cough may occur minutes or hours after extubation. Congenital subglottic stenosis is often the underlying lesion in patients in whom: (1) removal of an endotracheal tube is difficult after ill-managed, prolonged intubation; or (2) tracheotomy tube extubation fails after tracheotomy has been performed for prolonged or recurrent croup.

Endoscopic examination

Lateral airway radiography usually shows the congenital subglottic stenosis clearly (Fig. 16-21). However, the diagnosis is confirmed at endoscopy; the diameter of the subglottic region is assessed carefully and gently, especially if the airway is marginal. The usual finding is an isolated circumferential subglottic stenosis, the diameter of which is then measured. The outside diameter of a bronchoscope or an endotracheal tube that passes comfortably through the subglottic region represents the internal diameter of the cricoid, which is therefore calibrated and recorded for future reference. Endoscopic findings are less severe than those in patients with acquired subglottic stenosis.

Occasionally, diagnostic endoscopy results in minimal but significant mucosal swelling in the subglottic region, caused by the trauma of excessive manipulation, the passage of too large a bronchoscope, or repeated manipulation. This is more significant when there is preexisting subglottic stenosis. Subglottic edema occurs within the limits of the inexpansible cricoid cartilage in the immediate postendoscopic period. There may be croupy cough, stridor, and increased airway obstruction. Careful technique should minimalize the incidence of this complication.

Management

Management is based on the knowledge that many children outgrow congenital subglottic stenosis. Most cases produce few or minimal symptoms, and no definitive management is required unless acute inflammation or trauma from intubation or endoscopy precipitates serious obstruction. However, when congenital subglottic stenosis is severe or when acquired fibrous tissue granulations and edema produce a serious obstruction, a tracheotomy may be required. Small patients with stenosis severe enough to require a tracheotomy may require repeated endoscopic examination over months or years, awaiting sufficient relative improvement of the subglottic diameter to allow decannulation. This conservative management prevents the potential complications of external laryngeal surgery in the infant. However, Cotton and Evans,[13] among others, advocated a more aggressive approach by laryngotracheal surgical reconstruction to obtain a lumen large enough to permit decannulation. Repeated dilation management of hard cartilaginous stenosis is not successful, and ill-judged forced dilations inevitably cause further trauma and scarring. Laser resection has limited application and should be restricted to management of soft-tissue swelling in selected cases in which stenosis is less than 5 mm thick. There is no uniform management of subglottic stenosis and no universally successful endoscopic or external surgical technique. The tracheotomy tube usually should be worn for an extended time to allow the cartilaginous stenosis to grow at the child's general growth rate until the problem is overcome. Decannulation is usually possible, even in difficult cases, by the age of 3 or 4 years. Cricoid split procedures and laryngotracheoplasty are discussed in Chapter 18.

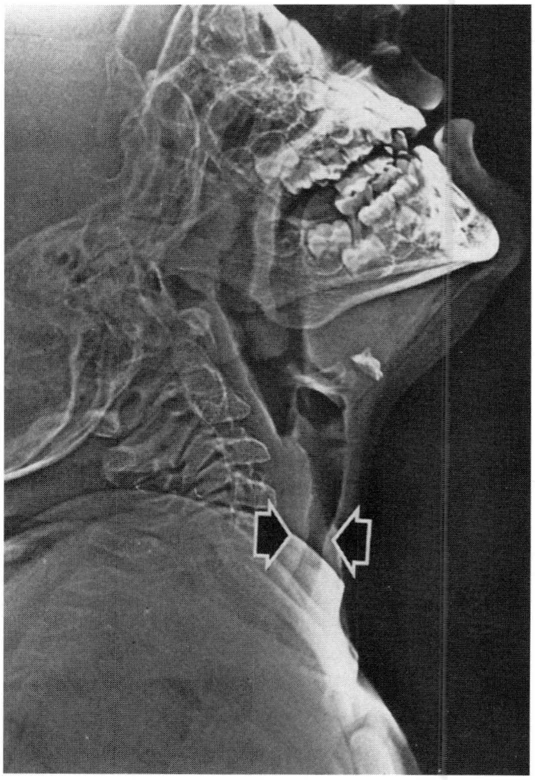

Fig. 16-21. Congenital subglottic stenosis *(arrows)* in a patient who had repeated attacks of atypical croup.

Laryngeal hemangiomas

Hemangiomas are congenital malformations that form from mesodermal rests of vasoformative tissue. In most anatomic sites they can be managed conservatively, but narrowing of the airway is an exception. Congenital hemangioma in the larynx usually occurs in the subglottic region, developing in the submucosa and following a typical growth pattern, with increased size usually causing symptoms within the first 8 weeks of life. A review of autopsy cases[7] showed that the lesion sometimes extends into the perichondrium and even into surrounding tissues between the tracheal rings and beyond the trachea, showing the possibility of regrowth after management. More extensive lesions may require an alternate management plan. About half of patients have cutaneous hemangiomas of the head, face, or neck, but no correlation exists with the site or size of the laryngeal lesion. All patients have some form of respiratory distress, which is usually variable and fluctuant. The clinical features are more clearly defined as inspiratory stridor (intermittent at first and then persistent), a harsh 'barking' cough, altered cry or hoarseness, and failure to thrive. An initial erroneous diagnosis of croup is often made. A 2:1 female-to-male preponderance exists. Most cases appear by 6 months of age.

Diagnostic evaluation

Lateral radiography of the upper airway shows subglottic soft-tissue swelling and usually clearly shows a subglottic abnormality consistent with hemangioma (Fig. 16-22).

Diagnosis is made by endoscopic examination. The appearance is sufficiently characteristic for an experienced observer to make a macroscopic diagnosis without biopsy, especially if there are associated cutaneous hemangiomas. The lesion is usually localized to the subglottic region on one side as a sessile, fairly firm, and compressible pink, red, or bluish lesion that is poorly delineated from the surrounding tissues. A biopsy may be performed when the diagnosis is uncertain, with precautions taken to maintain the airway in the unlikely event of excessive bleeding. Although infantile subglottic hemangioma has generally been regarded as a unilateral lesion, this is not always so. With modern anesthesia and sophisticated endoscopic techniques using magnification, evaluation of the site and distribution of the lesion can be exact. Classification of congenital laryngeal hemangiomas by anatomic site[5] includes lesions that are unilateral, bilateral, unilateral with posterior extension, and upper tracheal (see Fig. 16-22).

Management

The airway obstruction is usually severe and life threatening. Some patients have acute obstruction and require immediate relief by tracheotomy at the time of diagnostic endoscopy or by temporary intubation followed by tracheotomy. Most cases require a tracheotomy to ensure the patient's safety and to enable management to be performed.

Many forms of management have been advocated. They include tracheotomy and no active management, awaiting

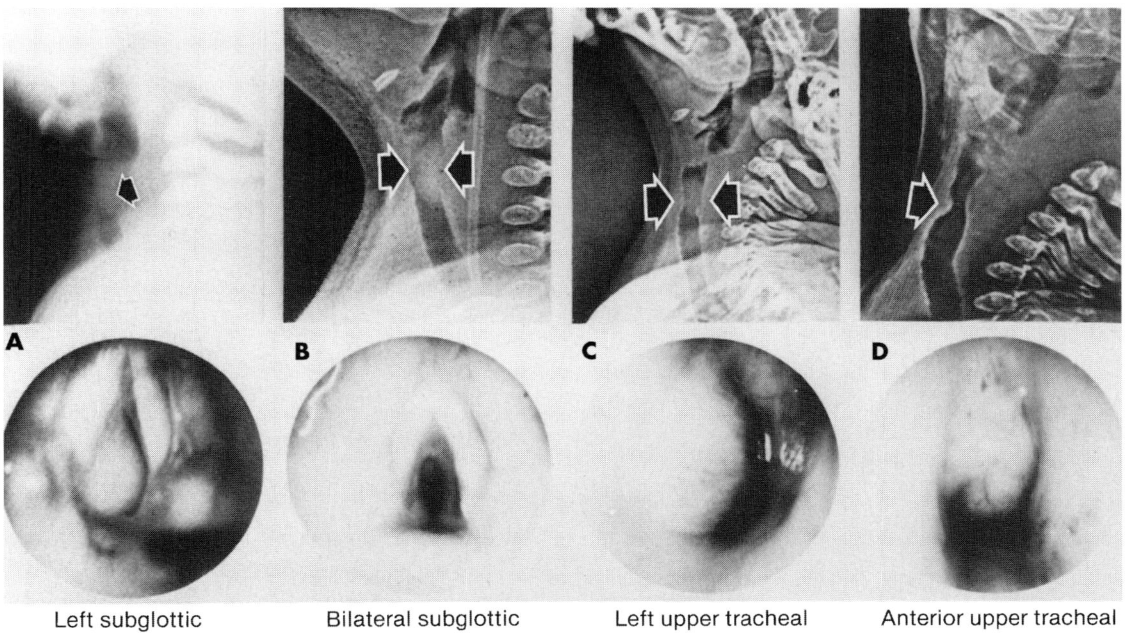

Fig. 16-22. Radiography and endoscopy. **A,** Radiography shows the subglottic soft-tissue mass of unilateral hemangioma. **B,** Xeroradiography shows radiopaque bilateral hemangiomas. **C,** Xeroradiography shows an upper tracheal lesion on the left side. **D,** Xeroradiography shows an upper tracheal lesion on the anterior wall. (From Benjamin B, Carter P: *Ann Otol Rhinol Laryngol* 92:448, 1983.)

spontaneous regression; temporary, intermittent, or prolonged endotracheal tube intubation with or without corticosteroids; injection of sclerosant: injection of intralesional corticosteroids for prolonged or repeated periods: use of interferon; excisional surgery; cryosurgery; external beam irradiation; or laser endoscopic surgery or endoscopic placement of a radioactive gold grain. Because of the relatively few patients managed and the varying attitudes to therapy, controlled studies have been impossible.

Success has been reported with each management modality, but generally, expectant management, corticosteroid management, or laser excision is favored. Radiotherapy was reliably used for many years to achieve resolution of the lesion and removal of the tracheotomy tube. A tracheotomy combined with external irradiation has a 93% cure rate.[7] There are no reports of untoward effects, despite the theoretic possibility of radiation-induced malignancy of the thyroid gland. For this reason, external radiotherapy is no longer generally favored. With placement of a radioactive gold grain in the substance of the hemangioma, the radiation dose to surrounding tissues (including the thyroid gland) is minimal. A unilateral lesion can usually be satisfactorily managed with the carbon dioxide laser with minimal chance of causing subglottic stenosis. The choice of management may depend on the variation in anatomic exposure, surgical visibility in the subglottic region, and age of the patient. Unrecognized, unmanaged, or poorly managed cases have a high mortality; active management, although it may be a tracheotomy alone, is always justified.

REFERENCES

1. Belmont JR, Grundfast K: Congenital laryngeal stridor (laryngomalacia): aetiologic factors and associated disorders, *Ann Otol Rhinol Laryngol* 93:430, 1984.
2. Benjamin B: Xeroradiography of the upper airways in paediatrics, *Australas Radiol* 23:214, 1975.
3. Benjamin B: Congenital laryngeal webs, *Ann Otol Rhinol Laryngol* 92:317, 1983.
4. Benjamin B: Anesthesia for laryngoscopy, *Ann Otol Rhinol Laryngol* 93:338, 1984.
5. Benjamin B, Carter P: Congenital laryngeal hemangioma, *Ann Otol Rhinol Laryngol* 92:448, 1983.
6. Benjamin B, Inglis A: Minor congenital laryngeal clefts: diagnosis and classification, *Ann Otol Rhinol Laryngol* 98:417, 1989.
7. Brodsky L, Yoshpe N, Ruben RJ: Clinical-pathological correlates of congenital subglottic hemangiomas, *Ann Otol Rhinol Laryngol (Suppl)* 105:4, 1983.
8. Chen J-C, Holinger LD: Congenital laryngeal lesions: pathology study using several macrosections and review of the literature, *Pediatr Pathol* 14:301, 1994.
9. Cohen SR: Arytenoidectomy in children, *Laryngoscope* 83:1293, 1973.
10. Cohen SR: Cleft larynx, *Ann Otol Rhinol Laryngol* 84:747, 1975.
11. Cohen SR, Isaacs H: Otolaryngological manifestations of arthrogryposis multiplex congenita, *Ann Otol Rhinol Laryngol* 85:484, 1976.
12. Cohen SR and others: Laryngeal paralysis in children, *Ann Otol Rhinol Laryngol* 91:417, 1982.
13. Cotton RT, Evans JNG: Laryngotracheal reconstruction in children: 5-year follow-up, *Ann Otol Rhinol Laryngol* 90:516, 1981.
14. Cox DJ, Simmons FB: Midline vocal cord fixation, *Arch Otolaryngol Head Neck Surg* 100:219, 1974.
15. Friedman EM and others: Paediatric endoscopy: a review of 616 cases, *Ann Otol Rhinol Laryngol* 93:517, 1984.
16. Gacek RR: Hereditary abductor vocal cord paralysis, *Ann Otol Rhinol Laryngol* 85:90, 1976.
17. Reference deleted in pages.
18. Holinger LD, Holinger PC, Holinger PH: Etiology of bilateral abductor vocal cord paralysis: a review of 389 cases, *Ann Otol Rhinol Laryngol* 85:428, 1976.
19. Holinger LD and others: Laryngocele and saccular cysts, *Ann Otol Rhinol Laryngol* 87:675, 1978.
20. Holinger PH and others: Subglottic stenosis in infants and children, *Ann Otol Rhinol Laryngol* 75:591, 1976.
21. Kelly SM, Gray SD: Unilateral supraglottic epiglottoplasty for severe laryngomalaria, *Arch Otolaryngol Head Neck Surg* 121:1351, 1995.
22. Plott D: Congenital laryngeal abductor paralysis due to nucleus ambiguus dysgenesis in three brothers, *N Engl J Med* 271:593, 1964.
23. Rizer FM, Schechter GL, Richardson MA: Macroglossia: etiologic considerations and management techniques, *Int J Pediatr Laryngol* 8:225, 1985.
24. Silberman HD, Tucker JA, Hampel A: Flexible neonatalscope, *Ann Otol Rhinol Laryngol* 93:468, 1984.
25. Tucker GF: Personal communication, 1982.
26. Tucker GF and others: Histopathology of congenital subglottic stenosis, *Laryngoscope* 89:866, 1979.
27. Ward PH, Engel E, Nance WE: The larynx in the cri-du-chat syndrome, *Laryngoscope* 78:1716, 1968.

SUGGESTED READINGS

Benjamin B: *Atlas of paediatric endoscopy: upper respiratory tract and oesophagus,* London, 1981, Oxford University Press.

Benjamin B: *Laryngoscopy: pediatric endoscopy,* New York, 1983, Grune & Stratton.

Benjamin B: *Diagnostic laryngology: adults and children,* Philadelphia, 1990, WB Saunders.

Cox DJ, Simmons FB: Midline vocal cord fixation, *Arch Otolaryngol Head Neck Surg* 100:219, 1974.

Desnos J and others: Vascular strictures of the respiratory tract in children, *Int J Pediatr Otolaryngol* 2:269, 1980.

Ferguson CG: Congenital anomalies of the infant larynx, *Otolaryngol Clin North Am* 3:185, 1970.

Healy GB, Holt GP, Tucker JA: Bifid epiglottis: a rare laryngeal anomaly, *Laryngoscope* 86:1459, 1976.

Holinger PH: Clinical aspects of congenital anomalies of the larynx, trachea, bronchi, and esophagus, *J Laryngol Otol* 65:1, 1961.

Holinger PH, Brown WT: Congenital webs, cysts, laryngoceles, and other anomalies of the larynx, *Ann Otol Rhinol Laryngol* 76:744, 1967.

Holinger PH, Schild JA, Weprin L: Pediatric laryngology, *Otolaryngol Clin North Am* 3:625, 1970.

Holinger PH, Schiller F, Johnston KC: Congenital anomalies of the larynx, *Ann Otol Rhinol Laryngol* 63:581, 1954.

McMillan WG, Duvall HA: Congenital subglottic stenosis, *Arch Otolaryngol Head Neck Surg* 87:70, 1968.

Chapter 17

Stridor and Airway Management

David Albert
Susanna Leighton

"When I use a word" Humpty Dumpty said in a rather scornful voice "it means precisely what I want it to mean, nothing more and nothing less."

The term *stridor* is often used loosely. Stridor should suggest a stridulous or harsh and attacking sound, but it may be soft and almost tuneful although no less worrying despite its musical quality. The term *stridulation* describes the vibration of the wings or legs in insects that supposedly attracts the opposite sex, which may explain why this term is not used to describe the production of pediatric stridor.

STRIDOR

Stridor is an abnormal or unwanted noise made by turbulent airflow in the airway. Most physicians exclude from this definition the snoring type of noise made by naso- and oropharyngeal obstruction, which is usually termed *stertor*. Clinically, stertor can occasionally be produced by the supraglottic larynx, so rigid differentiation between stridor and stertor is artificial and can wrongly limit the differential diagnosis (Boxes 17-1 through 17-3). Stridor may be characteristic of a particular pathology but is never diagnostic; the diagnosis can only be confirmed after endoscopy. However, not every child with stridor requires endoscopy because a thorough history and a limited physical examination can in some conditions (e.g., mild laryngomalacia) provide sufficient diagnostic probability to avoid initial endoscopy. Although important, preendoscopy assessment can only be a guide to the type and degree of pathology discovered at endoscopy. In about 5% of cases, a secondary pathology is present. In most children seen in a secondary and tertiary referral center, endoscopy is required and is usually the gold standard. However, dynamic conditions such as vocal cord palsy and tracheobronchomalacia often prove difficult to confirm or exclude at routine endoscopy.

AIRWAY OBSTRUCTION

For many otolaryngologists and anesthetists, management of the airway-compromised child represents a challenge. This chapter describes a safe approach to assessing and managing the airway of the stridulous child. The main techniques available for endoscopy are dealt with in some detail. Management includes medical treatment (e.g., corticosteroids), intubation, endoscopy, tracheotomy, and surgery. A few specified conditions (e.g., vocal cord palsy) are covered. For many conditions, tracheotomy is avoided using medical and adjuvant therapy and surgical techniques such as single stage laryngeal reconstruction. Tracheotomy and its complications are presented with techniques for ward and surgical decannulation.

Assessment

A physician dealing with a stridulous child should "stop, look, and listen." Note the child's breathing, listen to the parent while taking the history, and think about the differential diagnosis during the history and examination and prior to contemplating further investigations.

History

"Begin at the beginning" the King said gravely, "and go on till you come to the end; then stop."

(*From* ALICE IN WONDERLAND, Lewis Carroll.)

The obstetric and perinatal history is often relevant, especially in a premature child who requires ventilation. Few neonates of greater than 32 weeks' gestation require ventilation for respiratory distress syndrome, whereas ventilation is almost always required in neonates of less than 28 weeks' gestation, even with the administration of surfactant. Parents may fail to mention intubation in neonates admitted to intensive care for short periods. The term *intubation* may be mis-

Box 17-1. Nasopharyngeal causes of airway obstruction

Common

Neonates
- Neonatal rhinitis
- Choanal atresia or stenosis
- Craniofacial abnormalities
- Micrognathia

Children
- Allergic rhinitis
- Adenoiditis
- Adenotonsillar hypertrophy
- Foreign bodies

Acquired

Neonates
- Syphilis
- Neonatal rhinitis

Children
- Allergic rhinitis
- Adenoiditis
- Adenotonsillar hypertrophy
- Foreign bodies
- Nonallergic rhinitis
- Nonallergic rhinitis with eosinophilia
- Retropharyngeal abscess
- Glandular fever
- Ludwig's angina
- Thermal and caustic burns

Congenital

- Choanal atresia
- Choanal stenosis
- Midnasal stenosis
- Piriform aperture stenosis
- Nasal glioma
- Encephalocele
- Meningocele
- Nasopharyngeal mass
  - Hairy polyp
  - Teratoma
- Craniofacial abnormalities with small nasopharynx
- Micrognathia
  - Pierre Robin syndrome
  - Treacher Collins syndrome
- Macroglossia
  - Down syndrome
  - Cystic hygroma
  - Lingual thyroid

Box 17-2. Laryngeal causes of airway obstruction

Common

Neonates
- Laryngomalacia
- Intubation trauma
- Reflux laryngitis
- Laryngotracheal stenosis
- Vocal cord palsy

Children
- Croup
- Hemangiomas
- Papillomatosis
- Intubation trauma
- Vocal cord palsy

Acquired

Neonates
- Intubation trauma
- Surgical trauma (e.g., laser)
- Laryngotracheal stenosis
- Arytenoid fixation
- Reflux laryngitis

Children
- Epiglottitis
- Croup
- Bacterial tracheitis
- Hereditary angioedema
- Epidermolysis bullosa
- Foreign bodies
- Dislocated arytenoid
- Intubation trauma
- Fracture
- Caustic and thermal burns
- Hemangiomas
- Cystic hygroma
- Papillomatosis
- Rhabdomyosarcoma
- Wegener's granulomatosis

Congenital

- Laryngomalacia
- Posterior laryngeal cleft
- Vallecula cyst
- Laryngeal cysts
- Webs
- Laryngeal atresia
- Laryngotracheal stenosis
- Arytenoid fixation
- Vocal cord palsy

Box 17-3. Tracheal causes of airway obstruction

Common	***Acquired***	***Congenital***
Neonates	Neonates	Stenosis
Tracheobronchomalacia	Postintubation and endoscopy	Atresia
Tracheal stenosis	Tracheal stenosis	Trapped first tracheal ring
Vascular compression	Reflux tracheitis	Complete cartilage rings
Children	Children	Micro (stove pipe) trachea
Foreign bodies	Laryngotracheitis	Tracheal cysts
Tracheal stenosis	Bacterial tracheitis	Hemangiomas
	Foreign bodies	Tracheobronchomalacia (with tracheoesophageal fistula)
	Localized malacia secondary to tracheostomy or tracheoesophageal fistula repair	Vascular compression
		Aberrant innominate
		Pulmonary artery sling
	Thyroid	Double aortic arch
	Cystic hygroma	
	Mediastinal tumors	

taken for the passage of nasogastric tubes or for nasal and oral mucus extraction.

Stridor at birth is unusual and generally denotes fixed congenital narrowing (e.g., a laryngeal web, subglottic stenosis, tracheal narrowing).[88] Dynamic conditions such as laryngomalacia and congenital vocal cord palsy become evident in the first few weeks of life. A gradual increase in severity of stridor or airway compromise implies growth of an obstruction, which may be luminal as in a subglottic hemangioma or extrinsic as with a mediastinal mass.

Stridor is seldom constant; any diurnal or other variation can help pinpoint the cause, although asking parents about the timing of stridor in the respiratory cycle is seldom profitable. Typically, laryngomalacia is better in a child at rest and asleep but is made worse by crying, feeding, and distress. Airway obstruction with the baby supine can occur with a pedunculated laryngeal mass but is more often caused by, at least in part, a degree of supralaryngeal obstruction, such as micrognathia and resultant tongue base occlusion. Improvement in the airway with crying occurs in gross nasal obstruction, such as bilateral choanal atresia.

Airway obstruction produces several symptoms (Table 17-1) along with stridor, including recession, apnea or dying spells, cyanosis, dyspnea, tachypnea, cough, and hoarseness. Recession, even if severe, can be missed by parents but is a clear sign of inspiratory obstruction. Apnea with cyanosis is typical of severe tracheobronchomalacia and is sometimes termed a *dying spell*. Parents usually attempt resuscitation if apnea is severe, but it is often unclear how many of these attacks are otherwise self-limiting. Tachypnea and dyspnea are not limited to upper airway obstruction, but exertional dyspnea in an older child provides a useful functional assessment of severity. Cough is typical of tracheoesophageal fistula and tracheomalacia and is rarely caused by infant asthma. Hoarseness suggests a laryngeal lesion, such as laryngeal papillomatosis, but also occurs in vocal cord palsy.

Feeding is closely connected with breathing, particularly in the infant; an accurate picture of the feeding pattern should be obtained. Breast-fed babies with airway obstruction characteristically "come up for air," whereas bottle-fed babies may require thickened feeds or a "slow teat" (i.e., one with small holes). Aspiration suggests vocal cord palsy, tracheoesophageal fistula, or rarely, a cleft larynx with recurrent chest infections, usually accompanying significant aspiration. Regurgitation is common in neonates and by itself may not represent significant gastroesophageal reflux. The end result of poor feeding may be slow feeding, which troubles the mother more than the child, or failure to thrive with demonstrably poor weight gain. As laryngomalacia is common, it is important not to assign failure to thrive to this without first having considered and excluded other causes.

General medical history may explain a vocal cord palsy resulting from neurologic disease or cardiac surgery or may suggest vascular compression associated with congenital cardiac disease. The presence of birthmarks may be associated with a subglottic hemangioma.

In acute airway obstruction, history-taking is simultaneously with examination and resuscitation; in particular, any possible foreign body ingestion or concurrent illness should be noted. Rapidly progressing airway obstruction and drooling are the hallmarks of acute epiglottitis, which still occurs occasionally despite a dramatic reduction with immunization. The course of bacterial tracheitis or laryngotracheobronchitis is more prolonged.

Examination

He thought he saw a Banker's Clerk
Descending from a bus
He looked again, and found it was
A Hippopotamus

(*From* SYLVIE AND BRUNO, Lewis Carroll.)

Table 17-1. Symptoms associated with varying causes of airway obstruction

Symptoms	*Typical diagnosis*
Stertor	Nasopharyngeal obstruction (e.g., neonatal rhinitis)
Inspiratory stridor	Laryngeal and subglottic obstruction (e.g., laryngomalacia subglottic stenosis)
Biphasic stridor	High or midtracheal obstruction (e.g., tracheomalacia or stenosis)
Prolonged expiratory phase	Tracheal and bronchial obstruction (e.g., tracheobronchomalacia or stenosis)
Cough	Tracheoesophageal fistula (e.g., foreign body)
	Vocal cord palsy (e.g., tracheomalacia)
	Cleft larynx (e.g., reflux)
Aspiration	Tracheoesophageal fistula (e.g., cleft larynx)
	Vocal cord palsy
Hoarseness	Laryngeal lesion (e.g., vocal cord palsy)
Acute airway obstruction	Retropharyngeal abscess (e.g., epiglottitis)
	Tonsillitis (e.g., croup)
	Glandular fever (e.g., baterial tracheitis)
	Foreign bodies
Dysphagia and feeding difficulties	Epiglottitis (e.g., feeding affected with many causes of severe airway obstruction and aspiration)
	Tonsillitis
	Retropharyngeal abscess
Apnea or dying spell	Tracheobronchomalacia (e.g., reflex apnea)

The art of examination is in observing not just seeing. As discussed, a general impression can be obtained while taking a history, but careful general examination is necessary to avoid missing subtle features of related syndromes or of general pediatric disease. This examination is conducted with a search for the cause of airway obstruction and an estimation of its severity.

Observing the child at rest provides initial assessment of the degree of respiratory distress and the characteristics of any stridor, and it allows the physician to gain the child's confidence before further examination.

Typically, inspiratory stridor is caused by extrathoracic obstruction (Fig. 17-1), such as larynx or high trachea; bronchial obstruction causes expiratory stridor. Biphasic stridor can occur with obstruction anywhere in the tracheobronchial tree. Expiratory stridor may be absent, but a prolonged expiratory phase indicates intrathoracic obstruction (Fig. 17-2). The sound of stridor, even in a common condition such as laryngomalacia,[86] is variable and of little diagnostic use. Laryngomalacia has a musical quality, vocal cord palsy has a breathy quality, and the cough in tracheomalacia is barking. The site of the abnormal vibration is rarely found by stethoscope because of the variable transmission of sound through the thorax. However, auscultation is useful to detect heart murmurs and wheeze.

Subcostal, intercostal, and suprasternal recession may occur separately or together and may be associated with seesaw respiration. The severity of recession is a better indicator of the severity of airway compromise than the degree of stridor, which can paradoxically become less obvious as obstruction worsens because of diminishing airflow. Cyanosis is a late event and the child may still look pink.

If a supralaryngeal component is suspected, nasal patency should be assessed with a mirror, a wisp of cotton wool, or the bell end of a stethoscope. The jaw and tongue size should also be assessed.

Both stridor and recession will vary as the child rests, cries, and sleeps, but it is rare to demonstrate a similar repeatable change with position. Observing the child feeding is valuable, particularly if poor feeding or aspiration is a significant feature in the history. The ears, nose, throat, and neck should be examined last, being cautious not to examine the throat of a child in whom epiglottitis is suspected.

Special investigations

Because investigations in the management of the airway-compromised child are often unnecessary, unhelpful, or not cost-effective, they should be carefully selected on the basis of the history and examination.

A child in a tertiary referral center may have undergone several investigations, which can help in the initial assessment, although it is difficult to know how much weight to put on a normal echocardiogram or reflux study performed at another institution. If in doubt, reserve judgement and if necessary repeat.

In acute airway obstruction, oxygen (O_2) saturation monitoring is extremely helpful because it is noninvasive (unlike arterial blood gases) and more sensitive than clinical estimation (as described, cyanosis is a very late event). However, considerable airway obstruction can occur without desaturation as long as the child continues to have the energy to overcome the obstruction. Desaturation occurs with tiredness more often than with progression of the underlying ob-

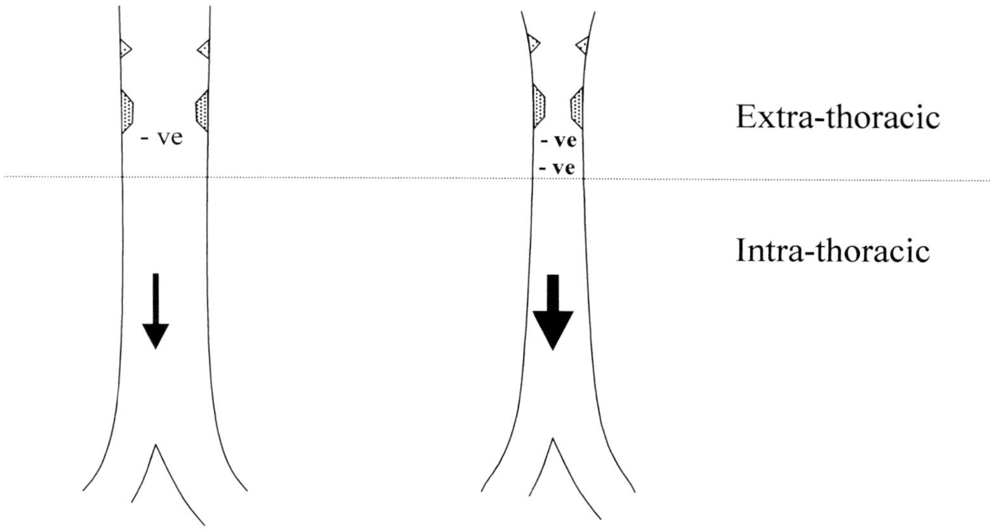

Fig. 17-1. Extrathoracic obstruction: collapse and increasing obstruction on inspiration.

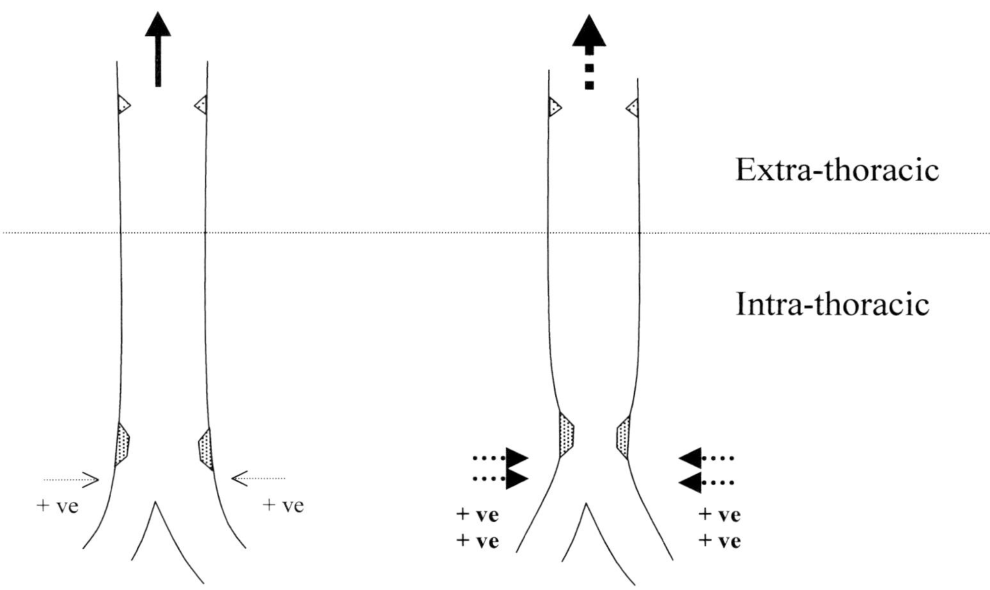

Fig. 17-2. Extrathoracic obstruction: collapse and increasing obstruction on expiration.

struction. Carbon dioxide (CO_2) build up can develop without desaturation, especially if O_2 is being administered. Transcutaneous CO_2 is unreliable, particularly in the shocked patient, so there is still a place for arterial blood gases. Some centers recommend that all suspected cases undergo endoscopy and intubation if appropriate, whereas other centers allow lateral radiograph of the neck as long as strict precautions are followed (e.g., the patient is accompanied by an anesthetist and surgeon in case of rapid deterioration). The result of the radiograph may not influence management.[25]

The value of radiology has been reviewed retrospectively by Tostevin and others.[113] A plain chest radiograph and a Cincinnati view are appropriate for screening; further radiography (e.g., contrast studies) is useful if abnormalities are found at endoscopy. A plain chest radiograph may show the ground glass appearance of bronchopulmonary dysplasia or mediastinal shift with obstructive emphysema of a foreign body, but it does not show the major airways well. A penetrated filtered film (the Cincinnati view) combined with a lateral view shows the subglottis, oropharynx, and nasopharynx and may be the only radiology technique required. If a foreign body is suspected, a more sensitive technique is diphragmatic screening; videofluoroscopy in young children or inspiratory and expiratory films in older children show diphragmatic immobility on the side of the obstruction. Videofluoroscopy is also an excellent way of demonstrating tracheomalacia and can be combined with a contrast swallow to detect vascular compression[5,42] and aspiration.

Bronchography is enjoying something of a renaissance after the introduction of safer nonionic contrast media. Bronchography of the lower airway is particularly useful for showing tracheobronchial stenosis and malacia.

Pediatric lung function tests[46] are seldom used because most children with suspected upper or lower airway obstruction are too young to undergo these tests.

Computed tomography (CT) and magnetic resonance imaging (MRI)[48,116,117] are usually insufficiently sensitive to fully characterize a stenotic segment, which can be more accurately assessed with endoscopy. If available, helical CT with multiplanar reconstruction may offer better definition of tracheal lesions.[94,120] However, CT and MRI can show extrinsic compression, particularly abnormal vasculature. Echocardiography can be used to screen for vascular compression and shows most of the abnormal vasculature and coincidental or symptomatic congenital heart disease.

Gastroesophageal reflux[12,21,65,83] can be assessed with a contrast study, milk scan, pH probe study, or lower esophageal biopsy. Contrast studies have low specificity and sensitivity and are very dependent on the radiologist for appropriate positioning and interpretation. The other investigations are more sensitive but are usually interpreted by gastroenterologists looking for reflux into the lower esophagus. The laryngologist is interested in the pH in the upper esophagus and pharynx, which can be measured using a second probe in the upper esophagus. Double-probe pH studies are used more for research because of technical difficulties and little in the way of normative data. Cotton (personal communication) recently suggested the use of tracheal biopsies, which may prove worthwhile.

Even if reflux is detected, it is difficult to determine if the reflux is primary or secondary to airway obstruction with negative intrathoracic pressure drawing gastric contents into the esophagus. Occasionally, the reflux may be the primary factor with secondary reflux laryngitis.

Ultrasonography of the vocal cords can show vocal cord palsy with reasonable accuracy to complement the endoscopic findings. Transcutaneous electromyography is helpful in adults, especially if the nerve has been severed. In children, the nerve is usually intact, and action potentials can be identified even in the presence of established bilateral cord palsy. Technical problems have limited the use of electromyography in children, even under the controlled conditions of anaesthetized endoscopy.

A sleep study is rarely used to assess the stridulous child because airway obstruction that worsens during sleep is usually a feature of pharyngeal obstruction, such as adenotonsillar obstruction or craniofacial anomaly. Laryngomalacia[15] and almost any laryngotracheal pathology are rarely worse with sleep.

Lung function tests (e.g., flow volume loops) help localize the site of obstruction but require a degree of patient cooperation. Other lung function tests (e.g., peak flows, ventilation or perfusion scans) are selected with the advice of a pulmonologist.

Acoustic assessment is clinically unreliable and does not seem to offer any great advantage because stridor from a particular cause is not associated with a characteristic type of noise.

In summary, a careful history, examination, and special investigations may suggest the diagnosis, but only endoscopy confirms the diagnosis.

Endoscopy

The two objectives in pediatric airway endoscopy are safety and accuracy. Achievement of these objectives requires a full range of specialized pediatric endoscopy equipment and a high level of experience of the endoscopist, anesthesiologist, and nursing staff. Too often a unit will perform an inadequate evaluation, which will only need to be repeated. Referral to a center with sufficient experience to perform a single comprehensive and definitive evaluation may be necessary. A systematic approach is diagnostic in most cases.[122]

Flexible endoscopy. Ultrathin endoscopes[4,26,85] with good optics and a diameter of less than 2 mm allow assessment in neonates without the need for a general anesthetic. This is usually considered a screening procedure because the view (particularly of the larynx) is often suboptimal. Also, no invasive diagnostic or therapeutic procedure can be undertaken. Even if an abnormality is shown (e.g., laryngomalacia), there is a 5% chance of a second pathology, which can easily be missed. In the ward, flexible endoscopy without anesthesia is particularly useful to assess dynamic abnormalities (e.g., vocal cord palsy) before formal endoscopy in the operating room, which is superior in assessing structural abnormalities. Flexible endoscopy under sedation in an endoscopy suite is widely practiced by pediatricians and pulmonologists[30,95,111] and is becoming more popular with otolaryngologists as an adjunct to rigid endoscopy.[43]

Laryngotracheobronchoscopy. Laryngotracheobronchoscopy[93,109] is a highly technical surgical procedure; the management team (surgeon, anesthetist, nursing assistant) needs to fully understand the equipment to perform the examination safely and to optimize assessment. Ideally, the surgeon, anesthetist, and nurse should routinely work together.

The advent of video has been invaluable for training and has made assessment safer because the anesthetist can monitor the endoscopy on the screen and the nurse can prepare equipment for the next stage. Accurate records should be kept to allow comparison with future examinations. This is facilitated by using a standardized form within a department.[47] Use of a recognized staging system (see Fig. 17-1) is important for publication of results. Polaroid prints from the video are a valid record for static conditions, whereas video is unparalleled for dynamic conditions. The most recent digital image recording systems allow multiple rapid images to be stored during the procedure, with only a selected few printed on Polaroid or converted to slide format.

Anaesthetic. An atropine premedication offers a dry surgical field and improves the efficacy of topical anesthetic, but to be effective does need to be given by intramuscular injection. Intravenous induction is preferable for older children, although gas induction may be needed in infants, those with poor venous access, and those with a precarious airway. Intravenous suxamethonium can be given if the patient is stable and may be given prior to lidocaine spray to avoid laryngeal spasm and to facilitate intubation if required. It is the pediatric use of lidocaine designed for adults that can result in overdosage.[2,105]

Centers vary as to whether to use intubation at the start of the procedure and whether respiration is spontaneous or maintained with jet ventilation in a paralyzed child.

Intubation. Once intubated, the child can be quickly ventilated to a level of anesthesia that will allow the passage of endoscopes without gagging while maintaining spontaneous respiration. The laryngoscope can be adjusted while the child is still intubated. Nasotracheal intubation allows the endotracheal tube to be withdrawn into the nasopharynx once the child is breathing spontaneously.

Nonintubation. After induction, the child is ventilated to the same level as above, which can take time in the presence of any obstruction. The advantage is that the view of the airway has not been altered by the passage of an endotracheal tube. Airway control can be regained at any time with intubation or an endoscope.

Jet ventilation. Jet ventilation[28,33,104] allows the child to be paralyzed, preventing coughing or gagging; gas exchange is maintained with short pulses of injected anesthetic gas, simulating normal respiration. The pressures required[56] are higher than physiologic levels, with a risk of pneumothorax in neonates and smaller children.

Laryngeal mask. The laryngeal mask[7,118] is useful for fiberoptic bronchoscopy if the patient is difficult to intubate because of mandibular hypoplasia.

Tracheotomy tube anesthesia. A tracheotomy tube in a child should be changed prior to anesthesia,[112] and a metal tube should be used if use of the laser is considered.

Halothane and O_2 maintain a level of anesthesia that allows thorough examination in a child who is breathing spontaneously. Halothane has the advantage that it is relatively nonirritant to the airway. Sevoflurane[57] is also nonirritant but has the advantage of rapid onset and no pungency, allowing immediate delivery of high concentrations. Experience with this new drug is limited, but the advantage of rapid induction may be offset by rapid termination of effect during relative hypoventilation or airway obstruction. The anesthetist should be able to control anesthesia in response to surgical conditions; a video monitor is invaluable. Preoperative corticosteroids are a good safeguard if significant stenosis is suspected. Peroperative O_2 monitoring is routine[62]; in time, CO_2 monitoring may also become routine.[36]

With any anesthetic technique, a microscope and laryngoscope are traditionally used to examine the larynx and a ventilating bronchoscope is used to examine the tracheobronchial tree. Continual improvement in optics of rigid telescopes and their ability to examine the subglottis in a retrograde fashion have prompted several centers to use telescopes over microscopes unless manipulation such as laser excision is required.

Microlaryngoscopy. A small sandbag under the shoulders is usually required to prevent hyperextension of the neck; sandbags are placed laterally to support the long thin heads of ex-premature neonates. A Mayo table supports the laryngostat clear of the chest.

It is important to prepare and check all equipment before endoscopy so that the endoscopist is fully prepared for all eventualities. A 400-mm lens allows the use of standard laryngeal instruments, but a 350-mm lens brings the patient closer, allowing easier manipulation of larynx, particularly in small neonates. The age-appropriate bronchoscope should be checked, and a bronchoscope at least one size smaller should also be instantly available. Antifog solution is only effective if freshly applied to the telescope lens.

Laryngeal examination is usually begun with the endotracheal tube in place by gently inserting the lubricated laryngoscope, taking care to protect the teeth and lips and keep the tongue central to provide a well-centered view. As in adults, it is important to check the overall appearance of the supraglottis and laryngopharynx during introduction of the laryngoscope. The endotracheal tube, if present, is followed to the tip of the epiglottis, gently lifting the epiglottis forward, making certain that the epiglottis does not curl up in front of the laryngoscope, preventing a complete view of the anterior commisure. Overall assessment of the larynx can be made with the tube *in situ*, providing a degree of stability that is particularly welcome in the child with a compromised airway.

Laryngeal examination with the endotracheal tube removed provides a superior view; using a probe to move the arytenoids independently, the physician can assess the mobility of the cricoarytenoid joints. If an interarytenoid scar is present, the arytenoids will not move independently. A posterior laryngeal cleft is excluded by passing the probe between the arytenoids, comparing the lower limit of the interarytenoid groove with that of the posterior commissure. Finally, the cords should be gently moved apart to inspect the subglottis.

The time available for the examination depends on the airway. In a child breathing spontaneously with a normal airway and normal lung function, anesthesia can be maintained solely by inhalational agents with the endotracheal tube withdrawn into the pharynx. In other cases, the time may be very limited; it is essential to be prepared to move ahead with bronchoscopy at any stage. If anesthesia is stable, a sucker can be placed in the laryngeal inlet to mimic laryngomalacia (the Narcy test). Photographs can be taken with a wide Storz telescope. If subglottic stenosis is significant, an ultrafine telescope passed through the laryngoscope causes less trauma than a bronchoscope.

Bronchoscopy. An appropriate size bronchoscope is used unless stenosis is suspected. Neonates pose particular problems if manipulation of the airway is required.[54,71] An anesthetic laryngoscope can be used in the vallecula to lift the larynx forward while passing the bevel of the bronchoscope through the vocal cords under video control on the monitor. The main bronchi, the carina, the trachea, and the subglottis are systematically examined, and videographs or digital images are recorded. Tracheomalacia should be observed with a small bronchoscope withdrawn from the area in question and without positive airway pressure to avoid splinting. The ratio of cartilage to trachealis is significant in recording the type of malacia and if aortopexy is likely to be successful.

Dynamic assessment of larynx on recovery from anesthesia. Typically, dynamic assessment of the larynx on recovery from anesthesia can be achieved by withdrawing the bronchoscope to just posterior to the tip of the epiglottis. This affords a good view of the vocal cords to exclude a cord palsy and of the arytenoids to exclude the common posterior form of laryngomalacia, although anterior collapse of the epiglottis may be masked. In this case, a 30° or 70° telescope should be used. The anesthetist should indicate the phase of respiration to check for paradoxic vocal cord movements.

An excellent technique for dynamic assessment of vocal cord movement is to insert a laryngeal mask with a fiberoptic broncoscope passed through to just above the laryngeal inlet.[119] If a bilateral vocal cord palsy is suspected and structural abnormalities have been excluded with full microlaryngoscopy and rigid bronchoscopy, it is sometimes necessary to reschedule the patient for further examination in which a laryngeal mask and fiberoptic scope are used from the outset, reducing the influence of prolonged anesthesia on cord function. An alternative is to use a 30° scope, which gives a view of the larynx without splinting the supraglottis.

Therapeutic microlaryngoscopy and bronchoscopy. Phonosurgery in children requires skill, patience, and specially designed microinstruments. Laser laryngoscopy is most useful for small postintubation granulomas and for laryngeal papillomatosis, although it has been used for many conditions, including laryngeal cysts, cystic hygroma, neurofibromas subglottic hemangioma, and tracheal or subglottic stenosis.[6] Attempts to use the laser for anterior webs or subglottic stenosis are usually unsuccessful.

A laser-safe tube should be used, or a conventional tube is withdrawn into the pharynx for lasering of the unintubated larynx. Great care should be taken not to damage healthy tissues and produce a secondary stenosis. Modern carbon dioxide laser bronchoscopes offer a reasonable view of lesions in the trachea and bronchi, which can then be lasered. However, the optics are vastly inferior to those of normal telescopes, and the technique is different. A 3.5-mm scope is the smallest available. Smaller children with tracheal papillomas often have a tracheotomy through which the laser bronchoscope can be passed. The potassium-titanyl-phosphate (KTP) laser solves some of these problems of tracheal laser therapy beause the fibers are sufficiently thin to be passed alongside a sucker of a conventional ventilating bronchoscope, providing an excellent view, hemostats, and controlled vaporization.

Summary. The operative record should clearly show the results of microlaryngoscopy, bronchoscopy, and the dynamic assessment on waking and should clearly state the plan for the patient based on these results. Appropriate management is best decided immediately after endoscopy. Alternative plans, if considered, should be discussed with the parents, and a final decision made before the patient's discharge. Diagnostic endoscopy is not an end in itself but a means to select the best management for the patient.

Management

Medical management

Acute management. Assessment, history-taking, and active resuscitation are simultaneous to stabilize the airway as expeditiously as possible. In a child who arrives in the emergency department with suspected laryngotracheobronchitis, the physician should assess the degree of airway obstruction by gauging the recession and dyspnea while asking the parent about the history and whether foreign body inhalation is a possibility. The nurse should check the O_2 saturation and set up humidified O_2. Another member of the team should call and alert the operating room that the child may need intubation and call the anesthesiologist and otolaryngologist. Most centers have a protocol for how to deal with the stridulous airway-compromised child. The protocols vary considerably, with some centers insisting on the presence of an otolaryngologist at intubation in case a tracheotomy is needed.

With an obstruction to airflow but normal alveolar function, increasing the concentration of inspired O_2 reduces the ventilatory requirement to maintain adequate O_2 saturation in the blood but does nothing to aid CO_2 excretion. As long as chronic hypercarbia is a possibility, O_2 is useful in the management of airway obstruction.

There is little objective evidence that increasing the humidity of inspired air is beneficial, although many centers use humidity tents or croupettes that have the disadvantage of decreased visibility and do little to allay the fears of a frightened child.

Intravenous corticosteroids (e.g., dexamethasone) are beneficial in croup. Inhaled corticosteroids have a similar effect. In carefully controlled circumstances, epiglotittis has been managed with appropriate intravenous antibiotics (e.g., chloramphenicol, co-amoxyclav).

Intubation. Intubation is increasingly used as an alternative to tracheotomy in acute airway obstruction, partly because of technologic advances in anesthesia and partly because of the realization that even short-term pediatric tracheotomy has numerous problems. Even with a skilled anesthetist and careful monitoring, unexpected pathology may be encountered, making intubation impossible. Severe subglottic stenosis, impacted foreign bodies, and advanced epiglottitis are obvious examples; a rare example is laryngeal aplasia, with ventilation achieved via a tracheoesophageal fistula. This uncertainty and the precipitate nature of pediatric airway obstruction require that an otolaryngologist be informed if a child with airway obstruction of unknown cause is to be intubated. Depending on the circumstances, it may be necessary to have an emergency tracheotomy set open with the correct size tube already selected.

Slow gasseous induction is followed by inspection of the larynx to exclude epiglottitis. If this approach is sufficient, the child can be managed on a nasal prong, perhaps with continuous positive airway pressure (CPAP). If intubation is required, it is important to minimize any damage to the already inflamed subglottic mucosa by gentle intubation with a soft tube just large enough for adequate ventilation and suction of secretions. If an oral tube is used for initial intubation, which tends to be easier, it should be replaced with a nasal tube, which is more secure if prolonged intubation is expected. The fit of the tube can be assessed by checking for a leak, and the tracheobronchial secretions can be sucked clear. If the secretions are very tenacious or there is an element of airway obstruction, a ventilating bronchoscope should be passed to exclude bacterial tracheitis[59,102] or a foreign body. In other clinical circumstances, the benefit of seeing the degree of pathology on endoscopy is usually outweighed by the trauma that occurs, particularly with the passage of a bronchoscope as opposed to the smaller diameter of a fine telescope.

Nonacute management. Because gastroesophageal reflux may play a part in several types of airway compromise, use of antireflux management to improve symptoms, avoid surgery, and improve surgical results is increasing. In many cases, antireflux management is empirical but well tolerated; at worst, it is a harmless placebo that allays a physician's fears.

In many series, systemic corticosteroids have been used alone or in combination with laser ablation to manage subglottic hemangiomas. Prophylactic antibiotics are sometimes useful in reducing the number of attacks of recurrent croup during winter, despite that most attacks have a viral origin.

Surgery

Endoscopy of the larynx and tracheobronchial tree. The microsurgical techniques and equipment needed in pediatric laryngology are closer to those of adult phonosurgery than those of general adult laryngology. Any damage to the delicate vocal fold can produce dysphonia that may be difficult to correct. Small subglottic cysts and vocal cord nodules can be resected with microinstruments having the same minimal degree of damage as a laser. In inexperienced hands, the laser probably has greater potential for damage. Injected corticosteroids have shown encouraging results for subglottic hemangiomas with a short postoperative intubation. Several techniques to endoscopically insert a laryngeal keel for laryngeal webs may be superseded by the recent technique of temporary cord lateralization. Minor laryngeal clefts (e.g., type 1 clefts, which only affect part of the cricoid) can be repaired endoscopically using specially designed needle holders. Aryepiglottic trimming for larygomalacia[61] was originally described using sharp dissection, taking a small wedge of the aryepiglottic mucosa on each side to prevent forward prolapse of the posterior larynx and arytenoids, which is typical of the condition.

The carbon dioxide laser for the larynx and more recently the KTP laser for the trachea and bronchi have become essential for management of the pediatric airway. Several improvements, including superpulsing, have reduced collateral damage around the intended area of vaporization, making the laser safe and effective in experienced hands. Subglottic cysts and granulations can be accurately vaporized with good hemostats and minimal postoperative edema. Similarly, aryepiglottoplasty for laryngomalacia is quick and bloodless using the laser. A subglottic hemangioma can be controlled with regular management, although the time to resolution is unchanged. With a large subglottic hemangioma, the laser can be combined with systemic corticosteroids to try to avoid tracheotomy. In laser arytenoidectomy for vocal cord palsy, the arytenoid and posterior vocal cord are removed to provide a posterior airway while preserving anterior functioning vocal cord apposition for vocalization. The laser is well suited for laryngeal and tracheal papillomatosis because vaporization may help reduce the survival of viable viral particles that can seed down the trachea. The KTP laser is a great advance on the carbon dioxide laser bronchoscope previously used to control tracheal papillomatosis.

Foreign body removal has been greatly facilitated by the introduction of foreign body extraction forceps that have a central channel for an extra-long Hopkins rod telescope.

Different forceps are available to remove friable foreign bodies such as peanuts and solid material such as plastic. The use of adrenaline before any attempt at removal shrinks the mucosa and reduces bleeding.

Tracheotomy. The indications for pediatric tracheotomy are usually relief of airway obstruction or long-term ventilation. The airway obstruction is typically at the laryngeal level, although occasionally an extended tracheotomy tube is used to support tracheomalacia or to pass through a tracheal stenosis. Informed consent requires that parents be fully apprised of the implications of caring for a child with a tracheotomy, preferably by meeting another family with a child with a tracheotomy. The family circumstances should be assessed and support offered if needed. Home suctioning equipment can be ordered at this stage.

The operation is usually conducted under general anesthesia with the child supine. An adhesive tape under the chin helps hold up any dewlap. A horizontal or short vertical incision can be used. The child is usually intubated or has a laryngeal mask in place. In very scarred necks or when finding the trachea may be difficult, a ventilating bronchoscope can be used as an illuminated landmark. In children, the thyroid isthmus can be simply divided using diathermy. A vertical incision should be made through the third and fourth tracheal rings with stay sutures placed on either side of the incision. If laryngetracheal reconstruction is planned, it may be worth trying to place the incision even lower. Occasionally, a high innominate vein should be protected from the tracheotomy tube by a small inferiorly based flap instead of vertical incision. Local policy dictates tube type, but beware of inserting too long a tube, particularly in neonates, for whom special short tubes are available. Tube lengths should be checked on the operating table by listening to the right lung with the head flexed. Some surgeons use a suture from the lower trachea to the skin, which closes the space in front of the trachea inferior to the stoma. This prevents a dislodged tracheotomy tube from being incorrectly reinserted in a false passage anterior to the trachea. Other surgeons use a suture from the skin inferiorly around the tube to prevent initial dislodgment. Any special techniques should be carefully described in the operative notes. Any skin sutures should not close the wound too tightly to prevent subcutaneous emphysema.

Customized tubes can be used for particular problems. A longer tube will support tracheomalacia or a tracheal stenosis; bifurcated tubes are available to perform the same function for the main bronchi. Occasionally, cuffed tubes are used to protect the airway in the presence of aspiration.

Complications Early tube dislodgment can be a serious emergency in small children and should be prevented by careful tape adjustment and by stay sutures through the trachea on either side of the incision. In the event of a tube dislodgment, these can be pulled apart to open the incision and bring the trachea to the surface. Conventional adult tracheal dilators are usually too large, but a small curved artery clamp is ideal and should be at the child's bedside with two spare tracheotomy tubes (one a size smaller). Tube blockage is avoided by frequent suctioning and an awareness of the problem.

Postoperative chest radiography checks the tube length and excludes a rare pneumothorax, which can occur from puncturing the lung apex or, in neonates, from high pressure ventilation. Hemorrhage is rarely a complication in children if the thyroid isthmus has been divided with electrocautery rather than between clamps and then ligated. Subcutaneous emphysema should be avoided by fitting the tube tightly in the trachea and not closing the wound too tightly. It is more likely if high pressure ventilation is required.

Tube dislodgment and blockage remain the most important late complications and have a mortality of 1% to 2%. Suprastomal granulation is almost universal.[96] It is probably caused by a combination of physical factors (e.g., movement, the effect of plasticizers in the tube) and infective factors from the skin and airway. The use of antibiotic ointment around the tube may improve but not remove the granulations. Long-standing suprastomal granulations are probably responsible for the development of suprastomal collapse, which is commonly responsible for difficult decannulation that requires further surgery.

Tracheal erosion can occur because of a poorly fitting tracheotomy tube, particularly if metal. The erosion can affect the mediastinum, esophagus, or a major vessel. An acquired tracheoesophageal fistula requires closure with an open operation and interposition of muscle. Small bleeds around the tracheotomy tube often occur before dramatic erosion of a major vessel.[110] Although suprastomal granulations can give rise to minor bleeding, any bleeding should be taken seriously and investigated radiologically or endoscopically. In very long-standing tracheotomy, the tube can migrate and require repositioning.

Tracheotomy decannulation. After appropriate assessment, adults and children with very short-duration tracheotomy (less than 1 month) can be decannulated[92] by removing the tube and covering the stoma with an occlusive dressing. However, most children, are more difficult to decannulate because of many factors, including suprastomal collapse and granulation, the relative size of the airway, and possibly psychologic attachment to the tracheotomy tube. A more controlled process, ward decannulation, is used in these children.

Before ward decannulation is attempted, a recent endoscopy[66] with suprastomal granulation removal is required. Significant suprastomal collapse is a common cause of failed decannulation and should be excluded. The tracheotomy tube is downsized in a controlled stepwise manner, usually one size smaller each day. The child should be kept on the ward during this process and carefully observed at night. Once the smallest tracheotomy tube has been tolerated, the tracheotomy tube can be blocked for 12 hours during the day and for 24 hours the next day and night. The tube can

Box 17-4. Management of the neonate who is difficult to extubate

Reflux management
Tube placement for at least 1 week between trials of extubation
Corticosteroids to cover extubation
Nasal prong and continuous positive airway pressure postextubation
Endoscopy with laser for small granulations, cysts, and other problems
Cricoid split
Single-stage laryngeal reconstruction
?Tracheotomy with stent to maintain airway

Box 17-5. Recent techniques to avoid tracheostomy

Type of Obstruction	*Technique*
Subglottic stenosis	Active medical management Cricoid split Single-stage laryngotracheoplasty
Subglottic hemangioma	Systemic or intralesional corticosteroids
Laryngomalacia	Aryepiglottoplasty
Tracheobronchomalacia	Continuous positive airway pressure via an endotracheal or tracheotomy tube

be safely removed and the stoma covered, although the child still needs to be kept on the ward for observation for about 5 days. If this approach fails, the child needs to undergo endoscopy again to exclude cord fixation, cord palsy, stomal granuloma, stomal collapse, and tracheomalacia.[37]

Surgical decannulation. If endoscopy before decannulation shows significant suprastomal collapse, surgical decannulation is required. This formal closure of the stoma, sometimes with additional support from cartilage, is followed by intubation. At the beginning of the operation, the child is intubated nasally with an age-appropriate tube. The tracheocutaneous fistula is excised preserving the tracheal wall unless a cartilage graft is required. If cartilage is not required (mild to moderate collapse only), the stoma is closed and sutured laterally to the sternomastoid to prevent collapse of the repair. If cartilage is required, it is harvested from a rib and carved to a boat shape as for laryngotracheal reconstruction. The malacic wall is excised until nonmalacic cartilage is exposed, which is sutured in place with minimal or no air leak. If the trachea is very malacic, an oversize graft can be supported on the sternomastoids, lifting the graft and anterior tracheal wall forward. Postoperatively, the patient is intubated for 24 to 48 hours.

Surgical procedures to avoid tracheotomy. In recent years, there has been a trend to avoid tracheotomy because of mortality, morbidity, and the effect on the family. This is particularly true in neonates who are difficult to extubate (Box 17-4). Medical management can help, but in many cases there is a clear decision between tracheotomy and a surgical procedure such as a cricoid split or single-stage laryngeal reconstruction (Box 17-5).

Cricoid split. Cricoid split is designed to decompress the complete cricoid ring and expand the lumen without grafting. Intubation is required. Of note is the histologic appearance of a child with a successful cricoid split who died of other causes. There is no significant gap filled with fibrous tissue, suggesting that any expansion is temporary.

Cricoid split is indicated in neonates who fail extubation because of subglottic edema or soft immature stenosis. It is contraindicated in patients less than 1.5 kg and in those with other medical problems, particularly an O_2 requirement greater than 35% because of bronchopulmonary dysplasia. However, determining the relative components of upper and lower airway compromise can be difficult.[91] The operation consists of a midline laryngofissure from the first tracheal ring to halfway up the thyroid cartilage. The child is then re-intubated with an age-appropriate tube or a tube one size larger. The tracheal incision is not closed, and a wound drain to avoid surgical emphysema is essential. Postoperative intubation is usually for 1 week; this rest period is probably important in the success of the operation. Long-term paralysis produces lung atelectasis and neuromuscular weakness and should be avoided. Most patients can be managed with minimal sedation.

Single-stage laryngeal reconstruction. In patients who fail extubation, single-stage laryngeal reconstruction is indicated as an alternative to tracheotomy if a mature subglottic stenosis is present. It is contraindicated in patients greater than 2 kg and in those with any medical problem that can prejudice a successful result (e.g., increased O_2 requirement, tracheobronchomalacia, cardiac anomalies).

The operation consists of a midline laryngofissure with an incision from the first tracheal ring to halfway up the thyroid cartilage, which allows re-intubation with an age-appropriate tube or a tube one size larger. Cartilage is harvested from the rib or ear and carved into a boat shape with beveled edges for security. Postoperatively, the patient is intubated and maintained with minimal sedation and no paralysis for 5 to 10 days (longer if younger). Antireflux management is provided empirically. The result is examined 1 week postintubation with a laser available for minor granulations. A patient in whom re-intubation is necessary requires, great care.

Long-term management of specific conditions

Vocal cord palsy. The etiology and management of vocal cord paralysis differs significantly in children and adults. Vocal cord paralysis is rare in children; the incidence is unknown, but a prevalence of 0.75 cases per million per year has been reported.[78] It is probably the second most common cause of neonatal stridor,[17] accounting for 10% of all congenital laryngeal anomalies.[52] It can result from lesions of the nucleus ambiguus or its supranuclear tracts or from injury to the main trunk of the vagal nerve or its branches. There is bilateral innervation of each nucleus ambiguus from the cerebral cortex, so supranuclear lesions do not commonly cause vocal cord paralysis. Central lesions are more frequently associated with bilateral cases, and peripheral lesions with unilateral cases.[60]

Congenital vocal cord paralysis typically presents within the first month of life.[27] Stridor, cyanosis, and apnea are the most frequent symptoms of bilateral paralysis; unilateral paralysis usually presents with dysphonia. Feeding problems and sternal recession are equally common in both types.[14,39] In most series, vocal cord paralysis occurs slightly more frequently in male than female infants[39,50] and is more commonly bilateral than unilateral.[18,39,52] This may result from underreporting of unilateral cases because the relatively innocuous clinical course leads to failure of diagnosis. Vocal cord paralysis has been predominantly right-sided in some series[13,17] and left-sided in others,[27,52,97] presumably depending on referral patterns.

Vocal cord paralysis is diagnosed at endoscopy, by observing one or both cords to be fixed in a median or paramedian position during inspiration and expiration, or by observing paradoxical inspiratory adduction of the cords with passive movement to a paramedian position with expiration. If diaphragmatic movement is not assessed in order to show the inspiratory and expiratory phases of respiration, paradoxical movement can be mistaken for normal movement. The position of the paralyzed cord may depend on residual innervation of the larynx and therefore the specific branches of the vagus nerve or parts of the nucleus ambiguus affected by a lesion. The posterior cricoarytenoid muscle is the sole vocal cord abductor and is innervated by neurons in the ventral division of the ipsilateral nucleus ambiguus via the recurrent laryngeal nerve; the laryngeal adductors are innervated by neurons in the more extensive dorsal division of the nucleus via the recurrent and superior laryngeal nerves. Rigid endoscopy, under general anesthesia with the patient breathing spontaneously, is preferable to flexible fiberoptic laryngoscopy because it permits manual palpation of the cords to distinguish true paralysis from cricoarytenoid joint fixation.[27] It also permits observation of the cords, even in the presence of laryngomalacia when it is important to ensure that the blade of the laryngoscope is not limiting vocal cord mobility; furthermore, it allows examination of the airway below the cords to exclude dual pathology.[50,108] Diagnosis of vocal cord paralysis may be confirmed by laryngeal ultrasonography.[38]

Management of pediatric vocal cord paralysis is influenced by the severity of symptoms and a knowledge of the etiology and the likelihood of spontaneous recovery. Patients may tolerate a marginal airway until a minimal change in status (increasing demand or further limitation of the airway) renders it inadequate. Decompensation occurs with stridor, dyspnea, sternal retraction, nasal flaring, use of accessory muscles, cyanosis, and eventual asphyxia. Early intervention with endotracheal intubation or tracheotomy to secure the airway should be undertaken if symptoms are severe or progressive. Reported tracheotomy rates vary from 0% to 36% for unilateral cases[18,97] and from 0% to 73% for bilateral cases.[18,78]

Causes of unilateral and bilateral vocal cord paralysis in children include neurologic disease (18%), meningomyelocele with Arnold-Chiari malformation and hydrocephalus (14%), birth trauma (19%), other trauma (11%), malignant disease (1%), familial disease (1%). In the remaincer and of cases (36%), no cause can be found.[18] Idiopathic congenital vocal cord paralysis is often associated with other congenital anomalies, mainly pulmonary, cardiovascular, and esophageal.[18,50,108] A familial congenital laryngeal abductor paralysis has been reported in which spontaneous improvement in function occurred over 1 to 2 years.[24]

Neurologic disorders associated with vocal cord paralysis include benign congenital hypotonia, Möbius syndrome, cerebral palsy, arthrogryposis multiplex congenita, leukodystrophy, hypoxic encephalopathy, and Charcot-Marie-Tooth disease.[18,50] Intracranial space-occupying lesions are another cause.[98] Neurotoxic effects of vinca alkaloids used in the management of childhood leukemia may induce unilateral or bilateral vocal cord paralysis; this is a dose-related complication and is reversible over 4 to 6 weeks after adjusting the dose or withdrawing medication.[3]

Meningomyelocele with Arnold-Chiari malformation, and hydrocephalus may cause bilateral vocal cord paralysis that presents with stridor. Early relief of the hydrocephalus by shunting usually allows recovery of the paralysis, suggesting that the condition is caused by compression of the vagus nerve or traction on its cervical rootlets. Patients with this condition are subject to episodic apnea and cyanosis, possibly related to hydrocephalus and brainstem compression. These symptoms should be distinguished from airway obstruction because they will not respond to tracheotomy.[51]

Birth trauma may cause congenital vocal cord paralysis. There is an association with difficult delivery using forceps, with a prolonged second stage of labor, with undue traction of the cervical spine, and with cesarean section.[18] Surgical trauma, particularly tracheoesophageal fistula repair[50] and repair of congenital cardiac defects,[34] is an important cause in infants; the former is more likely to cause bilateral paralysis.[18,52] The role of intubation trauma is controversial, but the recurrent laryngeal nerve may be susceptible to pressure injury between the endotracheal tube and the superior portion of the thyroid cartilage.[14] Blunt trauma, either closed head trauma causing central pathology or cervical trauma (e.g., strangulation injury), is a recognized cause of laryngeal paralysis.[79]

Spontaneous recovery is unpredictable in children. The value of laryngeal electromyography in establishing prognosis is uncertain.[9,63] Recovery usually occurs within 6 months and rarely after 36 months,[13,31,108] but it has been described up to 9 years after the onset of symptoms.[31] Late recovery may be incomplete because of laryngeal muscle atrophy, synkinesis, and cricoarytenoid joint fixation.[121] Spontaneous recovery is more likely in acquired (64%) than congenital (29%) vocal cord paralysis; the recovery rate in the latter group is better if no other congenital anomalies are present.[31] Spontaneous recovery is more common when vocal cord paralysis is unilateral (approximately 70%) than when bilateral (approximately 50%).[27,97] A neurologic etiology is associated with a poor recovery.[27]

Infants with unilateral vocal cord paralysis requiring tracheotomy can usually be decannulated, following growth of the airway, between 1 and 2 years of age without further surgical intervention even if the paralysis persists. Persistent dysphonia is unusual in children with unilateral vocal cord paralysis, but it may be managed by voice therapy, medialization using injection[70] or thyroplasty,[55] or selective reinnervation of the laryngeal adductors.[115] Vocal cord medialization may also improve aspiration.[70]

In patients with bilateral vocal cord paralysis, vocal cord lateralization can improve the airway permanently and permit decannulation when spontaneous recovery of function does not occur. Various techniques have been advocated, including arytenoidectomy (external via laryngofissure, or endoscopic using a laser technique[10]), arytenoidopexy,[81] and posterior cricoid grafting in patients who have residual adductor vocal fold motion.[40] Success rates as high as 80% have been achieved. However, lateralization procedures usually improve the airway at the expense of residual voice and risk causing or exacerbating aspiration. Persistent aspiration secondary to bilateral vocal cord paralysis may be severe enough to warrant laryngeal diversion. Reinnervation of the posterior cricoarytenoid muscles may be successful in permitting decannulation in up to 50% of suitable children[84,115] and has theoretical advantages over lateralization procedures: it does not precipitate dysphonia or aspiration, does not preclude other surgical procedures, and does not fix the vocal cord, so spontaneous recovery can still follow.

The complications of interventions designed to hasten decannulation should be weighed against the risks of prolonged pediatric tracheotomy in the management of patients with bilateral vocal cord paralysis. Irreversible surgical decisions should be delayed until little hope remains of spontaneous recovery of function and, preferably, until the child is old enough to participate in such decisions.

Subglottic hemangioma. Capillary hemangiomas are actually hamartomatous rather than neoplastic malformations. They are rare but have a caucasian preponderance and are twice as common in female as in male infants; 50% affect the head and neck. The true incidence of hemangiomas affecting the airway is unknown, but in one series they comprised 13 of 846 congenital laryngeal anomalies (1.5%).[52] In 50% of cases, they are associated with cervicofacial cutaneous hemangiomas. Benjamin and Carter[8] classified airway hemangiomas according to site. Subglottic hemangioma was first described by Mackenzie in 1864[71a]; this site is the most common, and 50% are left lateral. On occasion, airway hemangiomas may be multiple.

Presentation peaks at the age of 6 weeks and is nearly always within the first 6 months of life (85%). The most common symptom is stridor, often initially intermittent and misdiagnosed as recurrent croup, but it usually progresses to become constant, may be inspiratory or biphasic, and is exacerbated by crying or upper respiratory tract infections. Other symptoms such as dyspnea, feeding difficulties, failure to thrive, and hoarseness or abnormal cry may also be present.

Definitive diagnosis of airway hemangioma is by direct laryngoscopy. The classical appearance is of a pink or bluish smooth sessile mass (soft and compressible) arising from the lateral wall of the subglottis and often extending up to involve the undersurface of the cord; it only rarely extends into the trachea. This capillary hemangioma may be safely biopsied without risk of torrential hemorrhage. Practice varies, but many believe biopsy is unnecessary because the appearance is pathognomonic and up to 50% of biopsies may be too superficial and therefore not diagnostic. Airway imaging may be normal or may show subglottic narrowing, but the differential diagnosis includes subglottic stenosis and thus does not preclude endoscopy.

The natural history of the lesion is rapid proliferation up to the age of about 1 year followed by spontaneous involution; the time to completion of involution varies. Classic cutaneous hemangiomas regress by 5 to 8 years, but adequate involution, when combined with growth of the larynx, allows resolution of airway symptoms by the age of 2 to 3 years in most cases. After diagnosis and before involution, active management of the airway may be necessary in extensive disease. In a series of untreated cases reported in 1961, there was 50% mortality from respiratory obstruction.[35]

Maintenance of the airway may be achieved by bypassing the obstruction with a tracheotomy. A review in 1984 estimated that 50% to 70% of patients with airway hemangioma require tracheotomy and that the mean age at which growth of the airway and involution of the hemangioma will allow decannulation is 17 months[100] (other estimates range from 11 to 25 months). However, during cannulation, patients are subject to the morbidity and mortality risk associated with pediatric tracheotomy.

An alternative approach to management is to hasten involution of the lesion, ideally obviating the need for tracheotomy but at least shortening the period of cannulation. Any acceptable technique should be safe and free of sequelae because there are no sequelae after natural involution. Local and systemic management have been used to hasten involution, but there is no general agreement on the best approach.

Radiotherapy, whether by low-dose external beam[82] or by implantation with a radioactive gold grain,[49] successfully causes involution within 9 months but has largely been superseded by other techniques because of an association with thyroid malignancy. Surgical excision via laryngofissure was first described by Mawson[72] in 1961; however, it was associated with subglottic stenosis. A successful approach combining excision of the hemangioma with laryngotracheoplasty to expand the subglottis and avoid stenosis was subsequently reported,[32] but use of the carbon dioxide laser in the management of airway hemangiomas was more popular. Primary submucosal surgical excision with or without subglottic expansion is coming back into vogue. [77,101] Local management by injection of sclerosants[90] and cryotherapy[99] has been reported but is associated with later subglottic stenosis.

Katz and Askin[60] in 1968 observed that systemic corticosteroids caused cutaneous hemangiomas to regress in a patient being treated for thrombocytopenia. The mechanism of action of corticosteroids is uncertain, but they may increase the sensitivity of blood vessels to endogenous circulating vasoconstrictors. Successful management of a subglottic hemangioma with systemic corticosteroids was initially associated with high doses (2 to 5 mg/kg/day) for several weeks.[19] The frequency and severity of complications (e.g., growth retardation, spontaneous fractures, glycosuria, Cushing's syndrome) were later reduced by strategies such as alternating daily doses and intermittent courses,[80] but some cases are apparently resistant to therapy and management may be required for as long as 12 to 18 months in responders. Successful management of airway hemangioma by intralesional corticosteroid injections and prolonged intubation for several weeks has been reported to avoid tracheotomy in some cases,[73] but these results have not been easily reproducible.

In 1980, Healy and others[45] reported successful carbon dioxide laser vaporization of hemangioma in 11 cases within one or two applications and with no complications, but later reports were less encouraging. Some patients required repeated laser management up to 11 times,[11] and nearly 1 year's delay between the first application of the laser and decannulation has been reported.[16] Furthermore, subglottic stenosis has become recognized as a complication of carbon dioxide laser management of large hemangiomas.[8,22] The technique is probably only to be recommended in the management of small lesions.

Konior and others[64] reported successful selective embolization of hemangiomas in 1988. The risks of this procedure include injury to healthy tissue, sepsis, hemorrhage, and stroke, and it requires the dedication of a skilled interventional radiologist. It is not widely practiced.

Systemic management with interferon-α2a, an antiviral agent, was noted to improve Kaposi's sarcoma in clinical trials for acquired immunodeficiency syndrome (AIDS). It probably inhibits angiogenesis by blocking fibroblast growth factor and thus accelerates regression of hemangioma. A trial of management for severe multiple airway hemangiomas showed promising results.[87] In patients having daily subcutaneous injections until the airway was stable (2 to 31 months; mean, 11 months), no long-term morbidity was reported, although recognized side effects included elevated liver transaminases, leukopenia, thrombocytopenia, alopecia, neurotoxicity, and growth retardation. These complications are reversed on cessation of management.

The search continues for an effective involutional agent that has no sequelae and obviates the need for tracheotomy. Although local management may be useful for small lesions, subglottic stenosis is a potential complication with extensive lesions. A systemic approach holds more promise in these patients. Management with a combination of interferon-α2a and systemic corticosteroids, keeping the dose of each low enough to avoid complications but high enough to maintain the airway, is probably the best option at the present time. The need for close monitoring of the airway and of potential complications in patients undergoing such management cannot be overemphasized.

Respiratory papillomatosis. Recurrent respiratory papillomatosis is a diffuse diathesis of the respiratory mucosa. It is characterized by benign nonkeratinizing squamous papillomas that may be sessile or pedunculated, single or multiple, but are typically recurrent. They occur most commonly in the larynx but may affect the nose, mouth, pharynx, and esophageal inlet. They have a predilection for squamociliary junctions in the airway, either physiologic (e.g., in the margins of the vocal folds) or iatrogenic (e.g., where there has been squamous metaplasia along a tracheotomy tract).[58] The tracheobronchial tree is not often affected unless the patient has undergone tracheotomy. The pulmonary parenchyma is rarely involved and only in those with a tracheotomy.

The disease is caused by epithelial infection with human papillomavirus (HPV) types 6 and 11 (formerly 6c).[76] Sampling from clinically healthy respiratory tract tissue of patients shows viral deoxyribonucleic acid (DNA) incorporated into the cellular genome.[106] This explains recurrences and why a cure cannot be effected by mechanical removal of lesions. Remission may occur spontaneously but is more likely in limited disease and less likely if onset is very early in life. There is no association with the onset of puberty.[29] The duration of remission varies; relapse may be precipitated by laryngeal trauma[44] or immunosuppression.[89]

There is a worldwide prevalence of recurrent respiratory papillomatosis, although the incidence varies among countries; it has been estimated as 7 million per year in the United States.[107] There is a bimodal age distribution; 66% of new cases affect children younger than 16 years, and the peak incidence occurs between 2 and 5 years of age. Recurrent respiratory papillomatosis affects males and females equally, and racial and socioeconomic factors do not alter prevalence. It is likely that children become infected *in utero* or intrapartum from maternal genital papillomas in some cases,[103] but transmissibility is low and infection has never been recorded in siblings.

Presenting symptoms depend on the extent of disease. They vary from hoarseness or abnormal cry to dyspnea and stridor or acute respiratory obstruction. Management is primarily directed toward maintenance of the airway, although preservation of voice and avoidance of tracheotomy are also desirable. The most common complication of management is recurrence of papillomas. Development of a laryngocele if a papilloma obstructs the air exit from the laryngeal ventricle has been reported. Pulmonary papillomatosis with multiple cyst formation is a rare but progressive complication that carries a 50% mortality from cardiorespiratory failure. Malignant degeneration caused to laryngotracheal carcinoma or squamous cell carcinoma of the bronchus is also recognized; predisposing factors for malignant change include radiotherapy, smoking, and possibly, the use of cytotoxic drugs. HPV 11 is more likely than HPV 6 to be associated with extensive anatomic spread of disease, the need for tracheotomy, and therefore pulmonary papillomatosis, and malignant degeneration.[75]

Maintenance of the airway. Removal of lesions and reduction of viral burden do not induce remission of recurrent respiratory papillomatosis, so surgery is for airway rescue alone. Several techniques have been advocated. Traditional surgical resection may be complicated by bleeding and postoperative edema compromising the airway. Inhalation of papilloma may occur, obstructing the airway or seeding the virus further down the tracheobronchial tree. Ultrasonography, suction diathermy, and cryosurgery have been described but have been superseded by carbon dioxide laser vaporization,[107] which minimizes hemorrhage and trauma to adjacent structures with resulting scarring and deformity. Immediate complications of the carbon dioxide laser in the airway are well-recognized. Delayed complications of vocal fold fibrosis, web formation at the anterior and posterior commissures of the glottis, interarytenoid scarring, arytenoid fixation, and laryngeal stenosis[23] can be avoided by attention to laser emission parameters, depth of vaporization, and surgical technique, sparing the anterior commissure. Debulking rather than total extirpation of lesions is recommended. Nevertheless, the frequency and severity of complications increase with more severe disease, requiring many laser procedures. The introduction of the KTP laser has improved access for vaporization of lesions in the trachea and bronchial tree.

Various topical adjuvant therapies for maintenance of the airway have been assessed. Podophylum painted onto lesions induced remission in 41% of cases.[53] Photodynamic therapy can decrease the growth rate of lesions by 50%.[1] Diethylstilbestrol, fluorouracil, tetracycline, and idoxuridine showed promising initial results but no long-term advantage over surgery alone.

Tracheotomy for airway maintenance may be required in severe cases. The rate of tracheotomy varies among hospitals from 1.8% to 64% according to the referral pattern and the patient population. The presence of a tracheotomy results in an increased risk (50%) of developing tracheal papillomatosis. Risk factors for tracheal spread include the presence of subglottic disease at the time of tracheotomy and prolonged cannulation.[20] Diversionary tracheotomy has been described[114] but does not prevent distal spread of disease. Furthermore, complications are associated with subsequent reanastomosis of the trachea.

Eradication of disease. Because surgery cannot manage infection in visually healthy tissue, many physicians have sought effective systemic adjuvant therapy. Reported results of management are mainly anecdotal or of only a few patients; their significance is questionnable in the context of a disease with a notoriously variable course.

Cytotoxic drugs, autogenous vaccine, *cis*-retinoic acid, lysozyme, and acyclovir have shown no benefit. Adenine arabinoside is also probably ineffective. Ribavirin is a broad-spectrum antiviral drug that can be administered orally or by nebulizer. It causes significant regression of papillomas without major adverse reactions but is associated with anemia and with teratogenicity in rodents.[74]

Human leukocyte interferon has a well-documented benefit in respiratory papillomatosis.[41] Interferons act by effects on viral replication, cell growth, cell surface antigen expression, levels of cytotoxic effector cells, and antibody production. Up to 80% of patients respond to management; remission may be partial or complete but is dose-related. Any response will be sustainable and repeatable, but there is a rebound effect on cessation of treatment and no increase in prolonged remissions.[67,68] Side effects include inflammatory symptoms (fatigue, headache, nausea, fever, chills) on initial administration in 92% of recipients, these side effects become less severe with repeated doses. Delayed effects include leukopenia, elevated liver transaminase levels, thrombocytopenia, alopecia, neurotoxicity, polymyalgia and arthralgia, and growth retardation. All are generally tolerable, controllable, and reversible on cessation of management. Polyriboinosinic-polyribocytidylic acid stabilized with polylisine in carboxymethyl cellulose, a synthetic polynucleotide inducing interferon production *in vivo*, slows disease progression but is too toxic for long-term administration.[69]

There is no effective systemic treatment for eradication of HPV causing recurrent respiratory papillomatosis. The search for such a management, with acceptable side effects, should continue; immunomodulation may be the key to future developments. In the meantime, the aim of management should be to maintain the airway, avoiding complications resulting from overmanagement and reserving tracheotomy for severe disease. When tracheotomy is unavoidable, every effort should be made to keep the duration of cannulation as short as possible.

REFERENCES

1. Abramson AL and others: Clinical effects of photodynamic therapy on recurrent laryngeal papillomas, *Arch Otolaryngol Head Neck Surg* 118:25, 1992.

2. Amitai Y and others: Serum lidocaine concentrations in children during bronchoscopy with topical anesthesia, *Chest* 98:1370, 1990.
3. Annino DJ Jr, MacArthur CJ Friedman EM: Vincristine-induced recurrent laryngeal nerve paralysis, *Laryngoscope* 102:1260, 1992.
4. Arnold JE: Advances in pediatric flexible bronchoscopy, *Otolaryngol Clin North Am* 22:545, 1989.
5. Backer CL and others: Vascular anomalies causing tracheoesophageal compression: review of experience in children, *J Thorac Cardiovasc Surg* 97:725, 1989.
6. Bagwell CE: CO_2 laser excision of pediatric airway lesions, *J Pediatr Surg* 25:1152, 1990.
7. Baraka A, Choueiry P, Medawwar A: The laryngeal mask airway for fibreoptic bronchoscopy in children, *Paediatr Anaesth* 5:197, 1995.
8. Benjamin B, Carter P: Congenital laryngeal haemangioma, *Ann Otol Rhinol Laryngol* 92:157, 1983.
9. Berkowitz RG: Laryngeal electromyography findings in idiopathic congenital bilateral vocal cord paralysis, *Ann Otol Rhinol Laryngol* 105:207, 1996.
10. Bower CM, Choi SS, Cotton RT: Arytenoidectomy in children, *Ann Otol Rhinol Laryngol* 103:271, 1994.
11. Brodsky L, Yoshpe N, Ruben RJ: Clinicopathological correlates of congenital subglottic haemangiomas, *Ann Otol Rhinol Laryngol* 92: 4, 1983.
12. Burton DM and others: Pediatric airway manifestations of gastroesophageal reflux, *Ann Otol Rhinol Laryngol* 101:742, 1992.
13. Cavanagh F: Vocal palsies in children, *J Laryngol Otol* 69:399, 1995.
14. Cavo JW Jr: True vocal cord paralysis following intubation, *Laryngoscope* 95:1352, 1985.
15. Chetty KG and others: Acquired laryngomalacia as a cause of obstructive sleep apnea, *Chest* 106:1898, 1994.
16. Choa DI and others: Subglottic haemangioma in children, *J Laryngol Otol* 100:447, 1986.
17. Cohen SR and others: Endoscopy and tracheotomy in the neonatal period: a 10-year review, *Ann Otol Rhinol Laryngol* 86:577, 1977.
18. Cohen SR and others: Laryngeal paralysis in children: a long-term retrospective study, *Ann Otol Rhinol Laryngol* 91:417, 1982.
19. Cohen SR, Wang CJ: Steroid treatment of haemangioma of the head and neck in children, *Ann Otol Rhinol Laryngol* 81:584, 1972.
20. Cole RR, Myer CM III, Cotton RT: Tracheotomy in children with recurrent respiratory papillomatosis, *Head Neck* 11:226, 1989.
21. Contencin P and others: Gastroesophageal reflux and ENT disorders in childhood, *Int J Pediatr Otorhinolaryngol* 32(suppl):S135, 1995.
22. Cotton RT, Tewfik TL: Laryngeal stenosis following carbon dioxide laser in subglottic hemangioma: report of three cases, *Ann Otol Rhinol Laryngol* 94:494, 1985.
23. Crockett DM, McCabe BF, Shive CJ: Complications of laser surgery for recurrent respiratory papillomatosis, *Ann Otol Rhinol Laryngol* 96:639, 1987.
24. Cunningham MJ, Eavey RD, Shannon DC: Familial vocal cord dysfunction, *Pediatrics* 76:750, 1985.
25. Dawson KP, Steinberg A, Capaldi N: The lateral radiograph of neck in laryngo-tracheobronchitis (croup), *J Qual Clin Pract* 14:39, 1994.
26. de Blic J, Delacourt C, Scheinmann P: Ultrathin flexible bronchoscopy in neonatal intensive care units, *Arch Dis Child* 66:1383, 1991.
27. de Gaudemar I and others: Outcome of laryngeal paralysis in neonates: a long term retrospective study of 113 cases, *Int J Pediatr Otorhinolaryngol* 34:101, 1996.
28. Depierraz B and others: Percutaneous transtracheal jet ventilation for paediatric endoscopic laser treatment of laryngeal and subglottic lesions, *Can J Anaesth* 41:1200, 1994.
29. Doyle DJ and others: Recurrent respiratory papillomatosis: juvenile versus adult forms, *Laryngoscope* 104:523, 1994.
30. Eber E, Zach M: Flexible fiberoptische bronchoskopie in der padiatrie: eine analyse von 420 untersuchungen, *Wien Klin Wochenschr* 107: 246, 1995.
31. Emery PJ, Fearon B: Vocal cord palsy in paediatric practice: a review of 71 cases, *Int J Pediatr Otorhinolaryngol* 8:147, 1984.
32. Evans JNG, Todd GB: Laryngotracheoplasty, *J Laryngol Otol* 88: 589, 1974.
33. Evans KL, Keene MH, Bristow AS: High-frequency jet ventilation: a review of its role in laryngology, *J Laryngol Otol* 108:23, 1994.
34. Fan LL, and others: Paralyzed left vocal cord associated with ligation of patent ductus arteriosus, *J Thorac Cardiovasc Surg* 98:611, 1989.
35. Ferguson CF, Flake CG: Subglottic haemangioma as a cause of respiratory obstruction in infants, *Ann Otol Rhinol Laryngol* 70:1095, 1961.
36. Franchi LM, Maggi JC, Nussbaum E: Continuous end-tidal CO_2 in pediatric bronchoscopy, *Pediatr Pulmonol* 16:153, 1993.
37. Friedberg J, Giberson W: Failed tracheotomy decannulation in children, *J Otolaryngol* 21:404, 1992.
38. Garel C and others: Laryngeal ultrasonography in infants and children: a new way of investigating. Normal and pathological findings, *Int J Pediatr Otorhinolaryngol* 23:107, 1992.
39. Gentile RD, Miller RH, Woodson GE: Vocal cord paralysis in children 1 year of age and younger, *Ann Otol Rhinol Laryngol* 95:622, 1986.
40. Gray SD, Kelly SM, Dove H: Arytenoid separation for impaired pediatric vocal fold mobility, *Ann Otol Rhinol Laryngol* 103:510, 1994.
41. Haglund S and others: Interferon therapy in juvenile laryngeal papillomatosis, *Arch Otolaryngol Head Neck Surg* 107:327, 1981.
42. Han MT, and others: Double aortic arch causing tracheoesophageal compression, *Am J Surg* 165:628, 1993.
43. Handler SD: Direct laryngoscopy in children: rigid and flexible fiberoptic, *Ear Nose Throat J* 74:100, 1995.
44. Harries ML, Juman S, Bailey CM: Recurrent respiratory papillomatosis in the larynx: re-emergence of clinical disease following surgery, *Int J Pediatr Otorhinolaryngol* 31:259, 1995.
45. Healy GB and others: Treatment of subglottic haemangioma with the carbon dioxide laser, *Laryngoscope* 90:809, 1980.
46. Hira HS, Singh H: Assessment of upper airway obstruction by pulmonary function testing, *J Assoc Physicians India* 42:531, 1994.
47. Hoeve LJ, Rombout J: Pediatric laryngobronchoscopy. 1332 procedures stored in a data base, *Int J Pediatr Otorhinolaryngol* 24:73, 1992.
48. Hofmann U and others: Magnetic resonance imaging as a new diagnostic criterion in paediatric airway obstruction, *Prog Pediatr Surg* 27:221, 1991.
49. Holborow CA, Mott TJ: Subglottic haemangioma in infancy, *J Laryngol Otol* 87:1013, 1973.
50. Holinger LD, Holinger PC, Holinger PH: Etiology of bilateral abductor vocal cord paralysis: a review of 389 cases, *Ann Otol Rhinol Laryngol* 85:428, 1976.
51. Holinger PC and others: Respiratory obstruction and apnea in infants with bilateral abductor vocal cord paralysis, mengingomyelocele, hydrocephalus and Arnold-Chiari malformation, *J Pediatr* 92:368, 1978.
52. Holinger PH, Brown WT: Congenital webs, cysts, laryngocoeles and other anomalies of the larynx, *Ann Otol Rhinol Laryngol* 76:744, 1967.
53. Hollingsworth JB, Kohlmoos HW, McNaught RC: Treatment of juvenille papilloma of the larynx with resin of podophyllum: a preliminary report, *Arch Otolaryngol Head Neck Surg* 52:82, 1950.
54. Holmes DK: Expanding the envelope of neonatal endoscopic tracheal and bronchial surgery, *South Med J* 88:571, 1995.
55. Isaacson G: Extraluminal arytenoid reconstruction: laryngeal framework surgery applied to a pediatric problem, *Ann Otol Rhinol Laryngol* 99:616, 1990.
56. Janzen PR, Neasham J, Daniel M: Pressure reducing valve prevents barotrauma during jet ventilation for microlaryngeal surgery, *Anaesthesia* 50:831, 1995 (letter).
57. Johannesson GP, Floren M, Lindahl SG: Sevoflurane for ENT-surgery in children: a comparison with halothane, *Acta Anaesthesiol Scand* 39:546, 1995.

58. Kashima H and others: Sites of predilection in recurrent respiratory papillomatosis, *Ann Otol Rhinol Laryngol* 102:580, 1993.
59. Kasian GF and others: Bacterial tracheitis in children, *Can Med Assoc J* 140:46, 1989.
60. Katz HP, Askin J: Multiple haemangiomata with thrombopaenia: an unusual case with comments on steroid therapy, *Am J Dis Child* 115: 351, 1968.
61. Kelly SM, Gray SD: Unilateral endoscopic supraglottoplasty for severe laryngomalacia, *Arch Otolaryngol Head Neck Surg* 121:1351, 1995.
62. Kessler G, Rauchfuss A, Werner C: Pulsoximetrie bei Eingriffen im Bronchialsystem, *HNO* 37:216, 1989.
63. Koch BM, Milmoe G, Grundfast KM: Vocal cord paralysis in children studied by monopolar electromyography, *Pediatr Neurol* 3:288, 1987.
64. Konior RJ, Holinger LD, Russell EJ: Superselective embolization of laryngeal hemangioma, *Laryngoscope* 98:830, 1988.
65. Krishnamoorthy M and others: Diagnosis and treatment of respiratory symptoms of initially unsuspected gastroesophageal reflux in infants, *Am Surg* 60:783, 1994.
66. Lee TS, Wu Y: Bedside fiberoptic bronchoscopy for tracheostomy decannulation, *Respir Med* 89:571, 1995.
67. Leventhal BG and others: Long-term response of recurrent respiratory papillomatosis to treatment with lymphoblastoid interferon alfa-N1: papilloma study group, *N Engl J Med* 325:613, 1991.
68. Leventhal BG and others: Randomized surgical adjuvant trial of interferon alfa-n1 in recurrent papillomatosis, *Arch Otolaryngol Head Neck Surg* 114:1163, 1988.
69. Leventhal BG and others: Recurrent respiratory papillomatosis, *J Biol Response Mod* 4:525, 1985.
70. Levine BA and others: Vocal cord injection in children with unilateral vocal cord paralysis, *Arch Otolaryngol Head Neck Surg* 121:116, 1995.
71. Lindahl H and others: Bronchoscopy during the first month of life, *J Pediatr Surg* 27:548, 1992.
71a. Mackenzie M: *Essay on growths of the larynx*, Philadelphia 1871, Linsay and Blakeston.
72. Mawson S: Subglottic ha(e)mangioma of the larynx treated by excision, *J Laryngol Otol* 75:1076, 1961.
73. Meeuwis J and others: Subglottic hemangiomas in infants: treatment with intralesional corticosteroid injection and intubation, *Int J Pediatr Otorhinolaryngol* 19:145, 1990.
74. Morrison GA, Kotecha B, Evans JN: Ribavirin treatment for juvenile respiratory papillomatosis, *J Laryngol Otol* 107:423, 1993.
75. Mounts P, Kashima H: Association of human papilloma virus subtype and clinical course in respiratory papillomatosis, *Laryngoscope* 94: 28, 1984.
76. Mounts P, Shaw KV, Kashima H: Viral aetiology of juvenile and adult onset squamous papilloma of the larynx, *Proc Natl Acad Sci U S A* 79:5425, 1982.
77. Mulder JJ, Van Den Broek P: Surgical treatment of infantile subglottic hemangioma, *Int J Pediatr Otorhinolaryngol* 17:57, 1989.
78. Murty GE, Shinkwin C, Gibbin KP: Bilateral vocal fold paralysis in infants: tracheostomy or not? *J Laryngol Otol* 108:329, 1994.
79. Myer CM III, Fitton CM: Vocal cord paralysis following child abuse, *Int J Pediatr Otorhinolaryngol* 15:217, 1988.
80. Narcy P and others: Treatment of infantile subglottic hemangioma: a report of 49 cases, *Int J Pediatr Otorhinolaryngol* 9:157, 1985.
81. Narcy P, Contencin P, Viala P: Surgical treatment for laryngeal paralysis in infants and children, *Ann Otol Rhinol Laryngol* 99:124, 1990.
82. New GB, Clark CM: Angioma(s) of the larynx: report of three cases, *Ann Otol Rhinol Laryngol* 28:1025, 1919.
83. Nielson DW, Heldt GP, Tooley WH: Stridor and gastroesophageal reflux in infants, *Pediatrics* 85:1034, 1990.
84. Nunez DA, Hanson DR: Laryngeal reinnervation in children: the Leeds experience, *Ear Nose Throat J* 72:542, 1993.
85. Nussbaum E: Usefulness of miniature flexible fiberoptic bronchoscopy in children, *Chest* 106:1438, 1994.
86. Nussbaum E, Maggi JC: Laryngomalacia in children, *Chest* 98:942, 1990.
87. Ohlms LA and others: Interferon alfa-2a therapy for airway hemangiomas, *Ann Otol Rhinol Laryngol* 103:1, 1994.
88. Pedraza Pena LR, Rodriguez Santana JR, Sifontes JE: Neonatal stridor: a life-threatening condition, *P R Health Sci J* 13:33, 1994.
89. Perrick D and others: Evaluation of immunocompetency in juvenile laryngeal papillomatosis, *Ann Allergy* 65:69, 1990.
90. Pierce MK: Subglottic haemangioma in infants, *Ann Otol Rhinol Laryngol* 71:1057, 1962.
91. Pransky SM: Evaluation of the compromised neonatal airway, *Pediatr Clin North Am* 36:1571, 1989.
92. Prescott CA: Factors that influence successful decannulation after surgery for laryngo-tracheal stenosis in children, *Int J Pediatr Otorhinolaryngol* 30:183, 1994.
93. Puhakka H and others: Pediatric bronchoscopy: a report of methodology and results, *Clin Pediatr (Phila)* 28:253, 1989.
94. Quint LE and others: Stenosis of the central airways: evaluation by using helical CT with multiplanar reconstructions, *Radiology* 194: 871, 1995.
95. Raine J, Warner JO: Fibreoptic bronchoscopy without general anaesthetic, *Arch Dis Child* 66:481, 1991.
96. Rosenfeld RM, Stool SE: Should granulomas be excised in children with long-term tracheotomy? *Arch Otolaryngol Head Neck Surg* 118: 1323, 1992.
97. Rosin DF and others: Vocal cord paralysis in children, *Laryngoscope* 100:1174, 1990.
98. Ross DA, Ward PH: Central vocal cord paralysis and paresis presenting as laryngeal stridor in children, *Laryngoscope* 100:10, 1990.
99. Schechter GL, Biller HF: The limitations of corticosteroids and cryotherapy for subglottic hemangioma, *Trans Am Acad Ophthalmol Otolaryngol* 76:1360, 1972.
100. Sebastian B, Kleinsasser O: Zur behandlung der kehlkopfhamangiome bei kindern, *Laryngol Rhinol Otol (Stuttg)* 63:403, 1984.
101. Seid AB, Pransky SM, Kearns DB: The open surgical approach to subglottic hemangioma, *Int J Pediatr Otorhinolaryngol* 26:95, 1993 (letter).
102. Seigler RS: Bacterial tracheitis: recognition and treatment, *J S C Med Assoc* 89:83, 1993.
103. Shah K and others: Rarity of cesarean delivery in cases of juvenile-onset respiratory papillomatosis, *Obstet Gynecol* 68:795, 1986.
104. Shikowitz MJ, Abramson AL, Liberatore L: Endolaryngeal jet ventilation: a 10-year review, *Laryngoscope* 101:455, 1991.
105. Sitbon P and others: Lidocaine plasma concentrations in pediatric patients after providing airway topical anesthesia from a calibrated device, *Anesth Analg* 82:1003, 1996.
106. Smith EM and others: Human papillomavirus infection in papillomas and nondiseased respiratory sites of patients with recurrent respiratory papillomatosis using the polymerase chain reaction, *Arch Otolaryngol Head Neck Surg* 119:554, 1993.
107. Strong MS and others: Recurrent respiratory papillomatosis: management with the CO_2 laser, *Ann Otol Rhinol Laryngol* 85:508, 1976.
108. Swift AC, Rogers J: Vocal cord paralysis in children, *J Laryngol Otol* 101:169, 1987.
109. Teitelbaum DH: Bronchoscopy and esophagoscopy in children, *Curr Opin Pediatr* 5:341, 1993.
110. Terada Y and others: A case report of surgically treated tracheobrachiocephalic artery fistula following tracheostomy, *Kyobu Geka* 46:862, 1993 (in Japanese).
111. Todres ID, Noviski N: Flexible fiberoptic bronchoscopy: a practical guide to examining infants and children, *Mt Sinai J Med* 62:36, 1995.
112. Tom LW and others: Endoscopic assessment in children with tracheotomies, *Arch Otolaryngol Head Neck Surg* 119:321, 1993.

113. Tostevin PM and others: The value of radiological investigations in pre-endoscopic assessment of children with stridor, *J Laryngol Otol* 109:844, 1995.
114. Tucker HM: Double-barreled (diversionary) tracheostomy in the management of juvenile laryngeal papillomatosis, *Ann Otol Rhinol Laryngol* 89:504, 1980.
115. Tucker HM: Vocal cord paralysis in small children: principles in management, *Ann Otol Rhinol Laryngol* 95:618, 1986.
116. Vogl T and others: MR imaging in pediatric airway obstruction, *J Comput Assist Tomogr* 14:182, 1990.
117. Vogl T and others: MRI in tracheal stenosis by innominate artery in children, *Pediatr Radiol* 21:89, 1991.
118. Watanabe I and others: Anesthetic management for bronchofiberoscopy and esophageal manometric study in a patient with CHARGE association, *Masui* 44:1010, 1995 (in Japanese).
119. Wengen DF, Probst RR, Frei FJ: Flexible laryngoscopy in neonates and infants: insertion through a median opening in the face mask, *Int J Pediatr Otorhinolaryngol* 21:183, 1991.
120. Whyte RI and others: Helical computed tomography for the evaluation of tracheal stenosis, *Ann Thorac Surg* 60:27, 1995.
121. Woodson GE, Miller RH: The timing of surgical intervention in vocal cord paralysis, *Otolaryngol Head Neck Surg* 89:264, 1981.
122. Zalzal GH: Stridor and airway compromise, *Pediatr Clin North Am* 36:1389, 1989.

Chapter 18

Glottic and Subglottic Stenosis

George H. Zalzal
Robin T. Cotton

Chronic laryngeal stenosis is a partial or complete cicatricial narrowing of the endolarynx and may be congenital or acquired. The condition is rare and presents multiple problems affecting soft tissue and cartilage. Iatrogenic injuries and road traffic accidents account for most cases. Chronic laryngeal stenosis in pediatric patients often should be managed differently from that in adult patients. Of all laryngeal stenoses, chronic subglottic stenosis is the most common and the most difficult to manage (Fig. 18-1).

ETIOLOGY AND PATHOPHYSIOLOGY

Congenital laryngeal stenosis

Congenital stenosis is secondary to inadequate recanalization of the laryngeal lumen after completion of normal epithelial fusion at the end of the third month of gestation.[163] The final pathologic findings depend on the degree of recanalization; thus, if the laryngeal lumen is not recanalized and remains completely obliterated, it will result in complete laryngeal atresia, whereas if it is partially recanalized, incomplete atresia, stenosis, or web will occur. The cricoid cartilage is usually abnormally developed.

Congenital laryngeal atresia and web

Laryngeal atresia can occur at any laryngeal level or combination of levels. The clinical picture depends on the severity of the lesion. In incomplete atresia, the glottis is closed at or above the vocal cords by a firm fibrous membrane; the neonate is aphonic, tries vigorously to breathe, rapidly deteriorates and becomes cyanotic despite continued respiratory efforts, and soon dies of asphyxia unless immediate tracheotomy is performed.[37,66,94] The condition is incompatible with life unless an emergency tracheotomy is performed or there is an associated tracheoesophageal or bronchoesophageal fistula. The most severe type of congenital laryngeal atresia presents as stillbirth and may not be recognized.

Congenital laryngeal webs account for about 5% of congenital anomalies of the larynx.[93] About 75% occur at the glottic level, and the rest are supraglottic or subglottic.[13] Most webs present at birth or in the first few months of life. The severity of the web varies; only a few are severe enough to require airway support by intubation or tracheotomy. A laryngeal web is often an abnormality of the glottis and the subglottic-cricoid region (Fig. 18-2). The differential diagnosis includes bilateral vocal cord paralysis and congenital interarytenoid fixation. It is important to detect associated anomalies of the larynx, the respiratory tract, and other organ systems.

Different classifications of webs have been suggested, but the most useful is that of Benjamin.[13]

Glottic:	Thin and membranous; thick at the anterior commissure; or severe with subglottic involvement
Subglottic:	With or without cricoid cartilage involvement
Congenital:	Interarytenoid fixation
Supraglottic:	Extremely rare

Management

The immediate management of laryngeal atresia is by establishing an airway at birth through an emergency tracheotomy. Rarely, it may be possible to pass a small bronchoscope through an incomplete atresia into the trachea followed by a tracheotomy.[120] It is extremely difficult to insert a large-bore needle into the highly mobile trachea of infants, and a neck incision with tracheotomy is the preferable method of establishing an emergency airway. Occasionally, tracheal agenesis coexists. After adequate airway is maintained, the elective surgical correction of laryngeal atresia generally restores re-

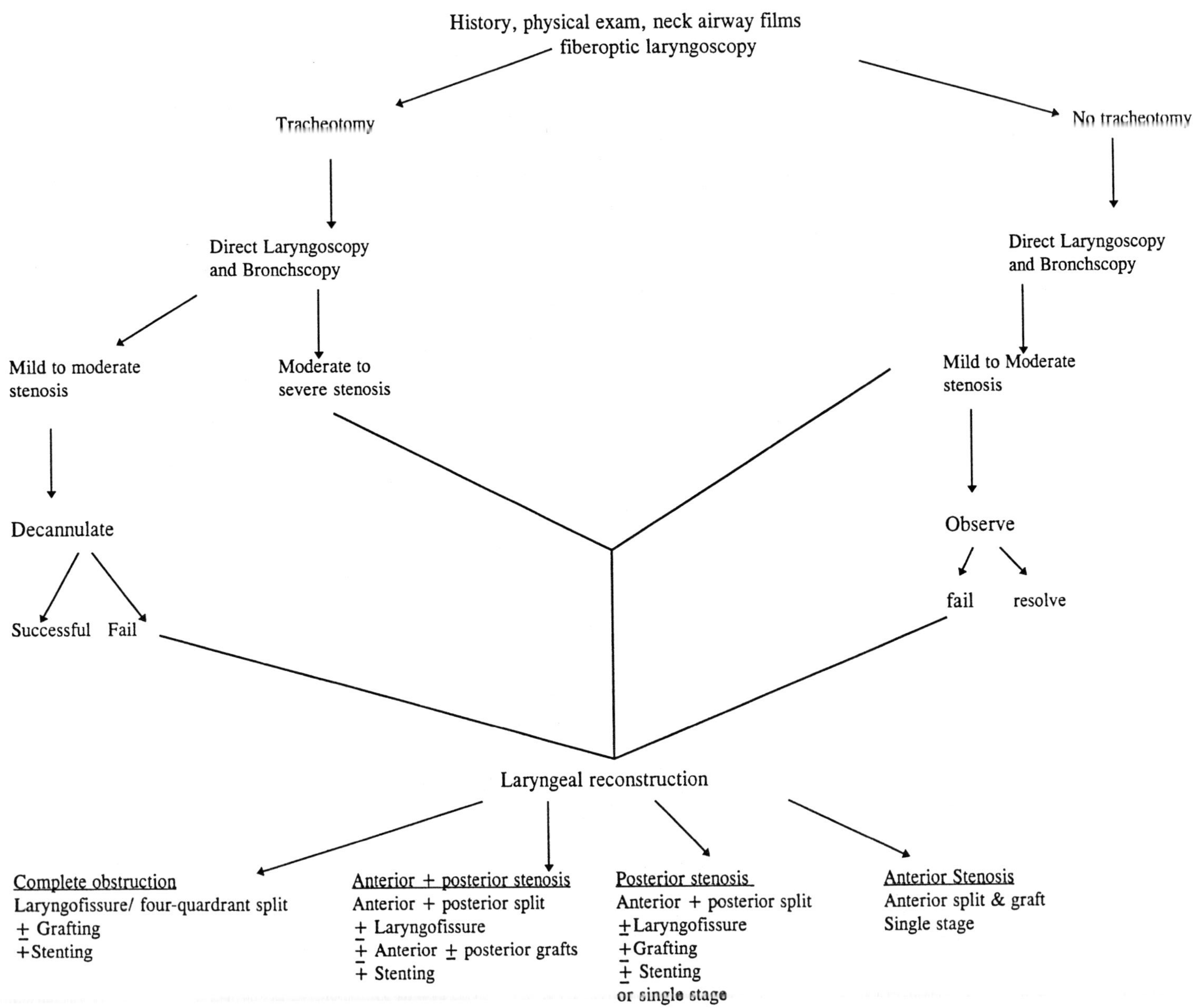

Fig. 18-1. Algorithm for management of laryngeal stenosis.

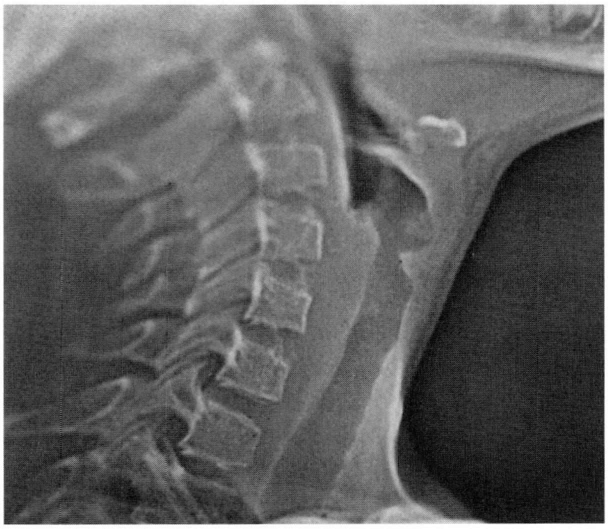

Fig. 18-2. Xeroradiography of neck shows a congenital glottic web with subglottic extension, having a triangular configuration like a sail.

spiratory function, but the phonatory and protective functions remain significantly impaired after surgery. Padovan[143] discussed methods of repairing laryngeal atresia.

Treatment of laryngeal webs depends on the thickness of the web.[39,120] A thin web may be broken down by passage of the bronchoscope or incised with a surgical knife, scissors, or the carbon dioxide (CO_2) laser. An attempt should be made to incise the web along one vocal cord, followed 2 weeks later by incision along the opposite side (to prevent further web formation). However, the smaller the larynx, the more difficult this is to achieve.

The less common thick glottic webs are more difficult to manage. They may be difficult or impossible to incise or dilate because of the associated subglottic-cricoid abnormality. Tracheotomy is required, followed by surgical excision of the glottic web and cartilaginous abnormality via a laryngofissure approach, followed by stenting with a glottic keel or placement of an anterior autogenous costal cartilage graft. The optimum age for surgery is unknown, and the possibility of aggravating the situation with an ill-judged operation should be considered. However, infants with severe obstruction above the tracheotomy are at greater risk of dying of cannula obstruction because of their decreased reserve airway above the tracheotomy. In such cases, earlier reconstruction should be considered. Endoscopic placement of a keel in children is difficult, and the external approach is recommended for best results.

Congenital subglottic stenosis

The normal subglottic lumen diameter in the full-term neonate is 4.5 to 5.5 mm and in premature babies about 3.5 mm. A subglottic diameter of 4 mm or less in a full-term neonate is considered to be narrowed.

Table 18-1. Histopathologic classification of congenital subglottic stenosis

Cartilaginous stenosis	Soft-tissue stenosis
Cricoid cartilage deformity	Submucosal fibrosis
Normal shape	Submucosal gland hyperplasia
Small for infant's size	Granulation tissue
Abnormal shape	
Large anterior lamina	
Oval (elliptic shape)	
Large posterior lamina	
Generalized thickening	
Submucous (occult) cleft (incomplete laryngeal cleft)	
Other congenital cricoid stenosis	
Trapped first tracheal ring	

Subglottic stenosis is considered to be congenital in the absence of a history of endotracheal intubation or other apparent acquired causes of stenosis. The diagnosis may be difficult to confirm, and it is unknown how many intubated premature infants who fail extubation have underlying congenital stenosis. Thus, by best approximation, congenital subglottic stenosis is the third most common congenital disorder of the larynx after laryngomalacia and recurrent laryngeal nerve paralysis. Acquired subglottic stenosis is more common than congenital stenosis because of increased use of prolonged endotracheal intubation for respiratory support.

Congenital subglottic stenosis can be divided into membranous and cartilaginous types.[35,62,173] The membranous type is a fibrous soft-tissue thickening of the subglottic area caused by increased fibrous connective tissue or hyperplastic, dilated mucous glands with no inflammatory reaction. It is usually circumferential, with the narrowest area 2 to 3 mm below the true vocal cords, sometimes extending upward to include the true vocal cords.[95]

The cartilaginous types are more variable, but the most common type is a thickening or deformity of the cricoid cartilage causing a shelf-like plate of cartilage, partially filling the concave inner surface of the cricoid ring and extending posteriorly as a solid rigid sheet, leaving only a small posterior opening.[62,122] It is less common than the membranous type.

Congenital subglottic stenosis is a clinical endoscopic diagnosis describing various histopathologic conditions that produce narrowing of the subglottic airway.[136,173] Table 18-1 lists one histopathologic classification of subglottic stenosis. From a management perspective, a combined classification of congenital and acquired subglottic stenosis in infants is useful (Fig. 18-3).

Symptoms depend on the degree of subglottic narrowing. In severe cases, respiratory distress and stridor are present at birth, whereas in milder cases the symptoms become evident

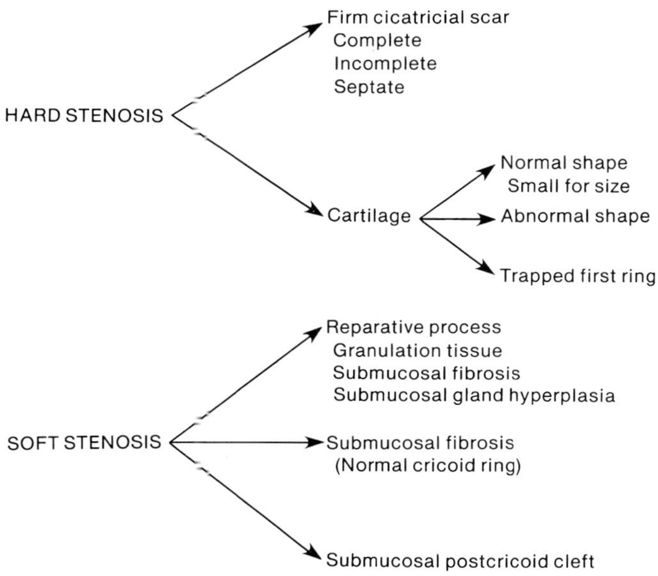

Fig. 18-3. Clinicopathologic classification of subglottic stenosis in infants.

during the first few weeks or months of life, presenting as prolonged or recurrent croup. Infants usually become symptomatic within 3 months of birth because of increased activity and increased ventilation requirements.[36,37]

Minimal laryngeal swelling secondary to infection or endoscopy may precipitate airway obstruction because the cricoid cartilage limits the swelling of tissue in any direction except toward the laryngeal lumen at the expense of the airway. Therefore great care is needed when endoscopy is performed on these children to prevent trauma to the subglottic mucosa.

Endoscopic diagnosis is essentially by means of flexible fiberoptic endoscopy to assess vocal cord function and rigid endoscopy to assess the degree of anatomic obstruction. Postendoscopic edema is avoided by operating on a quiet, relaxed infant who is well-oxygenated. Cooperation between the endoscopist and anesthesiologist is essential, as is gentle instrumentation, preferably with the rigid rod lens system telescope alone without the sheath. If postoperative edema occurs, aggressive management should be started with cool mist in a croup tent, racemic epinephrine by aerosol or intermittent positive-pressure breathing, and a short course of high-dose intravenous corticosteroids.

Management. Congenital subglottic stenosis is most often less severe than is acquired stenosis and may therefore be managed more conservatively. Some patients outgrow the condition.[28] Management depends on the degree of stenosis, shape (circumferential, partial, horizontal, or vertical) and size of stenosis, whether the cricoid cartilage is normal or abnormal, and whether there are associated congenital anomalies.[172]

Mild cases of stenosis are managed conservatively by watchful waiting and regular follow-up because many children will outgrow the problem. During observation, vigorous medical management of viral infection is recommended.[120]

For more severe cases, gentle periodic endoscopic dilation with well-lubricated, round, tracheal dilators is recommended to enhance the subglottic airway.[64] Although this may offer some benefit for soft subglottic stenosis, it has not shown any benefit for the cartilaginous type. More severe cases requiring airway support may be managed by tracheotomy and reconstructive repair.

Acquired laryngeal stenosis

External laryngeal trauma

Trauma is the most common cause of acquired laryngeal stenosis in children and adults. The laryngeal spaces are important in the creation of stenosis after injury. These spaces are readily distended by blood after trauma; if the blood is not evacuated, absorption of the hematoma by macrophage invasion or organization with deposition of fibrous tissue may occur. The collagen in fibrous tissue later contracts, causing stenosis and loss of mobility. External trauma was found to have the best outcome in a study to assess prognostic factors.[116]

Blunt trauma to the neck sustained during motor vehicle accidents injures the larynx when the anterior surface of the extended neck strikes the dashboard or steering wheel, causing a laryngeal framework fracture. This is more common in adults than in children, in whom the prominent mandible and the relatively high position of the larynx protect the latter from injury. Chronic acquired laryngeal stenosis is a sequela of severe laryngeal trauma with fracture of the cricoid cartilage with or without displacement or of inadequately managed early stages of laryngeal trauma.[114]

Another mechanism of blunt laryngeal trauma, the so-called clothesline injury, occurs when a person riding a bicycle hits the anterior neck on a branch or clothesline, sustaining laryngeal fracture and thyrotracheal or cricotracheal separation. A patient may have a separation of the cricoid and trachea and still survive the injury. Penetrating wounds of the larynx are usually less common than blunt trauma and are more common in adults than in children.

Internal laryngeal trauma

Endotracheal tube injury. Most cases of internal laryngeal injury are iatrogenic, secondary to prolonged endotracheal intubation, which is the most common cause of chronic laryngeal stenosis. Approximately 90% of cases of acquired chronic subglottic stenosis in infants and children occur secondary to endotracheal intubation.[32,95] The reported incidence of stenosis after intubation ranges from 0.9% to 8.3%.* This rate is much lower than the 12% to 20% reported in the late 1960s and early 1970s[69,111,166] because of recogni-

* Refs. 6, 82, 86, 97, 145, 146, 177.

tion of the problem and institution of preventive methods. These figures may underestimate the true incidence of the disease in the pediatric population because many infants who are intubated do not survive the primary illness; in addition, some acquired subglottic stenosis may not be recognized unless an infection of the upper respiratory tract develops or the patient requires reintubation later in life. The areas most commonly injured are the subglottic region in children and the posterior endolarynx in adults.[178]

In children, the subglottic region is especially prone to injury from endotracheal tube intubation for various reasons: (1) The cricoid cartilage is the only area in the upper airway that has a complete circular cartilaginous ring, preventing the outward extension of traumatic edema. (2) The pseudostratified, ciliated, columnar respiratory epithelium lining this region is delicate and tends to deteriorate under the stress of an indwelling tube. (3) The subglottic submucosa is made up of loose areolar tissue that allows edema to develop easily and quickly. (4) The subglottic region is the narrowest portion of the pediatric airway.[91,95] In adults, traumatic intubation denudes the mucosa in the posterior commissure, causing ulceration that heals by secondary intention. Collagen is deposited and contracts to form posterior glottic scarring, fixing the arytenoids toward the midline.

The pathophysiology of acquired subglottic stenosis is well-described in the literature.[39,65,86] The endotracheal tube causes pressure necrosis at the point of interface with tissue, leading to mucosal edema and ulceration. As ulceration deepens, normal ciliary flow is interrupted, with mucociliary stasis leading to secondary infection and perichondritis.[158] With further infection, chondritis and cartilaginous necrosis occur, especially with collapse of the airway during inspiration. Posterior cricoid chondritis may lead to the formation of a tracheoesophageal space abscess.[65] Healing occurs by secondary intention with granulation tissue proliferation in the areas of ulceration and deposition of fibrous tissue in the submucosa. Primary healing of laryngeal injury is hindered by the presence of loose and mobile subglottic mucosa, poor blood supply of the cartilage, and constant motion of the larynx associated with swallowing and head movement.[87] Gould and Young[76] studied intubated larynges from infants of 22 to 40 weeks' gestation who survived a few hours to 300 days. Acute injury was almost invariable and up to 100% of the subglottic epithelium was lost within a few hours of intubation, but progression of injury was relatively short lived. Ulcer healing started after a few days, rapidly progressed from day 10, and, in most cases, was complete after 30 days. This study suggests that long-standing acute injury of the subglottis is the exception rather than the rule, even with the endotracheal tube remaining in place.[76]

Duration of intubation is the most important factor in the development of laryngeal stenosis. There is no definite safe time limit for endotracheal intubation, and severe injury has been reported after 17 hours of intubation in adults[15] and 1 week in neonates.[105] Several studies in adults have shown that a 7- to 10-day period is acceptable, after which prolongation of intubation is accompanied by an increased incidence of laryngotracheal complications.[178] Premature infants tolerate more prolonged intubation (weeks rather than days). Explanations, include (1) relative immaturity of the laryngeal cartilage in the neonates (more hypercellular with scant gel-like matrix) rendering it more pliable, thus yielding to pressure,[86] and (2) the high location of the neonatal larynx in the neck with its posterior tilt and funnel shape.[87]

Insertion of an oversized endotracheal tube increases the risk of laryngeal injury. It has been suggested that to avoid subglottic injury, intubation should use tubes with a maximum internal diameter of 7 or 8 mm in adult male patients and 6 to 7 mm in female patients.[101] In children, the tube size should allow an air leak at 20 cm H_2O pressure if possible. Polymeric silicone and polyvinyl chloride are considered the safest materials for prolonged intubation.

Shearing motion of the tube causes abrasive traumatic action on the mucosa, especially in patients who are restless, those on respirators, and those with orotracheal intubation.[147] Superimposed bacterial infection compounds the mechanical mucosal trauma by increasing the inflammatory response and scar tissue formation.[158] Repeated intubations cause increased trauma and increase the risk of sequelae.[85,86,105] Nasogastric tubes can cause pressure necrosis and cricoid chondritis if placed in the midline.[71] Coexistence of endotracheal and nasogastric tubes may increase laryngeal complications.

When inexperienced personnel care for intubated patients, intubation complications may increase. Education of physician and nursing personnel caring for intubated patients markedly increases the expertise of that care. Systemic factors including chronic illness, general disability, immunosuppression, anemia, neutropenia, toxicity, avitaminosis, dehydration, hypoxemia, poor perfusion, radiotherapy, and the presence of gastric acid reflux encourage the vulnerability of laryngeal mucosa to injury by decreasing tissue resistance and increasing infection rate.

Other causes of internal laryngeal trauma. Laryngeal stenosis may occur secondary to laryngeal injury resulting from laryngeal surgery. Emergency cricothyroidotomy through the cricothyroid membrane[19,73] and high tracheotomy can produce severe stenosis, particularly in children. Acquired anterior glottic web can occur after excision of a laryngeal polyp or papilloma in the anterior commissure area if the anterior portions of both vocal cords are denuded simultaneously.[152,168] Laryngeal stenosis can also occur after partial vertical or horizontal laryngectomy, especially if excess tissue is removed without internal stenting.[165] Laryngeal stenosis also is described after endoscopic microsurgery with modalities such as electrocautery or laser.[40]

Chondroradionecrosis can lead to scarring and stenosis shortly after radiotherapy or as long as 20 years later.[133]

Intralaryngeal burns from fumes, smoke inhalation, or caustic lye ingestion can give rise to chronic laryngeal stenosis.[46]

Chronic infection. Laryngeal stenosis secondary to chronic infection is rare except in isolated endemic geographic areas. It has been described in tuberculosis, syphilis, leprosy, glanders, typhoid fever, scarlet fever, diphtheria, mycosis, and laryngeal scleroma.[84,170]

Chronic inflammatory diseases. Laryngeal stenosis has been described secondary to sarcoidosis, lupus erythematosus, Behçet's syndrome, Wegener's granulomatosis,[68,103] relapsing polychondritis, pemphigoid,[125] epidermolysis bullosa,[25] amyloidosis[81] and major aphthous ulceration.[165] Management of laryngotracheal stenosis in Wegener's granulomatosis is complex, requiring individualized frequent mutimodality interventions to achieve satisfactory results. Microvascular laryngotracheal reconstruction may be needed.[104]

Chronic inflammation secondary to gastroesophageal reflux,[12,100] may cause laryngeal stenosis. Gastroesophageal reflux in children can be classified as physiologic or pathologic. Many airway manifestations have been attributed to gastroesophageal reflux, including stridor, recurrent croup, exacerbation of subglottic stenosis, and chronic cough. Diagnosis is difficult unless the index of suspicion is high.[21] Pediatric laryngotracheal reconstruction outcome may not be related to the presence or management of gastroesophageal reflux.[185]

Laryngeal neoplasm. Chondroma, fibroma, hemangioma, and carcinoma can cause laryngeal stenosis because of tumor infiltration or secondary to infective perichondritis, postradiation perichondritis, or postsurgical scarring and stenosis.

Types of stenosis

Acquired glottic stenosis may be anterior, posterior, or complete. Anterior glottic stenosis can be a thin glottic web, which is a bridge of scar tissue covered by epithelium located between the vocal cords involving the anterior commissure. This usually results from enthusiastic endoscopy involving both true cords simultaneously. Thick, anterior glottic scarring is usually more extensive and results in true vocal cords, false cords, and laryngeal ventricles adhering to one another without any intervening web. The cause is often unmanaged severe external laryngeal trauma. Posterior glottic stenosis usually results from prolonged endotracheal tube intubation. Pressure necrosis of the mucosa overlying the vocal process of the arytenoid occurs, followed by ulceration and granulation tissue formation on the medial surface of the body of the arytenoid cartilage. A similar process occurs to a variable degree in the interarytenoid area with involvement of the interarytenoid muscle, causing fibrous ankylosis of one or both cricoarytenoid joints.[17,49] Posterior glottic scar frequently extends downward to the subglottic region. It is important to differentiate between a complete posterior glottic

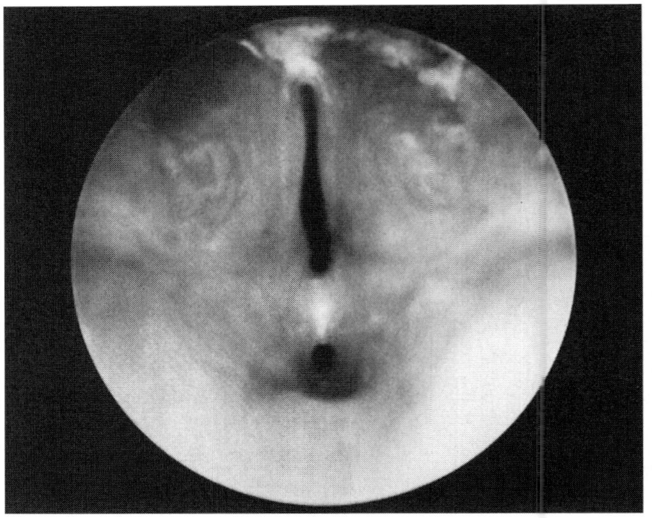

Fig. 18-4. Endoscopic view of interarytenoid adhesion shows a posterior fistula tract resulting from a scar tissue band between the vocal process of the arytenoid cartilages.

stenosis, in which the scar is located in the interarytenoid space and posterior commissure, and an interarytenoid adhesion, in which the scar is between the vocal processes of the arytenoids with a small posterior, mucosally lined sinus tract in the posterior commissure area (Figs. 18-4 and 18-5, *A*). The scarring of the posterior commissure may be confined to the submucosa (Fig. 18-4, *B*) or extend into one (Fig. 18-5, *C*) or both (Fig. 18-5, *D*) cricoarytenoid joints.

The voice is generally good because of the adducted position of the vocal cords. The major symptoms are referable to the airway. In mild or moderate cases, the patient may be able to ventilate without a tracheotomy and may experience only exercise intolerance. Patients who have a more severe stenosis may need a tracheotomy for adequate respiratory exchange. Diagnosis by indirect laryngoscopy is difficult and may be confused with bilateral abductor vocal cord paralysis. This condition has been named *pseudolaryngeal paralysis*.[24] Diagnosis at direct laryngoscopy is made by careful observation of the posterior commissure. The true vocal cords are closely approximated because the vocal processes and occasionally the arytenoid bodies are tethered together by heavy scar. A posterior sinus tract should be carefully sought and is particularly difficult to see in the pediatric larynx. Unlike in vocal cord paralysis, in posterior glottic stenosis the cricoarytenoid joints are partially or completely immobile on a passive motion test. Palpation of the arytenoids shows that they may be rocked in an anteroposterior direction but will not slide from side to side. Electromyography helps differentiate vocal cord fixation from nerve paralysis.

Complete total glottic stenosis rarely occurs in isolation and is usually accompanied by supraglottic or subglottic stenosis. In adults, it usually results from external laryngeal

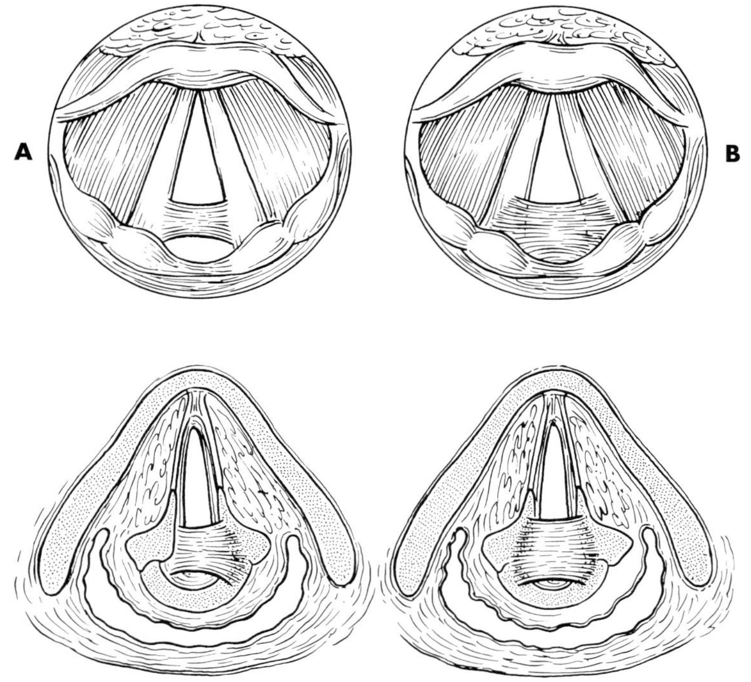

Fig. 18-5. Posterior glottic stenosis. **A,** Interarytenoid adhesion with a mucosally lined tract posteriorly. **B,** Posterior commissure and interarytenoid scar without a mucosally lined tract posteriorly. **C,** Posterior commissure scar extending into the right cricoarytenoid joint. **D,** Posterior commissure scar extending into both cricoarytenoid joints.

trauma with extensive cartilaginous fracture when early repair and stenting have not been performed. In children, it is a sequela of endotracheal intubation. Rare causes include severe inflammatory and infectious diseases, such as relapsing polychondritis,[47] tuberculosis, lye ingestion, and thermal burn.[132]

Prevention. Factors important in reducing the incidence of laryngotracheal stenosis include:

1. Early exploration of laryngeal fractures is advocated to minimize serious sequelae.
2. High tracheotomy and cricothyroidotomy should be avoided except in extreme emergencies. If it is suspected that a high tracheotomy or cricothyroidotomy has been performed, endoscopy is indicated. If the suspicion is confirmed, the neck should be explored, and the tracheotomy site should be relocated to a lower position to prevent chronic subglottic stenosis.[44]
3. When performing a tracheotomy, the surgeon should avoid extensive resection of the tracheal wall and use the smallest size tracheotomy tube compatible with ventilation and suctioning.
4. Aggressive endoscopy for benign laryngeal lesions should be avoided, especially for those from the anterior commissure area, to prevent formation of an anterior glottic web. The procedures should be staged 2 weeks apart for each side. Different principles may be appropriate for malignant lesions.
5. Intubation and endoscopy should be performed gently on relaxed patients.
6. Circumstances contributing to laryngeal trauma secondary to prolonged intubation should be recognized and avoided whenever possible.

DIAGNOSIS OF CONGENITAL AND ACQUIRED LARYNGEAL STENOSIS

Laryngeal stenosis is diagnosed by a thorough history and physical examination, radiologic evaluation, and endoscopic examination.[39] Other investigations such as pulmonary function tests also may be helpful.

History and physical examination

Mild-to-moderate laryngeal stenosis is usually asymptomatic until an infection of the upper respiratory tract causes additional narrowing of the airway, resulting in respiratory distress. These patients usually have a tendency toward prolonged courses of upper respiratory tract infections.

In acquired stenosis, there is a history of laryngeal insult. Symptoms usually occur 2 to 4 weeks after the original insult, although the latent period can occasionally be longer. In congenital stenosis, symptoms usually appear at or shortly after birth, suggesting the possibility of a laryngeal anomaly.

The main symptoms of laryngeal stenosis relate to airway, voice, and feeding. Progressive respiratory difficulty is the prime symptom of airway obstruction with biphasic stridor, dyspnea, air hunger, and vigorous efforts of breathing with suprasternal, intercostal, and diaphragmatic retraction. Abnormal cry, aphonia, or hoarseness occurs when the vocal cords are affected. Dysphagia and feeding abnormality with recurrent aspiration and pneumonia can occur.

Complete physical examination of the upper aerodigestive tract should be performed to rule out associated congenital anomalies or acquired injuries.

Radiologic evaluation

Radiologic evaluation is performed after stabilization of the airway. Radiography helps assess the exact site and length of the stenotic segment, especially for totally obliterated airways.[57]

The lateral soft-tissue radiograph is the single most important view in children. The anteroposterior high-kilovoltage technique increases visibility of the upper airway by enhancing the tracheal air column while deemphasizing the bony cervical spine.[53] In acquired stenosis, small areas of calcification may be seen, denoting the site of previous injury. Fluoroscopy is helpful in studying tracheal dynamics.

In xeroradiography (see Fig. 18-2), a selenium-coated, charged plate is substituted for the usual radiographic cassette before filming.[124] It has a better tissue-air interface and therefore enhances the edge and better documents soft-tissue details than does computed tomography (CT). However, it requires longer exposure time than conventional techniques and thus exposes the patient to higher radiation. Although xeroradiography is the best method for evaluating chronic airway problems in the young child,[45,115,137] its use should be reserved for the more difficult and unusual cases in which conventional techniques have been inadequate.

In adults, linear CT enhances anatomic details at critical levels; it is impractical for pediatric patients because it is a positive-contrast laryngogram with tantalum dust, liquid barium, or propyliodone. Linear CT shows mucosal details, length and thickness of a stenotic area and vocal cord fixation. Because it is highly viscous, linear CT compromises the airway in patients with a marginal airway; therefore, caution is advised unless a safe airway has been established.

CT and magnetic resonance imaging (MRI)[157] are useful in adults, especially after external trauma. They are difficult to perform in infants and children. High-speed CT has reduced imaging time and is becoming more popular in the assessment of airway lesions. MRI still requires a significant amount of time, necessitating sedation in younger patients; its use is not very common.[90]

Endoscopic examination

Indirect laryngoscopy alone is inadequate for diagnosis. Direct endoscopic visualization of the larynx is essential to study the stenosis carefully. Flexible fiberoptic endoscopy assesses the dynamics of vocal cord function and the upper airway, including the trachea.[174] In patients with severe burns with neck contractures, flexible endoscopy may be the only method to visualize the larynx. Flexible retrograde tracheoscopy through the tracheotomy site may provide useful information in some cases.

Rigid endoscopy should be performed in the operating room with the patient under general anesthesia. Additional magnification is helpful with the operating microscope or the rigid rod lens system telescope with both straight and angled lenses. The rigid telescope is especially important in the examination of children because it better visualizes the small larynx. However, it is important to recognize that the airway should be measured by passing bronchoscopes or endotracheal tubes of known sizes and cannot be gauged by the use of telescopes alone. It is important that the surgeon measure the outside diameter of the bronchoscope or endotracheal tube and not rely on the manufacturer's specification.

VOICE ASSESSMENT

Psychoacoustic evaluation and acoustic analysis of the voice may be used to establish the degree of vocal abnormality before surgery and compare it after surgery.[49,191] Videostrobolaryngoscopy helps assess vocal cord function in adults.

Although assessment of pre- and postoperative vocal quality in young children may be frustrating, improvement in technology has made the task easier over the past 3 to 4 years, and several reports have been published regarding specific voice issues. In general, the voice results are unsatisfactory, with the vocal parameters suggesting a pattern of lower-than-optimum pitch and a restricted pitch range. Vocal quality appears to be disturbed in most patients; however, laryngeal reconstruction makes oral communication possible.[11,117,164,189]

Pulmonary function tests with the spirometric maximum inspiration and expiration flow rates, flow volume loops, or pressure flow loops show characteristic changes in upper airway stenosis and can be used to compare the postoperative results with preoperative values.[20,78,83,190]

MANAGEMENT

Management should be individualized according to pathologic findings, patient age, degree and consistency of stenosis (hard or soft and percentage of stenosis), and general condition of the patient. Management of adults differs from that of children, and some operations useful in children are not applicable to adults.

All cases of moderate or severe laryngeal stenosis require a tracheotomy at or below the third tracheal ring to establish a safe airway. Stenosis that does not require a tracheotomy constitutes a mild case. A suggested grading scale of subglot-

Table 18-2. Grading of laryngeal stenosis

Grade	Percentage of laryngeal lumen obstruction
I	Less than 70%
II	70% to 90%
III	More than 90%; identifiable lumen is present (no matter how narrow)
IV	Complete obstruction; no lumen present

tic stenosis has been introduced (Table 18-2).[29] Classification of laryngeal stenosis to predict the probability of decannulation in adults has been suggested; use of four clinical stages of stenosis based on site of lesion effectively predicted the likelihood of successful decannulation. The only factors significantly affecting outcome were site and diameter of stenosis.[118] Massoud and McCullough[116] found that the anatomic site of stenosis and its length were independent determinants of outcome, whereas the diameter was not.

Severe cases of congenital subglottic stenosis or marked cartilaginous cricoid deformity need a tracheotomy to maintain an adequate airway. When a tracheotomy is performed, the smallest tube that permits adequate ventilation should be used. The tube should allow air leakage to occur to avoid injury to the tracheal mucosa and simultaneously preserve phonatory potential.[115]

Tracheotomy was required in congenital subglottic stenosis in less than half of a large series of patients.[95] Normal growth and development of the child may allow decannulation within 2 years. If the subglottic lumen does not enlarge during this 2-year period, other alternative methods to repair the airway should be considered. Watchful waiting is not advised because of morbidity and mortality associated with tracheotomy. Once the airway is secured, two basic management modalities are considered: endoscopic or external. Endoscopic methods include traditional dilation and newer techniques that use laser excision of stenotic areas. Open surgical methods have generally stressed excision of the stenotic lesion followed by reconstruction. The morbidity of open reconstruction is higher, but this is balanced against the multiplicity and futility of endoscopic procedures when inappropriately used. In general, less severe cases respond to endoscopic methods, and more severe cases require external reconstruction. If the cartilaginous framework of the larynx is significantly deficient, endoscopy is contraindicated.

Endoscopic management

Dilation is sometimes useful early in the development of stenosis. It is not recommended for mature, firm stenoses or cartilaginous stenoses. Dilation is usually performed with round, smooth dilators and can be done alone or supplemented with local or systemic corticosteroids[142] or intralaryngeal stenting.[75,99] Balloon dilatation has been reported to relieve tracheal strictures in children[89] and has been recently reported to be successful in subglottic stenosis.[10]

The use of corticosteroids in all stages of acquired subglottic stenosis is controversial. Corticosteroids tend to decrease scar formation by their anti-inflammatory action of delaying synthesis of collagen in early stages of wound healing and increasing collagen lysis in the later phases. Corticosteroids also delay wound healing by delaying the epithelial migration necessary to resurface the denuded area, thus increasing scar formation and predisposing to infection.

Corticosteroids may be used systemically or locally. Local injection into subglottic scar is technically difficult and may be ineffective if a pressure injection system is not used. Resorption of cartilage secondary to the presence of local corticosteroids is a serious complication. Inhalation corticosteroids are believed to reduce granulation tissue formation after stent removal or early after endotracheal tube injury.

Endoscopic scar excision with microcauterization,[98] cryosurgery,[153,167] and serial electrosurgical resection[52,96] have been used. CO_2 laser is popular because it allows the surgeon to vaporize scar tissue with precision, producing minimal damage to healthy areas.[92,161,162] Tissue destruction is directly related to the amount of energy delivered by the laser and the duration of exposure.[123] If minimal energy of short duration is delivered, damage to the underlying and normal surrounding structures is minimal. However, if the laser is used at high energy levels for long times, it acts similar to any other uncontrolled method of tissue destruction (e.g., diathermy, cryoprobe).

The laser is useful for managing early stenosis with granulation tissue and may improve the airway without causing significant bleeding or edema, thus avoiding the need for a tracheotomy. Many authors have reported adequate results in managing early or mild subglottic stenosis using the CO_2 laser,* generally with multiple procedures. Flaps elevated with laser have been reported to be successful in the repair of subglottic stenosis in children.[176]

Endoscopic management has not been successful in the presence of the following conditions:

1. Circumferential cicatricial scarring
2. Abundant scar tissue greater than 1 cm in vertical dimension
3. Fibrotic scar tissue in the interarytenoid area of the posterior commissure
4. Severe bacterial infection of the trachea after tracheotomy
5. Exposure of perichondrium or cartilage during CO_2 excision, predisposing to perichondritis and chondritis
6. Combined laryngotracheal stenosis
7. Failure of previous endoscopic procedures
8. Significant loss of cartilaginous framework

* Refs. 51, 55, 70, 87, 88, 102, 110, 162, 169.

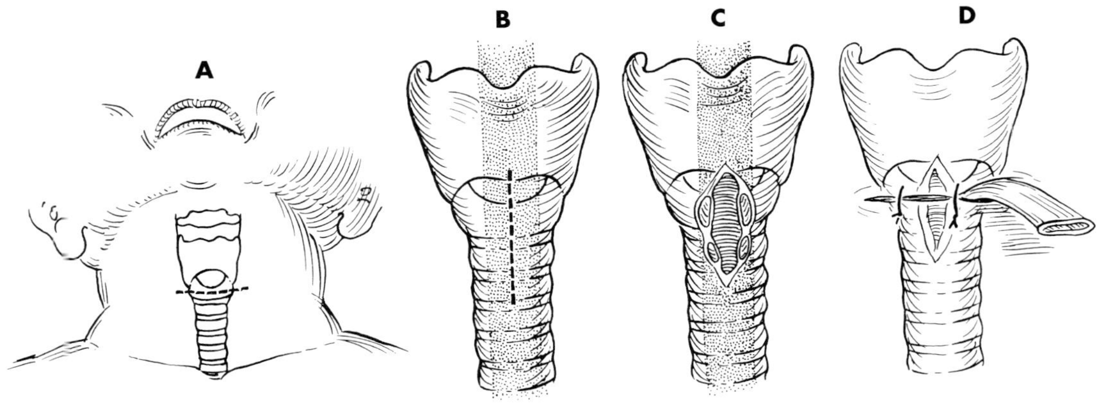

Fig. 18-6. Anterior cricoid split. **A,** Skin incision. **B,** Midline laryngeal incision through cartilage and mucosa. **C,** With the cricoid cartilage decompressed, the endotracheal tube is ghosted in **B** and **C. D,** Loose skin closure with a drain inserted.

External surgical reconstruction

Surgical reconstruction is recommended when conservative efforts to establish a satisfactory airway are inappropriate or have failed. In weighing the advantages of open reconstruction versus endoscopic management, the surgeon should consider his or her personal expertise and the severity of the lesion. In general, grades III and IV lesions require external methods. Grade II may be amenable to either method. Only rarely is open surgery required when the stenosis is of such a degree that tracheotomy has not been required.

Before surgery is performed, vocal cord paralysis should be ruled out and should be no reason for the patient to continue to be tracheotomy-dependent despite adequate patency of the airway (e.g., in neurologic damage or chronic pulmonary disease). The goal and rationale of open reconstructive surgery are to achieve early decannulation with minimal detrimental effect on the voice.[63]

External surgical repair should be directed at the site and severity. Each case should be individualized.[119] Expansion surgery is a collection of techniques that aim to widen the glottic and subglottic lumen. These techniques combine the use of laryngeal and cricoid splits, cartilage and bone grafts, and stenting. Many techniques for correction of stenosis are available, but choosing the most appropriate procedure and achieving a successful outcome are problematic.[33]

Splits

Anterior cricoid split operation. The anterior cricoid split operation (Fig. 18-6) was described by Cotton and Seid[38] as an alternative to tracheotomy in the management of acquired subglottic stenosis in premature infants. The procedure has subsequently been used in the management of congenital subglottic stenosis.[30] The concept is to split the cricoid and upper first and second tracheal rings in the midline anteriorly, thus allowing expansion of the cricoid ring. It is indicated in cases of congenital subglottic stenosis caused by a small cricoid ring (that is not otherwise seriously deformed) or extensive submucosal fibrosis with healthy cricoid cartilage. It should be used only in patients whose condition is severe enough to require airway support and in whom lung function is adequate to permit decannulation.

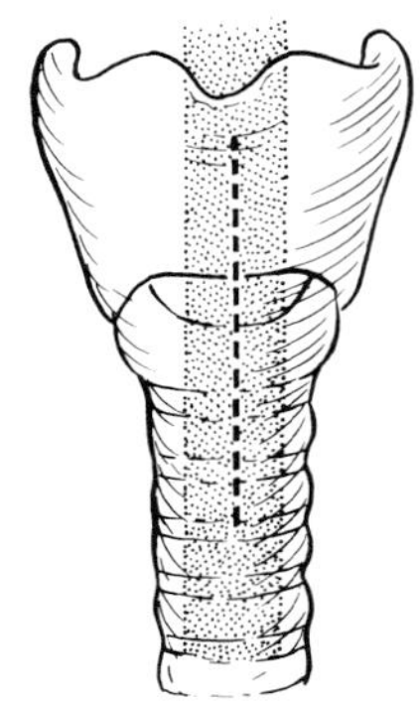

Fig. 18-7. Incision for an anterior cricoid split in the management of subglottic stenosis in infants (compare with Figure 18-6).

With the patient under general endotracheal anesthesia, a horizontal skin incision is made over the cricoid to expose the cricoid and upper two tracheal rings. A single vertical incision is made through the anterior cartilaginous ring of the cricoid and through the mucosa to expose the endotracheal tube. The incision is extended inferiorly to divide the upper two tracheal rings in the midline. When the incision is made through the cricoid, the cricoid springs open, and the endotracheal tube is readily visible in the lumen. The incision in the larynx is extended superiorly in the midline to include the lower third of the thyroid cartilage to a level just inferior to the anterior commissure, but it can be extended to within 2 mm of the thyroid notch (Fig. 18-7).[41] Stay sutures of 3-0 Prolene are placed on each side of the

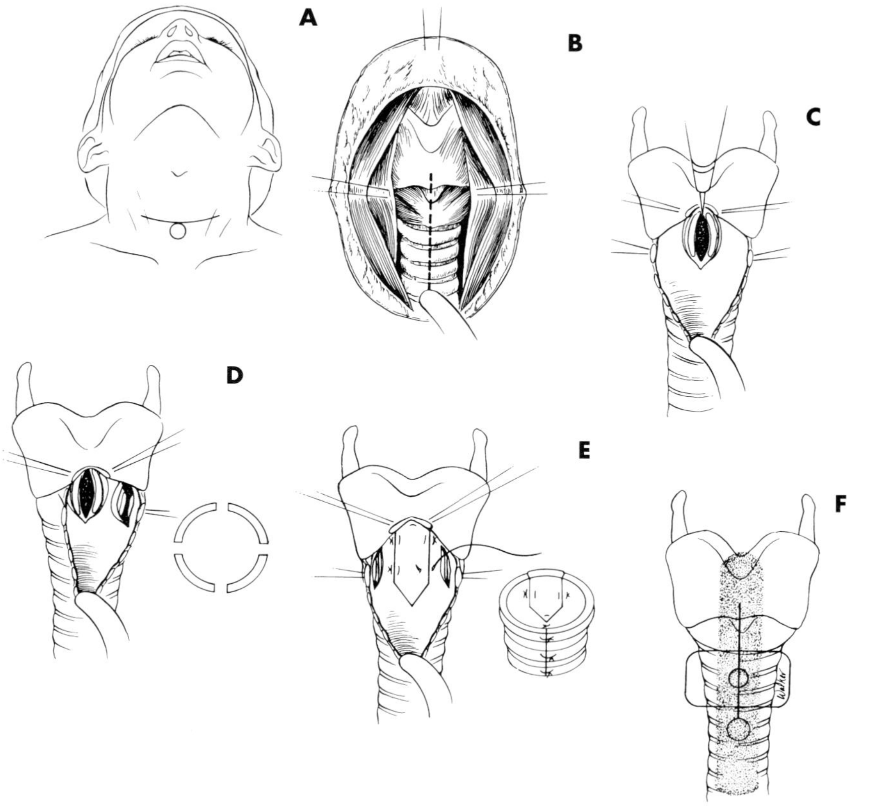

Fig. 18-8. Anterior laryngofissure with division of the posterior and lateral lamina of cricoid, together with posterior cricoid cartilage graft insertion. **A,** Horizontal skin incision incorporates the superior aspect of tracheotomy. **B,** Skin flap elevated in the neck and laryngofissure. **C,** Division of the posterior lamina of cricoid. **D,** Bilateral division of the cricoid cartilage. **E,** Autogenous cartilage graft interposed posteriorly between divided ends of the cricoid lamina and sutured in place. **F,** Laryngofissure closed anteriorly with a Cotton-Lorenz stent in place.

incised cricoid. These can be used as retractors in the postoperative period if the endotracheal tube becomes dislodged and cannot be reinserted. The skin is loosely approximated around an elastic band drain. The endotracheal tube is left in place around 7 days and acts as a stent while the mucosal swelling subsides and the split cricoid and tracheal rings heal. Endoscopy is not performed at extubation. Corticosteroids are administered before extubation and continued for 5 days.

Combined laryngofissure and posterior cricoid division. Division of the posterior cricoid lamina through a laryngofissure with prolonged stenting without resection of the posterior scar was first described by Rethi[150] in 1956. Good results also were obtained by others in adults and children.* This is the method of choice for combined posterior glottic and subglottic stenoses, for moderate subglottic and upper tracheal stenoses with loss of cartilaginous support, and for complete glottic and subglottic stenoses. The operation is effective in patients of all ages. Cartilage grafts can augment the lumen. Scar removal is unnecessary in this procedure.

With the patient under general anesthesia administered via the tracheotomy, a horizontal skin incision is made incorporating the upper portion of the stoma (Fig. 18-8). Subplatysmal flaps are elevated superiorly and inferiorly, and the strap muscles are retracted laterally, exposing the thyroid, cricoid, and upper tracheal rings. A midline anterior incision is made in the larynx and upper trachea, extending from the superior thyroid notch to the tracheotomy site. After injection of 1% lidocaine with epinephrine 1/100,000 into the posterior larynx, the posterior scar and full length of the posterior lamina of the cricoid are divided, taking care to cut strictly in the midline, down to the level of the hypopharyngeal mucosa. The laryngeal scar should not be excised. The incision is carried superiorly into the interarytenoid area through the interarytenoid muscle (when fibrosed) and inferiorly for about 1 cm into the membranous tracheoesophageal septum. The divided halves of the posterior cricoid lamina are distracted laterally; approximately 1 mm of distraction per year of age up to 10

* Refs. 29, 37, 43, 44, 64, 77, 134.

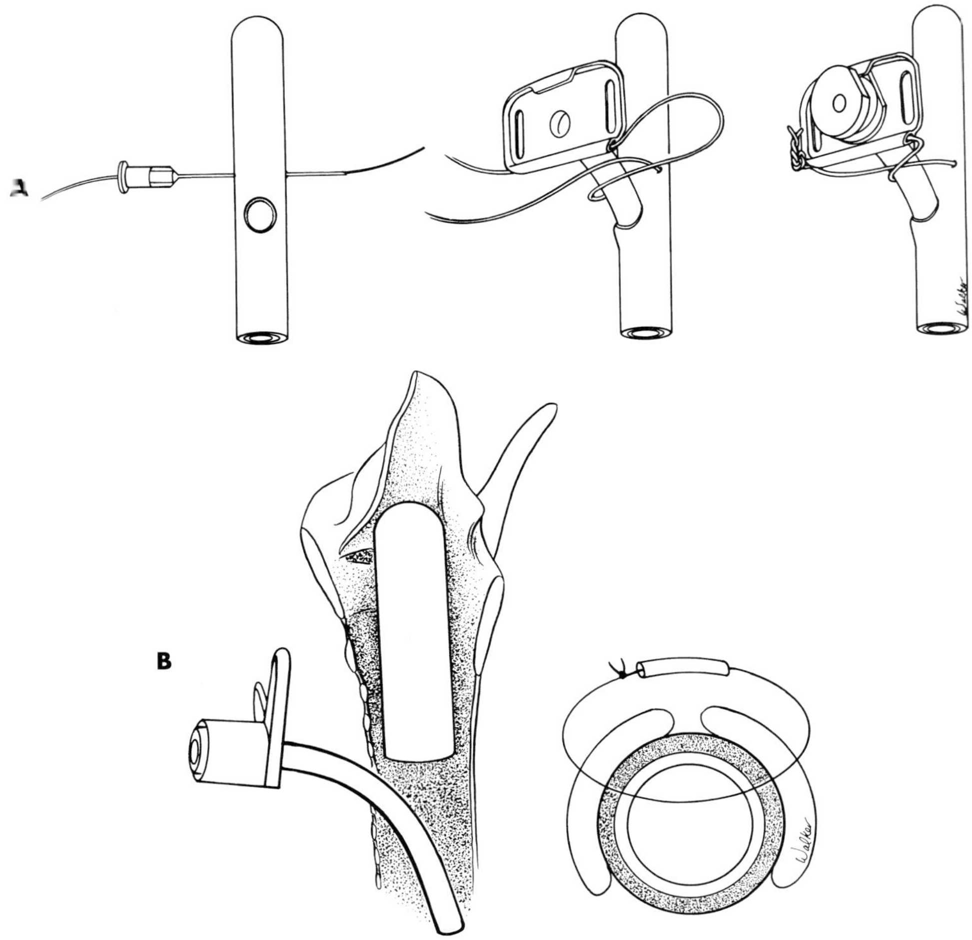

Fig. 18-9. A, Technique of inserting and attaching Holinger metal tracheotomy tube in a Cotton-Lorenz hollow polytef laryngeal stent. **B,** A short Cotton-Lorenz stent in the laryngeal lumen and placement of anchoring suture.

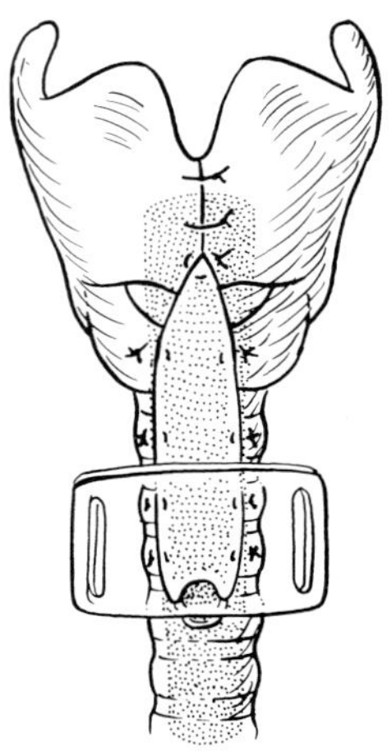

Fig. 18-10. Anterior costal cartilage graft in place after laryngofissure, division of the posterior plate of the cricoid, and placement of a Cotton-Lorenz stent.

years is obtained between the cut edges of the divided cricoid lamina. The Cotton-Lorenz stent, a variation of the Aboulker stent,[5] is the stent of choice in children and is inserted to maintain the diastasis of the divided cricoid lamina. In adults, Cotton-Lorenz and Montgomery laryngeal stents can be used. In the presence of tracheal lesions, a metal tracheotomy tube should be wired through the Cotton-Lorenz stent (Fig. 18-9). If cartilage loss is significant, autogenous costal cartilage (Fig. 18-10) (in children) or a hyoid-sternohyoid myo-osseous flap (in adults) is used to give support. In severe cases of subglottic stenosis, lateral cuts in the cricoid with anterior and posterior splits are needed (see Fig. 18-8).[34]

Grafts

In children, autogenous costal cartilage is the graft material of choice, especially when there is little identifiable cricoid cartilage remaining anteriorly.[28,29,61,63] Because of the abundance of available costal cartilage, any length of cartilage can be obtained to graft the subglottis and trachea.[112]

The use of costal cartilage and ear cartilage[108] offers advantages over free thyroid cartilage grafts[135] and composite nasal cartilage grafts, which can be used in adults.[54] The use of vascularized hyoid interposition techniques should be discouraged in children because the hyoid is too small to augment effectively the subglottic lumen, bone is too hard to sculpture, and the muscle pedicle tends to ossify, causing secondary compression of the larynx. Cartilage graft survival has been proven experimentally and clinically in children and adults.[186,193] Although costal cartilage may be used in adults, vascularized hyoid interposition techniques are preferred because the donor site is already in the operative field.

Looper[106] first reported on the interposition of a composite-free hyoid bone–muscle flap anteriorly to augment the airway in laryngeal stenosis. Bennett[14] reported the use of free hyoid bone graft for the management of subglottic stenosis. Alonso and others[8] revived the use of free hyoid bone grafts in canine experiments, with subsequent clinical application in humans.[9] Although results of free hyoid grafts were good, attempts to minimize bone resorption led to the development of vascularized hyoid-sternohyoid myo-osseous flaps, in which the sternohyoid muscle attachment to the hyoid bone was not severed.[67,171,175,180] Other variations on this theme have been described.[1,2]

Autogenous costal cartilage reconstruction. The patient is positioned in an extended neck position. The tracheotomy tube is replaced with an endotracheal tube to allow easy access to the neck and adequate anesthesia. The lower face, neck, and chest are scrubbed and draped. A 3-cm horizontal skin incision is made just inferior to the right mammary gland and is deepened to include the subcutaneous tissue and muscle. Costal cartilage is identified (Fig. 18-11), and the longest straight segment is removed without considering the rib to which it belongs. The cartilage is removed with overlying lateral perichondrium, and the medial perichondrium is kept intact. The cartilage is fashioned to fit the intended site of transplantation. If the stenosis is anterior, cartilage is trimmed to a modified boat shape (Fig. 18-12).[187,186] Flanges at the edges of the cartilage graft prevent prolapse into the lumen and allow maximum use of the width of the graft for distraction of the anterior cricoid. The regular boat-shaped graft is used for distraction of posteriorly cut cricoid segments in the management of posterior glottic and subglottic stenosis.[181] Indications for use of a cartilage graft in the posterior glottis and subglottis are (1) posterior glottic or subglottic stenosis, (2) isolated subglottic shelves, (3) circumferential subglottic stenosis, and (4) total or near total obstruction at the glottic or subglottic level. Posterior glottic or subglottic cartilage implantation is contraindicated in the absence of a rigid posterior cricoid lamina.

After a Rethi procedure is performed, a boat-shaped piece of cartilage with the perichondrium facing the lumen is sutured in the posterior cricoid incision, stenting the cricoid lamina open (see Fig. 18-8). Sutures are used through the mucosa, cricoid lamina, and cartilage graft. Despite suturing, the graft is not stable enough to remain in place and stenting is needed.

Cotton[31] reported a large series of posterior cartilage grafting with animal study documentation of survival of posteriorly placed cartilage grafts.[31] In cases of severe subglottic stenosis, anterior and posterior grafts have yielded success rates greater than 90% after a single procedure within a short time after removal of the stent.[183]

Free hyoid bone or hyoid-sternohyoid myo-osseous flap reconstruction. In a free hyoid graft, the hyoid bone is dissected free from its muscular attachments and its midportion is removed.

In a composite hyoid-sternohyoid myo-osseous flap, the suprahyoid muscular attachment to the hyoid bone is freed, preserving the superior laryngeal and hypoglossal nerves, while the hyoid bone is pedicled on the sternohyoid muscle below. The hyoid bone can be trimmed with the drill or bone-cutting instruments to bevel the edges, thus providing a proper fit into the anterior laryngotracheal defect. The hyoid bone is then interposed between the cut edges of the cricoid, with the convexity of the hyoid bone facing toward the outside to avoid creating a bulge into the laryngeal lumen. The hyoid bone is anchored in place with 3-0 Prolene sutures tied extraluminally. The incision is closed in layers, and a Penrose drain is inserted. The endolarynx is resurfaced with a dermal graft over an indwelling stent anchored to the larynx for 4 to 8 weeks.[7] The denuded area can be covered with a superiorly based mucosal flap from the posterior lateral wall of the subglottis without the use of a stent.[23] Decannulation usually occurs 3 months after granulation tissue is controlled.

Stents

Stents are used to counteract scar contractures and promote a scaffold for epithelium to cover the lumen of the airway. Stents also hold the reconstructed area in place and prevent mechanical disruption secondary to movement of the laryngotracheal complex during breathing, swallowing, and attempts at phonation. Stenting is necessary when using grafts to expand stenosed areas of the airway. Grafts provide rigidity and support and fill gaps in the incised and distracted segments to avoid the formation of fibrous tissue with subsequent contraction. If the grafts are dislodged, failure to correct the stenosis will follow. Several reports support the use of stents;[113] other reports do not recommend stenting.[141]

When choosing stents, the physician should focus on the material, size, location, and duration of stenting. Many types of stents have been used, including finger cots, endotracheal tubes,[16] Montgomery laryngeal stents, and T-tubes[128] (Fig. 18-13), polymeric silicone sheet rolls,[60] and Aboulker prostheses (see Fig. 18-9).[3-5]

T-tubes continue to be used successfully in adults; however, in children mixed results are obtained with potential complications of blockage.[72] Although far from ideal, the Alboulker stent remains the most useful in the pediatric age

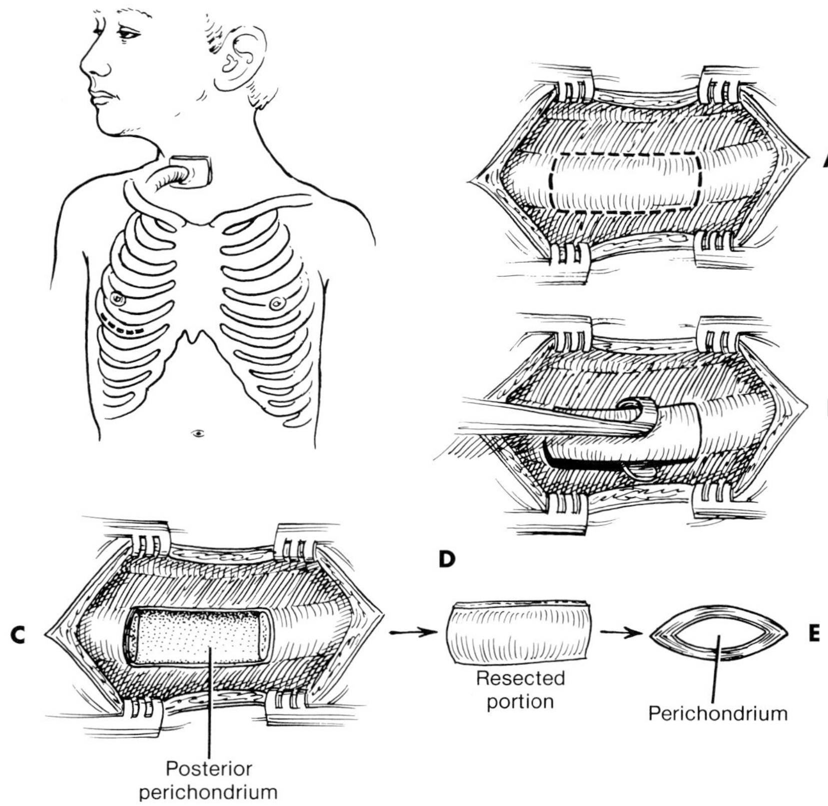

Fig. 18-11. Donor site of a costal cartilage graft used for anterior augmentation of stenotic cricotracheal area. **A,** Incision over the fifth costal cartilage to obtain a costal cartilage graft. **B,** Perichondrial incisions are made along the superior and inferior borders of the rib, with care taken not to injure underlying cartilage. **C,** Dissection in the subperichondrial plane is accomplished so that the perichondrium on the posterior part of the rib remains *in situ* on the chest wall of the patient. **D,** A 4-cm length of costal cartilage is removed and placed in physiologic saline solution. Lining perichondrium remains only on the anterior aspect of the graft. **E,** Costal cartilage graft is shaped into an ellipse and beveled to prevent the graft from settling into the lumen.

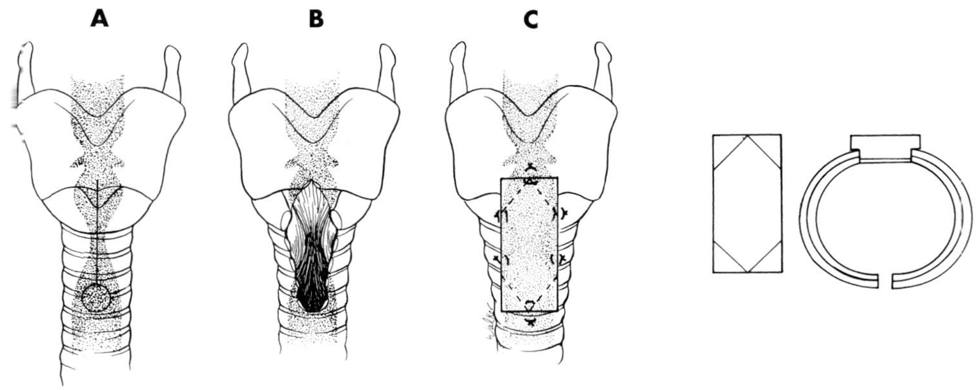

Fig. 18-12. Anterior cartilage graft. **A,** Vertical incision is made in the thyroid cartilage from a point immediately below the anterior commissure through the upper tracheal rings, with care taken to remain in the midline. **B,** Intraluminal scar and lining mucosa are incised along the length of the stenotic segment. **C,** Costal cartilage graft is shaped into a modified boat and placed in position with the lining of the perichondrium facing internally.

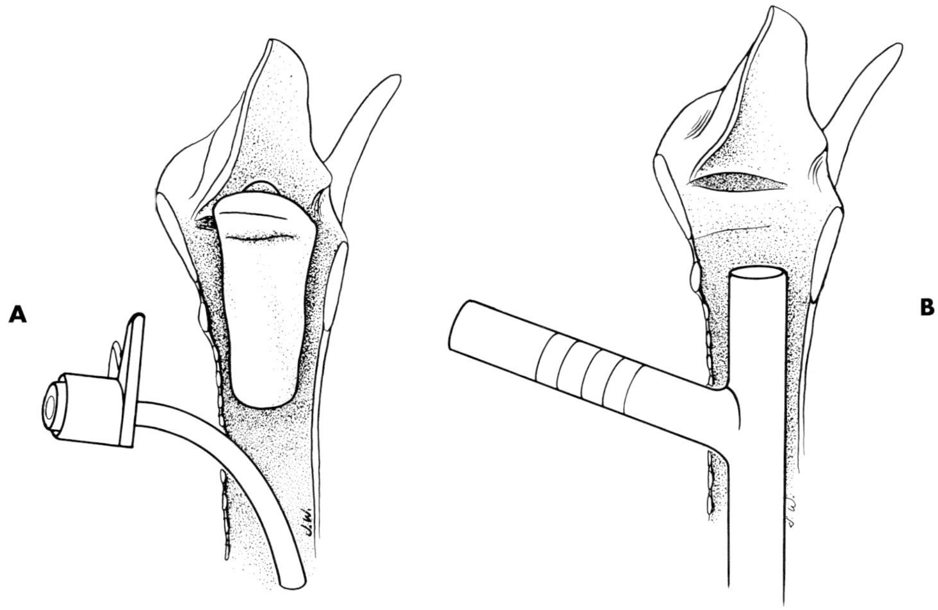

Fig. 18-13. A, Montgomery laryngeal stent. **B,** T-tube.

group.[182] A recent modification of the Aboulker stent is the Cotton-Lorenz stent. In children, the Cotton-Lorenz stent is used because it has several advantages over other available stents. It is available in several sizes with an outer diameter ranging from 7 to 16 mm, which makes it appropriate for all ages. Its 120-mm length is easily shortened by cutting with a knife. The stent is made of highly polished polytef, which is harder, provides better support, is more inert than silicone, and does not adhere to tissue. It has proven its superiority over polymeric silicone laryngeal stents.[32] Repair of laryngotracheal stenosis in almost all cases, except the anterior subglottis, requires stenting to keep the grafts in place, lend support to reconstructed areas, and create a rigid structure around which scar contracture can occur.

The Cotton-Lorenz stent can be used in the short form and the long form (see Fig. 18-9).[184] Short stents are indicated when a stenosis does not involve the trachea and when cartilage grafts are sufficient to act against scar contracture, necessitating brief stenting for 6 weeks or less. If possible, short stents should not be used for longer duration because there is risk of developing stenosis at the lower tip of the stent, above the tracheotomy. Long stents are used when there is tracheal stenosis or tracheostomal narrowing and collapse or when long-term stenting is needed. Long-term stenting (more than 2 months) is indicated when (1) keloids form; (2) the anatomy is severely altered by stenosis or surgical procedures; (3) cartilage grafts are not stable; (4) there is no rigidity of the walls of the airway, and cartilage is being used to build up rigid support; or (5) posterior cricoid split is performed without cartilage grafting.

A laryngofissure may be required for short and long stents because the superior tip of the stent should be inserted at the level of the superior edge of the arytenoid. The long segment is surgically placed by continuing the laryngofissure incision through the stenotic area to the level of the tracheal stoma. The inferior tip of the stent is placed about 1.5 cm above the carina. The diameter of the stent is gauged by placing several stents into the lumen until one fits snugly. A hole is made in the stent at the level of the tracheal stoma, and an appropriate Holinger silver tracheotomy tube is inserted. Before the trachea and larynx are closed, endoscopic examination of the superior tip of the stent should be performed. If the tip is low, glottic and supraglottic granulation tissue can occur. If the tip of the stent is high, aspiration may occur.

A short stent is measured in widths similar to a long stent, but the lower end of the short stent lies above the tracheotomy tube. It is anchored in place using a 0 Prolene suture passed through the strap muscles and trachea and stent, trachea, and muscle of the opposite side and then threaded through a small polyethylene tube and tied over the strap muscles under the skin. Both forms of the Cotton-Lorenz stent are removed endoscopically.

Cricoid resection with thyrotracheal anastomosis. Surgical resection of the anterior arch of the cricoid cartilage together with a portion of the posterior cricoid lamina below the cricothyroid articulation with thyrotracheal anastomosis was first suggested by Conley.[26] Several authors* subsequently reported good results.

The procedure is more difficult in patients younger than 10 years. In children with isolated tracheal stenosis, repair with resection and end-to-end anastomosis yields excellent

* Refs. 22, 42, 74, 81, 139, 140, 148, 160.

results.[179] When the stenosis involves the subglottis, the resection becomes technically difficult, but excellent results have been reported by Monnier and others.[126,127]

The procedure is limited to the few patients in whom the stenosis is entirely subglottic or upper tracheal with a normal lumen of at least 10 mm below the glottis. In such cases, this method is an alternative to stenting. With the patient under general anesthesia through the tracheotomy, the recurrent laryngeal nerve is identified on each side, following it upward to the posterolateral aspect of the cricoid cartilage, where it passes immediately posterior to the cricothyroid joint. In cases of severe external trauma, identification of the nerve in scar tissue is impossible, and dissection is performed on the cricoid in a subperichondrial plane to avoid injury to the nerve. The superior resection line starts at the inferior border of the thyroid cartilage and passes obliquely posteroinferiorly to cross the lower margin of the cricoid plate below the level of the exposed recurrent laryngeal nerve or below the cricothyroid joints (Fig. 18-14). The distal resection line is made immediately below the inferior border of the stenosis. To compensate for the disparity in the diameters between the tracheal and subglottic lumen, the superior cut of the tracheal lumen is beveled, and the membranous trachea may need to be plicated. Primary thyrotracheal anastomosis is accomplished by advancement of the distal segment superoanteriorly to the residual posterior shell of the cricoid cartilage and suturing them together with interrupted 3-0 polyglactin 910 sutures tied extramucosally. The anastomosis should be kept free of tension; this is best accomplished by the suprahyoid laryngeal mobilization tech-

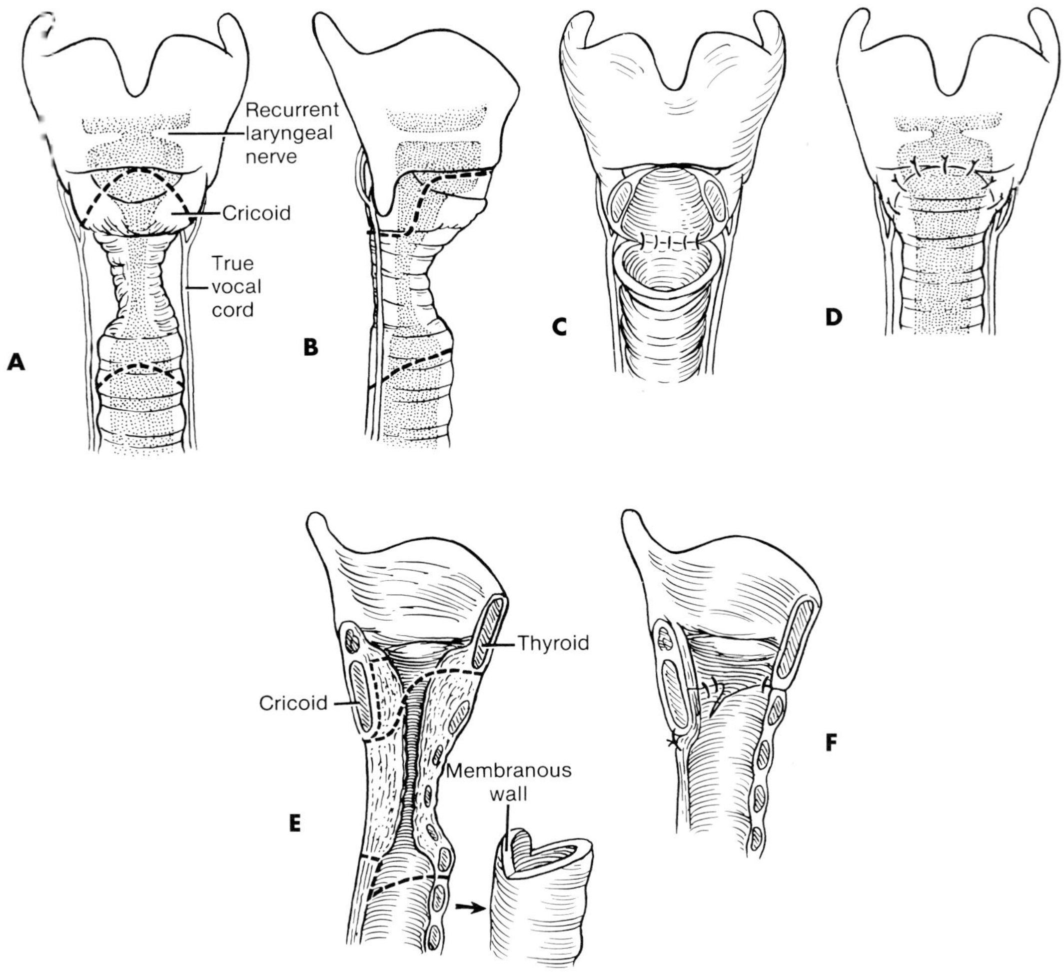

Fig. 18-14. Partial cricoid resection with thyrotracheal anastomosis. **A,** Anterior view of the stenotic area to be resected, including the anterior cricoid lamina. **B,** Lateral view of the same area. Note the preservation of the posterior cricoid lamina and the location of the recurrent laryngeal nerve. **C,** After resection. The trachea is beveled and approximated to the subglottis. **D,** Suturing is completed (3-0 polyglactin 910). **E,** If a posterior subglottic thick scar is present, it is resected with preservation of the posterior cricoid cartilage, and a mucosal flap is developed from the posterior tracheal wall. **F,** Suturing of the mucosal flap is performed, and coverage of raw areas is achieved.

nique.[131] After surgery, extension of the neck is to be avoided for 10 days by placing three sutures from the chin to the upper chest area. Stenting is not required. The tracheotomy is maintained until the anastomotic site is stable; this generally occurs within 4 weeks.

The rotary door flap technique has been reported in adults and children.[56,58,59] It involves the use of a sternohyoid myocutaneous flap to provide epithelial surfacing of the larynx and trachea along with luminal support without the need for cartilage or bone grafts.

MANAGEMENT OF SPECIFIC DISORDERS

Anterior glottic stenosis

Small anterior webs less than 2 to 3 mm wide produce minimal or no symptoms, and surgery is usually unnecessary. Thin anterior webs can be managed by microendoscopic incision of the web with a microsurgical knife[85] or CO_2 laser,[121,162,169] staging the procedure for each side separately (if possible) to avoid recurrence. A keel may be placed endoscopically in adults;[48] however, if this technique fails or longer thick anterior glottic scars are present, an external approach is needed. Tracheotomy is performed, followed by laryngofissure and incision of the stenotic area or web with the surgical knife. Resection of scar tissue should be minimized because this creates further mucosal loss. The Montgomery umbrella keel gives reliable results and should be inserted for 2 weeks. The keel prevents restenosis in the anterior commissure during reepithelialization; if the keel is used for 2 weeks or less, granulation tissue formation is minimal.[129,130,132] The design of the keel is such that contact with the posterior glottis is avoided, thus minimizing scarring secondary to the keel itself.

Stenosis and vocal cord paralysis

Vocal cord paralysis can accompany anterior, posterior, or complete glottic stenosis.[129,132] Bilateral vocal cord paralysis, associated with acquired glottic stenosis, needs an arytenoidectomy with lateralization of the true cord in addition to the above operation for correction of glottic stenosis. This is generally required unilaterally and only rarely bilaterally. Arytenoidectomy is reliably performed through the anterior thyrotomy approach. If done as a separate and later operation, an endoscopic laser arytenoidectomy is a valid alternative.[18]

Posterior glottic stenosis

Management of posterior glottic stenosis varies with the degree of pathologic findings. A simple interarytenoid adhesion requires a different approach from scarring involving both cricoarytenoid joints (see Fig. 18-5). It is a major challenge because the voice is generally excellent.

Endoscopic division of the adhesion is sufficient if a mucosally lined sinus tract is present posteriorly. This is easily accomplished with a microsurgical knife while the posterior surface of the mucosally lined sinus is protected by inserting a microsuction tip. In the absence of a mucosally lined sinus tract, simple endoscopic incision of the scar results in restenosis. In mild cases of posterior commissure stenosis, some authors advocate the laser using linear cuts[24] or a trapdoor flap.[51,55]

Laryngofissure, however, is the most common approach for such cases and is required for more advanced cases with cricoarythenoid joint fixation. After vertical incision of the posterior web, several techniques are used to cover the denuded posterior area. In adults, a superiorly based advancement mucosal flap from the interarytenoid area above the stenotic site[129,130] is recommended. A mucosal flap can also be taken from one aryepiglottic fold.[50] If the interarytenoid muscle is fibrosed, thus preventing lateral excursion and abduction of the arytenoid, division is necessary. If the mobility of both arytenoids is impaired, removal of the least mobile arytenoid may be necessary. Internal stenting is not needed if the vocal cords are mobile, but if there is associated vocal cord paralysis or cricoarytenoid joint fixation or if a free mucosal graft has been used, an indwelling laryngeal silicone stent is necessary for at least 2 weeks.[129,130,132] Some authors use a soft stent made of polymeric silicone sheets, applying gentle pressure on the mucosal flap or graft to the denuded surface.[17,177]

In adults and children with severe posterior glottic scarring with cricoarytenoid joint fixation or subglottic extension, a division of the posterior cricoid lamina in the midline with insertion of a free autogenous costal cartilage graft (see Fig. 18-8) is recommended. In children, the larynx is too small to create mucosal flaps endoscopically or by laryngofissure, and the posterior cricoid division operation is recommended initially. Complete glottic stenosis is difficult to manage, and voice results are usually poor because of severe scarring involving the vocal cords. Also, it is associated with a decrease in the anteroposterior diameter of the larynx. Management involves incising the scar in an anteroposterior manner and placing a stent for a long time. Cartilage grafts should never be used in the anterior commissure area.

Anterior subglottic stenosis is managed by incising the scar anteriorly and placing a modified boat-shaped cartilage graft (see Fig. 18-12) to keep the segments of the cricoid distracted. The perichondrium of the graft should be at the level of the mucosa. At the end of the procedure, endoscopic examination of the subglottic airway is recommended to check for possible poor placement or partial collapse of the graft. The cartilage graft can usually be extended inferiorly to cover the tracheostomy. The patient is intubated for several days depending on complexity of stenosis and method of repair. The results are best when the stenosis is located anteriorly.

The technique of intubating the patient after cartilage grafting instead of placing a stent and removing it later is termed *single-stage laryngotracheoplasty*. The goal is to avoid a second general anesthetic for removal of the stent.

During intubation, the patient is heavily sedated or paralyzed. Although anterior subglottic stenosis in neonates can be resolved by the cricoid split operation, use of costal cartilage grafts to keep the distracted segment of the cricoid open results in fewer complications and a higher success rate when extubating patients with acquired subglottic stenosis.[151] Auricular cartilage can be used for the same purpose.[109]

As more experience is gained using this procedure for more advanced stenosis, its use has become more prevalent; however, mixed results continue to be reported and are plagued by the unavailability of a uniformed classification system of laryngotracheal stenosis for comparison of data between centers.[27,107,159] Endotracheal intubation after a single-stage laryngotracheoplasty can range from 1 day for simple anterior cartilage grafting to 2 weeks for moderately severe stenosis repaired with anterior and posterior grafts. Postoperative complications can be serious, and sedation is preferred to paralysis.[144,155,192]

Posterior subglottic stenosis is managed in a similar manner to posterior glottic stenosis by placing a posterior cartilage graft. Circumferential and lateral subglottic stenoses are managed by incising the scar anteriorly and posteriorly and placing cartilage grafts between the anterior and posterior distracted segments, thus widening the subglottic lumen. This procedure necessitates stenting following the guidelines described.

Complete subglottic stenosis is treated with anterior, posterior, and lateral cuts in the cricoid. Cartilage grafts can be used anteriorly, posteriorly, or in both locations but cannot be used laterally. Stents used to manage this condition should be maintained for a long time.

Postoperative management

Postoperative management[79] is affected by whether a stent was used. In patients in whom stents were not used, antibiotics for 2 to 3 weeks after the surgery are recommended and endoscopy is indicated once the patient is ready for decannulation. In cases in which stenting has been used, long-term, low-dose antibiotics are recommended for the duration of stenting to prevent infection. Periodic endoscopy with a fiberoptic scope (every 4 weeks) also is recommended to assess the location of the stent and monitor for granulation tissue formation. Appropriate tracheotomy care is extremely important. The caregiver should be proficient and knowledgeable about routine and emergency care, especially when a long Cotton-Lorenz stent is needed. Patients with long Cotton-Lorenz stents are supplied with an endotracheal tube that can go through the Holinger silver tracheotomy tube in case the tracheotomy tube becomes blocked and suction catheters cannot open it. Possible complications that can occur with the use of the Cotton-Lorenz stent include infection, granulation tissue formation at both ends of the stent, subcutaneous emphysema, stent migration, and broken stents.

Broken Cotton-Lorenz stents are potentially serious and possibly life-threatening. To avoid this complication,[188] (1) insert the tracheotomy tube through the smallest hole possible in the stent; (2) avoid trauma from suctioning and manipulation; (3) use an endotracheal tube during mechanical ventilation instead of a direct connection between the tracheotomy and anesthesia tubes; (4) use the shortest possible duration of stenting; and (5) meticulously remove the tracheotomy tube without applying any force to the tracheotomy tube–stent complex.

A long Cotton-Lorenz stent is removed endoscopically by grasping the stent firmly, using an alligator forceps, through the hole in its proximal end while an assistant cuts and removes the wire attaching the tracheotomy tube to the stent. The tracheotomy tube is removed to release the anchorage. The short Cotton-Lorenz stent is also removed endoscopically after a small skin incision is made overlying the 0 Prolene suture knot, which is cut to release the anchorage. After stent removal, endoscopic inspection of the larynx and tracheal lumen is performed. Postoperative management after stent removal includes oral antibiotics and oral inhalation of beclomethasone dipropionate while plugging the tracheotomy by finger. Beclomethasone may help decrease buildup of granulation tissue. Two to three endoscopies may be required before decannulation is achieved. Granulation tissue should be removed only when pedunculated.

Decannulation. In adults, once the airway has been endoscopically assessed to be adequate, the tracheotomy tube is gradually downsized and eventually plugged and removed. The decannulation process in children is different from that in adults. Children should always be under adult supervision.[156] Once a child is ready for decannulation, endoscopy should be performed to ensure the airway is clear and the factors that influence successful decannulation after surgery have been well described.[149] Occasionally suprastomal granulomas are seen. If the child is being considered for decannulation, these granulomas should be removed; however, if the child is not ready for decannulation, removal of suprastomal granulomas is not indicated unless they are completely obstructing the airway. Therefore, interval bronchoscopies are unnecessary.[154]

The presence of suprastomal collapse can prevent decannulation, and further management may be needed.[138] When the child can tolerate the tracheotomy plugging for as long as he or she is awake, the decision for decannulation is made and the child is admitted to the hospital where the tracheotomy is plugged overnight with continuous monitoring (including oxygen monitoring). If there is no oxygen desaturation or apnea, the tracheotomy tube is removed the following morning, the stoma is covered with an occlusive dressing, and the child is kept for an additional night, again with continuous monitoring. Tracheotomy tube fenestration is not performed. Occasionally, tracheocutaneous fistulas should be surgically closed.

SUMMARY

Glottic and subglottic stenoses, although rare, are difficult to manage. Surgical goals are to produce an adequate airway, an acceptable voice, and a competent larynx to avoid aspiration. The keys to successful outcome depend on (1) accurate pre- and intraoperative assessment, (2) correct choice of surgical procedure, (3) meticulous surgery directed at site of lesion, and (4) close postoperative care and monitoring.

REFERENCES

1. Abedi E, Frable MA: Conjoint hyoid bone segments for the repair of severe laryngeal stenosis, *Arch Otolaryngol Head Neck Surg* 109A: 482, 1983.
2. Abedi E, Frable MA: Severe laryngeal stenosis repair: long term follow-up using conjoint hyoid bone segments, *Laryngoscope* 93B:745, 1983.
3. Aboulker P: *Chirurgie de la trachee: problems actuels d'proto-rhino-laryngologie*, Paris, 1962, Librairie Maloine.
4. Aboulker P: *Treitement des stenoses tracheals: problems actuels d'proto-rhino-laryngologie*, Paris, 1968, Librairie Maloine.
5. Aboulker P, Sterkers JM, Demaldent JE: Modifications apportees a l'printervention de Rethi, interest dans les stenoses laryngo-tracheales et tracheales, *Ann Otolaryngol Chir Cervicofac* 83:98, 1966.
6. Allen TH, Steven IM: Prolonged nasotracheal intubation in infants and children, *Br J Anaesth* 44:835, 1972.
7. Alonso WA: Hyoid arch transposition, *Otolaryngol Clin North Am* 12:903, 1979.
8. Alonso WA and others: Cricoid arch replacement in dogs: further studies, *Arch Otolaryngol Head Neck Surg* 101:42, 1975.
9. Alonso W, Druck N, Ogura J: Clinical experience in hyoid arch transposition, *Laryngoscope* 86:617, 1976.
10. Axon TR, Hartley C, Rothera MP: Endoscopic balloon dilatation of subglottic stenosis, *J Laryngol Otol* 109:876, 1995.
11. Bailey CM and others: Voice quality following laryngotracheal reconstruction, *Int J Pediatr Otorhinolaryngol* 32(suppl):S93, 1995.
12. Bain WM and others: Head and neck manifestations of gastroesophageal reflux, *Laryngoscope* 93:175, 1983.
13. Benjamin B: Chevalier Jackson lecture: congenital laryngeal webs, *Ann Otol Rhinol Laryngol* 92:317, 1983.
14. Bennett T: Laryngeal strictures, *South Med J* 53:1101, 1960.
15. Bergstrom J: Laryngologic aspects of the treatment of acute barbiturate poisoning, *Acta Otolaryngol (Stockh)* 173(suppl):1, 1962.
16. Birck HG: Endoscopic repair of laryngeal stenosis, *Trans Am Acad Ophthalmol Otolaryngol* 74:140, 1970.
17. Bogdasarian RS, Olson NR: Posterior glottic laryngeal stenosis, *Otolaryngol Head Neck Surg* 88:765, 1980.
18. Bower CM, Choi SS, Cotton RT: Arytenoidectomy in children, *Ann Otol Rhinol Laryngol* 103:271, 1994.
19. Boyd AD and others: A clinical evaluation of cricothyroidotomy, *Surg Gynecol Obstet* 149:365, 1979.
20. Brookes GB, Fairfax AJ: Chronic upper airway obstruction: value of the flow volume loop examination in assessment and management, *J R Soc Med* 75:425, 1982.
21. Burton DM and others: Pediatric airway manifestations of gastroesophageal reflux, *Ann Otol Rhinol Laryngol* 101:742, 1992.
22. Bryce DP: Subglottic stenosis, *Laryngoscope* 89:320, 1979.
23. Close LG, Lozano AJ, Schaefer SD: Sternohyoid myo-osseous flap for acquired subglottic stenosis in children, *Laryngoscope* 93:433, 1983.
24. Cohen SR: Pseudolaryngeal paralysis: a postintubation complication, *Ann Otol Rhinol Laryngol* 90:483, 1981.
25. Cohen SR, Landing BH, Isaacs H: Epidermolysis bullosa associated with laryngeal stenosis, *Ann Otol Rhinol Laryngol* 87(suppl):25, 1978.
26. Conley JJ: Reconstruction of subglottic air passage, *Ann Otol Rhinol Laryngol* 62:477, 1953.
27. Cotton RT: Management of laryngotracheal stenosis and tracheal lesions including single stage laryngotracheoplasty, *Int J Pediatr Otorhinolaryngol* 32(suppl):S89, 1995.
28. Cotton RT: Management of subglottic stenosis in infancy and childhood: review of a consecutive series of cases managed by surgical reconstruction, *Ann Otol Rhinol Laryngol* 87:649, 1978.
29. Cotton RT: Pediatric laryngotracheal stenosis, *J Pediatr Surg* 19:699, 1984.
30. Cotton RT: Prevention and management of laryngeal stenosis in infants and children, *J Pediatr Surg* 20:845, 1985.
31. Cotton RT: The problem of pediatric laryngotracheal stenosis: a clinical and experimental study on the efficacy of autogenous cartilaginous grafts placed between the vertically divided halves of the posterior lamina of the cricoid cartilage, *Laryngoscope* 12(suppl 56):1, 1991.
32. Cotton RT, Evans JNG: Laryngotracheal reconstruction in children: five year follow up, *Ann Otol Rhinol Laryngol* 90:516, 1981.
33. Cotton RT, Gray SD, Miller RP: Update of the Cincinnati experience in pediatric laryngotracheal reconstruction, *Laryngoscope* 99:111, 1989.
34. Cotton RT, Mortelliti AJ, Myer CM III: 4-Quadrant cricoid cartilage division in laryngotracheal reconstruction, *Arch Otolaryngol Head Neck Surg* 118:1023, 1992.
35. Cotton RT, Myer CM: Contemporary surgical management of laryngeal stenosis in children, *Am J Otolaryngol* 5:360, 1984.
36. Cotton RT, Richardson MA: Congenital laryngeal anomalies, *Otolaryngol Clin North Am* 14:203, 1981.
37. Cotton RT, Richardson MA, Seid AB: Panel discussion: the management of advanced laryngotracheal stenosis. Management of combined advanced glottic and subglottic stenosis in infancy and childhood, *Laryngoscope* 91:221, 1981.
38. Cotton RT, Seid AB: Management of the extubation problem in the premature child: anterior cricoid split as an alternative to tracheostomy, *Ann Otol Rhinol Laryngol* 89:508, 1980.
39. Cotton RT, Silver P, Nuwayhid NS: *Chronic laryngeal and tracheal stenosis.* In Paparella MM, Shumrick DA, editors: *Otolaryngology*, ed 2, vol 3, Philadelphia, 1980, WB Saunders.
40. Cotton RT, Tewfik TL: Laryngeal stenosis following carbon dioxide laser in subglottic hemangioma, *Ann Otol Rhinol Laryngol* 94:494, 1985.
41. Cotton RT and others: Anterior cricoid split, 1977–1987: evolution of a technique, *Arch Otolaryngol Head Neck Surg* 114:1300, 1988.
42. Courand L and others: Interet de la resection cricoidienne dans le traitment des stenoses cricotracheales apres intubation, *Ann Chir Thorac Cardiovasc* 33:242, 1979.
43. Crysdale W: Subglottic stenosis in children: a management protocol plus surgical experience in 13 cases, *Int J Pediatr Otorhinolaryngol* 6:23, 1983.
44. Crysdale WS: Laryngeal and tracheal stenosis in children, *Otolaryngol Clin North Am* 12:817, 1979.
45. Crysdale WS, Crepeau J: Surgical correction of subglottic stenosis in children, *J Otolaryngol* 11:209, 1982.
46. Cudmore RE, Vivori E: Inhalation injury to the respiratory tract of children, *Prog Pediatr Surg* 14:173, 1981.
47. Daly JF: Relapsing polychondritis of the larynx and trachea, *Arch Otolaryngol Head Neck Surg* 84:570, 1966.
48. Dedo HH: Endoscopic Teflon keel for anterior glottic web, *Ann Otol Rhinol Laryngol* 83:467, 1979.
49. Dedo HH, Rowe LD: Laryngeal reconstruction in acute and chronic injuries, *Otolaryngol Clin North Am* 16:373, 1983.
50. Dedo HH, Sooy FA: Surgical repair of late glottic stenosis, *Ann Otol Rhinol Laryngol* 77:435, 1968.
51. Dedo HH, Sooy CD: Endoscopic laser repair of posterior glottic, subglottic and tracheal stenosis by division or microtrapdoor flap, *Laryngoscope* 94:445, 1984.

52. Downing TP, Johnson DG: Excision of subglottic stenosis with the urethral resectoscope, *J Pediatr Surg* 14:252, 1979.
53. Dunbar JS: Upper respiratory tract obstruction in infants and children, *Am J Roentgenol* 109:227, 1970.
54. Duncavage J, Ossoff RH, Toohill RJ: Laryngotracheal reconstruction with composite nasal septal cartilage grafts, *Ann Otol Rhinol Laryngol* 98:581, 1989.
55. Duncavage J and others: The microtrapdoor technique for the management of laryngeal stenosis, *Laryngoscope* 97:825, 1987.
56. Eliachar I: Rotary door flap: a breakthrough in tracheal reconstruction, *Ear Nose Throat J* 71:584, 1992.
57. Eliachar I, Levin JS: Imaging evaluation of laryngotracheal stenosis, *J Otolaryngol* 22:265, 1993.
58. Eliachar I, Tucker HR: Reconstruction of pediatric larynx and upper trachea with the sternohyoid rotary door flap, *Arch Otolaryngol Head Neck Surg* 117:316, 1991.
59. Eliachar I and others: Advantages of the rotary door flap in laryngotracheal reconstruction: is skeletal support necessary? *Ann Otol Rhinol Laryngol* 98:37, 1989.
60. Evans JNG: Laryngotracheoplasty, *Otolaryngol Clin North Am* 10: 119, 1977.
61. Fearon B, Cinnamond M: Surgical correction of subglottic stenosis of the larynx: clinical results of the Fearon-Cotton operation, *J Otolaryngol* 5:475, 1976.
62. Fearon B, Cotton RT: Subglottic stenosis in infants and children: the clinical problem and experimental surgical correction, *Can J Otolaryngol* 1:281, 1972.
63. Fearon B, Cotton RT: Surgical correction of subglottic stenosis of the larynx in infants and children: progress report, *Ann Otol Rhinol Laryngol* 83:428, 1974.
64. Fearon B, Crysdale WS, Bird R: Subglottic stenosis of the larynx in the infant and child: methods of management, *Ann Otol Rhinol Laryngol* 87:645, 1978.
65. Fee WE Jr, Wilson GG: Tracheoesophageal space abscess, *Laryngoscope* 89:377, 1979.
66. *Congenital malformation in pediatric otolaryngology*. In Ferguson CF, editor: *Disorders of the respiratory tract in children*, vol 2, Philadelphia, 1972, WB Saunders.
67. Finnegan DA, Wong ML, Kashima HK: Hyoid autograft repair of chronic subglottic stenosis, *Ann Otol Rhinol Laryngol* 84:643, 1975.
68. Flye MW, Mundinger GH Jr, Fauci AS: Diagnostic and therapeutic aspects of the surgical approach to Wegener's granulomatosis, *J Thorac Cardiovasc Surg* 77:331, 1979.
69. Freeman GR: A comparative analysis of endotracheal intubation in neonates, children and adults: complications, prevention and treatment, *Laryngoscope* 82:1385, 1972.
70. Friedman EM, Healy GB, McGill TJ: Carbon dioxide laser management of subglottic and tracheal stenosis, *Otolaryngol Clin North Am* 16:871, 1983.
71. Friedman M and others: Laryngeal injuries secondary to nasogastric tubes, *Ann Otol Rhinol Laryngol* 90:469, 1981.
72. Froehlich P and others: Role of long-term stenting: treatment of pediatric subglottic stenosis, *Int J Pediatr Otolaryngol* 27:273, 1993.
73. Gaudet PT and others: Pediatric tracheostomy and associated complications, *Laryngoscope* 88:1633, 1978.
74. Gerwat J, Bryce DP: The management of subglottic laryngeal stenosis by resection and direct anastomosis, *Laryngoscope* 84:940, 1974.
75. Goode RL, Shinn JB: Long term stenting in the treatment of subglottic stenosis, *Ann Otol Rhinol Laryngol* 86:795, 1977.
76. Gould SJ, Young M: Subglottic ulceration and healing following endotracheal intubation in the neonate: morphometric study, *Ann Otol Rhinol Laryngol* 101:815, 1992.
77. Grahne B: Operative treatment of severe chronic traumatic laryngeal stenosis in infants up to three years old, *Acta Otolaryngol (Stockh)* 77:134, 1971.
78. Grahne B and others: Surgical treatment of chronic laryngeal stenosis secondary to vocal cord paralysis: pre and postoperative evaluation of ventilatory function, *Laryngoscope* 93:163, 1983.
79. Gray S and others: Adjunctive measures for successful laryngotracheal reconstruction, *Ann Otol Rhinol Laryngol* 96:509, 1987.
80. Gray SB, Kelly SM, Dov H: Arytenoid separation for impaired pediatric vocal cord mobility, *Ann Otol Rhinol Laryngol* 103:510, 1994.
81. Grillo HC: Primary reconstruction of airway after resection of subglottic laryngeal and upper tracheal stenosis, *Ann Thorac Surg* 33:3, 1982.
82. Grundfast KA and others: Prospective study of subglottic stenosis in intubated neonates, *Ann Otol Rhinol Laryngol* 99:390, 1990.
83. Hallenborg C and others: Severe upper airway obstruction caused by bullous pemphigoid: diagnostic usefulness of the flow-volume curve, *Otolaryngol Head Neck Surg* 90:20, 1982.
84. Hashash M and others: Local acriflavine in laryngoscleromatous subglottic stenosis, *J Laryngol Otol* 97:745, 1983.
85. Hawkins DB: Glottic and subglottic stenosis from endotracheal intubation, *Laryngoscope* 87:339, 1977.
86. Hawkins DB: Hyaline membrane disease of the neonate: prolonged intubation in the management. Effects on the larynx, *Laryngoscope* 88:201, 1978.
87. Healy GB: An experimental model for the endoscopic correction of subglottic stenosis with clinical applications, *Laryngoscope* 92:1103, 1982.
88. Healy GB and others: The use of the carbon dioxide laser in the pediatric airway, *J Pediatr Surg* 14:735, 1979.
89. Hebra A and others: Balloon tracheoplasty in children: results of a 15-year experience, *J Pediatr Surg* 26:957, 1991.
90. Hermans R, Verschakelen JA, Baert AL: Imaging of laryngeal and tracheal stenosis, *Acta Otorhinolaryngol Belg* 49:323, 1995.
91. Hilding AC, Hilding JA: Tolerance of the respiratory mucous membrane to trauma: surgical swabs and intratracheal tubes, *Ann Otol Rhinol Laryngol* 71:455, 1962.
92. Holinger LD: Treatment of severe subglottic stenosis without tracheotomy: a preliminary report, *Ann Otol Rhinol Laryngol* 91:407, 1982.
93. Holinger PH, Brown WT: Congenital webs, cysts, laryngoceles and other anomalies of the larynx, *Ann Otol Rhinol Laryngol* 76:744, 1967.
94. Holinger PH, Johnston KC: Congenital anomalies of larynx, *Ann Otol Rhinol Laryngol* 63:581, 1954.
95. Holinger PH and others: Subglottic stenosis in infants and children, *Ann Otol Rhinol Laryngol* 85:591, 1976.
96. Johnson DG, Stewart DR: Management of acquired tracheal obstructions in infancy, *J Pediatr Surg* 10:709, 1975.
97. Jones R and others: Subglottic stenosis in newborn intensive care unit graduates, *Am J Dis Child* 135:367, 1981.
98. Kirchner FR, Toledo PS: Microcauterization in otolaryngology, *Arch Otolaryngol Head Neck Surg* 99:198, 1974.
99. Kotton B: The treatment of subglottic stenosis in children by prolonged dilatation, *Laryngoscope* 89:1983, 1979.
100. Koufman JA: The otolaryngologic manifestations of gastreoesophageal reflux disease (GERD): a clinical investigation of 225 patients using ambulatory 24 pH monitoring. Experimental investigation of the role of acid and pepsin in the development of laryngeal injury, *Laryngoscope* 4(suppl 53):1, 1991.
101. Koufman JA, Forston JK, Strong MS: Predictive factors of cricoid ring size in adults in relation to acquired subglottic stenosis. *Otolaryngol Head Neck Surg* 91:177, 1983.
102. Koufman JA, Thompson JN, Kohut RI: Endoscopic management of subglottic stenosis with the CO_2 surgical laser, *Otolaryngol Head Neck Surg* 89:215, 1981.
103. Lampman JH, Querubin R, Kondapalli P: Subglottic stenosis in Wegener's granulomatosis, *Chest* 79:230, 1981.
104. Lebovics RS and others: The management of subglottic stenosis in patients with Wegener's granulomatosis, *Laryngoscope* 102:1341, 1992.

105. Lindholm CE: Prolonged endotracheal intubation, *Acta Anaesthesiol Scand Suppl* 33:1, 1970.
106. Looper EA: The use of hyoid bone as graft in laryngeal stenosis, *Arch Otolaryngol Head Neck Surg* 28:106, 1938.
107. Lusk RP, Gray S, Muntz HR: Single stage laryngotracheal reconstruction, *Arch Otolaryngol Head Neck Surg* 117:171, 1991.
108. Lusk RP, Kang DR, Muntz HR: Auricular cartilage grafts in laryngotracheal reconstruction, *Ann Otol Rhinol Laryngol* 102-4, 1993.
109. Lusk RP, Kang DR, Muntz HR: Auricular cartilage grafts in laryngotracheal reconstruction, *Ann Otol Rhinol Laryngol* 102:247, 1993.
110. Lyons GD and others: Carbon dioxide laser treatment of laryngeal stenosis, *Arch Otolaryngol Head Neck Surg* 106:255, 1980.
111. MacDonald RE, Smith C, Mitchell D: Airway problems in children following endotracheal intubation, *Ann Otol Rhinol Laryngol* 75:975, 1966.
112. Majeski JA and others: Tracheoplasty for tracheal stenosis in the pediatric burned patient, *J Trauma* 20:81, 1980.
113. Maran AGD, Geissler PR: A new material for laryngeal prosthesis, *J Laryngol Otol* 84:1174, 1970.
114. Maran AG and others: Early management of laryngeal injuries, *J R Soc Med* 74:656, 1981.
115. Marshak G, Grundfast KM: Subglottic stenosis, *Pediatr Clin North Am* 28:941, 1981.
116. Massoud EA, McCullough BW: Adult acquired laryngeal stenosis: a study of prognostic factors, *J Otolaryngol*, 24:234, 1995.
117. McArthur CJ, Kearns GH, Healy GD: Voice quality after laryngotracheal reconstruction, *Arch Otolaryngol Head Neck Surg* 120:641, 1994.
118. McCaffrey TV: Classification of laryngotracheal stenosis, *Laryngoscope* 102:133, 1992.
119. McCaffrey TV: Management of laryngotracheal stenosis on the basis of site and severity, *Otolaryngol Head Neck Surg* 109:468, 1993.
120. McGill T: Congenital diseases of the larynx, *Otolaryngol Clin North Am* 17:57, 1984.
121. McGuirt WF, Salmon J, Blalock D: Normal speech for patients with laryngeal webs: an achievable goal, *Laryngoscope* 94:1176, 1984.
122. McMillan WG, Duvall AJ: Congenital subglottic stenosis, *Arch Otolaryngol Head Neck Surg* 87:272, 1968.
123. Mihashi S and others: Laser surgery in otolaryngology: interaction of CO_2 laser and soft tissue, *Ann N Y Acad Sci* 267:263, 1976.
124. Mills RP: The value of xeroradiography in the management of subglottic stenosis in children, *J Laryngol Otol* 95:1255, 1981.
125. Mills RP, O'Conner MJ, Shin GA: Mucous membrane pemphigoid: a preventable cause of laryngeal stenosis, *J Laryngol Otol* 97:761, 1983.
126. Monnier P, Savary M, Chapuis G: Cricotracheal resection for pediatric subglottic stenosis: update of Lausanne experience, *Acta Otorhinolaryngol Belg*, 49:373, 1995.
127. Monnier P, Savary M, Chapuis G: Partial cricoid resection with primary tracheal anastomosis for subglottic stenosis in infants and children, *Laryngoscope* 103:1273, 1993.
128. Montgomery WW: T-tube tracheal stent, *Arch Otolaryngol Head Neck Surg* 82:320, 1965.
129. *Laryngeal stenosis.* In Montgomery WW, editor: *The surgery of the upper respiratory system*, vol 2, Philadelphia, 1973, Lea & Febiger.
130. Montgomery WW: Posterior and complete laryngeal (glottic) stenosis, *Arch Otolaryngol Head Neck Surg* 98:170, 1973.
131. Montgomery WW: Suprahyoid release for tracheal anastomosis, *Arch Otolaryngol Head Neck Surg* 99:255, 1974.
132. Montgomery WW: Management of glottic stenosis, *Otolaryngol Clin North Am* 12:841, 1979.
133. Montgomery WW: Subglottic stenosis, *Int Surg* 67:199, 1982.
134. Montgomery WW: Chronic subglottic stenosis, *Otolaryngol Clin North Am* 17:107, 1984.
135. Morgenstein KM: Composite auricular graft in laryngeal reconstruction, *Laryngoscope* 82:844, 1972.
136. Morimitsu T and others: Congenital cricoid stenosis, *Laryngoscope* 91:1356, 1981.
137. Noyek AM and others: Xeroradiography in the assessment of the pediatric larynx and trachea, *J Otolaryngol* 5:468, 1976.
138. Ochi JW, Bailey CM, Evans JN: Pediatric airway reconstruction at Great Ormond Street: a ten year review. III.: Decannulation and suprastomal collapse, *Ann Otol Rhinol Laryngol* 101:656, 1992.
139. Ogura JH, Biller HF: Reconstruction of the larynx following blunt trauma, *Ann Otol Rhinol Laryngol* 80:492, 1971.
140. Ogura JH, Powers WE: Functional restitution of traumatic stenosis of the larynx and pharynx, *Laryngoscope* 74:1081, 1964.
141. Olson NR: Wound healing by primary tension in the larynx: symposium on reconstruction of the larynx and trachea, Milwaukee, 1977, *Otolaryngol Clin North Am* 12:735, 1979.
142. Othersen HB: Steroid therapy for tracheal stenosis in children, *Ann Thorac Surg* 17:365, 1974.
143. Padovan IF: Surgical treatment of laryngeal stenosis, *J Otolaryngol* 5:131, 1976.
144. Palasti S and others: Anterior cricoid split for subglottic stenosis: experience at the Children's Hospital of New Jersey, *Laryngoscope* 102:997, 1992.
145. Papsidero MJ, Pashley NR: Acquired stenosis of the upper airway in neonates: an increasing problem, *Ann Otol Rhinol Laryngol* 89:512, 1980.
146. Parkin JL, Stevens MH, Jung DL: Acquired and congenital subglottic stenosis in the infant, *Ann Otol Rhinol Laryngol* 85:573, 1976.
147. Pashley NR: Risk factors and prediction of outcome in acquired subglottic stenosis in children, *Int J Pediatr Otorhinolaryngol* 4:1, 1982.
148. Pearson FG and others: Primary tracheal anastomosis after resection of cricoid cartilage with preservation of recurrent laryngeal nerve, *J Thorac Cardiovasc Surg* 70:806, 1975.
149. Prescott CA: Factors that influence successful decannulation after surgery for laryngotracheal stenosis in children, *Int J Pediatr Otorhinolaryngol*, 30:183, 1994.
150. Rethi A: An operation for cicatricial stenosis of the larynx, *J Laryngol Otol* 70:283, 1956.
151. Richardson MA, Inglis AF Jr: A comparison of anterior cricoid split with and without costal cartilage graft for acquired subglottic stenosis, *Int J Pediatr Otolaryngol*, 22:187, 1991.
152. Rinne J, Grahne B, Souijarvi AR: Laryngeal stenosis following papillomatosis: a report of 3 severe cases, *Int J Pediatr Otolaryngol* 5:309, 1983.
153. Rodgers BM, Talbert JL: Clinical applications of endotracheal cryotherapy, *J Pediatr Surg* 13:662, 1978.
154. Rosenfeld RM, Stool SE: Should granulomas be excised in children with long term tracheotomy, *Arch Otolaryngol Head Neck Surg*, 118:1323, 1992.
155. Rothschild MA, Cotcamp D, Cotton RT: Postoperative medical management in single stage laryngotracheoplasty, *Arch Otolaryngol Head Neck Surg*, 121:1175, 1995.
156. Runton N, Zalzal GH: The decannulation process in children, *J Pediatr Nurs* 4:370, 1989.
157. Sakai F and others: T_1 MRI imaging of the larynx at 1.5 T, *J Comput Assist Tomogr* 14:10, 1990.
158. Sasaki CT, Horicuchi M, Koss N: Tracheostomy related subglottic stenosis: bacteriologic pathogenesis, *Laryngoscope* 89:857, 1979.
159. Seid AB, Pransky SM, Kearns DB: One stage laryngotracheoplasty, *Arch Otolaryngol Head Neck Surg* 117:408, 1991.
160. Shaw RR, Paulson DL, Kee JL Jr: Traumatic tracheal rupture, *J Thorac Cardiovasc Surg* 42:281, 1961.
161. Simpson GT and others: Benign tumors and lesions of the larynx in children, surgical excision by CO_2 laser, *Ann Otol Rhinol Laryngol* 88:479, 1979.
162. Simpson GT and others: Predictive factors of success or failure in the endoscopic management of laryngeal and tracheal stenosis, *Ann Otol Rhinol Laryngol* 91:384, 1982.

163. Smith II, Bain AD: Congenital atresia of the larynx: a report of nine cases, *Ann Oto Rhinol Laryngol* 74:338, 1965.
164. Smith ME and others: Voice problems after pediatric laryngotracheal reconstruction: videolaryngostroboscopic, acoustic and perceptual assessment, *Int J Pediatr Otolaryngol*, 25:173, 1993.
165. Stell PM and others: Chronic laryngeal stenosis, *Ann Otol Rhinol Laryngol* 94:108, 1985.
166. Striker TW, Stool S, Downes JJ: Prolonged nasotracheal intubation in infants and children, *Arch Otolaryngol Head Neck Surg* 85:210, 1967.
167. Strome M, Donahoe PK: Advances in management of laryngeal and subglottic stenosis, *J Pediatr Surg* 17:591, 1982.
168. Strong MS and others: Recurrent respiratory papillomatosis: management with the CO_2 laser, *Ann Otol Rhinol Laryngol* 85:508, 1976.
169. Strong MS and others: Endoscopic management of laryngeal stenosis, *Otolaryngol Clin North Am* 12:797, 1979.
170. Taha A and others: Surgical management of cicatricial post scleromatous subglottic stenosis, *J Laryngol Otol* 95:827, 1981.
171. Thawley SE, Ogura JH: Panel discussion: the management of advanced laryngotracheal stenosis. Use of the hyoid graft for treatment of laryngotracheal stenosis, *Laryngoscope* 91:226, 1981.
172. Toohill RJ and others: *Treatment of acquired and congenital subglottic stenosis*. In English GM, editor: *Otolaryngology*, vol 3, Philadelphia, 1984, Harper & Row.
173. Tucker GF and others: Histopathology of congenital subglottic stenosis, *Laryngoscope* 89:866, 1979.
174. Vauthy PA, Reddy R: Acute upper airway obstruction in infants and children: evaluation by the fiberoptic bronchoscope, *Ann Otol Rhinol Laryngol* 89:417, 1980.
175. Ward PH and others: Composite hyoid sternohyoid muscle grafts in humans: its use in reconstruction of subglottic stenosis and the anterior tracheal wall, *Arch Otolaryngol Head Neck Surg* 103:531, 1977.
176. Werkhaven JA, Weed DT, Ossoff RH: Carbon dioxide laser serial micro trap door flap excision of subglottic stenosis, *Arch Otolaryngol Head Neck Surg*, 119:676, 1993.
177. Whited RE: Posterior commissure stenosis post long-term intubation, *Laryngoscope* 93:1314, 1983.
178. Whited RE: A prospective study of laryngotracheal sequelae in long-term intubation, *Laryngoscope* 94:367, 1984.
179. Wiatrak BJ, Cotton RT: Anastomosis of the cervical trachea in children, *Arch Otolaryngol Head Neck Surg* 118:58, 1992.
180. Wong ML and others: Vascularized hyoid interposition for subglottic and upper tracheal stenosis, *Ann Otol Rhinol Laryngol* 87:491, 1978.
181. Zalzal GH: Rib cartilage grafts for the treatment of posterior glottic and subglottic stenosis in children, *Ann Otol Rhinol Laryngol* 97A:506, 1988.
182. Zalzal GH: Stenting for pediatric laryngotracheal stenosis, *Ann Otol Rhinol Laryngol*, 101:651, 1992.
183. Zalzal GH: Treatment of laryngotracheal stenosis with anterior and posterior cartilage grafts: a report of 41 children, *Arch Otolaryngol Head Neck Surg*, 119:82, 1993.
184. Zalzal GH: Use of stents in laryngotracheal reconstruction in children: indications, technical considerations, and complications, *Laryngoscope* 98B:849, 1988.
185. Zalzal GH, Choi SS, Patel KM: The effect of gastroesophageal reflux on laryngotracheal reconstruction, *Arch Otolaryngol Head Neck Surg* 122:297, 1996.
186. Zalzal GH, Cotton RT: A new way of carving cartilage grafts to avoid prolapse into the tracheal lumen when used in subglottic reconstruction, *Laryngoscope* 96:1039, 1986.
187. Zalzal GH, Cotton RT, McAdams AJ: The survival of costal cartilage graft in laryngotracheal reconstruction, *Otolaryngol Head Neck Surg* 94:204, 1986.
188. Zalzal GH, Grundfast KM: Broken Aboulker stents in the tracheal lumen, *Int J Pediatr Otorhinolaryngol* 16:125, 1988.
189. Zalzal GH, Loomis SR, Fischer M: Laryngeal reconstruction in children: assessment of vocal quality, *Arch Otolaryngol Head Neck Surg* 119:504, 1993.
190. Zalzal GH and others: Pulmonary parameters after laryngotracheal reconstruction in children, *Ann Otol Rhinol Laryngol* 99:386, 1990.
191. Zalzal GH and others: Vocal quality of decannulated children following laryngeal reconstruction, *Laryngoscope* 101:425, 1991.
192. Zeitouni AG, Manoukian J: Severe complications of the anterior cricoid split operation and single stage laryngotracheoplasty, *Arch Otol Rhinol Laryngol* 103:723, 1994.
193. Zohar Y, Hadar H, Laurian N: Computed tomography evaluation of the nasal septal reconstructed larynx, *Head Neck* 7:357, 1985.

Chapter 19

Gastroesophageal Reflux and Laryngeal Disease—Aspiration and Swallowing Disorders

Philippe Narcy
Philippe Contencin
Thierry Van Den Abbeele

GASTROESOPHAGEAL REFLUX AND LARYNGEAL DISEASE

There is good evidence that a relationship exists between gastroesophageal reflux (GER) and chronic or recurrent otorhinolaryngologic disorders, but the link is poorly understood and controversial. More than a century ago, hiatal hernia was clinically shown to aggravate disorders of the lower airway.[12] GER-related otolaryngologic disorders, formerly called *atypical manifestations of GER*, are now included in the disease.[2] However, even when pathologic GER is shown, other causes should be sought because GER also can result from airway obstruction.

GER is an abnormal and repeated rise of gastric contents into the esophagus. There are three main forms:[6] (1) Physiologic GER occurs in the postprandial period. Small amounts of refluxed material cause burping at any age and a small degree of emesis in the infant. Esophageal pH monitoring is normal. (2) Functional GER is seen when frequent (at least daily) emesis occurs, with an esophageal pH less than 4 for more than 5% of the recorded time. Patients report no complications. This form is difficult to differentiate from silent GER, which can hide related respiratory disorders. (3) GER disease (GERD) is believed to have gastrointestinal (GI) or extra-GI signs. GI signs include emesis, dysphagia, choking, gagging, and failure to thrive in children. Extra-GI signs are chronic coughing, wheezing, hoarseness, sore throat, stridor, recurrent croup, and obstructive apnea. Heartburn is extremely rare.

Every pathogenic aspect of GER is caused by inappropriate, transient relaxation of the lower esophageal sphincter and by motor disturbances of the esophagus leading to a poor esophageal clearance. In addition, delayed gastric emptying and increased gastric acidity may contribute to the reflux. According to gastroenterologists, at least 20% of infants experience clinical GERD.[3] Screening is important for patients who experience silent GER with respiratory symptoms because major complications can occur.[4] However, GER is so frequent in children that other causes of chronic inflammation of the airway should not be forgotten.[4]

Pathogenic mechanism

Two main hypotheses have been proposed for the airway-GER relationship.

Direct contact and microaspiration

Regurgitated gastric contents climb to the laryngeal inlet where they can stagnate or pass through the glottis into the tracheobronchial tree. This has been shown by esophageal nuclide scintiscan. Simultaneous esophageal and pharyngeal pH probes and two-channel recording for 18 to 24 hours have detected refluxed material in the esophagus of most patients and in the pharynx of some patients.[9,10] The same findings have been reported in children with recurrent croup.[5] Pepsin and biliary salts plus other components of GI origin found in the refluxed liquid are considered harmful to the laryngeal epithelium.[13]

Vagal reflex

Chemoreceptors located in the lower esophagus may send neurovegetative signals through the vagus nerve to the central nervous system and produce bronchial dilation and hypersecretion with submucosal edema, which may extend up to the larynx.

Direct contact between gastropharyngeal reflux material and the larynx is the most likely mechanism, although both hypotheses could be involved.

However, even if there is a correlation, GER should still be considered a potential consequence of the airway disorder.

Disorders

The most frequent GER-related disorders in the airway of children of any age seems to be laryngeal diseases (Box 19-1). In older children and adults, dysphonia is the most frequently reported pathologic sign along with pharyngeal symptoms (e.g., pain, globus sensation). Recurrent subglottic laryngitis with dyspnea (croup) is the most common way in which GER influences the airway in pediatric patients. A statistically significant correlation with GER was found in patients with recurrent croup using two-channel pH monitoring.[5] Successful anti-GER therapeutic trials and recurrences after stopping management also were noted in these patients.[13] GER seems to be important in the development of subglottic stenosis. Long-term endotracheal intubation leads to increased acid pharyngeal reflux. Animal studies have shown that acid placed on the subglottic mucosa after local trauma leads to granulation tissue and fibrous scarring with subsequent stenosis. Some believe that the successful surgical management of subglottic stenoses in children depends on the control of GER.[8] This topic is controversial,[14] but GER should be sought and managed in cases of surgery for this and other laryngeal abnormalities (e.g., posterior cleft).[7]

However, the most important GER-associated laryngeal phenomena in babies are motor disorders. GER is found in more than 80% of cases of laryngomalacia.[1] It may cause edema at the laryngeal inlet. GER also may be induced by the negative endothoracic pressure resulting from the airway obstruction. It is probably only associated with pharyngoesophageal motor anomalies that are caused by the neurologic dysfunction that determines laryngomalacia.[1] Glottic and pharyngoesophageal dysfunctions that occur with GER lead to aspiration. Laryngeal adductor responses seem to coincide with reflux in the premature newborn, with subsequent obstructive reflex apnea.[11] Reflex apnea is considered to be a cause of sudden infant death syndrome (SIDS) in nonpremature children. A laryngeal adductor response, a central apnea

Box 19-1. Likely gastroesophageal reflux–related laryngeal disorders in infants and children

Recurrent croup (shown by pH monitoring)
Laryngospasm (shown by pH monitoring)
Laryngomalacia
Hoarseness
Subglottic stenosis (and laryngeal surgery)
Aspiration
Chronic cough

linked to esophagitis and obstruction of the nasopharyngeal airway, also may be one of the etiologies of SIDS. GER-induced stimulation from chemoreceptors at the laryngeal inlet seems to enhance the risk of apnea in infants with a central hyposensitivity to hypercapnia or hypoxia. But the etiology of SIDS is multifactorial. Lastly, a chronic cough at any age may be a GER-related disorder.

Diagnosis

A patient history of digestive and respiratory symptoms provides rapid, low-cost diagnosis of GERD (Fig. 19-1). When otolaryngologic symptoms are found, other respiratory signs and symptoms should be noted by careful questioning and examination. Classic GI signs and symptoms should be ruled out. In infants, feeding difficulties with tears, apparent life-threatening events with hypotonia, and paleness or cyanosis (near-miss SIDS) while supine should be recorded. A family history of GER is also significant. Radiographic studies with barium swallow are unreliable for diagnosis of GER. An esophageal and full thoracic scintiscan with ingestion of nuclide elements detects contamination of the lower airway with ingested materials. However, microaspiration is not necessary to produce a GER-related airway disorder. In addition, this technique is not routinely available in many centers. Finding lipid-laden macrophages at bronchial lavage confirms microaspiration down to the bronchi. Esophagoscopy with a flexible fiberscope may contribute to diagnosis because it can show esophagitis and large hiatal hernia. These abnormalities are rare in extra-GI manifestations of GER. Laryngoscopy and bronchoscopy also can point to the risk of aspiration when erythema in the posterior glottis and subglottis are found associated with cobblestoning of the posterior supraglottic area.[4]

Esophageal pH monitoring is considered by gastroenterologists to be the gold standard for diagnosing GER. Acid periods recorded over 18 to 24 hours can be correlated with airway manifestations (e.g., cough, stridor). An abnormal percentage of the recorded time at a pH less than 4 allows the physician to manage the GER. However, a negative test does not rule out GER. Combined pharyngeal and esophageal pH records showed that brief refluxes can reach the laryngeal inlet and cause problems, whereas classic stan-

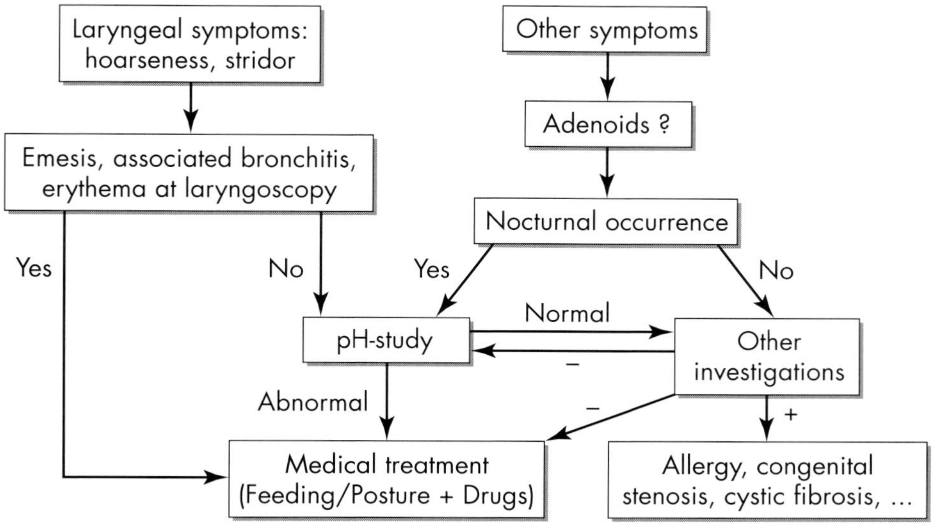

Fig. 19-1. Diagnosis of gastroesophageal reflux in ear, nose, throat.

dards for this pH test are considered normal with a poor total acid time. Thus, no single test is perfect for diagnosing GER, and it is difficult to prove that GER is responsible for a disorder. Other factors causing epithelial inflammation can lead to similar symptoms and endoscopic findings. The clinician should correlate one or more diagnostic tests with the clinical picture to correctly define the pretherapeutic procedure. A therapeutic trial is recommended if there is any doubt about whether GER is responsible for a laryngeal disorder (e.g., chronic laryngitis, recurrent croup).

Management

The first step in antireflux management is to ensure that the patient has a healthy diet and lifestyle. Fat, chocolate, coffee, tea, alcoholic beverages, orange juice, and tobacco release the lower esophageal sphincter and should be avoided. Small meals at regular times and avoidance of any food or drink 1 hour before bedtime are prophylactic. Infants should be given milk thickened with rice, and fruit juice should be avoided. The posture of the patient at rest also is extremely important. Gravity reduces the frequency and strength of reflux episodes. Raising the head of the bed by 10° to 15° is recommended for children, whereas babies up to 10 kg can be placed on a special mattress with a 30° to 45° slope. Pillows should be avoided. When not in bed, infants should be as upright as possible, even when physiotherapy is applied.

Recommended antireflux drugs (prokinetics) stimulate esophageal and gastric motility, while reinforcing the tonicity of the lower esophageal sphincter. Cisapride is the management of choice. Domperidone is usually less efficient and metoclopramide (sometimes more efficient than cisapride) is accompanied by a higher risk of adverse side effects (extrapyramidal syndrome). Alginates coat the gastric content and prevent its reascension. H_2 blockers inhibit gastric acid secretion and have been successfully used in some difficult cases, but some pediatric patients are nonresponders. Proton pump inhibitors (omeprazole, lansoprazole) are used in adult and pediatric practice. They prevent the release of hydrogen ions and are useful in severe forms resistant to other management. Proton pump inhibitors should be limited to these restricted indications. Management usually continues for years. However, drugs can be limited to 2- to 3-month cycles because the spontaneous course of the disease is typically episodic, except in the infant in whom management may be continued for longer periods. Surgery (Nissen fundoplication) is appropriate in cases in which severe disorders recur as soon as drugs are withdrawn or in which medical control is impossible to achieve.

REFERENCES

1. Belmont JR, Grundfast K: Congenital laryngeal stridor (laryngomalacia): etiologic factors and associated disorders, *Ann Otol Rhinol Laryngol* 93:430, 1984.
2. Burton DM and others: Pediatric airway manifestations of gastroesophageal reflux, *Ann Otol Rhinol Laryngol* 101:742, 1992.
3. Chouhou D and others: Le reflux gastro-oesophagien dans les centres de bilan de santé de l'enfant de moins de 4 ans, *Arch Fr Pediatr* 49: 839, 1992.
4. Contencin PH and others: Gastroesophageal reflux and ENT disorders in childhood, *Int J Pediatr Otorhinolaryngol* 32(suppl):S135, 1995.
5. Contencin PH, Narcy PH: Gastropharyngeal reflux in infants and children: a pharyngeal pH monitoring study, *Arch Otolaryngol Head Neck Surg* 118:1028, 1992.
6. Deschner WK, Benjamin SB: Extraesophageal manifestations of gastroesophageal reflux, *Am J Gastroenterol* 84:1, 1989.
7. Evans KL and others: Management of posterior laryngeal and laryngotracheoesophageal clefts, *Arch Otolaryngol Head Neck Surg* 121:1380, 1995.
8. Fligny I and others: Sténoses sousglottiques et reflux gastro-oesophagien, *Ann Otolaryngol Chir Cervicofac*, 106:193, 1989.

9. Katz PO: Ambulatory esophageal and hypopharyngeal pH monitoring in patients with hoarseness, *Am J Gastroenterol* 85:38, 1990.
10. Koufman JA: The otolaryngologic manifestations of gastroesophageal reflux disease (GERD): a clinical investigation of 225 patients using ambulatory 24-hour pH monitoring and an experimental investigation of the role of acid and pepsin in the development of laryngeal injury, *Laryngoscope* 101(suppl 53):1, 1991.
11. Orenstein SR and others: Stridor and gastroesophageal reflux: diagnostic use of intraluminal esophageal acid perfusion (Bernstein test), *Pediatr Pulmonol* 3:420, 1987.
12. Osler WB: *The principles and practice of medicine*, New York, 1892, Appleton.
13. Waki EY and others: The incidence of gastroesophageal reflux in recurrent croup, *Int J Pediatr Otorhinolarygol* 32:223, 1995.
14. Zalzal GH, Choi SS, Patel KM: The effect of gastroesophageal reflux on laryngotracheal reconstruction, *Arch Otolaryngol Head Neck Surg* 122:297, 1996.

SWALLOWING DISORDERS

Respiration and feeding share certain anatomic features. The central nervous system separates the functions by coordinating highly specialized structures, especially the pharynx. This complexity often makes it difficult to diagnose the etiology of swallowing disorders in children because the number of causes may be misleading. Thus, upper airway obstruction is often exacerbated by feeding, with the risk of inappropriate diagnosis of swallowing disorder. A detailed history and thorough physical examination are always necessary.

Physiology

Normal swallowing

Swallowing is divided into three stages:

1. The oral stage is the sucking reflex in infants; it consists of a sequence of labial and buccal constrictions, with elevation of the tongue similar to a piston in a cylinder. This pump-like reflex is associated with other archaic reflexes, such as the rooting reflex, which is excited by stroking around the mouth and results in movement of the head toward the stimulus. These reflexes gradually disappear after 3 to 4 months and are replaced by voluntary control. The development of swallowing skills seems to parallel the types of food eaten.[15] Bottle- or breast-feeding of liquids occurs from birth to 4 months, spoon-feeding of pureed food occurs after 4 months, and chewing of solid food occurs after 12 months. This first phase in 1-year-olds comprises the independent functions of chewing and moving food by combined movements of the tongue and the mandible (the oral preparatory phase).
2. The pharyngeal stage is the most complex. It starts when the bolus reaches the oropharynx, where there are tactile receptors. Many safety mechanisms ensure that the bolus is directed toward the esophagus. One is elevation and a posterior bulging of the tongue base, while its anterior portion plates against the palate, followed by elevation of the soft palate to close the nasopharyngeal inlet. Also, the larynx elevates, the cricoid tilts forward, the glottis tilts backward, and the laryngeal inlet closes. Lastly, there is contraction of the pharyngeal constrictor muscles with simultaneous relaxation of the superior sphincter of the esophagus. At the same time, breathing is inhibited.

   This second phase is short, less than 0.5 second, and occurs during apnea. The lower airway is protected by closure of the vocal folds and by elevation of the larynx combined with the bulging of the base of the tongue. The rise of the larynx under the overhanging tongue is critical for airway protection. The epiglottis plays only a secondary role, by dividing the bolus into two lateral currents toward the pyriform sinuses. This pharyngeal phase of deglutition is a reflexive function, but it can be released voluntarily; once initiated, it cannot be arrested.
3. The esophageal stage is a wave of peristaltic contractions that propagates downward in 7 to 8 seconds. Liquids cross the esophagus more rapidly when gravity is favorable, taking about 2 seconds.[3]

Neurologic control

The neurologic coordination of swallowing, which involves many groups of muscles, is under brainstem control (nuclei of the cranial nerves (CN) and swallowing center situated in the reticular formation). The CNs concerned are the trigeminal nerve (V) for labial and bucco-lingual sensitivity and for mandibular and palatal motricity; the facial nerve (VII) for lingual sensitivity and for bucco-facial motricity; and CN IX and X for palatal, pharyngeal, and laryngeal sensitivity and for pharyngeal and laryngeal motricity. Lastly, CN XI and XII are involved in pharyngeal, laryngeal, and lingual motricity.

The pharyngeal phase of swallowing depends totally on the integrity of the central nervous system. A deficit of the swallowing center or cranial nerve nuclei may result in aspiration caused by decreased pharyngeal contraction or laryngeal elevation, or decreased pharyngolaryngeal sensitivity. However, the functioning of esophageal peristaltic waves is independent of the brainstem and is only slightly affected in central nervous system deficiencies.

Neurologic maturation

The maturation of swallowing mechanisms is extremely complex and requires the structural integrity of the central nervous system. Swallowing begins during fetal life, as early as 4 months' gestation; even at this stage, swallowing is essential for the regulation of amniotic fluid volume. About half the total amniotic fluid volume is swallowed per 24 hours at the end of the gestation.[11] Although sucking movements appear early in fetal development after palatal closure at 10 weeks' gestation, they are not efficient and readily tire in the premature newborn. In contrast, they are immediately efficient and robust in full-term newborns.[9] However, because the tongue has piston-like movements, it is difficult to introduce solid food until the third or fourth month after birth. Youngers babies plate solid food against the palate and then regurgitate it. The pharyngeal stage is entirely reflexive and is already present in the premature infant. This reflex is mainly initiated by the sensitivity of the pharyngeal walls, but it is also the consequence of the buccal phase of swallowing.

Relaxation of the upper esophageal sphincter occurs at the same time as the contraction of the pharyngeal constrictor muscles and starts the esophageal phase. This stage is purely reflexive and is mature before birth. Relaxation of the gastroesophageal inferior sphincter occurs after 0.5 seconds instead of after 1.5 to 2 seconds because the esophagus of infants is shorter than that of adults.[3] Feeding development is greatly influenced by anatomic changes during growth. In the healthy infant, swallowing is purely reflexive and under brainstem control; gradually it comes under voluntary control by the suprabulbar centers and the cortex. The oral stage becomes voluntary, but the pharyngeal and esophageal phases remain involuntary.[15]

Diagnosis

Clinical examination

A thorough clinical examination is indispensable for diagnosis (Fig. 19-2), and should include observation of the child during eating or drinking. For a newborn or an infant, the examiner can put a finger into the baby's mouth to check for the presence of archaic reflexes and to test the suction strength. The mandible, mouth, tongue, and palate should be carefully examined, including the mobility of the soft palate. This minimal clinical examination should be completed by a pharyngolaryngeal fibroscopy to study the dynamic sequence of swallowing, laryngeal mobility and coordination, and the accumulation of pharyngolaryngeal secretions.

Clinical features

The most frequent and most typical clinical problem is aspiration, with bursts of coughing, apnea, or cyanosis at each attempt at feeding or with unremitting coughing and bronchoalveolar infection caused by the chronic aspiration of saliva. Less typical clinical features include dyspnea starting at or increasing during feeding. It may occur during every airway obstruction because sucking or swallowing induces an exertion dyspnea. It can sometimes reveal tracheal compression that increases during the filling of the esophagus by an anterior bulging of the posterior tracheal wall. It can also reveal an esophageal stenosis or dyskinesia by compression of the posterior tracheal wall during suprastenotic dilation of the esophagus. There also may be apparent life-threatening events during or just after feeding (e.g., cyanosis, apnea, bradycardia, hypotonia). These symptoms can be related to an airway abnormality, such as tracheal compression that increases during swallowing or a peptic esophagitis caused by GER.

The third possibility is a nasal reflux. It is not pathologic if it occurs during vomiting, but it is if it occurs during swallowing. The main cause is usually an abnormal palate or paralysis of the soft palate, but it can also be caused by achalasia of the superior esophageal sphincter.[13] Lastly, there are sometimes no swallowing movements because of the absence of suction or the second phase of swallowing without elevation of the larynx during attempts at feeding. These features are commonly seen in developmentally delayed children or in those with cerebral palsy.[17]

Instrumental evaluation

Several techniques have been used to assess swallowing disorders in children, including ultrasonography, videofluoroscopy, scintigraphy, fiberoptic endoscopic examination of swallowing, manometry, and electromyography. Most of these techniques were developed for adults and are difficult to adapt to children; there also is often a lack of normative data.[1]

Fiberoptic examination of swallowing is the most informative examination because it provides direct observation of the swallowing process. It should be routinely performed when swallowing disorders are suspected. It provides much information on the anatomy of the tongue, pharynx, larynx, and esophagus and on the dynamic functioning of the soft palate and the pharynx and the larynx during phonation and deglutition. However, analysis of laryngeal elevation during swallowing remains difficult. When clinical, radiologic, and endoscopic procedures fail to identify a precise etiology for swallowing disorders, other investigations are needed.

Imaging

Cineradiography and videofluoroscopy are the primary imaging techniques used to investigate swallowing disorders. Barium-contrast liquids (glasses or bottles) or solids (cookies, pudding) are administered to the child. Both methods provide dynamic study of the pharyngeal and esophageal phases of deglutition. Cineradiography is recorded on motion picture films and provides high-resolution images at 50 frames per second, but it is time-consuming and expensive and involves high radiation exposure. Videofluoroscopy has become the method of choice because of its lower cost, easier storage (standard videotapes with 25 frames per second), and lower radiation exposure. The main information obtained is the presence of a nasal reflux (velopharyngeal incompetence), laryngeal elevation, and precise timing of the stages of deglutition. However, the differential diagnosis between laryngeal aspiration and tracheo-esophageal fistula is sometimes difficult in infants. This examination covers a limited sample of swallowing movements and does not necessarily include the whole functioning of deglutition.[1]

Ultrasonography has been recently used to study the real-

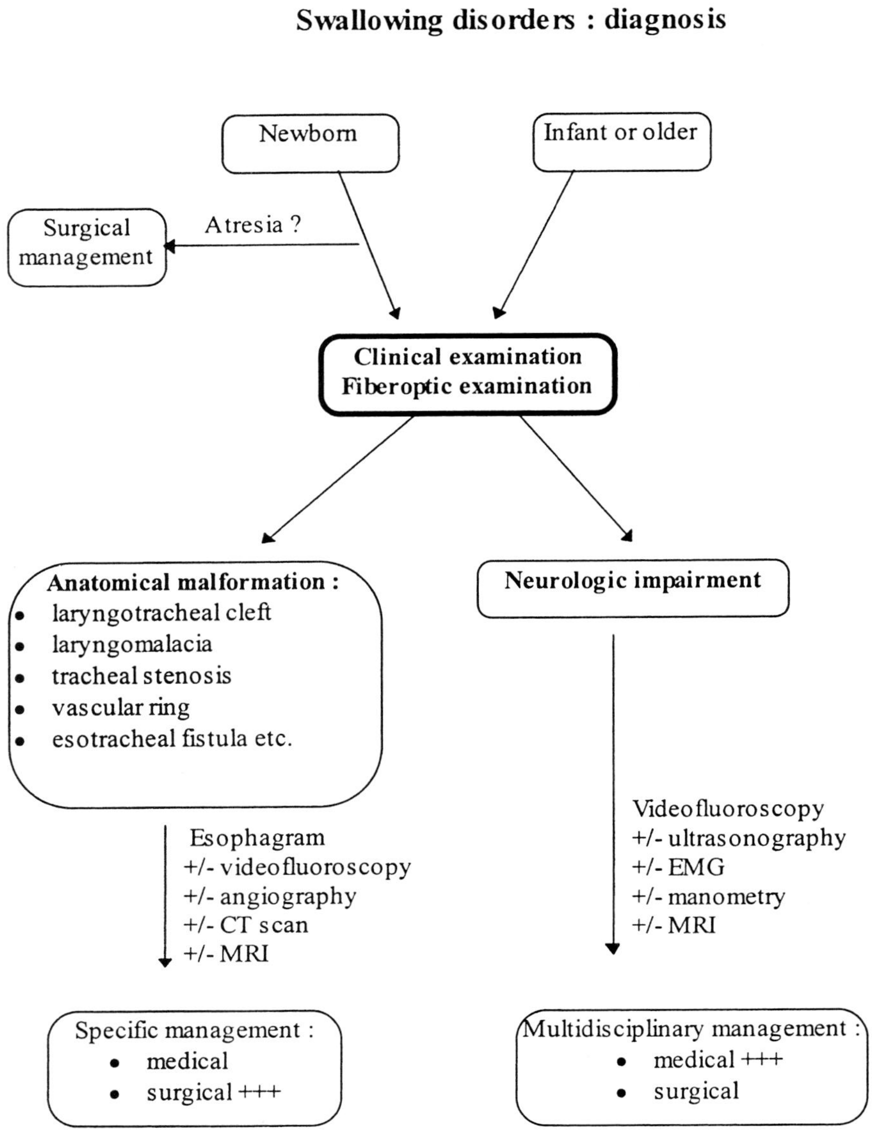

Fig. 19-2. Diagnosis of swallowing disorders.

time motion of the tongue and the floor of the mouth during swallowing in infants.[16] It is a low-cost, safe, fast method, that can be repeated several times without radiation damage. The ultrasound images can be stored on videotapes for frame-by-frame analysis and compared between examinations. A standard feeding procedure with the child in the mother's arms can be used. However, the mouth and the larynx cannot be visualized simultaneously, and laryngeal aspirations are not detected.[1]

Pharyngo-esophageal manometry has recently been improved for adults by the development of new pressure transducers, but manometry of the pharyngoesophageal sphincter remains difficult in children. This method is useful when a neuromuscular disease or an abnormal esophageal motility (achalasia) is suspected. This technique can be associated with videofluoroscopy for comparison with the transit time and can correlate manometric and videoscopic events.[1,8]

Electromyography of the pharyngolaryngeal muscles with surface or hooked-wired electrodes is not used routinely in children. However, it may be indicated in selected cases in which a neurologic or myogenic origin is suspected (myotonia, myasthenia) or in cases of delayed maturation.[12] Auditory, visual, and somesthetic evoked potentials are useful for testing brainstem function, especially in neurologically impaired children or in those with polymalformative syndromes. Magnetic resonance imaging is a useful complementary investigation in these children, especially if Arnold-Chiari malformation is suspected.[8]

Box 19-2. Classification of causes of swallowing disorders

I. Anatomic defects

A. OROPHARYNGEAL MALFORMATIONS

Nasal obstruction: e.g., choanal atresia, deviated septum, obstructive neonatal rhinitis
Cleft palate, submucous cleft
Laryngomalacia
Robin syndrome
Macroglossia: Beckwith-Wiedemann syndrome
Pharyngeal diverticula or tumors

B. ESOPHAGEAL DISORDERS

Esophageal atresia
Tracheosophageal fistula
Congenital stenosis
Secondary stenosis (anastomotic, caustic, peptic esophagitis)
External compression (vascular, tumor)
Esophageal tumors (e.g., leiomyomas, hamartomas)

II. Neuromuscular or brain disorders

Mental retardation
Cerebral palsy
Cranial nerve palsy (V, VII, IX, X, XI, XII)
Brainstem disorders: e.g., immaturity, Möbius' syndrome, Guillain-Barré syndrome, poliomyelitis
Muscle disorders: e.g., myasthenia, myotonia, Duchenne's syndrome, dermatomyositis
Congenital pharyngeal dysfunction
Cricopharyngeal achalasia
Polymalformative syndromes: e.g., CHARGE (coloboma, hearing deficit, choanal atresia, retardation of growth, genital defects, endocardial cushion defect) association, Cornelia de Lange's syndrome, Prader-Willi syndrome, Hallerman-Streiff (oculomandibulofacial) syndrome, fetal alcohol syndrome

III. Inflammatory disorders

Cricopharyngeal spasm
Swallowed corrosives
Infections: candidiasis, herpes stomatitis or esophagitis, Stevens-Johnson, acquired immune deficiency syndrome

IV. Trauma

Foreign bodies
Traumatic pseudodiverticula of pharynx
Perforation of esophagus

Etiologies

Swallowing disorders in newborns

Esophageal atresia is the first earliest diagnostic possibility, before the appearance of salivary aspiration. It is easy to eliminate immediately after birth by gently catheterizing the esophagus. However, swallowing disorders that appear after surgery for esophageal atresia are more difficult to manage. Many possible mechanisms (Box 19-2) include a second esophageal fistula, a posterior laryngeal cleft previously undiagnosed, repermeation of an initial fistula, esophageal stenosis, esophageal dyskinesia, tracheal compression, or tracheomalacia.[4] Several causes are often involved, and it is always difficult to choose which to manage first. Besides the problem of atresia, if aspiration occurs, the first diagnosis is an anomalous communication between the airway and the digestive tract, a tracheoesophageal fistula, or a posterior laryngeal or laryngotracheal cleft.

Tracheoesophageal fistulas cause aspiration during swallowing and coughing and are rapidly followed by bronchopulmonary infections. Clinical and radiologic examinations usually show aerogastric and aeroileic inflation. Clinical findings are often diagnostic: during endotracheal insufflation, abdominal auscultation or the bubble test with the proximal end of the esophageal tube placed in saline solution can show the communication. This diagnosis is confirmed by radiologic examination: videofluoroscopy is better than barium esophagraphy, but in some cases the differential diagnosis between fistula and aspiration is difficult. These cases require examination with an esotracheal rigid endoscope with rigid optics.

Posterior laryngeal or laryngotracheal clefts are rare malformations that may vary in depth; the intensity of the symptoms is often proportional to the extent of the cleft. The main symptoms are early swallowing aspirations and bronchopulmonary infections. Stridor, obstructive dyspnea, and dysphonia are variable. Diagnosis is often difficult and requires training in pediatric endoscopic procedures. Radiologic examinations and videofluoroscopy often fail to show the precise location of the communication between the airway and the digestive tract. Endoscopic examination is the only reliable procedure for diagnosing and staging the cleft, provided that the endoscopist remembers this diagnosis and performs instrumental palpation of the posterior commissura.

Congenital esophageal stenosis is often revealed by swallowing and regurgitation difficulties. This malformation is rare and should be differentiated from acquired stenosis secondary to GER. It usually affects the lower part of the esophagus, forming a membranous web or a segmental stenosis. Diagnosis is made by endoscopy and standard barium esophagography.

The many other causes of swallowing disorders are difficult to classify (see Box 19-2). Laryngeal palsy, especially unilateral, can cause swallowing disorders as a result of incomplete glottic closure, the association of a deficient pharyngolaryngeal sensitivity, or a pharyngeal palsy. Severe laryngomalacia is caused by insufficient laryngeal elevation during swallowing or associated central nervous system abnormalities. Gastroesophageal reflux is responsible for acute painful esophagitis, and it sometimes causes pre- or postprandial lethargy, superior esophageal sphincter dyskinesia, and esophageal peptic stenosis. Achalasia of the superior esophageal sphincter is related to an asynchronism between the release of the permanent tonus of the sphincter and the

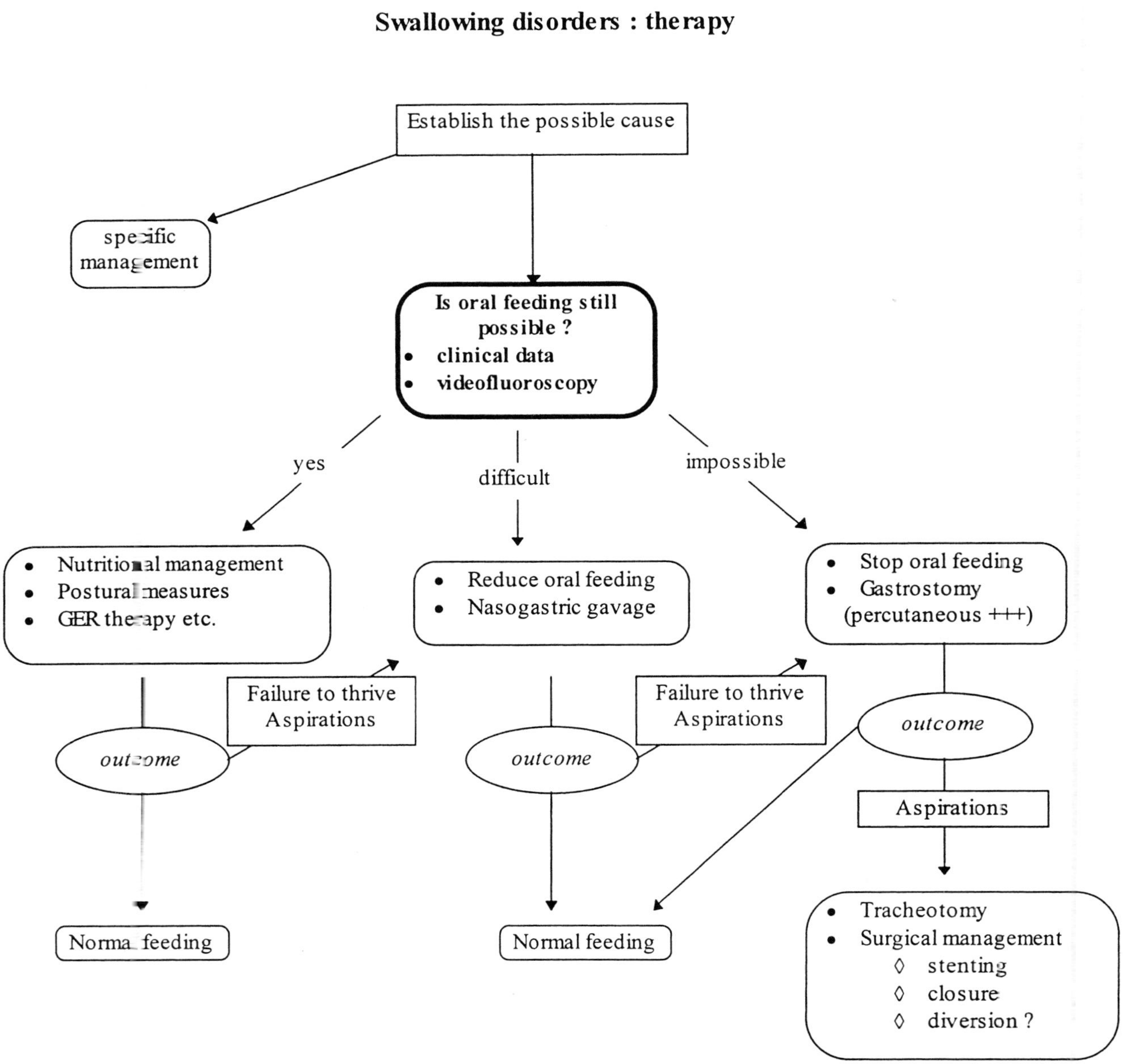

Fig. 19-3. Management of swallowing disorders.

contraction of the pharyngeal constrictor muscles.[13] The retro-esophageal right subclavicular artery is often believed to be responsible for swallowing disorders because this malformation is frequent and easily diagnosed. However, clinicians should be careful before opting for surgery because the vascular compression is generally not significant enough to explain the swallowing disorders. Management of other associated causes (e.g., GER) can ameliorate the symptoms and avoid surgery.

When the configuration of the upper respiratory-digestive tract is normal, most swallowing disorders have a neurologic origin. Immaturity of the neurologic command is often retained after clinical, radiologic, and endoscopic procedures fail to find a precise cause. In some cases, dysphagia is caused by congenital pharyngeal dysfunction, which recovers spontaneously after a few months.[10]

Swallowing disorders in infants and children

Swallowing disorders generally occur in neurologically impaired children (genetics, cerebral palsy, neuromuscular diseases) and are usually revealed by coughing during feeding and recurrent bronchopneumonitis or wheezing rather than by bradycardia or choking. However, the appearance of swallowing disorders is rare in infants and children and can reveal previously unknown neurologic disorders. Neurologic compression of the brainstem or the posterior fossa by tumors or malformations (Arnold-Chiari) should first be ruled out,[8] but infectious diseases including poliomyelitis, Guillain-Barré disease, Lyme disease, and other forms of viral neuritis or polyradiculoneuritis are probably more frequent. Occult pharyngeal or esophageal foreign bodies can be discovered after a long period of swallowing disorders. Peptic stenosis complicating occult GERD or achalasia is rarely diagnosed.

Management

Management of esophageal atresia (Fig. 19-3) and related malformations requires neonatal repair, with closure of the tracheoesophageal fistula and establishment of esophageal continuity by anastomosis of the upper and lower segments. Pre- and postoperative management is essential for a successful outcome and requires close cooperation between intensive care units and surgeons. The only postoperative complications that require a second surgical procedure are recurrent fistulas and early anastomotic leakage. Anastomotic strictures are often managed conservatively by recurrent dilations. Almost half of the patients have feeding difficulties often associated to GER with esophagitis or esophageal incoordination.[4] This makes it difficult for patients to swallow lumpy food, and they tend to have recurrent aspirations or have foreign bodies. All children should be given minced, thickened food. GER is probably not responsible in itself for the feeding difficulties but is likely to aggravate them; medical management should be considered before an antireflux procedure.[7]

Cases of central neurologic disorders or immaturity are more frequent in older children; management requires a multidisciplinary approach. The methods depend greatly on the severity of the swallowing problems (see Fig. 19-2). They may include oxygen therapy, GER therapy, antibiotics, and other pharmacologic management. The possibility of oral feeding should be evaluated first, together with water, caloric, and protein requirements. If possible, minimal oral feeding should be preserved with less liquids, thickening of food, plus supplemental tube feeding and hydration.

Physiotherapy for deglutition with adjustment of the feeding positions, reinforcement of the pharyngeal phase, and self-control of the laryngeal elevation are helpful and can be checked by videofluoroscopic recordings.[14] Oral feedings should be stopped if recurrent aspirations occur despite this management. Gastrostomy, especially with the endoscopic percutaneous technique, seems to be preferable to long-term nasogastric feeding.[2,8] Indeed, nasogastric tubes increase the incidence and the consequence of GER and salivary aspirations. They are often removed by the children, so they require repeated and traumatizing replacement.

Aspirations rarely persist once oral feeding is stopped. There is no universal agreement as to management of these children. Tracheotomy is the most simple technique, but it often increases swallowing disorders by reducing the laryngeal elevation. Other surgical procedures have been proposed to separate the airway and the oral tract.[5,6] They include epiglottopexy, laryngeal diversion, supraglottic or subglottic laryngeal closure, or stenting; all require a tracheotomy. The disadvantages of such procedures should be carefully weighed before any decision for surgery. Subglottic closure with a prosthesis seems to be the most simple and reversible technique.[6]

REFERENCES

1. Arvedson JC, Christensen S: *Instrumental evaluation.* In Arvedson JC, Brodsky L, editors: *Pediatric swallowing and feeding,* San Diego, 1993, Singular Publishing Group.
2. Benkov K and others: Percutaneous endoscopic gastrostomies in children, *Pediatrics* 77:248, 1986.
3. Carré IJ: *Some physiologic mechanisms of the upper gastrointestinal tract.* In Gracey M, Burke V, editors: *Pediatric gastroenterology and hepatology,* Boston, 1993, Blackwell Scientific Publications.
4. Carré IJ: *Disorders of the oropharynx and esophagus.* In Gracey M, Burke V, editors: *Pediatric gastroenterology and hepatology,* Boston, 1993, Blackwell Scientific Publications.
5. Eisele DW: Indications for the tracheoesophageal diversion procedure and the laryngotracheal separation procedure, *Ann Otol Rhinol Laryngol* 97:471, 1988.
6. Gilbert RW: Management of patients with long-term tracheotomies and aspiration, *Ann Otol Rhinol Laryngol* 96:561, 1987.
7. Holder TM and others: Care of infants with esophageal atresia, tracheoesophageal fistula and associated anomalies, *J Thorac Cardiovasc Surg* 94:828, 1987.
8. Loughlin GM, Lefton-Greif MA: Dysfunctional swallowing and respiratory disease in children, *Adv Pediatr* 41:135, 1994.
9. Matthew OP: Science of bottle feeding, *J Pediatr* 119:511, 1991.

10. Mbonda E and others: Prolonged dysphagia caused by congenital pharyngeal dysfunction, *J Pediatr* 126:923, 1995.
11. Pritchard JA: Deglutition by normal and anencephalic fetuses, *Obstet Gynecol* 25:289, 1965.
12. Renault F, Raimbault J: Electromyographie faciale, linguale et pharyngée chez l'enfant: une méthode d'étude des troubles de succion-déglutition et de leur physiopathologie, *Neurophysiol Clin* 22:249, 1992.
13. Schapiro J, Healy GB: Dysphagia in infants, *Otolaryngol Clin North Am* 21:737, 1988
14. Sorin R and others: The influence of videofluoroscopy on the management of the dysphagic patient, *Dysphagia* 2:127, 1988.
15. Stevenson RD, Allaire JH: The development of normal feeding and swallowing, *Pediatr Clin North Am* 38:1439, 1991.
16. Weber F, Woolridge MW, Baum JD: An ultrasonographic study of the organization of sucking and swallowing by newborn infants, *Dev Med Child Neurol* 28:19, 1986.
17. Weiss MH: Dysphagia in infants and children, *Otolaryngol Clin North Am* 21:727, 1988.

Chapter 20

Voice Disorders

Sukgi S. Choi
George H. Zalzal

Voice production starts with the expiration phase of respiration, which provides the air pressure to vibrate the vocal cords. The lowest periodic component of vocal fold vibration is termed *fundamental frequency* and is perceived as pitch.[58] Harmonics are integer multiples of fundamental frequency in voiced sounds. The energy or intensity in the harmonic components decreases as frequency increases.

Sound waves generated by vocal fold vibration are modified by the size, shape, and tenseness of the resonating chamber, which consists of the oropharynx, nasopharynx, and the nasal cavities. The resonance of the vocal tract is termed *formant*.[58] Although an infinite number of formants exist, only the first four formants (F1, F2, F3, F4) are of clinical interest; the lowest frequency formant is F1. Each formant is characterized by its center frequency and bandwidth. Constriction of the vocal tract near a volume velocity maximum or minimum can lower or raise the formant frequency, respectively. The resulting sound wave is further modified by the articulators (lips, teeth, tongue), resulting in voice and speech production. A normal voice should be pleasing in quality and have appropriate balance of oral and nasal resonance, intensity, fundamental frequency level, and prosody. Voice disorder can result in a voice that is unpleasant for the listener or can interfere with effective communication.

The underlying etiology of a voice disorders can be organic or functional. Organic voice disorders are secondary to congenital or acquired anatomic abnormalities. Functional disorders are caused by emotional or psychologic problems but may lead to anatomic alterations. However, even when a voice disorder results primarily from an organic cause, there is often a psychologic overlay.[86]

Although the reported incidence of voice disorders in children varies greatly, most voice surveys of children show a 6% to 9% incidence of voice disorders.[96] Voice disorders are categorized depending on the area of problem: voice quality, resonance, loudness, and pitch. This classification is arbitrary, and a voice disorder often has several problem areas. Any anatomic abnormality involving the free edge of the vocal cord can affect voice quality and result in harshness, breathiness, or hoarseness. Disturbances in resonance can be caused by hyper- or hyponasality. Loudness or intensity problems occur when a child speaks too loudly or too softly. Deviations in pitch occur with inappropriate speaking fundamental frequency, narrow pitch range, or excessive pitch breaks. An algorithm for evaluation and management of voice disorder is outlined in Figure 20-1.

EVALUATION

Evaluation of a child with voice disorder requires a systematic approach. Detailed history, including medical, birth, growth and development, and speech and language history, is obtained, followed by detailed voice history to determine the cause of the voice disorder and its contributing factors, including pulmonary diseases. Typically, voice history should include a description of the disorder, time of onset, any known causes, severity of the disorder and exacerbating or alleviating factors, voice use history, and any previous history of voice or speech therapy.

Physical examination should concentrate on the head and neck areas. Ears are examined for evidence of previous and current ear disease. Nasal examination should reveal any deviation of the septum and turbinate abnormalities. Oropharyngeal examination should concentrate on the structural integrity and mobility of the soft and hard palates and be followed by flexible fiberoptic nasopharyngolaryngoscopy. This technique was introduced in 1976 by Silberman, Wilf,

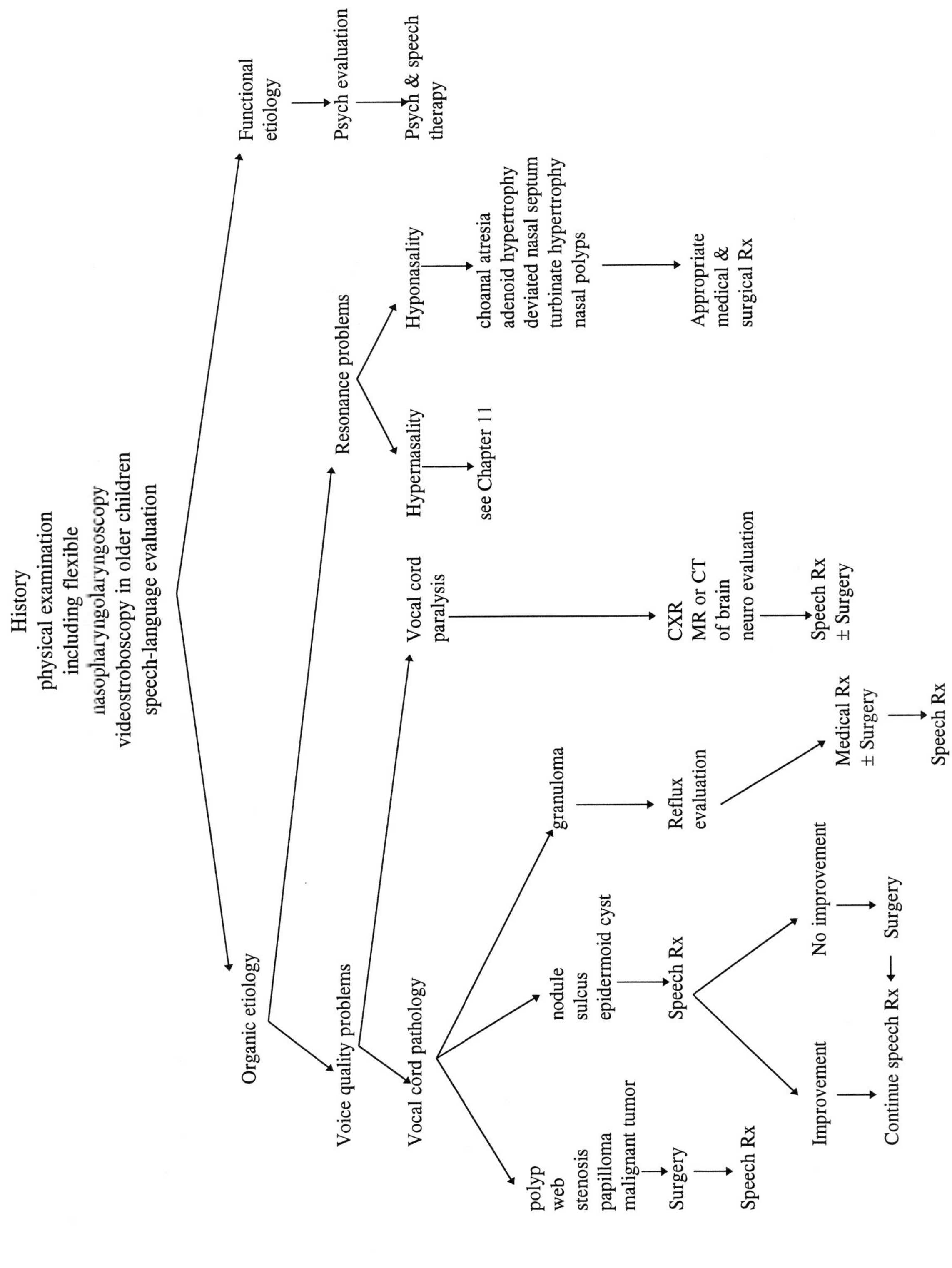

Fig. 20-1. Evaluation and management of voice disorder.

and Tucker[79] for use in the pediatric population, and has gained wide acceptance because of the high rate of success.[42,79] Flexible fiberoptic scopes determine the size of the adenoid, velopharyngeal function, and any pathology in the supraglottic and glottic areas.

Stroboscopic examination, which uses short burst of light in synchrony with vocal cord motion, can seemingly slow down the movement of the vocal cords and allow more careful examination of the vocal cords and their motion.[10] It is particularly useful in differentiating superficial from deep lesions.[2] Laryngeal stroboscopy can delineate vocal cord symmetry, periodicity, vibratory amplitude, mucosal wave, glottal closure, and rigidity[10] but is not possible in many children. Bouchayer and Cornut[15] found that stroboscopic examination in children often had to be quick; therefore, their results tended to be inconclusive. Hirschberg and others[45] found that stroboscopy was possible only in children older than 6 or 7 years. McAllister and others[67] completed stroboscopic examination in only half of 60 patients aged 10 years and older. Therefore, although stroboscopic examination can be instrumental in accurate diagnosis of a voice disorder, it is often of limited use in the pediatric population.

The child's voice is evaluated by a speech-language pathologist, usually in a voice laboratory (Fig. 20-2). A typical voice evaluation consists of perceptual, acoustic, and aerodynamic analyses carried out as the child performs several speaking tasks. There are no universally accepted standards for speech and voice evaluation, and the speaking tasks, the speech parameters measured, and the method of measurement vary greatly.[85]

There are several commonly used speaking tasks.[96] The first is oral reading, which is possible only in older children. Children who can read at third grade level or better are given a specific passage to read; younger children are allowed to select the reading material. The second task is conversational speech or connected speech at least 1 minute long. The child is asked to tell a story about a picture or talk about a specific topic (e.g., pets, a vacation, a hobby). Based on these two tasks, the speech-language pathologist can perceptually and acoustically analyze the child's speech for most voice parameters, including prosody.

The remaining speaking tasks are designed to evaluate more isolated aspects of the child's voice. The next task consists of counting from 1 to 10, 60 to 70, and 90 to 100.[66,96] The counting is done carefully, once slowly and then as rapidly as possible. This is repeated for three levels of loudness (soft, average, loud) and pitch (low, modal, high). This task will reveal any problems with laryngeal tone, resonance, pitch, and loudness.

The fourth speaking task is the production of isolated speech sounds. This consists of sustaining certain vowel sounds (e.g., /ā/, /ī/) for at least 5 seconds and repeating them three times to determine laryngeal tone, resonance, and fundamental frequency. The child should then sustain /ā/ at a comfortable pitch and loudness for as long as possible after a deep inspiration and repeat this three times with a break in between each attempt to determine the maximal phonation time and whether the child had adequate respiratory drive to maintain continuous voice.[96] This same procedure is repeated with /s/ and /z/. In a normally functioning larynx, the s:z ratio should be close to 1. However, a lesion in the vocal cord margins, (e.g., vocal cord nodules) increases the amount of airflow and decreases the time on /z/, resulting in a ratio of 1.4 or greater 95% of the time.[31]

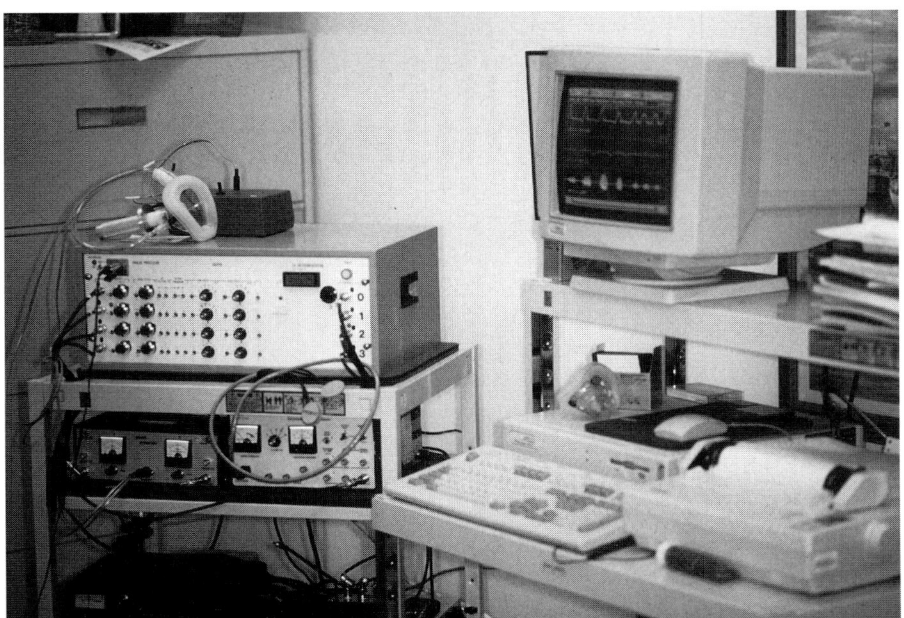

Fig. 20-2. A voice laboratory.

Finally, the examiner should instruct the child to repeat certain consonants, words, and short sentences to assess the child's articulation abilities and speech intelligibility. The words and sentences are typically chosen to bring out specific problems such as velopharyngeal insufficiency.

The speech samples are analyzed, and a voice profile is developed using the Buffalo III voice profile.[96] The voice profile classifies voice abnormalities as 1—normal, 2—mild, 3—moderate, 4—severe, or 5—very severe. This profile evaluates laryngeal tone, pitch, loudness, nasal resonance, oral resonance, breath supply, muscles, voice abuse, rate, speech anxiety, speech intelligibility, and overall voice rating.

Aerodynamic analysis provides objective measures of the velopharyngeal and vocal cord functions. The Oral Nasal Acoustic Ratio and Palatal Efficiency Rating Computed Instantaneously have been used to evaluate velopharyngeal function.[34,94] Laryngeal airway resistance can be measured to assess the effective closure of the vocal cords to airflow. This is measured noninvasively using an anesthesia mask, a pressure-sensing catheter, and a flow-sensing pneumotachometer. Values below 30 cm H_2O/l/sec indicate inadequate closure, whereas values greater than 60 cm H_2O/l/sec are associated with hyperkinetic voice disorders.[81] These techniques of aerodynamic analysis are being replaced by computerized voice analysis programs.

Computer-assisted analysis of voice disorder was recently introduced and is being used with increasing frequency.[85] This new technology presents the opportunity to supplement perceptual evaluation of voice disorders and may replace many traditional methods of evaluation. Evaluation of naturalness and intelligibility of speech will still require the human ear.

Computerized voice analysis can provide the mean fundamental frequency, intensity, and amplitude of voice based on a small voice sample (0.5 sec) for comparison with existing normative values for age and sex (Figs. 20-3 and 20-4).[85] There are no normative data for children in these analysis systems, and normative data in literature are used.[4] Other provided information includes harmonics : noise ratio, amplitude perturbation (shimmer), frequency perturbation (jitter), and electroglottography. Acoustic measures can be obtained in less than 60 seconds using the pneumotachographic mask. Parameters that can be measured include subglottal pressure; transglottal airflow; inspiratory, expiratory, and pause aerodynamics; oral pressure; airflow; resistance and efficiency; nasal flow; and nasal and velopharyngeal resistance.

SPEECH AND VOICE THERAPY

Voice therapy entails two stages.[97] The first stage consists of 10 exploratory sessions, each lasting 35 to 40 minutes. This stage helps determine the goals and specific procedures to be used in stage two, which consists of regular voice therapy sessions for 2 to 5 months. The frequency of therapy is determined by the severity of the dysphonia. Therapy should be supplemented by practice at home to hasten resolution of dysphonia. The total therapy duration is approximately 4 to 5 months; improvement or resolution of dysphonia should be significant.

During the initial phase of voice therapy, the mechanisms of voice production and voice problems are explained to the child in simple terms and a list of rules regarding good and bad voice are provided.[96,97] A main goal of therapy is to eliminate vocal abuse by decreasing the total amount of talking; however, even in highly motivated children, total voice rest may not be feasible. Listening training and auditory feedback are essential in voice therapy because, to correct a voice disorder, the patient should learn to differentiate normal and abnormal voices for comparison with their own voice.[96]

Problematic muscular tonus, loudness, pitch, and rate require therapy. These areas are often closely interrelated and should be managed simultaneously. The child is taught the following steps to correct a problematic voice parameter:[96] correct rules of specific voice parameters; identification of incorrect and correct voice habits in others; recognition of personal use of incorrect voice and modification of this habit; recognition of personal use of correct voice; recognition of situations that cause personal use of poor voice habits and good voice habits; and an increase in the amount of time that correct habits are used. These steps can be applied to any problematic voice parameter.

Voice production depends on well-coordinated movement of muscles involved in phonation. Hyperfunction or excessive muscular tonus frequently occurs in children with benign laryngeal pathology, whereas hypofunction with flaccid muscular tonus occurs in those with functional dysphonia. For both problems, control of muscular tonus and proper positioning of the laryngeal, pharyngeal, and oral structure should be taught. To correct hyperfunctional states, posture instruction, breathing exercises, relaxation procedures, muscle tension reduction technique, chewing method, muscle stretching exercises, and biofeedback can be used.* Wilson[96] found that the chewing method and progressive relaxation are particularly useful in reducing muscular tension. For hypofunctional states, the pushing method increases muscular tension.[18]

Excessive loudness of voice is accompanied by high pitch, rapid rate of speaking, and hyperfunctional state. Therefore, it is often necessary to manage these problems simultaneously. Eliminating loud speaking is particularly important in children with vocal nodules. Correct training for loudness, pitch, and rate involves teaching the child to listen and to monitor various voice parameters. Often, modifying loudness will lower pitch, and attention to loudness and pitch will normalize the rate of speaking.

* Refs. 5, 13, 17, 19, 40, 89.

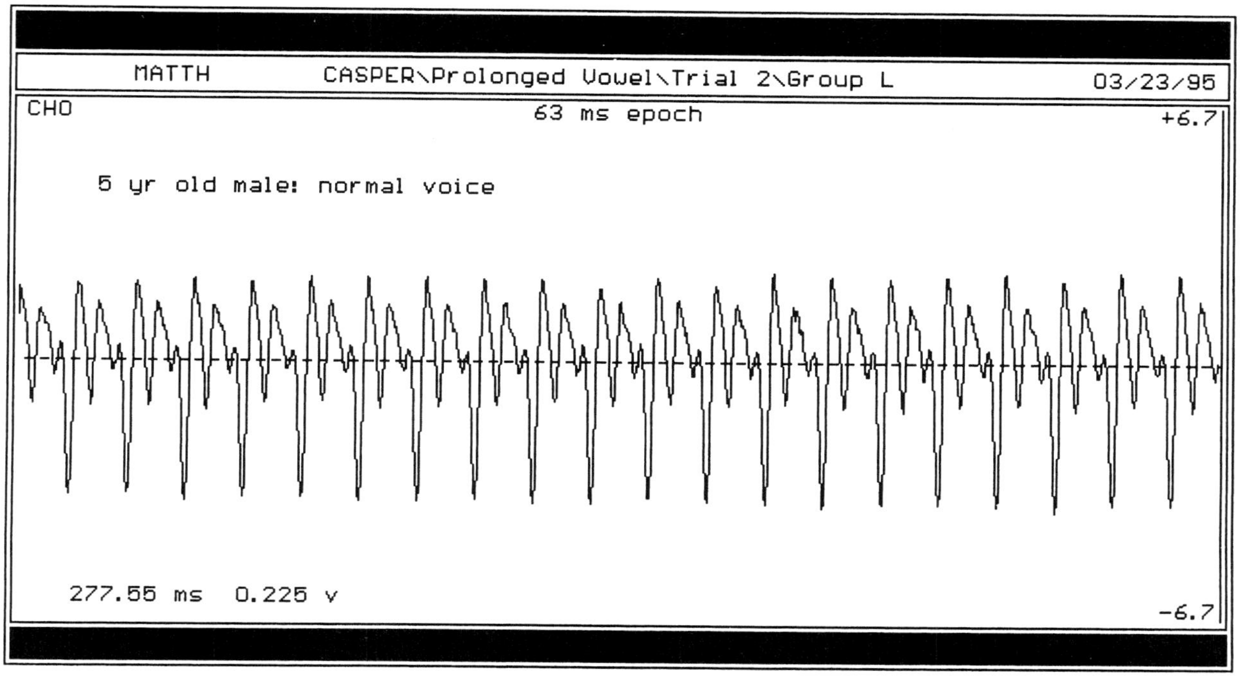

Fig. 20-3. Voice tracing of a normal voice sustaining a prolonged vowel: mean fundamental frequency, 332.53 Hz; jitter, 0.36%; shimmer, 1.9%; harmonic:noise ratio, 12.37 dB.

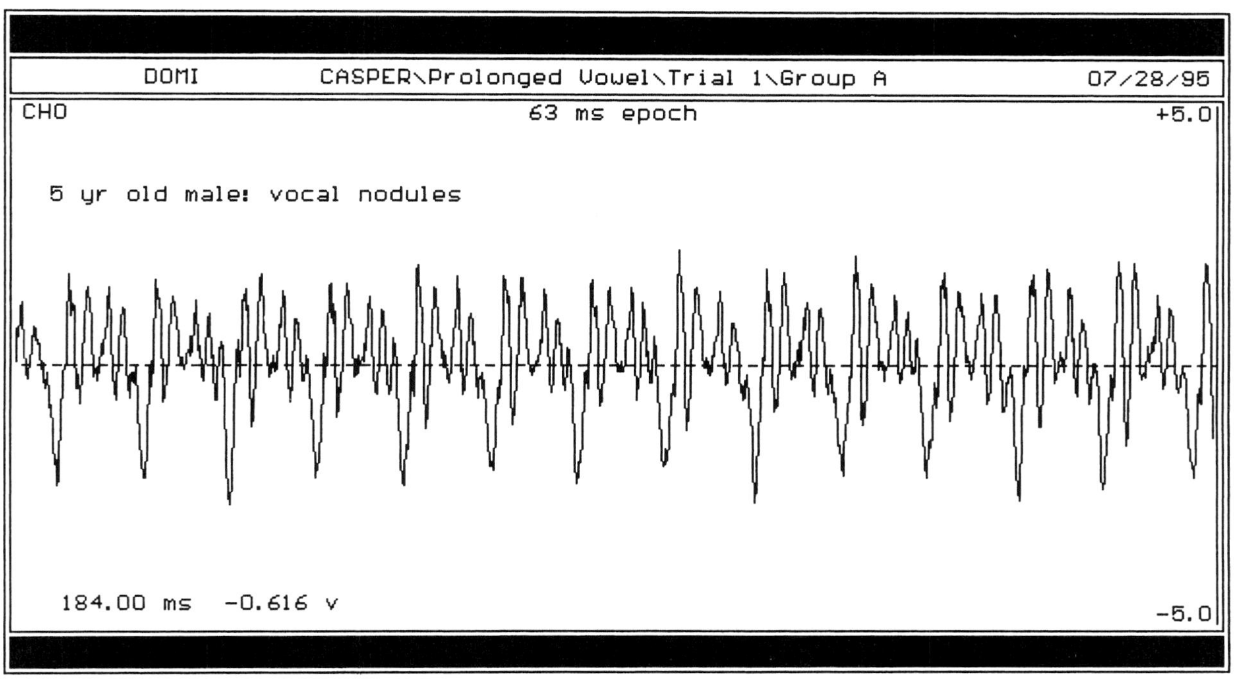

Fig. 20-4. Voice tracing of a hoarse voice (caused by vocal nodules) sustaining a prolonged vowel: mean fundamental frequency, 220.60 Hz; jitter, 2.26%; shimmer, 4.34%; harmonic : noise ratio, 7.84 dB.

FUNCTIONAL VOICE DISORDERS

Functional voice disorder is diagnosed when no anatomic or organic cause can be found. Functional dysphonia is categorized as disturbed mutation, psychologic dysphonia, imitation, and faulty learning.[96] Mutation is the change of voice that occurs during puberty. Pitch lowers in males and, to a lesser extent, females. Mutation can be delayed, prolonged, or incomplete. High pitch, hoarseness, and voice breaks are characteristic. Mutational voice disorder can be secondary to endocrine pathology.[96]

Functional dysphonia resulting from psychologic causes seldom occurs in children; only isolated case reports can be found in the literature.[35] The underlying psychologic problems are related to or part of tensional symptoms, adjustment, anxiety, or personality disorders.[70] Functional dysphonia may be a form of conversion hysteria. The disorder may be complete aphonia or partial loss of voice. The dysphonia is often variable, with effortful voice production and easy fatigue. Laryngeal examination may show ventricular band approximation, bowed vocal cords, or hypoadducted vocal cords (hysterical aphonia). Vocal cord movement is normal with inhalation and cough.

Faulty learning[?2] occurs when a child imitates cleft palate or hearing-impaired speech or learns to talk louder than normal because of the presence of hearing-impaired persons in the household.

In adults, several approaches have been used to manage functional dysphonia, including behavior therapy, hypnosis, speech therapy, psychotherapy, and a combination of speech therapy and psychotherapy. In children, the optimal management is unknown but psychotherapy or psychologic counseling is often carried out in conjunction with speech therapy.

ORGANIC VOICE DISORDERS

Resonance problems

Resonance problems include hypernasality and hyponasality. Hypernasality is usually caused by velopharyngeal insufficiency from underlying palatal abnormalities. For details on diagnosis and management, see Chapter 11.

Hyponasality can result from any underlying condition that causes nasal or nasopharyngeal obstruction. The underlying pathology may be choanal atresia, deviated nasal septum, turbinate hypertrophy, nasal polyps, or, most frequently, adenoid hypertrophy. In performing adenoidectomy, particular attention should be paid to the structural integrity of the palate to decrease the incidence of postoperative velopharyngeal incompetence. Appropriate medical and surgical management of these underlying conditions is discussed in Chapters 7, 8, 12, and 13.

Vocal cord paralysis

Vocal cord paralysis in children is secondary to birth trauma and congenital anomalies of the central nervous system and the heart and great vessels. Any infant or child diagnosed with vocal cord paralysis should be evaluated with chest radiograph and imaging of the central nervous system.[11,16,46,77] Vocal cord paralysis is the second most common cause of congenital stridor in children and represents 10% of congenital anomalies of the larynx.[47] Prognosis for spontaneous recovery is better for acquired, right-sided, and unilateral paralysis.[28,29,33]

Greater than 50% of vocal cord paralysis in children is bilateral.[24,46] Because arytenoid fixation can be mistaken for bilateral vocal cord paralysis, the cricoarytenoid joint should be palpated at rigid endoscopy. Laryngeal electromyography may be the most specific and sensitive test to determine the presence of vocal cord paralysis. Bilateral vocal cord paralysis more than 50% of the time requires tracheotomy for establishment of an airway; however, the voice is often normal. Although spontaneous recovery of vocal cord function is possible after 2 to 3 years, late recovery is often incomplete because of laryngeal muscle atrophy, synkinesis, and cricoid fixation.[100] If vocal cord function does not return spontaneously after 10 to 12 months, surgery to decannulate the child should be considered.[16,72]

Surgical options to correct bilateral vocal cord paralysis consist of reinnervation with a nerve-muscle flap, lateralization procedures (e.g., arytenoidopexy), arytenoidectomy through a posterolateral external approach, arytenoidectomy through laryngofissure, or endoscopic arytenoidectomy.[16,72,84,88,99] Reinnervation of the posterior cricoarytenoid muscle is not universally successful,[24] although Tucker[87] reported it to be the management of choice in children. Because of the small size of the laryngeal structure, endoscopic techniques can be more difficult and less successful in children.[16,37] Narcy, Contencin, and Viala[72] found Woodman's procedure to have a higher failure rate and recommended arytenoidopexy by an external posterolateral approach. However, Bower, Choi, and Cotton[16] recommended arytenoidectomy through a laryngofissure because it provided better exposure, better control over the final cord position, and a high rate of success (84%). Although most patients have adequate voice postoperatively, breathiness, hoarseness, and pitch change are seen, and patients may require speech therapy. The resulting voice disorder is inversely proportional to the adequacy of the airway

Unilateral vocal cord paralysis rarely requires airway intervention and often goes unrecognized until the child is older. The voice in unilateral vocal cord paralysis is hoarse, weak, and breathy. It usually improves spontaneously over 6 to 12 months by contralateral cord compensation; recovery may be hastened by the use of speech therapy. However, in a few patients, persistent problems with dysphonia or aspiration require surgical intervention.[65] Surgical options include vocal cord injection, surgical medialization, and reinnervation. Surgical interventions should be done in conjunction with pre- and postoperative speech therapy

Polytef injection immediately improves voice; however, it is irreversible, changes vocal cord vibratory characteristics, and thus results in poor vocal quality. Furthermore, in children, determining the amount of polytef to inject is difficult because general anesthesia is often necessary and airway obstruction is possible because of the small size of the larynx.[87] Levine and others[65] recommended injection of an absorbable gelatin sponge, which is similar to polytef injection except its effects are temporary. Fat injection was recently introduced and appears to be well tolerated by the body, does not cause the vocal cord to become stiff, and is not absorbed extensively.[68]

Several surgical techniques are available for medialization of the vocal cord.[50-52,87] Isshiki type I thyroplasty is theoretically reversible and does not change the vibratory characteristics of the vocal cord; however, it does not restore tensioning capability of the vocal cords and requires external incision and a temporary tracheotomy in most cases. In children, this procedure is technically more difficult and may cause airway compromise. Experience with thyroplasty in children has been limited because of a lack of knowledge about the effect of this technique on thyroid cartilage growth.[65] Although voice quality improves using objective measurement, the resulting voice is not ideal.[41]

Selective reinnervation of the adductors of the larynx does not compromise potential spontaneous recovery, necessitate tracheotomy, or preclude eventual use of other techniques; it also restores tensioning capability, thereby providing better pitch control. However, it is an open procedure, and motion may not be observed for up to 6 months.[87] Excellent results have been reported by Crumley[27] and Tucker.[87] Tucker[87] advocated it to be the procedure of choice in children.

Vocal cord pathology—surgical

Polyps

Vocal cord polyps occur infrequently in children and adolescents.[55,71] They arise from chronic abuse of the larynx or from a single traumatic episode. Hoarseness is the most common presenting symptom. The polyps occur at the junction of the anterior and middle third of the vocal cord and may be fusiform, pedunculated, or generalized.[59] A recent study showed that polyps are caused by circulation impediment, thrombosis, exudation, and edema of the lamina propria. Inflammation and secondary atrophy of the vocal cord epithelium occur.[21] Baker reported similar findings in 1963.[6]

Management of vocal cord polyps is surgical removal.[15,59,91] Pedunculated polyps are removed at the base using carbon dioxide (CO_2) laser or microscissors. For generalized polyps, an incision is made over the superior surface of the vocal cord and the fibrous exudate is suctioned out or vaporized.[15,95] The resulting voice quality depends on the degree of irreversible damage to the superficial layer of the lamina propria by fibrous or hyaline infiltration. Speech therapy is recommended before and after surgery to prevent recurrences.[15,97]

Web

Smith and Caitlin[80] reported that glottic web and atresia account for 5% of congenital anomalies; however, some consider the true incidence of congenital web of larynx to be more common, whereas others consider it more rare. Web occurs because of failure of the epithelium, which temporarily obliterates the developing laryngotracheal lumen, to reabsorb during the eighth week of embryogenesis. Glottic web is classified depending on its severity.[23] Type 1 is an anterior web involving 35% or less of the glottis. True cords are visible within the web, and there is little or no subglottic extension. Although there is usually no airway obstruction, voice dysfunction is common. Type 2 is an anterior web involving up to 50% of the glottis. True cords are usually visible within the web, and subglottic involvement is minimal. Voice disorder is the common presenting symptom. However, airway compromise can be seen with upper respiratory tract infections. Type 3 involves up to 75% of the glottis, and the anterior portion of the web is solid and extends into the subglottis. Most of the true cords are visible within the web. Airway obstruction and voice disorder are moderately severe. Type 4 involves up to 90% of the glottis, and the web is uniformly thick and extends into the subglottic area with resulting subglottic stenosis. The infant is aphonic with severe airway compromise.

In 1985, Cohen and others[23] reviewed 51 children with laryngeal web and recommended that surgery be tailored according to web severity.[23] A type 2 web was divided with a knife, microsurgical scissors, or laser followed by dilations. Types 3 and 4 were managed by tracheotomy and insertion of a laryngeal keel through a laryngofissure. The anterior commissure is not adequately reconstructed by any surgical procedure, and the resulting voice continues to be abnormal and requires vocal rehabilitation.

Recommended management of a thin laryngeal web involves endolaryngeal division of the web with a knife or CO_2 laser with temporary placement of a keel to prevent readhesion. Thick glottic webs are approached through precise midline thyrotomy, a laryngofissure with removal of excess tissue under direct vision using a fiberoptic laryngoscope, and placement of a mucosal graft fixated with fibrin glue or stenting.[53] The use of CO_2 laser in cases of thick web is not recommended. The resulting voice is reportedly satisfactory, but objective postoperative analysis of voice is unavailable.

Posterior glottic stenosis and cricoarytenoid joint fixation

Posterior glottic stenosis in children may be congenital (e.g., caused by interarytenoid web or cricoarytenoid fixation). More commonly, posterior glottic stenosis is secondary to airway trauma from intubation. Bogdasarian and Olson[12] classified posterior glottic stenosis into four types. This classification was later modified for the pediatric population by Irving, Bailey and Evans.[48] Type I is vocal process adhesion, type II is posterior commissure or interarytenoid scar, type III is congenital or acquired unilateral cricoarytenoid fixation with or without interarytenoid scar, and type IV is congenital or acquired bilateral cricoarytenoid fixation with or without interarytenoid scar.

With interarytenoid web and scarring, there is bilaterally impaired abduction but normal adduction; these patients tend to have a normal voice.[7] The main presenting symptom in these cases is airway compromise. In cricoarytenoid joint fixation, adduction and abduction of the vocal cord are limited, which may also cause dysphonia. To distinguish cricoarytenoid joint fixation from vocal cord paralysis, palpation of the cricoarytenoid joint at rigid endoscopy is necessary. Laryngeal electromyography may be necessary for definitive diagnosis.

Benjamin and Mair[9] noted that interarytenoid webs are often associated with other airway abnormalities. They recommend that interarytenoid web be managed by long term watchful waiting or by tracheotomy if associated abnormalities of the airway exist. In pediatric posterior glottic stenosis, arytenoidectomy should be avoided to prevent the possibility of aspiration, deterioration of voice, and difficulty with future airway repair.[102] Although many techniques have been tried, anterior and posterior cricoidotomy with posterior graft appears to give the most consistent results and is considered the procedure of choice in children.[48,102] Improved vocal cord mobility has been observed postoperatively.[39,102]

The postoperative voice is considered to be functional in most children; a voice disorder consisting of hoarseness and breathiness often persists.[102] Bogdasarian and Olson[12] noted in adult patients that final voice results depended on the severity of stenosis; the same applies to children.

Recurrent respiratory papillomatosis

Recurrent respiratory papillomatosis is the most common benign neoplasm of the larynx. Papilloma patients present with hoarseness or airway obstruction. Papillomas have a predilection for anatomic sites where ciliated and squamous epithelium are juxtaposed. Common sites in the larynx are the midzone of the laryngeal surface of the epiglottis, the upper and lower margins of the ventricle, and the undersurface of the vocal cords.[36] Recurrent respiratory papillomatosis is most often diagnosed between ages 2 and 3 years (usually before age 5).[82] Juvenile and adult-onset forms of the disease are possible; the juvenile form has a more aggressive clinical course. The need for tracheotomy in juvenile recurrent respiratory papillomatosis is reportedly 14% to 21%.[25,30]

An association between cervical human papillomavirus (HPV) types 6 and 11 in the mother and recurrent respiratory papillomatosis in the child has been established.[1,26,57,75,83] HPV is found in the genital tract of approximately 25% of women of child-bearing age and is clinically apparent in 2% to 5%. Shah and others[78] estimate the risk of HPV transmission to be 1 in 400 vaginal births in mothers with active *condylomata*.

Surgery is the management of choice, although it is only palliative because the natural history of recurrent respiratory papillomatosis is one of recurrence. The goal of surgery is to establish a stable airway and a serviceable voice. Surgical options are CO_2 laser ablation and microlaryngoscopy with forceps removal; CO_2 laser ablation is generally accepted as the procedure of choice.[30] Papillomas are removed to the level of the mucosa or submucosa avoiding the deeper muscular and ligamentous levels. Caution should be exercised in removing papillomas from the anterior and posterior commissure areas because irreversible scarring may result. Although removal of recurrent respiratory papillomatosis temporarily improves the voice, the increasing number of required procedures results in scarring of the vocal cords and deteriorating voice.

Leventhal and others[64] recommended the use of interferon in any patient requiring surgery every 2 to 3 months. The duration of management should be 6 months. If there is no response or complete response, management should be discontinued, but if there is a partial response, management should be continued. However, the results of interferon management of recurrent respiratory papillomatosis have been disappointing.[43] After the cessation of interferon therapy, there is a rebound effect and papillomas recur at an increased rate.[95] Other adjuvant therapies (e.g., photodynamic therapy, acyclovir, ribavirin, isotretinoin, indole 3-carbinol) are infrequently used.[30]

Malignant tumors

Malignant tumors of the pediatric larynx are rare. Isolated case reports are seen in the literature, but more extensive experience is lacking. A 15-year review of malignant laryngeal tumors at a tertiary pediatric referral center revealed only four cases.[73] These laryngeal tumors are usually in the sarcoma group, most commonly rhabdomyosarcoma Other malignancies include squamous cell carcinoma, lymphoma, mucoepidermoid carcinoma, metastatic carcinoma, neuroectodermal tumor, and metastatic carcinoma.[22,38,69,101] Spontaneous malignant degeneration of long-standing recurrent respiratory papillomatosis has an incidence of 2% to 3%.[36] In addition, squamous cell carcinoma may be seen in recurrent respiratory papillomatosis patients with a history of radiotherapy.

Patients with laryngeal tumors present with voice change (often hoarseness), stridor, and progressive airway obstruction. Delay in diagnosis is common because of a low suspicion for malignancy. Any child with persistent hoarseness should thus be fully evaluated. Management goals are patient survival and preservation of laryngeal function when possible. Management depends on the tumor histology and consists of combination surgery, radiotherapy, and chemotherapy.

Radiotherapy of a prepubescent larynx can result in a fibrotic infantile larynx with no useful voice, airway, or swallowing function.[73] This should be considered when deciding on a management protocol. Ohlms, McGill, and

Healy[73] provide an example of a prepubescent child with a laryngeal rhabdomyosarcoma. Although radiotherapy may have provided adequate local control, total laryngectomy was chosen to improve local control. Total laryngectomy was justified because it provided a better chance of cure, whereas the larynx may have been useless after undergoing radiotherapy.

Vocal cord pathology—medical

Granuloma

Patients with vocal cord granuloma commonly present with hoarseness. Granuloma is often secondary to intubation trauma. Habitual throat clearing, excessive glottal attacks, and reflux esophagitis are important causal factors.[44,93] Inflammation over the vocal process of arytenoid progresses to infection involving the perichodrium and formation of granuloma. Histologically, the granulomas are nonspecific reparative granulation tissue covered by hyperplastic squamous epithelium.[8]

Children with vocal cord granuloma should be evaluated for GERD. The most reliable means of diagnosing GERD is prolonged (24-hour) pH-manometry study.[60] A reflux event is defined as a drop in the pH to less than 4. Normally, the time that pH is less than 4 is approximately 6.3% upright, 1.2% supine, and 4.2% total.[20] Other less specific and sensitive methods are barium esophagography, radionuclide scanning, and lipid-laden macrophage testing for aspiration.

The primary management of vocal cord granuloma is management of underlying GERD. Most granulomas resolve on medical management. Management of GERD involves[76] (1) dietary and lifestyle modifications and the use of antacids; (2) H_2 blockers (cimetidine, ranitidine, famotidine), prokinetic agents (bethanechol, metoclopramide, cisapride), and mucosal cytoprotectants (sucralfate) in combination; and (3) hydrogen ion blocker (omeprazole) combined with surgical repair of hiatal hernia and reestablishment of lower esophageal sphincter function.

Surgical removal (CO_2 laser or sharp incision with microlaryngeal instruments) of the vocal cord granuloma is reserved for lesions causing airway obstruction.[8,60] Regardless of the surgical technique used, recurrence is frequent. Although voice therapy has been recommended, it does not appear to be an effective primary management modality for vocal cord granulomas.

Vocal cord pathology—speech therapy with or without surgery

Opinions about the management of cysts, sulcus vocalis, and nodules differ widely. Traditionally, surgery was discouraged in children because of the small size of the larynx, difficulty in reinforcing voice rest postoperatively, and high recurrence when underlying vocal behavior is not modified. Surgery was recommended for only the most recalcitrant and severe dysphonia. However, some surgeons have reported that surgery of the pediatric larynx is safe and technically feasible with good results as seen in a series by Bouchayer and Cornut[15] of 191 children who underwent microsurgery. However, advocates of surgery recommend waiting until the child is 8 to 9 years old.[9,15] In addition, a highly motivated patient and involved parents are prerequisites to surgery.

Pre- and postoperative voice therapy is essential. Surgical intervention is most often by microsurgical technique, although CO_2 laser is infrequently used. The principles of surgery are to remove the pathology with maximal preservation of normal mucosa and to avoid injury to the anterior commissure and vocal ligament.

Cysts and sulcus vocalis

It is unclear whether epidermoid cysts and sulcus of the vocal cords are congenital or acquired lesions. Van Caneghem[90] and others[49,54] support the view that these lesions are acquired, whereas Bouchayer and others[14] theorize that they are congenital. In a series of 2334 patients, Bouchayer and Camut[15] found that congenital lesions of the vocal cords were the most frequently seen benign lesions requiring surgical intervention; they believe these congenital lesions are often overlooked or misdiagnosed.

Patients with either lesion often present with hoarseness, voice breaks, and vocal fatigue. With epidermoid cysts, unilateral submucosal swelling of the superior mid-third surface often occurs with associated edema of the contralateral vocal cord. Reduced mucosal waves are seen on stroboscopy. Epidermoid cysts are lined with stratified keratinizing squamous epithelium and contain keratin debris. With sulcus vocalis, the surface epithelium invaginates into Reinke's space and adheres to the vocal ligament, resulting in a longitudinal furrow parallel to the edge of the vocal cord and an oval glottic chink. Stroboscopy shows incomplete closure of the free edges of the vocal cords.

Cysts and sulcus vocalis usually do not resolve spontaneously.[15] Epidermoid cysts are often mistaken for vocal nodules, and patients are thus referred for speech therapy. Referral to the otolaryngologist occurs when the voice disorder does not resolve after several months of speech therapy. Sulcus vocalis is often difficult to diagnose in children because careful examination of the larynx with a stroboscope is often impossible. These children are referred for voice abnormality that fails to improve with speech therapy.

Epidermoid cyst and sulcus vocalis are managed by microsurgery. For cysts, a mucosal incision is made on the superior surface of the vocal cord, parallel to the free edge, and the cyst is dissected. Bouchayer and Camut[15] recommend intracordal injection of the surgical site with corticosteroid to decrease the inflammation. Woo and others[98] recently reported improved laryngeal microsurgery results using 6-0 chronic endo-knot sutures to close the microflaps of the vocal cord. Sulci are resected by making incisions in the superior and inferior edges of the pocket and dissecting the pocket from the vocal ligament. A slicing mucosa surgical technique that detaches the mucosa of the sulcus and interrupts the longitudinal fibrotic tension line has been used with good results.[74] Although the resulting voice is improved compared with the preoperative state, it is not perfect. Postoperative speech therapy is important and has significant effect on voice results. Therapy is recommended for at least 3 to 6 months.

Nodules

Most voice disorders in children are secondary to vocal cord nodules. Vocal cord nodules occur frequently, often as a result of misuse or overuse of the larynx (hyperfunctional state). The incidence of hoarseness, a symptom of dysphonia, in school children is estimated to be approximately 5%.[92] Of children evaluated by an otolaryngologist for chronic hoarseness, 38% to 78% have vocal cord nodules. Thus, more than 1 million children in the United States have vocal cord nodules. Vocal nodules are most often seen as a child enters a group activity. They are more common in boys. Patients with vocal nodules present with hoarseness and breathiness. Stroboscopic examination shows decreased mucosal waves and incomplete approximation of the free edges.[92]

Vocal nodules develop secondary to mechanical trauma and occur at the free edge of the anterior and middle third of the vocal cord. Often, vocal cord nodules are bilateral, although unilateral nodules can occur. Vocal nodules develop in three stages[91]: (1) an inflammatory phase with increased vascularity and protein accumulation; (2) localized swelling on the edge of the vocal that appears as grayish, translucent thickening (nodules are reversible within 24 to 48 hours if trauma is eliminated); and (3) replacement of thickening by fibrotic tissue which appears gray or white. Histologically, circumscribed hyperplasia or hyperkeratinization and secondary hyaline degeneration in the lamina propria are seen.[21]

Management options include speech therapy, surgery, speech therapy plus surgery, and no intervention.[3,9,15,61-63,92] It is difficult to determine the success of differing modes of management because follow-up of control groups (no management) is rare. Because of the benign nature of nodules, patients who undergo medical or surgical management are often lost to follow-up evaluation. The fact that vocal nodules in children often resolve spontaneously by puberty may also influence management. The most widely accepted management option for vocal cord nodules in children is speech therapy. According to von Leden,[92] most nodules resolve or show significant improvement within 3 to 6 months with speech therapy. Surgery is considered in children who fail to show improvement with speech therapy and in whom severe hoarseness interferes with daily functioning.[9,92]

Surgical management of choice is microsurgical excision, although CO_2 laser has been used. The nodule is stretched medially and removed at its base with microscissors without excessive mucosal removal. Bilateral nodules can usually be removed in one sitting; however, care should be taken to avoid injuring the anterior commissure. Some surgeons recommend removing bilateral nodules in stages that are 4 weeks apart.[9] Voice rest is recommended for 7 to 10 days. Long-term results depend on the quality of speech therapy, but they are generally good. Recurrences are frequent without speech therapy.

REFERENCES

1. Abramson AL, Steinbert BM, Winkler B: Laryngeal papillomatosis: clinical, histopathologic and molecular studies, *Laryngoscope* 97:678, 1987.
2. Alberti PW: The diagnostic role of laryngeal stroboscopy, *Otolaryngol Clin North Am* 11:347, 1978.
3. Allen MS, Pettit JM, Sherblom JC: Management of vocal nodules: a regional survey of otolaryngologists and speech-language pathologists, *J Speech Hear Res* 34:229, 1991.
4. Andrews ML: *Manual of voice treatment: pediatrics through geriatrics,* San Diego, 1995, Singular Publishing Group.
5. Aronson AE: *Clinical voice disorders: an interdisciplinary approach,* ed 2, New York, 1985, Thieme.
6. Baker DC: Polypoid vocal cord, *N Y State J Med* 63:3096, 1963.
7. Benjamin B, Croxson G: Vocal cord granulomas, *Ann Otol Rhinol Laryngol* 94:538, 1985.
8. Benjamin B, Croxson G: Vocal nodules in children, *Ann Otol Rhinol Laryngol* 96:530, 1987.
9. Benjamin B, Mair EA: Congenital interarytenoid web, *Arch Otolaryngol Head Neck Surg* 117:1118, 1991.
10. Bless DM, Hirano M, Feder RJ: Videostroboscopic evaluation of the larynx, *Ear Nose Throat J* 66:289, 1987.
11. Boey HP, Cunningham MJ, Weber AL: Central nervous system imaging in the evaluation of children with true vocal cord paralysis, *Ann Otol Rhinol Laryngol* 104:76, 1995.
12. Bogdasarian RS, Olson NR: Posterior glottic laryngeal stenosis, *Otolaryngol Head Neck Surg* 88:765, 1980.
13. Boone DR: *The voice and voice therapy*, ed 3, Englewood Cliffs, NJ, 1983, Prentice-Hall.
14. Bouchayer M and others: Epidermoid cycts, sulci and mucosal bridges of the true vocal cord: a report of 157 cases, *Laryngoscope* 95:1087, 1985.
15. Bouchayer M, Cornut G: Microsurgical treatment of benign vocal fold lesions: indications, technique, results, *Folia Phoniatr (Basel)* 44:155, 1992.
16. Bower CM, Choi SS, Cotton RT: Arytenoidectomy in children, *Ann Otol Rhinol Laryngol* 103:271, 1994.
17. Brodnitz FS: Voice problems of the actor and singer, *J Speech Hear Disord* 19:322, 1954.
18. Brodnitz FS: *Vocal rehabilitation*, ed 4, Rochester, Minn, 1971, American Academy of Ophthalmology and Otolaryngology.
19. Cacciotti T: *The Cacciotti method: the feel good about yourself workout*, New York, 1983, Villard Books.
20. Castell DO: Ambulatory monitoring in esophageal disease, *Viewpoints on Digestive Diseases* 21:1, 1989.
21. Chen X: Comparative research on vocal polyps and nodules, *Chung Hua Erh Pi Yen Hou Ko Tsa Chih* 24:53, 1989.
22. Cohen SR: Congenital glottic webs in children: a retrospective review of 51 patients, *Ann Otol Rhinol Laryngol* 14:2, 1985.
23. Cohen SR and others: Laryngeal paralysis in children: a long-term retrospective study, *Ann Otol Rhinol Laryngol* 91:417, 1982.

24. Cohen SR, Thompson JW, Siegel SE: Non-Hodgkin's lymphoma of the larynx in children, *Ann Otol Rhinol Laryngol* 96:357, 1987.
25. Cole RR, Myer CM, Cotton RT: Tracheotomy in children with recurrent respiratory papillomatosis, *Head Neck* 11:226, 1989.
26. Corbitt G and others: Human papillomavirus (HPV) genotypes associated with laryngeal papilloma, *J Clin Pathol* 41:284, 1988.
27. Crumley RL: Teflon versus thyroplasty versus nerve transfer: a comparison, *Ann Otol Rhinol Laryngol* 99:759, 1990.
28. Dedo DD, Dedo HH: *Neurogenic diseases of the larynx.* In Bluestone CD, Stool SE, Scheetz MD, editors: *Pediatric otolaryngology*, ed 2, Philadelphia, 1990, WB Saunders.
29. Dedo DD: Pediatric vocal cord paralysis, *Laryngoscope* 89:1378, 1979.
30. Derkay CS: Task force on recurrent respiratory papillomas, *Arch Otolaryngol Head Neck Surg* 121:1386, 1996.
31. Eckel FC, Boone DR: The s/z ratio as an indicator of laryngeal pathology, *J Speech Hear Disord* 46:147, 1981.
32. Eisenson J, Ogilvie M: *Speech correction in the schools*, ed 4, New York, 1977, Macmillan.
33. Emery PJ, Fearon B: Vocal cord palsy in pediatric practice: a review of 71 cases, *Int J Pediatr Otorhinolaryngol* 8:147, 1984.
34. Fletcher SG: Theory and instrumentation for quantitative measurement of nasality, *Cleft Palat Craniofac J* 7:601, 1970.
35. Froese AP, Sims P: Functional dysphonia in adolescence: two case reports, *Can J Psychiatry* 32:389, 1987.
36. Gaylis B, Hayden R: Recurrent respiratory papillomatosis: progression to invasion and malignancy, *Am J Otolaryngol* 12:104, 1991.
37. Gentile RD, Miller RH, Woodson GE: Vocal cord paralysis in children 1 year of age and younger, *Ann Otol Rhinol Laryngol* 95:622, 1985.
38. Gindhart TD and others: Carcinoma of the larynx in childhood, *Cancer* 46:1683, 1980.
39. Goodwin WJ and others: Vocal cord mobilization by posterior laryngoplasty, *Laryngoscope* 98:846, 1988.
40. Gordon MT, Morton FM, Simson IC: Air flow measurements in diagnosis, assessment and treatment of mechanical dysphonia, *Folia Phoniatr (Basel)* 30:161, 1978.
41. Gray SD and others: Vocal evaluation of thyroplastic surgery in the treatment of unilateral vocal fold paralysis, *Laryngoscope* 102:415, 1992.
42. Hawkins DB, Clark RW: Flexible laryngoscopy in neonates, infants, and young children, *Ann Otol Rhinol Laryngol* 96:81, 1987.
43. Healy GB and others: Treatment of recurrent respiratory papillomatosis with human leukocyte interferon: results of a multicenter randomized clinical trial, *N Engl J Med* 319:401, 1988.
44. Hill FT: Granuloma of larynx following endotracheal anesthesia, *Ann Otol Rhinol Laryngol* 57:910, 1948.
45. Hirschberg J and others: Voice disorders in children, *Int J Pediatr Otorhinolaryngol* 32:S109, 1995.
46. Holinger LD, Holinger PC, Holinger PH: Etiology of bilateral abductor vocal cord paralysis: a review of 389 cases, *Ann Otol Rhinol Laryngol* 85:428, 1976.
47. Holinger PH, Brown WT: Congenital webs, cysts, laryngoceles and other anomalies of the larynx, *Ann Otol Rhinol Laryngol* 76:744, 1967.
48. Irving RM, Bailey CM, Evans JNG: Posterior glottic stenosis in children, *Int J Pediatr Otorhinolaryngol* 28:11, 1993.
49. Ishii H, Baba T, Kawabata J: Clinical observations on the sulcus vocalis, *J Otolaryngol (Japan)* 70:911, 1967.
50. Isshiki N and others: Recent modifications in thyroplasty type I, *Ann Otol Rhinol Laryngol* 98:777, 1989.
51. Isshiki N and others: Surgical treatment of laryngeal web with mucosa graft, *Ann Otol Rhinol Laryngol* 100:95, 1991.
52. Isshiki N, Tanabe M, Sawada M: Arytenoid adduction for unilateral vocal cord paralysis, *Arch Otolaryngol Head Neck Surg* 104:555, 1978.
53. Isshiki N and others: Thyroplasty as a new phonosurgical technique, *Acta Otolaryngol (Stockh)* 78:451, 1974.
54. Itoh T and others: Vocal fold furrows: a 10 year review of 240 patients, *Auris Nasus Larynx* 10:S17, 1983.
55. Kambic V and others: Vocal cord polyps: incidence, histology and pathogenesis, *J Laryngol Otol* 95:609, 1981.
56. Kashima HK and others: Polymerase chain reaction identification of human papillomavirus DNA in CO_2 laser plume from recurrent respiratory papillomatosis, *Otolaryngol Head Neck Surg* 104:191, 1991.
57. Kashima HK and others: Sites of predilection in recurrent respiratory papillomatosis, *Ann Otol Rhinol Laryngol* 102:580, 1993.
58. Kent RD, Read C: *The acoustic analysis of speech*, San Diego, 1992, Singular Publishing Group.
59. Kleinsasser O: Pathogenesis of vocal cord polyps, *Ann Otol Rhinol Laryngol* 91:378, 1982.
60. Koufman JA: The otolaryngologic manifestations of gastroesophageal reflux disease (GERD): a clinical investigation of 225 patients using ambulatory 24-hour pH monitoring and an experimental investigation of the role of acid and pepsin in the development of laryngeal injury, *Laryngoscope* 101:1, 1991.
61. Lancer JM and others: The outcome of different management patterns for vocal cord nodules, *J Laryngol Otol* 102:423, 1988.
62. Krecicki T, Zalesska-Krecicka M: Clinical aspects of vocal cord nodules, *Acta Otorhinolaryngol Belg* 47:339, 1993.
63. Lancer JM and others: Vocal cord nodules: a review, *Clin Otolaryngol* 13:43, 1988.
64. Leventhal B and others: Long-term response of recurrent respiratory papillomatosis to treatment of lymphoblastoid interferon α-n1, *N Engl J Med* 325:613, 1991.
65. Levine BA and others: Vocal cord injection in children with unilateral vocal cord paralysis, *Arch Otolaryngol Head Neck Surg* 121:116, 1995.
66. Maddern BR, Campbell TF, Stool S: Pediatric voice disorders, *Otolaryngol Clin North Am* 24:1125, 1991.
67. McAllister A and others: Relations between voice range profiles and physiological and perceptual voice characteristics in ten-year-old children, *J Voice* 8:230, 1994.
68. Mikaelian DO, Lowry LD, Sataloff RT: Lipoinjection for unilateral vocal cord paralysis, *Laryngoscope* 101:465, 1991.
69. Mitchell DB, Humphreys S, Kearns DB: Mucoepidermoid carcinoma of the larynx in a child, *Int J Pediatr Otorhinolaryngol* 15:211, 1988.
70. Morrison MD, Nichol H, Rammage LA: Diagnostic criteria in functional dysphonia, *Laryngoscope* 94:1, 1986.
71. Nagata K and others: Vocal fold polyps and nodules: a 10-year review of 1156 patients, *Auris Nasus Larynx* 10:S27, 1983.
72. Narcy P, Contencin P, Viala P: Surgical treatment for laryngeal paralysis in infants and children, *Ann Otol Rhinol Laryngol* 99:124, 1990.
73. Ohlms LA, McGill T, Healy GB: Malignant laryngeal tumors in children: a 15-year experience with four patients, *Ann Otol Rhinol Laryngol* 103:686, 1994.
74. Pontes P, Behlau M: Treatment of sulcus vocalis: auditory, perceptual and acoustical analysis of the slicing mucosa surgical technique, *J Voice* 7:365, 1993.
75. Quiney RG and others: Laryngeal papillomatosis: correlation between severity of disease and presence of HPV 6 and 11 detected by in situ DNA hybridization, *J Clin Pathol* 42:694, 1989.
76. Richter JE: A critical review of current medical therapy for gastroesophageal reflux disease, *J Clin Gastroenterol* 8(suppl 1):72, 1986.
77. Ross DA, Ward PH: Central vocal cord paralysis and paresis presenting as laryngeal stridor in children, *Laryngoscope* 100:10, 1990.
78. Shah K and others: Rarity of cesarean delivery in cases of juvenile onset respiratory papillomatosis, *Laryngoscope* 68:795, 1986.

79. Silberman HD, Wilf H, Tucker JA: Flexible fiberoptic nasopharyngolaryngoscope, *Ann Otol Rhinol Laryngol* 85:640, 1976.
80. Smith RJH, Catlin FI: Congenital anomalies of the larynx, *Am J Dis Child* 138:35, 1984.
81. Smitheran JR, Hixon TJ: A clinical method for estimating laryngeal airway resistance during vowel production, *J Speech Hear Disord* 46: 138, 1981.
82. Strong MS and others: Recurrent respiratory papillomatosis: management with the CO_2 laser, *Ann Otol Rhinol Laryngol* 85:508, 1976.
83. Terry RM and others: Demonstration of human papillomavirus types 6 and 11 in juvenile laryngeal papillomatosis by in situ DNA hybridization, *J Pathol* 153:245, 1987.
84. Thornell WC: Intralaryngeal approach for arytenoidectomy for bilateral abductor vocal cord paralysis, *Arch Otolaryngol Head Neck Surg* 47:505, 1948.
85. Till JA: Computer-assisted evaluation of speech disorders: rationale and directions for future development, *J Comput Use Speech Hear* 6:134, 1990.
86. Toohill, RJ: The psychosomatic aspects of children with vocal nodules, *Arch Otolaryngol Head Neck Surg* 101:591, 1975.
87. Tucker HM: Human laryngeal reinnervation, *Laryngoscope* 86:769, 1976.
88. Tucker HM: Vocal cord paralysis in small children: principles in management, *Ann Otol Rhinol Laryngol* 95:618, 1986.
89. Van Riper C, Irwin JV: *Voice and articulation,* Englewood Cliffs, NJ, 1958, Prentice-Hall.
90. Van Caneghem D: L'etiologie de la corde vocale a sillon, *Annales des malades de l'oreille, du larynx, de nez et du pharynx* 47:121, 1928.
91. Vaughan CW: Current concepts in otolaryngology: diagnosis and treatment of organic voice disorders, *N Engl J Med* 307:863, 1982.
92. von Leden HV: Vocal nodules in children, *Ear Nose Throat J* 64: 473, 1985.
93. Ward PH and others: Contact ulcers and granulomas of the larynx: new insights into their etiology as a basis for more rational treatment, *Otolaryngol Head Neck Surg* 88:262, 1980.
94. Warren DW: Perci: a method for rating palatal efficiency, *Cleft Palate J* 16:279, 1979.
95. Werkhaven J, Ossoff RH: Surgery for benign lesions of the glottis, *Otolaryngol Clin North Am* 24:1179, 1991.
96. Wilson DK: Management of voice disorders in children and adolescents, *Semin Speech Lang* 4:245, 1983.
97. Wilson DK: *Voice problems of children,* ed 3, Baltimore, 1987, Williams & Wilkins.
98. Woo P and others: Endoscopic microsuture repair of vocal fold defects, *J Voice* 9:332, 1995.
99. Woodman D: A modification of the extralaryngeal approach to arytenoidectomy for bilateral abductor paralysis, *Arch Otolaryngol Head Neck Surg* 43:63, 1946.
100. Woodson GE, Miller RH: The timing of surgical intervention in vocal cord paralysis, *Otolaryngol Head Neck Surg* 89:264, 1981.
101. Zalzal GH, Cotton RT, Bove K: Carcinoma of the larynx in a child, *Int J Pediatr Otorhinolaryngol* 13:219, 1987.
102. Zalzal GH: Posterior glottic fixation in children, *Ann Otol Rhinol Laryngol* 102:680, 1993.

Chapter 21

Congenital Disorders of the Trachea

Gerald B. Healy
Cheryl S. Cotter

Anomalies of the trachea can become apparent at any age and can range from complete agenesis to minor malformations that are completely asymptomatic. The tracheal lumen can be compressed externally or can be narrowed by an intrinsic developmental abnormality. Most infants with significant anomalies present with stridor and respiratory symptoms in the perinatal period. Classically, biphasic stridor with a marked expiratory component is described. Associated symptoms may include cough, wheezing, episodic cyanosis, apnea, recurrent pneumonia, atypical or repeated croup, and feeding difficulties. Hyperextension of the neck may reflect an attempt by the patient to straighten the airway (e.g., in vascular compressions of the trachea).

Initial evaluation of the patient with minimal respiratory distress should include flexible laryngoscopy because laryngeal anomalies can accompany any tracheal abnormality. Careful evaluation of the laryngeal anatomy and dynamics is warranted.

Information regarding airway anatomy can be obtained through anteroposterior and lateral radiographs of the neck and chest. Contrast fluoroscopy of the upper aerodigestive tract should be considered in a patient with feeding difficulties. Abnormalities of the esophagus may help diagnose vascular compressions, tracheoesophageal fistulas, and neurologic conditions leading to aspiration or pharyngeal discoordination. Computed tomography (CT) and magnetic resonance imaging (MRI) delineate intrathoracic anatomy. Despite the availability of many radiographic techniques, most patients with suspected airway pathology should undergo complete assessment with rigid endoscopy (Table 21-1). Tracheal anomalies include agenesis or atresia, stenosis, deformities, and tumors.

TRACHEAL AGENESIS OR ATRESIA

Tracheal agenesis is a rare anomaly in which there is no continuity between the larynx and bronchi. The trachea may be completely or partially absent, and the infant may survive a short time if there is a connection between the esophagus and bronchi for the passage of air.[13] The condition is ultimately fatal, and no suitable options are available for tracheal prostheses or transplants.

TRACHEAL WEBS

A tracheal web is usually a thin band of tissue spanning the tracheal lumen without deformity of the underlying cartilage. Management depends on the thickness and firmness of the web. Most webs are amenable to dilation or laser transection. Resection and reanastomosis are reserved for thicker and longer strictures.

TRACHEAL STENOSIS

Congenital tracheal stenosis is a rare but serious anomaly often associated with anomalies of the respiratory tract, esophagus, cardiovascular system, and skeleton.[2] The association with H-type tracheoesophageal fistula, pulmonary hypoplasia, and vascular sling is well documented.[2,6,12] Recent literature has shown an association between midtracheal stenosis (hourglass trachea) and trisomy 21 (Down syndrome).[17]

Malformation of the trachea is most commonly secondary

A

B

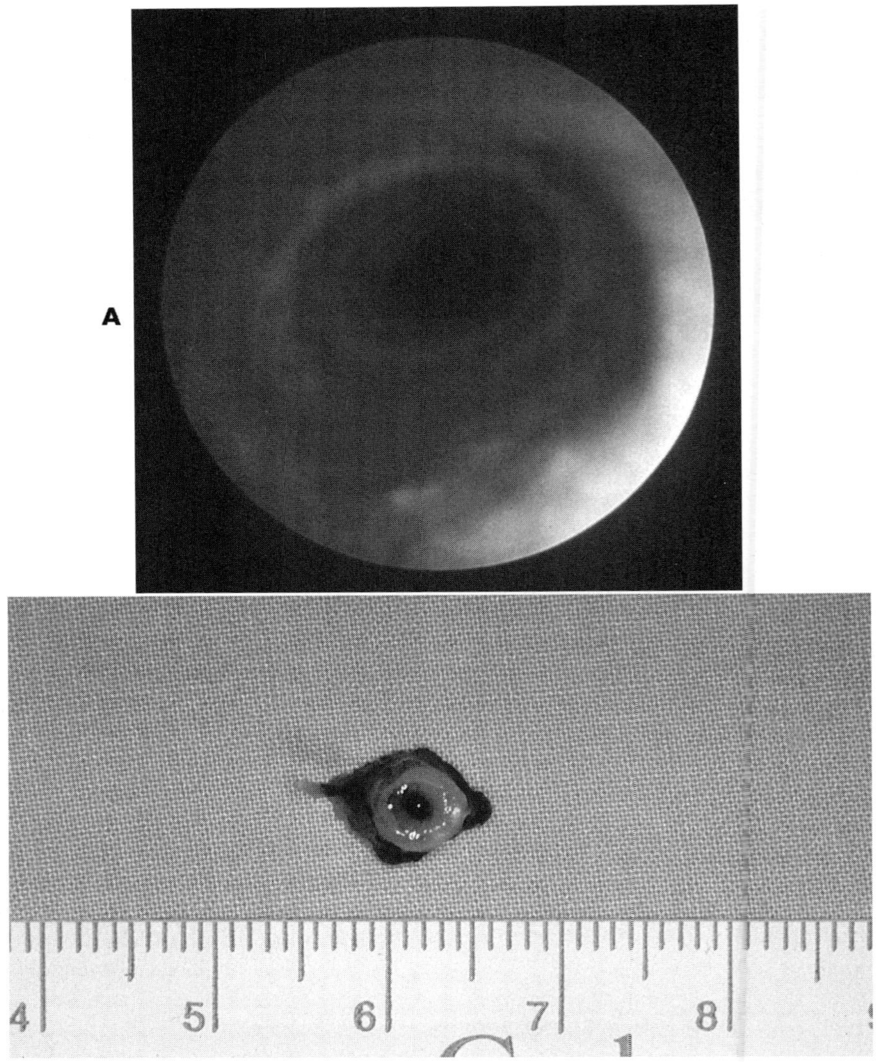

Fig. 21-1. A, Endoscopic view of tracheal stenosis caused by complete tracheal rings. **B,** A surgical specimen of the trachea shows segmental stenosis secondary to complete tracheal rings. Note the internal diameter of the airway of 2 mm.

Table 21-1. Evaluation of congenital tracheal lesions

Symptoms
Stridor, classically biphasic
Wheezing
Recurrent pneumonia, bronchitis, or croup
Cyanosis
Apnea or dying spells
Diagnosis
Auscultation
Flexible fiberoptic laryngoscopy
Anteroposterior and lateral neck films and chest radiography
Barium esophagography
Rigid endoscopy
Computed tomography or magnetic resonance imaging: intrathoracic anatomy

to complete tracheal rings. Tracheal cartilage is smaller than normal and nonflexible, and the trachea lacks the posterior membranous portion (Fig. 21-1 *A, B*). In 1964, Cantrell and Guild[5] classified the morphology of congenital tracheal stenosis as segmental stenosis, funnel-shaped stenosis, and generalized hypoplasia (Fig. 21-2).

Symptoms usually are present in the neonatal period and reflect the severity of the tracheal and often associated bronchial stenosis (Box 21-1). Some patients have distress at birth, whereas others develop symptoms months later, often precipitated by an upper respiratory infection. The presenting symptoms include stridor, cyanosis, apnea, wheezing, recurrent pneumonia, and recurrent or atypical croup or bronchitis. The expiratory phase of respiration is usually prolonged. In patients who are intubated for respiratory distress, the presence of an endotracheal tube may lead to further airway obstruction if granulation tissue or edema forms at the tip of the tube. Removal of the endotracheal tube

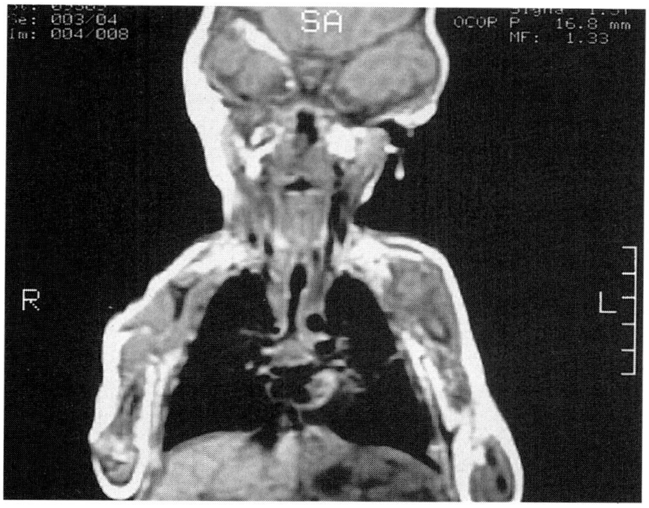

Fig. 21-2. Magnetic resonance imaging shows funnel-shaped tracheal stenosis in an infant with Pfeiffer's syndrome. Note the normal caliber of the upper third of the trachea.

Box 21-1. Evaluation of tracheal stenosis

Symptoms

Respiratory distress
Cyanosis
Biphasic stridor with prolonged expiratory phase
Wheezing
Recurrent or atypical croup or bronchitis
Rule out associated anomalies, including tracheoesophageal fistula, pulmonary hypoplasia, vascular sling, and trisomy 21

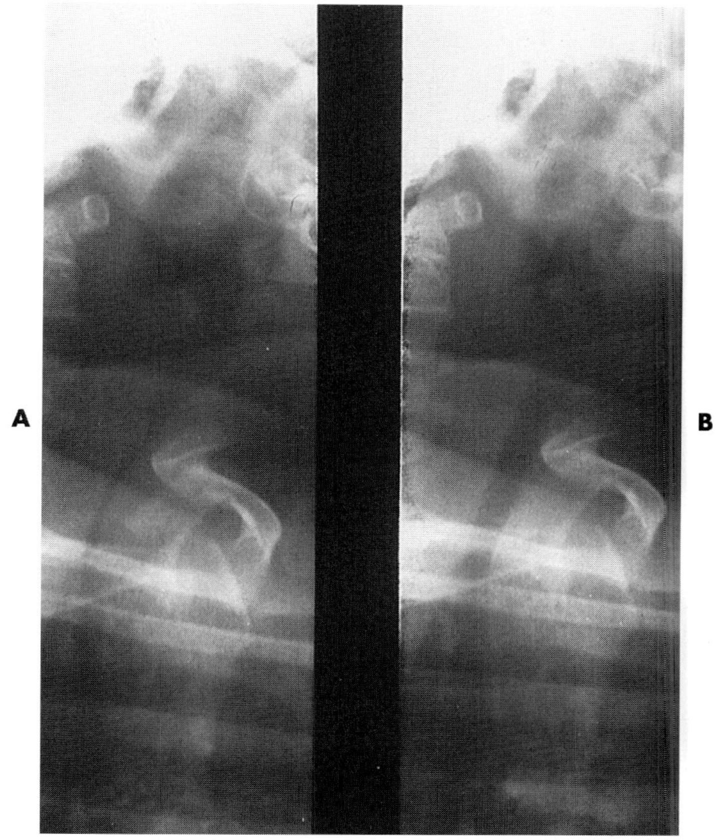

Fig. 21-3. Lateral chest radiography shows tracheomalacia. **A,** Expiratory radiography shows anteroposterior collapse of the trachea with a resultant tracheal lumen of 8 mm. **B,** Inspiratory radiography shows a more normal tracheal lumen.

should be performed as early as possible, maximizing medical therapy with humidification of inspired air, chest physiotherapy, antireflux measures, corticosteroids, and antibiotics, if appropriate.

Endoscopic assessment of the airway is the best method to diagnose and characterize the suspected congenital tracheal stenosis. The procedure is best performed under general anesthesia with rigid instrumentation.[10] Even in ideal conditions, the procedure should be carried out with great caution. In severe stenoses, the smallest bronchoscope often cannot be advanced, and evaluation requires the apneic technique using small 2.2-mm telescopes without a ventilating sheath. Examination of the lower trachea and bronchi is important for surgical planning and prognosis. If the nature of the stenosis cannot be ascertained endoscopically, contrast tracheobronchography can be considered, although this technique carries a potential risk of airway obstruction associated with the contrast material. CT and MRI can be used in conjunction with endoscopy to identify intrathoracic relationships and associated anomalies. Several studies have shown the ability of three-dimensional CT and MRI to describe tracheal and bronchial anatomy.[14,15]

In many cases, conservative management is possible. Severe stenoses have been managed with resection and reanastomosis of short segment lesions and tracheoplasty for more diffuse lesions. Tracheoplasty with autologous grafts using costal cartilage or pericardium facilitated by cardiopulmonary bypass is currently the preferred surgical technique. Prognosis is based on the degree of distal tracheal and bronchial disease and on associated anomalies. Mortality ranges from 20% to 80% in the recent literature.[8,12,19]

TRACHEOMALACIA

Tracheomalacia is a weakness of the tracheal wall resulting in marked exaggeration of movement with respiration. With forced respiration, crying, or coughing, the posterior membranous tracheal wall approximates the anterior wall and may touch it, reducing the tracheal lumen. Tracheomalacia can often be diagnosed with airway fluoroscopy (Fig. 21-3). Histologically, deficient cartilage and increased width of the membranous tracheal wall result in less cartilage sup-

Box 21-2. Evaluation of tracheomalacia

Symptoms

Expiratory stridor, wheezing
Brassy, barking cough
Hyperextension of neck
Reflex apnea, dying spells
Rule out vascular compression and congenital cardiovascular disease

port, allowing the wide, floppy posterior wall to balloon forward with expiration.

Primary tracheomalacia is a rare congenital deformity of the tracheal rings that can be seen in premature infants, in otherwise healthy full-term infants, and in infants with connective tissue disorders. Secondary tracheomalacia occurs with external compression of the trachea (e.g., in vascular anomalies, after surgical repair of tracheoesophageal fistula).[3]

The clinical presentation typically includes expiratory stridor, often reminiscent of asthmatic wheezing, and varying degrees of respiratory distress. The cough may have a peculiar barking quality, and the neck may be hyperextended. Patients with severe tracheomalacia may have dramatic episodes of respiratory or cardiac arrest, termed *reflex apnea* or *dying spells* (Box 21-2).[9]

Primary tracheomalacia

Premature infants with respiratory distress syndrome at birth are often managed with prolonged endotracheal intubation and ventilation. Tracheal enlargement and distension may be an acquired condition secondary to prolonged positive pressure ventilation. Mature infants may have similar presentation in the first few weeks of life, suggesting a congenital tracheomalacia. In both groups, diagnosis can be made with rigid endoscopy showing the characteristic findings of a widened posterior wall with expiratory collapse (Fig. 21-4). Endoscopy should be performed with the patient breathing spontaneously because positive pressure ventilation may mask the severity of the collapse. The condition usually improves with growth; most symptoms resolving by 18 to 24 months of age. Tracheotomy with or without continuous positive airway pressure is sometimes required to stent the airway in severe cases.

Secondary tracheomalacia

Tracheomalacia is a major cause of pulmonary complications after surgical repair of tracheoesophageal fistula and esophageal atresia. Symptoms can be mild to severe. Rigid endoscopy reveals tracheal cartilages having indented semicircular rather than the normal horseshoe shape and a wide posterior membranous wall, which narrows the anteroposterior lumen (Fig. 21-5).[3] These abnormalities typically affect the lower third of the trachea.

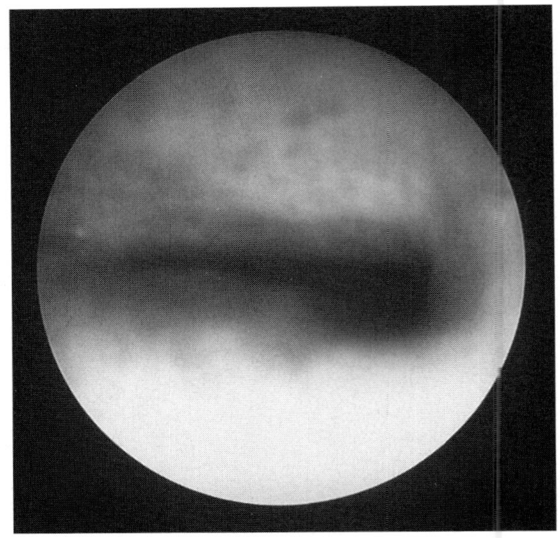

Fig. 21-4. Endoscopic view of tracheomalacia. There is a widened posterior wall with collapse of the tracheal lumen.

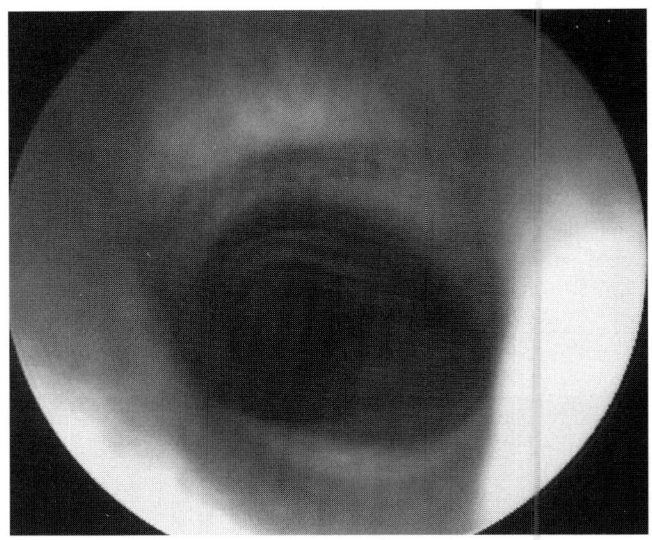

Fig. 21-5. Endoscopic view of tracheomalacia in a patient who underwent repair of a tracheoesophageal fistula. Note the indented semicircular rather than normal horseshoe shape of the tracheal cartilages.

Innominate artery compression of the trachea can result in secondary tracheomalacia, which involves a shorter segment of the trachea than does tracheoesophageal fistula. The posterior membranous trachea may be normal in appearance.

External compression of the trachea by vascular anomalies can result in a localized area of tracheal wall, which remains weak after surgical removal of the cause. This area may be subject to collapse with increased intrathoracic pressure. Rarely, surgical suspension of the weakened area is required if the patient has severe symptoms, (e.g. dying spells). The condition usually resolves in months to years as the area becomes firm.

DEFORMITY CAUSED BY VASCULAR ANOMALIES

Malformations of the heart and great vessels can result in compression of the trachea or esophagus. The more severe the compression, the earlier the symptoms present. The patient is often prone to recurrent respiratory infections resulting from difficult clearing of secretions past the narrowed area. Infection accentuates the symptoms, which are often described as expiratory wheezing and a brassy, barking cough. The patient may lie with the head extended, putting the trachea on stretch, to lift the compressing vessel forward. Difficulty with feeding occurs with vascular rings caused by esophageal compression. Laryngomalacia is common in patients with tracheobronchial compression by vascular anomalies.[10]

The terms *reflex apnea* and *dying spells* describe dramatic episodes of respiratory arrest and cyanosis, usually with spontaneous recovery.[9] These attacks occur in patients with tracheobronchial compression caused by congenital cardiovascular anomalies. Reflex apnea is present in many patients with double aortic arch and innominate artery compression and is an indication for surgical correction.[9]

Radiography of the chest is used in conjunction with contrast esophagography to delineate the compression. The vascular anomaly may completely encircle the trachea and esophagus, producing obstruction, or may compress the anterior wall of the trachea alone. CT and MRI[15] can delineate vascular compression of the tracheobronchial tree (Fig. 21-6). Rigid and flexible laryngoscopy, bronchoscopy, and esophagoscopy are essential to assess the degree of compression and associated laryngotracheomalacia.

Innominate artery compression

Innominate artery compression of the trachea occurs when the artery arises more to the left than usual, passing from left to right and compressing the anterior wall of the trachea. It is the most common cause of vascular compression of the tracheobronchial tree.[9] Signs and symptoms gradually disappear over months to years in most patients. The esophagogram is normal. Chest radiography may show persistent indentation of the anterior trachea at the thoracic inlet in the lateral projection (Fig. 21-7).

Bronchoscopy reveals an anterior, pulsatile compression of the trachea, running obliquely downward from right to left, approximately 2 cm from the carina. Pressure with the tip of the bronchoscope may decrease the right radial and temporal pulses, not altering the left radial pulse. Tracheal compression is more pronounced in the expiratory phase, often obliterating the tracheal lumen when the child coughs.

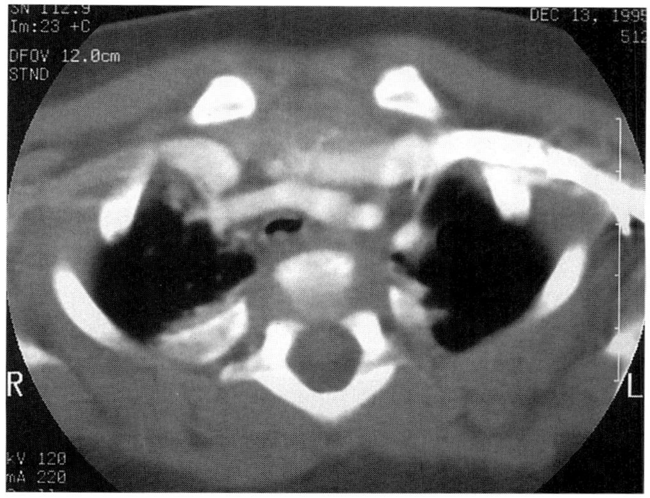

Fig. 21-6. Computed tomography of the chest shows anterior tracheal compression by an aberrant innominate artery. The innominate artery is arising more from the left than usual, resulting in anterior tracheal compression. This patient presented with wheezing and reflex apnea.

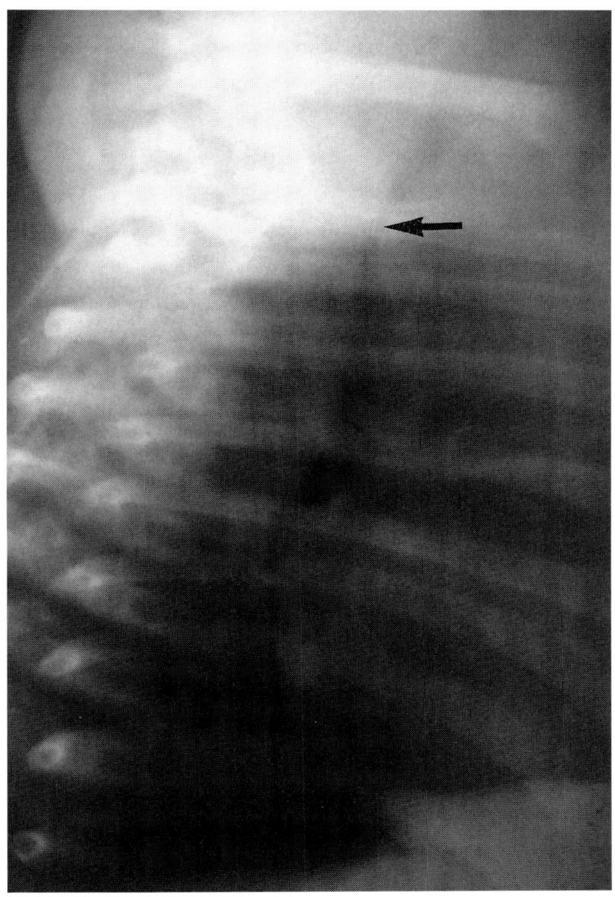

Fig. 21-7. Lateral chest radiography shows innominate artery compression of the anterior trachea at the thoracic inlet.

In patients with severe symptoms or reflex apnea, aortopexy is indicated to suspend the aortic arch (with its attachment to the anterior tracheal wall) to the sternum. This relieves the vascular compression and suspends the weakened trachea.

Double aortic arch

Double aortic arch, also known as the *complete vascular ring*, encircles the trachea and esophagus and joins to form the descending aorta. It is the second most common cause of vascular compression of the tracheobronchial tree.[9] Diagnosis can be made with contrast fluoroscopy, which characteristically shows posterior esophageal compression (Fig. 21-8). Usually one arch is larger, although both may be the same size. Bronchoscopy reveals anterior and posterior pulsatile compression of the trachea just above the carina, usually involving one or both main bronchi. Compression with the bronchoscope does not affect the radial pulse. Management consists of division of the smaller arch.

Right aortic arch

With a right aortic arch, the aorta courses over the right main bronchus, to the right of the trachea, curving downward to lie just right of the midline posteriorly. It can be similar to a vascular ring if a persistent ligamentum arteriosum or ductus arteriosum is present. There is usually mild anterior pulsatile compression of the trachea, anteriorly near the carina, with marked compression of the right main bronchus. Alternatively, there can be anterior tracheal compression by the left subclavian artery. Compression with the bronchoscope has little effect on the peripheral pulses. Management consists of division of the ligamentum arteriosum or ductus arteriosum to relieve the obstruction.

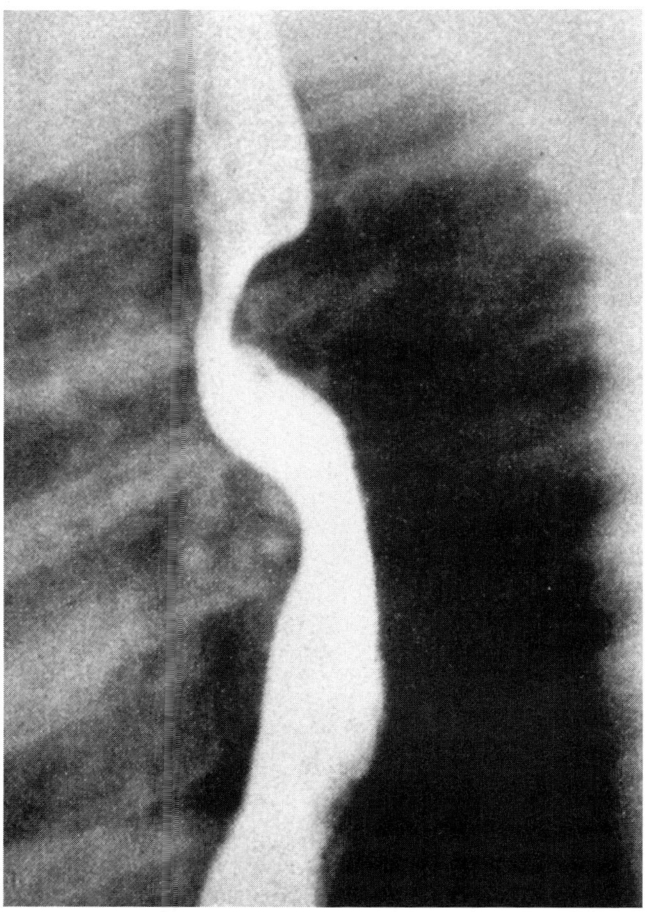

Fig. 21-8. Contrast esophagography shows posterior esophageal compression by a double aortic arch.

Anomalous subclavian artery

An aberrant right subclavian artery passes behind the esophagus causing posterior compression of the esophagus seen on contrast esophagography. There are usually no airway symptoms. Dysphagia, termed *dysphagia lusoria*, can occur if esophageal compression is significant. Anomalous subclavian arteries have also been reported to cause anterior tracheal compression or to pass between the trachea and esophagus.

Pulmonary artery sling

The aberrant left pulmonary artery, termed the *pulmonary artery sling*, arises from the right pulmonary artery, curves to the right, and passes between the trachea and esophagus to the left lung. Compression of the posterior trachea and anterior esophagus by a mass separating the two is diagnostic of this condition. There is a strong association with tracheal stenosis resulting from complete cartilaginous rings.[6] If the trachea is normal, there is usually marked compression of the right main bronchus. Surgical reanastomosis of the aberrant vessel may not relieve the respiratory symptoms unless the tracheal abnormality is addressed.

Pulmonary artery dilation

Dilated, hypertensive pulmonary arteries in association with cardiac defects with large left-to-right shunts can result in compression of the trachea and bronchi. Cardiac anomalies that predispose to this condition are ventricular septal defect, patent ductus arteriosus, interrupted aortic arch, and tetrology of Fallot.[4] The dilated pulmonary arteries can cause bronchial compression directly or can displace the aorta against the left wall of the trachea. Left atrial enlargement in conjunction with dilated pulmonary arteries pushes on both bronchi, worsening the compression. Pulmonary arteriopexy may relieve the compression.

TRACHEOESOPHAGEAL FISTULA

Tracheoesophageal fistula can occur in various forms, the most common of which is proximal esophageal atresia with distal tracheoesophageal fistula. A less common form is the H-type fistula, in which a small communication exists between the upper trachea and upper third of the esophagus. There may be an association with other severe anomalies vertebral, anal, cardiac, tracheal, esophageal, renal, and limb anomalies (VACTERL) of the cardiovascular, genitourinary, and musculoskeletal systems.

Tracheoesophageal fistula should be suspected in the infant who has difficulty with feeding, aspiration, and respiratory distress soon after birth. The infant with esophageal atresia has severe problems with mucous and aspiration and may develop fatal problems if fed. Infants with H-type fistula are often the least symptomatic because only small amounts of secretions are diverted into the trachea to cause symptoms (Box 21-3).

Box 21-3. Evaluation of tracheoesophageal fistula

Symptoms

Aspiration, coughing, apnea, or respiratory distress with feeding

Failure to pass a feeding catheter beyond the upper esophagus

H-type fistula may be relatively asymptomatic

Rule out associated anomalies of the cardiovascular, genitourinary, and musculoskeletal systems (vertebral, anal, cardiac, tracheal, esophageal, renal and limb anomalies).

Esophageal atresia can be diagnosed by failure to pass a catheter beyond the upper esophagus or by contrast esophagography. Care is taken to avoid aspiration of contrast by instilling only a small amount of thin radioopaque material through a small feeding tube placed distal to the larynx in the esophagus. In a small H-type fistula, contrast esophagography may be repeatedly negative (Fig. 21-9, *A*). Bronchoscopy may be necessary to identify the opening in the posterior membranous wall of the trachea. Cannulation of the depression confirms the connection to the esophagus and facilitates surgical repair of the fistula (Fig. 21-9, *B*). Management includes surgical repair and, often, dilation of esophageal strictures at the site of the anastomosis.

Postoperatively, patients often have symptoms of tracheomalacia, esophageal dysmotility, and gastroesophageal reflux. Tracheomalacia is related to tracheal cartilages having an indented semicircular rather than a normal horseshoe shape and a wide, flaccid, posterior membranous wall.[13] Most respiratory symptoms resolve with time.

A

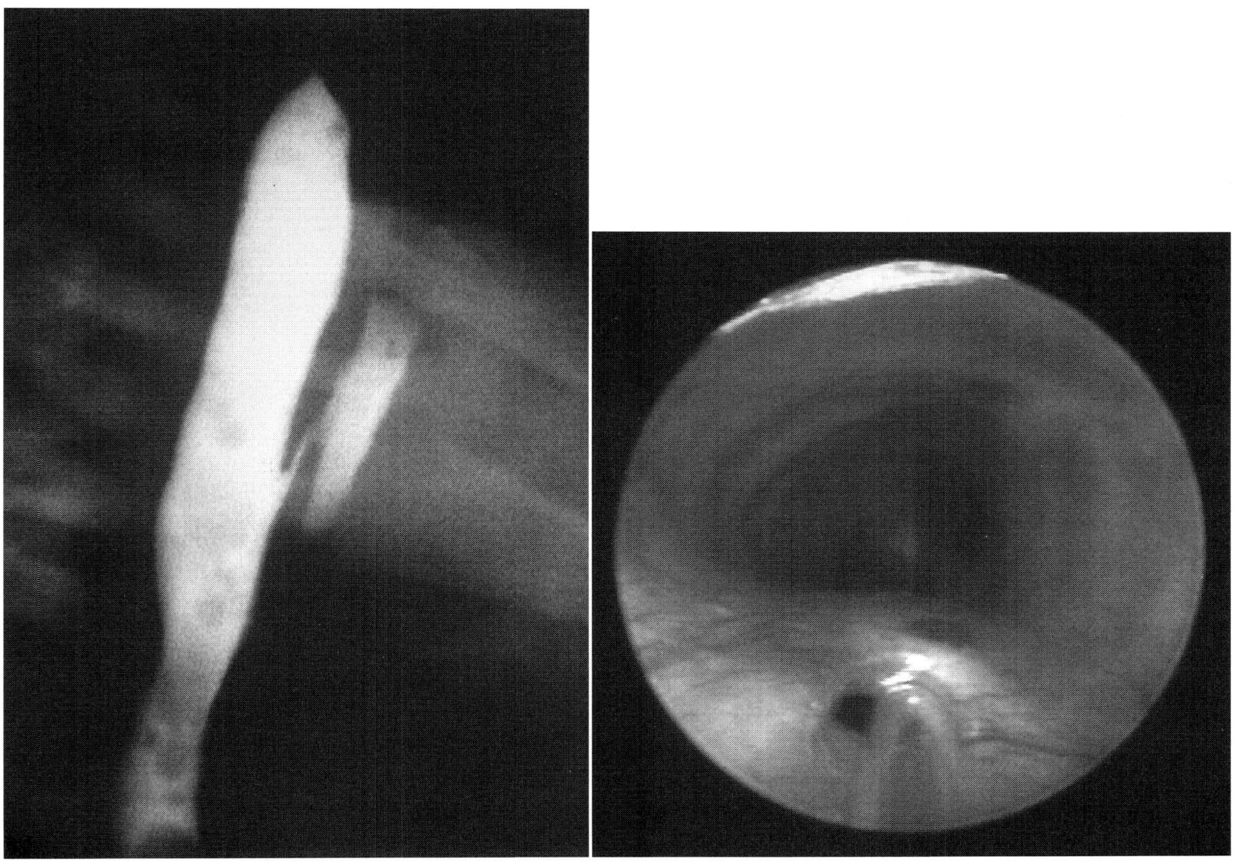

B

Fig. 21-9. A, Contrast esophagography shows an H-type tracheoesophageal fistula. Note retrograde flow of contrast into the trachea. **B,** Endoscopic view of the same patient before repair of the fistula. Cannulation of the fistula confirms connection to the esophagus.

TRACHEAL ENLARGEMENT

Congenital enlargement of the trachea is extremely rare. It has been associated with Mounier-Kuhn syndrome, an atrophy or absence of elastic fibers of the muscle of the trachea and bronchi, allowing for flaccidity and marked dilation.[16,18] Tracheal enlargement has also been associated with bronchiectasis or other organomegaly.

TRACHEAL EVAGINATION

Tracheogenic cysts are evaginations of the primitive trachea similar to bronchogenic cysts. They can be located anywhere from the trachea to the carina and can contain any elements of the tracheobronchial wall.[7,11] They can be asymptomatic or can cause respiratory symptoms based on their location and airway compression. Radiography may show a cystic mass in the mediastinum and airway deviation. Bronchoscopy may be necessary to determine the degree of airway obstruction. Management is with surgical excision to remove the cyst and alleviate the airway distortion.

ABNORMAL TRACHEAL BIFURCATION

Abnormal bifurcation of the trachea is common. This occurs when the takeoff of the bronchus is above the level of the carina. It is most common on the right side and can be associated with recurrent pneumonias. The right upper lobe bronchus gives rise to three normal divisions in most cases. Rarely, complete duplication of the right upper bronchus and lobe is seen.[11] Most patients are asymptomatic. Treatment is not usually necessary.[16]

REFERENCES

1. Benjamin B: Endoscopy in esophageal atresia and tracheoesophageal fistula, *Ann Otol Rhinol Laryngol* 90:376, 1981.
2. Benjamin B, Pitkin J, Cohen D: Congenital tracheal stenosis, *Ann Otol Rhinol Laryngol* 90:364, 1981.
3. Benjamin B: Tracheomalacia in infants and children, *Ann Otol Rhinol Laryngol* 93:438, 1984.
4. Berlinger NT and others: Tracheobronchial compression in acyanotic congenital heart disease, *Ann Otol Rhinol Laryngol* 92:387, 1983.
5. Cantrell JR, Guild HG: Congenital stenosis of the trachea, *Am J Surg* 108:297, 1964.
6. Cohen SR, Landing BH: Tracheostenosis and bronchial abnormalities associated with pulmonary artery sling, *Ann Otol Rhinol Laryngol* 85: 582, 1976.
7. Cohen SR and others: Foregut cysts in infants and children: diagnosis and management, *Ann Otol Rhinol Laryngol* 91:622, 1982.
8. Dunham M and others: Management of severe congenital tracheal stenosis, *Ann Otol Rhinol Laryngol* 103:351, 1994.
9. Fearon B, Shortreed R: Tracheobronchial compression by congenital cardiovascular anomalies in children: syndrome of apnea, *Ann Otol Rhinol Laryngol* 72:949, 1963.
10. Healy GB: *Congenital anomalies of the aerodigestive tract.* In Bailey BJ, editor: *Head and neck surgery*: otolaryngology, Philadelphia, 1993, JB Lippincott.
11. Holinger PH and others: Congenital malformation of the trachea, bronchi, and lung, *Ann Otol Rhinol Laryngol* 61:1159, 1952.
12. Loeff DS and others: Congenital tracheal stenosis: a review of 22 patients from 1965 to 1987, *J Pediatr Surg* 23:744, 1988.
13. Manschot HJ, van den Anker JN, Tibboel D: Tracheal agenesis, *Anesthesia* 49:788, 1994.
14. Manson D and others: Three-dimensional imaging of the pediatric trachea in congenital tracheal stenosis, *Pediatr Radiol* 24:175, 1994.
15. Myer CM III and others: Magnetic resonance imaging in the diagnosis of innominate artery compression of the trachea, *Arch Otolaryngol Head Neck Surg* 116:314, 1990.
16. Schild JA: *Congenital malformations of the trachea and bronchi.* In Bluestone C, Stool S, Kenna N, editors: *Pediatric otolaryngology*, ed 3, Philadelphia, 1996, WB Saunders.
17. Wells TR and others: Association of Down syndrome and segmental tracheal stenosis with ring tracheal cartilages: a review of nine cases, *Pediatr Pathol* 12:673, 1992.
18. Woodring JH, Howard RS II, Rehm SR: Congenital tracheobronchomegaly (Mounier-Kuhn syndrome): a report of 10 cases and review of the literature, *J Thorac Imaging* 6:1, 1991.
19. Yamaguchi M and others: Concomitant repair of congenital tracheal stenosis and complex cardiac anomaly in small children, *J Thorac Cardiovasc Surg* 100:181, 1990.

Chapter 22

Tracheal Stenosis

Mark A. Richardson
Greg R. Licameli

Diagnosis and surgical management of tracheal stenosis, whether acquired or congenital, remain a challenge. In infants and children, tracheal stenosis is frequently a fatal disease process that is often associated with other congenital anomalies and in which definitive means of surgical repair are poorly defined for patients with the most severe disease. Diagnosis, evaluation, and development of a logical management plan for a patient with tracheal stenosis are complex.

EMBRYOLOGY

The trachea develops as an evagination of foregut mesochyme in the fourth week of gestation. This gradually expands caudally to form the developing lungs and joins together posteriorly to form the common membranous wall of the esophagus and trachea. Initially this evagination has an extensive communication with the ventrocaudal part of the pharynx. From this primordial outgrowth the trachea extends caudad ventral to and roughly parallel with the esophagus. Only the epithelial lining and the glands of the trachea are derived from the original entodermal outgrowth from the pharynx. The cartilage, connective tissue, and muscle of its wall are formed by mesenchymal cells that migrate to become massed around the growing entodermal tube. Usually by the ninth week developing cartilaginous rings can be identified.

DIAGNOSIS

The severity of tracheal stenosis probably determines the age at presentation, which can be quite variable, ranging from days to weeks or even months. A long-segment stenosis with a markedly limited tracheal diameter would ordinarily present in early infancy with evidence of respiratory obstruction, especially when the airway may be compromised by additional secretions or infection, which produce additional incremental difficulties in adequate respiration (Fig. 22-1). Shorter segments, with a more moderate degree of obstruction in terms of tracheal diameter, may present later in infancy or early childhood when the increasing respiratory demands of growing infants outstrip the capacity of the narrow airway to provide adequate levels of air and gas exchange (Fig. 22-2).

Any child who is being considered for bronchoscopy and who has atypical asthma, inspiratory and expiratory stridor, and recurrent respiratory disease should also have a potential diagnosis of tracheal stenosis. Poor weight gain and sometimes poor feeding are also associated with tracheal stenosis. Chest radiography may be helpful but is often nondiagnostic due to the dynamic aspects of the pediatric trachea. In some cases, however, a suggestion of the stenosis may be evident on close examination of the radiograph.

Endoscopy

Endoscopic evaluation with a rigid bronchoscope is clearly the most accurate means of diagnosing tracheal stenosis and assessing its length, degree, and character. Due to the limited diameter of the trachea, however, endoscopy must be approached expertly and with full availability of the smallest equipment possible. In some cases placement of an endotracheal tube through the larynx to the level of the stenosis may in fact cause a loss of ventilatory capability as a result of obstruction of the tube at the site of the stenosis. Additionally, even the smallest bronchoscope (4-mm outer diameter) may not pass through the stenosis and, in some cases, the telescope alone may be the only means of visualization of the length of the stenosis and identification of any distal abnormalities in the tracheobronchial tree. The length

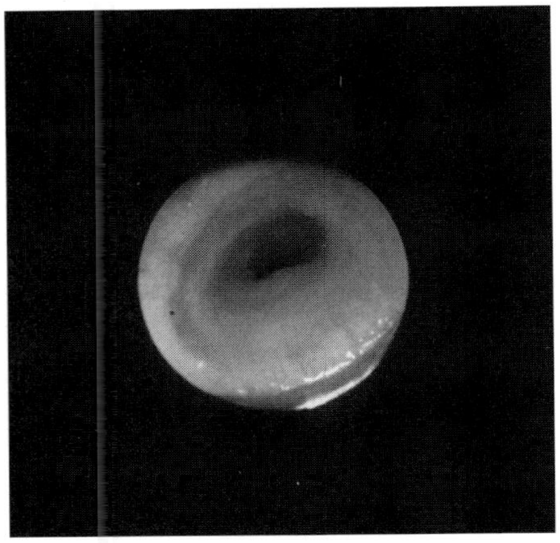

Fig. 22-1. Long-segment tracheal stenosis (complete rings).

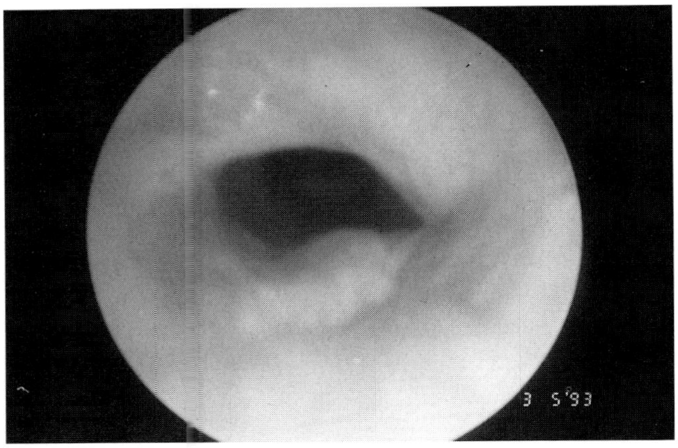

Fig. 22-2. Short-segment tracheal stenosis.

of the stenotic segment should always be estimated during the course of endoscopy, and is frequently underestimated. Commonly, the congenital stenotic tracheal segment is associated with a somewhat longer trachea than the native and normal trachea of newborns.

Endoscopic evaluation of the airway with rigid instrumentation with the patient under general anesthetia is, however, accompanied by the greatest risk and requires skilled anesthesia, expert endoscopic skills, and a full complement of pediatric endoscopic instruments and photographic documentation capability. Once the patient has been given general anesthesia, additional anesthesia can be obtained by using lidocaine topically to the tracheal mucosa. Hopefully the patient has been able to maintain spontaneous ventilation so that the adequacy of neuromuscular movement in the larynx can be assessed. It is generally wise to use the telescope as an initial form of evaluation without the accompanying bronchoscope for tracheoscopy to identify whether there is a significant stenosis, its approximate location, and the nature of the tracheal rings (i.e., whether they are complete or incomplete). In some cases, even the smallest 2.5-mm pediatric bronchoscope (4-mm outer diameter) will not pass through the stricture, and again the 2.2-mm bronchoscopic telescope may be the only instrument able to pass through the stenosis to visualize the carina and distal bronchi. Obviously, the patient must be hyperventilated in order to permit such an examination, but in doing so the length of the trachea affected can be gauged and a potential surgical procedure designed.

At the completion of the endoscopic evaluation, some conclusion should be reached as to the actual nature of the stenosis as well as the degree of involvement of the trachea and main bronchi. The determination that a tracheal stenosis is congenital versus acquired is an important one. Congenital problems are often associated with other abnormalities of vascular structure and genetic defects. Acquired stenoses are accompanied by irregular scarring, perichondritis, and loss of cartilaginous support, which complicate surgical resection and reanastomosis.

Radiology

Computed tomography and magnetic resonance imaging (MRI) provide accurate evaluations of the airway, with magnetic resonance images having a slight edge as to detail and the actual nature of the stenosis. There is of course an inherent risk for infants, who may require sedation or general anesthesia in order to accomplish the examination.

Because some cases of congenital tracheal stenosis are often associated with a vascular ring or pulmonary artery sling, some means of determining whether there are abnormalities in the great vessels of the heart should be performed. Cardiac ultrasound examination or MRI may be satisfactory in some cases, although arteriography or heart catheterization may be necessary in order to fully identify or rule out the possibility of aberrant vasculature.

If additional information must be obtained, contrast bronchography may be performed with a thin solution of contrast material in order to outline the tracheal dimensions and bronchial branchings. This contrast material must be thinned because the secretions themselves and inflammation—which is sometimes stimulated by the contrast—may cause significant problems in ventilation for the patient. Despite the inherent danger in contrast bronchography, it does provide a measurable evaluation of long-segment tracheal stenosis and any accompanying bronchial abnormalities, which are often seen in congenital stenoses.

SURGERY

Surgery for tracheal stenosis can be categorized generally in the following way: (1) endoscopic, using laser or dilation; (2) resection and reanastomosis, including slide tracheoplasty; or (3) augmentive procedures using cartilage, perichondrium, or vascularized tissue.

Surgical management involves two options: endoscopic

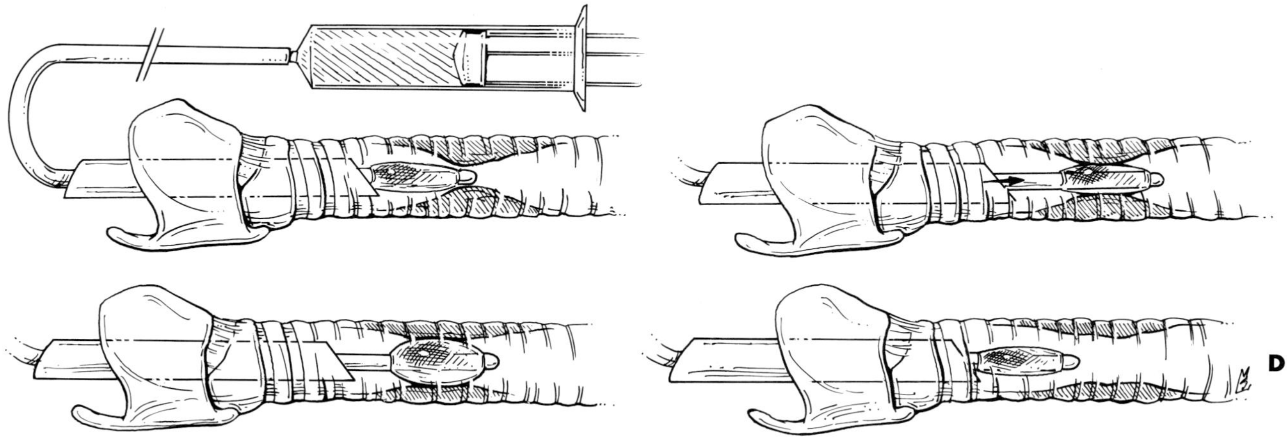

Fig. 22-3. **A** to **D**, Pneumatic dilation of short-segment, acquired stenosis.

tracheoplasty and open tracheal reconstruction. Endoscopic options include tracheal dilation, intraluminal stent placement, and laser ablation. Biopsies may be performed if there is suspicion of systemic disease such as amyloidosis or sarcoidosis. Open tracheal reconstruction may include the use of autologous, homologous, or inert stenting material to enlarge the airway diameter or to remove stenotic segments. The morbidity of an endoscopic approach is less than that of an open procedure but often involves repeated surgeries. Selection of a therapeutic approach depends on the type of airway anomaly and may involve a variety of endoscopic modalities either alone or combined with an open approach to the trachea.

Dilation

Dilation of strictures has traditionally been performed with Jackson or Maloney rigid dilators. This method involves serial dilation with progressively larger-diameter bougies but has a tendency to shear tissue, which may create more scarring and further stricture formation.[27] In comparison, balloon tracheoplasty imparts only radial forces to the lesion and is less traumatic to the surrounding tissues. Balloon devices range from catheters developed for percutaneous transluminal angioplasty to specially designed balloons that fit over the tip of a rigid bronchoscope. Balloon-tipped catheters are connected to an inline pressure gauge and a water-filled syringe that delivers a steady, constant dilation. Serial dilation is performed with increasingly larger balloons. Balloon-tipped catheters may also be placed under radiologic guidance to confirm placement (Fig. 22-3).[9]

A 15-year experience of balloon tracheoplasty in 37 patients was reported by Hebra, Powell, and Smith.[27] Short-term improvement for both congenital and acquired lesions was seen in 90% of patients, with long-term improvement in 54%. Complications were infrequent and included tracheitis, atelectasis, and pneumomediastinum. This method appears to be most useful in the management of soft granulation tissue or to aid in delaying open reconstruction in premature or medically unstable infants.

Messino and others[42] and Bagwell, Talbert, and Tepas[3] have described aggressive balloon dilation of complete tracheal rings with endotracheal stenting in children younger than 2 years of age. The posterior wall of a complete ring is the weakest point, as demonstrated by their postmortem studies, and allows disruption of the trachea with subsequent fibrotic healing. This method should be reserved for critically ill patients because complications can be life threatening.

Laser therapy

Laser therapy is often combined with dilation procedures in the endoscopic management of tracheal strictures or obstructing masses. Use of the laser allows precise tissue ablation with less trauma to the surrounding tissue compared with cryosurgery and electrocautery.[52] Early reports described the use of the carbon dioxide laser with a bronchoscopic coupler and a rigid bronchoscope to manage tracheal lesions.[53] With the development of improved optics and laser micromanipulators mounted directly to the microscope, visualization and precision have improved. Lesions most amenable to this technique are soft granulation and short segments of mature fibrosis. Simpson and others[52] and Ossoff and others[47,48] listed the following factors as contributing to laser therapy failure: circumferential scarring, fibrosis greater than 1 cm in vertical length, tracheomalacia, and severe bacterial infection in the presence of a tracheostomy.

A method employing radial incisions and dilation with a rigid bronchoscope for moderate to severe subglottic and tracheal stenosis was described by Shapshay and others.[51] Success was attributed to the preservation of islands of epithelium between the radial incisions. Results were good at 1 year follow-up (Fig. 22-4). Mucosal preservation was also advocated by Dedo and Sooy,[12] who described the use of the carbon dioxide laser in the elevation of mucosal flaps.

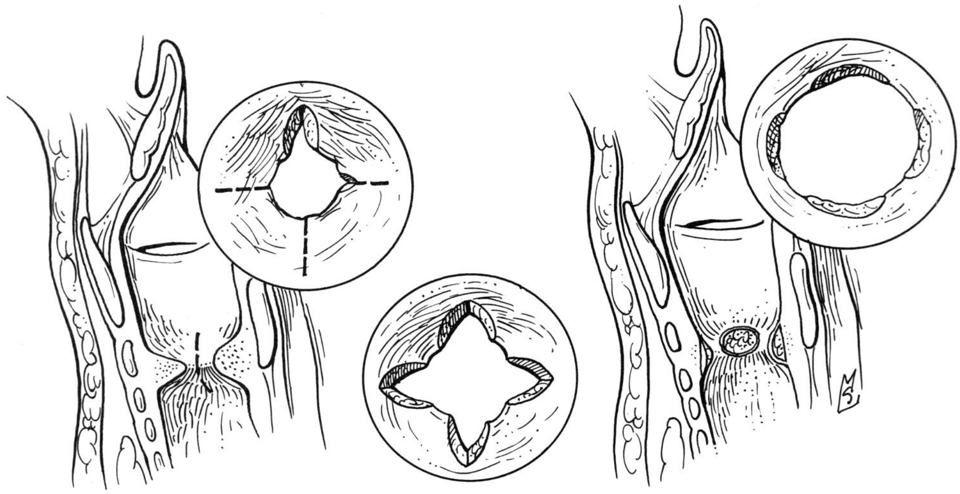

Fig. 22-4. Star-shaped laser incision and dilation (Shapshay).

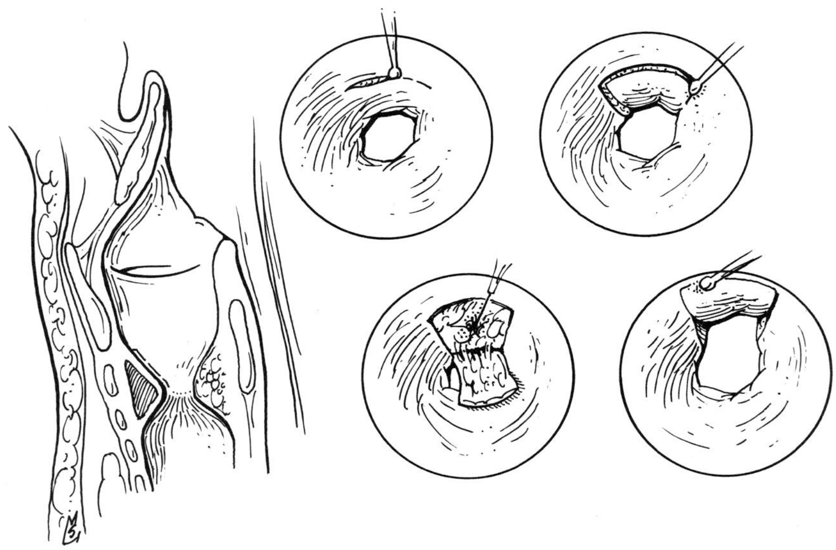

Fig. 22-5. Laser trapdoor flap.

An incision is made into the superior surface of the scar, creating a trapdoor flap, and the underlying fibrous tissue is ablated with the laser with replacement of the mucosal flap (Fig. 22-5). Success with these techniques appears to be dependent on re-epithelialization before scar formation, avoidance of extensive tissue damage, preservation of mucosa, and careful patient selection.

Intralesional and systemic corticosteroids have been suggested by some authors to aid in the prevention of scar formation. However, corticosteroids may act to reduce epithelial migration, increase scar formation, or weaken existing cartilaginous support.[28] Other adjunctive measures include the use of antibiotics and antireflux medications.

Stents

Stents are important in the management of tracheal stenosis and may be employed in either endoscopic or open approaches. Montgomery[44] first described the use of a polymeric silicone (Silastic) T-tube (Boston Medical Products) in 1965. This type of stent allows ventilation, support for soft tissue grafts and cartilage, and tracheal lumen suctioning. This tube is used in conjunction with a tracheostomy and is placed under endoscopic guidance. Maniglia[40] reported on the use of the T-tube stent in 53 adult patients with tracheal stenosis, subglottic stenosis, or both, with good results in 85%. Problems associated with stents include obstruction, granulation tissue formation, infection, and malposition.

A

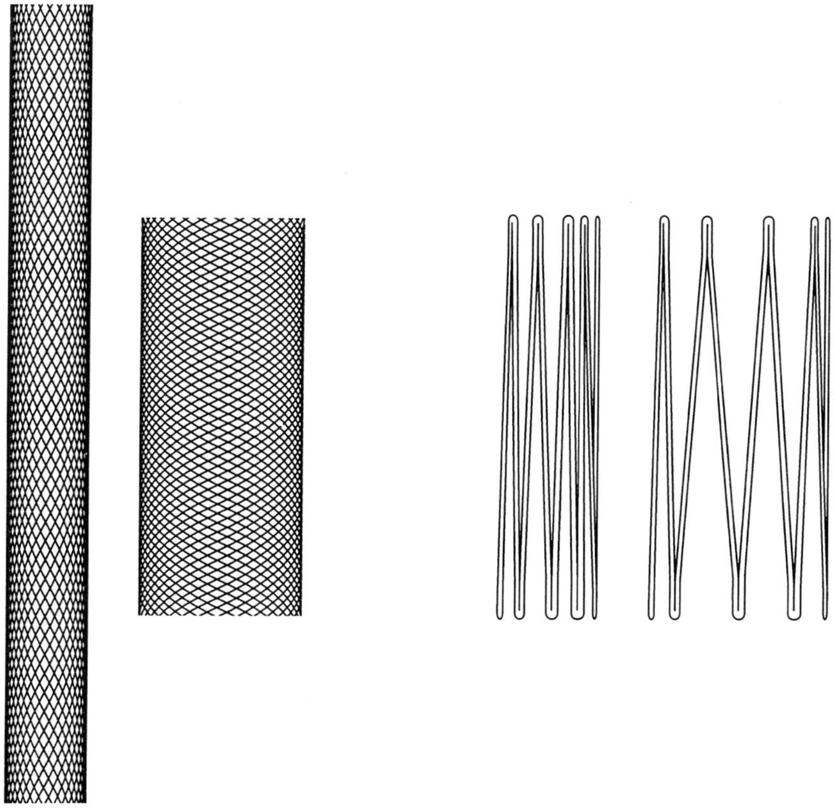

B

Fig. 22-6. A and **B,** Polymer and wire stents in unexpanded and expanded forms.

Experience with indwelling expandable stents in children has been limited, and to date these devices have been used primarily in adults with advanced tracheobronchial malignancies.[14] Materials currently in use include self-expanding woven polymers and stainless steel wire, which are placed bronchoscopically. Mair, Parsons, and Lally[39] demonstrated faster mucosalization and improved tracheal patency with polymer stents versus stainless steel stents both in a piglet model and in children. Bugmann and others[6] reported on the successful use of an expandable Z-shaped wire stent in a 6-month-old patient with severe tracheomalacia. No complications were reported at 2-year follow-up. In adults, Nashef and others[3] found that the most common complication of stent placement was the formation of granulation tissue.[46] Concerns raised by the authors regarding their use in children include the uncertainty of long-term tolerance of these stents, mucosal hypersecretion, and the risk of perforation and migration (Fig. 22-6).

Open repair

Acquired stenoses are often further complicated by scarring, poor vascular supply, and chronic infection. Tracheal resection and reanastomosis have been widely used in hundreds of adult patients for tracheal stenosis since the 1960s; however, Halsband[24] found only 26 reports of these procedures in children between 1969 and 1984. In general, surgical therapy should be pursued when conservative or nonsurgical therapy fails or is deemed inappropriate. A variety of techniques are available for the surgical management of tracheal stenosis, including tracheoplasty with autologus material, wedge resection, slide tracheoplasty, total resection with end-to-end anastomosis, tracheal homograft reconstruction, and stenting with bioinert materials. Often, multiple techniques must be employed.

Tracheoplasty may be performed with rib cartilage as described by Kimura and others.[35] Cartilage is a rigid autologous tissue that derives its nutritional support through diffusion and can survive without a direct vascular supply. Because of this, cartilage has been widely used as a tracheal graft material. The surgical technique involves securing the airway either by a previously placed tracheostomy or by endotracheal intubation, which is performed orally and then converted to a transtracheal site once the trachea is exposed. The area of stenosis is exposed anteriorly and the extent of the stenosis is outlined bronchoscopically, either by palpation with the bronchoscope or using the light of the telescope. The external appearance of the trachea can underestimate the extent of the stenosis.[34] Intraluminal granulation tissue is removed and the scar is incised. A rib graft is harvested (usually a fifth or sixth rib on the right is used) and fashioned

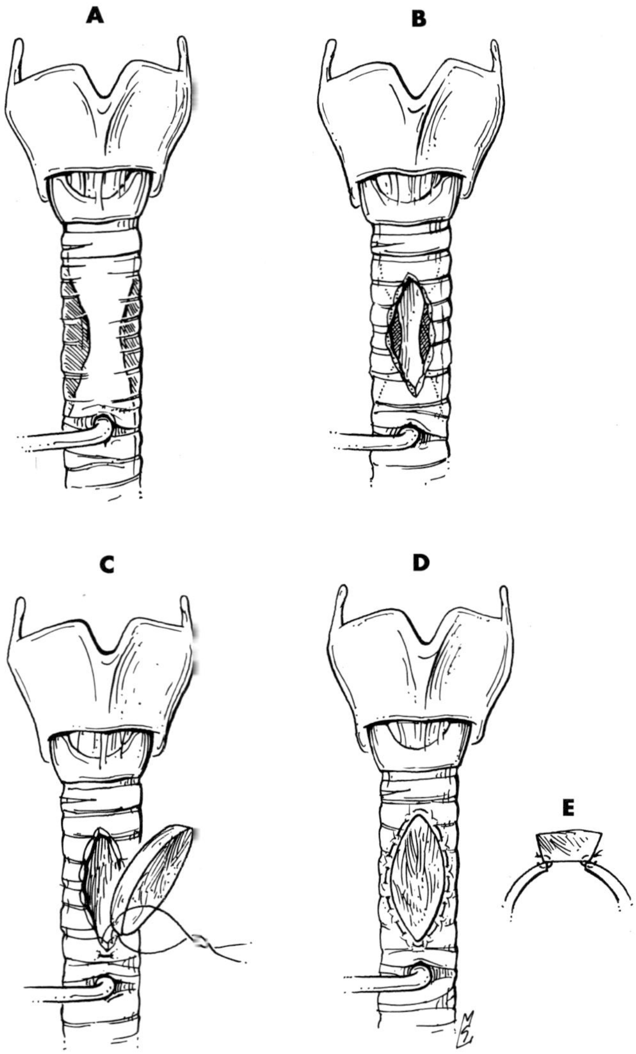

Fig. 22-7. **A** to **E,** Cartilage graft placement for augmentation of tracheal stenosis. Note the graft placement in lumen **E**.

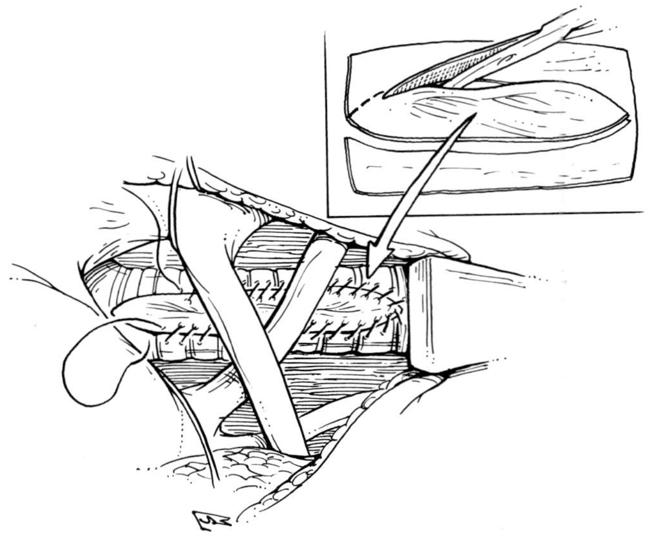

Fig. 22-8. Pericardial patch sewn in position.

as described previously. Perichondrium is preserved on the anterior surface of the rib graft and becomes the luminal surface of the airway. The graft is held in place by interrupted suture material and, depending on the extent of the stenosis, is supported with an endotracheal tube for 5 to 7 days (Fig. 22-7). For longer-term stenting, an Aboulker or T-tube stent may be used. The decision of whether to use cardiopulmonary bypass, extracorporeal membrane oxygenation, or distal tracheal intubation during the procedure is controversial and depends on the site of the lesion and the surgeon's personal preference. Pericardium is the most commonly used alternative to rib augmentation and also has good long-term survival (Fig. 22-8).[10,15,29,31] Other autologous materials that may be used include periosteum,[37] pedicled muscle flaps,[17,23] composite grafts,[7] the esophagus,[16,50] omentum,[56] and solvent-preserved dura.[36]

Kimura and others[35] were the first to report successful repair of a 1-year-old with complete stenosis of the trachea using costal cartilage.[35] Their experience was updated with an additional four patients in 1988.[55] Long-term survival was 80%, with one death due to respiratory distress 10 months after repair. Complications related to this procedure include anastomotic breakdown, stenosis, and granulation tissue formation at the suture line. Jaquiss and others[27] described six patients who underwent rib tracheoplasty (mean age, 14 weeks), with an average stenosis of 70% of the total length of the trachea.[34] All patients had survived by a follow-up of 6 months to 7.6 years. Bronchoscopy was performed three times or fewer postoperatively in all but one patient. These authors advocated cardiopulmonary bypass to obtain an unobstructed view of the airway during repair. Lobe and others[36] reported on seven infants with congenital tracheal stenosis, four of whom were repaired with costal cartilage.[26] One death secondary to pneumonia occurred 5 weeks postoperatively.

Troublesome to repair is the formation of granulation tissue at the graft site. One advantage of rib graft in contrast to pericardial grafts is that the endotracheal tube does not need to be beyond the proximal edge of the graft for stenting purposes and subsequently decreases granulation tissue formation.[34] DeLorimier and others[13] have suggested that the formation of granulation tissue is more likely if the graft involves 30% or more of the luminal surface. Epithelialization of costal cartilage grafts in the trachea has been demonstrated in both animals and humans.[28] Grillo, Zannini, and Michelassi[20] have stated that the use of absorbable (polyglycolic acid polymer) versus nonabsorbable suture material reduces the amount of granulation seen at the anastomotic site.

The technique of wedge resection is most useful for a

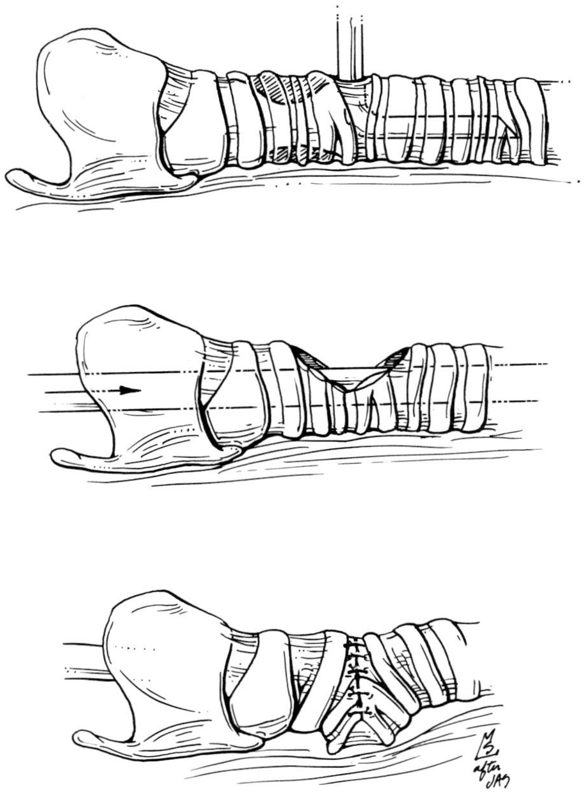

Fig. 22-9. Wedge resection and closure.

localized stenosis involving one or two tracheal rings. This method may be useful in small infants in whom the recurrent laryngeal nerve may be difficult to identify. After oral intubation the lesion is defined and an anterior wedge of trachea is removed. The defect is closed primarily with interrupted sutures. Weber, Connors, and Tracy[57] used this procedure successfully in four patients with localized stenosis (Fig. 22-9).

Segmental resection is successful for repair of long-segment tracheal stenosis comprising less than 50% of the tracheal length. In children this operation uses the principles of tracheal repair that were developed for adults.[21] Following endoscopy to outline the extent of the lesion, the stenotic segment is excised. Dissection beyond the stenosis is kept to a minimum in order to preserve the vascular supply to the trachea. Sutures are placed submucosally and tied extraluminally. Important to the success of the repair is the ability to achieve a tension-free anastomotic suture line. Various techniques may be applied, including suprahyoid release, infrahyoid release, peritracheal mobilization, intercartilaginous incisions, perihilar release, dissection of the pulmonary vasculature, transplantation of the left mainstem bronchus, and neck flexion with chin-to-chest suturing (Fig. 22-10).[5,25,43]

The results of several authors have been encouraging.[25,41,49,57] Nakayama and others[45] reported on 10 patients, four of whom underwent tracheal resection. They emphasized the association of multiple tracheobronchial and vascular anomalies in these patients and the need for a detailed preoperative evaluation. Healy[26] reported on three children, ages 4 weeks to 3 years, who were successfully resected. The author felt that three to five tracheal rings could be resected in children without a laryngeal release. He also commented that postoperative endotracheal intubation can often be avoided in adults but in children the cartilage is still very pliable and may not offer sufficient resistance to tracheal collapse at the anastomotic site. Two patients who required postoperative nasotracheal intubation were not mechanically ventilated but allowed to breathe spontaneously in an intensive care unit setting and were successfully extubated several days later. DeLorimier and others[13] detailed their experience with 45 patients with tracheobronchial stenoses. Seventeen patients underwent segmental resection, with three anastomotic strictures developing postoperatively. These strictures were resected with success in two patients. In their series of 52 patients ranging in age from 7 weeks to 15 years, Grillo and Zannini[19] undertook segmental resection in 20. Good results were obtained in 17 patients. The remaining 32 patients were treated conservatively, with 24 requiring either a T-tube or tracheotomy. In their series of 21 patients with congenital tracheal stenosis, Benjamin, Pitkin, and Cohen[4] also treated 12 patients without surgery. This experience lends support to the individualized treatment options and the nonsurgical management of selected patients.

Segmental resection is often not possible due to the length of trachea to be resected. First described by Tsang and others,[59] slide tracheoplasty involves dividing the stenosis transversely in the midportion and then incising the upper segment vertically posteriorly and the lower segment vertically anteriorly. The two ends are then placed over each other, effectively halving the stenotic segment while doubling the circumference. The distance that the tracheal ends need to move is half that of a resection and primary reanastomosis. This fact aids in reducing tension along the suture line—which may be more critical in children than in adults.[38] Grillo[22] described two children, ages 3 months and 3 years, and two young adults, all of whom had complete cartilaginous rings. The stenotic areas were 36% and 50% of the total tracheal length for each group. Short-term results were deemed good. An advantage to this technique is decreased granulation tissue that is often seen at the site of the cartilage graft reconstruction. Other advantages to this procedure are the avoidance of graft materials, decreased tracheal mobilization, and a good success rate (Fig. 22-11).

Tracheal homograft transplantation with cadaveric human tracheal homograft is an exciting new modality for the repair of severe long-segment tracheal stenosis in children. Initially described in 1980 in adult patients,[30] 24 children were recently reported by Jacobs and others.[32] An 83%

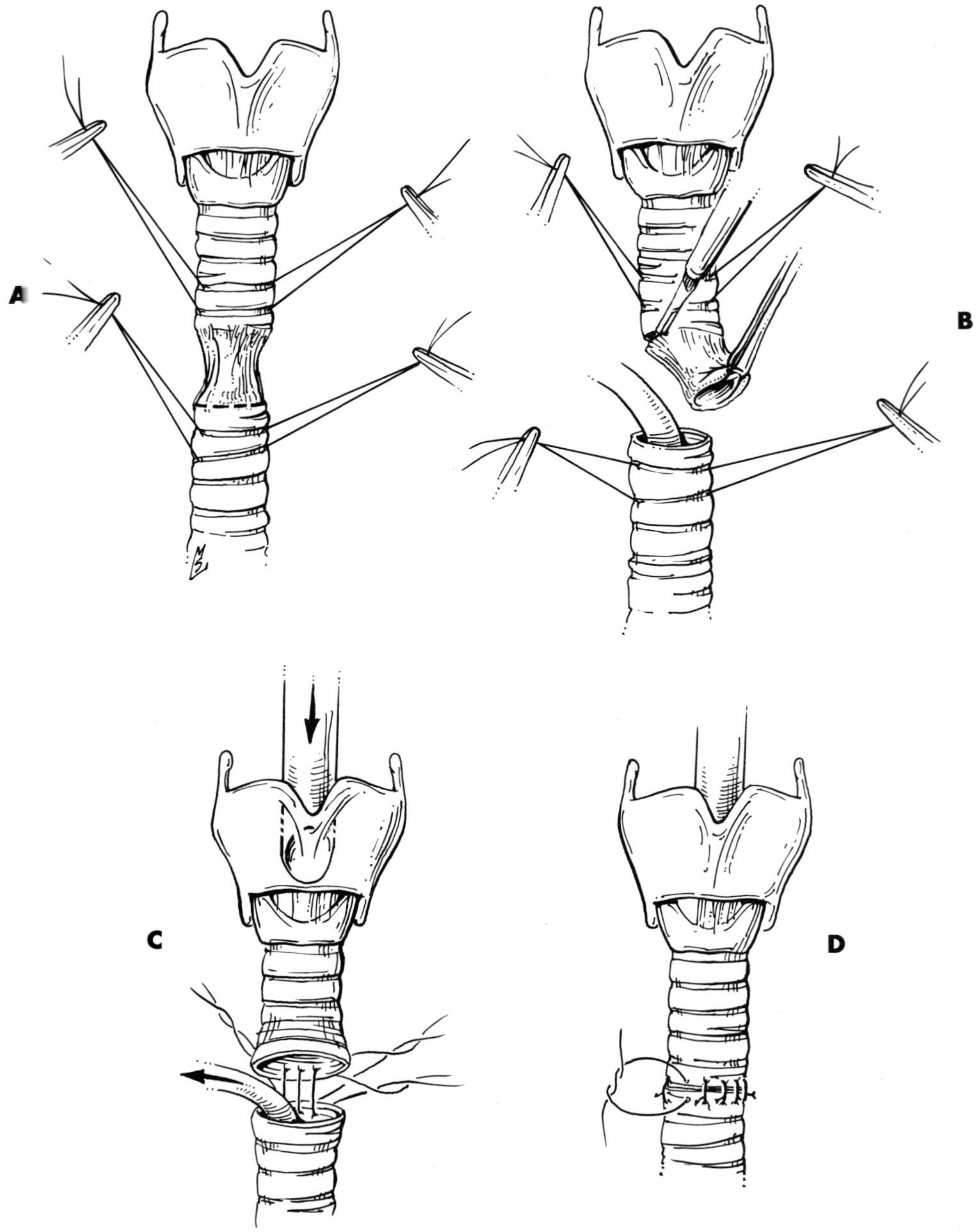

Fig. 22-10. A to **D,** Interrupted absorbable sutures placed circumferentially and reintubated from above.

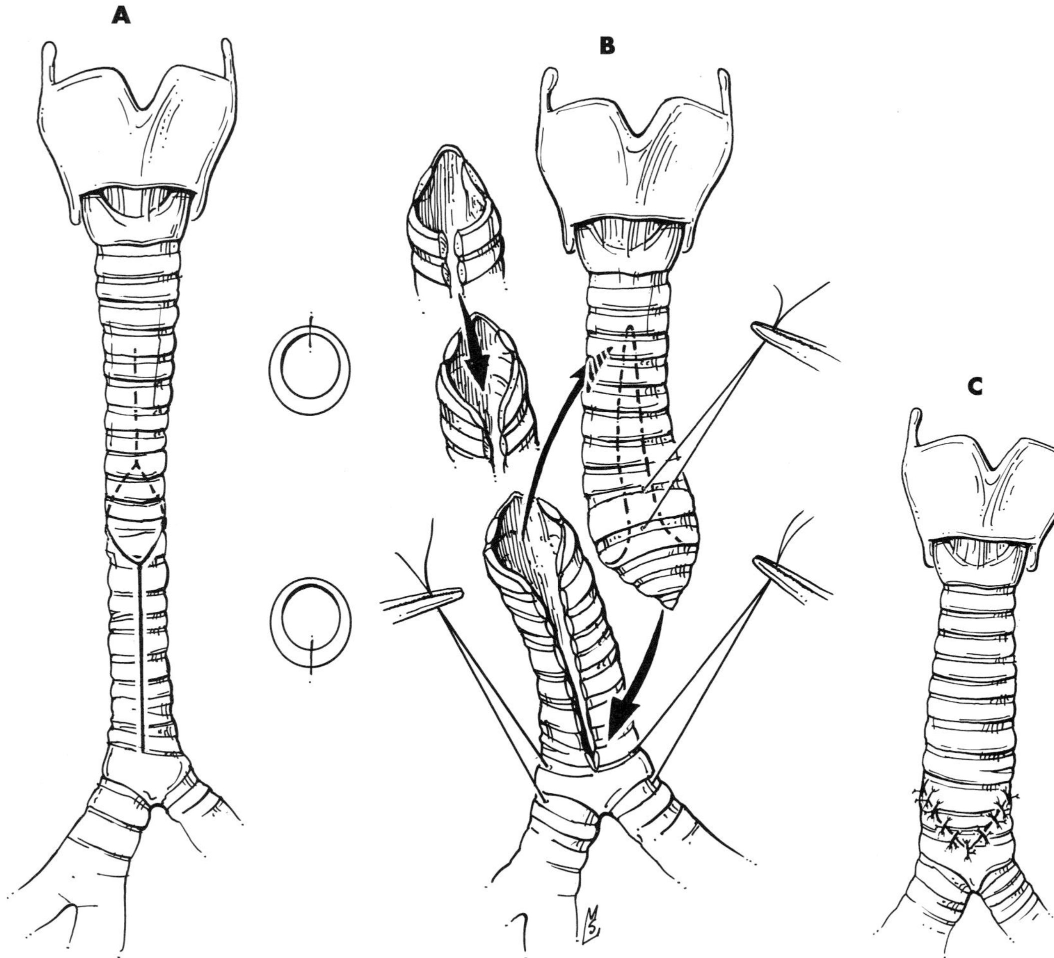

Fig. 22-11. **A** to **C,** Slide tracheoplasty. The trachea is divided on an angle and then vertically anteriorly and posteriorly.

survival rate was achieved, with follow-up ranging from 5 months to 10 years. Tracheal homograft banks exist in Europe, and specimens are fixed in formalin, washed in thimerosal (sodium ethylmercurithiosalicylate), and stored in acetone. The trachea is exposed through a neck incision, a median sternotomy, or both. Cardiopulmonary bypass is used to facilitate the operative field. The anterior part of the trachea is removed, leaving only a posterior tracheal wall intact. Dumon stents are then sutured into the native trachea to provide support for the homograft for 10 to 12 weeks until the graft hardens and re-epithelialization occurs. The endotracheal tube is positioned to lie within the lumen of the Dumon stent. The homograft is fashioned to the defect and sutured in place with interrupted sutures (Fig. 22-12).

Postoperative care includes 2 weeks of intravenous antibiotics followed by 4 weeks of oral trimethoprim as well as inhaled albuterol and corticosteroids. No immunosuppression is needed as the thimerosal used in the preparation of the homograft destroys antigenicity. Frequent bronchoscopy is required to remove granulation tissue at the site of the stents.

Advantages to the tracheal homograft include an adequate supply of tissue, which can be placed without suture-line tension, and the presence of a carina, which is needed for distal reconstruction. Ciliated columnar epithelium has been shown to coat the homograft. Tracheal homograft reconstruction is an exciting new approach to severe or recurrent tracheal stenosis.

Synthetic tracheal prostheses have not enjoyed the success of prosthetic devices used elsewhere in the head and neck because the trachea is much more susceptible to infection. Synthetic devices that have been employed include ceramic rings, marlex mesh, and Silicone stents.[33] These are complicated by dense granulation tissue reaction, migration of the prosthesis recurrent stenosis, and the risk of vascular erosion (Fig. 22-13).

Complications related to open surgical resection have

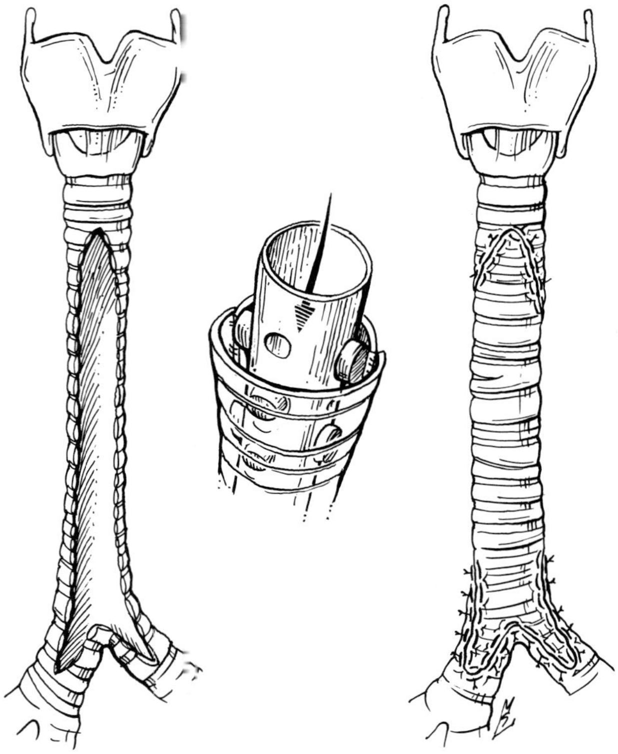

Fig. 22-12. Homograft transplant with a Dumon stent.

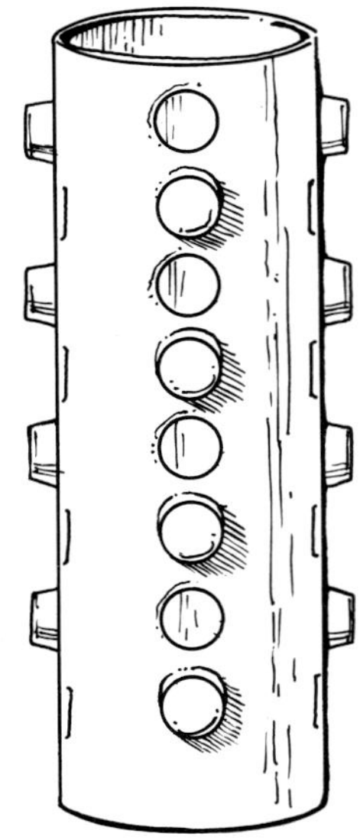

Fig. 22-13. Silastic Dumon stent.

been addressed by several authors.[11,20,24,55] The most common complication of tracheal reconstruction is the formation of granulation tissue at the anastomotic site or around the stent. This problem is usually managed with bronchoscopic-guided laser removal and with intravenous or intralesional injection of corticosteroid. Anastomotic leak or separation is often caused by excessive tension at the site of resection. Several techniques have been described to lessen the tension, including the supralaryngeal-, tracheal-, and hilar-releasing maneuvers mentioned earlier. Recurrent laryngeal nerve injury is rare and is usually managed conservatively if it is unilateral. Aspiration may also complicate recurrent laryngeal nerve injury and may be seen after thyrohyoid or suprahyoid release.

Complications may be avoided by ensuring several factors prior to surgery.[18] Ideally, the surgical resection candidate should not be mechanically ventilated, should not be on steroids, and should not have prior radiotherapy to the area. Muscle flaps between the esophagus and trachea can reduce the incidence of fistula formation. Glottic competence should be evaluated, especially in neurologically compromised patients.

CONCLUSION

Evaluation and management of tracheal stenosis is a complex undertaking, as evidenced by the numerous methods available for reconstruction. In general, short-segment tracheal stenoses can be managed endoscopically, whereas longer stenoses are better corrected through an open approach. No one surgical method is appropriate for every setting and often the surgeon must employ several therapeutic options. Furthermore, the surgeon must recognize the limitations and complications of each of the various management options in order to ensure a successful outcome.

REFERENCES

1. Amedee RG, Mann WJ, Lyons GD: Tracheomalacia repair using ceramic rings, *Otolaryngol Head Neck Surg* 106:270, 1992.
2. Anand VK, Alemar G, Warren T: Surgical considerations in tracheal stenosis, *Laryngoscope* 102:237, 1992.
3. Bagwell CE, Talbert JL, Tepas JJ III: Balloon dilatation of long segment tracheal stenoses, *J Pediatr Surg* 26:153, 1991.
4. Benjamin B, Pitkin J, Cohen D: Congenital tracheal stenosis, *Ann Otol Rhinol Laryngol* 90:364, 1981.
5. Biller HF, Munier MA: Combined infrahyoid and inferior constrictor muscle release for tension-free anastomosis during primary tracheal repair, *Otolaryngol Head Neck Surg* 107:430, 1992.
6. Bugmann P and others: Use of Gianturco Z stents in the treatment of vascular compression of the tracheobronchial tree in childhood, *Chest* 106:1580, 1994.
7. Burstein FD, Canalis RC, Ward PH: Composite hyoid-sternohyoid interposition graft revisited: UCLA experience 1974-1984, *Laryngoscope* 96:516, 1986.
8. Cantrell JR, Guild HG: Congenital stenosis of the trachea, *Am J Surg* 108:297, 1964.
9. Cohen MD, Weber TR, Rao CC: Balloon dilatation of tracheal and bronchial stenosis, *Am J Roentgenol* 142:477, 1984.
10. Cosentino CM and others: Pericardial patch tracheoplasty for severe tracheal stenosis in children: intermediate results, *J Pediatr Surg* 26:879, 1991.
11. Couraud L and others: Prevention and treatment of complications and sequelae of tracheal resection anastomosis, *Int Surg* 67:235, 1982.
12. Dedo HH, Sooy CD: Endoscopic laser repair of posterior glottic, subglottic and tracheal stenosis by division or microtrapdoor flap, *Laryngoscope* 94:445, 1984.

13. deLorimier AA and others: Tracheobronchial obstructions in infants and children: experience with 45 cases, *Ann Surg* 212:277, 1990.
14. Dumon JF: A dedicated tracheobronchial stent, *Chest* 97:328, 1990.
15. Dunham ME and others: Management of severe congenital tracheal stenosis, *Ann Otol Rhinol Laryngol* 103:351, 1994.
16. Ein SH and others: Tracheoplasty: a new operation for complete congenital tracheal stenosis, *J Pediatr Surg* 17:872, 1982.
17. Friedman M, Mayer AD: Laryngotracheal reconstruction in adults with the sternocleidomastoid myoperiosteal flap, *Ann Otol Rhinol Laryngol* 101:897, 1992.
18. Grillo HC, Mathisen DJ: Surgical management of tracheal strictures, *Surg Clin North Am* 68:511, 1988.
19. Grillo HC, Zannini P: Management of obstructive tracheal disease in children, *J Pediatr Surg* 19:414, 1984.
20. Grillo HC, Zannini P, Michelassi F: Complications of tracheal reconstruction: incidence, treatment, and prevention, *J Thorac Cardiovasc Surg* 91:322, 1986.
21. Grillo HC: Reconstruction of the trachea, *Thorax* 28:667, 1973.
22. Grillo HC: Slide tracheoplasty for long segment congenital tracheal stenosis, *Ann Thorac Surg* 58:613, 1994.
23. Gustafson RA, Hrabovsky EE: Intercostal muscle and myoosseous flaps in difficult pediatric thoracic problems, *J Pediatr Surg* 17:541, 1982.
24. Halsband H: Long distance resection of the trachea with primary anastomosis in small children, *Prog Pediatr Surg* 21:76, 1987.
25. Har-El G and others: Resection of tracheal stenosis with end-to-end anastomosis, *Ann Otol Rhinol Laryngol* 102:670, 1993.
26. Healy GB: An experimental model for the endoscopic correction of subglottic stenosis with clinical applications, *Laryngoscope* 92:1103, 1982.
27. Hebra A, Powell DD, Smith CD: Balloon tracheoplasty in children: results of a 15-year experience, *J Pediatr Surg* 26:957, 1991.
28. Heatly DG and others: Auricular cartilage versus costal cartilage as a grafting material in experimental laryngotracheal reconstruction, *Laryngoscope* 105:983, 1991.
29. Heimansohn DA and others: Anterior pericardial tracheoplasty for congenital tracheal stenosis, *J Thorac Cardiovasc Surg* 102:710, 1991.
30. Herberhold C, Franz B, Bripohl W: Chemish-konservierte menschliche Trachea als Prothesenmaterial zur Deckung trachealer Defekete, *Laryngorhinootologie* 59:453, 1980.
31. Idriss FS and others: Tracheoplasty with pericardial patch for extensive tracheal stenosis in infants and children, *J Thorac Cardiovasc Surg* 88: 527, 1984.
32. Jacobs JP and others: Pediatric tracheal homograft reconstruction: a novel approach to complex tracheal stenoses in children, *J Thorac Cardiovasc Surg* 112:1549, 1996.
33. Jacobs JR: Investigations into tracheal prosthetic reconstruction, *Laryngoscope* 98:1239, 1988.
34. Jaquiss RDB and others: Repair of long segment tracheal stenosis in infancy, *J Thorac Cardiovasc Surg* 110:1504, 1995.
35. Kimura K and others: Tracheoplasty for congenital stenosis of the entire trachea, *J Pediatr Surg* 17:869, 1982.
36. Lobe TE and others: Successful management of congenital tracheal stenosis in infancy, *J Pediatr Surg* 22:1137, 1987.
37. Loeff DS and others: Congenital tracheal stenosis: a review of 22 patients from 1965 to 1987, *J Pediatr Surg* 23:744, 1988.
38. Maeda M, Grillo HC: Effect of tension on tracheal growth after resection and anastomosis in puppies, *J Thorac Cardiovasc Surg* 65:658, 1973.
39. Mair EA, Parsons DS, Lally KP: Treatment of severe bronchomalacia with expanding endobronchial stents, *Arch Otolaryngol Head Neck Surg* 116:1087, 1990.
40. Maniglia AJ: Conservative surgical management of tracheal stenosis, *Otolaryngol Head Neck Surg* 86:380, 1978.
41. Mattingly WT, Belin RP, Todd EP: Surgical repair of congenital tracheal stenosis in an infant, *J Thorac Cardiovasc Surg* 81:738, 1981.
42. Messino A and others: The balloon posterior tracheal split: a technique for managing tracheal stenosis in the premature infant, *J Pediatr Surg* 27:1142, 1992.
43. Montgomery WW: Suprahyoid release for tracheal anastomosis, *Arch Otolaryngol Head Neck Surg* 99:255, 1974.
44. Montgomery WW: T-tube tracheal stent, *Arch Otolaryngol Head Neck Surg* 82:320, 1965.
45. Nakayama DK and others: Reconstructive surgery for obstructing lesions of the intrathoracic trachea in infants and small children, *J Pediatr Surg* 17:854, 1982.
46. Nashef SM and others: Expanding wire stents in benign tracheobronchial disease: indications and complications, *Ann Thorac Surg* 54:937, 1992.
47. Ossoff RH and others: Limitations of bronchoscopic carbon dioxide laser surgery, *Ann Otol Rhinol Laryngol* 94:498, 1985.
48. Ossoff RH and others: Efficacy of bronchoscopic carbon dioxide laser surgery for benign strictures of the trachea, *Laryngoscope* 95:1220, 1985.
49. Peskind SP, Stanley RB, Thangathurai D: Treatment of the compromised trachea with sleeve resection and primary repair, *Laryngoscope* 103:203, 1993.
50. Sasaki S and others: Esophageal tracheoplasty for congenital tracheal stenosis, *J Pediatr Surg* 27:645, 1992.
51. Shapshay SM and others: Endoscopic treatment of subglottic and tracheal stenosis by radial laser incision and dilation, *Ann Otol Rhinol Laryngol* 96:661, 1987.
52. Simpson GT and others: Predictive factors of success or failure in the endoscopic management of laryngeal and tracheal stenosis, *Ann Otol Rhinol Laryngol* 91:384, 1982.
53. Strong MS and others: Bronchoscopic carbon dioxide laser surgery, *Ann Otol Rhinol Laryngol* 83:769, 1974.
54. Tsang V and others: Slide tracheoplasty for congenital funnel shaped tracheal stenosis, *Ann Thorac Surg* 48:632, 1989.
55. Tsugawa C and others: Congenital stenosis involving a long segment of the trachea: further experience in reconstructive surgery, *J Pediatr Surg* 23:471, 1988.
56. Tsugawa C and others: The use of the omental pedicle flap for tracheobronchial reconstruction in infants and children, *J Pediatr Surg* 26: 762, 1991.
57. Weber TR, Connors RH, Tracy TF: Acquired tracheal stenosis in infants and children, *J Thorac Cardiovasc Surg* 102:29, 1991.

Chapter 23

Caustic Ingestion

J. Dale Browne
James N. Thompson

The challenges of caring for the patient with a presumed caustic ingestion are multiple. They include accurately predicting the severity of an unseen injury to the larynx, esophagus, and stomach; appropriately addressing any mucosal injury to prevent the complications of airway obstruction, perforation, and stricture formation; and adequately dealing with any long-term sequelae resulting from a circumferential esophageal injury. Medical literature is replete with retrospective evaluations of hundreds of patients, old and young, with varying forms of caustic ingestion. Taken collectively, a consensus approach cannot be found in the literature for this not uncommon problem. However, if patient age and the circumstances and type of ingestion are considered, the clinician can approach this injury rationally.

Caustic ingestions have been reported since the turn of the century when cleaning solutions composed of strong alkalis or acids were conveniently packaged and widely available to the average household. An alarming number of serious pediatric injuries from alkali ingestions led physicians such as Jackson, developer of the first distal lighted esophagoscope, to support successful 1927 legislation that controlled the sale of these potential toxins. In 1921, Jackson noted in the *Journal of the American Medical Association*:[21]

> The fact is that not one of the caustic alkalis sold for cleansing purposes, so far as I have been able to discover, has a sufficient warning of the dangerous nature of the contents. In 1910 I called attention to this fact and mentioned that poison sold by druggists to the laity are subject to legal regulations as to labeling, and such drugs go into the medicine cupboard while the caustic alkalis sold by the grocer go into the kitchen. . . .

With the introduction of liquid drain cleaners 40 years later, further legislation brought about a reduction in the concentration of 35% sodium hydroxide. In the 1970s, the Poison Prevention Packaging Act and the Hazardous Substances Act mandated concentration restrictions (less than 10%), child-resistant containers, and conspicuous warning labels for all caustic cleaning agents available for home use. Despite these measures, serious injuries secondary to the ingestion of these products continue.

In general, caustic ingestions are accidental in the pediatric population and intentional in adults. The offending agent is usually representative of the more prevalent cleaning agents: alkali drain cleaner in the United States, acid-base agents in India.[24] Anecdotal reports of esophageal burns from concentrated laundry detergent, concentrated ammonia, dishwashing detergent, alkali hair straighteners, and nail-decorating liquids have been reported.[11,23,30,42] Sodium hydroxide–containing glucose test tablets have given rise to alkaline burns when ingested, especially if they lodge in the esophagus. Similarly, small disk-shaped batteries are easily swallowed by the unsuspecting child and subsequently may lodge, leading to a significant mucosal electrolyte damage with potential esophageal perforation.[40] In farming households, liquid and solid alkalis have been accidentally ingested by children causing significant injury. These agents have been exempt from protective packaging legislation and are used as disinfectants, for clearance of residual milk from pipelines and drains, and to remove residual horns from cattle.[29]

Strong acids lead to a protective coagulum of damaged mucosa that limits the degree of esophageal injury from the passing caustic, thereby placing the stomach at much greater risk from pooling and prolonged contact with the compound. More damaging is the liquefactive necrosis from strong alkalis, occurring within seconds after contact with a mucosal surface. Alkalis combine with fats to form soaps and with proteins to form proteinates, thereby disrupting cell membranes. Because alkalis are soluble, the damaged tissues separate and allow even deeper penetration of the caustic agents. Damage ceases only when the alkali is neutralized by its reaction with tissue. The extent of the injury depends on the strength of the alkali ingested and on the amount and form of the product. Detailed characterization of caustic injuries has centered around the liquefactive necrosis of alkaline burns because they are the most severe and generally the most common, especially among the pediatic population. Histologically, Bosher, Burfard, and Ackerman[2] outlined in 1951 the basic pathologic events after a 10% sodium hydroxide burn of esophageal mucosa: edema of the submucosa, inflammation of the submucosa with thrombosis, sloughing of the superficial layers, necrosis of the muscular layer, fibrosis of the deep layers, and ultimately, delayed re-epithelialization.

DIAGNOSIS AND INITIAL ASSESSMENT

Patients with caustic ingestion present with many symptoms, ranging from asymptomatic to overtly stridorous secondary to laryngeal edema (Box 23-1). Paramount in the initial assessment of these patients is verification of the ingested agent, with note made of its pH and concentration, physical form (i.e., granular, liquid), approximate time of ingestion, and volume swallowed. Significant esophageal injuries may follow ingestion of only a few milliliters of a strong alkali, whereas strong acids generally require much larger volumes. The social setting of the ingestion may provide clues to the amount of caustic involved in the injury and should be explored in the history because children ingest a caustic accidentally, whereas adults generally do so in greater volumes as an act of suicide. Although the amount of titratable base is a more accurate predictor of a strong alkaline substance,[16] pH is a more practical, rapid method of estimating the risk of mucosal injury in the clinical setting. Vancura and others[47] showed that a pH of 12.5 or greater is a reasonable threshold to produce esophageal ulceration, whereas significant mucosal damage in cats occurred with sodium hydroxide concentrations as low as 0.4%.

Box 23-1. Signs and symptoms of caustic ingestion

Pharyngeal or laryngeal
Odynophagia
Mucosal erythema, ulceration
Drooling
Tongue edema
Stridor
Hoarseness

Esophageal
Dysphagia
Odynophagia
Chest or back pain

Gastric
Epigastric pain or tenderness
Vomiting
Hematemesis

The initial physical examination of patients suspected of having ingested a caustic should focus on immediate complications. Patients with significant oral mucosal burns, tongue edema, hoarseness, stridor, and dyspnea should be monitored closely for possible airway obstruction. Fiberoptic laryngoscopy in the awake patient can be valuable to assess hypopharyngeal damage and the risk of airway compromise. In the patient with an injured but stable airway, dexamethasone (adult 20 to 30 mg intravenous bolus, pediatric 0.5 to 1 mg/kg) can help prevent further deterioration. In the setting of acute airway obstruction, blind nasotracheal intubation should be avoided because it may lead to bleeding of an already inflamed mucosa and further worsening of an already marginal airway. If direct visualization of the larynx for intubation is not possible because of edema and exudate, emergent cricothyrotomy or tracheotomy is a safer choice. Dyspnea associated with rales and ronchi may be indicators of aspiration of caustic material; chest and abdominal radiography should be obtained to rule out pulmonary infiltrates or free air. Associated epigastric pain and findings suggestive of peritonitis (e.g., abdominal wall rigidity, tenderness) are highly correlated with gastric injury.[37] All patients suspected of a severe injury should have large-bore intravenous catheters for early fluid resuscitation and medication.

After ingestion of extremely alkaline substances, the bulk of the injury occurs almost instantly. In contrast, the time frame to produce severe injury in the upper gastrointestinal mucosa after acid ingestion is more prolonged; the reflex pylorospasm that occurs after entry of acid into the stomach contributes to increased exposure and a predominance of gastric mucosal injuries in these patients. The use of emetics is condemned because they do not lessen the injury and increase the risk of aspiration. Likewise, buffering ingested alkali with weak acids (e.g., acetic acid) or acid burns with antacids is impractical and risks emesis with aspiration. Burns of the oral mucosa can be cleansed with water to dilute any remaining caustic, and any visible lye granules can be removed to lessen continuing injury.

Although the acute crises of esophageal perforation and upper airway obstruction are more dramatic, the most common complications from strong alkaline burns result from the more protracted courses of fibrosis and delayed epithelialization. Superficial burns generally heal without sequelae; however, deeper injuries involving the muscular layer and submucosa are associated with a more extensive loss of mucosa with subsequent fibrosis. A characteristic esophageal stricture develops in four stages: (1) An intense inflammatory response with associated dysmotility occurs in the area of the burned mucosa and deeper layers. (2) Granulation tissue with fibroblasts brings a matrix of collagen fibers to the newly formed connective tissue. (3) Three or 4 weeks after the initial injury, these collagen fibers begin to contract, with irregular formation of this collagen matrix, which enables the formation of adhesive bands. (4) Pseudodiverticula form between these adhesions as the contracting process continues until a dense inflexible fibrous scar replaces the destroyed submucosa and muscular layers. Circumferential burns are much more likely to lead to a symptomatic stricture than are noncircumferential injuries.[48]

ENDOSCOPY

Accurately predicting which injuries are prone to rapid, inconsequential healing and which are prone to stricture formation or perforation is the principal diagnostic challenge for the clinician. Among physicians who routinely care for patients injured by caustic ingestion, there is little disagreement that endoscopy is the most useful method of assessing whether esophageal injury has occurred. Radiographic studies such as barium swallow rely on motility disturbance and mucosal irregularities to detect injury. False-negative rates of up to 30% to 60% have been reported in some series of radiographic assessment of lye burns.[25,41] Therefore, heavily depending on low-sensitivity radiography for guidance may lead the clinician to underestimate the degree of injury.

Although there is little disagreement that endoscopy is the most useful diagnostic study, there is significant controversy regarding the setting in which to best use this diagnostic procedure. The argument for endoscopy within 24 hours in all cases of caustic ingestions is supported by retrospective reviews detailing instances of significant esophageal injury despite the absence of symptoms or signs of mucosal burns.[10,13,32] In citing the poor correlation of signs, symptoms, and esophageal injury, such studies frequently do not differentiate the form of the ingested substance (liquid or granular) and whether the asymptomatic burns were from more potent liquid alkalis. This association may thereby lead to the conclusion that any form of an ingested caustic may cause significant distal injury even in the absence of signs or symptoms of mucosal burns. Although conservative and cautious, this approach may subject patients (and parents) to occasionally unneeded procedures, worry, and expense. In a retrospective study of 41 ingestions that noted the type of lye ingested, the granular form did not cause significant mucosal injury, whereas all strictures resulted from liquid alkalis.[10]

An alternative view of when to apply endoscopy considers several factors: form and strength of the caustic, presence or absence of multiple signs and symptoms, and the age of the patient. Most adult patients ingest caustic agents as a suicide attempt, which is easy to diagnose; the volume of agent swallowed is usually great, commonly causing dysphagia, stridor, or oropharyngeal burns. Suicidal adults may be unreliable historians, which forces the clinician to rely on physical findings to direct therapy, especially since oral mucosal injury may be absent when a strong alkali is quickly swallowed. Consequently, endoscopy is advisable for any adult having ingested a strong alkali or acid (sodium hydroxide, potassium hydroxide, or HCl, H_2SO_4), regardless of the lack of presenting symptoms or signs. In suicidal ingestions, the physician should examine the stomach for necrosis through endoscopy, laparoscopy, or laparotomy because a large volume of caustic may have been swallowed.

In contrast, toxic agents are accidentally swallowed in the pediatric population as a result of innocent curiosity and confusion with food and drink. Children will not swallow a great deal of any distasteful food or medicine nor any noxious, bitter acid or unpalatable granular lye. These compounds rarely are associated with significant esophageal burns because the volume ingested is generally very small.[5,7,10] Exceptions have been reported, but these cases are associated with presenting combinations of oral burns, drooling, and dysphagia that easily raise suspicion that a significant amount of the compound has been swallowed. In cases of pediatric ingestion of acids or granular lye, endoscopy can be reserved for children with significant oral burns, dysphagia, or stridor. However, the glucose test tablet and disk-shaped watch battery need to be endoscopically removed as quickly as possible because they cause localized transmural necrosis and esophageal perforation.

Nonetheless, most severe pediatric esophageal injuries are the result of just a few milliliters of a strong liquid alkali, usually sodium hydroxide. Some investigators have found that the presence of two or more signs and symptoms (oral burns, drooling, dysphagia, vomiting, stridor) reliably indicates esophageal injury significant enough to lead to stricture formation or perforation, thus requiring endoscopy.[5-7] Although these criteria are helpful in evaluating the child with a questionable history of liquid alkali ingestion, prudent evaluation of the pediatric patient with known ingestion of a strong liquid alkali should consider reported cases of an otherwise silent, significant injury appreciated only through endoscopy. In cases of known pediatric liquid alkali ingestion, endoscopy offers a direct assessment with low morbidity for the presence or absence of injury. Therefore, in children who lack a strong history and have only one presenting sign or symptom, the risk of significant injury is low and endoscopy can be deferred. Otherwise, it is safer to endoscope all children with known ingestion of a strong liquid alkali.

Although any portion of the esophageal wall may be involved with the burn, the areas with the greatest extrinsic compression are most prone to injury. These are the cricopharyngeus, the aortic arch and left main stem bronchus compression sites, and the distal esophagus at the esophagogastric junction. As for other foreign bodies, this site is where solid caustics or batteries may lodge causing severe localized injuries. When evaluating a significant burn of the esophagus, the endoscopist should be aware of the potential for a tracheoesophageal fistula resulting from the injury, especially at the upper and midesophageal narrowings. Tracheoscopy should be included when extensive burns are seen in these areas to examine the posterior tracheal wall for injury.

STAGING

Methods of staging and reporting esophageal burns endoscopically vary. Historically, a classification borrowed from thermal burns has been used with references to first-, second-, and third-degree injuries that range from mild mucosal edema to partial thickness necrosis to transmural necrosis, respectively.[17] Variations on this method have noted whether the lesion was circumferential. Recurrent difficulties accurately and consistently applying this method include a failure to appreciate the true burn depth through the endoscope because of a necrotic exudate. Also contributing to endoscopic inaccuracy is difficulty in the assessment of the true amount of surface area burned because mucosal edema may obscure a complete circumferential examination and sometimes subtle changes of an evolving submucosal necrosis are underestimated in marginally burned areas.

Using modified classifications, four stages can provide the endoscopist with a consistent format for describing caustic injury to the esophageal lumen: First degree—mucosal erythema; second degree—erythema plus noncircumferential exudate; third degree—circumferential exudate; fourth degree—circumferential exudate with esophageal wall perforation (Fig. 23-1).[9] Additional reference to the site and length of the burn can be documented. In this staging system, only first-degree burns consistently heal uneventfully. Second-degree injuries occasionally form strictures, and generally, all third-degree burns form strictures. Fourth-degree burns carry the additional risk of sepsis and mediastinitis. Because it is difficult to accurately predict the true depth, there is the potential for a third-degree burn to eventually extend into a fourth-degree burn, hence the need for close follow-up.

Several days after a caustic esophageal injury, any necrotic mucosa, submucosa, and muscular layer will have sloughed. At this point, the esophageal wall is at its weakest and may be prone to perforation, either spontaneously or secondary to an endoscope or nasogastric tube. The same is true for a transmural injury to the gastric wall. Thus, close observation in all patients with third-degree esophageal burns is mandatory in a hospitalized setting for several days. Although antibiotics have not been shown to prevent strictures, broad-spectrum antibiotics are prudent in extensive third-degree burns that may lead to perforation.[10]

Additionally, endoscopy in the first 24 hours is safer to minimize the risk of perforation and for early identification of patients at risk for a fourth-degree injury. Although traditionally endoscopy has been aborted at the first significant burn,[10,17] the value and safety of full-length esophagoscopy has been shown, especially in identifying patients with significant distal injury extending into the stomach.[8,39,43,44] Endoscopy should be aborted when there is no definable lumen. Whereas rigid and flexible endoscopes have been used to successfully examine the full length of esophagus, the flexible model is necessary for adequate visualization of the stomach. If necrosis is identified extending into the gastric mucosa, direct visualization of the outer gastric wall should be strongly considered to rule out a transmural necrosis; visualization may be by laparoscopy or laparotomy depending on surgeon preference.

THERAPY

Once esophagogastic mucosal injury is diagnosed, the choice of therapy depends on the degree of injury. Injuries limited to first-degree burns of the esophageal mucosa require

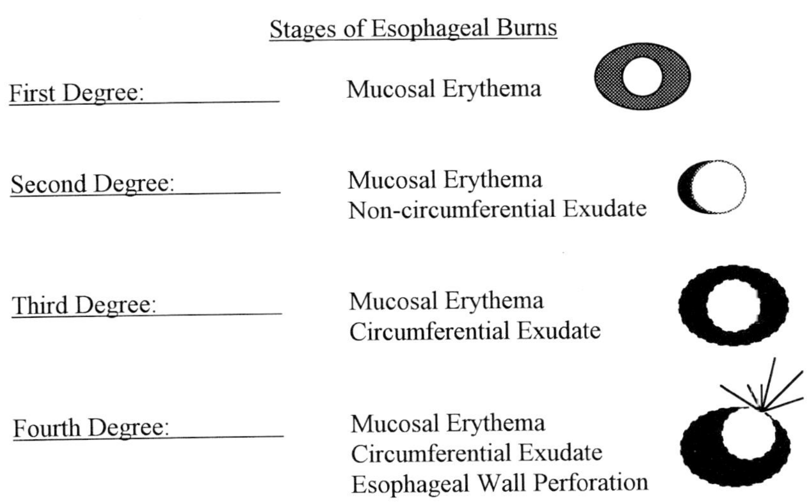

Fig. 23-1. The four stages of esophageal burns.

no further therapy. Blunt esophagectomy after identification of fourth-degree and even selected extensive third-degree esophageal burns reduces the expected mortality from leaving a necrotic esophagus in place.[9,12] Identifying a perforation makes the decision for esophagectomy relatively straightforward. For extensive third-degree burns, however, a thoracotomy for direct examination of the esophageal wall may be indicated to assess for transmural necrosis; such decisions may be difficult and may require the judgement and experience of the endoscopist. Débridement at the time of lapartomy or laparoscopy is dictated by the injury; in cases of gastric perforation, débridement of omentum, small bowel, and other intra-abdominal structures may be necessary.

The major controversy in therapeutic choices involves intermediate esophageal burns (i.e., second- and localized third-degree injuries without transmural necrosis). The goals of therapy are to maintain the esophageal lumen by the pharmacologic reduction or prevention of stricture formation and to maintain a conduit from the hypopharynx to the stomach by esophageal dilation, stenting, or reconstruction.

PHARMACOLOGIC THERAPY

In 1950, Howes and others[19] and Spain, Molomut, and Haber[40a] documented the retarding effect of corticosteroids on wound healing in separate laboratory studies.[19] In 1951, Rosenberg and others[36] noted decreased stricture formation with corticosteroid therapy after alkali burns of rabbit esophageal mucosa. Although infection leads to a high mortality rate, the supposed benefit from corticosteroids seemed clear. The addition of antibiotics reduced mortality, and the subsequent regimen of corticosteroids and antibiotics reduced esophageal strictures in the laboratory setting.[14,35,49] These findings led to the empiric therapeutic combination of corticosteroids and broad-spectrum antibiotics for significant second- and third-degree esophageal injuries. Retrospective analyses produce conflicting results; some studies show benefit in reducing strictures, whereas others do not.[4,38]

In an attempt to resolve this controversy Anderson, Rouse and Randolph[1] reported on a prospective analysis over 18 years of 60 children with esophageal burns secondary to strong caustics (80% alkali). Patients were randomly assigned to receive 21 days of corticosteroids or no therapy, with the degrees of injury stratified equally in both groups. Of 21 patients identified as having circumferential burns, 20 developed strictures; only 1 of 20 patients with a noncircumferential burn developed a stricture. Corticosteroids had no effect in the circumferential group. Ironically, the only stricture in the noncircumferential injury occurred in a child who received corticosteroids.

Lathyrogenic drugs that reduce collagen crossbonding have been used in attempts to decrease stricture formation.[45] Compounds such as β-aminopropionitrile, *N*-acetylcysteine, and penicillamine decrease stricture formation in laboratory settings, but their benefit in humans is unproven. Of these medications, penicillamine is the least toxic and may potentially play a limited role.

Contact with acid and pepsin retards the healing of lye-induced esophageal burns in rabbits.[26] Efforts to decrease the effects of stomach acid on injured esophageal mucosa may be very useful clinically. Sucralfate therapy for caustic esophageal burns has shown promise in the healing of ulcers without stricture formation.[27,33] Although unproven clinically, the low toxicity of reducing gastroesophageal reflux with H_2 blockers or proton pump inhibitors provides an attractive adjunctive measure in controlling strictures that is worthy of a prospective study.

MECHANICAL THERAPY

The simplest mechanical method for maintaining a lumen in a third-degree esophageal burn is to place a nasogastric tube at the time of initial endoscopy. The true benefit of nasogastric tube stenting varies, with results ranging from spectacular to no benefit.[28,50] In a patient with a third-degree burn and dysphagia, a nasogastric tube provides a convenient stent and a means of nutritional support. Other types of stents have used polymeric Silicone tubes in the esophagus with mixed success; any clear benefit over serial dilations has not been shown.[34] Ideally, if this philosophy is used in guiding therapy, stents should remain in place long enough to allow re-epithelialization (2 to 3 weeks).

Mild strictures can be serially dilated in a prograde fashion through an esophagoscope with filiform dilators. Cooperative patients (generally adults) may tolerate the periodic swallowing of weighted dilators in the office. Once identified, multiple strictures are most safely managed with retrograde dilators popularized by Tucker[46] in the 1920s. A gastrostomy is necessary for the passage of an endless loop of silk exiting the mouth to allow slow, serial increases in caliber while maintaining a secure position within the narrowed lumen and minimizing the risks of perforation (Fig. 23-2). If a significant, lengthy third-degree burn is identified at initial endoscopy, consideration should be given to the placement of a gastrostomy tube and retrograde silk during the same anesthesia or before discharge to avoid a delay in safe dilation in the outpatient setting.

The timing of stricture dilation depends on the severity of the injury. In second-degree injuries, prophylactic dilation is not recommended, although periodic follow-up is important. Stricture formation may occur up to 6 weeks from the time of injury and may become evident only when obstructed with food. Generally, a barium swallow at 3 weeks will serve as a baseline in asymptomatic patients and as an initial study before prophylactic dilations in patients with lengthy third-degree injuries who are at high risk for stricture development. Routine barium esophagography is useful over the course of 1 year to monitor progress of a managed stricture and to rule out the development of an occult one. For symptomatic patients, the frequency of dilations depends on patient response. Weekly dilations may be necessary to maintain a viable lumen in severe injuries (Fig. 23-3).

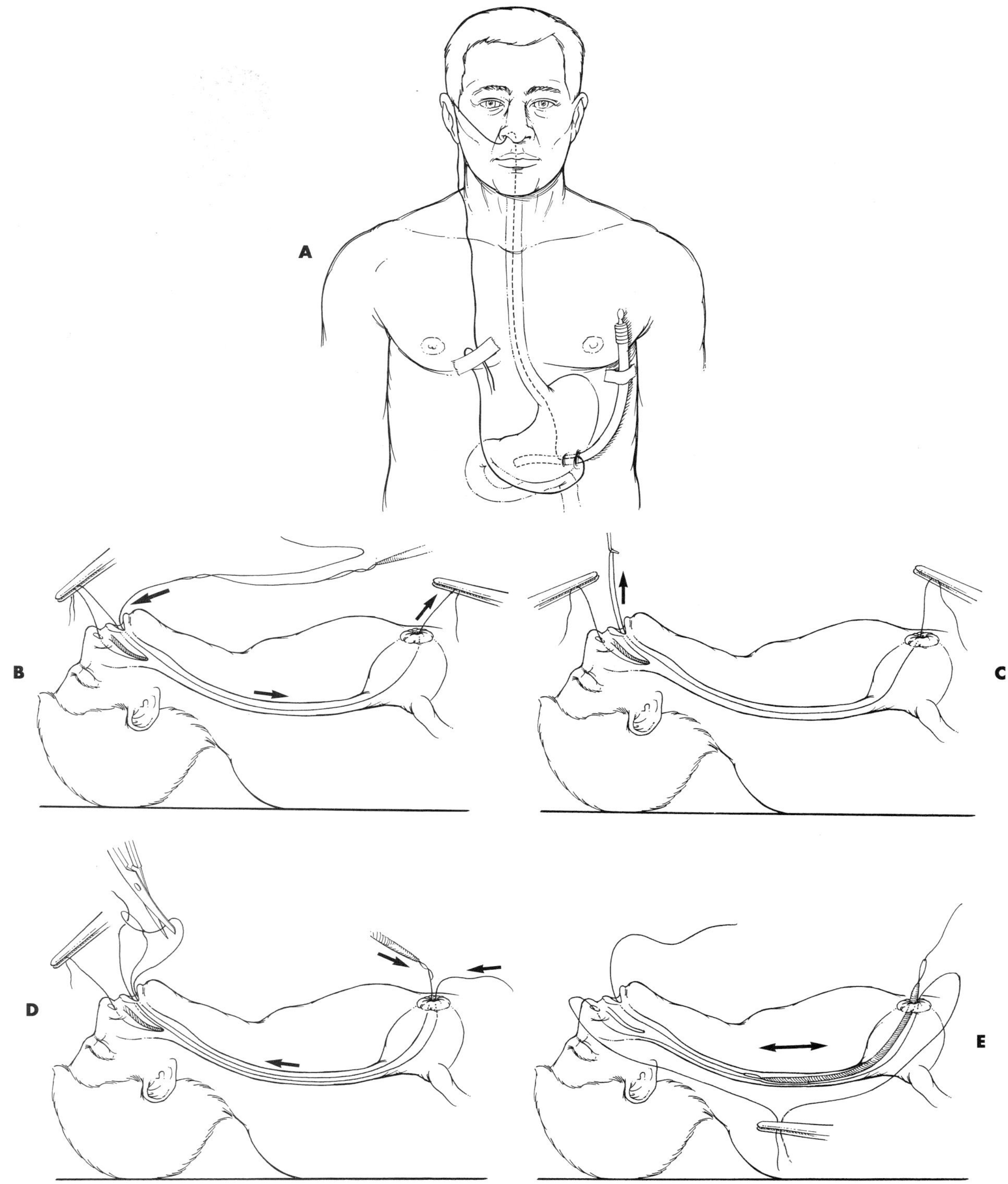

Fig. 23-2. A, Appearance of a typical patient undergoing chronic retrograde dilations via gastrostomy. A guide string enters the nasal cavity, loops behind the ear, and enters alongside the gastrostomy tube. **B,** String (heavy silk) is retrieved from the posterior pharynx. **C,** A dilator is secured to silk exiting the mouth for gentle progressive prograde dilation. Care is taken to clamp the loop exiting the mouth and nose. **D,** A dilator is secured to silk exiting the gastrostomy tube for gentle progressive retrograde dilations. **E,** Once the dilator is within the lumen of the strictures, a gentle to-and-fro prograde or retrograde dilation may be accomplished. For security, a second heavy silk loop can be passed before any dilation in case the dilator string should break.

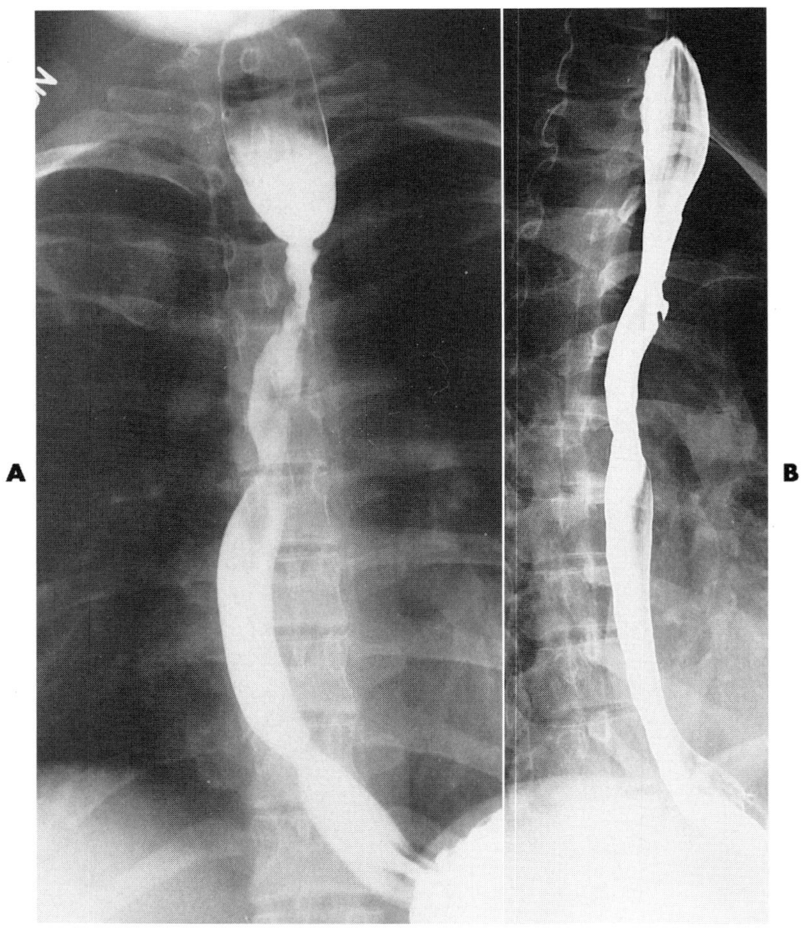

Fig. 23-3. **A,** A barium swallow shows a midesophageal stricture after lye ingestion in an adolescent 4 weeks after ingestion and at the beginning of retrograde dilations. **B,** The same patient 5 years later after 4 years of repetitive dilations; the patient has a stable stricture and is generally nonsymptomatic.

A B

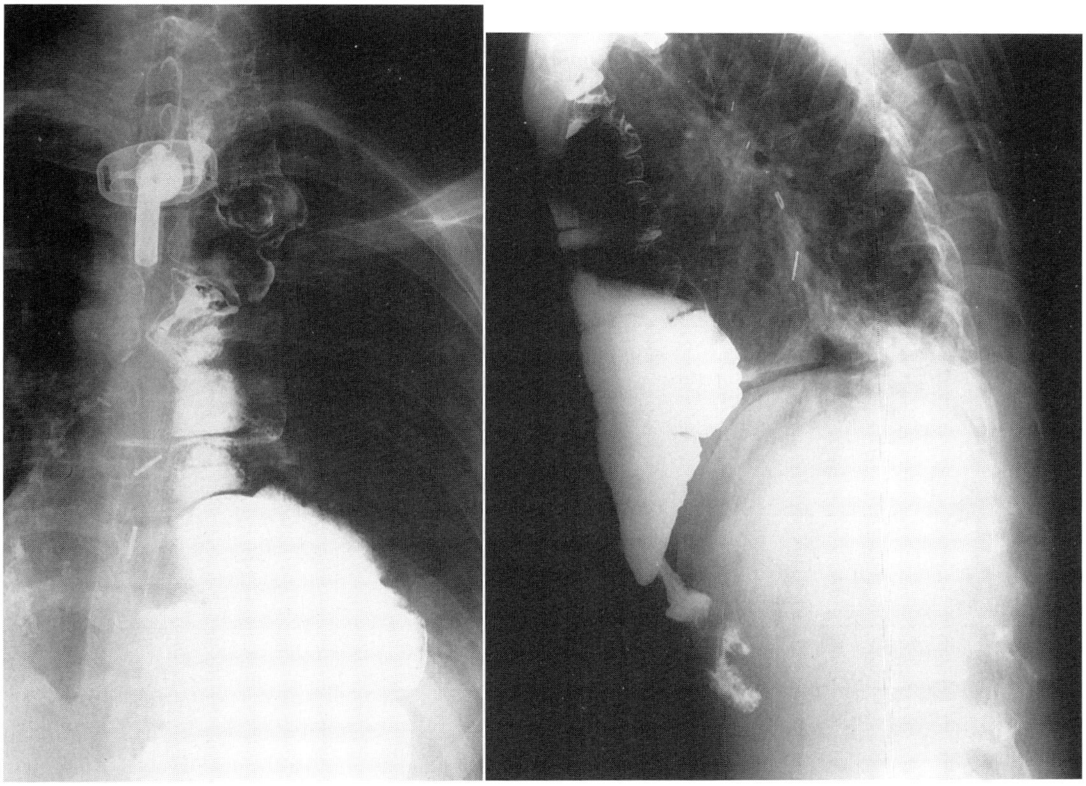

Fig. 23-4. **A,** Anterior view of a barium swallow of a patient with a fourth-degree burn necessitating a total blunt esophagectomy with subsequent reconstruction using the right descending colon. The tracheotomy was originally placed emergently because of laryngeal obstruction secondary to supraglottic necrosis or edema. **B,** Lateral view of the same patient. Note the position of colon transfer in the anterior mediastinum.

When repetitive dilations fail to relieve symptoms or when severe esophageal strictures render dilation impossible or fruitless, more aggressive techniques are indicated to reconstruct the conduit from hypopharynx to stomach. Esophageal replacement with gastric tubes, right colon, transverse colon, and descending colon was described; right colon was the most useful conduit (Fig. 23-4).[15,31] When possible, blunt esophagectomy is preferable to thoracotomy. For isolated strictures, local resection with end-to-end reanastomosis and colon patch esophagoplasty were reported in successful attempts to preserve an injured esophagus.[3,22]

The benefits from esophagectomy are not limited to the reconstruction of a swallowing conduit. In large series of esophageal carcinomas, a 1% to 4% incidence of caustic ingestion is typical. Although the true increased risk of carcinoma is unknown, it has been estimated at 1000-fold. Fortunately, the tendency for local extension of these malignancies is lower than expected with a higher potential rate of cure because they develop in the stenotic scar.[18] With this in mind, long-term follow-up is essential in any patient with a caustic esophageal stricture. The redevelopment of dysphagia after years of minimal difficulties should prompt an investigation with at least barium esophagography and, if abnormal, esophagoscopy with appropriate biopsies.

In selected patients with a severely strictured esophagus requiring a lifetime of repetitive dilations to maintain any useful lumen, elective esophagectomy with subsequent reconstruction may be reasonable. Additionally, a hiatal hernia, esophagitis, and peptic stricture may develop decades after a severe caustic injury, with resultant progressive fibrosis and dysfunction of the gastroesophageal sphincter. In this setting, the use of traditional dilation techniques as primary chronic therapy only worsens the situation and the reflux.[20] Aggressive prophylactic antireflux measures with proton pump inhibitors may improve the outlook for these patients by increasing the long-term success of dilation, thereby avoiding the need for aggressive surgery.

CONCLUSION (Fig. 23-5)

Caustic ingestion is a common injury that has wide variability in severity, ranging from minimal mucosal erythema to frank transmural necrosis of the esophagus and stomach with viscous perforation. After appropriate identification

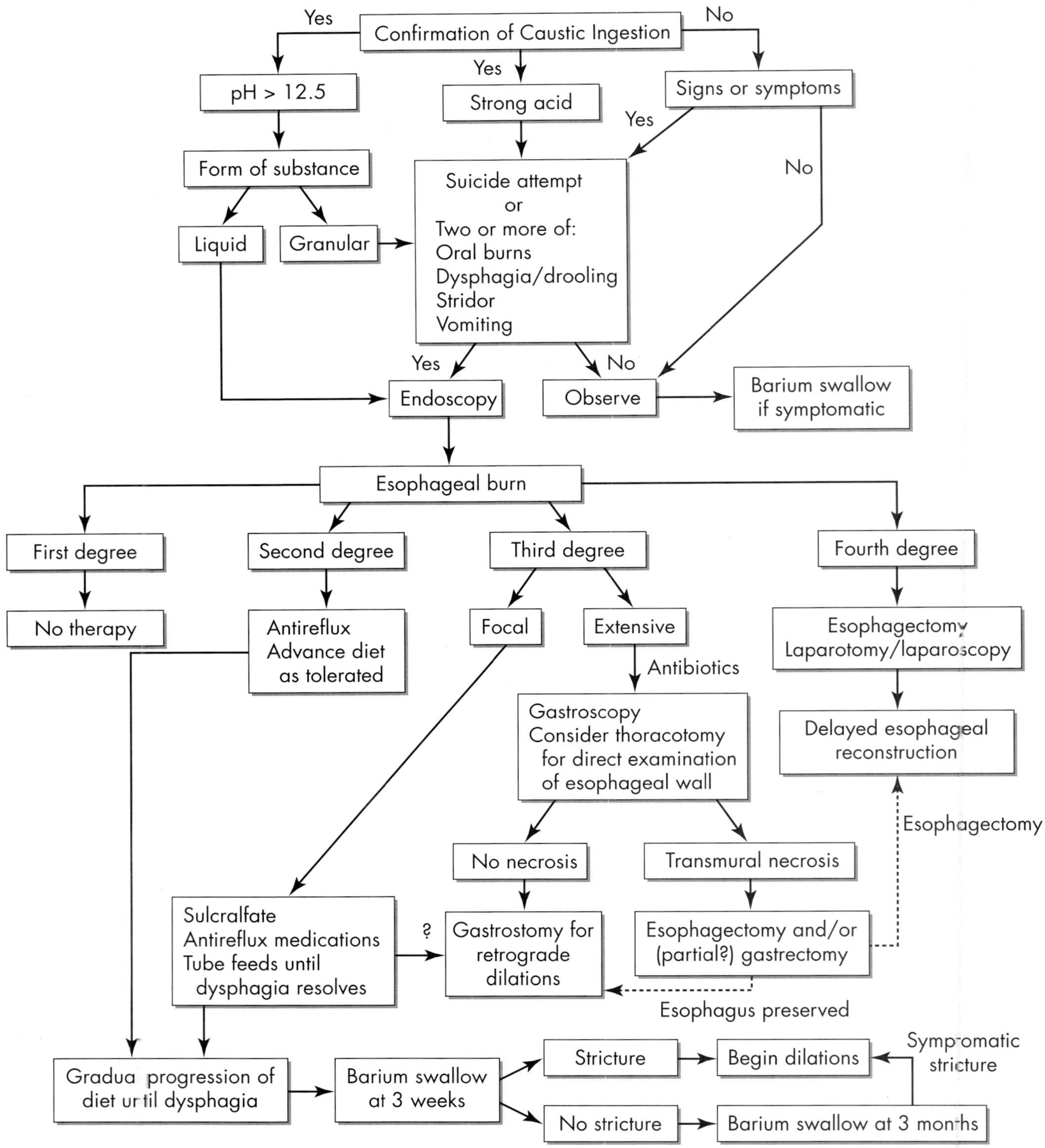

Fig. 23-5. Confirmation of caustic ingestion.

of concentration, pH, and form of the ingested substance, the clinician should decide whether to further evaluate the upper aerodigestive tract. Full-length esophageal endoscopy is the most accurate initial method of examination and is indicated after any ingestion of a strong liquid alkali. The need for endoscopy in other settings depends on the strength, volume, and form of the ingested caustic and associated signs and symptoms. Esophageal stricture formation is the chief complication with a potential devastating impact on quality-of-life. Although repetitive stricture dilations are the mainstay of management, prevention or reduction in the severity of this complication is promising. Extensive necrotic esophageal injuries are doomed to fibrosis, but protocols emphasizing mucosal protectants with aggressive antireflux management may provide a means to minimize stricture formation in second- and localized third-degree injuries.

REFERENCES

1. Anderson KD, Rouse TM, Randolph JG: A controlled trial of corticosteroids in children with corrosive injury of the esophagus, *N Engl J Med* 323:637, 1990.
2. Bosher LH Jr, Burford TH, Ackerman L: The pathology of experimentally produced lye burns and strictures of the esophagus, *J Thorac Surg* 21:483, 1951.
3. Burrington JD: Clinitest burns of the esophagus, *Ann Thorac Surg* 20: 400, 1975.
4. Campbell GS and others: Treatment of corrosive burns of the esophagus, *Arch Surg* 112:495, 1977.
5. Christesen HBT: Prediction of complications following unintentional caustic ingestion in children: is endoscopy always necessary? *Acta Paediatr* 84:1177, 1995.
6. Clausen JO, Nielsen TL, Fogh A: Admission to Danish hospitals after suspected ingestion of corrosives, *Dan Med Bull* 41:234, 1994.
7. Crain EF, Gershel JC, Mezey AP: Caustic ingestions: symptoms as predictors of esophageal injury, *Am J Dis Child* 138:863, 1984.
8. Di Constenza J and others: New therapeutic approach to corrosive burns of the upper gastrointestinal tract, *Gut* 21:370, 1980.
9. Estrera A and others: Corrosive burns of the esophagus and stomach: a recommendation for an aggressive surgical approach, *Ann Thorac Surg* 41:276, 1986.
10. Ferguson MK and others: Early evaluation and therapy for caustic esophageal injury, *Am J Surg* 157:116, 1989.
11. Forsen J, Muntz H: Hair relaxer ingestion: a new trend, *Ann Otol Rhinol Laryngol* 102:781, 1993.
12. Gasset D, Sarfati E, Celervier M: Early blunt esophagectomy in severe caustic burns of the upper digestive tract: report of 29 cases, *J Thorac Cardiovasc Surg* 94:188, 1987.
13. Gaudreault P and others: Predictability of esophageal injury from signs and symptoms: a study of caustic ingestion in 378 children, *Pediatrics* 71:767, 1983.
14. Haller JA Jr, Bachman K: The comparative effect of current therapy on experimental caustic burns of the esophagus, *Pediatrics* 34:236, 1964.
15. Heimlich HJ: Esophagoplasty with reversed gastric tube: review of fifty-three cases, *Am J Surg* 123:80, 1972.
16. Hoffman RS and others: Comparison of titratable acid/alkaline reserve and pH in potentially caustic household products, *Clinical Toxicology* 27:241, 1989.
17. Hollinger PH: Management of esophageal lesions caused by chemical burns, *Ann Otol Rhinol Laryngol* 77:819, 1968.
18. Hopkins RA, Postlewhait RW: Caustic burns and carcinoma of the esophagus, *Ann Surg* 194:146, 1981.
19. Howes EL and others: Retardation of wound healing by cortisone, *Surgery* 28:177, 1950.
20. Imre J, Kopp M: Arguments against long-term conservative treatment of oesophageal strictures due to corrosive burns, *Thorax* 27:594, 1972.
21. Jackson C: Esophageal stenosis following the swallowing of caustic alkalis, *JAMA* 77:22, 1921.
22. Kennedy AP, Cameron BH, McGill CW: Colon patch esophagoplasty for caustic esophageal stricture, *J Pediatr Surg* 30:1242, 1995.
23. Klein JD, Olson KR: Caustic ingestion from household ammonia, too, *J Pediatr* 108:328, 1986 (letter).
24. Lahoti D, Broor S: Corrosive injury to the upper gastrointestinal tract, *Indian J Gastroenterol* 12:135, 1993.
25. Mansson I: Diagnosis of acute corrosive lesions of the esophagus, *J Laryngol Otol* 92:499, 1978.
26. Messner AH, Browne JD, Geisinger KR: Effect of intermittent acid and pepsin exposure on burned esophageal mucosa, *Am J Otol* 17:45, 1996.
27. Mittal PK and others: Sucralfate therapy for acid induced upper gastrointestinal tract injury, *Am J Gastroenterol* 84:204, 1989 (letter).
28. Moore WR: Caustic ingestions: pathophysiology, diagnosis, and treatment, *Clin Pediatr* 25:192, 1986.
29. Neidich G: Ingestion of caustic alkali farm products, *J Pediatr Gastroenterol Nutr* 16:75, 1993.
30. Nuutinen M and others: Consequences of caustic ingestions in children, *Acta Paediatr* 83:1200, 1994.
31. Postlewhait RW and others: Colon interposition for esophageal substitution, *Ann Thorac Surg* 12:89, 1971.
32. Previtera C, Giusti F, Guglielmi M: Predictive value of visible lesions (cheeks, lips, oropharynx) in suspected caustic ingestion: may endoscopy reasonably be omitted in completely negative pediatric patients? *Pediatr Emerg Care* 6:176, 1990.
33. Reddy AN, Budjraja M: Sucralfate therapy for lye esophagitis, *Am J Gastroenterol* 83:71, 1988.
34. Reyes HM and others: Experimental treatment of corrosive esophageal burns, *J Pediatr Surg* 9:317, 1974.
35. Rosenberg N and others: Prevention of experimental esophageal strictures by cortisone II: control of suppurative complications by penicillin, *Arch Surg* 66:593, 1953.
36. Rosenberg N and others: Prevention of experimental lye strictures of the esophagus by cortisone, *Arch Surg* 63:147, 1951.
37. Ruppert P and others: Diagnostic and therapeutic management of esophageal and gastric caustic burns in childhood, *Eur J Pediatr Surg* 3:202, 1993.
38. Sarfarti E and others: Management of caustic ingestion in adults, *Br J Surg* 74:146, 1987.
39. Sellars SL, Spence RAI: Chemical burns of the esophagus, *J Laryngol Otol* 101:1211, 1987.
40. Sigalet D, Lees G: Tracheoesophageal injury secondary to disc battery ingestion, *J Pediatr Surg* 23:996, 1988.

40a. Spain DM, Molomut N, Haber A: The effect of cortisone on the formation of granulation tissue in mice, *Am J Pathol* 26:710, 1950.

41. Stannard MW: Corrosive esophagitis in children: assessment by the esophagram, *Am J Dis Child* 132:596, 1978.
42. Stenson K, Gruber B: Ingestion of caustic cosmetic products, *Otolaryngol Head Neck Surg* 109:821, 1993.
43. Sugawa C, Lucas CE: Caustic injury of the upper gastrointestinal tract in adults: a clinical and endoscopic study, *Surgery* 106:802, 1989.

44. Sugawa C and others: The value of early endoscopy following caustic ingestion, *Surg Gynecol Obstet* 153:553, 1981.
45. Thompson JN: Corrosive esophageal injuries: II. An investigation of treatment methods and histochemical analysis of esophageal strictures in a new animal model, *Laryngoscope* 97:1191, 1987.
46. Tucker G: Cicatricial stenosis of the esophagus, with particular reference to treatment of continuous string retrograde bougienage with the author's bougie, *Laryngoscope* 3:1180, 1924.
47. Vancura EM and others: Toxicity of alkaline solutions, *Ann Emerg Med* 9:118, 1980.
48. Waggoner LG: Diagnosis and management of chemical burns of the esophagus, *Laryngoscope* 68:1790, 1958.
49. Weisskopf A: Effects of cortisone on experimental lye burns of the esophagus, *Ann Otol Rhinol Laryngol* 61:681, 1952.
50. Wilburg FA and others: Nasogastric intubation as sole treatment of caustic esophageal lesions, *Ann Otol Rhinol Laryngol* 94:337, 1985.

Chapter 24

Foreign Bodies of the Airway and Esophagus

Alan D. Murray
Eileen M. Mahoney
Lauren D. Holinger

Airway foreign bodies continue to be a diagnostic and therapeutic challenge for the practicing otolaryngologist. Despite improvement in public awareness and emergency care, foreign bodies result in approximately 3000 deaths per year caused by asphyxiation.[24] Most deaths occur before hospital intervention. Although the role of the otolaryngologist begins after the child is evaluated initially by emergency room or primary care physicians, both otolaryngologists and primary physicians should have a high index of suspicion for foreign body aspiration. Because foreign body aspiration can mimic other conditions, particularly without a witnessed event or history of aspiration, there can be a delay in management, which may lead to complications.

Before the twentieth century, bronchotomy was the method of choice for airway foreign body removal. Most victims of foreign body aspiration died from the initial event, the bronchotomy for removal, or complications thereof. Although intubation of the airway was suggested as far back as the time of Hippocrates, Killian in 1895 was the first to use a hollow tube to evaluate the tracheobronchial airway.[4] He used this technique to remove a bone from the right main bronchus in 1897, becoming the first to perform endoscopic removal of an airway foreign body.

Endoscopic illumination was initially used in esophagoscopy and was incorporated into a bronchoscope[4] by Chevalier-Jackson who revolutionized the field of bronchoesophagology with the development of sound principles and instruments for foreign body removal.[18] Their techniques and equipment were paramount in reducing the mortality associated with airway foreign bodies and are still the basis of foreign body removal today.

The introduction of the rod-lens telescope in the 1970s greatly improved the visualization of bronchoscopic removal of foreign bodies. Foreign body removal has been performed with topical anesthesia and sedation, but with new, safer anesthetic agents and improved anesthesia techniques, general anesthesia is now used routinely.

Children frequently swallow objects that pass through the gastrointestinal tract without problems. This also may occur in adults. Foreign bodies occasionally become lodged in the esophagus because of the object's size or shape, narrowing of the esophageal lumen, or extrinsic compression or anatomic abnormalities.

Before the mid-1850s, the most common management for suspected esophageal foreign body impaction was to attempt to push the object into the stomach. Various instruments, including curved hooks, forceps, and even a walking cane, were used. Dupuytren was reported to vigorously pinch the neck of patients to crush a food impaction in the cervical esophagus, allowing it to pass to the stomach.[4] The first esophagoscope used in 1890 by Mackenzie was later improved by Jackson, Ingals, and Mosher. The earliest rigid esophagoscopies for foreign body extraction by Jackson and Ingals were performed on awake patients in a sitting position. Because anesthesia risks have decreased and instrumentation for endoscopic removal of esophageal foreign bodies has improved, these procedures are performed with the patient supine under general endotracheal anesthesia.

EPIDEMIOLOGY

The incidence of airway and esophageal foreign bodies has not changed significantly, but the safety in removal has increased dramatically. Most airway foreign body aspirations occur in patients younger than 15 years of age. The highest incidence occurs between 1 and 3 years of age; up to 25% of patients are younger than 1 year.[7,13,15,16,29] The reasons toddlers are most susceptible are (1) they lack molars necessary for proper grinding of food; (2) they have less-controlled coordination of swallowing and immaturity in laryngeal elevation and glottic closure; (3) there is an age-related tendency to explore the environment by placing objects in the mouth; (4) they are often running or playing at the time of ingestion.[22] Accidental aspiration or ingestion of objects tends to be twice as common as in boys. Vegetative matter is seen in approximately 70% to 80% of airway foreign bodies, the most common are peanuts in the United States, watermelon seeds in Egypt,[8] and pumpkin seeds in Greece.[12] The percentage of aspirated metallic foreign bodies, especially safety pins, has decreased, primarily because of the widespread use of disposable diapers. Plastic pieces comprise approximately 5% to 15% of airway foreign bodies and tend to remain longer because they are inert and radiolucent.

By far, the most common esophageal foreign bodies are coins[7,13,15,16,25] (in up to 75% cases).[13] Meat and vegetable matter impactions are less common in children, and round objects, trinkets, disk batteries, and sharp objects comprise less than 20% of impacted esophageal foreign bodies. The duration of impaction before endoscopic removal is less than 24 hours in most patients, more than 1 week in 6%, and of unknown duration in 10%.[13,15]

Of patients with multiple esophageal foreign body impactions, 80% have an esophageal anomaly on further evaluation.[13] Of patients with recurrent esophageal foreign bodies, 14% have esophageal anomalies that previously required surgical repair.

LOCATION

Most airway foreign bodies become lodged in the bronchi because their size and configuration allow passage through the larynx and trachea (Fig. 24-1). Larger objects become impacted in the larynx or trachea, at times causing complete obstruction, an acute emergency. Bronchial foreign bodies are more common in the right bronchus in adults, which is thought to be caused by the position of the carina to the left of the midline and its lesser angle of divergence from the tracheal axis.[9] Several authors report airway foreign bodies in children with equal frequency in the right and left main bronchi, with no clear explanation for this occurrence.[1,5,17]

Most esophageal foreign body impactions occur in the cervical esophagus just below the cricopharyngeus (Fig. 24-2).[7,13,16] Another 4% to 5% of esophageal foreign bodies become lodged at the mid or distal esophagus, often caused by extraluminal compression by the aortic arch or left main bronchus (Fig. 24-3). Esophageal foreign body impactions also can occur above an esophageal stricture site.[13]

ACUTE AIRWAY OBSTRUCTION

Complete airway obstruction resulting from a foreign body is an absolute emergency. Food (e.g., hot dogs, candies) and nonfood objects (e.g., toys, balloons) commonly become lodged in the larynx and trachea. Increased public awareness, availability of emergency personnel, and the widespread use of the Heimlich maneuver have greatly reduced the mortality of acute obstruction.[14] The most important factor in reducing mortality is recognition of the person in acute airway distress. Coughing and gagging indicate partial obstruction. Older children and adults may signal choking by grasping the neck.

The Committee on Accident and Poison Prevention of the American Academy of Pediatrics developed guidelines in accord with the American Red Cross and the American Heart Association for Management of choking victims.[6] For children younger than 1 year, back blows and chest thrusts are recommended. Children older than year require gentle abdominal thrusts while supine. Older children and adults are positioned standing, sitting, or recumbent for the Heimlich maneuver. Back blows or abdominal thrusts in only partially obstructed persons could lead to complete obstruction and are not recommended.

SYMPTOMS

Foreign body aspiration is suspected when a victim develops acute choking or severe coughing with respiratory distress. At times, the diagnosis is obscured if the event is unwitnessed in the young child. Some children do not admit to aspiration because of fear of punishment. Symptoms of foreign body aspiration can mimic conditions such as asthma, croup, and pneumonia. Onset of wheezing in an otherwise healthy child should prompt suspicion of foreign body aspiration.

There are three clinical phases of foreign body aspiration.[9] The initial phase consists of choking, gagging, and paroxysms of coughing or airway obstruction, which occur at the moment of aspiration. This subsides during the asymptomatic phase when the foreign body becomes lodged and the reflexes fatigue. The asymptomatic phase can last for hours to weeks. Complications occur in the third phase, when obstruction, erosion, or infection causes pneumonia, atelectasis, abscess, or fever.

In general, a careful history and physical examination are most important in diagnosing foreign body aspiration. Determining the site of the obstruction is important in the management of the problem.

Laryngeal foreign bodies

A foreign body in the larynx may constitute an airway emergency that requires lifesaving first aid before transport to the hospital. Irregular foreign bodies or orientation in the sagittal plane may produce only partial obstruction, allowing

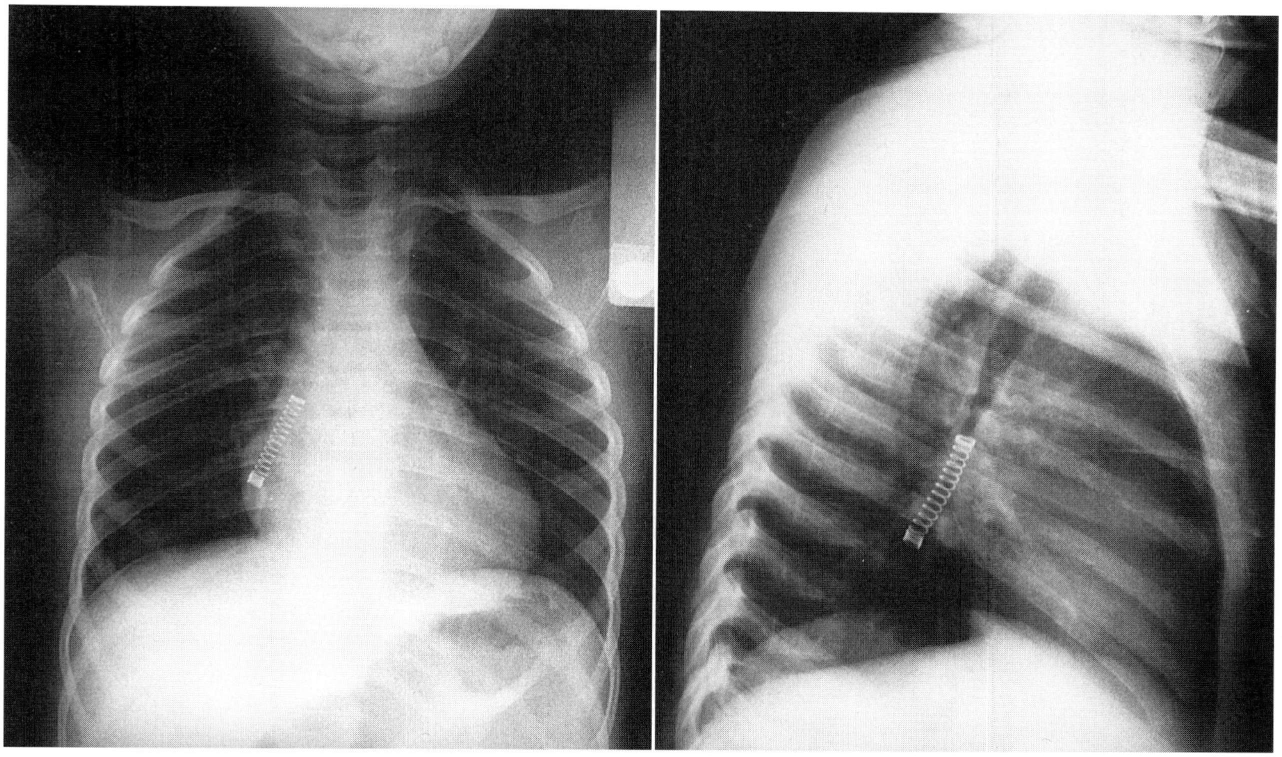

Fig. 24-1. Posteroanterior and lateral view of pen spring in right main bronchus.

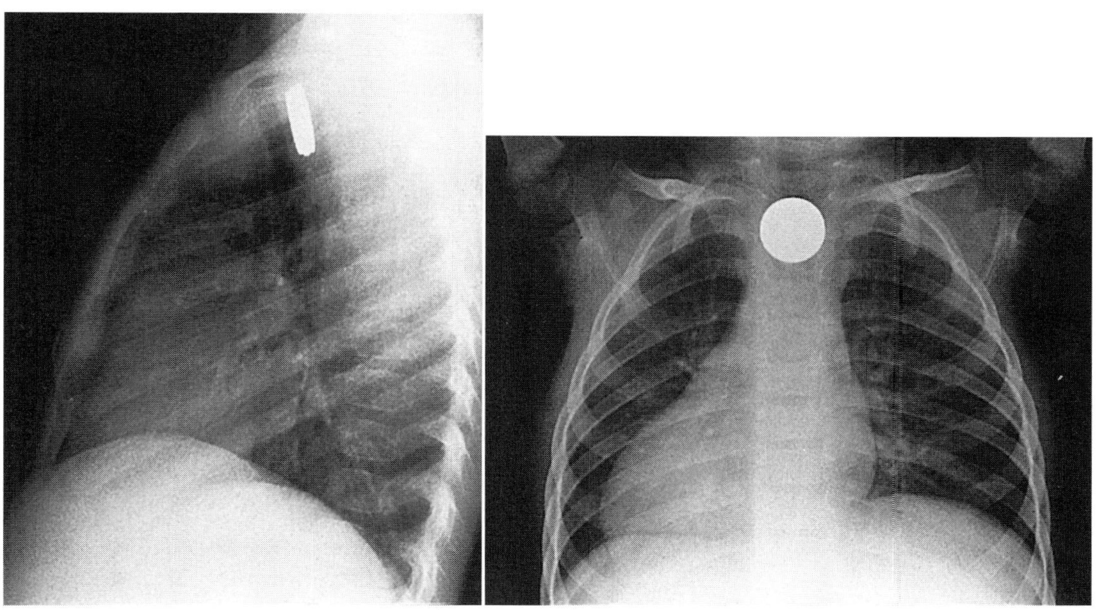

Fig. 24-2. Posteroanterior and lateral film of multiple coins in a typical esophageal location immediately below cricopharyngeus.

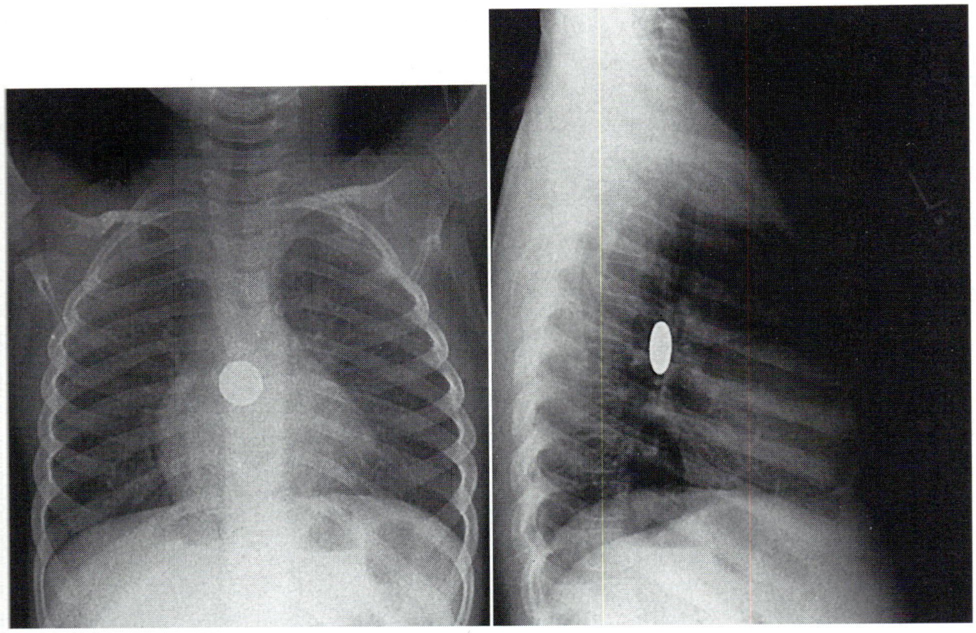

Fig. 24-3. Posteroanterior and lateral chest films of a coin in the midesophagus.

adequate air movement around the obstruction. Resulting laryngeal edema can lead to complete obstruction. Typically, these patients present with symptoms of obstruction and hoarseness. Some symptoms can mimic croup.[18] Delayed diagnosis may lead to complications.

Tracheal foreign bodies

Patients with tracheal foreign bodies present in similar fashion but typically do not have hoarseness. Jackson and Jackson[18] described three signs associated with tracheal foreign bodies: the "asthmetoid wheeze," the "audible slap" produced from foreign body contact with the trachea, and the "palpable thud" over the trachea. As with laryngeal foreign bodies, edema can progress to complete obstruction.

Bronchial foreign bodies

Of airway foreign bodies, 80% to 90% are found in the bronchi.[11] These patients typically present with a triad of cough, wheezing, and decreased breath sounds. One large series reported that 65% present with the classic triad[17] but that up to 95% present with at least one finding.[1]

The asymptomatic phase may give a false sense of security that the problem has resolved and lead to a delay in diagnosis. Chest auscultation may reveal decreased breath sounds or wheezing. Sudden onset of wheezing is particularly suggestive of a bronchial foreign body. Occasionally, bronchial foreign bodies can cause respiratory compromise as a result of swelling of dried vegetable matter or edema around the object, producing complete obstruction and lobar collapse. Movement of the foreign body from one main bronchus to the other produces respiratory distress, resulting from obstruction of the previously normally ventilating lung.

Esophageal foreign body impaction is most frequently associated with vomiting, odynophagia, dysphasia, and ptyalism.[7,13,15,16] If the ingestion is witnessed, gagging or choking may be reported. A large foreign body may cause symptoms of airway obstruction and cough caused by compression or irritation of the upper airway. In long-standing esophageal foreign body impaction, fever and other symptoms of respiratory infection may be present.[13]

A careful history and physical examination are the first steps necessary to diagnose esophageal foreign body impaction. Appropriate radiographic evaluation further aids diagnosis and management.

RADIOGRAPHIC EVALUATION

Laryngotracheal foreign bodies

Airway films—high-kilovolt posteroanterior and lateral soft-tissue radiography of the neck—are the radiographic examination of choice to identify laryngeal and tracheal foreign bodies. Chest radiography is ordered before intervention. Neck radiography may show subglottic narrowing. Esclamado and Richardson[11] reported that 92% of patients with tracheal foreign bodies had abnormal neck radiographs, whereas 50% had normal chest films. When such children do not respond rapidly to medical management, foreign body aspiration must be ruled out.

Bronchial foreign bodies

Children with bronchial foreign bodies can be radiographically normal and may show obstructive emphysema (air trapping or hyperinflation—an early finding) and atelectasis

A

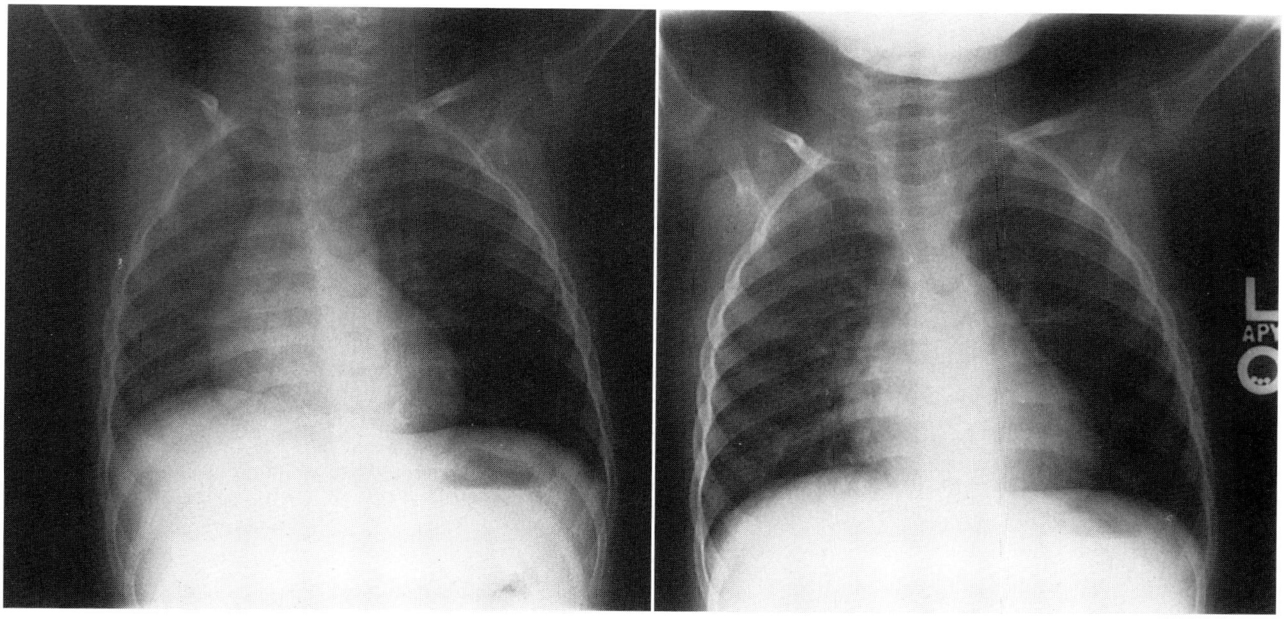

B

Fig. 24-4. A, Inspiratory and **B,** expiratory chest films show hyperinflation on side of left bronchial foreign body (a peanut fragment).

or consolidation (late findings). Even if the diagnosis is strongly suspected by history and physical examination, posteroanterior and lateral chest radiography is performed. In general, chest radiography is an adjunctive procedure because the history and physical examination are sufficient to suspect a bronchial foreign body.

During normal respiration, the airway dilates with inspiration and contracts on expiration. This respiratory cycle can be altered by the presence of bronchial foreign bodies.[3] Small objects may cause no radiographic abnormalities. Foreign bodies that obstruct only on expiration cause a check valve effect, resulting in hyperinflation of the affected side and mediastinal shift to the opposite side (Fig. 24-4). A ball-valve effect is produced when foreign bodies obstruct on inspiration and open on expiration, producing atelectasis on the affected side and a mediastinal shift toward the affected side (Fig. 24-5). When the object completely obstructs the bronchus, a stop-valve effect occurs, leading to consolidation of the lobe involved.

Inspiratory and expiratory chest films can aid in the diagnosis, showing hyperinflation on expiratory films or atelectasis on inspiratory films. In younger children who cannot cooperate, lateral decubitus films may help. The dependent lung should collapse normally but remain inflated in bronchial obstruction. Fluoroscopic evaluation is of little benefit; decreased diaphragmatic movement on the side of the obstruction is helpful in only 50% of cases.[1] Simultaneous biplane fluoroscopy is used for extraction of radiopaque foreign bodies in the lung periphery.

Radiographic findings often suggest but do not diagnose

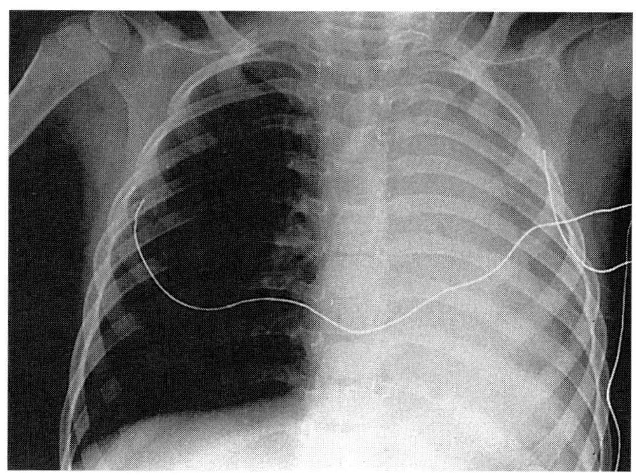

Fig. 24-5. Anteroposterior chest film of left lobar collapse secondary to candy corn in the left main bronchus.

foreign body aspiration. Asthma and mucous plugging can simulate foreign body aspiration. Mu, He, and Sun[23] reported that 35% of patients having normal radiographic studies were later found to have bronchial foreign bodies. Svedstrom, Puhakka, and Kero[27] found that 24% of patients with normal radiographic studies had foreign bodies and concluded that "plain film radiography is neither a sufficiently sensitive nor is it a specific method for the diagnosis of foreign body aspiration."

Table 24-1. Guidelines for selection of bronchoscope, esophagoscope, and laryngoscope for diagnostic endoscopy by age

Mean age (range)	Bronchoscope size*	mm*	Laryngoscope size*	Esophagoscope size*
Premature infant	2.5	3.7	8	4
Term newborn (newborn to 3 mo)	3	5.8	8	4 to 5
6 mo (3 to 18 mo)	3.5	5.7	9	5 to 6
18 mo (1 to 3 yr)	3.7	6.3	10.5	6
3 yr (2 to 6 yr)	4	6.7	10.5 to 12	6 to 7
7 yr (5 to 10 yr)	5	7.8	12	7
10 yr (older than 10 yr to adolescent)	6	8.2	16	8

* Outside diameter given in millimeters

Esophageal foreign bodies

When an esophageal foreign body is suspected by history and physical examination, a radiologic evaluation is performed to assess its location and size and to anticipate the possibility of multiple foreign bodies. Posteroanterior and lateral airway films and posteroanterior and lateral chest films including the abdomen are obtained. Flat objects in the esophagus usually lie in the coronal plane on a posteroanterior radiograph and parallel to the vertebral column on lateral film.[29]

In rare cases in which an esophageal foreign body was not found on initial endoscopy and migrated extraluminally, fluoroscopy with contrast may aid in preoperative location of the object. Open surgical exploration may be required to retrieve the foreign body.[29]

MANAGEMENT

Most patients who arrive at the hospital with airway foreign bodies have passed the acute phase and are no longer in respiratory distress. With rare exceptions, esophageal foreign body impactions are not dire emergencies. There is time to obtain a history regarding the ingestion and a pertinent medical history. An inadequate diagnostic workup and hasty preparation of the operating suites likely lead to a poor outcome. The standard radiographic posteroanterior and lateral airway and chest films may give adequate information for foreign body removal. If the foreign body is sharp or irregularly shaped, a radiograph in the plane of the greatest dimension of the foreign body may help plan removal. If a suspected esophageal foreign body is radiolucent, a swallow study should be avoided because it will delay endoscopy in that the patient can no longer take anything by mouth, and the foreign object may be obscured by the material swallowed. In general, the patient should take nothing by mouth for 6 hours and then be adequately hydrated.

The basic principles of endoscopic foreign body removal have not changed since the days of Chevalier-Jackson.[16,18] The type and size of endoscope depend on the age of the patient and the location of the object. Foreign body forceps are selected based on practice with a similar object, preferably a duplicate brought in by the patient's family. It is important that the operating room personnel be familiar with the planned procedure and that communication with the anesthesiologist regarding the anesthetic and endoscopy plan has occurred.

Equipment

Age-appropriate equipment for endoscopic foreign body removal is carefully selected before the patient is brought to the operating room (Table 24-1). Equipment should be in good working order. All members of the endoscopy team should be familiar with the location, set up, and use of the instrumentation. If there is inadequate equipment or a lack of trained personnel, transfer of the patient to an adequately equipped center with an experienced endoscopy team is considered.

Laryngoscopy visualizes laryngeal foreign bodies and facilitates passing the bronchoscope. Preferred bronchoscopes with a rod-lens telescope are the Doesel-Huzly bronchoscopes (Karl Storz) (Fig. 24-6). Age-appropriate sizes minimize laryngeal edema. For airway foreign bodies, two bronchoscopes are prepared so that if one fails, another is immediately available. For esophageal foreign bodies, an esophageal speculum and appropriate-sized esophagoscope for the patient's age and size are chosen (Fig. 24-7). Suctions and forceps should be checked to ensure they are of adequate length to be used with the endoscopy equipment. Active or passive action forceps may be used; in many situations, the improved visualization achieved with optical forceps is helpful. With bronchial foreign bodies, these optical forceps reduce the amount of ventilation space within the bronchoscope, therefore alternate forceps should be readily available.[15,16,18] A Fogarty catheter may be considered only for objects in the airway that are round or smooth.[19] With all endoscopic foreign body procedures, safety glasses should be worn by the endoscopy team and a tooth protector worn by the patient.

Anesthesia

Foreign body removal is done under general anesthesia unless the patient is in extremis. General anesthesia is preferred for optimal airway control and patient comfort. Excel-

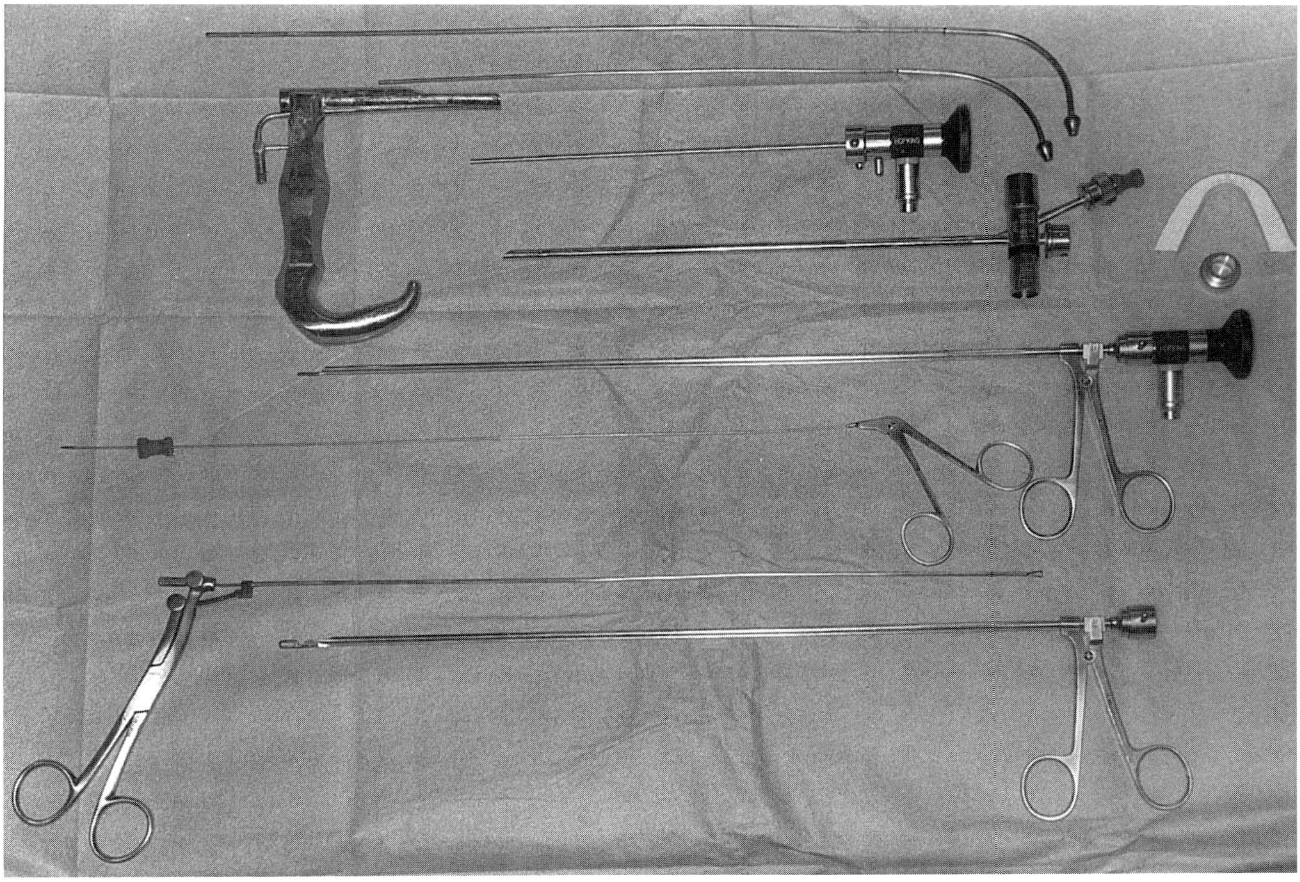

Fig. 24-6. Instruments for endoscopic removal of airway foreign body.

lent communication between the endoscopist and anesthesiologist, preoperatively and during the procedure, is necessary. Patients are given nothing by mouth for an adequate time to reduce the risk of aspiration. Patients are placed supine for mask induction using halothane for children. Eye protection prevents corneal abrasions. Preoperative atropine (0.02 mg/kg intramuscularly) prevents arrhythmia and bradycardia. Spontaneous respiration is maintained. The larynx is sprayed with 1% to 4% lidocaine to inhibit laryngeal reflexes and reduce the incidence of laryngospasm.

For a suspected laryngeal foreign body, patients are preoxygenated. After mask induction, anesthesia is maintained with an insufflation catheter through the nares into the hypopharynx. For tracheobronchial foreign body removal, the laryngoscope tip is placed in the vallecula to expose the larynx for passage of the bronchoscope. The patient breathes through the bronchoscope until the conclusion of the procedure. For esophageal foreign bodies, the patient undergoes endotracheal intubation. The endotracheal tube prevents inadvertent aspiration of the foreign body into the airway during attempted removal and minimizes any tracheal compression caused by a rigid esophagoscope.

Technique

For bronchial foreign bodies, the healthy bronchus is examined first. The bronchoscope is positioned above the foreign body and gently suctions secretions to fully expose the object. One hundred percent oxygen is given before and during the attempt at removal. The forceps are placed through the bronchoscope, and the foreign body is engaged. The bronchoscope, forceps, and foreign body are removed as a unit, and the bronchoscope is returned immediately to the airway for ventilation and assessment for other foreign bodies.

Occasionally, endoscopic attempts at retrieval fail, and thoracotomy is required. If the foreign body is too large to be extracted through the larynx, (1) the foreign body may be broken into small fragments and removed through the bronchoscope or (2) a tracheotomy is performed, and the foreign body is removed through the neck, maintaining the airway and delivering the object with bronchoscopic guidance.[28]

For esophageal foreign body removal, an esophageal speculum or esophagoscope is passed through the right side of the mouth and directed toward the pyriform sinus. It is

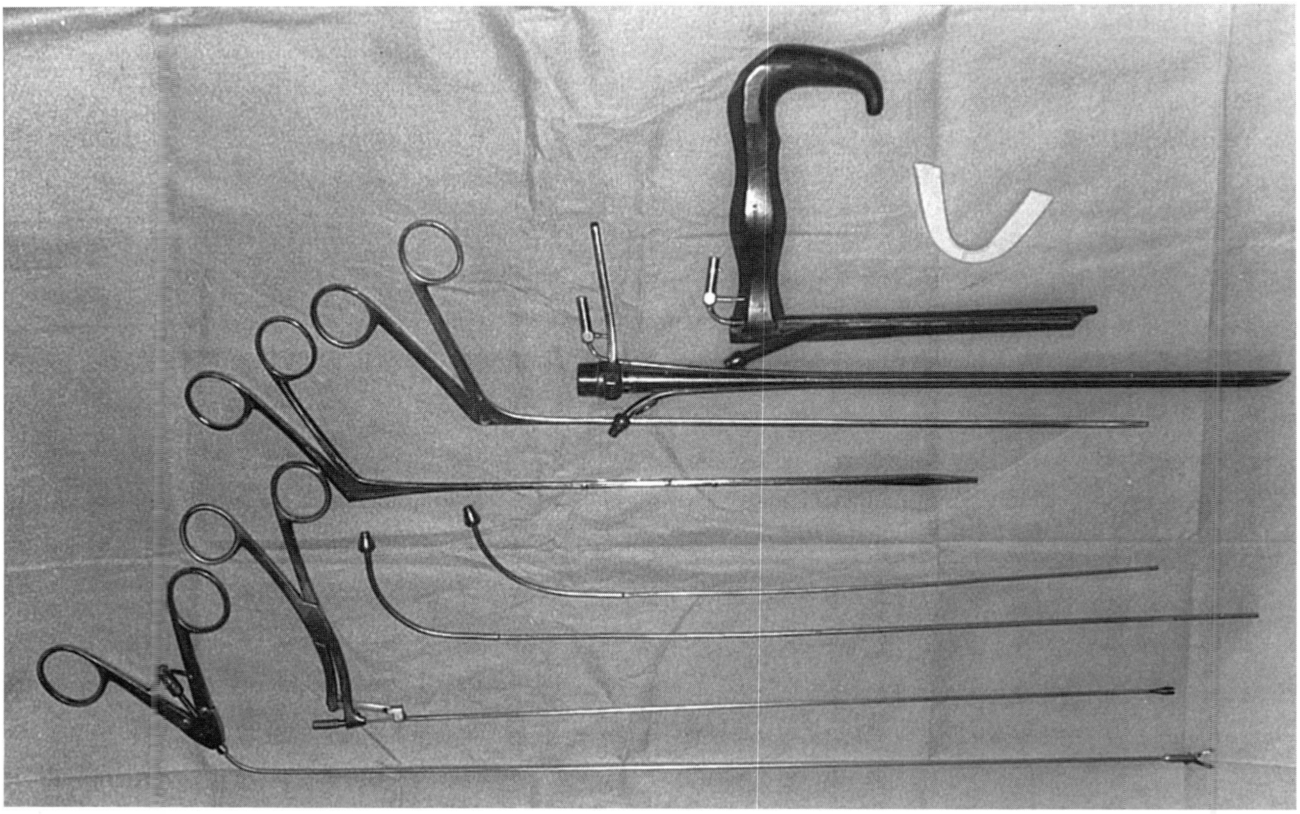

Fig. 24-7. Instruments for removal of an esophageal foreign body.

then angled forward the sternal notch. Gentle pressure at the cricopharyngeus allows passage of the esophagoscope into the esophagus. The esophageal lumen is kept in view at all times while the esophagoscope is gently passed until the foreign body is visualized. The foreign body is engaged with the forceps, the esophagoscope is advanced toward the object, and the foreign body, forceps, and esophagoscope are removed as a single unit. If multiple foreign bodies are suspected, the esophagoscope is reinserted to assess the condition of the esophageal mucosa and to identify additional foreign bodies below the primary one. Multiple foreign bodies are found in up to 5% of patients (Fig. 24-8).[13]

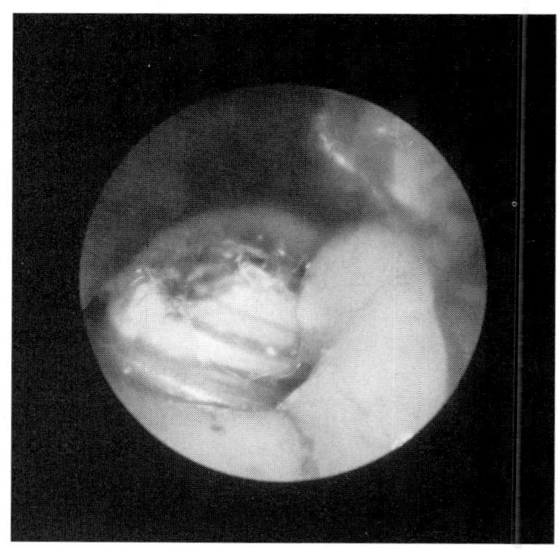

Fig. 24-8. Multiple coins in the esophagus of a patient with a history of tracheoesophageal fistula.

Removal of sharp objects

Extraction of sharp or pointed objects can be extremely challenging.[15] Locating the point is crucial. Usually, the tip of a pointed object engages the mucosa, causing the object to tumble and proceed with the point trailing. Pointed objects are bendable or breakable; analysis of a duplicate may aid in this determination. The endoscope is aligned parallel to the long axis of the airway or esophagus to minimize the likelihood of damage to the surrounding mucosa. During the extraction, the object first is moved distally to disengage the point.

Pin-bending forceps may be used for bendable objects; this reconfigures the object's point to trail on removal. Safety pins are uniquely challenging; those that become lodged are invariably open. The incidence of safety pins as foreign bodies has decreased with the introduction of disposable diapers. Two methods of removal are suggested: (1) sheathing the point within the endoscope while locking the forceps closed to hold the keeper against the outside of the tube particularly during extraction through the larynx, and (2) gastric version (under fluoroscopic control) of esophageal safety pins, using rotation forceps to flip the safety pin point down within the stomach. The Clerf-Arrowsmith pin-closing forceps risk entanglement with the safety pin, which becomes virtually impossible to remove. This dangerous tool is not recommended. If a sharp object is severely impacted or embedded, an open surgical approach may be the safest method of foreign body removal.[7,15] Tetanus immunization status is determined in all patients with sharp or penetrating foreign bodies.

Long or large objects in children younger than 2 years may not pass through the duodenum. It is preferable to remove these objects from the stomach endoscopically before they migrate further or perforate a bowel wall. If a disk battery traverses beyond the esophagus and the patient remains asymptomatic, parents are advised to check the patient's stools for passage and to return immediately to the hospital if fever or abdominal pain occurs.[15,20] An abdominal film is obtained. Children younger than 6 years with a battery 15 mm in diameter or larger that has not passed out of the stomach within 48 hours should undergo endoscopic removal. Many batteries 15 mm or greater do not pass out of the stomach and cause corrosive injury in an acid environment.

Disk battery ingestions

A patient with a history of ingestion and esophageal lodging of disk batteries (e.g., found in hearing aids, calculators, and certain toys) needs prompt attention.[15,20,21] The peak incidence occurs at 1 to 2 years of age. In 33% of cases, the ingested battery is from the child's hearing aid.[21] In as little as 1 hour, the esophageal mucosa may be damaged; in 4 hours, leakage of caustic battery contents may cause erosion through the muscular wall of the esophagus; and within 6 or more hours, an esophageal perforation leading to mediastinitis, tracheoesophageal fistula, or death may occur.[15,20,21] If esophageal lodging of a disk battery is suspected, radiography will aid in localizing the battery, and an immediate esophagoscopy is performed to remove the battery and assess the patient's esophageal mucosa. Most batteries of this type are 7.9 or 11.6 mm and usually traverse the gastrointestinal tract with only minor injury. Larger button batteries (at least 15 mm in diameter) are more likely to lodge in the esophagus or stomach, causing serious corrosive injury. Mercuric oxide–containing batteries can cause systemic mercury poisoning if they open in the gastrointestinal tract. The imprint code of a duplicate battery is related to a Poison Control Center or Button Ingestion Hotline for specific instructions.[21]

Esophageal perforation

Perforation of the esophagus in a patient with an impacted esophageal foreign body may be caused by the object itself, by the length of time that the object has been lodged, or by attempts to retrieve the object.* If perforation has occurred preoperatively, esophageal perforation may be diagnosed on preoperative radiographic evaluation. Mediastinal emphysema, a retroesophageal abscess, or an obvious extraluminal portion of the esophageal foreign body may be apparent.[7] The patient may be febrile with tachycardia, tachypnea, and increased pain. With early recognition and management, the mortality rate for esophageal perforation has decreased from 60% to 9%. After esophagography has been performed to locate and evaluate the extent of the injury, early institution of nothing by mouth and broad-spectrum antibiotics may be all that is necessary in pharyngoesophageal perforations,[10] the most common area injured in endoscopic removal of esophageal foreign bodies. In more severe injuries, drainage, closure, or more complex surgical repairs may be necessary.

POSTOPERATIVE MANAGEMENT

After esophagoscopy for foreign body extraction, children are observed and given nothing by mouth for at least 4 hours. The patients are monitored for fever, tachycardia, and tachypnea—signs of perforation. Antibiotics are not routinely given unless significant esophageal injury is evident.

When appropriate-sized bronchoscopes are used for brief procedures, racemic epinephrine or corticosteroids are not given. Chest physiotherapy helps clear secretions. A routine postoperative radiograph is not obtained unless the patient's symptoms persist or progress. When extraction attempts fail or are incomplete, patients are rested for several days, then returned to the operating room for repeat endoscopy.

COMPLICATIONS

Before the twentieth century, the mortality rate caused by foreign body aspiration was high, with most patients succumbing to complications. In 1882, Weiss[4] reported 937 cases for which bronchotomy was performed with a 27% mortality rate: 23% died without management and Jackson's techniques reduced the mortality rate to about 2%.[3] The present rate is 2% or less.[1,5,17]

Most complications are the result of delayed diagnosis.[17] Earlier diagnosis correlates with fewer complications. Of laryngotracheal foreign bodies, 45% were associated with major complications, 67% when the delay was longer than 24 hours.[11] The introduction of rod-lens telescopes has reduced the incidence of missed or incomplete removal of foreign bodies, further reducing complications.

Pneumonia and atelectasis are the most common complications after bronchial foreign body removal. Patients usually respond to intravenous antibiotics and chest physiotherapy. Bleeding can occur because of granulation tissue or erosion into a major vessel. Pneumothorax and pneumomediastinum can result from an airway tear. Small perforations typically heal spontaneously and do not require specific

* Refs. 2,10,16,21,25,29.

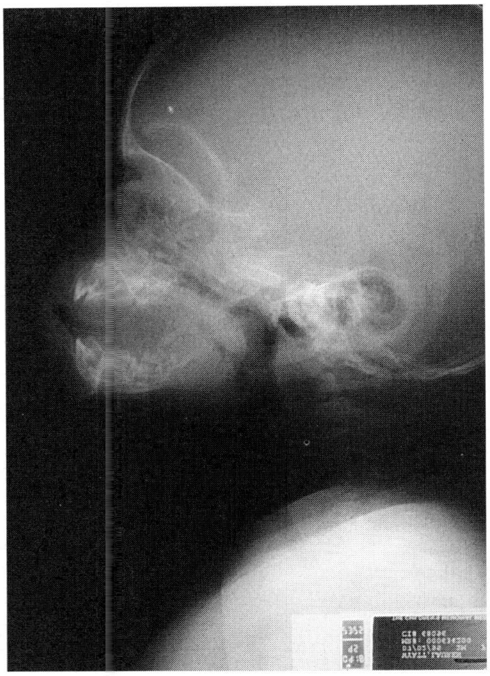

Fig. 24-9. Lateral neck film reveals retroesophageal abscess.

management. Impaction of the foreign body can cause airway obstruction converting a controlled situation into an emergency. Laryngeal inflammation and edema have decreased significantly with the use of appropriate-sized endoscopic equipment.

Long-term complications (e.g., granulation tissue, stricture formation) can occur at the site where the foreign body is lodged. Certain foreign bodies are more likely to cause more complications. The oils of nuts may contribute to edema and granulation tissue.[18]

The most frequent complications of endoscopic esophageal foreign body removal are categorized as those occurring before endoscopy, during endoscopy, and after endoscopy.[19]

Vomiting and respiratory distress are most common preoperatively. During esophagoscopy, the endotracheal tube may be dislodged, and the patient may have cricopharyngeal spasm, esophageal mucosal injury, or perforation. After esophagoscopy, vomiting, aspiration, a second missed foreign body, and fever are the most common complications. Esophageal perforation, retroesophageal abscess, mediastinitis, and death are rare (Fig. 24-9). In several large series of endoscopic esophageal foreign body removal, there were no life-threatening complications.[7,10,13,25]

CONTROVERSIES IN MANAGEMENT

Nonendoscopic means of foreign body extraction have been suggested. These methods have been detrimental in some cases, causing emergent situations and even death. Although chest physiotherapy and bronchodilators have been suggested as a management for airway foreign bodies, this proposal has been retracted.[26] Flexible bronchoscopic removal of airway foreign bodies seems attractive, with recent literature advocating its use in adults, particularly with peripherally located objects and patients with facial trauma. Flexible bronchoscopic foreign body removal in children is not recommended, especially in small children. The main problems are poor control of the airway and the foreign body itself.

For impacted esophageal foreign bodies, bougienage with esophageal dilators or a nasogastric tube has been proposed to push foreign bodies into the stomach.[4,26] This blind technique may cause esophageal injury and is not recommended. Foley catheter removal with fluoroscopic control of blunt radiopaque esophageal foreign bodies has been recommended for objects lodged below the cricopharyngeus for a short duration.[23,25] The advantages are reduced cost and avoidance of general anesthesia. Few serious complications have been reported when this technique was used in healthy children. Other authors[13,26,29] point out that the risks of general anesthesia in these patients are small. This technique does not allow a postretrieval assessment of the esophageal mucosa or a search for a nonradiopaque second foreign body. There is a risk of vomiting and aspiration with an unprotected airway; young patients who have this procedure performed while awake and restrained in a steep head-down position may suffer emotional trauma.

Another technique that had some transient popularity is the use of papain in patients with impacted esophageal meat boluses.[26] Papain was given as a 5% solution to adult patients, with the meat passing in most instances. However, there were at least two cases of mediastinitis and death in these patients caused by necrosis of the esophagus and perforation.

Careful endoscopic removal of foreign objects under direct vision is the safest management for patients with foreign bodies of the airway and esophagus. Prevention is ideal, with increased education of parents on age-appropriate foods and household objects and strict industry standards for toy part sizes and safe containers.

REFERENCES

1. Black RE, Johnson DG, Matlak ME: Bronchoscopic removal of aspirated foreign bodies in children, *J Pediatr Surg* 29:682, 1994.
2. Campbell JB, Condon VR: Catheter removal of blunt esophageal foreign bodies in children, *Pediatr Radiol* 19:361, 1989.
3. Chatterji S, Chatterji P: The management of foreign bodies in air passages, *Anesthesia* 27:390, 1972.
4. Clerf LH: Historical aspects of foreign bodies in the air and food passages, *South Med J* 68:1149, 1975.
5. Cohen SR and others: Foreign bodies in the airway: five year retrospective study with special reference to management, *Ann Otol Rhinol Laryngol* 89:437, 1980.
6. Committee on Accident and Poison Prevention: First aid for the choking child, *Pediatrics* 81:740, 1988.
7. Crysdale WS: Esophageal foreign bodies in children: 15 year review of 484 cases, *Ann Otol Rhinol Laryngol* 100:329, 1991.

8. Daniilidis J and others: Foreign body in the airways: a review of 90 cases, *Arch Otolaryngol Head Neck Surg* 103:570, 1977.
9. Darrow DH, Holinger LD: *Foreign bodies of the larynx, trachea and bronchi.* In Bluestone C, Stool S, editors: *Pediatric otolaryngology*, Philadelphia, 1996, WB Saunders.
10. Dolgin SR and others: Conservative medical management of traumatic pharyngoesophageal perforations, *Ann Otol Rhinol Laryngol* 101:209, 1992.
11. Esclamado RM, Richardson MA: Laryngotracheal foreign bodies in children: a comparison with bronchial foreign bodies, *Am J Dis Child* 141:259, 1987.
12. Gaffar H and others: The value of x-ray examination in the diagnosis of tracheobronchial foreign bodies in infants and children, *ORL J Otorhinolaryngol Relat Spec* 44:340, 1982.
13. Hawkins DB: Removal of blunt foreign bodies from the esophagus, *Ann Otol Rhinol Laryngol* 99:935, 1990.
14. Heimlich HJ: A life-saving maneuver to prevent food-choking, *JAMA* 234:398, 1975.
15. Holinger LD: Management of sharp and penetrating foreign bodies of the upper aerodigestive tract, *Ann Otol Rhinol Laryngol* 99:684, 1990.
16. Holinger PH: Foreign bodies of the air and food passages, *Trans Am Acad Ophthalmol Otol* 66:193, 1966.
17. Inglis AF, Wagner DB: Lower complication rates associated with bronchial foreign bodies over the last 20 years, *Ann Otol Rhinol Laryngol* 101:61, 1992.
18. Jackson C, Jackson CL: *Diseases of the air and food passages of foreign body origin*, Philadelphia, 1936, WB Saunders.
19. Kosloske AM: Tracheobronchial foreign bodies in children: back to the bronchoscope and a balloon, *Pediatrics* 66:321, 1980.
20. Litovitz T, Schmitz B: Ingestion of cylindrical and button batteries: an analysis of 2382 cases, *Pediatrics* 89:747, 1992.
21. Maves MD, Carithers JS, Birck HG: Esophageal burns secondary to disc battery ingestion, *Ann Otol Rhinol Laryngol* 93:364, 1984.
22. McGuirt WF and others: Tracheobronchial foreign bodies, *Laryngoscope* 98:615, 1988.
23. Mu L, He P, Sun D: Inhalation of foreign bodies in Chinese children: a review of 400 cases, *Laryngoscope* 101:657, 1991.
24. *Accident facts*, Chicago, 1995, National Safety Council.
25. Reeder LB, DeFilippi VJ, Ferguson MK: Current results of therapy for esophageal perforation, *Am J Surg* 169:615, 1995.
26. Ritter F: Questionable methods of foreign body treatment, *Ann Otol Rhinol Laryngol* 83:729, 1974.
27. Svedstrom E, Puhakka H, Kero P: How accurate is chest radiography in the diagnosis of tracheobronchial foreign bodies in children? *Pediatr Radiol* 19:520, 1989.
28. Swensson EE and others: Extraction of large tracheal foreign bodies through a tracheostoma under bronchoscopic control, *Ann Thorac Surg* 39:251, 1985.
29. Yee KF, Schild JA, Holinger PH: Extraluminal foreign bodies (coins) in the food and air passages, *Ann Otol Rhinol Laryngol* 84:619, 1975.

Chapter 25

Infections of the Airway

Newton O. Duncan, III
Robert C. Sprecher

Children may experience a variety of infections involving the upper respiratory tract and surrounding structures. Some infections occur commonly, may be self-limited, and may be relatively inconsequential. However, other infections, some of which are more rare, may be life threatening. The astute clinician often can identify the various airway infections by an accurate clinical history and targeted physical examination. Radiologic imaging, laboratory studies, or airway endoscopy also may be helpful for accurate diagnosis. Nevertheless, a keen understanding of the various signs and symptoms of airway infections is important. The signs and symptoms of the various airway infections may have many similarities because the anatomic structures and tissues involved are close in proximity. These similar airway findings also can be present in children with acute tonsillitis, infectious mononucleosis, diphtheria, peritonsillar abscess, congenital airway anomalies, subglottic stenosis of any etiology, and in those with airway foreign bodies. Therefore, great familiarity with the spectrum of childhood airway disease entities can be extremely important in their prompt diagnosis and management. This chapter will emphasize the current recognition and management of croup (laryngotracheitis), supraglottitis (epiglottitis), bacterial tracheitis, and retropharyngeal abscesses.

CROUP (LARYNGOTRACHEITIS)

Croup is a term from the ancient Scottish language that refers to the harsh, barking cough that may be present in those with a number of different acquired or congenital disorders.[17,60] There have been several terms used synonymously with croup, which have led to confusion concerning the exact nature of the disease. These terms include croup, viral croup, laryngotracheitis, laryngotracheobronchitis, pseudomembranous croup, spasmodic croup, and postintubation croup. This infectious disease primarily involves the vocal folds or glottis and the subglottis. Because viruses predominantly cause this entity, the most descriptive and widely used terms are either *viral croup* or, more properly, *viral laryngotracheitis*. Viral laryngotracheitis, or croup, is the most common form of infectious upper airway tract obstruction in children. It is estimated that this condition accounts for 90% of infectious airway obstructions and that 3% to 5% of children have at least one episode of croup. This condition can be recurrent in approximately 5% of children.[66] Some children (1.5% to 15%) with croup require hospital admission for airway obstructive symptoms, and during hospitalization 1% to 5% may require intubation.[4,18] Parainfluenza viruses 1 and 2 primarily are implicated in this disease (up to 75%), but influenza A and B, respiratory syncytial virus, measles, adenovirus, varicella, and herpes simplex virus type I all have been isolated. Measles involvement in those with croup historically leads to an aggressive form of the disease.[12,36]

Children most commonly are affected when aged between 6 months and 3 years, with a peak incidence at 18 to 24 months. Boys are more likely affected by more than a 2:1 ratio. Although croup can occur at any time of the year, there is a strong seasonal occurrence in late autumn and winter. Croup may be called atypical if it occurs in infants aged less than 6 months, lasts more than 7 days, or does not respond to appropriate treatment. Other etiologies besides acute viral laryngotracheitis should be considered in these atypical cases.

Viral croup transmission occurs by direct contact and exposure to nasopharyngeal secretions.[68] The incubation period before onset of clinical symptoms is 2 to 6 days for parainfluenza virus type I, and children may continue to shed the virus for up to 2 weeks.[2] After acquisition, the viral infection involves the nasopharynx, producing nasal symptoms. Local spread to the larynx and trachea ensues. The mucosae of the vocal folds and subglottis become erythematous and swollen. Lymphocytes, histiocytes, and polymorphonuclear leukocytes infiltrate the lamina propria, submucosa, and adventitia, and there is generalized mucosal edema. The duration of illness usually is from 3 to 5 days. The crucial factor in those with viral croup is the amount of swelling in the subglottic area. The subglottis is the narrowest portion of the upper respiratory tract, and because of the complete cartilaginous cricoid ring, any edema that occurs in the subglottis does so at the expense of the airway lumen. Because stridor does not occur until there already is significant airway obstruction and because any decrease in cross-sectional area is proportional to the square of the radius of the airway lumen, any further decrease in airway size caused by mucous plugging or crusting may lead to almost rapid and complete airway obstruction.

Clinical features

Characteristically, children with viral croup have a history of prodromal upper airway infection. Low-grade fever may be present. There also may be leukocytosis, although the leukocyte count in most patients is normal. Inspiratory stridor, hoarseness, and a barking cough are cardinal symptoms of viral croup. This cough is invariably present and may help distinguish croup from other illnesses. The presence of biphasic stridor, retractions, high respiratory rate, or oxygen desaturations indicates severe airway obstruction.

Viral croup may present with only mild symptoms of airway obstruction, but it also can be severe with life-threatening airway obstruction. Many different schemes have been developed to assess the spectrum and severity of croup in an effort to assist in determining how to best manage the different presentations of croup.[2,17,37] One best scheme has not been devised. Therefore, it is important to consider the following parameters when evaluating children with croup or airway obstruction in general: (1) stridor: inspiratory versus expiratory, (2) respiratory rate, (3) chest retractions, (4) air entry into the chest by auscultation (decreased with severe obstruction), (5) anxiety or restlessness, (6) color or cyanosis, (7) oxygen desaturation by pulse oximetry, and (8) level of consciousness.

Diagnosis

The diagnosis of croup is highly suggested by history and physical examination alone. Detailed questioning about possible foreign body ingestion should be made along with any previous intubation history. Radiographic imaging of the airway traditionally has been helpful in evaluating those with airway disorders (Figs. 25-1 and 25-2). The diagnosis can be confirmed radiographically by anteroposterior (AP) and lateral (high kilovoltage) films of the upper airway. The

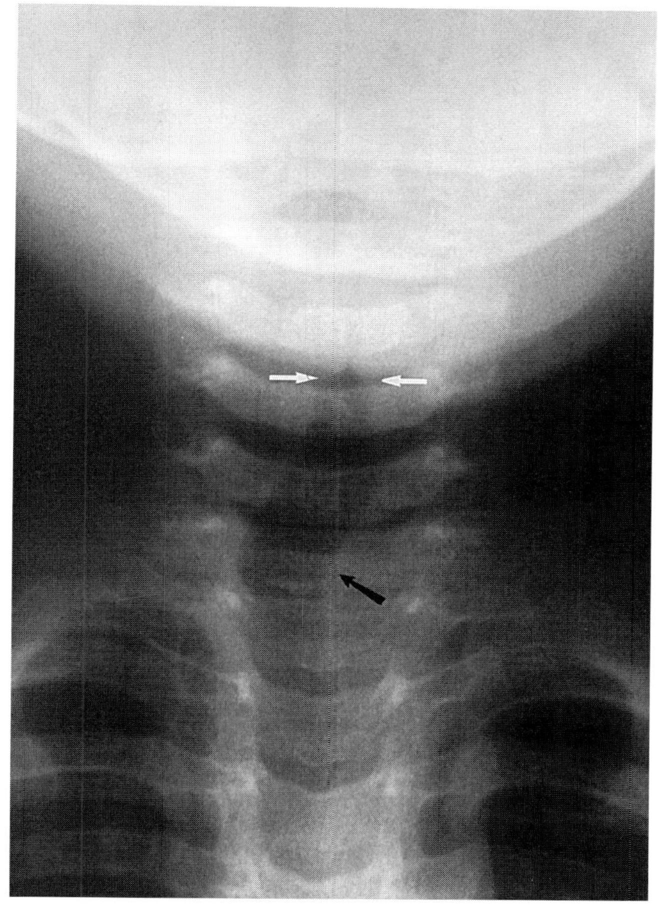

Fig. 25-1. Normal anteroposterior radiographic view of the soft tissues of the neck demonstrating the normal shouldering contours of the proximal trachea *(white arrows)*. Many children will show slight angulation of the trachea, which is a normal variant *(black arrow)*.

frontal AP view classically shows a "steeple sign" in the subglottic area, whereas the lateral view is characterized by haziness of the same area (Figs. 25-3 and 25-4). Flexible fiberoptic laryngoscopy occasionally may be helpful in establishing the correct diagnosis of viral croup. This procedure should be performed with utmost care if there are moderate-to-severe airway obstructive symptoms. In patients with severe airway obstruction, the diagnosis may be confirmed by direct laryngoscopy at the time of intubation (Figs. 25-5 and 25-6).

Differential diagnosis

The most important differential diagnosis to consider in children with suspected croup is epiglottitis (Table 25-1). Thereafter, the possible presence of any airway foreign body, particularly in the larynx or subglottis, must be considered. Subglottic hemangiomas may have similar symptoms in infants aged less than 6 months. Recurrent episodes of a croup-

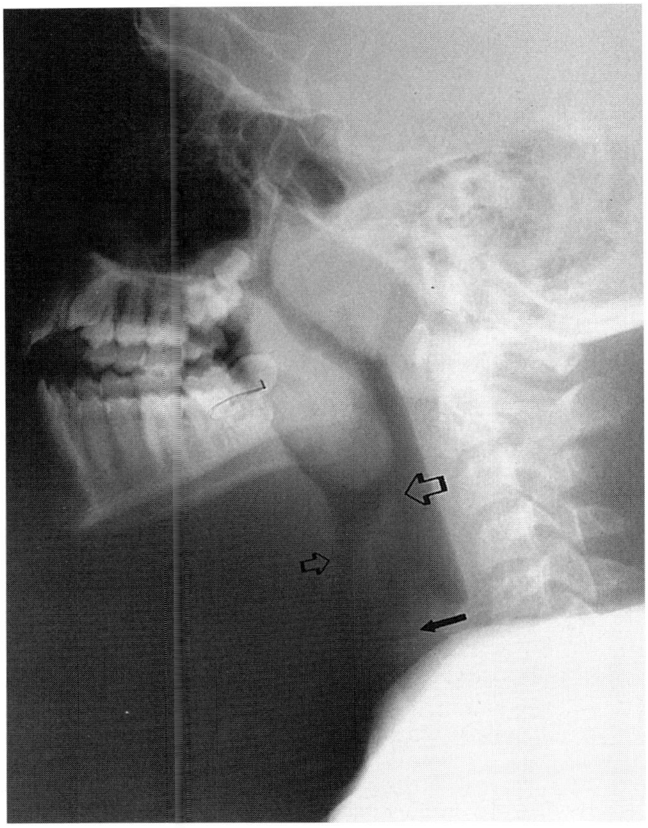

Fig. 25-2. Normal lateral soft-tissue radiograph of the airway with normal epiglottis *(larger open arrow)* and well-defined vallecula *(smaller open arrow)*. The *black arrow* shows the laryngeal ventricle.

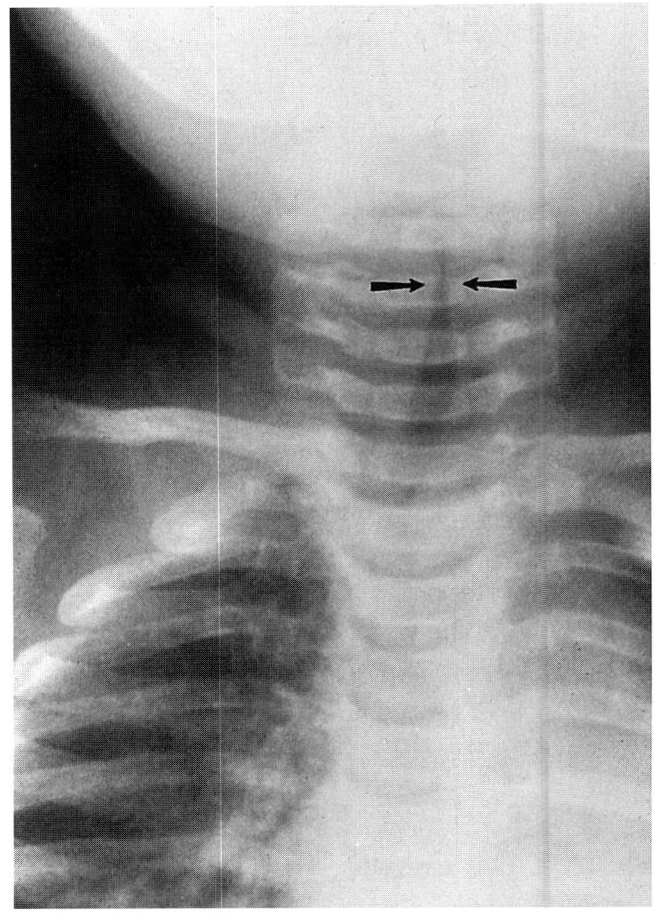

Fig. 25-3. Narrowed subglottis in viral croup *(arrows)* in the anteroposterior radiographic view.

Table 25-1. Differential diagnosis of upper airway infections in children

	Laryngotracheitis (viral croup)	**Supraglottitis (epiglottitis)**	**Bacterial tracheitis**	**Retropharyngeal abscess**
Prodrome	URI symptoms	None or mild URI	URI symptoms	URI symptoms
Onset	Slow	Rapid	Rapid	Slow
Age	6 months-3 years	1-8 years	6 months-8 years	1-5 years
Fever	Variable or none	High	Usually high	Usually high
Hoarseness/barky cough	Yes	No	Yes	No
Dysphagia	No	Yes	Yes	Yes
Toxic appearance	No	Yes	Yes	Variable

URI—Upper respiratory infection.

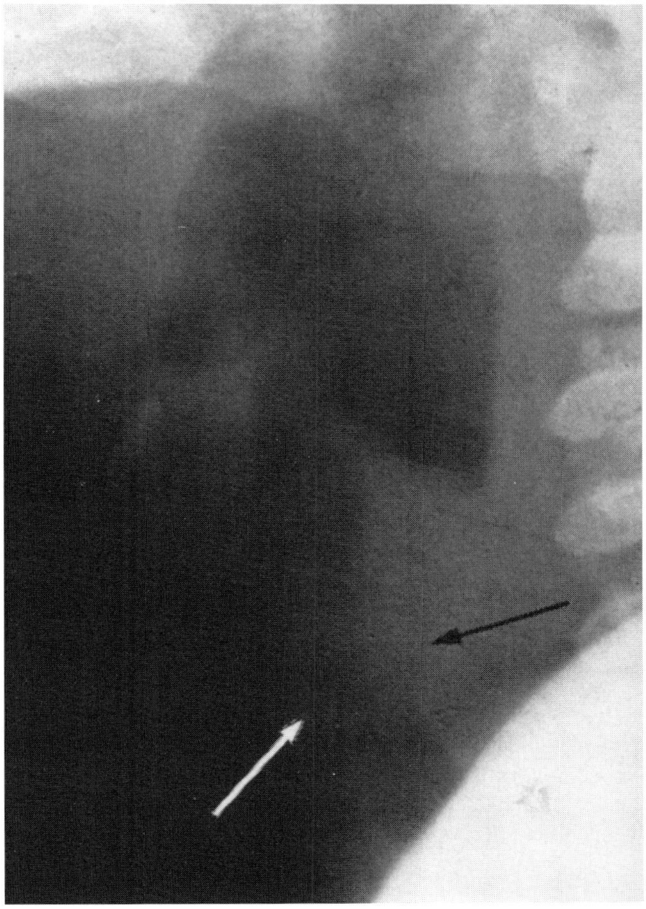

Fig. 25-4. Hazy subglottis in the lateral radiographic view *(arrows)* seen in viral croup.

like illness may occur not only in those with congenital subglottic narrowing, but also in children with acquired subglottic stenosis. Therefore, a history of intubation may be important. Viral croup in the presence of any preexisting laryngeal or subglottic narrowing may lead to early or recurrent stridor and symptoms of croup. Atypical or recurrent symptoms of croup always demand close attention for other etiologies of airway compromise in addition to viral croup. Gastroesophageal reflux also may be a contributing cause of recurrent croup.[67]

Spasmodic croup

Spasmodic croup is a poorly understood entity that is manifested by the sudden onset of stridor, usually at night, in a healthy child aged between 1 and 3 years with no concomitant upper respiratory tract infection. A barking cough and dyspnea accompany the stridor. These episodes may be recurrent in nature and usually resolve spontaneously or with cool humid air within several hours. The vocal folds may be involved with spasm and mild, pale transient vocal fold and subglottic edema may be present. Some of the same viruses that cause viral croup may be involved with causing spasmodic croup, but there is an increasing association between spasmodic croup and recurrent croup with nonspecific bronchial hyperactivity, asthma, and allergic disease.[51,54] Spasmodic croup and viral croup also may well represent two ends of a broad spectrum in the clinical presentation of a single disease.[59] Gastroesophageal reflux also has been implicated in recurrent croup.

When viral croup is not responding to appropriate therapy and when children exhibit an increasingly febrile or toxic appearance, bacterial superinfection in the subglottis or trachea should be suspected. This may occur in 10% to 15% of patients hospitalized with more severe croup. Bacterial tracheitis actually may originate as a complication of viral croup.[23]

Management

Most children with viral croup have symptoms within the mild spectrum of the illness and do not require a physician visit. The illness usually is self-limited, peaking in severity over 3 to 5 days with no specific treatment required at home. A quiet environment and parental comforting or support is universally important in the treatment of children with croup. Any stimulus or disturbance promotes crying and an increased respiratory rate. The airway is stabilized with less mucosal dryness when the child is quiet and when anxiety or crying is diminished.

Management strategies for viral croup have included mist, racemic epinephrine, and corticosteroids. Although viral croup is the most common form of airway obstruction in young children, there remains no consensus regarding optimal treatment.

Humidified air can be provided by portable humidifiers or by steaming a bathroom in the home environment or by mist tents in hospitals. Presumably humidified air moistens secretions, making it easier for children to expectorate them, and prevents drying or crusting that may further compromise a narrow airway. There also may be soothing of the involved mucosa, making children more comfortable and less likely to increase submucosal inflammation by vigorous coughing. There is no evidence showing any effect of humidified air on subglottic edema. Only several studies have looked at the effectiveness of moist air in the management of croup and have shown no benefit of treatment in a mist tent over control patients.[9] Furthermore, the issue of warm versus cool mist has not been settled.

Although there is no scientific evidence that humidified air is of benefit, there is strong anecdotal evidence to support its use in children with viral croup. It is prudent to maintain reasonably humidified air at home or in the hospital. A portable humidifier at home or a mist tent in the hospital may serve this purpose. When a mist tent is used, saline instead of water may provide heavier mist. The mist should not be so thick that the child cannot be easily observed, and a tent should not be used if the child is anxious or not tolerat-

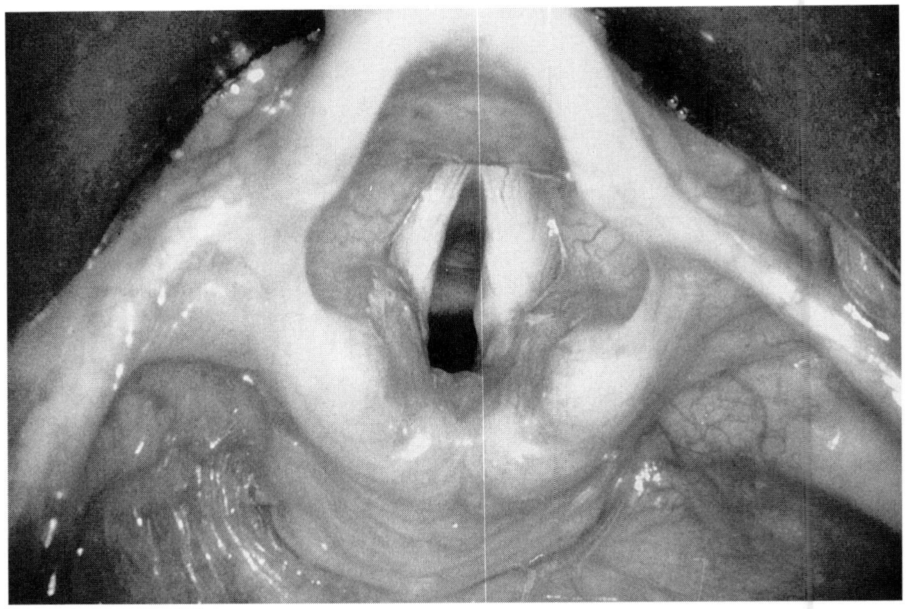

Fig. 25-5. Normal child larynx with crisp vocal folds and widely patent subglottis visualized by a rigid rod telescope.

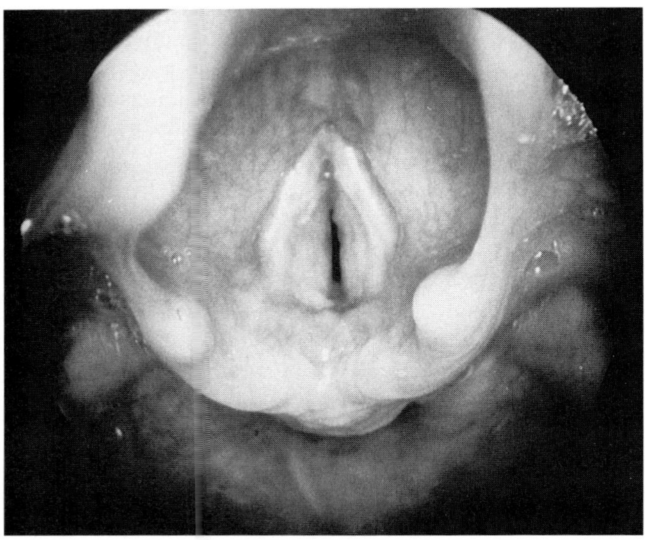

Fig. 25-6. Viral croup with severe vocal fold and subglottic edema as seen with a rigid rod telescope.

ing the tent for any reason. Blow-by mist may be used in these patients. Oxygen should be administered only if needed to maintain adequate oxygen saturations.

Racemic epinephrine is an equal mixture of the d- and l-isomers of epinephrine. It has been used in North America since 1971,[1] but it has been unavailable in other countries. It has been shown that l-epinephrine is at least as effective as racemic epinephrine, is readily available worldwide, has no increased side effects, and is less expensive.[65] The α-adrenergic effects of epinephrine cause mucosal vasoconstriction, leading to decreased edema in the subglottic region. Using 0.5 ml of a 2.25% solution diluted in 3 ml of saline delivered by a nebulizer results in rapid clinical improvement in moderate-to-severe respiratory distress within 10 to 30 minutes.[45,59] This effect wanes and disappears by 2 hours after administration with rebound subglottic mucosal edema in some patients. Because of this temporary effect and possible rebound, children should be observed closely after administering racemic epinephrine. In the past, racemic epinephrine use mandated hospitalization for overnight observation. Recent reports suggest the safe use of racemic epinephrine in an outpatient setting when administered with dexamethasone and mist. These children were observed for at least 3 hours, were significantly improved, could easily return to the hospital if needed, and were closely followed as outpatients.[11,48,56] Racemic epinephrine thus should be used cautiously in an outpatient setting. In an intensive care unit setting, it can be used every 30 minutes, but it usually is spaced every 3 to 4 hours in a regular hospital unit.

The use of corticosteroids in children with viral croup has been controversial since they were first used for management of croup in the 1960s. Controversy has originated from inadequacies of design in many clinical trials, although the evidence is mounting in an overwhelming fashion to support the use of corticosteroids in the management of moderate-to-severe croup.[39,61] The exact mechanism of action of corticosteroids in croup is unknown, but corticosteroids probably decrease capillary endothelial permeability, thus leading to decreased mucosal edema. This effect commonly takes at least 3 hours; therefore corticosteroids usually are combined with racemic epinephrine usage. If the symptoms of croup are severe enough to warrant the use of racemic epinephrine, then corticosteroids may be helpful. This is not only true for hospitalized patients but also for outpatients.[13] Dexamethasone, 0.6 mg/kg to 1.0 mg/kg, given as a single dose intramuscularly or intravenously has been well tolerated with no major adverse effects. Prednisolone, 2.0 mg/kg/day, or dexamethasone, 1.0 mg/kg/day, in divided doses may be used to sustain the corticosteroid effect in either outpatients or inpatients. The severity of symptoms and duration of hospitalization have been improved with these regimens. Nebulized corticosteroids (budesonide) also may prove to be a safe alternative to oral or parenteral corticosteroids.[43] Prolonged use of corticosteroids should be monitored carefully, particularly when antibiotics may be used, to prevent candida overgrowth in the subglottis and trachea.[3] In the absence of clinical evidence of an emerging bacterial process, there is no support for the use of antibiotics in management of viral croup.

When medical therapy fails to alleviate respiratory distress, endotracheal intubation (nasotracheal or orotracheal) may be needed. A tube at least 0.5 mm smaller than estimated for the child's size or age should be used. When possible, intubation should be done in a controlled situation in the operating room or intensive care unit while the child is spontaneously breathing. This also may allow for airway endoscopy at the same time. Optical rigid rod telescopes should be used to assess the airway, and rigid bronchoscopes should be avoided if possible to prevent further airway mucosal injury. Extubation can be performed when an air leak is detected. If no air leak is detected after 5 to 7 days, thorough airway endoscopy is indicated. Airway endoscopy also is important in recurrent, prolonged, or atypical cases of croup. Ideally, endoscopy should be performed 3 to 4 weeks after the acute episode has resolved so that acute inflammatory changes can be differentiated from previous existing anatomic abnormalities. A thorough evaluation of the larynx, subglottis, and trachea with rigid rod telescopes then should be performed.

SUPRAGLOTTITIS (EPIGLOTTITIS)

Since Michel's original description of "angina epiglottidea anterior" in 1878,[62] acute epiglottitis, or supraglottitis as it is more correctly called, has become recognized as a rapidly progressive, life-threatening airway emergency predominantly affecting children. It is a bacterial cellulitis of all the supraglottic structures (not just the epiglottis) that may completely obstruct the airway. As the supraglottic edema increases, the epiglottis curls posteriorly and inferiorly as a result of diffuse inflammatory infiltration of the lingual surface of the epiglottis (Fig. 25-7). With the airway partially occluded, mucous can easily complete obstruction of the airway. Diffuse infiltration of immature polymorphonuclear lymphocytes and inflammatory edema are seen histologically.[68] Progress is rapid, in terms of hours rather than days. The disease classically occurs in children aged 2 to 6 years; however, it may occur at any age, including in newborns.[8,57] A higher incidence may be seen in the winter or spring, although the disease may occur at any time of the year.[49]

The causative organism most commonly identified in more than 90% of supraglottitis is *Hemophilus influenzae* type b (HIB).[58] This bacterial species may be part of the normal nasopharyngeal flora, or it may be acquired by respiratory transmission from other intimate contact. These bacteria may become blood borne and subsequently seed the epiglottis, meninges, facial skin, lungs, or joints. Other pathogens have been isolated such as group-A β-hemolytic streptococcus,[29] staphylococcus,[14] pneumococcus,[16] klebsiella,[53] *Hemophilus parainfluenzae*,[21] pseudomonas,[47] viruses,[21] and candida.[47] Other rare causes have been reported, including crack cocaine,[42] Kawasaki disease,[40] and thermal epiglottis caused by hot food or drink.[46] With the appearance of the human immunodeficiency virus (HIV), chronic epiglottitis associated with lymphoid hyperplasia within the epiglottis of an HIV-infected child was recently reported.[19]

Acute supraglottitis is a rare infection. Its importance lies in its high mortality if the diagnosis is not made promptly. Before widespread HIB vaccination, the incidence among children ranged from 6 per 100,000 in Canada[69] to 34 per 100,000 in Switzerland.[10] Many centers are reporting dramatic declines in disease caused by HIB (notably meningitis and supraglottitis) after the initiation of HIB vaccinations.[28,58,64,70] Immunization produces protection by production of antibodies to the polysaccharide capsule of HIB.[68]

Clinical features

Regardless of the age at presentation, the three most common signs of supraglottitis are fever, difficulty breathing, and irritability. The children are toxic in appearance and have clinical evidence of major upper airway obstruction. The child exhibits shallow respiration, inspiratory stridor, retractions, and drooling. There is severe throat pain and dysphagia. Speech is limited because of pain. A cough or hoarseness usually is not present, but the voice may be muffled. Stridor occurs late when airway obstruction is almost complete. Activity is minimal, and the patient usually prefers sitting or leaning forward. The child may assume a "tripod" position, i.e., seated, with the hands braced against the bed and the head held in the sniffing position to maximize airflow through a narrowed laryngeal inlet. Sudden laryngospasm may occur with aspiration of secretions into an already compromised airway and produce respiratory arrest.

Diagnosis

Prompt recognition of this acute airway emergency is essential to prevent airway obstruction. The diagnosis of acute epiglottitis is made by direct inspection of the supraglottic structures in a controlled environment, usually in the operating room. In a cooperative patient with no imminent complete airway obstruction, the pharynx may be visualized without a tongue blade to rule out acute tonsil or peritonsillar infection. Attempts to visualize the epiglottis in the office or emergency room without the ability or equipment to manage an obstructed airway are strongly discouraged.

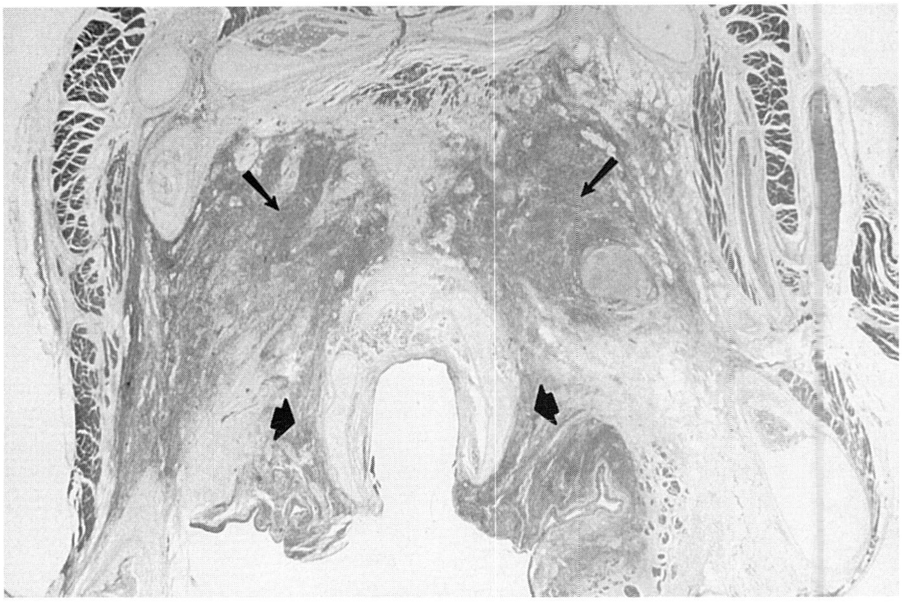

Fig. 25-7. Histologic section of a larynx (post-mortem) in supraglottitis showing posterior curling of the epiglottic cartilage *(arrowheads)* and severe inflammatory edema of the lingual surface of the epiglottis *(arrows)*.

The need for radiologic studies is controversial. Although there is no question that supraglottitis can be diagnosed on a lateral neck radiograph, the question arises whether this is a safe and necessary procedure. Most radiology suites lack the facilities to handle an obstructed pediatric airway. A child presenting with the previous signs and symptoms probably should forego radiologic testing and proceed directly to the operating room. If there is any question as to the correct diagnosis and if the child is not in respiratory distress, radiologic examination can confirm the diagnosis and exclude other causes of acute airway obstruction. Among the different diagnoses to be excluded are foreign bodies, retropharyngeal abscesses, and viral croup or laryngotracheitis.

Lateral neck radiographs in those with epiglottitis reveal swelling and rounding of the epiglottis with thickening and bulging of the aryepiglottic folds and distention of the hypopharynx (Fig. 25-8). In addition, the subglottic airway will appear normal on AP radiographs. Chest radiographs may reveal cardiac enlargement and pulmonary edema, resulting from upper airway obstruction. In the operating room, examination of the supraglottis reveals an edematous, erythematous epiglottis with variable degrees of obstruction of the airway (Fig. 25-9). The cartilaginous landmarks often are obscured. Mucosal changes range from erythema to frank ulceration or sloughing. Rarely, an abscess can be found in the lingual surface of the epiglottis. The differential diagnosis of inpatients with possible supraglottitis includes viral croup or laryngotracheitis, bacterial tracheitis, uvulitis, acute tonsillitis, retropharyngeal or peritonsillar abscess, and diphtheria. Diphtheria is a rare infection seen only in certain areas with nonimmunized patients. A history of diphtheria immunization and the absence of pharyngeal membranes make the diagnosis unlikely. Foreign body aspiration in a child with an acute upper respiratory infection also may mimic supraglottitis.

Management

Close cooperation between the otolaryngologist, pediatrician, and anesthesiologist is paramount in the management of supraglottitis. If the diagnosis of acute supraglottitis is suspected, care should be taken to avoid stimulating the child. The child naturally will assume a posture and breathing pattern that maximizes ventilation. Any intervention may convert a functional, albeit unstable airway into a nonfunctional, acutely obstructed airway. Anything that causes the child to cry may precipitate obstruction. Therefore, drawing blood, throat examination, establishing an intravenous line, restraining for a radiograph, undressing the child, or even separating from the parent may cause distress and lead to airway obstruction. Any of these procedures should wait until a stable airway has been established.

Once the diagnosis of acute supraglottitis is made, survival is closely related to the establishment of an artificial airway. For many years, this meant a tracheotomy was performed when the diagnosis was made. During the past 20 years, the safety of intubation has been established, and now endotracheal intubation by nasal or oral routes has become the standard method of managing acute supraglottitis.[71] The rationale for this change is based on the rapid response of the infectious process to appropriate antibiotic therapy. The edema of the supraglottic larynx usually subsides within 48 to 72 hours, allowing safe removal of the endotracheal tube. Despite this observation, if personnel skilled in endotracheal intubation will not be available postoperatively or if the airway can only initially be secured with a rigid bronchoscope, then a tracheotomy still may be the most appropriate choice.

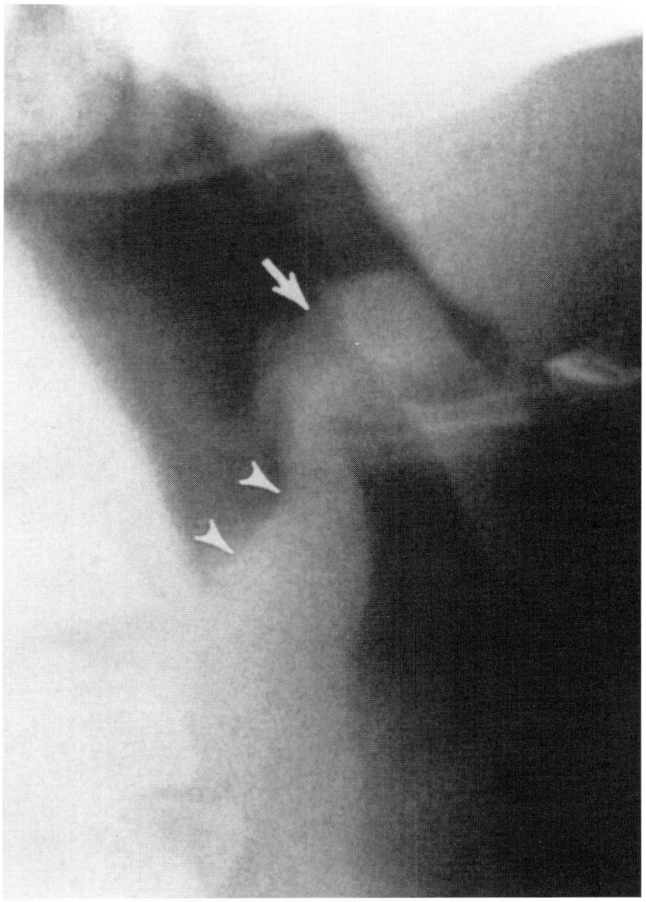

Fig. 25-8. Supraglottitis seen on lateral soft-tissue radiograph with a rounded epiglottis *(arrow)*, thickened aryepiglottic folds *(arrowheads)*, and distention of the hypopharynx.

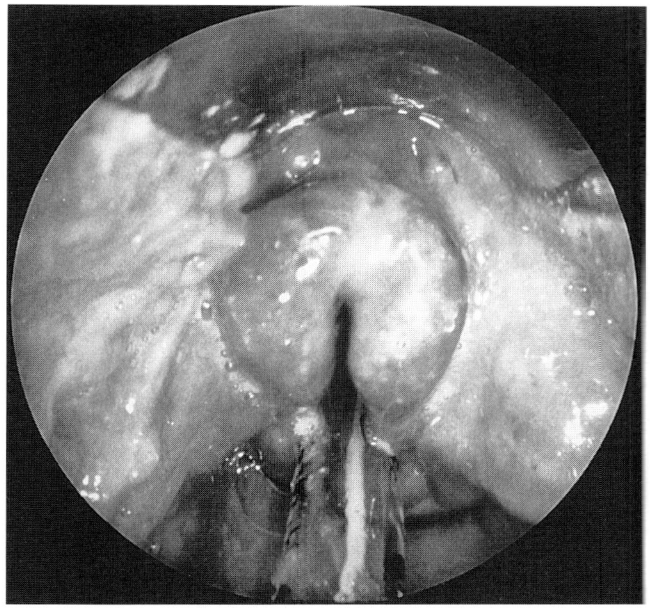

Fig. 25-9. Supraglottitis just after intubation, visualized by a rigid rod telescope.

If supraglottitis is suspected, the patient should be taken to the operating room accompanied by personnel experienced in the establishment of an emergency airway, including tracheotomy. Once in the operating room, the patient undergoes gentle, slow, inhalational induction of general anesthesia with a nonirritating inhalation agent. Muscle relaxants should be avoided until an airway is established. Only after adequate anesthesia is obtained should blood samples be taken or intravenous lines be established. A small 0° rigid rod telescope with an endotracheal tube threaded over it also may be useful in patients in whom the glottic airway cannot be visualized. The telescope is advanced through the larynx, and then the endotracheal tube is advanced over the telescope into the trachea. A rigid bronchoscope of the appropriate size and one size smaller should be available. In addition, equipment for a tracheotomy should be at hand. The larynx is examined by the otolaryngologist, and the diagnosis is confirmed. Temporary orotracheal intubation is performed; cultures are taken from the surface of the epiglottis, and simultaneous blood cultures are drawn. Blood cultures almost always are positive for HIB when this is the causative organism. Orderly nasotracheal intubation can be performed in most patients with removal of the orotracheal tube. Nasotracheal intubation is preferred because there is less motion and resultant irritation of the subglottis. Adequate sedation or restraint is essential to prevent accidental self-extubation.

Appropriate antibiotic therapy is begun with the first dose given in the operating room. Historically, HIB infections were managed with ampicillin or chloramphenicol. An increasing number of HIB strains have begun producing β-lactamase, and thus β-lactamase stable antibiotics have become standard. Ceftriaxone (100 mg/kg/day), cefotaxime (100 mg/kg/day), or ampicillin/sulbactam (200 mg/kg/day, ampicillin component) all are appropriate choices. The duration of antibiotic therapy depends on the clinical response of the child. Oral antibiotics indicated by culture results can be used to complete a 7- to 10-day course of therapy as soon as extubation has been accomplished and adequate oral intake is present. Adjunctive treatment with corticosteroids is controversial.

Extubation generally can be accomplished within 48 hours.[31] Criteria for extubation include decreased erythema and swelling of the epiglottis on laryngoscopy, and the development of an air leak around the endotracheal tube or after an empiric 48 hours of intubation. Visualization of the supraglottis offers the best guide to extubation. When there is no air leak at 48 hours, flexible fiberoptic laryngoscopy or even direct laryngoscopy can be performed safely and quickly in the intensive care units in effort to determine when extubation is safe and to shorten the direction of intubation.

Complications

Although the airway compromise in supraglottitis itself is a life-threatening illness, other infections may occur simultaneously, which may have an equally deleterious effect. In those with HIB supraglottitis, there is a 90% to 95% rate of positive blood culture for HIB.[30] Therefore, it is not surprising that hematogenous dissemination of the disease occurs. The most common infectious complication is pneumonia. Other concomitant HIB infections induce meningitis, cervical adenitis, pericarditis, septic arthritis, and otitis media.[25,30] Meningitis may be difficult to diagnose in a sedated patient, and therefore one must be cognizant of this manifestation of HIB disease. The dose of antimicrobial agent ordinarily given may be below that which is recommended for managing meningitis.

Noninfectious complications also may occur in patients with supraglottitis. Any patient with complete airway obstruction and respiratory arrest can suffer hypoxic damage of the central nervous system and other organ systems. Even patients who have had appropriate management of their airway obstruction can become hypoxic. The sudden relief of upper airway obstruction can result in postobstructive pulmonary edema with subsequent hypoxia.[7] This potential complication should be anticipated before the placement of an artificial airway, especially in those patients exhibiting a high degree of airway obstruction. Appropriate levels of positive end-expiratory pressure (PEEP) after endotracheal intubation can provide a protective mechanism against the development of pulmonary edema.

BACTERIAL TRACHEITIS

Bacterial tracheitis, also known as *bacterial laryngotracheobronchitis, membranous laryngotracheobronchitis*, and *pseudomembranous croup*, is a rare but potentially life-threatening disease. The disease was certainly described by C. L. Jackson in 1945, but it was not until 1979 that it was redescribed in detail.[15,38] Since then, there has been a growing consensus of opinion that bacterial tracheitis represents a secondary or complicating bacterial infection of viral croup or laryngotracheitis.[12,20] The secondary bacterial pathogens most often include *Staphylococcus aureus*, but also include *Streptococcus pyogenes, H. influenzae, Moraxella catarrhalis*, and more rarely gram-negative enteric bacteria.[68]

Bacterial tracheitis primarily occurs during the respiratory virus seasons of autumn and winter, similar to viral croup. It may be seen in those of a wider range of ages than typical croup, those aged 6 months to 8 years, with an average age of 5 years.[50] The infectious inflammatory process involves the subglottis and trachea with marked edema in the subglottis as in those with viral croup. Diffuse mucosal ulceration and pseudomembrane formation follow, with sloughing of these membranes into the tracheal lumen further contributing to airway obstruction. A purulent exudate commonly is present in copious amounts throughout the trachea and main bronchi as well.[34] Blood cultures usually are negative, but tracheal cultures reliably reveal the bacterial pathogen.[68]

Clinical features

The onset of bacterial tracheitis is variable. Some children become acutely ill and have severe respiratory distress within hours of the onset of illness. In other children, there is a several day prodromal period of stridor, barky cough, and hoarseness typical of viral croup that precedes the rapid, dramatic onset of higher fever, increasing respiratory distress, and toxic appearance. These patients often do not respond to racemic epinephrine because the disease rapidly progresses. High fever, cough, and stridor occur almost simultaneously over several hours. The rapid onset of the illness is similar to supraglottitis, but there usually is no dysphagia or drooling. Leukocytosis often is prominent in those with bacterial tracheitis as well.

Diagnosis

The diagnosis may be suspected on the basis of signs and symptoms, but it is confirmed by endoscopic examination of the airway. Plain radiographic imaging of the upper airway will show a ''steeple'' sign of the upper trachea or subglottis in anterior views, similar to viral croup, but it is the lateral view that can be most helpful. Diffuse haziness is present in the tracheal air column along with soft-tissue irregularities within the lumen, indicating pseudomembrane detachment (Fig. 25-10).

No clinical, radiologic, or laboratory feature alone or in combination is a reliable predictor of bacterial tracheitis. The only diagnostic procedure that distinguishes bacterial tracheitis promptly and accurately from other acute upper airway disease is airway endoscopy.[22]

Management

Airway endoscopy is not only diagnostic of bacterial tracheitis but also is therapeutic at the same time. Children should be taken to the operating room where induction of anesthesia with spontaneous ventilation is similar to that in children with supraglottitis. Direct laryngoscopy then is performed with careful examination of the larynx, subglottis, trachea, and main bronchi with a rigid rod telescope (Fig. 25-11). A rigid bronchoscope may be needed along with the rigid rod telescope to adequately suction and remove the copious secretions and pseudomembranes. Cultures and a Gram's stain should be obtained from the tracheal secretions. Orotracheal or nasotracheal intubation then can be performed to secure the airway. When rigid bronchoscopy is performed, this may induce further mucosal injury and edema in the subglottis, requiring a longer period of intubation. Tracheotomy rarely is necessary.

The majority of patients with bacterial tracheitis will require intubation and ventilatory support. While intubated, meticulous airway care with frequent saline administration

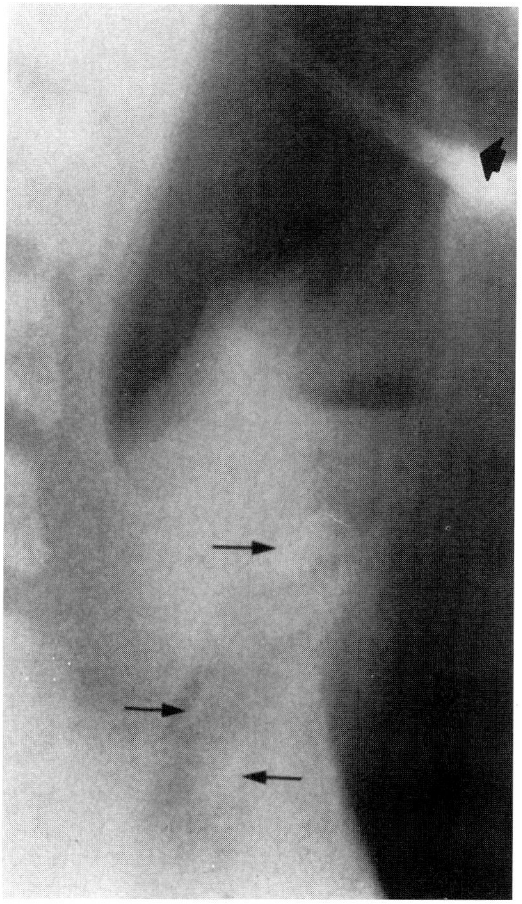

Fig. 25-10. Bacterial tracheitis in a lateral soft-tissue radiograph with obscured tracheal airway caused by sloughed mucosa *(arrows)*. The epiglottis *(arrowhead)* is normal.

and suctioning of the trachea should be performed to evacuate the thick and copious secretions. Occasionally, repeat rigid bronchoscopy may be needed to handle unusually tenacious secretions. The Gram's stain of tracheal secretions helps in directing initial parenteral antibiotic therapy. When gram-positive organisms are present, nafcillin is indicated, particularly because the most common organism cultured is *S. aureus*. Cefotaxime or ceftriaxone may be indicated in those with gram-negative organisms or mixed flora, but culture results will direct ultimate antibiotic choices. Parenteral antibiotics should be continued beyond extubation when the child has undergone major clinical improvement. Extubation can be safely performed when the temperature has returned to normal, when a leak is present around the endotracheal tube, and when the secretions have markedly decreased. Oral antibiotics then can be used to complete a 10- to 14-day course of therapy. Intubation may be needed for 6 to 7 days with a mean hospitalization of 10 days, which usually is longer than that of those with viral croup.[66]

The most common complication of bacterial tracheitis is

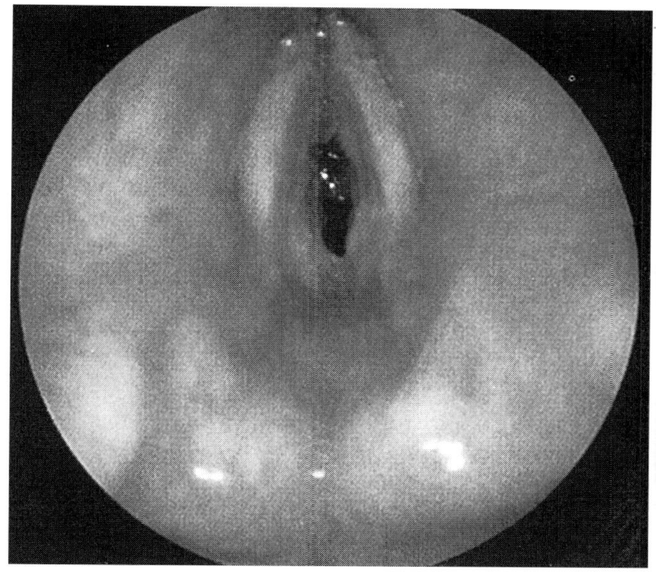

Fig. 25-11. Bacterial tracheitis with severe glottic and subglottic edema with sloughed mucosa in the lumen.

pneumonia, occurring in about 50% of children.[26] Severe hypoxia with death has occurred after respiratory arrest in severe cases of airway obstruction.[12]

RETROPHARYNGEAL ABSCESS

Retropharyngeal abscess primarily occurs in children, but it can be seen in adults when associated with penetrating trauma, granulomatous disease, and cervical spine osteomyelitis. In children, retropharyngeal abscess has been described since antiquity, but it has become less common as a result of antibiotic use during the past 50 years.[55] Because of its anatomic relations, it still can be a life-threatening illness that requires prompt diagnosis and treatment.

The retropharyngeal space extends from the skull base into the mediastinum as far as T6. It is limited posteriorly by the prevertebral fascia; anteriorly by the buccopharyngeal fascia, pharyngobasilar fascia over the three pharyngeal constrictor muscles, and the esophagus; and laterally by the carotid sheath. The space communicates directly with the parapharyngeal space anterolaterally. Within the retropharyngeal space are two vertical paramedian chains of lymph nodes, which drain potential infections in the nasopharynx, oropharynx, paranasal sinus, and possibly middle ear.[66] These lymph nodes are common in childhood, but they undergo atrophy by puberty. Suppuration of these nodes leads to abscess formation within the retropharyngeal space. Other sources of infection in this space include penetrating foreign bodies, endoscopy or intubation trauma, pharyngitis, pyogenic or mycobacterial vertebral body osteomyelitis, petrositis, and dental procedures.[27]

Retropharyngeal abscesses are most common in early childhood, with 70% of patients aged less than 6 years and

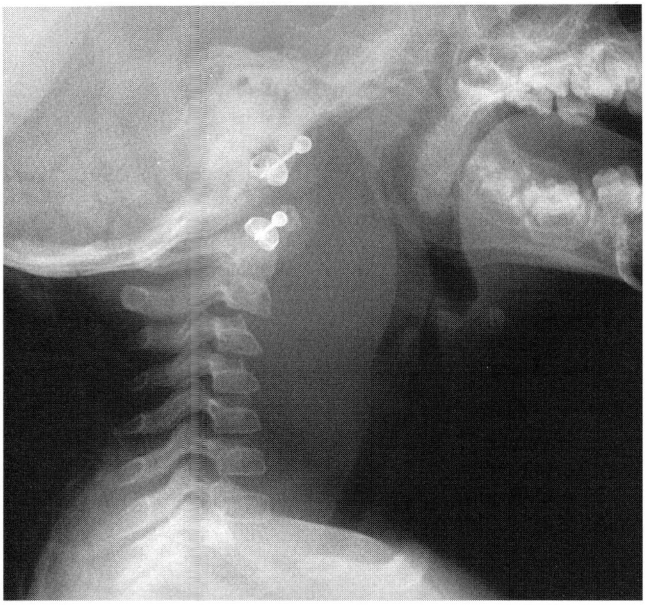

Fig. 25-12. Retropharyngeal cellulitis and abscess seen on a lateral radiographic view with widened soft tissue in the retropharynx compared with the adjacent vertebral bodies.

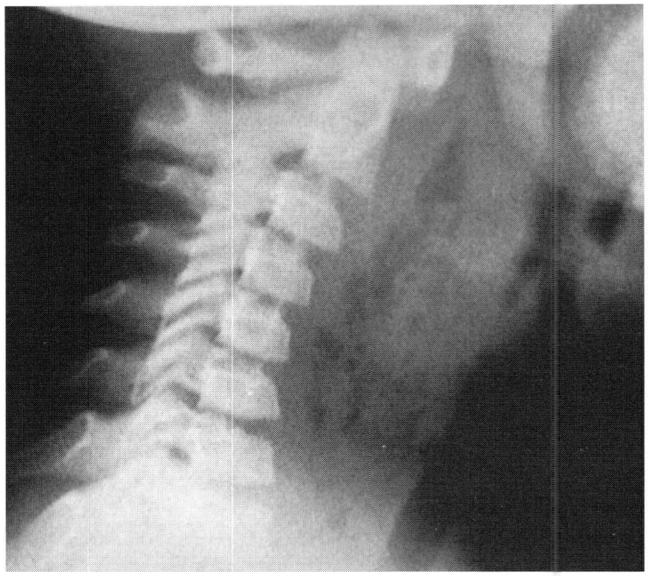

Fig. 25-13. Retropharyngeal abscess in a lateral view with gas production within the soft tissues of the retropharynx.

50% aged less than 3 years.[63] Coulthard and Isaacs[11] reported that 55% of their cases were aged less than 1 year, and 10% presented in the neonatal period.

Clinical features

The symptoms of retropharyngeal abscess often, but not always, begin insidiously after an antecedent mild upper respiratory infection. Children usually present with fever, sore throat, progressive dysphagia, and drooling. Neck stiffness and mild torticollis also may be present and may be suggestive of the diagnosis, distinguishing it from supraglottitis. Stridor is more prominent in younger children and increases as the abscess increases in size. Examination of the pharynx may reveal asymmetric swelling of the posterolateral oropharyngeal wall, but this may be difficult to assess in an uncooperative child with pooling of pharyngeal secretions. Examination of the pharynx must be performed with utmost care until supraglottitis is excluded. Cervical adenopathy also is common. Because of the presence of nonspecific signs and symptoms, a high degree of suspicion often is required to ultimately make the diagnosis of retropharyngeal abscess.

Diagnosis

To confirm the clinical suspicion of retropharyngeal abscess, a lateral soft-tissue radiograph of the neck should be obtained. The neck should be extended, and the radiograph should be taken in inspiration. The diagnosis of retropharyngeal cellulitis or abscess is suggested when the retropharyngeal space at the level of C2 is twice the diameter of the vertebral body (Fig. 25-12).[2] This criterion has a sensitivity of nearly 90%.[11] The lateral radiograph also may reveal gas caused by gas-producing bacteria within the widened retropharyngeal tissues (Fig. 25-13). The normal cervical spine lordosis may be lost or even reversed, and the radiograph should be examined carefully for vertebral or intervertebral disease. The radiographic technique is extremely important because retropharyngeal thickening may be seen when the neck is flexed or when the view is taken in expiration. A chest radiograph also should be performed to exclude mediastinitis or aspiration pneumonia.

When the lateral neck radiograph reveals widened retropharyngeal soft tissues, a computed tomography (CT) scan is extremely helpful in differentiating an abscess from retropharyngeal cellulitis (Fig. 25-14). The CT scan also defines the exact abscess location and any possible extension into other anatomic areas such as the parapharyngeal space. This is the most valuable information when incision and drainage of the abscess is performed.

Management

As in other airway infections, the airway should be secured in severe cases of respiratory distress before ever performing diagnostic procedures. Once the diagnosis is confirmed, initial antibiotic therapy is directed empirically toward aerobic and anaerobic flora of the nasopharynx. Alpha and γ hemolytic streptococci, *S. aureus*, and *Hemophilus* species are the aerobes. Bacteroides, peptostreptococci, and fusobacteria are the most commonly encountered anaerobes.[27] Initial antimicrobial therapy should include nafcillin combined with clindamycin or metronidazole, ampicillin or sulbactam, or ticarcillin or clavulanic acid. An aminoglycoside or third

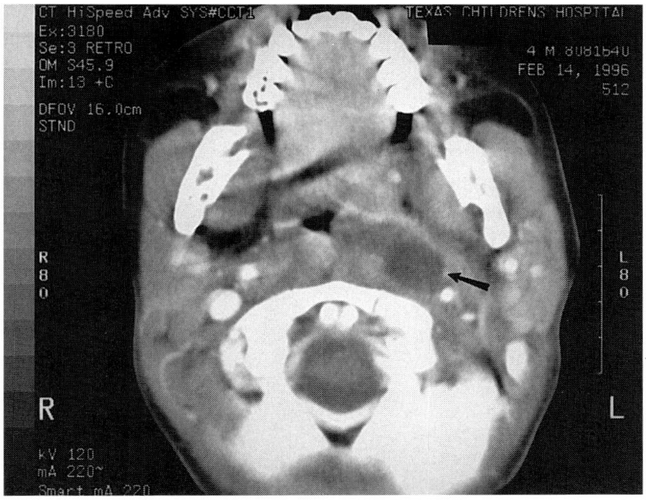

Fig. 25-14. Axial computed tomography showing a hypodense area in the left retropharynx, indicating a retropharyngeal abscess *(arrow)*.

generation cephalosporin also may be needed in neonates to provide management for gram-negative enterics.

With the availability of CT imaging to distinguish retropharyngeal cellulitis from abscess formation, the surgeon can best determine those children who will require abscess incision and drainage. When an abscess is found, incision and drainage should be performed. The transoral approach is indicated in most patients. Careful oral intubation should be performed to avoid abscess rupture and possible aspiration of purulent material. The pharyngeal incision is made over the most prominent bulging area, which almost always is located on one side of the posterior pharynx near the lateral pharyngeal wall. Blunt dissection may reveal thin secretions in early abscess formation but thicker mucopurulent secretions in a more defined abscess. Even when a CT scan indicates a hypodense area in the retropharynx compatible with a well-defined abscess, occasionally only thin secretions will be found at the time of incision and drainage. Gentle blunt lateral dissection can be performed via this approach and in cases where CT imaging indicates extension into the parapharyngeal space. A drain is not required. When a child presents with a major inflammatory lateral neck mass and a large parapharyngeal space abscess, in addition to retropharyngeal involvement, a lateral cervical incision and drainage procedure is indicated with drain placement. Cultures of the purulent drainage from either approach will help direct antibiotic therapy. When the child is afebrile, asymptomatic, and swallowing well, appropriate oral antibiotics (e.g., amoxicillin or clavulanic acid) can be used to complete a 10- to 14-day course of therapy.

Complications

Complications that should be considered in children with retropharyngeal abscesses include airway obstruction, spontaneous abscess perforation, aspiration pneumonia, mediastinitis, and sepsis. More rarely, retropharyngeal abscess can result in chest empyema, thrombosis of the internal jugular vein, erosion of the carotid artery, and atlantoaxial dislocation.[2,27] In the absence of complications, the morbidity and mortality rates from retropharyngeal abscesses are low.

REFERENCES

1. Adair J: Ten-year experience with IPPB in treatment of acute laryngotracheobronchitis, *Anesth Analg* 50:649, 1971.
2. Bank D, Krug S: New approaches to upper airway disease, *Emerg Med Clin North Am* 13:473, 1995.
3. Burton D and others: Candida laryngotracheitis: a complication of combined steroid and antibiotic usage in croup, *Int J Pediatr Otorhinolaryngol* 23:171, 1992.
4. Baugh R, Gillmore B: Infectious croup: a critical review, *Otolaryngol Head Neck Surg* 95:40, 1986.
5. Biern J and others: Infectious mononucleosis complicated by necrotizing epiglottitis, dysphagia, and pneumonia, *Chest* 96:204, 1989.
6. Bogger-Goren S: Acute epiglottitis caused by herpes simplex virus, *Pediatr Inf Dis J* 6:1133, 1987.
7. Bonadio W, Losek J: The characteristics of children with epiglottitis who develop the complication of pulmonary edema, *Arch Otolaryngol Head Neck Surg* 117:205, 1991.
8. Bos A and others: Streptococcal pharyngitis and epiglottitis in a newborn infant, *Eur J Pediatr* 151:874, 1992.
9. Bourchier D, Dawson K, Fergusson D: Humidification in viral croup: a controlled trial, *Aust Paediatr J* 20:289, 1984.
10. Bye M and others: Clinical candida supraglottitis in an infant with AIDS-related complex, *Ped Pulm* 3:280, 1987.
11. Coulthard M, Isaacs D: Retropharyngeal abscess, *Arch Dis Child* 66: 1227, 1991.
12. Cressman W, Myer C: Diagnosis and management of croup and epiglottitis, *Pediatr Clin North Am* 41:265, 1994.
13. Cruz M, Stewart G, Rosenberg N: Use of dexamethasone in the outpatient management of acute laryngotracheitis, *Pediatrics* 96:220, 1995.
14. Crysdale WS, Sendi K: Evolution in the management of acute epiglottitis: a ten year experience with 242 children, *Int Anesthesiol Clin* 26: 32, 1988.
15. Cunningham M: The old and new of acute laryngotracheal infections, *Clin Pediatr* 31:56, 1992.
16. Daum R and others: Nosocomial epiglottitis associated with penicillin- and cephalosporin-resistant steptococcus pneumoniae bacteremia, *J Clin Microbiol* 32:246, 1994.
17. DeBoeck K: Croup: a review, *Eur J Pediatr* 154:432, 1995.
18. Denny F and others: Croup. An 11 year study in a pediatric practice, *Pediatrics* 71:871, 1983.
19. Diamant E and others: Chronic epiglottitis in a child with acquired immunodeficiency syndrome, *Pediatr Inf Dis J* 11:770, 1992.
20. Donnelly B, McMillan J, Win L: Bacterial tracheitis: a report of eight new cases and review, *Rev Infect Dis* 12:729, 1990.
21. Dudley J: Supraglottitis and *Hemophilus parainfluenzae*: pathogenic potential of the organism, *Ann Otol Rhinol Laryngol* 96:400, 1987.
22. Eckel H and others: Airway endoscopy in the diagnosis and treatment of bacterial tracheitis in children, *Int J Pediatr Otorhinolaryngol* 27 147, 1993.
23. Edwards K, Dunden M, Alterneier W: Bacterial tracheitis as a complication of viral croup, *Pediatr Infect Dis J* 2:390, 1983.
24. Fearon B, Cinnamond M: Tracheotomy in acute supraglottitis (epiglottitis): the treatment of choice. *Laryngoscope* 87:975, 1977.
25. Friedman E and others: Supraglottitis and concurrent hemophilus meningitis, *Ann Otol Rhinol Laryngol* 94:470, 1986.
26. Friedman E and others: Bacterial tracheitis—a two year experience, *Laryngoscope* 95:9, 1985.

27. Gaglani M, Edwards M: Clinical indicators of childhood retropharyngeal abscess, *Am J Emerg Med* 13:333, 1985.
28. Gervaiz A, Suter S: Epidemiology of invasive hemophilus influenza type b infection in Geneva, Switzerland 1976–1989, *Pediatr Inf Dis J* 10:370, 1991.
29. Glenn G, Schofield T, Krober M: Group A streptococcal supraglottitis, *Clin Pediatr* 29:674, 1990.
30. Gonzalez C and others: Complications of acute epiglottitis, *Int J Pediatr Otolaryngol* 11:67, 1986.
31. Gonzalez C and others: Duration of intubation in children with acute epiglottitis, *Otolaryngol Head Neck Surg* 95:477, 1986.
32. Grattan-Smith T and others: Viral supraglottitis, *J Pediatr* 110:434, 1987.
33. *Hemophilus influenzae* infections. In Report of the Committee on Infectious Diseases, Chicago, American Academy of Pediatrics, 1991.
34. Henry R, Mellis C, Benjamin B: Pseudomembranous croup, *Arch Dis Child* 58:180, 1983.
35. Herman T, MacAlister W: Epiglottic enlargement: two unusual causes, *Pediatr Radiol* 21:139, 1991.
36. Inglis A: Herpes simplex virus infection: a rare cause of croup, *Arch Otolaryngol Head Neck Surg* 119:551, 1993.
37. Jacobs S and others: Validation of a croup score and its use in triaging children with croup, *Anesthesia* 49:903, 1994.
38. Jones R, Santos J, Overall J: Bacterial tracheitis, *JAMA* 242:721, 1979.
39. Kairys S, Olmstead E, O'Connor G: Steroid treatment of laryngotracheitis: a meta-analysis of the evidence from randomized trials, *Pediatrics* 83:683, 1989.
40. Kazi A and others: Uvulitis and supraglottitis: early manifestations of Kawasaki disease, *J Pediatr* 120:564, 1992.
41. Kelley P, Simon J: Racemic epinephrine use in croup and disposition, *Am J Emerg Med* 10:181, 1992.
42. Kharasch S, Vinci R, Reece R: Esophagitis, epiglottitis, and cocaine alkaloid (''crack''): ''accidental'' poisoning or child abuse? *Pediatrics* 86:117, 1990.
43. Klassen T and others: Nebulized budesonide for children with mild to moderate croup, *N Engl J Med* 331:285, 1994.
44. Kresch M: Pericarditis complication of *Hemophilus* epiglottitis, *Pediatr Inf Dis* 4:559, 1985.
45. Kristjansson S, Berg-Kelly K, Winso E: Inhaling racemic adrenaline in the treatment of mild and moderately severe croup, *Acta Paediatr* 83:1156, 1994.
46. Kulick R and others: Thermal epiglottitis after swallowing hot beverages, *Pediatrics* 81:441, 1988.
47. Lacroix J, Ahronheim G, Girouard G: *Pseudomonas aeruginosa* supraglottitis in a six month old child with severe combined immunodeficiency syndrome, *Pediatr Inf Dis J* 7:739, 1988.
48. Ledwith C, Shea L, Mauro R: Safety and efficacy of nebulized racemic epinephrine in conjunction with oral dexamethasone and mist in the outpatient treatment of croup, *Ann Emerg Med* 25:331, 1995.
49. Lepow M, Hetherington S: *Infections of the lower respiratory tract,* In Bluestone C, Stool S, editors: *Pediatric otolaryngology*, ed 2, Philadelphia, 1990, WB Saunders.
50. Liston S, Gehrz R, Jarvis C: Bacterial tracheitis, *Arch Otolaryngol* 107: 561, 1981.
51. Litmanovich M and others: The relationship between recurrent croup and airway hyperreactivity, *Ann Allergy* 65:239, 1990.
52. Mayo-Smith M and others: Acute epiglottis: an 18-year experience in Rhode Island, *Chest* 108:1640, 1995.
53. Murrage K, Janzen V, Ruby R: Epiglottitis: adult and pediatric comparisons, *J Otolaryngol* 17:194, 1988.
54. Pearlman D: The relationship between allergy and croup, *Allergy Proc* 10:227, 1989.
55. Pontell J, Har-El G, Lucente F: Retropharyngeal abscess: clinical review, *Ear Nose Throat J* 74:701, 1995.
56. Prendergast M, Jones J, Hartman D: Racemic epinephrine in the treatment of laryngotracheitis: can we identify children for outpatient therapy? *Am J Emerg Med* 12:613, 1994.
57. Rosenfeld R, Fletcher M, Marban S: Acute epiglottis in a newborn infant, *Pediatr Inf Dis J* 11:594, 1992.
58. Senior B and others: Changing patterns in pediatric supraglottitis: a multi-institutional review, 1980–1992, *Laryngoscope* 104:1314, 1994.
59. Skolnik NS: Treatment of croup: a critical review, *AJDC* 143:1045, 1989.
60. Stool S: Croup syndrome: historical perspective, *Pediatr Inf Dis J* 7: S157, 1988.
61. Super D and others: A prospective randomized double-blind study to evaluate the effect of dexamethasone in acute laryngotracheitis, *J Pediatr* 115:323, 1989.
62. Theisen CF: Angina epiglottidea anterior: report of three cases, *Albany Med Ann* 21:395, 1900.
63. Thompson J, Cohen S, Redd X: Retropharyngeal abscess in children, *Laryngoscope* 98:589, 1988.
64. Valdepena H and others: Epiglottitis and *Hemophilus influenzae* immunization: the Pittsburgh experience—a five year review, *Pediatrics* 96: 424, 1995.
65. Waisman Y and others: Prospective randomized double-blind study comparing l-epinephrine and racemic epinephrine aerosols in the treatment of laryngotracheitis (croup), *Pediatrics* 89:302, 1992.
66. Walker P, Crysdale W: Croup, epiglottitis, retropharyngeal abscess, and bacterial tracheitis: evolving patterns of occurrence and care, *Int Anesth Clin* 30:57, 1992.
67. Waki E and others: The incidence of gastroesophageal reflux in recurrent croup, *Int J Pediatr Otorhinolaryngol* 32:223, 1995.
68. Wald E: *Croup.* In Oski F and others editors: *Principles and practice of pediatrics*, Philadelphia, 1994, JB Lippincott.
69. Wurtele P: Acute epiglottitis in children and adults: a large scale incidence study, *Otolaryngol Head Neck Surg* 103:902, 1990.
70. Wurtele P: Acute epiglottitis in children: results of a large scale anti-*Haemophilus* type b immunization program, *J Otolaryngol* 24:92, 1995.
71. Zulliger J and others: Assessment of intubation in croup and epiglottitis, *Ann Otol Rhinol Laryngol* 91:403, 1982.

Chapter 26

Audiology: Early Identification and Management of Hearing Loss

Patricia G. Stelmachowicz
Michael P. Gorga

The audiologic management of pediatric patients differs from that of adults in many ways. Specialized test techniques are required to obtain valid and reliable results. The incidence of middle ear disease is high in this population, and disease recurrence is common. When sensorineural hearing loss occurs, its degree and configuration may differ substantially from typical adult patterns (i.e., sloping, high-frequency hearing loss caused by presbycusis or noise exposure). In children, sensorineural hearing loss may fluctuate or show signs of progression and often may be associated with other medical or developmental conditions. For example, Mace and others[62] and Karchmer[48] reported that approximately 30% of children with sensorineural hearing loss show at least one additional condition.

Most adults with hearing loss experience gradual progression during adulthood, long after the development of speech and language. The consequences of hearing loss in early childhood are different from those in adulthood, regardless of whether the loss is transient or permanent. For example, an adult with a mild-to-moderate high-frequency sensorineural hearing loss may show only minimal communication difficulties in quiet listening conditions. A young child with the same hearing loss is likely to show delays in speech and language development. Even under ideal listening conditions, communication may be difficult because the child cannot use contextual cues to "fill in the blanks" during conversation. Without appropriate intervention, even mild hearing loss in early childhood may have long-term consequences in terms of social, emotional, and academic performance.

Although early identification of hearing loss and early intervention were assumed to be critical for maximum speech, language, and psychosocial development, objective evidence to support this contention has been lacking until recently.[5,6,9,98,109] In a study of 109 deaf and hard-of-hearing children, Yoshinaga-Itano and others[109] found that children in whom hearing loss was identified and remediated before 6 months of age had significantly higher scores on tests of vocabulary, expressive language, and language comprehension than those diagnosed after 6 months (Fig. 26-1). The mean differences between the two groups in expressive language scores did not diminish as a function of age, at least up to 3 years. Similar trends were observed for receptive language and vocabulary scores. These data support the efficacy of universal hearing screening programs and early amplification.

Evidence also is increasing with respect to the long-term consequences of early chronic otitis media. Numerous studies have reported delays in speech and language development for this population.[24,27,28,35] At least one study found that children with chronic otitis media from low-socioeconomic households may be more at risk for speech and language delays than children from mid- or high-socioeconomic households.

These studies suggest that early identification of hearing

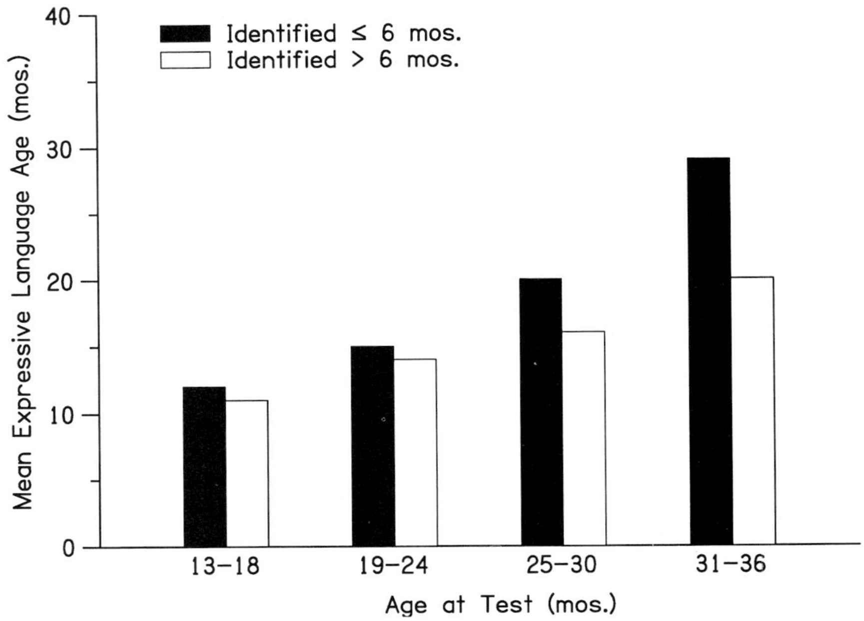

Fig. 26-1. Mean expressive language as a function of age for 109 deaf and hard-of-hearing children. The parameter is age of identification. (Adapted from Yoshinaga-Itano C and others: *The effect of early identification on the development of deaf and hard-of-hearing infants and toddlers.* Poster presented at American Academy of Audiology Conference, Salt Lake City, 1996.)

loss followed by timely and appropriate management is critical for the pediatric population. This chapter provides an overview of current audiologic procedures for identification and quantification of hearing loss in young children, discusses appropriate management strategies, and review current procedures and philosophies regarding amplification in this population.

EARLY IDENTIFICATION AND QUANTIFICATION OF HEARING LOSS

Electrophysiologic test techniques

Identification of hearing loss

Growing interest in early identification of hearing loss has resulted in the development of several programs that attempt to screen all newborns for hearing loss (e.g., National Institutes of Health, 1993). These programs range from high-risk registries to objective physiologic or acoustic measures, such as auditory brainstem responses (ABRs) and otoacoustic emissions (OAEs). This chapter provides an overview of some of these techniques and some preliminary data from studies that have used these measurements. Although technical problems with newborn hearing screening have been solved, unresolved issues include questions related to test performance, cost-effectiveness, and practicality. This chapter only addresses issues related to test performance.

High risk registry. High-risk registries were one of the earliest approaches to identifying infants with hearing loss. Such registries attempt to focus efforts on infants who present with conditions known to be associated with hearing loss.[2] Infants presenting with one or more risk factors undergo testing (e.g., ABR, OAE) to determine if they have hearing loss. If all babies confined to an intensive care nursery (ICN) for at least 3 days and babies having other obvious risk factors (e.g., a positive family history, ear pits, and other conditions that alone do not result in confinement in the ICN) are considered, approximately 10% of live births would qualify as having a condition that potentially places them at risk for hearing loss. Thus, there would be some cost advantage in screening only babies with one of these risk factors because fewer babies would be screened. However, there are reports that approximately 50% of newborns with hearing loss of moderate degree or greater present with no known risk factors.[67] Presumably, hearing loss in these babies would go undetected for some time unless all newborns were screened.

Objective tests. Although several objective tests have been used to identify newborn hearing loss (e.g., Crib-o-gram, acoustic reflex test), ABR or OAE measurements appear to be most promising in terms of identifying mild to profound hearing loss. One advantage of ABRs and OAEs is that they can be automated sufficiently to maintain high test performance while reducing costs. Also, both measures presumably have low failure rates, which is important given the incidence of neonatal hearing loss and the costs of follow-up testing.

ABR tests are performed by placing surface electrodes at several places on the head, playing brief-duration stimuli to the ear, and recording brain electrical activity across these electrodes in response to these sounds. Responses typically are amplified, filtered, and time averaged to resolve them from the background noise. These averaged waveforms are evaluated to determine if a response is present.

ALGO[79] may be the most widely recognized automated ABR system. Several descriptions of this system support its usefulness (e.g.,[42,52,79]). Herrmann, Thornton, and Joseph[38] compared the results of an automated ABR with those of conventional ABR techniques. The automated and conventional ABR provided the same test performance.

OAEs also have been used in newborn hearing screening programs. The two stimulus-related OAEs that have received the most attention are transient evoked OAEs and distortion product OAEs. Significantly more data are available on transient evoked OAEs in relation to newborn hearing screening. Data on distortion product OAE test performance in newborn hearing screening will be available over the next several years.

Transient evoked OAEs, first described by Kemp,[50] are low-level acoustic signals generated in the cochlea and reverse transmitted through the middle ear into the external ear where they can be measured with a sensitive microphone. To ensure that the measured waveform does not include stimulus artifact, transient evoked OAEs typically are measured several milliseconds after stimulation with a brief stimulus, most typically a click. Similar to ABRs, transient stimuli are used, and the response must be conditioned (filtered) and averaged. Unlike ABRS, a fast-Fourier transform (FFT) can be performed on the response waveform, thus providing information for a wide range of cochlear regions, although the response was elicited by a broad-band stimulus. If the response includes energy over some frequency region, the portion of the cochlea where these frequencies are represented is presumedly performing normally. All OAEs are a test of outer hair cell function. However, outer hair cell damage and hearing loss are sufficiently linked that it follows that if OAEs are absent, hearing loss is present, assuming external and middle ear function is normal.

There are several reports on OAE measurements in newborn hearing screening (e.g.,[13,47,51,105]). White, Vohr, and Behrens[106] and White and others[107] described the results of the universal newborn hearing screening program frequently referred to as the Rhode Island Hearing Assessment Project. They reported a low failure rate, indicating that transient evoked OAE screenings are not failing infants with normal hearing.

The technical aspects of screening newborns for hearing loss have essentially been solved. Every infant can be tested during the perinatal period using safe noninvasive test procedures. As mentioned, both ABRs and OAEs have relatively low failure rates, although this was not always the case. Failure rates in excess of 10% were not uncommon for both procedures. Efforts have been devoted to bringing these failure rates down to levels more comparable with the expected occurrence rates of congenital hearing loss.

However, without follow-up data, only the false-positive rate can be estimated. That is, follow-up testing of only the failures (the typical approach in newborn hearing screening programs) will help to determine how many babies with normal hearing failed initial perinatal screening. Although few babies with hearing loss are expected to pass a perinatal test (false-negatives), quantitative statements are not possible unless follow-up testing is performed on all infants. Such follow-up testing is needed to provide a comprehensive description of test performance in terms of true-positive, false-negative, and false-positive rates. The extent to which universal newborn hearing screening takes place throughout the United States has less to do with technical issues and more to do with financial and political issues. Screening for hearing loss is possible in most (if not all) infants.

Quantification of hearing loss

Although behavioral test techniques typically are successful with cooperative and developmentally normal children as young as 6 months, they are not appropriate for many persons at risk for hearing loss, including newborns, multiply handicapped persons, and developmentally delayed persons. As a result, techniques have been developed that attempt to circumvent the special problems associated with the audiologic evaluation of these difficult-to-test patients.

Auditory brainstem response. The ABR, which represents the sum of synchronous neural discharges from lower portions of the auditory nervous system, is the most accurate and sensitive objective test of hearing loss in difficult-to-test patients. Other evoked potential techniques, such as the middle latency response or the 40-Hz potential, are not discussed in this chapter because they have not proven to be reliable indicators of peripheral hearing loss in young children.

The most robust component of the ABR is wave V, and the lowest level at which this response is detected can be used to predict peripheral auditory sensitivity. The stimulus used to elicit the ABR strongly influences what can be said regarding hearing sensitivity. Although some disagreement exists, the general view is that click-evoked ABR thresholds correlate best with behavioral thresholds at 2000 and 4000 Hz.[33,45,103] A relationship exists between the slope of the wave V latency-intensity function and configuration of hearing loss.[32,33] Patients with high-frequency losses often have steep latency-intensity functions, whereas patients with flat audiometric configurations tend to have more shallow functions. These effects are attributed to an interaction between stimulus intensity and the place of excitation along the basilar membrane that dominates the response. With mild-to-moderate high-frequency hearing loss, intense stimuli can excite basal regions of the cochlea. Because latency is related to place of excitation, the latency of response may be normal or near normal under these circumstances. As level decreases, however, the response may not be as dominated by these high-frequency regions as it is in normal ears. Thus, response latency might be abnormally long at low-stimulus levels because of larger contributions from low-frequency regions and because it takes longer to reach the low-frequency places of representation in the cochlea. The resulting wave V latency-intensity function, therefore, would have a steeper-than-normal slope.

Although the click-evoked ABR correlates best with high-frequency sensitivity, there are reports that, under certain stimulus conditions, information can be obtained from a range of different frequencies. For example, Don, Eggermont, and Brackmann[22] reported on the use of the derived band technique for obtaining estimates of hearing at octave frequencies from 500 to 4000 Hz. Gorga, Kaminski, and Beauchaine[31] and Gorga and others[34] reported on obtaining ABRs to frequencies of 250 to 16,000 Hz using tone-burst stimuli. Stapells and others[94] and Stapells, Gravel, and Martin[93] recently reported on the relation between pure-tone hearing sensitivity and tone-burst ABR thresholds when the tone bursts were embedded in notched noise with the notch centered at the nominal tone-burst frequency. These reports suggest that although some special conditions may need to be met when attempting to predict the pure-tone audiogram, several techniques can achieve this goal.

The application of ABRs to predict hearing loss in multiply handicapped patients also has been shown.[96] These patients may be difficult to test using behavioral test techniques but are more likely to have hearing loss. ABR tests during sleep (sometimes sedation-induced) provide reliable information on auditory sensitivity for these patients.

Test techniques are available that quantify the magnitude and configuration of hearing loss in any patient, regardless of developmental level or cognitive skills. If reliable test information is obtained using behavioral test techniques, the use of objective tests (e.g., ABR) is obviated. However, ABR techniques can be used if reliable behavioral test data cannot be obtained.

Otoacoustic emissions. As discussed, OAEs can be measured in the ear canal with sensitive microphones, appropriate stimulus paradigms, and signal averaging. The fact that these responses are present in normal ears but absent in ears with hearing loss has led primarily to use of these techniques for early identification of hearing loss. OAEs appear to be of limited value in quantifying the magnitude of hearing loss.

However, OAEs are tests of cochlear function, primarily outer hair cell function. Thus, the combination of OAE and other objective measurements, such as acoustic immittance and ABR measurements, better identifies the site of dysfunction in patients with hearing loss. Measuring OAEs is valuable in pediatric patients with hearing loss because elevated auditory thresholds (whether measured behaviorally or electrophysiologically) may not be a consequence of cochlear damage. For example, extreme elevations in bilirubin may lead to kernicterus, a neurotoxic condition that might affect auditory brainstem pathways. Such a patient may not produce an ABR but may reveal robust OAEs. Traditional approaches to rehabilitation in such cases, including the use of amplification, should be considered cautiously because rehabilitative options are designed primarily to overcome peripheral hearing disorders. The peripheral auditory systems of these patients may be functioning normally, making such intervention inappropriate and potentially damaging (because of the presentation of unnecessarily loud sound). It is thus recommended that every child newly identified with hearing loss receive a comprehensive auditory assessment, including OAE, behavioral, immittance, and ABR evaluations. A combination of these measurements will assure an appropriate plan for intervention.

Behavioral test techniques

Audiogram

The audiogram is a grid that plots frequency on the x abscissa and hearing level on the y ordinate. The typical frequency range is 250 to 8000 Hz, with vertical lines denoting octave and some half-octave frequencies. Hearing level (HL) is expressed in decibels and is based on national standards appropriate for the test (e.g., supraaural earphones, insert earphones, bone vibrators, loudspeakers). With specialized instrumentation, thresholds can be measured for frequencies from 8000 to 20,000 Hz, which is thought to be useful when monitoring potential ototoxic effects during certain drug therapies. These thresholds, however, are not typically plotted on a standard audiogram form.

A standard audiogram form is shown in Figure 26-2, and the symbols commonly used to record thresholds are shown in Figure 26-3.[3] The appropriate symbol is recorded on the form at the intersection of frequency and the measured threshold. If no response is observed, an arrow pointing down at a 45° angle is plotted at the limits of the instrumentation. The most commonly used symbols describe air and bone conduction thresholds, but other symbols denote such things as aided thresholds or acoustic reflex thresholds.

Air-conduction testing. Air-conducted signals generally are transduced by a supraaural earphone, which is calibrated in a standard 6-cm^3 coupler, or an insert earphone, which is calibrated in a 2-cm^3 coupler. For certain test populations, however, alternative transducers are needed. For example, test signals may be presented in the sound field through a loudspeaker when testing young children who will not tolerate earphones. When properly calibrated, threshold measures (expressed in dB HL) should be equivalent for different transducers. Insert earphones are useful in cases of artifactual hearing loss caused by occlusion from collapse of the external auditory meatus under the pressure of a su-

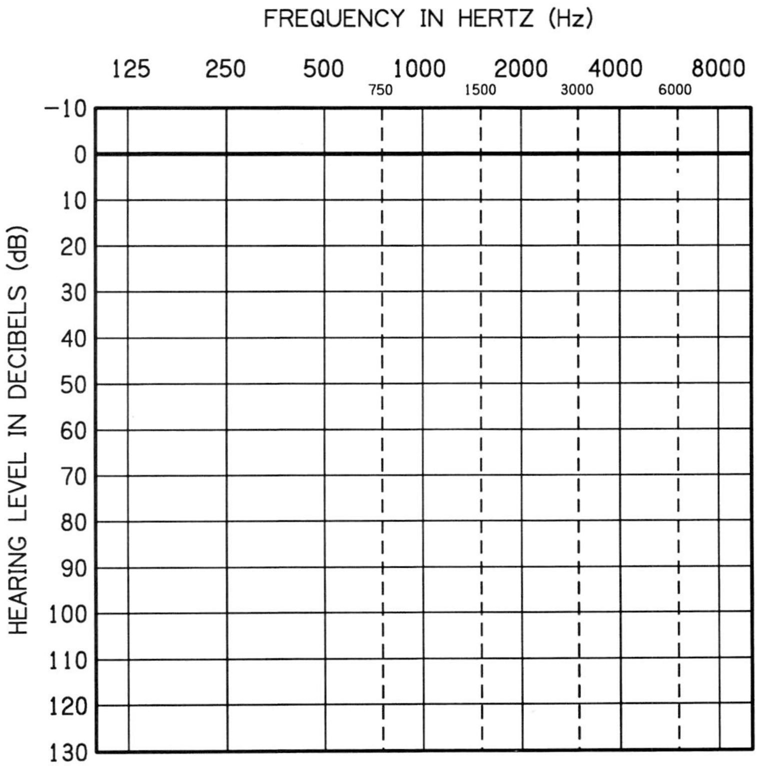

Fig. 26-2. Example of a standard audiogram form. (Adapted from *American Speech-Language-Hearing Association*: Guidelines for audiometric symbols, 32:25, 1990.)

Modality	Ear		
	Left	Unspecified	Right
Air conduction--earphones			
Unmasked	X		O
Masked	□		△
Bone conduction--mastoid			
Unmasked	>	^	<
Masked	]		[
Air conduction--sound field		S	
NR	↙	↓	↘

Fig. 26-3. Symbols used to represent different threshold responses on the audiogram. (Adapted from *American Speech-Language-Hearing Association*: Guidelines for audiometric symbols, 32:25, 1990.)

praaural earphone cushion, a condition that is relatively common in young children.[53] Insert earphones also provide an increase in interaural attenuation of air-conducted signals, which is useful when testing patients with maximum conductive hearing loss.[54]

Bone-conduction testing. Bone-conducted signals are presented through a bone vibrator, which should be coupled to the head with a force of 550 grams. Unlike air-conducted signals, a bone vibrator is calibrated using an artificial mastoid.[1] For clinical testing, the vibrator is most commonly placed on the mastoid process. Because of clinical test-retest reliability, differences in calibration procedures, and error tolerances for air- and bone-conduction signals, air and bone conduction thresholds will not always agree in patients with normal middle ear function. In some children, optimal placement of the bone vibrator may be difficult because of skull shape or prior operations, which can affect bone-conduction thresholds. In the low frequencies (250 and 500 Hz), supraaural earphones may not fit some children adequately, and air-conduction thresholds may be elevated at these frequencies, leading to the incorrect conclusion that a low-frequency conductive hearing loss is present.

Interpretation of results. Type and degree of hearing loss are based on an interpretation of thresholds as a function of frequency for different stimulus conditions. These interpretations typically are straightforward. If air- and bone-conduction thresholds are similar and within normal limits, hearing is normal. If air-conduction thresholds are poorer than bone-conduction thresholds, a conductive hearing loss is present. This is true even when air-conduction thresholds are normal provided that the bone-conduction thresholds are at least 10 dB better. If air- and bone-conduction thresholds are symmetrically elevated, a sensorineural hearing loss exists. If both threshold measures are elevated but air-conduction thresholds are poorer than bone-conduction thresholds, a mixed hearing loss, including conductive and sensorineural components, is present. As expected, this latter condition is common among young children with sensorineural hearing loss and middle ear disease.

Understanding the different audiometric symbols is important, particularly when considering conditions in which no response is observed. Specifically, it is important to recognize that a notation of "no response" does not mean no hearing. "No response" only indicates that no response was observed at the highest level that could be produced at the limits of the instrumentation. This upper limit depends on many factors, including the audiometer, the transducer, and the frequency being tested. For example, consider a child with a flat audiometric configuration with 100-dB HL air-conduction thresholds and concomitant middle ear dysfunction. In this case, it might be difficult to identify either the presence or magnitude of the conductive component because bone conduction has a lower maximum output (typically 70 dB HL at those frequencies at which it has the greatest dynamic range) than air conduction for which maximum outputs may be as high as 120 dB HL. Of course, acoustic immittance measurements and physical examination of the ear would alert the otolaryngologist to the presence of middle ear dysfunction.

Finally, magnitude of hearing loss is represented by the extent to which thresholds exceed the normal range. In general, the threshold for normal hearing is less than or equal to 25 dB HL, for mild hearing loss is 25 to 45 dB HL, for moderate hearing loss is 40 to 65 dB HL, for severe hearing loss is 66 to 85 dB HL, and for profound hearing loss is greater than 85 dB HL. In young children, borderline normal hearing sensitivity (15 to 25 dB thresholds) has been associated with speech, language, and academic problems.[10]

Pure-tone thresholds and audibility of speech. Figure 26-4 shows how hearing loss affects the audibility of average conversation. In this case, the hearing loss slopes from near normal in the low frequencies to severe in the high frequencies. The superimposed speech sounds were taken from Nerbonne and Schow[75] and represent the frequency and intensity at which these sounds occur in average conversation. Some sounds are represented at several places, reflecting that speech sounds have energy at more than one frequency. In this example, the low-frequency components of speech are heard at a near-normal sensation level (25 to 30 dB SL), but the high-frequency sounds occur near or below threshold. This child will miss many of the consonants of speech and, when listening in noise, the audibility of even low-frequency speech sounds may be reduced. The speech spectrum information in Figure 26-4 is extremely helpful in explaining the consequences of peripheral hearing loss.

Test techniques

Behavioral observation audiometry (BOA). For children who have a developmental age of less than 5 to 6 months, it is generally impossible to use operant conditioning techniques to assess auditory function. Historically, behavioral observation audiometry has been used to informally evaluate these patients. Various signals (e.g., noisemakers, calibrated signals presented in the sound field) are introduced, and the infant's behavior is observed. Responses include reflexive activity (e.g., Moro's reflex), eye widening, onset or cessation of crying, or other changes in the patient's state. Attempts have been made to increase the objectivity of behavioral observation audiometry by monitoring changes in infant activity via sensors in the base of an infant crib (Crib-o-gram).[91] Newer technology (ABR) has replaced this technique, and BOA generally is not recommended for the following reasons: (1) responses can only be observed at relatively high signal levels, thus mild to moderate hearing loss would be missed; (2) responses depend on patient state; (3) accuracy is subject to examiner bias and experience; (4) the most robust responses occur to broad-spectrum signals, which do not provide frequency-specific information; (5) the test technique cannot provide individual ear information; and (6) large intersubject variability makes it difficult to establish

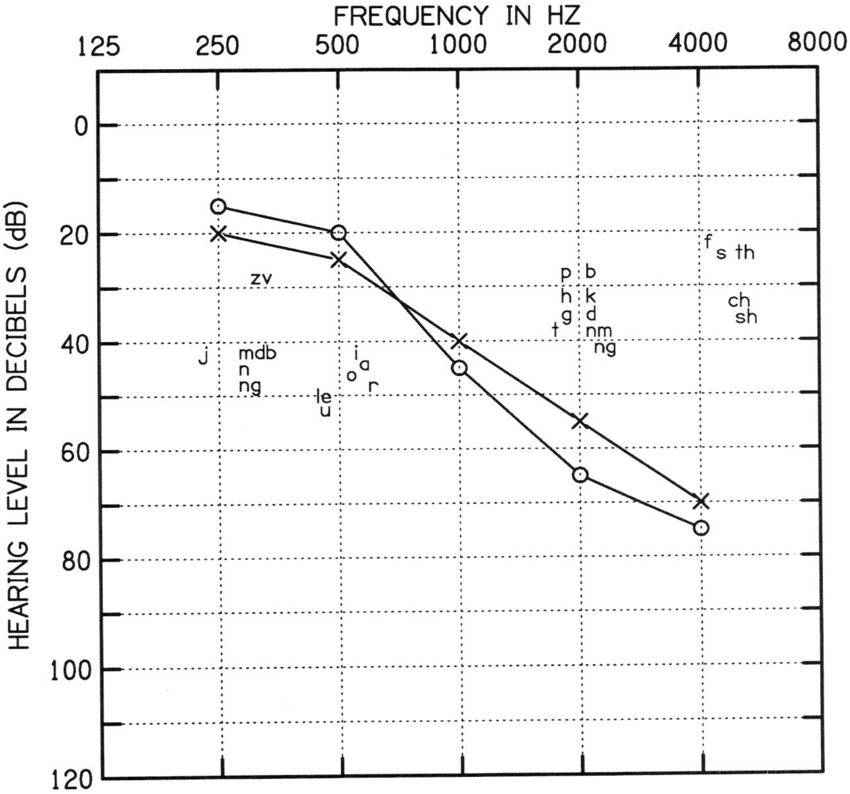

Fig. 26-4. Pure-tone air-conduction thresholds of a patient with a sloping high-frequency hearing loss. The superimposed speech sounds represent average conversational speech.

meaningful norms using this technique. Although behavioral observation audiometry should not be used to rule out significant hearing loss, it may be a useful adjunct to more objective measures on a long-term basis when dealing with multiply handicapped or neurologically impaired children.

Visual reinforcement audiometry (VRA). An operant conditioning technique known as VRA[60] is the most commonly used test procedure for children in the 6- to 24-month age range.[101] Signals generally are presented in the sound field and may be broadband (e.g., speech, music) or frequency specific (e.g., frequency-modulated sinusoids). The child is seated on the parent's lap, and a second examiner maintains the child's attention at midline with interesting toys. With this technique, a head-turn response toward the sound source is reinforced by illuminating or animating a toy that is located at the child's eye level near the loudspeaker. When signals are presented in the sound field, test results reflect hearing in the better ear only. For some children, it is possible to use VRA with test signals or masking noise presented via supraaural or insert earphones. In this way, behavioral thresholds may be obtained for each ear independently. Because this latter procedure is time consuming and may require repeated visits because of habituation and the child's limited attention span, ear information often is obtained only in cases in which knowledge of asymmetric thresholds may be important for management (known hearing loss, head trauma, significant visual impairment, pre- or postoperative audiologic assessment). Despite various potential problems (e.g., habituation, false-positive responses, examiner bias), behavioral thresholds obtained using VRA agree with adult values within approximately 10 dB.

Conditioned play audiometry (CPA). By a developmental age of 24 to 29 months, approximately 70% of children can be evaluated by CPA.[100] The child is required to perform a simple motor task (e.g., dropping blocks into a bucket) in response to auditory signals. Testing can be performed by having a second examiner in the test room or by using a portable audiometer. In the latter case, flexibility is compromised because the child must accept earphones and speech testing cannot be performed easily. By this age, social reinforcement generally is adequate to keep the child involved in the task long enough to obtain pure-tone air- and bone-conduction thresholds. Some variants of this procedure have been developed. Lloyd, Spradlin, and Reid[61] described a technique to use with difficult-to-test patients known as *tangible reinforcement operant conditioning audiometry*. With this procedure, tangible reinforcers such as cereal, candy, or small toys are used in conjunction with social reinforcement. This procedure may require a lengthy conditioning, and it may be difficult to find motivating reinforcers for some children. More recently, various computer graphics were used as reinforcers for CPA. This approach allows for rapid changes in reinforcers, thus making the task more interesting to the child, particularly if the evaluation is lengthy.

Conventional audiometry. By the time a child is at a developmental age of 42 to 48 months, they can often perform the same test techniques as adults. The instructional set may need to be altered, and social reinforcement continues to be important.

Tests of speech perception ability

Tests of speech perception are critical to the evaluation of auditory function. These tests can be divided into threshold and suprathreshold measures. The test used will depend on the developmental and language level of the child and on the specific purpose of the assessment.

Threshold tests

The speech reception threshold (SRT) is defined as the lowest level at which a listener can correctly identify 50% of test items from a set of two-syllable words (spondees). The spondees are familiar and are produced with equal stress on each syllable (e.g., cowboy, hot dog). A psychophysical procedure similar to that used for pure-tone testing is used to establish the SRT. Children are expected simply to repeat the test item. A closed-set, picture-pointing task can be used for children as young as 18 to 24 months. For younger children or persons developmentally delayed, a speech awareness threshold (SAT) or speech detection threshold (SDT) can provide similar information. The SAT/SDT is the lowest level at which 50% of test items can be detected (as opposed to identified).

In clinical practice, the primary purpose of the SRT or SAT is to corroborate the pure-tone thresholds. The audiometric calibration of speech signals allows these measures to be related to pure-tone thresholds expressed in dB HL, and the relation between pure-tone thresholds and the SRT is well understood.[37] The SDT (or SAT) is generally 5 to 6 dB lower than the SRT. The SRT should agree with the three-frequency (500, 1000, and 2000 Hz) pure-tone average (PTA) within 5 to 6 dB.[40] In cases of sloping hearing loss, however, a two-frequency average sometimes is used. A difference of 12 dB or more between the SRT and PTA suggests that the pure-tone thresholds may not be valid.

Suprathreshold tests

Clinical tests of suprathreshold speech recognition ability can be used (1) to provide an estimate of functional performance in everyday listening situations; (2) to monitor potential changes in speech perception over time; and (3) to quantify the ability to perceive speech processed by a child's hearing aids. The test materials and methodology depend on the purpose of the measurement. Many factors (e.g., presentation level, word familiarity, mode of presentation, type of competing signals) influence performance on speech perception tests.

Regardless of the test being used, the presentation level has a marked influence on performance. In general, performance (the percentage of correct responses) increases as a function of intensity. The slope of this function is steepest for test materials with high contextual cues (e.g., sentences) and increasingly shallow as the test materials become more difficult (e.g., nonsense syllables). To ensure maximum performance for a patient, assessment over a range of intensities may be necessary. In clinical practice, it is customary to use a presentation level that is 40 dB above the patient's SRT unless the hearing loss is steeply sloping in configuration. In these cases, the level should be elevated to ensure that the speech energy is audible at 2000 Hz if possible.

It is often desirable to compare the scores obtained across test conditions, across ears, or with previous test results. Thus, it is important that any test of speech recognition yield good test-retest reliability. Scores expressed as a percentage follow a binomial distribution; the reliability of a given test score is dependent, in part, on the absolute score.[23,102] The variability is greatest in the middle range of test scores and lowest at the two extremes of the scale. To determine if two scores are significantly different, the number of test items, the absolute scores, and the confidence level used to interpret results should be considered. Table 26-1 shows the critical differences needed for monosyllabic word lists with 25 and 50 test items at a 95% confidence level. For example, using a 25-word list, a score of 48% is not significantly different from a score of 24% or 72% (a range of ± 24%). At either extreme of the continuum, however, the critical differences are substantially smaller, and increasing the number of test items reduces the variability. It is important to understand the clinical implications of these relationships. Given the variability inherent in speech recognition testing, attempts

Table 26-1. Lower and upper limits of the 95% critical differences for discrimination scores. Values within the range shown are not significantly different from the scores shown in column 1

Percentage correct	50 Items (%)	25 Items (%)
0	0-4	0-8
12	4-26	4-32
24	10-42	8-48
36	20-54	16-60
48	30-66	24-72
60	42-78	36-84
72	54-86	48-92
84	68-94	60-96
100	96-100	92-100

From Thornton AR, Raffin MJM: Speech-discrimination scores modeled as a binomial variable, *J Speech Hear Res* 21:507, 1978.

to compare scores across various conditions should be approached with caution. It is impossible to directly compare scores across different types of tests. The same test items produced by male and female speakers produce mean differences in performance of 15% to 20%, depending on signal level.[108]

Many materials developed for testing speech perception abilities, ranging from nonsense syllables to sentence-length materials, are commercially available. The Pediatric Working Group of the Conference on Amplification for Children with Auditory Deficits[99] provided a comprehensive review of suprathreshold speech perception tests for children.

Children's materials

When assessing speech perception ability in young children, the type of speech materials and the mode of test administration will depend on the linguistic level of the child. For young children, the results of speech perception tests can yield information about the auditory system and about the language level of the child. For example, if a 3-year-old child who hears normally cannot identify familiar pictures accurately, a referral for a speech and language evaluation may be warranted.

A closed-set picture-pointing format is the most appropriate option for young children. The most commonly used tests are the Word Intelligibility by Picture Identification Test and the Northwestern University Children's Speech Perception Test (NU-CHIPS). The Word Intelligibility by Picture Identification Test[84] consists of 25 monosyllabic words (e.g., ball, boat) in a six-item multiple-choice format. The test is appropriate for children aged 4 to 6 years. The NU-CHIPS test[49] consists of 50 test items in a four-choice format. This test has been normalized on hearing-impaired children and is appropriate for children as young as 2.8 years. For children aged 6 to 9 years, Phonetically Balanced Kindergarten lists typically are used as a word-repetition task.

For children older than 10 years, the most commonly used tests of suprathreshold speech recognition ability are phonetically balanced word lists such as the CID W-22 word lists[39] or the NU-6 lists.[56] Each list is made up of speech sounds whose occurrence in the list parallels that in everyday speech. Test reliability can be maximized by the use of complete (50-word) lists and prerecorded materials on compact disk, audio tape, or digitized speech played back through a digital-to-analog converter. Test reliability and validity are severely compromised by the use of monitored live-voice presentation.[14,102]

Although performance in everyday conversation correlates with one's ability to perceive single words, these types of tests cannot predict the communication difficulty a listener may have outside the test environment. Factors such as the listening environment and the listener's linguistic and speech-reading abilities help determine communication skills. Sentence-length materials may be a better indicator of everyday performance. The Pediatric Speech Intelligibility Test developed by Jerger and others[46] is a closed-set sentence test designed for children aged 3 to 10 years.

Central auditory tests

The above speech recognition tests are intended to assess the function of the peripheral auditory system, including the cochlea and the primary auditory neurons. Accurate coding of acoustic information, however, involves various complex processes within the central auditory nervous system (CANS). To accurately represent acoustic information at the highest level of the CANS, the peripheral auditory system, brainstem, ascending auditory pathways and subcortical centers, interhemispheric connections, and the auditory cortex should be functioning properly. If the system is not functioning properly, difficulties in attention, recall, and processing of speech in quiet or in noise may occur, although performance on pure-tone tests and standard speech perception tests is within normal limits.

The current approach to assessment of central auditory function is based on the assumption that various levels of the CANS serve specific functions. Many tests have been developed to assess the functional integrity of a particular level of the CANS. At present. CANS testing is not routine in most audiologic clinics. Several factors limit the clinical usefulness of these tests. Most tests tend to be time-consuming, and the tasks can be complicated, generally involving competing signals or some form of degraded speech. As such, performance on these tests can be complicated by language level, attention span, and the age appropriateness of the task, thus limiting their usefulness in young children and elderly patients. In cases in which a peripheral hearing loss also exists, interpretation of test results is even more complicated. Finally, very little work in this area has been validated radiologically, surgically, or histologically, and the reliability of specific tests in various patients has not been investigated thoroughly, yet work in this area continues. Reviews of central auditory tests have been published by Musiek,[73] Musiek and Chermak,[74] Beasley and Rintelmann,[6] Noffsinger and Kurdziel,[76] Starr and others,[95] and Sloan.[92]

Acoustic immittance measures

Although routine pure-tone air- and bone-conduction measures can be used to identify and quantify the magnitude of a conductive component, they generally do not yield information about the nature of middle ear pathology. Acoustic immittance measures provide information about middle ear function that often cannot be derived without invasive measures (e.g., exploratory surgery). The currently available measurement systems are relatively inexpensive, easily tolerated by most patients, fast, and require no behavioral response. As a result, immittance measures have become a routine and indispensable part of the clinical audiologic battery.

Equipment and method

The middle ear system is not a perfect transducer of energy and thus offers some opposition to the flow of energy. This opposition is known as *acoustic impedance*. Alternatively, the flow of energy through the middle ear is known as *acoustic admittance*. The term *acoustic immittance* describes the transfer of acoustic energy through the middle ear system, regardless of whether the measurement is made in terms of impedance or admittance. The sound delivery and measurement system is coupled hermetically to the ear canal through a flexible rubber cuff. A known acoustic signal is introduced to the ear, and the sound pressure level (SPL) in the ear canal is measured under various conditions. This SPL is taken as an indirect measure of acoustic immittance. Block and Wiley[11] provided an overview of the basic principles of acoustic immittance. The clinical acoustic immittance battery consists of many tests to assess the integrity and function of the middle ear and the afferent portion of cranial nerve (CN) VIII and part of the motor portion of CN VII.

Tympanometry

Tympanometry is the most commonly used test in the acoustic immittance battery. A tympanogram is a graphic representation of how the immittance of the middle ear is altered by changes in air pressure in the ear canal. Tympanometry yields information about resting middle ear pressure (tympanometric peak pressure) and helps identify low-impedance conditions (e.g., ossicular disarticulation, tympanic membrane scarring) and high-impedance conditions (e.g., ossicular fixation, otitis media). Until recently, most acoustic immittance devices allowed measurements at only one or two probe frequencies (usually 226 and 678 Hz). Most data relating various tympanometric patterns to specific pathologic conditions are based on measures at these two frequencies. Multifrequency tympanometry has been under investigation for some time but its clinical usefulness has not been established.[36,66,88] Several schemes for classifying and interpreting tympanograms have been suggested. The most common was developed by Liden[58] and later modified.[43,44,59] A Type A tympanogram, designating normal middle ear function, has a normal height and peak pressure at or near 0 deka Pascal. A Type A_S tympanogram is shallow with normal peak pressure and may be indicative of ossicular fixation or certain types of middle ear effusion. A Type A_D tympanogram also has normal peak pressure but an unusually high amplitude, suggestive of a thin atrophic tympanic membrane or possible ossicular disarticulation. A Type B tympanogram is flat and indicative of middle ear effusion or, uncommonly, a cholesteatoma (if impacted cerumen, tympanic membrane perforation, or an improperly placed probe have been ruled out). A Type C tympanogram is characterized by a negative peak pressure and suggests eustachian tube dysfunction. This classification is appropriate only for single-component systems that use a low-frequency probe tone. Vanhuyse, Creten, and Van Camp[104] proposed a more complicated classification system that considers the reactive and resistive components of immittance.

Table 26-2. Suggested normative values for tympanometric width, static acoustic immittance (at 226 Hz), and equivalent ear canal volume for children and adults

	Mean (90% range)	Mean (90% range)	Mean (90% range)
	Tympanometric width (deka Pascal)	**Equivalent volume (cm^3)**	**Static immittance (cm^3)**
Children (3 to 5 yr)	100 (60-150)	0.7 (0.4-1)	0.5 (0.2-0.9)
Adults	80 (50-110)	1.1 (0.6-1.5)	0.8 (0.3-1.4)

Values from Margolis RH, Heller JW: Screening tympanometry criteria for medical referal, *Audiology* 26:197, 1987.

Attempts have been made to quantify the tympanometric shape in the region of the peak.[15,59] The clinical usefulness of various measures of tympanometric gradient has been investigated, and gradient appears to be a good indicator of middle ear effusion.[21,55,87] Using the measurement scheme described by Liden, Harford, and Hallen,[59] Margolis and Heller[64] reported the mean normal values and 90% ranges shown in Table 26-2. Abnormally wide tympanometric widths suggest middle ear effusion.

Regardless of the classification system used, there will always be patterns that do not fit well-defined criteria and will be difficult to interpret. In addition, the relationship between tympanometry and middle ear dysfunction is extremely complex. For example, tympanometry with a low-frequency probe tone is not extremely sensitive to ossicular fixation.[65] Tympanometric shape is influenced greatly by abnormalities of the tympanic membrane that may dominate the pattern, making it difficult to diagnose pathologic processes medial to the tympanic membrane. Tympanometry in infants younger than 6 to 7 months has a high false-negative rate,[78] possibly because of ear canal wall movement in response to pressure changes during the procedure. When possible, tympanometric results should be viewed within the context of the entire clinical picture.

Equivalent volume measures

An equivalent volume (V) measure of the external ear canal can be derived from the tympanogram. In ears with a tympanic membrane perforation or patent ventilating tube, this measure includes the middle ear space and mastoid air cells. The test is performed by introducing a high-negative or high-positive pressure (usually +200 deka Pascal into the hermetically sealed ear canal, thus creating a rigid-walled cavity. In such a cavity, there is a predictable relationship between cavity size and sound pressure level. In adult ears with a tympanic membrane perforation (and normal middle ear mucosa), normative values will increase by a factor of two or more. In young children, however, the increase is not as large and values of 1 cm^3 or greater (with a flat tympanogram) suggest a possible perforation or patent tympanostomy tube.[89] This test is particularly useful in diagnosing small perforations that may be missed otoscopically and in determining the patency of ventilation tubes, particularly in persons in whom pneumatic otoscopy may be difficult. For young children, the preoperative equivalent ear canal volume should be recorded for comparison with postoperative values. These measurements do not differ in children as much as they do in adults.

Static acoustic immittance

Peak-compensated static acoustic immittance refers to the height of the tympanogram relative to its tail. This value can be derived directly from the tympanogram. Although this information has not been used widely in clinical settings, it can provide important objective information used in conjunction with tympanometric shape. These measures allow for a direct comparison of data across clinics or across clinical instruments.

Eustachian tube function tests

The purpose of eustachian tube function (ETF) testing is to assess the ventilatory capability of the eustachian tube in passive and nonpassive states. The test requires perforation of the tympanic membrane or patent ventilating tube.

In the passive ETF test, positive pressure is gradually applied to the ear until the eustachian tube opens (usually at greater than 200 deka Pascal). A completely obstructed, eustachian tube usually will not open within the limits of the equipment; if the tube is abnormally patent, it will be impossible to pressurize the ear. This latter case can be difficult to differentiate from failure to seal the external ear hermetically. If a seal can be obtained with negative pressure only, a patulous eustachian tube should be suspected.

The function of the eustachian tube can be assessed under more physiologically relevant conditions. Bluestone[12] suggested that the ear be pressurized to +200 deka Pascal (or less if necessary) and that the patient swallow five times. The remaining pressure is known as the residual positive pressure. The procedure is repeated with a −200 deka Pascal. According to Bluestone,[12] positive and negative pressures should be equilibrated in a healthy ear. At present, the test-retest reliability and the long-term diagnostic significance have not been established.

Acoustic reflex measures

Although there are two middle ear muscles (tensor tympani and stapedius) in humans, only the stapedius muscle contracts in response to sound. Contraction of the stapedius causes a change in the axis of rotation of the stapes footplate, thus increasing the immittance of the middle ear system. This change in conductivity through the middle ear can be measured indirectly as changes in acoustic immittance. The neural pathway includes CN VIII, the ventral cochlear nucleus, the trapezoid body, the medial superior olivary complex, the medial portion of the facial motor nucleus, and the stapedius muscle. When either ear is stimulated by a loud signal (70 to 90 dB HL), the ipsilateral and contralateral stapedius muscles contract. Acoustic reflex tests are a very powerful clinical tool and can provide diagnostic information about CN VII and CN VIII function and about the reflex pathways in the lower brainstem.

Testing is performed with the external ear canal pressure set to the middle ear peak pressure. It requires only passive cooperation from the patient; measurements cannot be made in a very active or crying child or in the presence of a tympanic membrane perforation or patent tympanostomy tube. For each ear, reflex thresholds to stimulation can be measured ipsilaterally to assess the integrity of the uncrossed pathways and contralaterally to assess the crossed pathways, for a total of four test configurations. Stimuli may be pure tones, narrow bands of noise, or broad-band noise. Reflex threshold is defined as the lowest stimulus level that elicits a time-locked change in acoustic immittance. For children with normal hearing, acoustic reflex thresholds in response to pure-tone stimuli occur between 70 and 100 dB HL for frequencies of 500 to 2000 Hz. The presence or absence of acoustic reflexes at 4000 Hz is not clinically significant. In the presence of even mild conductive hearing loss, acoustic reflexes are usually absent with the probe in the ear with disease. In patients with cochlear hearing loss, acoustic reflexes may be present at normal or increased levels or absent depending on the degree of hearing loss. When the pure-tone thresholds exceed 75 dB HL, 90% of patients with cochlear hearing loss do not exhibit reflexes at any stimulus level.[90] This information can help identify children with nonorganic hearing loss; that is, if acoustic reflexes are present at levels near or below the voluntary behavioral thresholds, a functional hearing loss should be suspected. Historically, attempts have been made to use acoustic reflex measures to identify and quantify the magnitude of sensorineural hearing loss in young children for whom behavioral estimates of threshold could not be obtained.[80] Although this approach appeared promising in the mid-1970s, improved electrophysiologic techniques (e.g., frequency-specific ABRs) have replaced this method.

Acoustic reflex decay

Acoustic reflex decay testing can rule out a retrocochlear site of lesion. A sustained stimulus is presented at a suprathreshold level (typically 10 dB SL regarding acoustic reflex threshold), and the change in immittance is measured for 10 seconds.[4] If the magnitude of the response decays by more than 50% in this interval, the test is considered positive for retrocochlear abnormality. Although this test theoretically can be performed for many different stimuli, the observation of decay at 2000 or 4000 Hz is not considered clinically significant.[29] Thus, the test typically is performed only at 500 and 1000 Hz.

Tests for nonorganic hearing loss (pseudohypoacusis)

For various reasons, some children (typically aged 10 to 16 years) feign hearing loss or exaggerate the degree of an existing hearing impairment. The referral source, patient history, or interview often alerts the clinician to the potential of a nonorganic hearing loss even before testing begins. Although financial gain often is the motivation for adult patients, nonorganic hearing loss in children often is used as a means of getting attention or as an excuse for poor academic performance.

If initial pure-tone or speech testing yields results inconsistent with the child's observed communication abilities, a nonorganic loss should be suspected. As discussed, there is a predictable relationship between SRT and PTA; a significant SRT/PTA discrepancy suggests the need for further testing. Similarly, poor test-retest reliability may be indicative of nonorganic hearing loss.

Historically, many tests have been developed but few are used clinically. Rintelmann, Schwan, and Blakley[81] reviewed test procedures. These tests can be divided into those that confirm the existence of a nonorganic component and those that estimate auditory thresholds without the patient's cooperation.

Nonthreshold tests

Once a nonorganic hearing loss is suspected, the test approach should be altered immediately. Unless the hearing loss is unilateral, an SRT should be established using an ascending approach. These results should be compared with the voluntary pure-tone thresholds at 500 and 2000 Hz. Speech perception tests administered at a low sensation level relative to the voluntary thresholds (e.g., 10 dB SL) also can confirm nonorganic hearing loss. Children do not realize that monosyllabic words cannot be perceived with a high degree of accuracy at these low levels.

Threshold tests

In an uncooperative child, only two methods can estimate threshold. Frequency-specific ABR measures are the only method that can be used reliably in bilaterally symmetric nonorganic hearing loss. In unilateral or asymmetric hearing loss (a difference of greater than 20 dB between ears), the Stenger test can estimate threshold in the poorer ear. The test is based on the fact that a signal presented binaurally at different sensation levels will be heard in one ear only. For this test, a tone is introduced to the "good" ear at 10 dB SL and at a level considerably below the voluntary threshold in the "poorer" ear. The test signals are introduced simultaneously, and the patient is instructed to respond whenever a signal is heard. The intensity of the signal in the "poorer" ear is increased systematically. As soon as the sensation level of the signal in the "poorer" ear exceeds that in the "good" ear (10 dB SL), the patient will perceive the signal as being delivered to the "poor" ear only and will stop responding. Similar techniques can be used to establish an SRT. The Stenger test is the most expedient method for suspected nonorganic unilateral hearing losses and this approach has been shown to produce threshold estimates that agree with actual thresholds within 15 to 20 dB or less.

The need for additional recommendations and follow-up in cases of nonorganic hearing loss should be determined on an individual basis. In general, the parents or caregivers should be informed of the situation, and possible reasons for the child's behavior should be explored. In some instances, it will be enough to tell the child that their hearing is within normal limits. In other cases, referral to a school counselor, social worker, or psychologist may be needed.

MANAGEMENT STRATEGIES AND AMPLIFICATION

Conductive hearing loss

Transient middle ear disease

As mentioned, recent data from prospective studies have shown that children with a history of otitis media with effusion have difficulties with speech perception (particularly in noise), attentiveness, and higher-order language processes.[25,28,35,82] Because otitis media with effusion can be accompanied by hearing loss, an audiologic evaluation should be performed to determine the degree of hearing loss. Children with greater degrees of hearing loss should be managed more aggressively than children with normal hearing or minimal hearing loss. Recently, the United States Department of Health and Human Services[97] published guidelines for managing otitis media with effusion in children aged 1 to 3 years who are otherwise healthy. Cases of acute otitis media or additional medical problems (e.g., craniofacial anomalies, concomitant sensorineural hearing loss) do not fall under these guidelines. Briefly, these guidelines state that a combination of pneumatic otoscopy and tympanometry be used at the initial diagnosis. After 3 months of unresolved effusion, a hearing evaluation is suggested. Observation or antibiotic therapy is recommended for management of children with thresholds of 20 dB HL or less. For children with thresholds of 20 dB HL or greater, bilateral myringotomy with tympanostomy tubes is an additional management option. Thus, in an otherwise normal child, documentation of HL is the primary determinant of management. Because children with middle effusion generally are asymptomatic, otologic (and possibly audiologic) follow-up is critical to ensure that the effusion has resolved and that hearing has returned to normal.

Permanent conductive hearing loss

The most common causes of permanent conductive hearing loss among young children are congenital middle ear anomalies. Crabtree and Harker[20] and Glasscock and others[30] provided a detailed description of this issue. When surgery is not an option, some form of amplification should be considered. When possible, use of a conventional (air conduction) hearing aid is considered the best option. Compared with a bone-conduction hearing aid, a conventional hearing aid is more cosmetically appealing, has a much wider dynamic range, and provides a higher fidelity signal. When a bone-conduction hearing aid is used in an infant or young child, it is important to shift the placement of the vibrator periodically to minimize permanent distortion of the skull. A surgically implanted bone-anchored hearing aid was developed in the 1970s and became commercially available in the United States in 1986. It is approved by the United States Food and Drug Administration for use in children aged 3 years or older when conventional (air conduction) hearing aids cannot be used. Roland and Yellin[83] provided a discussion on the use of this implantable device in children.

Sensorineural hearing loss

Hearing aid candidacy

Regardless of a child's age or the test techniques used to diagnose the hearing loss, when an educationally significant hearing loss is confirmed, amplification and habilitation should begin immediately. If the diagnosis is made by ABR and the child is developmentally too young for VRA testing, it is not necessary or desirable to wait until reliable behavioral thresholds can be obtained. Various ABR measures can be used to estimate thresholds for selecting the initial hearing aid characteristics. The electroacoustic characteristics of hearing aids can be altered over a reasonably wide range, thus allowing for minor adjustments in hearing aid characteristics as more specific information about the degree and configuration of hearing loss becomes known.

As mentioned, even relatively mild sensorineural hearing loss can impact speech and language development in young children. As such, children with thresholds poorer than 20 to 25 dB HL should be considered potential candidates for amplification. Some school-age children with mild hearing loss or hearing loss restricted to the high frequencies may appear to hear relatively well, and academic performance may be uncompromised. This may be particularly true in the early elementary school years. Further exploration of these cases, however, often reveals that these children display behavioral problems in school or show frequent signs of inattentiveness. Some children need to concentrate so intensely to compensate for their hearing loss that they are completely exhausted by the end of the school day. Teachers and parents often do not attribute these behaviors to a peripheral hearing loss. Trial amplification should be considered whenever possible for a child with mild hearing loss.

Audiologic management of unilateral hearing loss is a matter of some debate. Several researchers[7,9,41,77] reported that children with unilateral hearing loss are at high risk for academic failure in the elementary school years. Approximately 30% of children in these studies failed at least one grade between kindergarten and sixth grade. In cases in which the poorer ear is anakusic or unaidable because of extremely poor speech recognition or intolerance, loudness amplification options are limited. A specialized hearing aid that routes signals from the poor ear into the good ear generally is not a successful option for children. Because these children are at risk for academic failure, use of an FM system or sound-field FM system in the classroom should be considered.

Types of hearing aids

The behind-the-ear (BTE) hearing aid is the most commonly used device in children. This style offers flexible electrocoustic characteristics and good durability and is appropriate for all degrees of hearing loss. This style also can be coupled to FM systems, and all current forms of advanced signal processing are available in these casings. The major disadvantage of the BTE hearing aid is cosmetic, although, depending upon the earmold style and hearing aid size, BTE hearing aids may be less noticeable than some other styles. In young children, proper retention of the BTE hearing aid behind the pinna may require tape or special devices. The in-the-ear (ITE) hearing aid has been used increasingly in older children, and some audiologists have advocated the use of an in-the-canal or completely in-the-canal hearing aid for this population. The hearing aid and earmold are combined into a single unit that may be more cosmetically appealing than a BTE hearing aid. However, because these devices are small, many advanced features may not be available, and the ability to couple the devices to FM systems is limited. For young children, who are typically very active, safety issues also are a concern. Even a minor fall may cause the hard case to shatter in the ear canal. These styles are not appropriate for severe to profound hearing loss. Furthermore, because the earmold and hearing aid are a single unit, frequent re-casing is necessary as the child's ear canal grows, and acoustic feedback (whistling) can be a recurrent problem.

In the past few years, several forms of advanced signal processing have been introduced in hearing aids. These hearing aids, often referred to as *programmable devices*, include several types of circuits or features. Sandlin[85] provided a discussion of programmable hearing aids.

Programmability. With specialized equipment, the audiologist can alter many hearing aid characteristics (e.g., gain, frequency response, compression parameters) and write the desired parameters to a memory in the hearing aid. These parameters may be changed as often as necessary, providing flexibility, which can be useful in cases in which the exact degree and configuration of hearing loss are unknown. When hearing loss is progressive, however, it may be necessary to replace the hearing aid with a more powerful model.

Directional microphones. Specialized dual microphone circuitry reduces noise coming from behind the listener. This circuitry may be used exclusively in a hearing aid, or a switch or remote control device may be used to alternate between a directional and nondirectional microphone. Because sounds from the rear are attenuated, safety concerns may arise in certain situations. Children also may have difficulty hearing speakers from the sides or the rear (e.g., classmates in school). If the child is old enough to know when a directional microphone would improve listening, use of a system that can be switched between a directional and nondirectional microphone may be the best option.

Multi-memory capabilities. Currently, hearing aids with two to seven memories are available. Different hearing aid characteristics can be programmed into the memory, and the user can switch to different memories depending on listening conditions. The efficacy of this technology in adults has not been proven, and studies have found that most users only use two to three memories. Evaluation time is greatly increased to program additional memories. In addition, the child should be old enough to operate a remote control or other switching method and should be able to evaluate when each memory is to be used. Alternatively, with young children, some manufacturers recommend that parents control the memories as the listening environment changes.

Wide dynamic range compression. Wide dynamic range compression provides greater gain for low-level signals than for high-level signals. The goal is to improve the audibility and comfort of speech for many signal levels. Wide dynamic range compression devices can be single- or multi-channel (typically two to three channels), allowing for different input and output characteristics in different frequency regions. To properly fit these devices, the user often is required to provide reliable judgments of loudness, comfort, or intelligibility. These tasks are impossible for young children, and fitting strategies should be based solely on threshold measures and consideration of speech audibility.

Hearing aid evaluation

Many types of hearing aid circuitry are available, and no single hearing aid processing strategy meets the needs of all patients. The goal of hearing aid evaluation is to select the most appropriate type of hearing aid circuitry and to individualize the many parameters for an optimal fit. An appropriately fit device should make speech audible and comfortable across a wide range of listening conditions. Figure 26-5 shows the gain and maximum output characteristics for an appropriate hearing aid for a child with moderate sloping sensorineural hearing loss. In this example, the high frequencies show greater gain than the low frequencies, consistent with the configuration of hearing loss. To ensure safety and comfort, all hearing aid circuits are designed to limit the amount of gain available for high-level input signals. In this example, the maximum output of the hearing aid is set so that amplified signals never exceed 120 dB SPL. Although there is a positive correlation between the pure-tone audiogram and these hearing aid characteristics, the exact strategies used to select these parameters for a given hearing loss is a matter of debate. When fitting hearing aids to adults and older children, subjective measures of loudness discomfort, clarity, comfort, and ease of listening can be used to optimize parameters. Young children cannot provide this type of information during the evaluation, so hearing aid selection is based on the pure-tone audiogram and the electroacoustic characteristic of the hearing aid. Numerous hearing aid selection procedures have been described,[16,19,68,86] which provide target values for hearing aid gain and maximum output.

Probe microphone measures. The electroacoustic characteristics shown in Figure 26-5 were measured in a standard coupler, which was designed primarily for quality control. The gain and maximum output of a hearing aid generally are greater when measured in a real ear. For a fixed set of hearing aid characteristics, there is a great deal of individual variability in the real ear measured values due primarily to differences in ear canal size and middle ear impedance. Individual differences as large as 15-20 dB are possible. Because of the small ear canal size in young children and infants, individual ear canal acoustics should be considered during the hearing aid evaluation process.[26] This can be accomplished using a probe microphone system. A small, flexible tube is placed in the ear canal adjacent to the earmold. This tube is connected to a miniature microphone. Signals processed by the hearing aid are picked up by the microphone and directed to a computerized hearing aid analysis system. These real ear measures have been in clinical use for more than a decade, and recent modifications have allowed this technique to be used in infants and adults.[11]

Assistive listening devices. The most commonly used assistive listening device is the FM system, in which the talker (e.g., a classroom teacher) wears a transmitter and microphone and the child wears a receiver. These systems can be used alone or in conjunction with a child's personal hearing aid. The primary advantage of an FM system is that the adverse effects of room noise, reverberation, and distance between the talker and listeners are greatly diminished. Although these systems are most commonly used in classroom situations, they can be used in the home environment.[63,70] Other types of assistive devices are available for various degrees of hearing loss and other purposes (e.g., to ensure safety, to foster independence).[17,18,57] For example, if a child cannot hear environmental sounds (e.g., telephone, doorbell, smoke alarm, alarm clock) with or without hearing aids, an appropriate alerting device should be considered. An amplifier can improve television viewing for children with mild-to-moderate hearing loss, and closed captioning can be used for children with severe-to-profound hearing loss. Telephone amplifiers can be useful for children with mild-to-severe losses, and Telephone Devices for the Deaf can be used in cases of profound hearing loss in a child who is old enough to read and type.

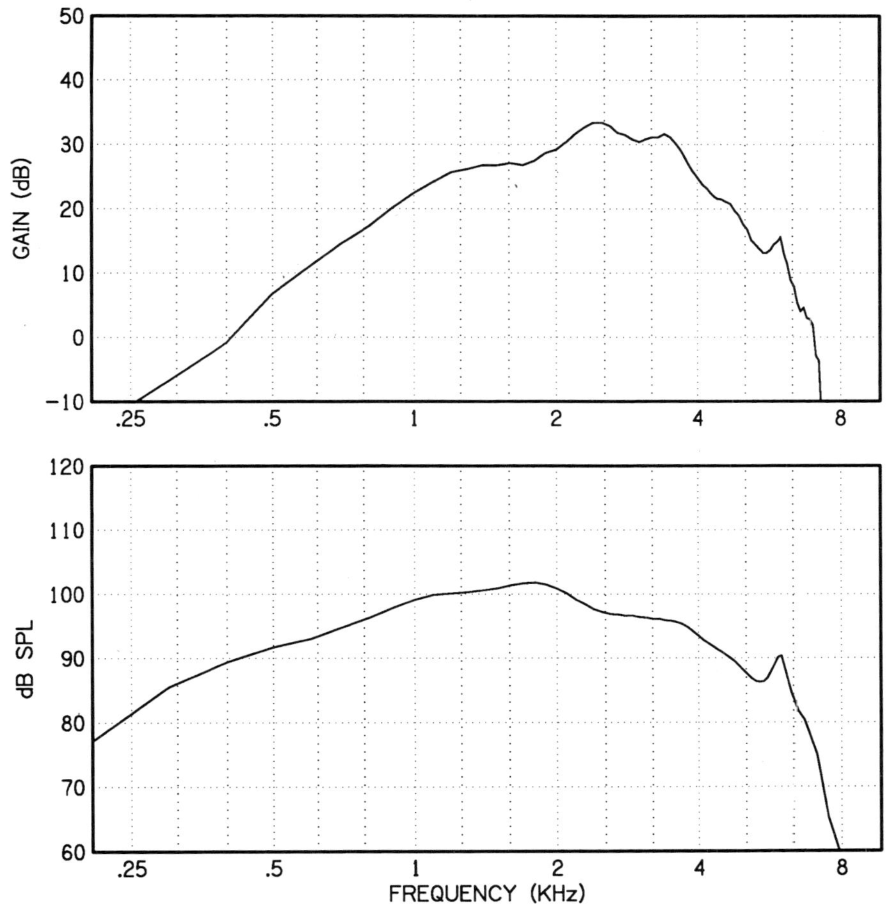

Fig. 26-5. Hearing aid gain as a function of frequency *(top panel).* Hearing aid maximum output (in dB sound pressure level) as a function of frequency (*bottom panel*).

Practical issues. In addition to the technical aspects of amplification, many practical details should be considered. Many details are unique to children (e.g., need for loaner hearing aids, frequent need to fabricate earmolds, methods of hearing aid retention, feedback control, battery ingestion precautions) and require the experience and expertise of a pediatric audiologist. In many cases, a team approach, involving many services (e.g., parent-infant specialists or educators, social workers, psychologists, geneticists, otolaryngologists) may be warranted. In addition, the pediatric audiologist should develop a comprehensive knowledge of local resources that may be of value to the family (e.g., funding agencies, preschools and schools for the hearing impaired, educational resources, advocacy groups, family support groups).

SUMMARY

Audiologic tests can provide the otolaryngologist with useful information for the identification and quantification of hearing loss and appropriate medical and nonmedical rehabilitation. Although audiologists typically manage nonmedical aspects of hearing loss, the otolaryngologist should understand basic principles related to these tests to integrate test results into the clinical picture and optimally serve their patients.

REFERENCES

1. American National Standards Institute: *Reference equivalent threshold levels for audiometric bone vibrators, ANSI S3.26–1981*, New York, 1981, Acoustical Society of America.
2. American Speech-Language-Hearing Association: Joint Committee on Infant Hearing 1994 position statement, *ASHA* 36:38, 1994.
3. American Speech-Language-Hearing Association: Guidelines for audiometric symbols, *ASHA* 32:25, 1990.
4. Anderson H, Barr B, Wedenberg E: *Intraaural reflexes in retrocochlear lesions.* In Hambarger C, Wasall J, editors: *Disorders of the skull base region*, Stockholm, 1969, Almquist and Wiksell.
5. Apuzzo ML, Yoshinaga-Itano C: Early identification of infants with significant hearing loss and the Minnesota child development inventory, *Semin Hear* 16:124, 1995.
6. Beasley DS, Rintelmann AK: *Central auditory processing.* In Rintelmann WF, editor: *Hearing assessment*, Baltimore, 1979, University Park Press.
7. Bess F: Children with unilateral hearing loss, *Journal of the Academy of Rehabilitative Audiology* 20:131, 1982.

8. Bess FH: The minimally hearing-impaired child, *Ear Hear* 6:43, 1985.
9. Bess F, Tharpe AM: An introduction to unilateral sensorineural hearing loss in children, *Ear Hear* 7:3, 1986.
10. Blair J, Peterson M, Viehweg S: The effects of mild sensorineural hearing loss on academic performance of young school-age children, *Volta Review* 87:87, 1985.
11. Block MG, Wiley TL: *Overview and basic principles of acoustic immittance measurement.* In Katz J, editor: *Handbook of clinical audiology*, ed 4, Baltimore, 1994, Williams & Wilkins.
12. Bluestone CD: *Otitis media with effusion atelectasis and eustachian tube dysfunction.* In Bluestone CD, Stool SE, editors: *Pediatric otolaryngology*, vol 2, Philadelphia, 1983, WB Saunders.
13. Bonfils P and others: Evoked otoacoustic emissions in newborn hearing screening, *Laryngoscope* 100:186, 1990.
14. Brandy WT: Reliability of voice tests of speech discrimination, *J Speech Hear Res* 9:461, 1966.
15. Brooks DN: The use of electroacoustic bridge in the assessment of middle ear function, *Audiology* 8:563, 1969.
16. Byrne D, Dillon H: The National Acoustic Laboratories' (NAL) new procedure for selecting the gain and frequency response of a hearing aid, *Ear Hear* 7:257, 1986.
17. Compton C: *Assistive devices: doorways to independence*, Washington DC, 1989, Gallaudet University.
18. Compton C: Innovations in assistive technology: a potpourri of exciting approaches, *The Hearing Journal* 49:10, 1996.
19. Cox RM: The MSU hearing instrument prescription procedure, *Hear Instr* 39:6, 1988.
20. Crabtree JA, Harker LA: *Developmental abnormalities of the ear.* In Cummings CW and others, editors: *Otolaryngology: head and neck surgery*, ed 2, vol 4, St Louis, 1993, Mosby.
21. de Jonge RR: Normal tympanometric gradient: a comparison of three methods, *Audiology* 25:299, 1986.
22. Don M, Eggermont JJ, Brackman DE: Reconstruction of the audiogram using brainstem responses and high-pass noise masking, *Ann Otol Rhinol Laryngol Suppl* 88:1, 1979.
23. Egan JP: Articulation testing methods, *Laryngoscope* 58:955, 1948.
24. Eimas PD, Clarkson RL: *Speech perception in children: are there effects of otitis media?* In Kavanaugh JF, editor: *Otitis media and child development*, Parkton, Md, 1986, York Press.
25. Feagans L and others: Relationship of middle ear disease in early childhood to later narrative and attentional skills, *J Pediatr Psychol* 12:581, 1987.
26. Feigin JA and others: Probe-tube microphone measures of ear-canal sound pressure levels in infants and children, *Ear Hear* 10:254, 1989.
27. Friel-Patti S, Finitzo T: Language learning in a prospective study of otitis media with effusion in the first two years of life, *J Speech Hear Res* 33:188, 1990.
28. Friel-Patti S and others: Language delay in infants associated with middle ear disease and mild, fluctuating hearing impairment, *Pediatr Infect Dis J* 82:104, 1982.
29. Givens GD, Seidemann MF: A systematic investigation of measurement parameters of acoustic reflex adaptation, *J Speech Hear Disord* 44:534, 1979.
30. Glasscock ME III and others: Management of congenital ear malformations, *Ann Otol Rhinol Laryngol* 92:504, 1983.
31. Gorga MP, Kaminski JR, Beauchaine KA: Auditory brain stem responses to high-frequency tone bursts in normal-hearing subjects, *Ear Hear* 8:222, 1987
32. Gorga MP, Reiland JK, Beauchaine KA: Auditory brainstem responses in a case of high-frequency conductive hearing loss, *J Speech Hear Disord* 50:346, 1985.
33. Gorga MP and others: Some comparisons between auditory brain stem response thresholds, latencies, and the pure-tone audiogram, *Ear Hear* 6:105, 1985.
34. Gorga MP and others: Auditory brainstem responses to tone bursts in normally hearing subjects, *J Speech Hear Res* 31:87, 1988.
35. Gravel JS, Wallace IF: Listening and language at 4 years of age: effects of early otitis media, *J Speech Hear Res* 35:588, 1992.
36. Hall JW III, Chandler D: *Tympanometry in clinical audiology.* In Katz J, editor: *Handbook of clinical audiology*, ed 4, Baltimore, 1994, Williams & Wilkins.
37. Harris JD, Haines HL, Meyers CK: A new formula for using the audiogram to predict speech hearing loss, *Arch Otolaryngol Head Neck Surg* 64:447, 1956.
38. Herrmann BS, Thornton AR, Joseph JM: Automated infant hearing screening using the ABR: development and validation, *Am J Audiology* 4:6, 1995.
39. Hirsh IJ and others: Development of materials for speech audiometry, *J Speech Hear Disord* 17:321, 1952.
40. Hodgson WR, editor: *Basic audiologic evaluation*, Baltimore, 1980, Williams & Wilkins.
41. Humes LE and others: Recognition of nonsense syllables by hearing-impaired listeners and by noise-masked normal hearers, *J Acoust Soc Am* 81:765, 1987.
42. Jacobson JT, Jacobson CA, Spahr RC: Automated and conventional ABR screening techniques in high-risk infants, *J Am Acad Audiol* 1: 187, 1990.
43. Jerger J: Clinical experience with impedance audiometry, *Arch Otolaryngol Head Neck Surg* 92:311, 1970.
44. Jerger JF, Jerger S, Mauldin L: Studies in impedance audiometry: I. Normal and sensorineural ears, *Arch Otolaryngol Head Neck Surg* 96:513, 1972.
45. Jerger J, Mauldin L: Prediction of sensorineural hearing level from the brainstem evoked response, *Arch Otolaryngol Head Neck Surg* 104:456, 1978.
46. Jerger S and others: Pediatric speech intelligibility test: I. Generation of test materials, *Int J Pediatr Otorhinolaryngol* 2:217, 1980.
47. Johnsen NJ and others: Evoked acoustic emissions from the human ear: IV. Final results in 100 neonates, *Scand Audiol* 17:27, 1983.
48. Karchmer MA: *A demographic perspective.* In Cherow E, editor: *Hearing impaired children and youth with developmental disabilities*, Washington, DC, 1985, Gallaudet Press.
49. Katz DR, Elliott LL: *Development of a new children's speech discrimination test.* Paper presented at the American Speech-Language-Hearing Association convention, Chicago, 1978.
50. Kemp DT: Stimulated acoustic emissions from the human auditory system, *J Acoust Soc Am* 64:1386, 1978.
51. Kemp DT, Ryan S: The use of transient evoked otoacoustic emissions in neonatal hearing screening programs, *Semin Hear* 14:30, 1993.
52. Kileny PR: ALGO-1 automated infant hearing screener: preliminary results, *Semin Hear* 8:125, 1987.
53. Killion M: New insert earphones for audiometry, *Hear Instr* 35:28, 1984.
54. Killion M, Wilber L, Gudmundsen G: Insert earphones for more interaural attenuation, *Hear Instr* 36:34, 1985.
55. Koebsell KA, Margolis RH: Tympanometric gradient measured from normal preschool children, *Audiology* 25:149, 1986.
56. Lehiste I, Peterson GE: Linguistic considerations in the study of speech intelligibility, *J Acoust Soc Am* 31:280, 1959.
57. Lewis D: *FM systems and assistive devices: selection and evaluation.* In Feigin J, Stelmachowicz P, editors: *Pediatric amplification: proceedings of the 1991 national conference,* Omaha, 1991, Boys Town National Research Hospital.
58. Liden G: The scope and application of current audiometric tests, *J Laryngol Otol* 83:507, 1969.
59. Liden G, Harford E, Hallen O: Tympanometry for the diagnosis of ossicular disruption, *Arch Otolaryngol Head Neck Surg* 99:23, 1974.
60. Liden G, Kankkunen A: Visual reinforcement audiometry, *Acta Otolaryngol (Stockh)* 67:281, 1969.
61. Lloyd L, Spradlin J, Reid M: An operant audiometric procedure for difficult-to-test patients, *J Speech Hear Disord* 33:236, 1968.

62. Mace AL and others: Relevant factors in the identification of hearing loss, *Ear Hear* 12:287, 1991.
63. Madell JR: FM systems as primary amplification for children with profound hearing loss, *Ear Hear* 13:102, 1992.
64. Margolis RH, Heller JW: Screening tympanometry: criteria for medical referral, *Audiology* 26:197, 1987.
65. Margolis RH, Shanks JE: *Tympanometry*. In Katz J, editor: *Handbook of clinical audiology*, ed 3, Baltimore, 1985, Williams & Wilkins.
66. Margolis RH and others: Multifrequency tympanometry in normal ears, *Audiology* 24:44, 1985.
67. Mauk G and others: The effectiveness of screening programs based on high-risk characteristics in early identification of hearing impairment, *Ear Hear* 12:312, 1991.
68. McCandless GA, Lyregaard PE: Prescription of gain/output (POGO) for hearing aids, *Hear Instr* 34:16, 1983.
69. Moeller MP: *Early intervention of hearing loss in children*. In Bess FH, editor: *Fourth international symposium on childhood deafness*, Nashville, Bill Wilkerson Center Press (in press).
70. Moeller MP and others: Longitudinal study of FM system use in nonacademic settings: effects on language development, *Ear Hear* 17:28, 1996.
71. Moodie KS, Seewald RC, Sinclair ST: Procedure for predicting real-ear hearing aid performance in young children, *Am J Audiology* 3: 23, 1994.
72. Reference deleted in pages.
73. Musiek FE: *Application of central auditory tests: an overview*. In Katz J, editor: *Handbook of clinical audiology*, ed 3, Baltimore, 1985, Williams & Wilkins.
74. Musiek FE, Chermak GD: Three commonly asked questions about central auditory processing disorders: management, *Am J Audiology* 4:15, 1995.
75. Nerbonne M, Schow R: *Auditory stimuli in communication*. In Nerbonne M, Schow R, editors: *Introduction to aural rehabilitation*, Baltimore, 1980, University Park Press.
76. Noffsinger PD, Kurdziel SA: *Assessment of central auditory lesions*. In Rintelmann WF, editor: *Hearing assessment*, Baltimore, 1979, University Park Press.
77. Oyler RF, Oyler AL, Matkin ND: Warning: a unilateral hearing loss may be detrimental to a child's academic career, *The Hearing Journal* 18:20, 1987.
78. Paradise JL, Smith CG, Bluestone CD: Tympanometric detection of middle ear effusion in infants and young children, *Pediatrics* 59:198, 1976.
79. Peters JG: An automated infant screener using advanced evoked response technology, *The Hearing Journal* 39:25, 1986.
80. Popelka GR: *The acoustic reflex in normal and pathologic ears*. In Popelka GR, editor: *Hearing assessment with the acoustic reflex*, New York, 1981, Grune & Stratton.
81. Rintelmann WF, Schwan SA, Blakley BW: Pseudohypacusis, *Otolaryngol Clin North Am* 24:381, 1991.
82. Roberts JE and others: Otitis media in early childhood, and cognitive, academic, and classroom performance of the school-aged child, *Pediatrics* 83:477, 1989.
83. Roland PS, Yellin W: Use of the Audiant bone conductor in children with congenital anomalies, *Semin Hear* 13:331, 1992.
84. Ross M, Lerman J: A picture identification test for hearing-impaired children, *J Speech Hear Res* 13:44, 1970.
85. Sandlin RE, editor: *Understanding digitally programmable hearing aids*, Boston, 1994, Allyn & Bacon.
86. Seewald RC: The desired sensation level method for fitting children: version 3.0, *The Hearing Journal* 45:36, 1992.
87. Shanks JE, Wilson RH: Effects of direction and rate of ear-canal pressure changes on tympanometric measures, *J Speech Hear Res* 29: 11, 1986.
88. Shanks JE, Wilson RH, Palmer CV: Multi-frequency tympanometry, *ASHA* 29:131, 1987.
89. Shanks J and others: Equivalent ear canal volumes in children pre- and post-tympanostomy tube insertion, *J Speech Hear Res* 35:936, 1992.
90. Silman S, Gelfand SA: The relationship between magnitude of hearing loss and acoustic reflex threshold levels, *J Speech Hear Disord* 46: 312, 1981.
91. Simmons FB, McFarland WH, Jones FR: An automated hearing screening technique for newborns, *Acta Otolaryngol (Stockh)* 87:1, 1979.
92. Sloan C: *Auditory processing difficulties in children*, San Diego, 1985, College-Hill Press.
93. Stapells DR, Gravel JS, Martin BA: Thresholds for auditory brain stem responses to tones in notched noise from infants and young children with normal hearing or sensorineural hearing loss, *Ear Hear* 16:361, 1995.
94. Stapells DR and others: Thresholds for short-latency auditory-evoked potentials to tones in notched noise in normal-hearing and hearing-impaired subjects, *Audiology* 29:262, 1990.
95. Starr A and others: Auditory neuropathy, *Brain Res* 119:741, 1996.
96. Stein L, Kraus N: *Auditory brainstem response measures with multiply handicapped children and adults*. In Jacobson JT, editor: *The auditory brainstem response*, San Diego, 1985, College-Hill Press.
97. Stool SE and others: *Managing otitis media with effusion in young children: quick reference guide for clinicians. AHCPR Publication No. 94-0623*, Rockville, 1994, Agency for Health Care Policy and Research, Public Health Service, US Department of Health and Human Services.
98. Strong CJ, Clark TC, Walden BE: The relationship of hearing-loss severity to demographic, age, treatment, and intervention-effectiveness variables, *Ear Hear* 15:126, 1994.
99. The Pediatric Working Group of the Conference on Amplification for Children with Auditory Deficits: Amplification for infants and children with hearing loss, *Am J Audiology* 5:53, 1996.
100. Thompson G, Weber B: Responses of infants and young children to behavior observation audiometry (BOA), *J Speech Hear Disord* 39: 140, 1974.
101. Thompson G, Wilson WR: Clinical application of visual reinforcement audiometry, *Semin Hear* 5:85, 1984.
102. Thornton AR, Raffin MJM: Speech-discrimination scores modeled as a binomial variable, *J Speech Hear Res* 21:507, 1978.
103. van der Drift JFC, Brocaar MP, van Zanten GA: The relation between the pure-tone audiogram and the click auditory brainstem response threshold in cochlear hearing loss, *Audiology* 26:1, 1987.
104. Vanhuyse VJ, Creten WL, Van Camp KJ: On the W-notching of tympanograms, *Scand Audiol* 4:45, 1975.
105. White KR, Behrens TR: The Rhode Island Hearing Assessment Project: implications for universal newborn hearing screening, *Semin Hear* 14:1, 1993.
106. White KR, Vohr BR, Behrens TR: Universal newborn hearing screening using transient evoked otoacoustic emissions: results of the Rhode Island Hearing Assessment Project, *Semin Hear* 14:18, 1993.
107. White KR and others: Screening all newborns for hearing loss using transient evoked otoacoustic emissions, *Int J Pediatr Otorhinolaryngol* 29:203, 1994.
108. Wilson RH and others: Normative data in quiet, broadband noise, and competing message for Northwestern University auditory test no. 6 by a female speaker, *J Speech Hear Disord* 55:771, 1990.
109. Yoshinaga-Itano C and others: *The effect of early identification on the development of deaf and hard-of-hearing infants and toddlers*. Poster presented at American Academy of Audiology Conference, Salt Lake City, 1996.

Chapter 27

Congenital Malformations of the Inner Ear

Robert K. Jackler

Development of the inner ear begins early in embryogenesis. By the end of the eighth week, the membranous labyrinth has assumed its characteristic convoluted shape.[123] Gradual ossification of the otic capsule develops around the membranous labyrinth and is essentially complete by birth.[124] Maturation of the sensory epithelium occurs long after formation of the membranous labyrinth, during the late second and early third trimesters. By the twenty-sixth to twenty-eighth weeks of gestation, hair-cell and auditory neural development are largely complete. Thus the normal human fetus may be able to hear 2.5 to 3 months before birth.

Most inner ear malformations arise when formation of the membranous labyrinth is interrupted during the first trimester of pregnancy.[42] This interruption may be either a result of inborn genetic error or a consequence of a teratogenic exposure during the period of inner ear organogenesis between the fourth and eighth weeks of gestation. Genetic errors may be either autosomal dominant or recessive and may manifest as sensorineural hearing loss (SNHL) alone or be associated with any of a number of syndromes.[28] A partial list of syndromes associated with radiologically detectable inner ear malformation includes Pendred's, Usher's, Waardenburg's, Wildervanck's (cervico-oculoacoustic), branchio-otorenal and Alagille's.[31,47,80,132] Nonsyndromic familial inner ear malformations have also been described.[14,29]

Teratogenic influences known to affect inner ear organogenesis include *in utero* viral infection (e.g., rubella, cytomegalovirus), chemical teratogens (e.g., thalidomide), and radiation exposure.[7,44] Abnormalities in otic capsule structure and deficiencies in the organ of Corti appear to arise as secondary effects of the earlier error in development of the membranous labyrinth. Derangement of the otic capsule ossification process alone does not appear to be a major mechanism in congenital hearing loss. Ossification of the labyrinthine lumen, however, is a common finding in early acquired deafness, typically arising as a consequence of meningitis.

Developmental damage to cochlear structure and function is not restricted to agents that cause gross structural malformations. Even in doses that are below those that would be ototoxic in adult species, aminoglycoside antibiotics administered in the animal equivalent of the human first trimester of pregnancy cause severe hearing losses in several species.[102] This time frame corresponds to the maturation of the outer hair cells and initiation of the cochlear potentials. Human studies also document this. In 35 of the infants delivered by 72 women who received streptomycin prophylaxis for tuberculosis during the first 4 months of pregnancy, auditory deficits ranging from minor high-frequency threshold elevations to severe bilateral deafness were noted.[120]

The risk is not restricted to the first trimester. Even at low doses, smaller hearing losses were seen when aminoglycoside antibiotics were administered during the human equivalent of the last two trimesters of pregnancy, which has obvious implications for use of these drugs in pregnant women and in premature infants who have not yet reached functional cochlear maturity.

Congenital anomalies of the inner ear may be considered in two broad categories: malformations with pathologic changes limited to the membranous labyrinth and malformations that involve both the osseous and membranous labyrinth. This division has been chosen because of its clinical relevance. Only patients with malformed otic capsules have abnormal inner ear radiographs and therefore may be diagnosed during life. By inference, children with congenital SNHL and radiographically normal inner ears may be assumed to possess anomalies limited to the membranous labyrinth or neural pathways. Although several types of membranous deformities have been described, their classification is not yet of clinical use because differentiation requires histopathologic examination. Among the deformities that affect the otic capsule, a variety of morphologic patterns may be recognized radiographically, and classification may have prognostic and even therapeutic importance.

INCIDENCE

It can be safely assumed that all children with congenital sensory hearing loss would have detectable abnormalities in their inner ears if they could be examined histologically. Because most children with profound bilateral deafness have radiographically normal inner ears, it can be inferred that malformations limited to the membranous labyrinth predominate. Jensen[41] studied 62 children enrolled in a school for the deaf with polytomography and detected cochlear malformations in only 15%. By contrast, Unger and Shaffer[130] evaluated a series of 104 deaf students with polytomography and found no cochlear anomalies that were clearly attributable to developmental arrest. In a recent series of 234 children who had SNHL of varying degrees of severity, Reilly[104] found cochlear anomalies in only 4% of those evaluated by high-resolution computed tomography (CT). In unilateral profound deafness, Everberg[19] detected only a 2% incidence of cochlear malformations among the 122 children studied. In analyzing each of these studies, children with radiographic signs of labyrinthine ossification were not included in the calculation of incidence of congenital malformation, because this finding is usually a marker for acquired deafness, typically due to meningitis.

The incidence of deformities of the semicircular canals (SCCs) and inner ear aqueducts has been less well studied than that of cochlear deformities. In a recent series of patients with radiographically detectable malformations of the inner ear, the cochlea was involved in 76%, the semicircular canals in 39%, and the vestibular aqueduct (VA) in 32% of ears.[42] These data total more than 100% because many cases demonstrate abnormalities of more than one portion of the inner ear. In recent years, a heightened awareness of VA enlargement, combined with the greater sensitivity of axial CT in demonstrating this deformity, has led to a substantial increase in its detection. The recent rapid accrual of cases by clinicians interested in inner ear malformations suggests that enlargement of the VA will ultimately prove to be the most common radiographically detectable inner ear anomaly.[39]

Among deaf children with radiographically normal inner ears, pathologic studies indicate that cochleosaccular dysplasia (Scheibe's dysplasia) is by far the most common deformity.[113] Due to the paucity of pathologic specimens available for examination, it is impossible to estimate the relative frequency of the various membranous malformations.

Box 27-1. Classification of congenital inner ear malformations

Malformations limited to the membranous labyrinth

- Complete membranous labyrinthine dysplasia (Siebenmann-Bing)
- Limited membranous labyrinthine dysplasia
  - Cochleosaccular dysplasia (Scheibe)
  - Cochlear basal turn dysplasia

Malformations of the osseous and membranous labyrinth

- Complete labyrinthine aplasia (Michel)
- Cochlear anomalies
  - Cochlear aplasia
  - Cochlear hypoplasia
  - Incomplete partition (Mondini)
  - Common cavity
- Labyrinthine anomalies
  - Semicircular canal dysplasia
  - Semicircular canal aplasia
- Aqueductal anomalies
  - Enlargement of the vestibular aqueduct
  - Enlargement of the cochlear aqueduct
- Internal auditory canal abnormalities
  - Narrow internal auditory canal
  - Wide internal auditory canal

CLASSIFICATION

The traditional nomenclature used to describe congenital anomalies of the inner ear involves a confusing array of eponyms that stem from the first reports, usually by eighteenth or nineteenth century authors, of the various morphologic patterns. In this chapter, a descriptive classification system is used along with the traditional eponyms in an attempt to make this topic more logical, easier to learn, and more clinically relevant (Box 27-1). In membranous malformations this classification is based on histopathologic changes in the inner ear, whereas in combined osseous/membranous deformities, radiographic appearance is used to distinguish among the various entities.[42] Correct use of the terminology used in pathoembryology is important because these terms are frequently applied imprecisely in the earlier literature. Key terms are *aplasia* (complete lack of development), *hypoplasia* (incomplete development), and *dysplasia* (aberration in development).

MALFORMATIONS LIMITED TO THE MEMBRANOUS LABYRINTH

In malformations limited to the membranous labyrinth, which account for over 90% of congenital deafness, the bony labyrinth is normal.[3,57,79,115] In its most severe form, membranous dysplasia involves the entire labyrinth, including the cochlea, SCCs, utricle, and saccule. Membranous labyrinthine dysplasia may also be limited, involving only a portion of the inner ear.

Complete membranous labyrinthine dysplasia (Bing-Siebenmann)

Complete membranous labyrinthine dysplasia was first described by Siebenmann and Bing,[117] and is extremely rare. It has been reported in association with cardioauditory (Jervell and Lange-Neilsen) and Usher's syndromes.[24]

Limited membranous labyrinthine dysplasia

Cochleosaccular dysplasia (Scheibe)

Incomplete development of the pars inferior is the most frequent histopathologic finding in congenital deafness. It was first described by Scheibe[108] and is commonly known as *cochleosaccular dysplasia*. The spectrum of its pathologic findings in this anomaly, which is confined to the cochlea and the saccule, has been well described.[8,10,23,75,79] The organ of Corti is either partially or completely missing. The cochlear duct is usually collapsed, with Reissner's membrane adherent to the limbus. Less commonly the duct is distended, presumably as a result of endolymphatic hydrops. The stria vascularis is typically degenerated and may contain colloidal inclusions. Schuknecht[119] described characteristic strial changes consisting of aplasia alternating with regions of hyperplasia and gross deformity. Cochlear changes may be severe in the base turn and gradually lessen in intensity toward the apex, or they may be severe throughout. The saccule is usually collapsed and has degenerated sensory epithelium. In cochleosaccular dysplasia, the SCCs and utricle are normal. Auditory neuronal survival is variable but may remain normal into adulthood, at least in some cases. Cochleosaccular dysplasia has also been demonstrated in a number of animal species, including the deaf white cat, dalmatian dogs, and various mouse mutants.[122]

Cochlear basal turn dysplasia

Dysplasia limited to the basal turn of the cochlea may be related to familial high-frequency SNHL. No description of membranous labyrinthine dysplasia limited to the pars superior was found in an extensive review of the literature. This outcome is not surprising as such individuals are probably minimally symptomatic. They would have normal hearing and presumably would have compensated for their congenital vestibular deficit.

MALFORMATIONS OF THE MEMBRANOUS AND OSSEOUS LABYRINTH

Congenital anomalies of the inner ear that deform the otic capsule are of special interest to the clinician because they may be recognized and differentiated during life through radiographic imaging. As discussed previously, only about 5% to 15% of congenitally deaf individuals demonstrate radiographically anomalous inner ears. The clinical manifestations and natural history of these deformities are highly variable. Although some individuals are deaf from birth, most maintain some residual hearing into adulthood. Slowly progressive deterioration of hearing during childhood, with eventual stabilization, is common. Sudden decrements in hearing are frequent and may appear to be spontaneous or may be triggered by head trauma, even minor in nature. Presumably, most of these cases are secondary to either internal fistulization secondary to membrane rupture within the cochlea with admixture of perilymph and endolymph or external fistulization to the middle ear. Fluctuant hearing loss is unusual in these patients, and endolymphatic hydrops is an atypical finding. In some patients, hearing may be best preserved in very high frequencies (>8000 Hz), which are not measured by conventional audiometry.[21] Residual ultra-audiometric hearing should be suspected in hearing-impaired children who manifest substantially better auditory function than would be predicted by pure tone results in the speech frequencies.[11] Occasionally, malformation of the inner ears may be associated with normal hearing.[52,66] Vestibular symptoms, which are occasionally severe, are present in about 20% of patients.[42] Retardation of motor development has been documented in some children with malformed inner ears, particularly those with absent semicircular canals.[128] A few patients experience vertigo when exposed to loud sounds, the so-called "Tullio phenomenon."[54]

A wide variety of morphologic patterns of inner ear malformation has been observed radiographically and may involve the cochlea, SCCs, or vestibular aqueduct (Fig. 27-1).* Similar diversity has been observed on histologic analysis.† The majority of combined osseous and membranous malformations appears to arise from a premature arrest in the development of one or more components of the inner ear (Fig. 27-2). The strongest evidence for this theory comes from the resemblance of most malformed inner ears to the appearance of the inner ear during embryogenesis, particularly between the fourth and eighth weeks of gestation. As a general rule, the earlier the developmental arrest the more severe the deformity and the worse the hearing will be.

Other anomalies cannot be explained by a premature arrest in development alone and appear to arise from an aberrant embryologic process. An example of this type of anomaly is a cochlea of normal length but abnormal size or coiling geometry.[48] In humans, the inner ear is adult size at birth and shows strikingly little variation in size among individuals. Pappas and others[85] suggested that some children with congenital SNHL and apparently normal inner ear morphology on CT possess subtle abnormalities in the dimensions of inner ear structures. They propose that such dimensional variations arise from a teratogenic insult during the second or third trimester, after the membranous labyrinth has formed but before it has reached adult size. Further study is

* Refs. 17, 42, 61, 70, 78, 94, 95.

† Refs. 48, 57, 69, 83, 107, 112.

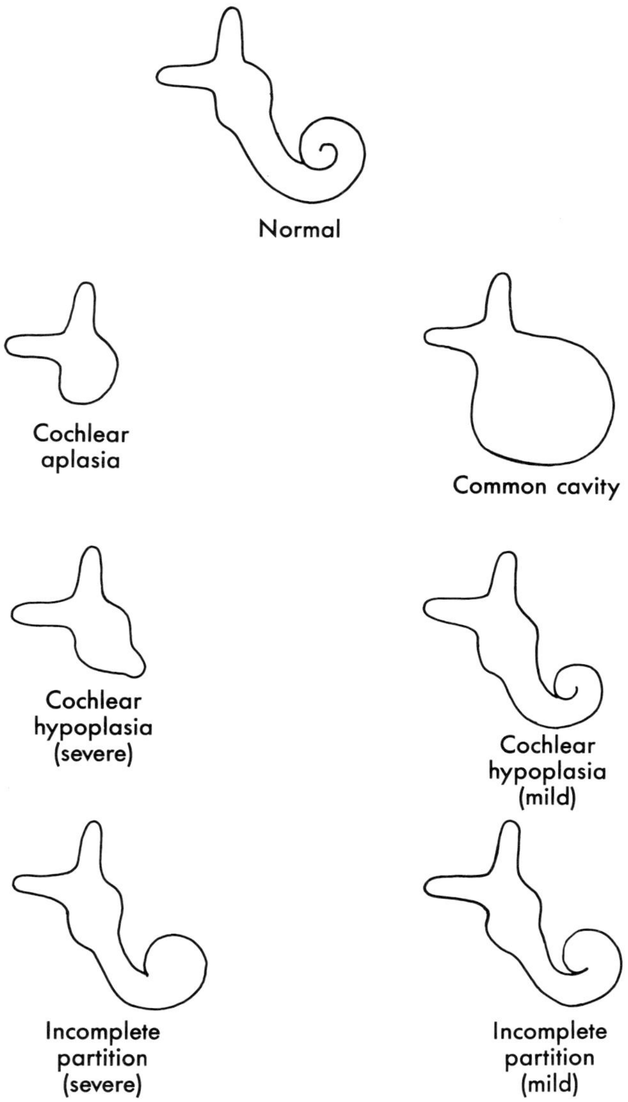

Fig. 27-1. Cochlear malformations as seen on coronal computed tomography. (From Jackler RK, Luxford WM, House WF: *Laryngoscope* 97[suppl 40]:2, 1987.)

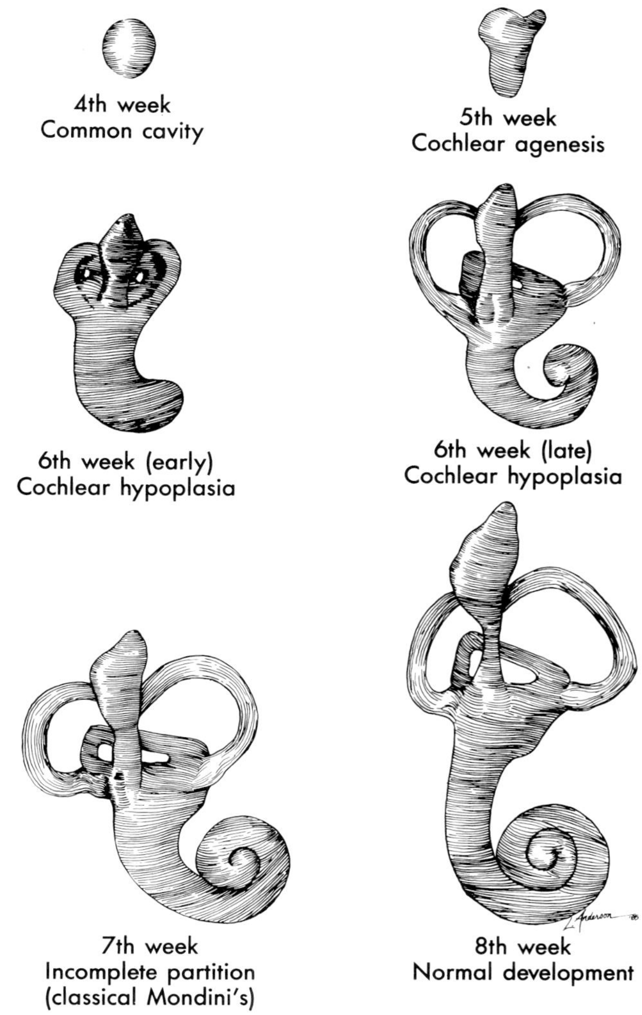

Fig. 27-2. Embryogenesis of cochlear malformations. (From Jackler RK, Luxford WM, House WF: *Laryngoscope* 97[suppl 40]: 2, 1987.)

needed to determine the clinical relevance of these observations.

Whereas some inner ear malformations involve only one portion of the inner ear, many patients have a combination of anomalies involving more than one component. Between the fourth and fifth weeks of development, the spheric otocyst develops three buds that ultimately form the cochlea, SCCs, and VA (see Fig. 27-2). An inner ear malformation may be limited to one of these anlages, may involve a combination of two, or may even affect all three.

The frequent coexistence of deformities involving the cochlea, SCCs, and VA has several possible explanations: (1) the anomaly is genetically predetermined, (2) an insult to the embryo occurred before the fifth week, or (3) each of the buds was susceptible to some teratogenic influence at a later stage of development. The majority of inner ear malformations are bilateral and symmetric. In cases in which radiographs detect an anomaly on only one side, the opposite ''normal'' inner ear has a hearing loss in approximately 50% of cases.[42]

Before the evolution of high-resolution imaging technology, clinicians and histopathologists alike tended to lump these malformations together under the term *Mondini's dysplasia*, after the first report by Carlo Mondini. An English translation of Mondini's original article has recently been published.[67a] Before the Academy of Sciences of the University of Bologna, Mondini described the inner ear findings in a deaf 8-year-old boy who was struck on the foot by a wagon and later died of gangrene.[68,90] The cochlea possessed only 1.5 turns and had a hollow apical cavity. An enlarged

Table 27-1. Relative incidence of cochlear malformations

Malformation	Incidence (%)
Incomplete partition (Mondini)	55
Common cavity	26
Cochlear hypoplasia	15
Cochlear aplasia	3
Complete labyrinthine aplasia (Michel)	1

From Jackler RK, Luxford WM, House WF: Congenital malformations of the inner ear: a classification based on embryogenesis, *Laryngoscope* 97(suppl 40):2-14, 1987.

vestibule and VA were also present. This deformity is the most common form of cochlear anomaly (Table 27-1). Although numerous other distinct anatomic patterns of inner ear malformation are discernible radiographically and histologically, many continue to use the term *Mondini's dysplasia* to describe them all. To avoid a confusing and overly broad nomenclature system, this term is best reserved for describing the particular subtype of cochlear malformation first described by Mondini, whether or not it is associated with other inner ear malformations.

Complete labyrinthine aplasia (Michel)

The severest deformity of the membranous and osseous labyrinth, complete labyrinthine aplasia, was first described by Michel.[63] This malformation is exceedingly rare. Presumably, a developmental arrest occurs before the formation of an otic vesicle, resulting in a complete absence of inner ear structures. Complete labyrinthine aplasia has been reported in association with anencephaly and thalidomide exposure.[49,57] An association with external-ear abnormalities also has been reported.[33] A recent purported case of Michel's dysplasia actually described a cystic inner ear of the common cavity type.[51] This is but one example of the inaccurate use of traditional eponyms—a frequent occurrence in the literature. The incidence of complete labyrinthine aplasia is overestimated in the radiographic literature because it is confused with labyrinthine ossification. In the latter condition, which is usually acquired during life, a sizable and dense otic capsule is present radiographically. In complete labyrinthine aplasia, the otic capsule is entirely absent (Figs. 27-3, 27-4, 27-5). Such ears are of course uniformly deaf.

Cochlear anomalies (see Fig. 27-1)

Cochlear aplasia

In cochlear aplasia the cochlea is completely absent, presumably as a result of an arrest in the development of the cochlear bud at the fifth week of gestation. This morphologic pattern is rare. Radiographically, only a vestibule and SCCs (usually deformed) are present. To differentiate this anomaly from labyrinthine ossification it is necessary to assess the amount of otic capsule bone anterior to the internal auditory canal (IAC). In cochlear aplasia, the otic capsule is absent,

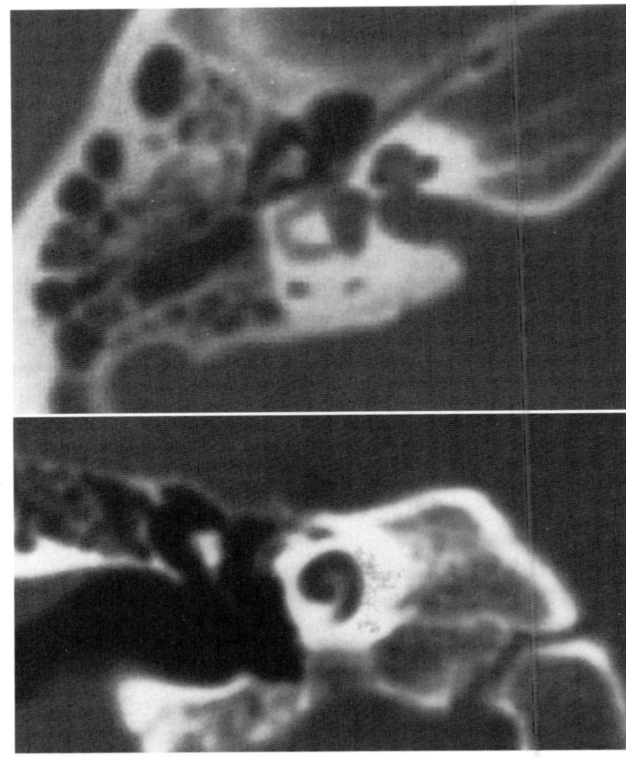

A

B

Fig. 27-3. A, Radiographically normal inner ear on axial and, **B,** coronal high-resolution computed tomography. Note that the normal cochlea appears to have only 1.5 turns on coronal scans as a result of the oblique angle of section in relation to the axial scans of the modiolus.

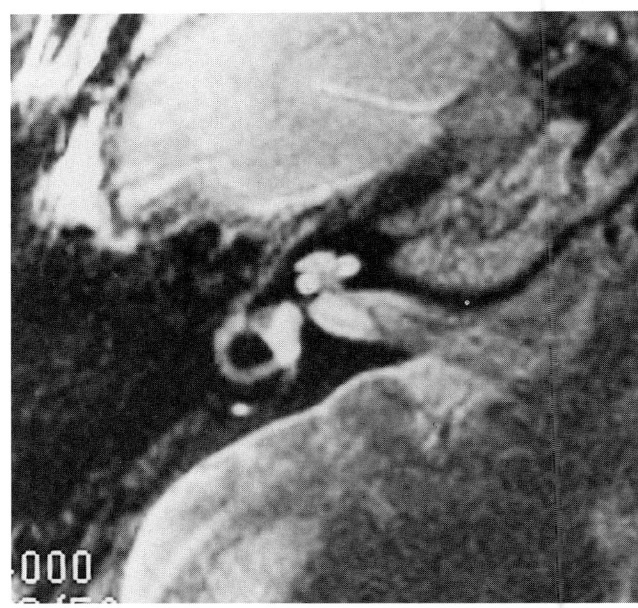

Fig. 27-4. Axial, high-resolution T2-weighted image (fast spin-echo) of a normal inner ear at the level of the mid- and apical cochlea and lateral semicircular canal. Note the internal detail of the cochlea, which includes visualization of the scalar partitions and the modiolus. The seventh and eighth cranial nerves can be seen in the internal auditory canal outlined by cerebrospinal fluid.

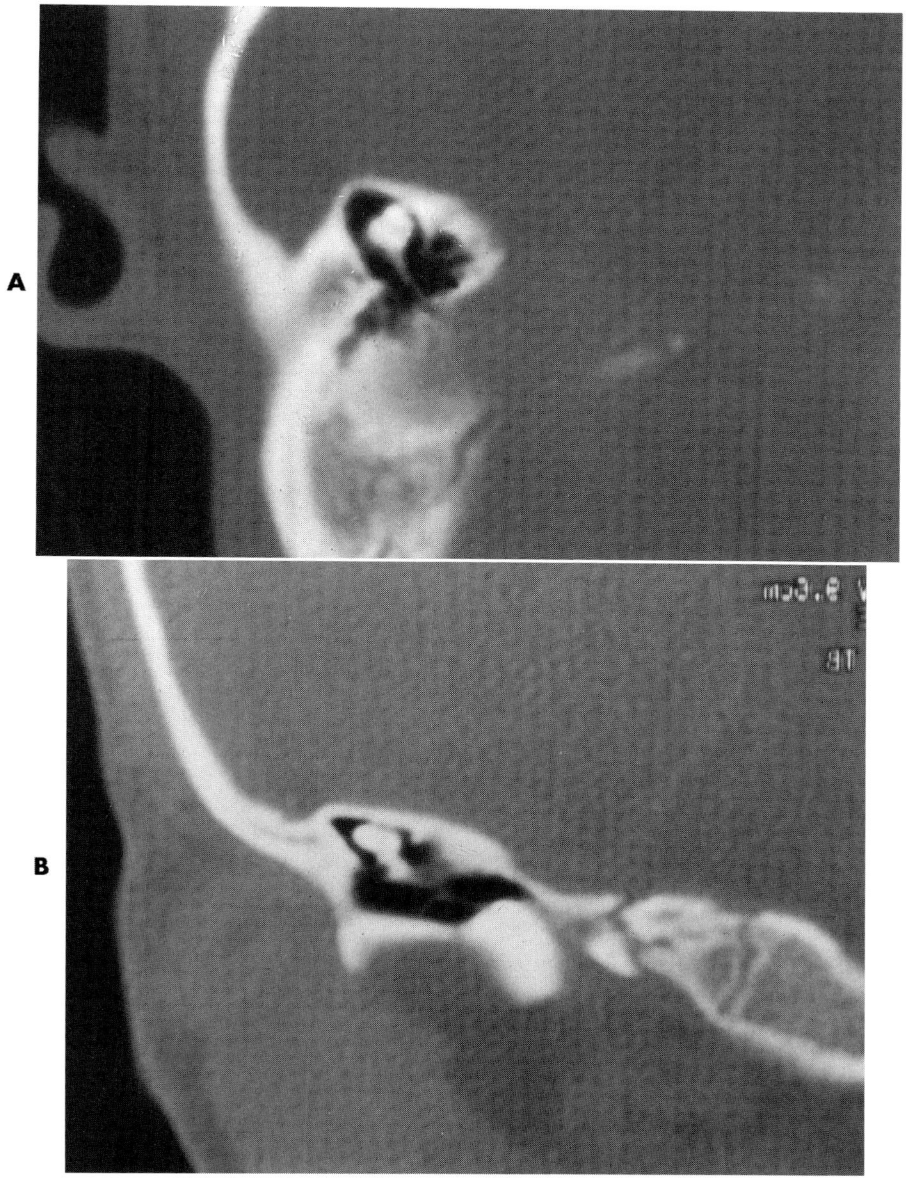

Fig. 27-5. Complete labyrinthine aplasia as seen on an **A,** axial and **B,** coronal computed tomography. Note the presence of an ear canal and middle ear but complete absence of the otic capsule. (Courtesy of Joel Swartz, MD.)

whereas in osseous obliteration it is dense and of normal dimensions. Ears with cochlear aplasia are devoid of auditory function.

Cochlear hypoplasia

An arrest during the sixth week of gestation results in a hypoplastic cochlea consisting of a single turn or less. This deformity comprises approximately 15% of all cochlear anomalies. Radiographically, a small bud of variable length (usually 1 to 3 mm) protrudes from the vestibule (Fig. 27-6). The vestibule is frequently enlarged with accompanying semicircular malformations in about half of the cases. Small cochleas lacking a modiolus or other internal architecture have been described histologically.[8,40,112] Hearing is variable in these ears and may be remarkably good considering the minute size of the cochlea. The variability of hearing presumably is accounted for by the degree of membranous labyrinthine development within the truncated cochlear lumen.

Incomplete partition (Mondini)

Arrest at the seventh week of gestation yields a cochlea that has only 1.5 turns. This is the most common type of cochlear malformation, accounting for over 50% of all such deformities. Radiographically, the cochlea is smaller than normal and partially or completely lacks an interscalar septum (Figs. 27-7 and 27-8). Although the cochlea usually measures 8 to 10 mm vertically, it is typically in the 5- to 6-mm range in incomplete partition deformity. Care must be exercised in

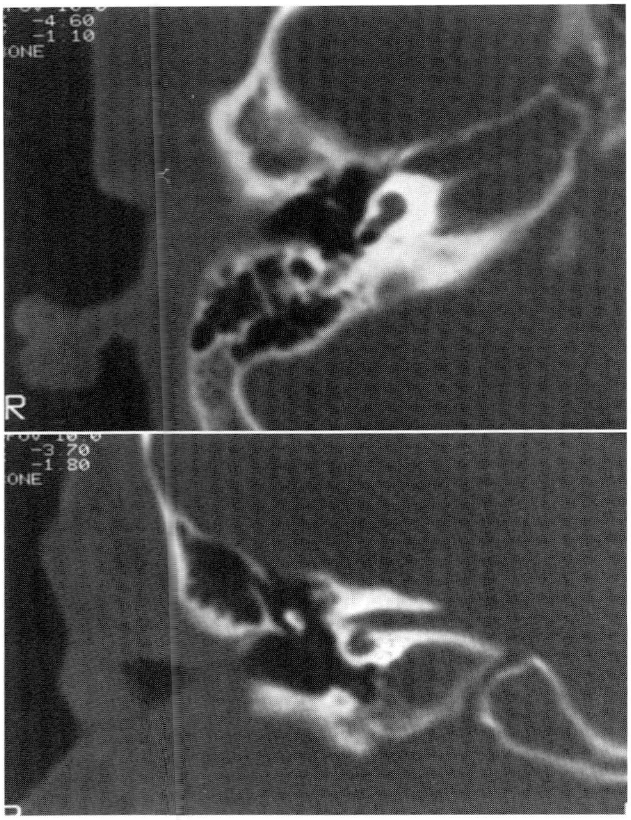

Fig. 27-6. **A,** Cochlear hypoplasia as seen on axial and **B,** coronal computed tomography. The cochlea consists only of a small bud off of the vestibule.

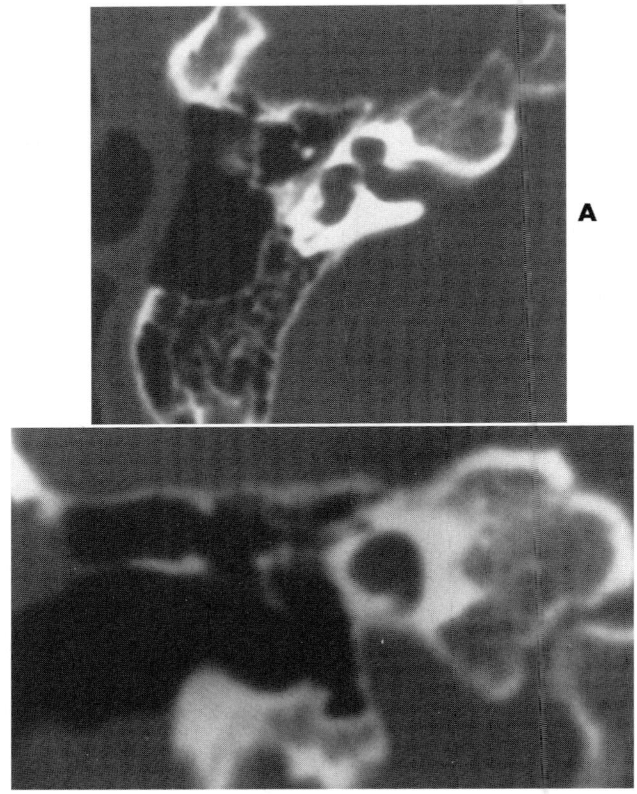

Fig. 27-7. **A,** Incomplete partition as seen on axial and **B,** coronal computed tomography. Note the absence of an interscalar septum, which is most evident on the coronal scan.

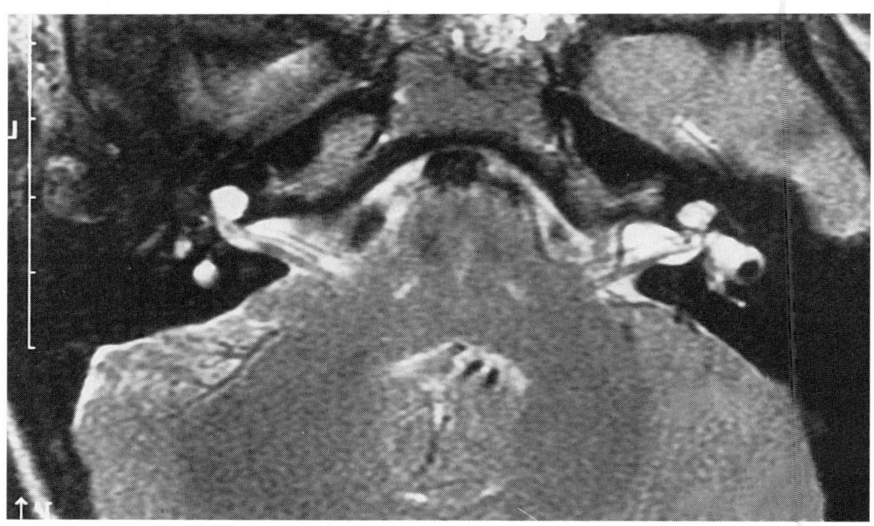

Fig. 27-8. High-resolution T2-weighted image (fast-spin-echo) of an incomplete partition deformity. Note the absence of intracochlear septation.

A

B

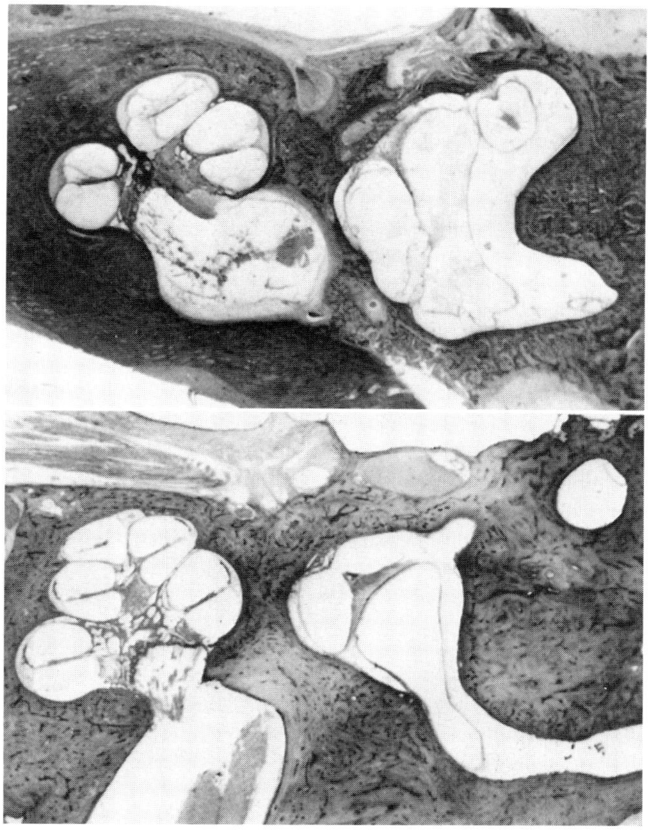

Fig. 27-9. A, Photomicrograph of a malformed cochlea with the typical features of Mondini's dysplasia. The cochlea has 1.5 turns and an apical scala communis. **B,** Midmodiolar section through a normal cochlea for comparison. (From Monsell EM and others: *Laryngoscope* 97[suppl 40]:18, 1987.)

counting the number of cochlear turns radiographically because this may be difficult to determine even using high-resolution CT. The radiographic diagnosis depends more on cochlear size and the absence of a scalar septum than on the number of cochlear turns perceived. Histologically, incomplete partition appears to be the radiographic correlate of classical Mondini's dysplasia (Fig. 27-9). In numerous reported cases a small cochlea with 1.5 turns possessing an apical scala communis due to deficiency in the osseous spiral lamina has been described.[8,48,83] Organ of Corti development is variable as is auditory neural population. As might be expected, auditory function is also variable, ranging from normal to profound deafness. The mean hearing threshold (three-tone average) in a group of 41 ears with incomplete partition was 75 dB.[42] SCC deformities accompany incomplete partition of the cochlea in approximately 20% of cases.

Common cavity

A deformed inner ear in which the cochlea and vestibule are confluent, forming an ovoid cystic space without internal architecture, may be explained by an arrest at the fourth-week otocyst stage. Alternatively, this deformity may result from aberrant development at a later stage. An empty ovoid space typically longer in its horizontal dimension is seen radiographically. Although the size of the cyst may vary, it averages 7 mm vertically and 10 mm horizontally. It is quite easy to misdiagnose a dysplastic lateral SCC as a common cavity deformity. The key to differentiating between the two is that a common-cavity cochlea lies predominantly anterior to the IAC on axial plane CT, and a dysplastic vestibular system lies posterior to it. Histologically, an ovoid or spherical smooth-walled cystic cavity containing a primordia of the membranous labyrinth has been described.[49,83,112] Sensory and supporting cells may be differentiated into recognizable organs of Corti that are scattered peripherally around the walls of the cyst. Neural population is usually sparse or absent. Hearing is usually, but not invariably, poor.

Labyrinthine anomalies (Fig. 27-10)

Semicircular canal dysplasia

Dysplasia of the lateral SCC is a common type of inner ear malformation. Approximately 40% of ears with a malformed cochlea will have an accompanying dysplasia of the lateral SCC.[42] Occasionally, dysplasia of the lateral SCC exists as the sole inner ear malformation. During the sixth week of development the budding SCC forms a semicircular evagination from the vestibular anlage. The central portion of the pocket-shaped protrusion adheres, leaving a peripheral semicircular tube. When this central adhesion fails to occur, SCC dysplasia results (see Figs. 27-2 and 27-11. SCC dysplasia occasionally takes the form of a small bud rather than the more common half-disk shape, presumably due to a slightly earlier timing of the developmental insult. The lateral SCC is deformed more often than the posterior or superior SCC, apparently because it forms earlier in embryogenesis. The typical radiographic appearance of SCC dysplasia is that of a short, broad cystic space confluent with the vestibule (Fig. 27-12).

There are numerous histologic descriptions of SCC dysplasia in the literature.[48,69,83,107,112] The half-disk–shaped cavity may contain a rudimentary crista ampullaris. The utricle and saccule may be distended, collapsed, or entirely absent. Caloric responses in SCC dysplasia are functionally absent or reduced in most cases, but a few may have normal responsiveness.[42] Ears with malformations limited to the vestibular system often have normal or near-normal hearing. Although conclusive data are lacking, SCC dysplasia appears to have an association with conductive hearing loss due to congenital stapes fixation.

Semicircular canal aplasia

SCC aplasia is only one fourth as common as SCC dysplasia.[42] It is usually associated with cochlear anomalies.[23] Presumably, SCC aplasia arises from a failure in the development of the vestibular anlage before the sixth week of gestation.

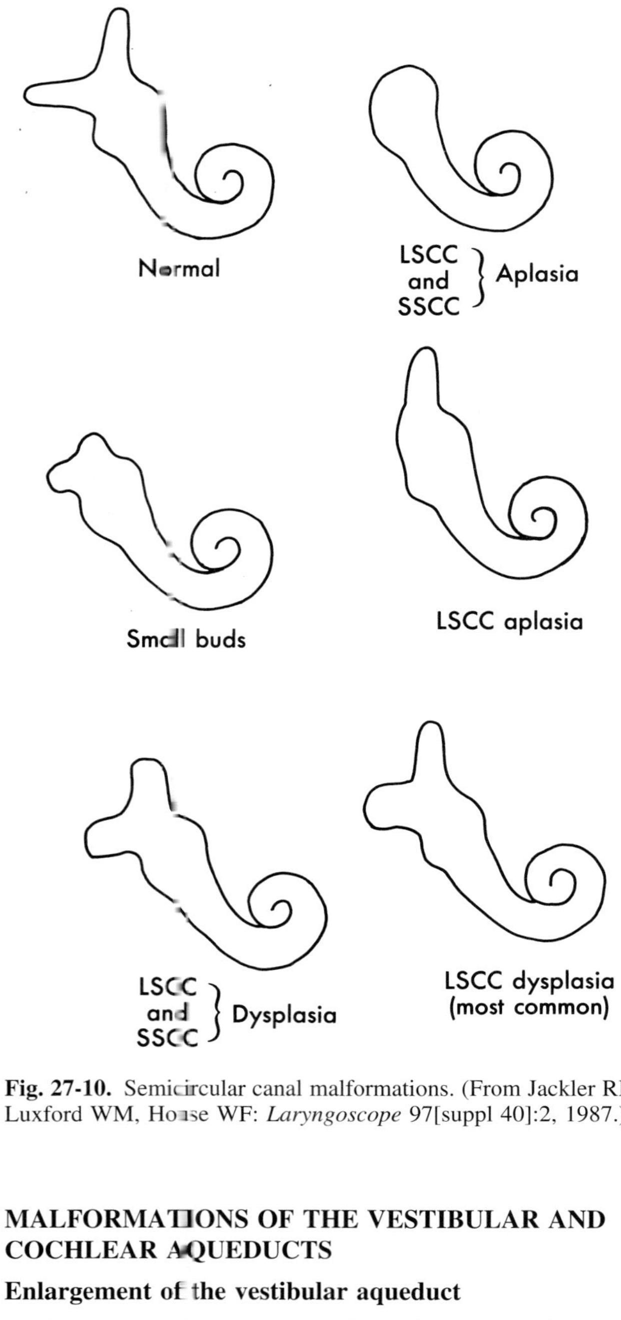

Fig. 27-10. Semicircular canal malformations. (From Jackler RK, Luxford WM, House WF: *Laryngoscope* 97[suppl 40]:2, 1987.)

MALFORMATIONS OF THE VESTIBULAR AND COCHLEAR AQUEDUCTS

Enlargement of the vestibular aqueduct

Recent experience suggests that enlargement of the VA is the most common radiographically detectable malformation of the inner ear.* In earlier literature its incidence was underestimated, partially because of a lack of awareness but mostly because it could only be visualized by lateral polytomography at a time when most studies were confined to the anteroposterior plane. The advent of high-resolution CT in the axial plane has made assessment of the VA much easier. The diameter of a normal VA, when measured halfway between the common crus and its external aperture, is between 0.4 and 1.0 mm. Enlargement of the VA is diagnosed when its diameter exceeds 2.0 mm, although enlarged VA's may exceed 6 mm in width. Whereas the VA is well visualized on axial CT (Fig. 27-13), the dilated endolymphatic sac is better seen with T2-weighted magnetic resonance imaging (MRI) (Fig. 27-14).[32,35] The sac is often seen to be enormously enlarged on MRI, sometimes measuring 2 cm or more in diameter.[105] In many cases, VA enlargement accompanies malformation of the cochlea and/or SCC. It also may be the sole radiographically detectable abnormality of the inner ear in a child with hearing loss. This condition is commonly referred to as the *large VA syndrome*, after Valvassori's and Clemis' first descriptions.[131,131a]

The VA derives from a diverticulum formed in the wall of the otocyst during the fifth week of gestation. It begins as a short, broad pouch but gradually elongates and thins until it achieves its characteristic "J" shape of adulthood (see Fig. 27-2). A premature arrest in development would be expected to produce a VA that is abnormally short and broad. However, an increasing body of evidence suggests that VA enlargement does not stem from an early arrest of sac development, but rather is an acquired deformity. Histologically, the sac and aqueduct are thin-walled and lack both vascularity and the rugose features thought to be important for physiologic function. Three observations suggest that a large VA stems from an abnormal communication between the subarachnoid space and the fluid chambers of the inner ear. The bone surrounding the VA may show signs of erosion, a finding that is inconsistent with a stable congenital deformity.[30] The existence of cerebrospinal fluid (CSF) pressure ("gusher") within the inner ear has been observed in ears with large VA during both cochlear implantation and stapedectomy.[116,119] Furthermore, the existence of abnormal CSF in the inner ear pathway has frequently been observed with CT or MRI; this typically consists of a defect of the cochlear modiolus at the distal end of the IAC.[35] For CSF to become confluent with the endolymphatic space, the CSF fistula (subarachnoid space to perilymph compartment) must be accompanied by a second fistula joining the endolymph and perilymph spaces.

The large VA syndrome is typically bilateral. Children are usually born with normal or mildly impaired hearing that gradually deteriorates through childhood into adolescence and early adulthood. Hearing levels are variable, although at least 40% eventually develop profound SNHL. As with other inner ear malformations, there is a tendency to suffer sudden decrements of hearing, particularly following head trauma. Conductive hearing loss due to stapes fixation may be present. Stapes surgery is best avoided because of the risk of CSF otorrhea.[116] Vestibular complaints in these patients have frequently been reported.[109] Large VA syndrome has recently been observed to occur in a familial clusters.[29]

Surgical manipulation of the endolymphatic sac has been attempted in patients with large VAs. In a sizable series of shunt procedures, there was a high incidence of postopera-

* Refs. 5, 39, 56, 60, 77, 131, 139.

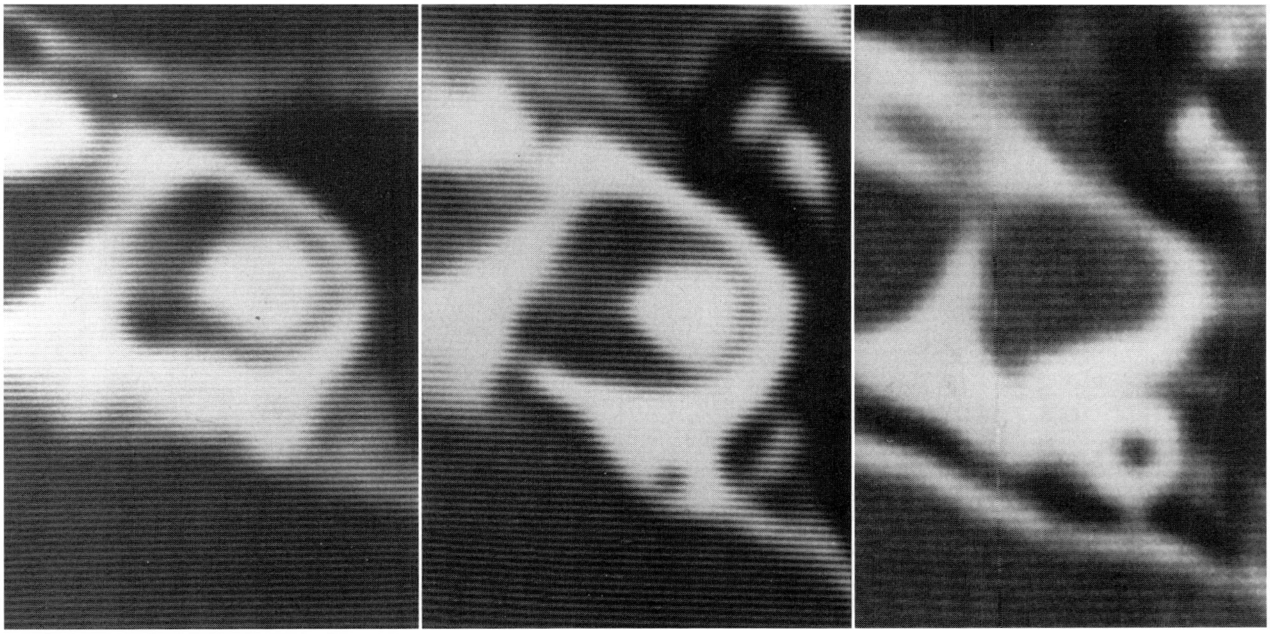

Fig. 27-11. A, Lateral semicircular canal dysplasia as seen on axial computed tomography. The normal appearance should be contrasted with **B,** mild, and **C,** severe dysplasia. These images illustrate how semicircular canal dysplasia may arise from a failure of adhesion of the central region of the vestibular evagination during development. (From Jackler RK, Luxford WM, House WF: *Laryngoscope* 97[suppl 40]:2, 1987.)

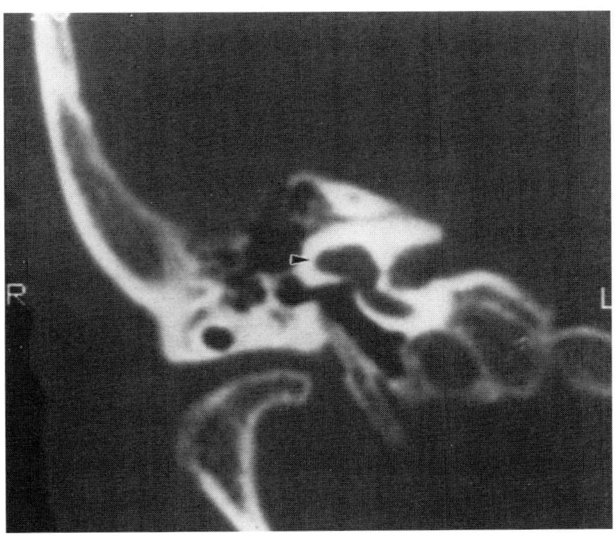

Fig. 27-12. Lateral semicircular canal dysplasia (*arrow*) as seen on coronal computed tomography. Note that the canal appears short, broad, and confluent with the vestibule.

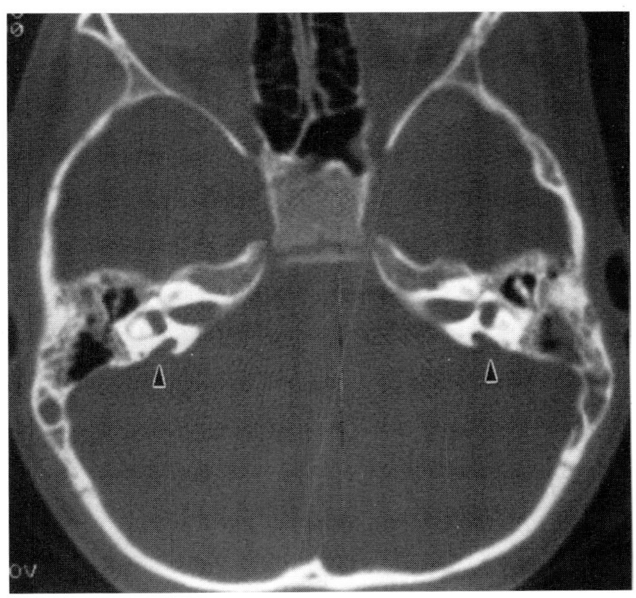

Fig. 27-13. Bilateral enlargement of the vestibular aqueducts *(arrows)* as seen on axial computed tomography.

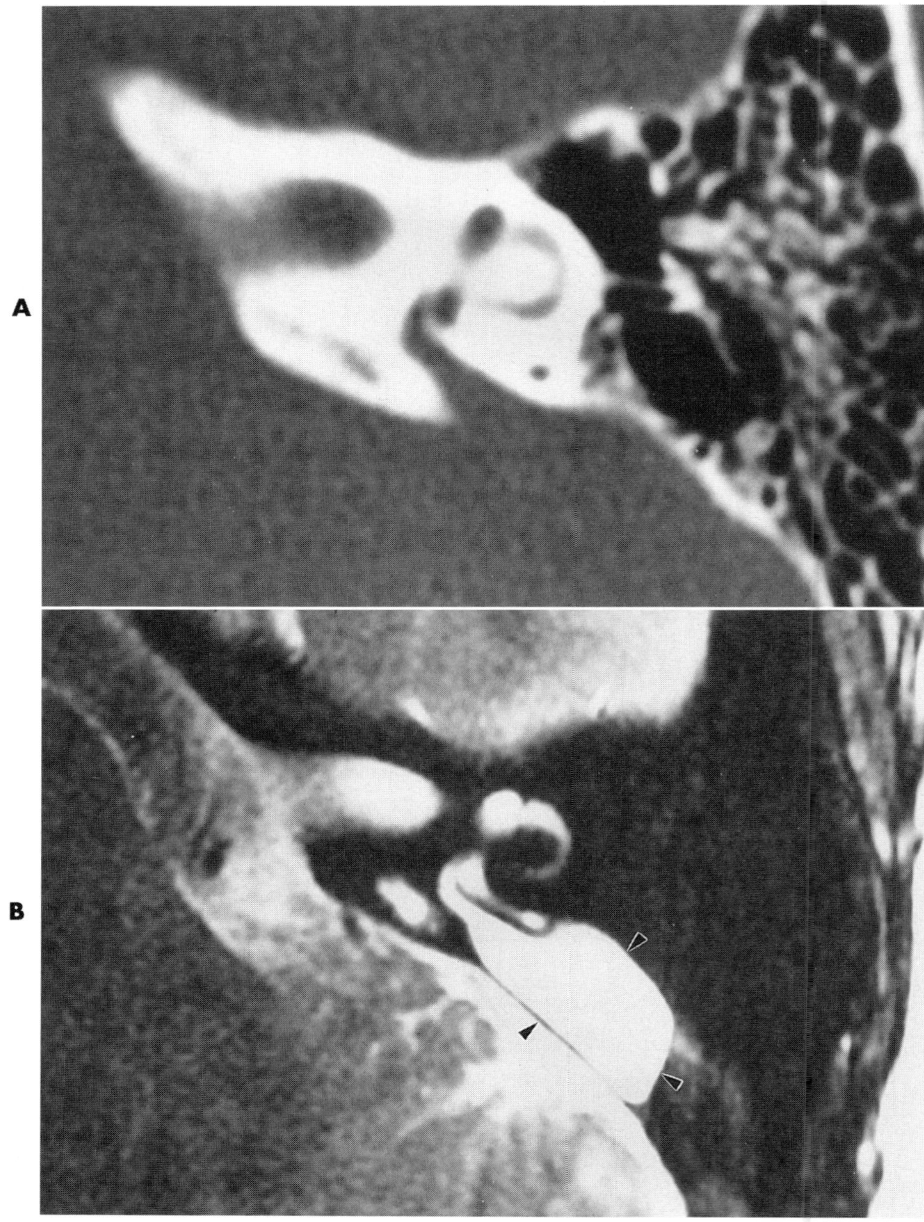

Fig. 27-14. A comparison between **A**, axial computed tomography and **B**, magnetic resonance imaging (MRI) (T2-weighted image, fast-spin echo) of a large vestibular aqueduct deformity. Note that only the MRI delineates the extent of the enormously enlarged endolymphatic sac *(arrows)*. (Courtesy of Joel Swartz, MD.)

tive hearing loss.[39] Furthermore, a comparison of the operated and contralateral unoperated ears revealed no evidence of hearing stabilization following surgery. Recently, surgical obliteration of the enlarged endolymphatic sac with muscle and fascia has been attempted in a small group of patients,[137] although it is too early to assess the result of these efforts.

Enlargement of the cochlear aqueduct

Enlargement of the cochlear aqueduct (CA) is frequently mentioned in the otologic literature because of its purported association with stapedectomy gusher and transotic CSF leak. Despite an active interest in the field and an extensive review of published radiographic images, the author has never seen a radiograph that convincingly demonstrated CA enlargement.[41] Most cases presented as enlargement of the CA are misinterpretations of the wide internal funnel that opens into the posterior fossa.[73,89] In healthy subjects, the radiographic diameter of this aperture averages 3 to 4 mm but ranges from radiographically invisible to over 10 mm (Figs. 27-15 and 27-16).[12,48,71,103] For enlargement of the CA to be diagnosed radiographically, the intraosseous portion coursing toward the vestibule must be enlarged beyond 1 mm, the practical resolution limit of contemporary CT scanners. If analogous criteria to enlargement of the VA are used, then an enlarged CA must have a diameter exceeding 2 mm throughout its course between the inner ear and posterior fossa.

The preponderance of evidence suggests that the human CA is functionally patent in most persons.[81,103] However, in most individuals it can neither transmit sudden large pressure changes to the inner ear nor allow free flow of spinal fluid in any significant quantity (e.g., when there is outflow of perilymphatic fluid from perilymphatic fistula or an open vestibule). This reflects two anatomic features of the aqueduct: a narrow diameter of the bony channel and the presence of a fibrous tissue meshwork occupying and baffling the lumen. Recently, Schuknecht and Reisser[114] evaluated over 1400 temporal bones in the Massachusetts Eye and Ear Infirmary collection and found no CA that exceeded 0.2 mm at its narrowest point. This series included 29 congenitally malformed inner ears. Notably, the CA was absent or nonpatent in 21 of these dysmorphic ears.

In some individuals there is less than normal or no fibrous tissue within the lumen and the bony diameter is wider than normal. An opportunity could then exist for free flow of CSF from the oval window via the CA. According to Poiseuille's law, fluid flow through a tube varies with the fourth power of the radius, suggesting the possibility of free flow in an individual with a large-diameter unimpeded channel, as discussed by Allen.[2] Several histologic studies of congenital inner ear malformations have detected slightly large CAs, particularly at their lateral orifice at the vestibule.[107,117] Even in these malformed inner ears, however, the aqueduct diameter remained well in the sub-millimeter range. From a clinical standpoint, a CA less than 1 mm in diameter is undetecta-

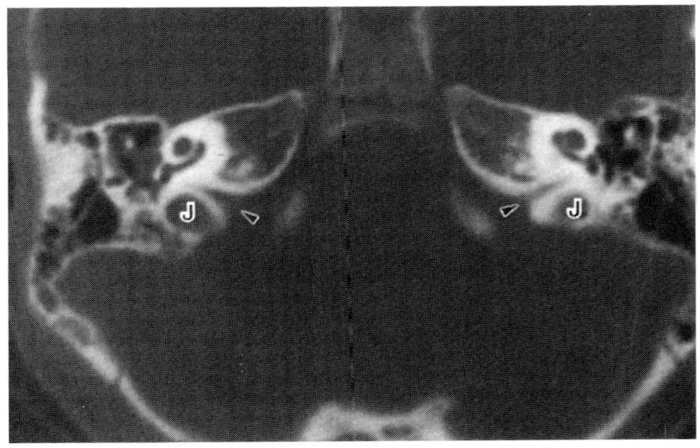

Fig. 27-15. Axial computed tomography demonstrating a normal cochlear aqueduct bilaterally *(arrows)*. The external aperture typically lies inferior to the internal auditory canal and just above the jugular bulb *(J)*.

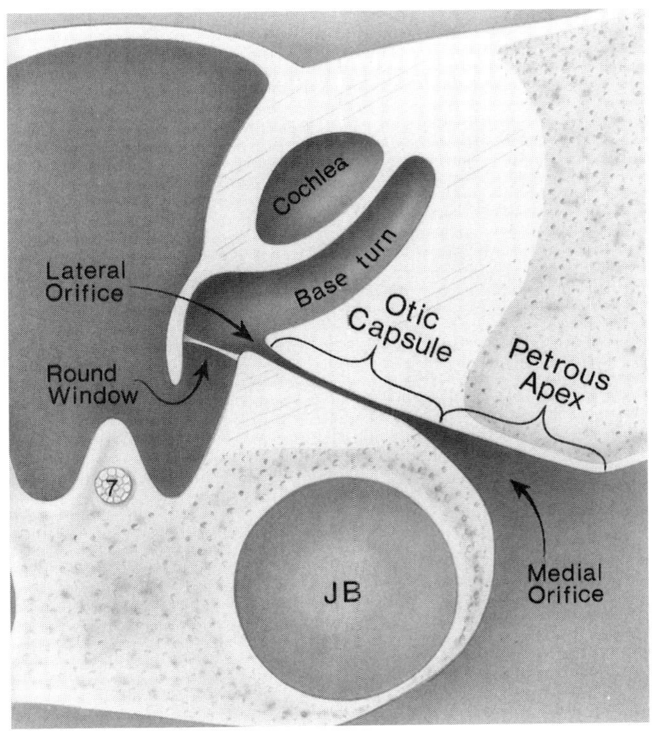

Fig. 27-16. Illustration of the cochlear aqueduct in the axial plane. The diameter of the medial orifice is highly variable but is often wide (as depicted here) in normal-hearing individuals. By contrast, the otic capsule portion is typically very narrow in both healthy and congenitally deaf individuals. (From Jackler RK, Hwang PH: Enlargement of the cochlear aqueduct: fact or fiction? *Otolaryngol Head Neck Surg* 109:14, 1993.)

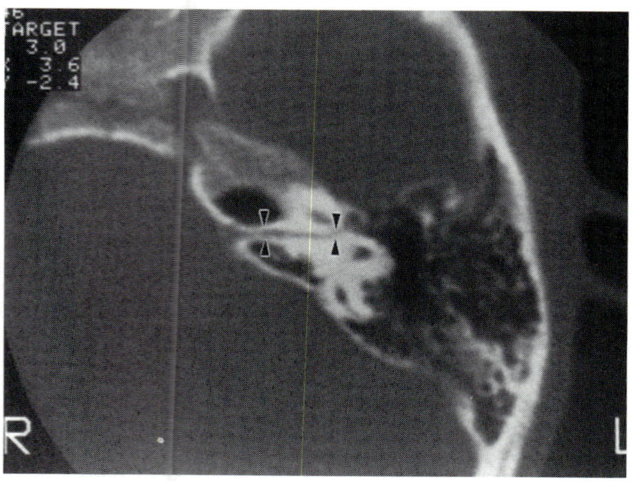

Fig. 27-17. A pathologically narrow internal auditory canal (IAC) as seen on axial computed tomography *(arrows)*. When the IAC is less than 3 mm in diameter, incomplete auditory nerve development is probable.

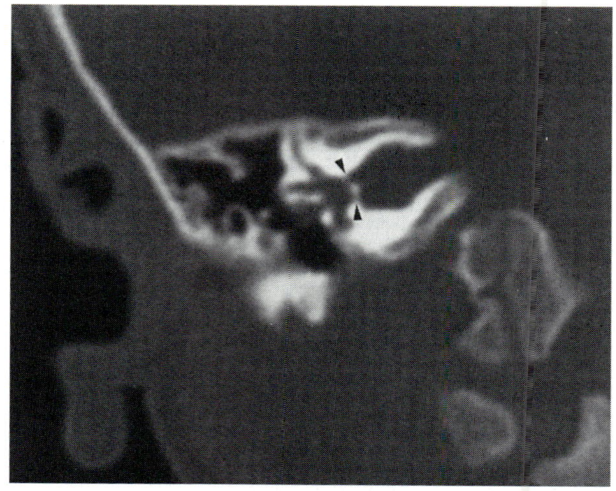

Fig. 27-18. Axial computed tomography of a bulbous internal auditory canal (IAC). Note the minimal separation between the lateral end of the IAC from the vestibule *(arrows)*. Such an ear may be prone to spontaneous cerebrospinal fluid leakage and to gusher during stapes surgery.

ble radiographically. Despite the theoretic possibility that a widely patent CA may cause a stapedectomy gusher, abnormal connections between the IAC and the vestibule appear to be etiologic in the majority of cases.[14,22,26,89]

DEVELOPMENTAL ANOMALIES OF THE INTERNAL AUDITORY CANAL

Narrow internal auditory canal

A narrow IAC may indicate a failure of eighth nerve development. When a patient has normal facial function and an IAC less than 3 mm in diameter, it is likely that the bony canal transmits only the facial nerve (Fig. 27-17). A narrow IAC may accompany inner ear malformations or may be the sole radiographically detectable anomaly in a deaf child. A narrow IAC has been considered a relative contraindication to cochlear implantation.[113,115] Experience with electric stimulation in several patients has shown that they develop facial pain and twitching without useful auditory sensation.

Wide internal auditory canal

Unlike congenital narrowness of the IAC, a congenitally large canal may be an incidental finding in healthy individuals (Fig. 27-18). When a large IAC (>10 mm in diameter) accompanies a malformation of the inner ear, it does not, as an independent variable, correlate with the level of hearing. The importance of detecting enlargement of the IAC is its association with spontaneous CSF leak and gusher during stapes surgery.[22] Because hearing after stapedectomy complicated by perilymphatic (CSF) gusher is frequently poor, a CT scan should be obtained before undertaking stapedectomy for congenital fixation. Dilation of the IAC, especially when the partition between the lateral end of the canal and inner ear appears deficient, should contraindicate stapedectomy.

CEREBROSPINAL FLUID LEAKAGE AND MENINGITIS

Congenitally malformed inner ears may be a source of CSF otorhinorrhea.[87,100] For CSF leakage to occur, two abnormal connections must be present: one between the subarachnoid space and the inner ear and a second between the inner ear and middle ear. The most common pathologic interconnection between the subarachnoid space and the inner ear is through the fundus of the IAC. Histologically, large defects in the modiolar end of the IAC have been shown to exist in 10% of dysplastic ears.[114] Leakage may occur less often around the facial nerve at the lateral end of the IAC.[6,25] The junction between the IAC and the inner ear may be evaluated with CT (Figs. 27-19 and 27-20). A well-defined bony plate normally partitions the distal IAC from the labyrinthine lumen. In a number of well-documented cases of CSF leakage, radiopaque contrast placed into the cerebellopontine angle cistern could be traced through the IAC into the inner ear.[6,13,50,87,106] The propensity of a dysplastic inner to leak CSF depends on its morphologic type. The common cavity deformity appears to be at particularly high risk. By contrast, Phelps and others[92,96] maintain that the incomplete partition deformity (Mondini's dysplasia) is not associated with a heightened risk of CSF leakage. In ears with CSF fistulae the SCCs are usually severely deformed. Although enlargement of the VA is a sign that CSF pressure is present within the inner ear, it does not necessarily imply the existence of an external leak into the middle ear. Rarely,

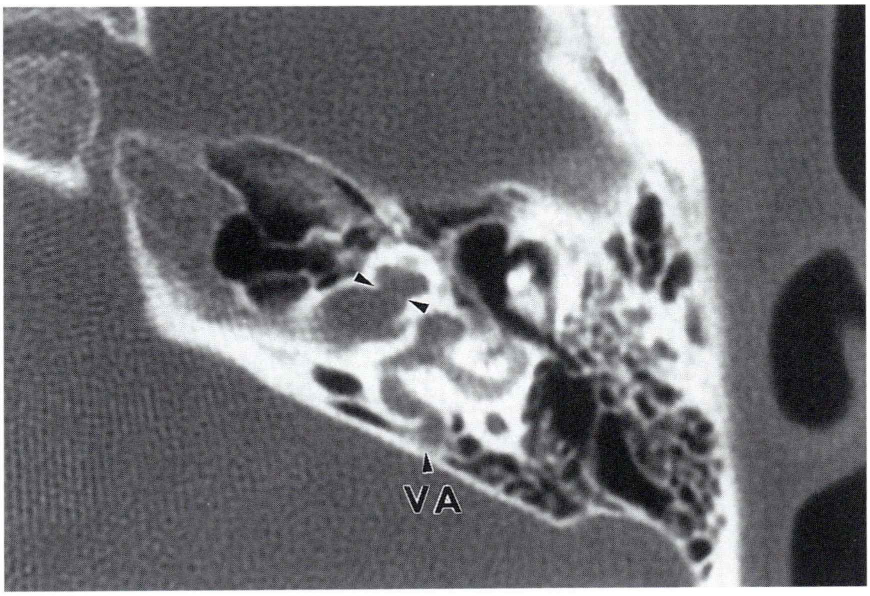

Fig. 27-19. Axial computed tomography of an abnormal interconnection between the lateral end of the internal auditory canal and the cochlea. Note the absence of the modiolus *(arrows)* and the large vestibular aqueduct (*VA*).

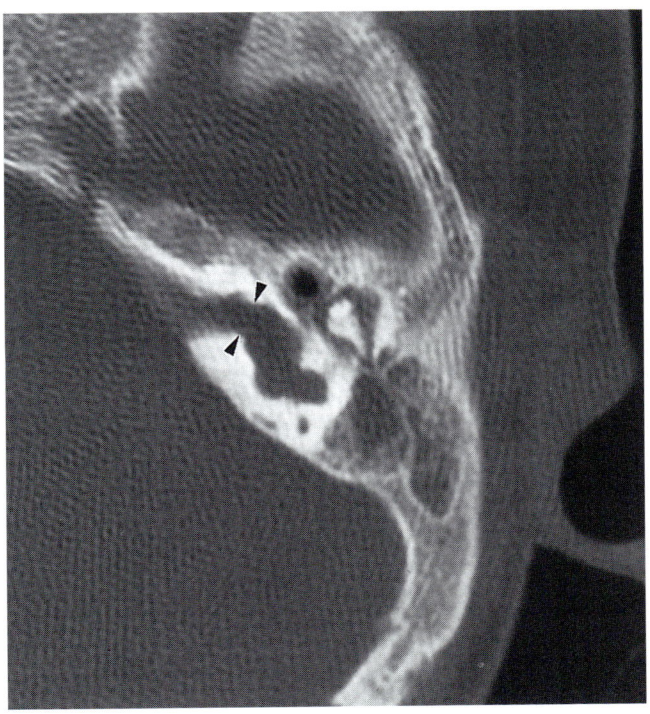

Fig. 27-20. Axial computed tomography of an abnormal interconnection between the lateral end of the internal auditory canal (IAC) and a dysplastic vestibular system. Note the junction between the IAC and the dilated vestibule *(arrows)*.

transotic CSF leakage may be accompanied by a second congenital fistula in the anterior skull base.[15]

A second potential pathway between the subarachnoid space and the inner ear is the CA. As discussed previously there is little evidence to suggest that this pathway is a source of vigorous CSF leakage. In one published report, a CT metrizamide cisternogram is said to have demonstrated a large CSF leak via the CA; however, the published image showed the defect to be far anterior and superior to the region of the CA.[87] A direct route between the subarachnoid space and middle ear, bypassing the inner ear, may exist in rare cases. Hyrtl's fissure, a congenital cleft that runs between the hypotympanum and posterior cranial fossa, passing in proximity to the jugular bulb has been reported to be a source of CSF leakage.[25]

The pathologic interconnection between the inner ear and middle ear most frequently is at the oval window. Numerous reports have described defects in the central portion of the footplate with a protruding membrane, most probably arachnoid (Fig. 27-21).* In other cases the defect is adjacent to the footplate, particularly just anterior to it. Much less frequently, leakage may occur via the round window or a fissure on the promontory.[100] Schuknecht and Reisser[114] evaluated the oval and round windows in 29 ears with congenital malformations of the inner ear. On histologic examination, the stapes were absent in 4, fixed in 6, and normal in 15 cases. In 4 cases the footplates were noted to have defects that were bridged by thin membranes only. The round windows were normal in 28 cases and abnormal in only 1 (bony closure). No deficiencies in the round-window membranes were noted.

* Refs. 6, 34, 58, 59, 76, 86, 100.

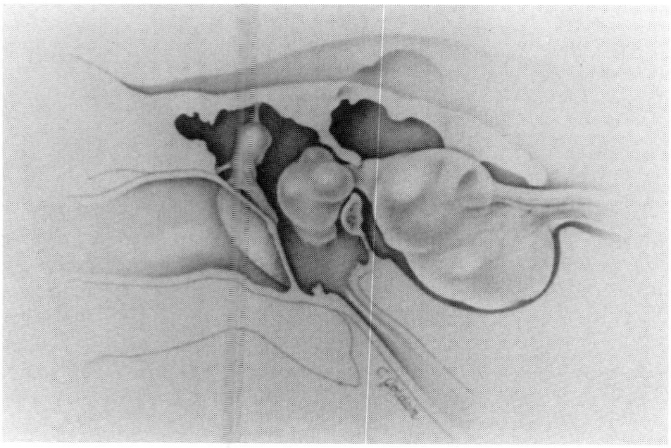

Fig. 27-21. Illustration of a dural hernia protruding through the oval window in a child with cochlear hypoplasia, chronic cerebrospinal fluid leakage, and recurrent meningitis. (From Herther C, Schindler RA: *Laryngoscope* 95:655, 1985.)

The primary clinical importance of CSF leakage is the risk of meningitis. There have been numerous reports of meningitis complicating congenital malformation of the inner ear.* Recurrent bouts of meningitis are typical and recognition of the inner ear as the source frequently comes only after several episodes have occurred. Acute otitis media appears to be the bacterial source in most cases. All children with recurrent meningitis without an obvious cause should undergo CT of the inner ear to exclude inner ear malformation. Even children with a single episode of meningitis should have a postrecovery audiogram followed by CT if unilateral or bilateral SNHL is discovered. The causative organisms in a review of 24 reported cases have been *Streptococcus pneumoniae* (71%), *Haemophilus influenzae* (33%), and β-hemolytic streptococcus (8%). The totals exceed 100% due to the incidence of polymicrobial infection.

Surgical closure of transotic CSF leakage may be attempted at four anatomic levels: (1) the posterior cranial fossa, (2) the dysplastic inner ear, (3) the middle-ear windows, and (4) the eustachian tube. In an ear with residual hearing, tympanotomy and overlay grafting of the site of leakage with a connective tissue graft is indicated as a first attempt. Unfortunately, recurrent leakage is common. When this technique fails and a useful amount of hearing persists, posterior fossa craniotomy with placement of a muscle plug in the IAC or connective tissue graft over the fistulous tract may prove successful and spare hearing.[87] When the hearing is poor, a direct approach to the dysplastic inner ear is indicated. After tympanotomy and removal of the footplate, an oversized piece of muscle may be used to obliterate the vestibule.[24,100,112,125] If the anatomy is unfavorable for this maneuver, a postauricular translabyrinthine approach to the IAC should prove effective. Farrior and Endicott[20] proposed a hypotympanic approach to ablation of the CA. However, this aqueduct has never been convincingly demonstrated to cause a high-volume CSF leak. The final option, closure of the eustachian tube, is not a good choice for children. Following this procedure the anomalous CSF pathway is still open to the middle ear—a disadvantageous situation at an age when acute otitis media is common. Subsequent to the repair of any CSF leakage, the patient is placed on bed rest with the head elevated 30% for several days. Acetazolamide (Diamox) is administered to reduce CSF production and fluids are restricted. Placement of a lumbar drain is a useful adjunctive measure, although it may be difficult to insert and maintain in young children.[12]

* Refs. 6, 34, 59, 76, 86, 87, 100.

X-linked stapes gusher syndrome

A form of hereditary mixed conductive and sensory hearing loss associated with CSF gusher during stapes surgery has recently been described.[16] Inheritance follows an X-linked pattern.[98] The characteristic inner ear deformity may be seen radiographically.[97,127] On CT, the cochlear modiolus is deficient and the lateral portion of the IAC is often bulbous (see Fig. 27-19). These observations provide strong evidence that the abnormal interconnection between the subarachnoid space and the inner ear is via the lateral terminus of the IAC. The labyrinthine segment of the fallopian canal may be dilated. In the vestibular system, the posterior semicircular canal is often deformed and the VA may be enlarged.

The occurrence of stapes fixation in X-linked gusher syndrome is questionable. It has been proposed that the observed air–bone gap may be accounted for by alteration in cochlear micromechanics rather than dysfunction of the conducting system.[121] Results of acoustic reflex testing and auditory evoked responses are more consistent with a pure sensory hearing loss than a mixed form. The outcome of stapes surgery in these patients is usually poor, with anacusis in the operated ear a frequent result. When contemplating surgery for a congenital conductive hearing loss, preoperative imaging is advisable to screen for inner ear malformation.

PERILYMPHATIC FISTULA

In contrast to CSF leakage, a perilymphatic fistula requires only one abnormal pathway: an interconnection of the inner ear with the tympanic cavity. In all probability, perilymph fistula and CSF leak are part of a spectrum of related disturbances of inner ear fluid homeostasis. Although separation of the two topics may be artificial pathophysiologically, it can be justified by the different clinical settings of the two problems. With CSF leakage, the cardinal clinical issues are gross fluid leakage and recurrent meningitis, whereas with perilymph fistulization, sudden or progressive hearing loss and vertigo are the primary manifestations.

Much controversy surrounds the diagnosis and management of perilymphatic fistula in children. The candidate group for exploratory tympanotomy is children with progressive or sudden SNHL. CT of the inner ear may demonstrate

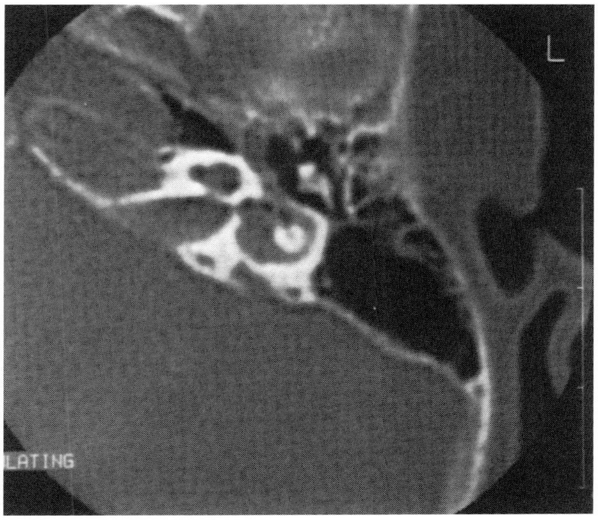

Fig. 27-22. Air bubbles in the inner ear (pneumolabyrinth) in a congenitally deaf child with a perilymphatic fistula.

pneumolabyrinth, although this is rare (Fig. 27-22). Conservative surgeons have advocated exploring only children with radiographically abnormal inner ears who have a clear antecedent event of head trauma or barometric pressure change.[84] Others have espoused the notion of exploring all children with unexplained SNHL.[88,104,126] There is great variability in the number of fistulas ''confirmed'' at surgery. Pappas, Simpson, and Goodwin[84] found only 4 fistulas in 36 ears (11%) explored for progressive SNHL during childhood. It is important to note that 50% of these ears had radiographically malformed inner ears. By contrast, Parnes and McCabe[88] found fistulas in 20 of 26 children's ears (77%), only 6 of whom had inner ear anomalies radiographically. A high incidence of fistulae among children with sensory hearing loss (64%), both with and without inner ear malformation, has been reported.[135,136] Furthermore, this group claims to have objective verification of the presence of perilymph in the middle ear through evaluation of β_2-transferrin levels in surgical aspirates.[134] It should be noted that there is considerable doubt as to whether this test is valid. A recent study in which perilymph samples were directly obtained during either stapedectomy or cochlear implant surgery failed to detect β_2-transferrin in this fluid.[55]

When performing a perilymph fistula exploration it is important to perform provocative maneuvers to render subtle perilymph flows more visible. These include performance of Valsalva's maneuver, using the Trendelenburg position, and compression of the jugular veins. Depending on one's point of view, many surgeons are missing either subtle or intermittent perilymphatic fistulas during explorations or overdiagnosing them by misinterpreting middle-ear secretions or local anesthetic as perilymph. Most surgeons patch both oval and round windows with connective tissue whether or not a perilymphatic fistula was identified during exploration.

Rather than dwell on the controversy about how many fistulas are found, the critical observer should judge the effectiveness of the therapeutic intervention by analyzing its outcome relative to the natural history of the disease. In this regard, results of perilymphatic fistula exploration in children have been disappointing. In one series of 36 patients, hearing was better in 3, unchanged in 21, and worse in 12.[84] Similar results have been obtained in other childhood perilymphatic fistula series. It would be difficult to argue that these data represent a significant improvement over the natural history of the inner ear disease. Congenital progressive SNHL is often characterized by long periods of stability interspersed with periods of rapid deterioration. Even a relative improvement in hearing may occur after an episode of sudden loss. It is apparent that most children with sudden or progressive SNHL have suffered from cochlear diseases other than perilymphatic fistula. Examples include hereditary progressive loss, viral labyrinthitis (e.g., measles, mumps, cytomegalovirus), autoimmune inner ear disease (e.g., Cogan's syndrome), and endolymphatic hydrops. Even in the situation of highest suspicion—sudden loss triggered by head trauma in a child with radiographically malformed inner ears—only a minority of patients demonstrate oval- or round-window fistulization. Many of these children probably lose hearing as a result of internal fistulization between the endolymphatic and perilymphatic space due to deficiencies of the osseous spiral lamina rather than due to external fistulization to the middle ear. A minority of children with sudden or progressive SNHL have prominent vestibular symptoms. Results of perilymphatic fistula repair in the relief of vertigo have been quite good, although spontaneous recovery from vestibulopathy is common in this age group.

INNER EAR MALFORMATIONS IN CONGENITAL AURAL ATRESIA

Development of the external and middle ears is embryologically distinct from that of the inner ear. Anomalies of the lateral portion of the temporal bone typically result from derangement of the first or second branchial arches. Despite their embryologic separateness, congenital aural atresia may coexist with malformation of the inner ear.[45] In one study of atresia patients, 12% (8 of 66) had a radiographically detectable inner ear abnormality.[74] In this group, SCC abnormalities were most common, including some ears with normal bone-conduction hearing. Cochlear anomalies were present in 5% (3 of 66) of these patients, all of whom had poor bone-conduction hearing. It is an embryologic enigma that one patient with unilateral atresia had a malformed inner ear only on the contralateral side. In another polytomographic study of atretic ears, 8% (4 of 48) had SCC anomalies, and 2% (1 of 48) had a deformed cochlea.[99] Based on a comprehensive review of the relevant literature, about 5% of atresia patients have cochlear deformities, whereas about 10% have malformed SCCs. As a general rule, it is not advisable to undertake surgical reconstruction of atretic ears when they are associated with malformation of the inner ear. The deformed cochlea is more vulnerable to injury from vibratory trauma, and there is an increased risk of inducing a sensory hearing loss. This surgery also carries with it a heightened risk of CSF leakage.

IMAGING

For the past two decades, CT has been the gold standard for imaging in patients suspected of having an inner ear malformation. In recent years, new MRI techniques have been developed that are capable of producing images superior to those obtained with CT. In contrast to CT, which depicts otic capsule bone, MRI displays inner ear morphology by imaging inner ear fluids. High-resolution, thin-section, T2-weighted sequences (e.g., fast-spin echo) provide exquisite detail of inner ear anatomy (see Fig. 27-4).[91] MRI is superior to CT in a number of ways. MRI can distinguish between a cochlea filled with fluid and one occluded by soft tissue. CT is unable to make this distinction—an observation of great importance when assessing scala tympani patency prior to cochlear implantation. MRI provides more information about large VAs than does CT.[32,35,82] It displays not only the dilated osseous canal but also the dimensions of the often impressively expanded endolymphatic sac. Direct visualization of the eighth nerve in the IAC, where it appears as a linear filling defect outlined by CSF, is yet another advantage of MRI. This capability is important in certain severe deformities in which neural agenesis may be found.

There are numerous causes of acute and chronic SNHL in children in addition to inner ear malformation. Whereas either CT or MRI would be normal in the great majority of these, there are a few disorders that can only be visualized by MRI. The obvious category is lesions of the cerebellopontine angle (e.g., tumors) and brainstem (e.g., adrenoleukodystrophy). On noncontrast T1-weighted MRI, acute hemorrhage results in hyperintensity of the inner ear. On gadolinium-enhanced studies, acute inflammation (e.g., viral infection) results in high signal in the inner ear or along the course of the eighth nerve.

When selecting MRI as an imaging study to screen for inner ear malformation it is important for the physician to be aware that standard MRI protocols designed to screen for central nervous system abnormalities provide only limited information concerning the inner ear. To be useful in screening for inner ear anomalies, specially designed protocols are needed.[92,93] One disadvantage of MRI is the difficulty young children have in tolerating the confined spaces of the magnet. In addition, fast-spin echo MRI requires considerably longer scan time than does CT. While simple sedation is usually sufficient for CT, acquiring quality magnetic resonance images may require general anesthesia in pediatric patients. Thus despite the numerous advantages of MRI (including the absence of ionizing radiation), CT is the pediatric examination of choice in many centers for this important practical reason.

EVALUATION AND MANAGEMENT

High-resolution CT or MRI of the inner ears is recommended for all children with suspected congenital malformation of the inner ear, including those with otherwise unexplained SNHL regardless of whether it has existed from birth or occurred later. Scans are usually obtained when hearing impairment is first recognized. To adequately image the minute inner ear structures, we use thin slices of 1- or 1.5-mm thickness with 0.5-mm overlap.[40] If only one plane of view is to be obtained, the axial orientation is preferred because it provides superior images of the VA, a frequently malformed structure that is difficult to visualize on coronal scans. When possible, both axial and coronal views should be obtained because certain subtle deformities, such as deficiency of the interscalar septum, are best seen in the coronal orientation. It is important to examine thoroughly all portions of the inner ear because anomalies are frequently multiple (Fig. 27-23).

No medical or surgical therapy has been shown to prevent the progressive hearing loss associated with congenital malformation of the inner ear. After a sudden decrease in hearing, a short course of oral corticosteroid (e.g., prednisone) is administered. Although no studies have assessed the efficacy of corticosteroids in children with inner ear deformities, studies of idiopathic sudden SNHL in adults suggest some benefit. Furthermore, autoimmune mechanisms may play a role in a few children with rapid hearing deterioration, a possibility that justifies a therapeutic trial. Of course, many patients have a spontaneous partial recovery after sudden losses, even without therapeutic intervention.

Few patients with congenitally malformed inner ears have a fluctuating pattern of hearing loss suggestive of endolymphatic hydrops. When fluctuations are encountered, however, a low-salt diet and diuretics are prescribed. Surgical intervention is indicated in a few well-defined circumstances. Obviously, CSF leakage and meningitis require in-

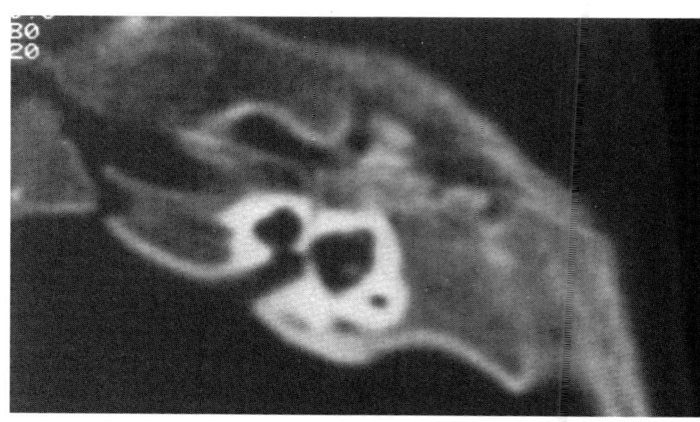

Fig. 27-23. Axial computed tomography demonstrating a cochlear deformity (incomplete partition) as well as dysplasia of the lateral semicircular canal. Many congenitally malformed inner ears have abnormalities of more than one portion of the inner ear.

tervention. Exploration for perilymphatic fistula is reserved for patients with radiographically abnormal inner ears who have suffered a sudden hearing deterioration temporally related to a precipitating event such as head trauma, rapid barometric pressure change, vigorous exercise, or sneezing. As discussed previously, even in these patients only a minority have a fistula, and those who do frequently continue to lose hearing despite repair. House and House[37] and later others advocated endolymphatic sac surgery for congenital malformations of the inner ear;[27,62,64] however, a careful analysis of the outcome in a large series revealed no benefit of this surgery in terms of hearing stabilization.[38] In fact, nearly 30% suffered a significant postoperative hearing deterioration. Patients with large VAs appear to be at particularly high risk for poor outcome after sac surgery. As mentioned earlier, surgical obliteration of the endolymphatic sac with muscle and fascia has been attempted in a small group of patients with enlargement of the VA.[137] It is too early to assess the result of these efforts.

Preventive measures are important in the management of patients with congenitally malformed inner ears. The risk of CSF leakage may be estimated by CT or MRI of the inner ear. Anatomic features of concern include a wide IAC, deficient partitioning between the IAC and inner ear, and enlargement of the vestibule in the horizontal plane. Parents should be made aware of the risk of meningitis and instructed in recognizing its early symptoms and signs. Because most episodes of meningitis associated with inner ear malformation are pneumococcal, use of the pneumococcal vaccine is recommended. Children with malformed inner ears should avoid head trauma and rapid barometric pressure changes because these risk provoking a sudden hearing loss or even CSF leakage. Activities such as contact sports and scuba diving are discouraged. Finally, establishing a prognosis for future auditory function in a hearing-impaired child serves as a guide for educational and rehabilitative efforts. Recognizing an inner ear malformation on CT may be helpful because certain morphologic patterns have more favorable prognoses than others.

COCHLEAR IMPLANTATION

Electric stimulation of the auditory nerve has proven useful in many forms of sensory deafness, including those associated with congenital malformations of the inner ear. The fundamental premise of cochlear implantation is that some of the cochlear neural population survives despite the absence of hair cells. In congenital malformations of the inner ear, the auditory nerve population is typically less than with other forms of sensory deafness. The normal human spiral ganglion cell count is usually 25,000 to 35,000. In eight congenitally dysplastic ears, Schmidt[110] reported cell counts that ranged from 7677 to 16,110, with an average of only 11,478. In contrast, ears profoundly deaf due to ototoxicity, otosclerosis, and sudden loss have ganglion cell populations in the 18,000 to 22,000 range. This observation suggests that malformed inner ears could be electrically stimulated but that improvements in speech discrimination would fall below average for the deaf population at large. A narrow IAC on preimplant CT (<3 mm diameter) is a strongly adverse predictor of neural survival.[115]

Cochlear implantation in deformities that involve both the membranous and osseous labyrinth raises several special considerations. Cochlear implantation in malformations limited to the membranous labyrinth is equivalent to implantation in the prelingually deaf child (see Chapter 149). Results of implantation with short, single-channel devices in patients with cochlear hypoplasia common cavity, and incomplete partition deformities appear in the literature.[43,66] In successful cases, sound detection levels are similar to those in other prelingually deaf children. Implantation of deformed cochleas with multichannel devices has also proven to be valuable in the majority of cases but has a high rate of complications.[36,67,118,119,129] Performance varies widely and appears, on average, to be somewhat below that realized in most other forms of deafness. The design of multichannel electrodes makes certain assumptions about the geometry of the scala tympani that affect the anticipated orientation of stimulating electrodes to neural elements. Although standard electrodes are not optimized for dysplastic cochleas, fabrication of custom electrodes for each malformed cochlea is not feasible with current technology. The degree of electrode insertion varies, in large part according to the size and geometry of the deformed cochlea. Only partial insertion may be realized, particularly in hypoplastic cochleas, whereas complete insertion is more common in milder deformities such as incomplete partition.

One complication of unpredictable electrode positioning is stimulation of the facial nerve at current levels lower than the threshold for auditory perception. Cross-stimulation of the facial nerve has been reported with both single-channel and multichannel designs and has prevented some patients from using the device. Multichannel systems have a distinct advantage in this regard because the offending electrode pair or pairs may be programmed out of the stimulation map, thus preserving the ability to provide auditory stimulation. The presence of a dysplastic inner ear may be a warning that the facial nerve is malpositioned.[101] An anomalous facial nerve course has been reported to occur in 16% of malformed inner ears.[36] In one patient with cochlear hypoplasia an anomalous facial nerve was injured immediately above the round-window niche, a highly vulnerable location during implant surgery.[119] Use of electrophysiologic facial nerve monitoring during implantation of patients with malformed inner ears is advisable. It is also possible for a persistent stapedial artery to traverse the round-window region and preclude implantation.[133]

Another complication of implantation in malformed cochleas is inadvertent penetration of the IAC by the electrode.[129] When such a malpositioned electrode is activated, vigorous facial twitching may occur at an extremely low stimulation threshold. To avoid this misadventure, postimplantation CT is advisable prior to undertaking stimulation to assess electrode position following implantation of a malformed cochlea. CSF leak has also been a frequent complication during implantation of the malformed cochlea, occurring with an incidence of approximately 40%.[36] This is typically evident immediately on opening the round window and presumably arises as a result of deficiencies in the partition between the modiolus and the dural envelope at the lateral end of the IAC. Leaks have been successfully handled by packing connective tissue around the electrode, but they may require temporary CSF diversion to obtain a lasting seal. In one unpublished case, bacterial meningitis occurred several days after a multichannel implantation complicated by CSF leakage.[18] Fortunately, the infection resolved with antibiotics and did not necessitate removal of the device.

REFERENCES

1. Alexander G: Zur pathologie und pathologischen anatomie der kongenitalen taubheit, *Arch Otor Nas Kohlk Heilk* 61:183, 1904.
2. Allen G: Fluid flow in the cochlear aqueduct and cochlea-hydrodynamic considerations in perilymph fistula, stapes gusher, and secondary endolymphatic hydrops, *Am J Otol* 8:319, 1987.
3. Altmann F: Malformations, anomalies, and vestigial structures of the inner ear, *Arch Otolaryngol Head Neck Surg* 57:591, 1953.
4. Anson BJ: The endolymphatic and perilymphatic aqueducts of the human ear: developmental and adult anatomy of their parietes and contents in relation to otological surgery, *Acta Otolaryngol (Stockh)* 59:140, 1965.
5. Arcand P and others: The large vestibular aqueduct syndrome and sensorineural hearing loss in the pediatric population, *J Otolaryngol* 20:247, 1991.
6. Barez DV and others: Subarachnoid space: middle ear pathways and recurrent meningitis, *Am J Otol* 6:157, 1985.
7. Bauman NM and others: Mondini dysplasia and congenital cytomegalovirus infection, *J Pediatr* 124:71, 1994.
8. Beal DD, Davey FR, Lindsay JR: Inner ear pathology of congenital deafness, *Arch Otolaryngol Head Neck Surg* 85:134, 1967.
9. Reference deleted in pages.
10. Bergstrom L: Pathology of congenital deafness: present status and future prospects, *Ann Otol Rhinol Laryngol* 89(suppl 74):31, 1980.
11. Berlin CI and others: Superior ultra-audiometric hearing: a new type of hearing loss which correlates highly with unusually good speech in the "profoundly deaf," *Trans Am Acad Ophthalmol Otolaryngol* 86:111, 1978.
12. Bhimani S, Virapongse C, Sarwar M: High resolution computed tomographic appearance of the normal human cochlear aqueduct, *Am J Neuroradiol* 5:715, 1984.
13. Burton EM and others: CSF fistula in a patient with Mondini deformity: demonstration by CT cisternography, *Am J Neuroradiol* 11:205, 1990.
14. Chan KH and others: Familial sensorineural hearing loss: a correlative study of audiologic, radiographic, and vestibular findings, *Ann Otol Rhinol Laryngol* 100:620, 1991.
15. Claros P and others: Association of spontaneous anterior fossa CSF rhinorrhea and congenital perilymphatic fistula in a patient with recurrent meningitis, *Int J Pediatr Otorhinolaryngol* 27:65, 1993.
16. Cremers C and others: X-linked progressive mixed deafness with perilymphatic gusher during stapes surgery, *Arch Otolaryngol Head Neck Surg* 111:249, 1985.
17. Curtin HD: Congenital malformations of the ear, *Otolaryngol Clin North Am* 21:317, 1988.
18. Daspit P: Personal communication, 1990.
19. Everberg G: Investigations into unilateral total deafness and absence of vestibular function with a particular view to the X-ray appearances in the inner ear, *Acta Otolaryngol Head Neck Surg* 52:47, 1960.
20. Farrior JB, Endicott JN: Congenital mixed deafness: cerebrospinal fluid otorrhea. Ablation of the aqueduct of the cochlea, *Laryngoscope* 81:684, 1971.
21. Feghali JG, Leone CA, Linthicum FH: Residual high frequency hearing in a patient with Mondini's deformity: clinical implications, *Am J Otol* 6:336, 1985.
22. Flood LM, Kernink JL, Karnish JM: Pneumocephalus following treatment of a stapes gusher, *Am J Otol* 6:508, 1985.
23. Friedmann I: *Pathology of the ear*, London, 1974, Blackwell Scientific.
24. Friedmann I, Fraser GR, Frogan P: Pathology of the inner ear in the cardioauditory syndrome of Servell and Lange-Neilsen, *J Laryngol* 80:451, 1966.
25. Gacek RR, Leipzig B: Congenital cerebrospinal otorrhea, *Ann Otol Rhinol Laryngol* 88:358, 1979.
26. Glasscock ME: The stapes gusher, *Arch Otolaryngol Head Neck Surg* 98:82, 1973.
27. Goin DW, Rasband RW, Mischke RE: Endolymphatic sac surgery in Mondini's dysplasia: a report of 16 cases, *Laryngoscope* 94:343, 1984.
28. Gorlin RJ, Toriello HV, Cohen MM: *Hereditary hearing loss and its syndromes*, 1995, Oxford University Press.
29. Griffith AJ and others: Familial large aqueduct syndrome. *Laryngoscope* 106:960, 1996.
30. Gussen R: The endolymphatic sac in Mondini disorder, *Arch Otorhinol Laryngol* 242:71, 1985.
31. Harada T, Takahara T, Ishii S: Three-dimensional reconstruction of the temporal bone from a case of E trisomy syndrome, *Laryngoscope* 103:541, 1993.
32. Harsberger HR and others: Advanced techniques in magnetic resonance imaging in the evaluation of the large endolymphatic duct and sac syndrome, *Laryngoscope* 105:1037, 1995.
33. Hersh JH, Ganzel TM, Fellows RA: Michel's anomaly, type I microtia and microdontia, *Ear Nose Throat J* 70:155, 1991.
34. Herther C, Schindler RA: Mondini's dysplasia with recurrent meningitis, *Laryngoscope* 95:655, 1985.
35. Hirsch BE and others: Magnetic resonance imaging of the large vestibular aqueduct, *Arch Otolaryngol Head Neck Surg* 118:1124, 1992.
36. Hoffman RA and others: Cochlear implantation in pediatric patients with Mondini deformities, *Am J Otol* 1997 (in press).
37. House WF, House JW: *Mondini deformity: surgical treatment.* Paper presented at IVth Pan-Pacific Surgical Association Congress, Honolulu, Hawaii, April, 1978.
38. Jackler RK and others: Endolymphatic sac surgery in congenital malformations of the inner ear, *Laryngoscope* 98:698, 1988.
39. Jackler RK, De La Cruz A: The large vestibular aqueduct syndrome, *Laryngoscope* 99:1238, 1989.
40. Jackler RK, Dillon WP: Computed tomography and magnetic resonance imaging of the inner ear. *Otolaryngol Head Neck Surg* 99:494, 1988.
41. Jackler RK, Hwang PH: Enlargement of the cochlear aqueduct: fact or fiction? *Otolaryngol Head Neck Surg* 109:14, 1993.
42. Jackler RK, Luxford WM, House WF: Congenital malformations of the inner ear: a classification based on embryogenesis, *Laryngoscope* 97(suppl 40):2, 1987.
43. Jackler RK, Luxford WM, House WF: Congenital malformations of the inner ear: sound detection with cochlear implant in five ears of four children with congenital malformations of the cochlea, *Laryngoscope* 97(suppl 40):15, 1987.
44. Jackler RK and others: Endolymphatic sac surgery in congenital malformations of the inner ear, *Laryngoscope* 98:698, 1988.
45. Jahrsdoerfer RA: Congenital atresia of the ear, *Laryngoscope* 88(suppl 13):1, 1978.

46. Jensen J: Malformations of the inner ear in deaf children, *Acta Radiol* (suppl 286):1, 1969.
47. Jonhsen T and others: Pendred's syndrome: acoustic, vestibular, and radiological findings in 17 unrelated patients, *J Laryngol Otol* 101: 1187, 1987.
48. Johnsson L and others: Four variations of the Mondini inner ear malformations as seen in microdissections, *Am J Otolaryngol* 5:242, 1984.
49. Jorgensen MB, Kristensen HK: Thalidomide induced aplasia of the inner ear, *J Laryngol Otol* 78:1095, 1964.
50. Kaufman B, Jordan VM, Pratt LL: Positive contrast demonstration of a cerebrospinal fluid fistula through the fundus of the internal auditory meatus, *Acta Radiol* 9:83, 1969.
51. Kavanagh KT, Magill HL: Michel dysplasia: common cavity inner ear deformity, *Pediatr Radiol* 19:343, 1989.
52. Komune S and others: Bilateral Mondini dysplasia with normal hearing, *J Otorhinolaryngol Relat Spec* 55:143, 1993.
53. Konigsmark BW, Gorlin RJ: *Genetic and metabolic deafness*, Philadelphia, 1976, WB Saunders.
54. Kwee HL: The occurrence of the Tullio phenomenon in congenitally deaf children, *J Laryngol Otol* 90:501, 1976.
55. Levenson MJ, Desloge RB, Parisier SC: Beta-2 transferrin: limitations of use as a clinical marker for perilymph, *Laryngoscope* 106:159, 1996.
56. Levenson MJ and others: The large vestibular aqueduct in children, *Arch Otolaryngol Head Neck Surg* 115:54, 1989.
57. Lindsay JR: Profound childhood deafness: inner ear pathology, *Ann Otol Rhinol Laryngol* 83(suppl 5):1, 1973.
58. Luntz M and others: Large perilymph fistulas, *Am J Otol* 7:282, 1986.
59. MacRae DL, Ruby RR: Recurrent meningitis secondary to perilymph fistula in young children, *J Otolaryngol* 19:222, 1990.
60. Mafee MF and others: Large vestibular aqueduct and congenital sensorineural hearing loss, *Am J Neuroradiol* 13:805, 1992.
61. Mafee MF and others: Congenital sensorineural hearing loss, *Radiology* 150:427, 1984.
62. Mangabeira-Albernaz PL and others: The Mondini dysplasia: a clinical study, *J Otorhinolaryngol Relat Spec* 43:131, 1981.
63. Michel EM: Memoires sur les anomalies congenitales de l'oreille interne, *Gaz Med Strasbourg* 3:55, 1863.
64. Mitchell DP, Rubin AM: Mondini dysplasia: late complications, *J Otolaryngol* 14:265, 1985.
65. Miyamoto RT and others: Cochlear implantation in the Mondini inner ear malformation, *Am J Otol* 7:258, 1986.
66. Mizuno M, Harada T: Labyrinthine anomalies with normal cochlear function, *J Otorhinolaryngol Relat Spec* 54:278, 1992.
67. Molter DW, Pate BR Jr, McElveen JT Jr: Cochlear implantation in the congenitally malformed ear, *Otolaryngol Head Neck Surg* 108: 174, 1993.
67a. Mondini C: The minor works of Carlo Mondini: the anatomical section of a boy born deaf, *Am J Otol* 18:288, 1997.
68. Mondini C: *Anatomia surdi nedi sectio,* De Bononiensi Scientiarum et Artium Instituto Arque Academia Commentarii, Bologna 7:419, 1791.
69. Monsell EM and others: Congenital malformations of the inner ear: histologic findings in five temporal bones, *Laryngoscope* 97(suppl 140):18, 1987.
70. Murata K and others: Quantitative analysis of inner ear anomalies by high resolution CT scanning of the temporal bone, *J Otolaryngol* 16: 133, 1987.
71. Muren C, Wilbrand H: Anatomic variations of the human cochlear aqueduct: a radioanatomic investigation. *Acta Radiol Diagn* 27:11, 1986.
72. Nadol JB, Young YS, Glynn RJ: Survival of spiral ganglion cells in profound sensorineural deafness: its implications for cochlear implantation, *Ann Otol Rhinol Laryngol* 98:411, 1989.
73. Narcy PH and others: Aqueduc Cochleaire et fistules peri-lymphatiques congenitales, *Ann Otol Laryngol (Paris)* 106:57, 1989.
74. Naunton RF, Valvassori GE: Inner ear anomalies: their association with atresia, *Laryngoscope* 78:1041, 1968.
75. Nomura Y, Kawabata I: Scheibe dysgenesis of the inner ear, *J Laryngol Otol* 94:1345, 1980.
76. Ohlms LA and others: Recurrent meningitis and Mondini dysplasia, *Arch Otolaryngol Head Neck Surg* 116:608, 1990.
77. Okumura T and others: Sensorineural hearing loss in patients with large vestibular aqueduct, *Laryngoscope* 105:289, 1995.
78. Olson JE, Dorwart RH, Brant WE: Use of high resolution thin section CT scanning of the petrous bone in temporal bone anomalies, *Laryngoscope* 92:1274, 1982.
79. Ormerod FC: The pathology of congenital deafness, *J Laryngol* 74: 919, 1960.
80. Ostri B, Johnsen T, Bergmann I: Temporal bone findings in a family with branchio-oto-renal syndrome (BOR), *Clin Otolaryngol* 16:163, 1991.
81. Palva T, Dammerr K: Human cochlear aqueduct, *Acta Otolaryngol Suppl (Stockh)* 246:1, 1969.
82. Papadopoulos A and others: Value of Gd-DTPA-enhanced MR imaging of the labyrinth in patients with sudden hearing loss, *Magn Reson Imaging* 13:387, 1995.
83. Paparella MM: Mondini's deafness: a review of histopathology, *Ann Otol Rhinol Laryngol* 89(suppl 67):1, 1980.
84. Pappas DG, Simpson LC, Godwin GH: Perilymphatic fistula in children with pre-existing sensorineural hearing loss, *Laryngoscope* 98: 507, 1988.
85. Pappas DG and others: High-resolution computed tomography: determination of the cause of pediatric sensorineural hearing loss. *Laryngoscope* 100:564, 1990.
86. Parisier SC, Birken EA: Recurrent meningitis secondary to idiopathic oval window CSF leak, *Laryngoscope* 86:1503, 1977.
87. Park TS and others: Spontaneous cerebrospinal fluid otorrhea in association with a congenital defect of the cochlear aqueduct and Mondini dysplasia, *Neurosurgery* 11:356, 1982.
88. Parnes LS, McCabe BF: Perilymph fistula: an important cause of deafness and dizziness in children, *Pediatrics* 80:524, 1987.
89. Phelps PD: Congenital cerebrospinal fluid fistulae of the petrous temporal bone, *Clin Otolaryngol* 11:79, 1986.
90. Phelps PD: Ear dysplasia after Mondini, *J Laryngol Otol* 108:461, 1994.
91. Phelps PD: Fast spin echo MRI in otology, *J Laryngol Otol* 108:383, 1994.
92. Phelps PD: Imaging for congenital deformities of the ear, *Clin Radiol* 49:663, 1994.
93. Phelps PD, King A, Michaels L: Cochlear dysplasia and meningitis, *Am J Otol* 15:551, 1994.
94. Phelps PD: Mondini and "pseudo Mondini," *Clin Otolaryngol* 15: 99, 1990 (editorial).
95. Phelps PD, Lloyd GAS: Radiological investigation of congenital deafness. In *Radiology of the ear*, Oxford, 1983, Blackwell Scientific.
96. Phelps PD and others: Congenital cerebrospinal fluid fistula through the inner ear and meningitis, *J Laryngol Otol* 107:492, 1993.
97. Phelps PD and others: X-linked deafness, stapes gushers and a distinctive defect of the inner ear, *Neuroradiology* 33:326, 1991.
98. Piussan C and others: X-linked progressive mixed deafness: a new microdeletion that involves a more proximal region in Xq21, *Am J Hum Genet* 56:224, 1995.
99. Potter GD: Inner ear abnormalities in association with congenital atresia of the external auditory canal, *Ann Otol Rhinol Laryngol* 78:598, 1969.
100. Quiney RE and others: Recurrent meningitis in children due to inner ear abnormalities, *J Laryngol Otol* 103:473, 1989.
101. Raine CH and others: Anomaly of the facial nerve and cochlear implantation, *Ann Otol Rhinol Laryngol Suppl* 166:430, 1995.
102. Raphael Y, Fein A, Nebel L: Transplacental kanamycin ototoxicity in the guinea pig, *Arch Otorhinolaryngol* 238:45, 1983.

103. Rask-Anderson H, Stahle J, Wilbrand H: Human cochlear aqueduct and its accessory canals, *Ann Otol Rhinol Laryngol* 86(suppl 42):1, 1977.

104. Reilly JS: Congenital perilymphatic fistula: a prospective study in infants and children. *Laryngoscope* 99:393, 1989.

105. Reussner LA, Dutcher PO, House WF: Large vestibular aqueduct syndrome with massive endolymphatic sacs, *Otolaryngol Head Neck Surg* 113:606, 1995.

106. Rockett FX and others: Pantopaque visualization of a congenital dural defect of the internal auditory meatus causing rhinorrhea, *Am J Roentgenol* 91:640, 1964.

107. Sando I, Takahara T, Owaga A: Congenital anomalies of the inner ear, *Ann Otol Rhinol Laryngol* 93(suppl 112):110, 1984.

108. Scheibe A: Ein fall von trubstummheit mit acusticus-atrophie und gildung sangomalien im hautigen labyrinth beiderseits, *Z Ohrenh* 22: 11, 1892.

109. Schessel DA, Nedzelski JM: Presentation of large vestibular aqueduct syndrome to a dizziness unit, *J Otolaryngol* 21:265, 1992.

110. Schmidt JM: Cochlear neuronal populations in development defects of the inner ear: implications for cochlear implantation, *Acta Otolaryngol (Stockh)* 99:14, 1985.

111. Schuknecht HF: *Pathology of the ear.* Cambridge, 1974, Harvard University Press.

112. Schuknecht HF: Mondini dysplasia: a clinical and pathological study, *Ann Otol Rhinol Laryngol* 89(suppl 65):1, 1980.

113. Schuknecht HF: Dysmorphogenesis of the inner ear. *Birth Defects* 16:47, 1980.

114. Schuknecht HF, Reisser C: The morphologic basis for perilymphatic gushers and oozers. *Adv Otorhinolaryngol* 39:1, 1988.

115. Shelton C and others: The narrow internal auditory canal in children: a contraindication to cochlear implants, *Otolaryngol Head Neck Surg* 100:227, 231, 1989.

116. Shirazi A, Fenton JE, Fagan PA: Large vestibular aqueduct syndrome and stapes fixation, *J Laryngol Otol* 108:989, 1994.

117. Siebenmann F, Bing R: Uber den labyrinth and Hirnbefund bei einem an Retinitis pigmentosa erblindeten angeboren taubstummen, *Z Ohrenheilk* 54:265, 1907.

118. Silverstein H, Smouha E, Morgan N: Multichannel cochlear implantation in a patient with bilateral Mondini deformities, *Am J Otol* 9:451, 1988.

119. Slattery WH, Luxford WL: Cochlear implantation in congenitally malformed cochlea. *Laryngoscope* 105:1184, 1995.

120. Snider DE and others: Treatment of tuberculosis during pregnancy, *Ann Rev Respir Dis* 122:65, 1980.

121. Snik A and others. Air-Bone gap in patients with X-linked stapes gusher syndrome, *Am J Otol* 16:241, 1995.

122. Steel KP, Bock GR: Hereditary inner ear abnormalities in animals: relationships with human abnormalities, *Arch Otolaryngol Head Neck Surg* 109:22, 1983.

123. Streeter GL: On the development of the membranous labyrinth and the acoustic and facial nerves in the human embryo, *Am J Anat* 6: 139, 1906.

124. Streeter GL: The histogenesis and growth of the otic capsule and its contained periotic tissue-spaces in the human embryo, *Carnegie Contrib Embryol* 7:5, 1918.

125. Stevenson DS, Proops DW, Phelps PD: Severe cochlear dysplasia causing recurrent meningitis: a surgical lesson, *J Laryngol Otol* 107: 726, 1993.

126. Supance JS, Bluestone CD: Perilymph fistulas in infants and children, *Otolaryngol Head Neck Surg* 91:663, 1982.

127. Talbot JM, Wilson DF: Computed tomographic diagnosis of X-linked congenital mixed deafness, fixation of the stapedial footplate, and perilymphatic gusher, *Am J Otol* 15:177, 1994.

128. Tsuzuku T, Kaga K: The relationship between motor function development and vestibular function tests in four children with inner ear anomaly, *Acta Otolaryngol (Stockh)* 481:443, 1991.

129. Tucci DL and others: Cochlear implantation in patients with cochlear malformations, *Arch Otolaryngol Head Neck Surg* 121:833, 1995.

130. Unger JM, Shaffer KA: The abnormal temporal bone in the normal deaf, *Head Neck Surg* 3:185, 1981.

131. Valvassori GE: The large vestibular aqueduct and associated anomalies of the inner ear, *Otolaryngol Clin North Am* 16:95, 1983.

131a. Valvassori GE, Clemis JD: Abnormal vestibular aqueduct in cochleovestibular disorders, *Adv Otorhinolaryngol* 24:100, 1978.

132. van Aarem A, Cremers WR, Benraad-van Rens MJ: Usher syndrome: a temporal bone report, *Arch Otolaryngol Head Neck Surg* 121:916, 1995.

133. Wardrop P, Kerr AI, Moussa SA: Persistent stapedial artery preventing successful cochlear implantation: a case report, *Ann Otol Rhinol Laryngol Suppl* 166:443, 1995.

134. Weber PC and others: Correlation of beta-2 transferrin and middle ear abnormalities in congenital perilymph fistula, *Am J Otol* 16:277, 1995.

135. Weber PC, Perez BA, Bluestone CD: Congenital perilymphatic fistula and associated middle ear abnormalities, *Laryngoscope* 103:160, 1993.

136. Weissman JL, Weber PC, Bluestone CD: Congenital perilymphatic fistula: computed tomography appearance of middle and inner ear anomalies, *Otolaryngol Head Neck Surg* 111:243, 1994.

137. Wilson DF, Hodgson RS, Talbot JM: Endolymphatic sac obliteration for large vestibular aqueduct, *Am J Otol* 1996 (in press).

138. Wilson JT and others: Mondini dysplasia: spontaneous cerebrospinal fluid otorrhea. New perspectives in management, *Pediatr Neurosurg* 16:260, 1990–91.

139. Zalzal GH and others: Enlarged vestibular aqueduct and sensorineural hearing loss in childhood, *Arch Otolaryngol Head Neck Surg* 121:23, 1995.

Chapter 28

Reconstruction Surgery of the Ear

Microtia Reconstruction

Craig S. Murakami
Vito C. Quatela

Microtia occurs in approximately 0.03% (1 in 10,000 to 20,000) of live births, and it is estimated that half of these patients have associated congenital syndromes.[16,17,19,21] Certain populations such as the Navaho Indians and the Japanese may have higher incidences of microtia.[1] Microtia deformities appear to have a right-ear preponderance and affect boys more often than girls at roughly a 2.5:1 ratio. Unilateral cases outnumber bilateral cases by a 4:1 ratio.[19] Despite this relatively low incidence, microtia is one of the more common congenital malformations presented to otolaryngologists. Auricular reconstruction of the microtia deformity is a complex and labor-intensive process that requires a great deal of preoperative planning and preparation. This chapter reviews some of the nuances of microtia reconstruction. Discussion of auricular atresia is presented elsewhere within this Chapter.

EMBRYOLOGY

The internal ear begins as the otic placode at approximately the third week of gestation, then forms into the otic pit and otic cyst. The external ear begins to form at the fifth week of gestation. The auricle begins as six small buds of mesenchyme (classically called the *auricular hillocks of His*) surrounding the dorsal end of the first pharyngeal cleft.[12,13,22,26] On either side of the first pharyngeal cleft are the first (mandibular) and second (hyoid) pharyngeal arches. Hillocks 1 to 3 arise from the first pharyngeal arch, and hillocks 3 to 6 arise from the second pharyngeal arch. Conventional teaching is that the first hillock forms the tragus, the second and third form the helix, the fourth and fifth form the antihelix, and the sixth hillock forms the antitragus. The majority of the central ear is derived from hillocks 4 and 5, and the lobule appears to be one of the last parts of the ear to develop (Fig. 28-1). It has been estimated that the hyoid arch forms about 85% of the auricle.[19] The exact embryology of each of these hillocks remains unclear, although it is apparent that they are not six independent anlagen. The position of the auricular complex begins at the anterior neck region, but as the mandible develops from gestational weeks 8 through 12 the auricular complex moves dorsal and cephalad. The etiology of most microtias remains unknown, although the inciting event that arrests development of the ear must occur in the first trimester between the 4th and 12th weeks and may be related to abnormal neural crest cell migration.

Known teratogens such as isotretinoin (Accutane, Roche; Nutley, NJ) can produce forms of microtia in conjunction with limb anomalies.* Thalidomide is another teratogen associated with anomalies of the first and second branchial arches.[31] Microtia is associated with other anomalies 50% of the time and is also found in a number of well-known congenital syndromes such as Treacher Collins syndrome, which has an autosomal dominant inheritance, and in other facial syndromes that fall under the broad classification of the facioauriculovertebral spectrum. Within the facioauriculovertebral spectrum are malformations and syndromes that affect the first and second branchial-arch derivatives such as Goldenhar's syndrome (preauricular nodes, epibulbar dermoids, mandibular hypoplasia), hemifacial microsomia,[3] and oculoauricular vertebral dysplasia (microtia, cervical spine anomalies, and epibulbar dermoids).[10,15] It may be that Goldenhar's syndrome, hemifacial microsomia, oculoauriculovertebral dysplasia, and microtia are simply variants of the same entity.[17]

EAR ANATOMY

To understand the nature and extent of microtic ear deformities, the anatomic contour of the normal ear must first be reviewed (Fig. 28-2). The auricle is an aesthetic sculpture

* Refs. 11, 14, 18, 24, 27, 29.

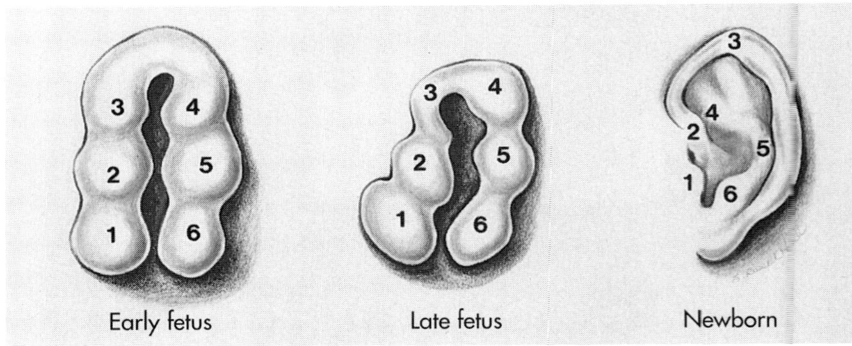

Fig. 28-1. Embryonic development. The ear develops from six hillocks of His. Hillocks 1 to 3 are from the first branchial arch, and hillocks 4 to 6 are from the second branchial arch. Hillock 1 forms the tragus, hillock 2 forms the root of the helix, and hillock 6 forms the antitragus. Hillocks 2 to 5 appear to form the helix and antihelix.

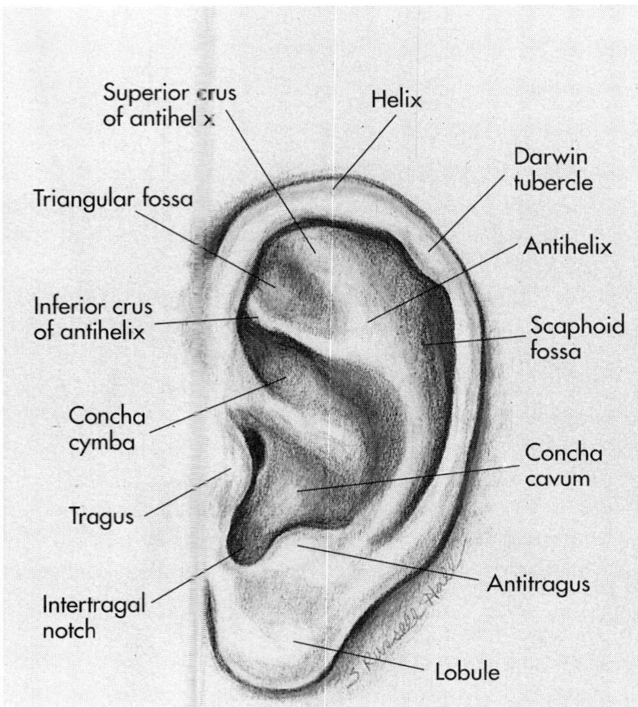

Fig. 28-2. Normal anatomic landmarks: helix, antihelix superior crus, antihelix inferior crus, tragus, antitragus, intertragal notch, scaphoid fossa, concha cavum, concha cymba, triangular fossa, and Darwinian tubercle

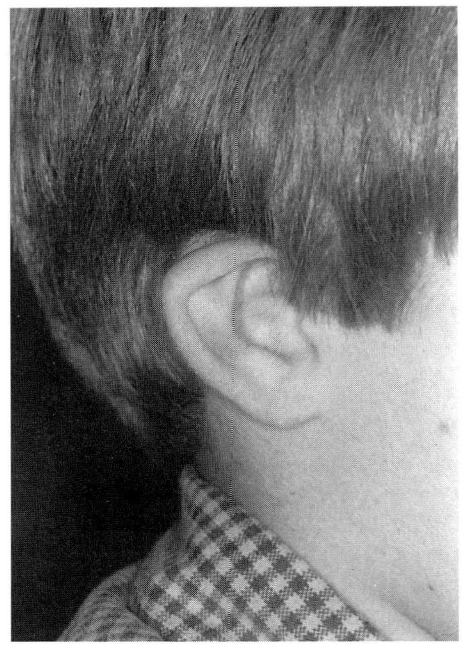

Fig. 28-3. Type I microtia: A constricted ear with minimal tissue deficiency.

of complex convexities, concavities, and curvilinear lines such as the helix and the antihelix, which are smooth and uninterrupted. The elastic cartilage framework is pliable yet structurally strong and extraordinarily resistant to trauma. The skin of the ear is fibrofatty and loose over the lobule and the margin of the helix and thin and fixed over the remaining cartilage framework.

Normal ear height ranges from 5.5 to 6.5 cm at maturity, which is typically attained at 15 years of age in boys and 13 years of age in girls. The horizontal width of the ear is achieved at an earlier age (10 years in boys and 6 years in girls). Protrusion of the ear from the surface of the mastoid should be 1.5 to 2.0 cm, creating an angle between 15° and 20°.[8] The superior margin of the helix is at the level of the tail of the eyebrow in 85% of people. Because the tail of the eyebrow is also quite variable, the level of the upper eyelid also may be used as a landmark if the patient has bilateral microtia.[23] The ear inclination is the angle formed by the vertical axis of the face and the longitudinal axis of the ear with the patient in the Frankfort horizontal position. This is approximately 24.8° with a standard deviation of 6.2°.[25] Therefore, the longitudinal

A

B

C

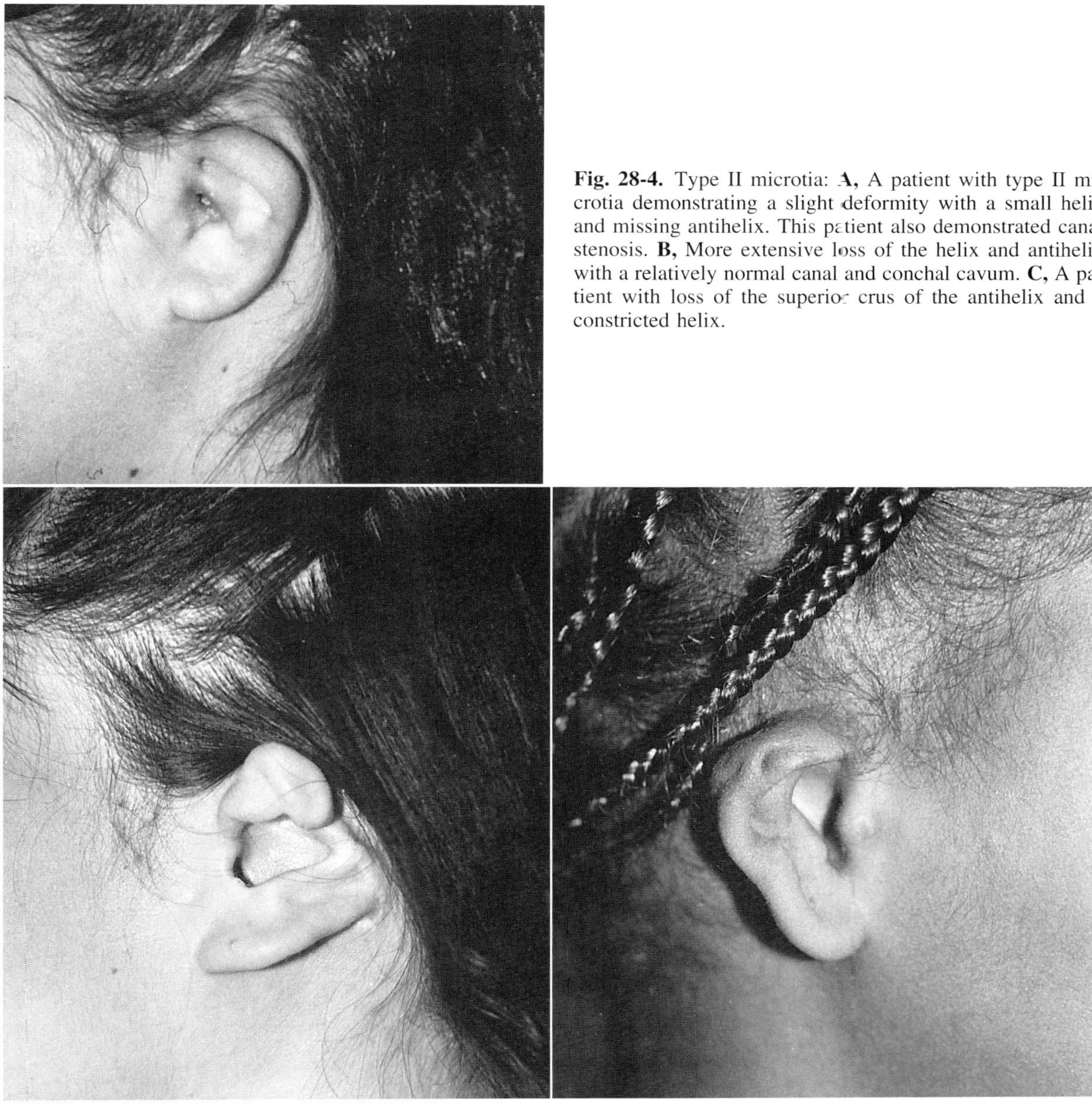

Fig. 28-4. Type II microtia: **A,** A patient with type II microtia demonstrating a slight deformity with a small helix and missing antihelix. This patient also demonstrated canal stenosis. **B,** More extensive loss of the helix and antihelix with a relatively normal canal and conchal cavum. **C,** A patient with loss of the superior crus of the antihelix and a constricted helix.

axis of the ear is not quite parallel with the dorsum of the nose as is commonly thought because the ear is in a slightly more vertical orientation.

MICROTIA

Microtia deformities come in various shapes and sizes, and, unfortunately, there is currently no universal, precise, and accurate classification scheme that is clinically useful in a statistical sense. Classification schemes are further complicated if the status of the external auditory canal (EAC) and middle-ear contents is included with the presence or absence of an associated syndrome.[19,20] Classification is usually simplified by evaluating the external auricular deformities alone. Perhaps *dysplasia* is a better term than microtia to describe ear deformities.

Dysplasia deformities are typically divided into three broad and simple categories that have a great deal of overlap.[2] Type I (Fig. 28-3) is used to designate ears with mild deformity that typically have a slightly dysmorphic helix and antihelix. This category includes prominent or lop-ear deformities, cupped ears, and mildly constricted ears. All major structures are present to some degree, and reconstruction does not require additional tissue. Type II (atypical microtia) dysplasia (Fig. 28-4) includes ears that

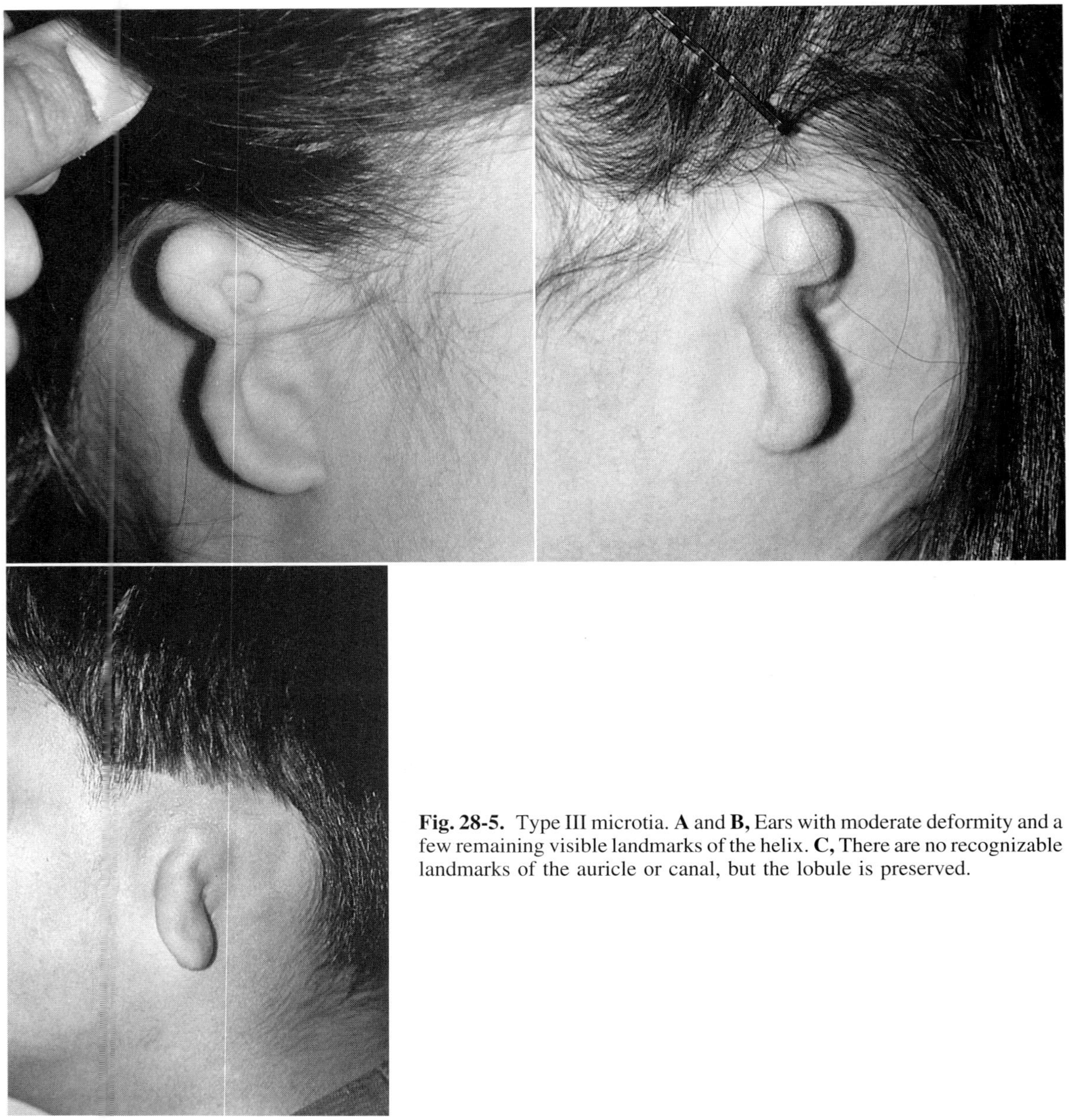

A B C

Fig. 28-5. Type III microtia. **A** and **B,** Ears with moderate deformity and a few remaining visible landmarks of the helix. **C,** There are no recognizable landmarks of the auricle or canal, but the lobule is preserved.

have all major structures present to some degree. There is an absolute deficiency of tissue, and surgical correction requires the addition of cartilage and skin. Mini-ear and severe cup-ear deformities are included in this category. The external auditory meatus is present but may demonstrate some degree of stenosis. Type III (classic microtia) dysplasia (Fig. 28-5) deformities have few or no recognizable landmarks of the auricle or canal, although the lobule is usually present and positioned anteriorly. Anotia is the complete absence of auricle and lobule. Reconstructive surgeons may find it more useful to simply note the status of the helix/antihelix, the conchal bowl, the lobule, the tragus, and the EAC because these are the landmarks that dictate the stages of ear reconstruction and the degree of surgical difficulty. When reconstructing third-degree dysplasia, the first stage generally begins with reconstruction of the helix/antihelix and conchal bowl, then progresses to the lobule, tragus, and EAC with each subsequent stage. When reconstructing type II dysplasias the emphasis is on unfurling or increasing the vertical height of the existing ear with composite grafts. In many cases more predictable results are found in type III dysplasia because the surgeon has complete control of the size, shape, and position of the cartilaginous framework.

EVALUATION

Children with microtia typically present to an otolaryngologist early in infancy because of parental concerns related to the child's hearing. The parents are usually concerned with the short- and long-term effects of monaural hearing on the child's speech and communication development and the possibility of learning disabilities. The external ear, EAC, and tympanic membrane are inspected and compared with the contralateral side. A thorough head-and-neck examination should be completed to rule out additional congenital abnormalities, which often occur in patients with microtia. Particular attention should be paid to the mandible, mouth, mouth opening, maxilla, eyes, and neck to rule out epibulbar dermoids, coloboma, maxillary or mandibular asymmetry, and vertebral anomalies, which may indicate that the microtia is part of a syndrome.

Patients with unilateral microtia typically have normal hearing in the contralateral ear, although this should be confirmed with an audiogram. If the child is younger than 7 months of age we obtain an auditory brain response (ABR) or an evoked otoacoustic emission (EOE) examination. In children 7 months to 2 years of age we first obtain behavioral audiograms using visual-reinforced audiometry; if this test is abnormal we proceed with the ABR or EOE because in this age group these tests usually require sedation.

At some point during the patient's childhood, fine-cut computed tomography (CT) of the temporal bone, base of skull, maxilla, mandible, and possibly the neck (if vertebral anomalies are suspected) is obtained. This is to evaluate the status of the middle-ear space, pneumatization of the mastoid, and symmetry or asymmetry of the facial skeletal growth as well as to rule out any vertebral anomalies that may be present in patients with microtia and other syndromes. In older patients with suspected hemifacial microsomia, a panorex is often helpful. If multiple anomalies are found, the child is usually evaluated by a multidisciplinary craniofacial team for a more comprehensive evaluation and coordination of nonsurgical and surgical plans.

PLANNING

Early evaluation by an otologist familiar with aural atresia is generally recommended. In most cases of unilateral microtia with canal atresia and a contralateral normal-hearing ear, canal reconstruction is not recommended because speech development will be normal and learning will not be impaired. Patients with bilateral microtia will require bone-conducting hearing aids. A decision regarding the possibility of an implantable hearing device is not recommended until auricular reconstruction is completed. The patient and family are presented the options of auricular reconstruction or observation. Generally, observation is recommended until the child is at least 5 to 8 years of age. This allows both growth of the donor rib cartilage and development of the contralateral normal ear; which will act as a template for the microtic side. Waiting until the child is older may reduce the risk of developing a thoracic deformity secondary to harvesting of cartilaginous rib graft, although the authors feel this risk is minimal.[9]

The child is included in all discussions and is allowed to participate to some degree in the decision-making process because compliance will have an impact on the perioperative management of these patients and the final success of the reconstruction as determined by the patient, the parents, and the surgeon. It is important to question the child about his or her personal concerns and to inquire about the effects of their microtia on social interaction with friends and classmates. Each child and parent will have different concerns that need to be voiced preoperatively.

During the planning stage of reconstruction, the surgical complications—infection, bleeding, graft loss, displacement or resorption, asymmetry, and pneumothorax—should be discussed in detail. The possibility of a less-than-optimal aesthetic result is also discussed, and the expectations of the patient, parents, and surgeon must be realistic and clearly defined. Providing postoperative photographs of previous patients is often helpful to patients if the pictures depict a realistic result of a similar deformity.

One option for older children or adults may include the temporary use of an auricular prosthesis. In some institutions a permanent auricular prosthesis with bone-anchored implants is recommended as the primary modality, and the aesthetic appearance is often excellent. However, most reconstructive surgeons discourage the use of bone-anchored implants for these patients as a primary modality for two reasons. The first is that the prosthesis is a synthetic appendage substitute that will forever require daily care to position and secure, and the patient may unnecessarily avoid situations that might accidentally dislodge the ear and cause embarassment. The second reason is that placement of the prosthesis violates the vascularity of the non–hair-bearing skin over the mastoid and complicates future reconstruction using the standard rib-grafting techniques should the patient become dissatisfied with the bone-implanted prosthesis.

RECONSTRUCTION

Although there have been attempts to use synthetic auricular framework implants, most surgeons have abandoned alloplastic implants because of the associated high rates of extrusion and infection, instead relying on autologous rib grafts for ear reconstruction. The use of rib cartilage in auricular reconstruction was pioneered by Tanzer[28] and perfected by the meticulous work and accomplishments of Brent.[4,6] Reconstruction using the standard rib-grafting technique requires three to four stages, each separated by 3 to 6 months beginning when the patient is approximately 5 to 8 years of age. The general health of the child is assessed, with particular attention to growth maturation and lung function. It is

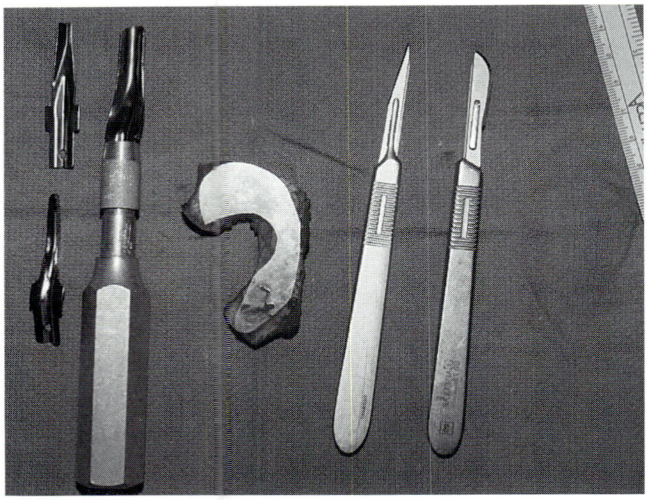

Fig. 28-6. Basic carving instruments for microtia reconstruction: a V-shaped gouge; #6 metal X-ACTO knife handles; assorted gouges, including $\frac{3}{8}$-inch and $\frac{3}{32}$-inch gouges, and assorted scalpels, including #11, #15, and #10.

important to assess lung function because there is a significant risk of pneumothorax and postoperative atelectasis and pneumonia.

A basic set of carving instruments is required (Fig. 28-6): two #6 X-ACTO (Hunt Manufacturer, NC) metal knife handles, one #155 X-ACTO $\frac{3}{8}$-inch U-shaped gouge, one #156 X-ACTO $\frac{3}{32}$-inch U-shaped gouge, two #3 scalpel handles, three to four #15 and #15c blade scalpels, three to four #10 blade scalpels, and two #11 blade scalpels. The X-ACTO carving tools can be obtained at any hobby shop. The #6 metal knife handles are autoclavable and reusable and the blades are disposable.

The surgeon must become facile with these instruments and develop carving and sculpting skills prior to undertaking a microtia reconstruction on a patient. For obvious reasons, fresh cadaveric rib cartilage is the best material with which to practice carving and harvesting grafts. If this cannot be obtained, carving the basic auricular framework can be practiced using wood, soap, or potatoes.

CLASSIC MICROTIA RECONSTRUCTION

Stage I: cartilage implantation

The first stage of microtia reconstruction is undoubtedly the most tedious and crucial of the entire process.[4] One of the most important objectives in the first stage is to place the auricular framework in a position that achieves the best symmetry with the patient's face. Placement of the reconstructed ear is determined by the position of the normal ear, and we do not alter this position to accomodate future reconstruction of the canal atresia or a low-lying hairline. If the hairline is low, the initial ear reconstruction is destined to have hair along the helix that will require depilation or excision at a later date. Preoperative tissue expansion to increase the amount of non–hair-bearing skin is not recommended because the expanded skin capsule does not contour well over the implanted cartilaginous framework.

A series of three templates must be made using radiographic film: a positioning template, a sizing template, and a carving template. The positioning template is made by carefully tracing the contour of the normal ear. It has the outline of the normal ear drawn in exact size and morphology, with the landmarks of the lateral palpebral fissure and the lateral commissure for reference points. The landmarks are etched onto the radiographic film with an 18-gauge needle or scalpel to avoid losing these reference points (Fig. 28-7). The distance from the lateral palpebral fissure to the root of the helix is also measured on the template and should approximate 6.5 cm or the length of the normal ear. The sizing template, which is drawn as a silhouette of the entire ear, is used to test the size of the skin pocket in which the cartilaginous framework is placed. The carving template is drawn from the sizing template to include the landmarks of the antihelix, the triangular fossa, the scaphoid fossa, the medial aspect of the helix, and the antihelix. It is drawn 1 to 2 mm smaller than the sizing template to compensate for the thickness of the overlying skin. It also is used to determine the best donor site during rib harvesting and as a template for sculpting the cartilaginous framework. Once the landmarks are permanently etched, the templates are autoclaved. The patient is placed on perioperative intravenous antibiotics and is maintained postoperatively on oral antibiotics for the first week after surgery.

Correct positioning and draping of the patient are required to provide simultaneous surgical access to both the donor chest site and the recipient ear site. The entire head-and-neck region is prepared so that the contralateral normal side can be easily visualized to evaluate symmetry. The contralateral chest is prepared because the contralateral rib graft has better contour characteristics. The chest incision is drawn just superior to the margin of the rib cage. The eyes and mouth are covered with a transparent drape to allow visualization of the lateral palpebral fissure and the lateral commissure and to facilitate placement using the positioning template. The recipient ear site is injected with lidocaine with epinephrine to assist with hemostasis, and the incision drawn along the anterior and superior margin of the rudimentary lobule.

The authors generally use two surgical teams to expedite the procedure and reduce operating time. The donor-site incision is made on the contralateral chest, and the inferior margin of the rib cage is exposed. The sixth, seventh, and eighth ribs are exposed and the synchondrosis between sixth and seventh ribs identified. The floating eighth rib is identified, and dissection is continued posteriorly to the bony–cartilaginous junction. The carving template is used to determine the best donor site for the cartilaginous auricular frame at the synchondrosis between the sixth and seventh ribs (Fig. 28-8). The rib cartilage is harvested with the perichondrium

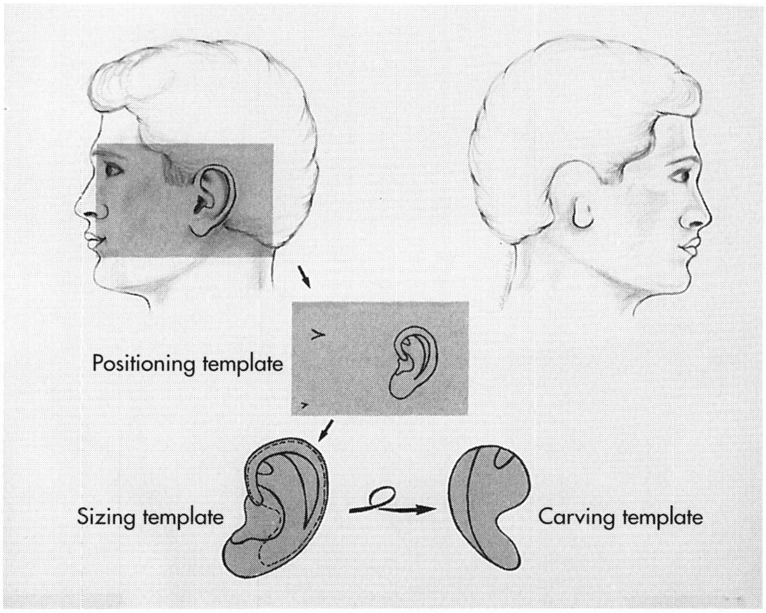

Fig. 28-7. Templates. The positioning template, which is drawn with reference landmarks, is used to create the sizing and carving templates. The sizing template is drawn to match the exact size of the normal ear. The carving template is slightly smaller than the sizing template to compensate for the thickness of the skin flap.

A

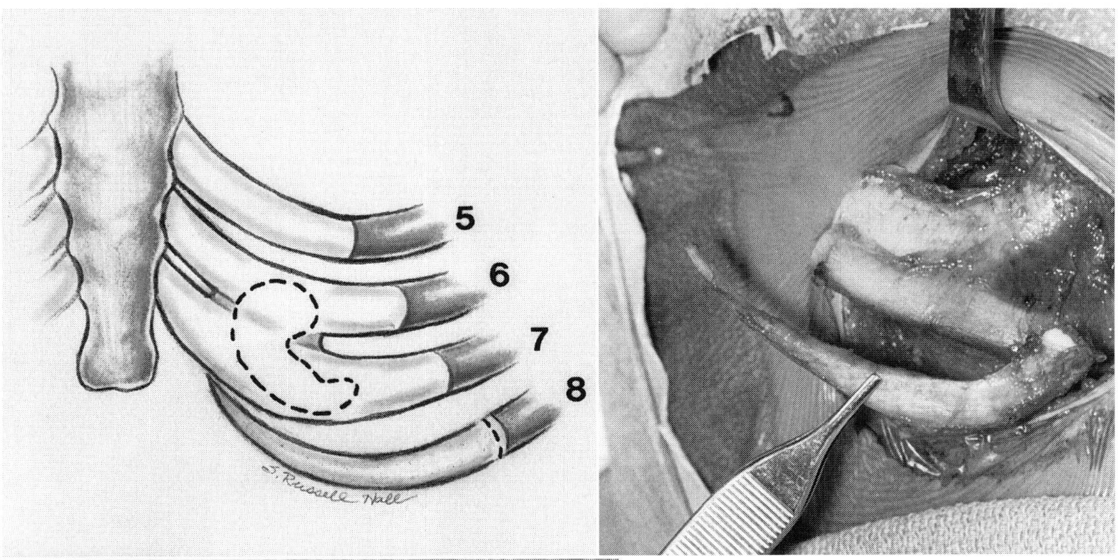

B

C

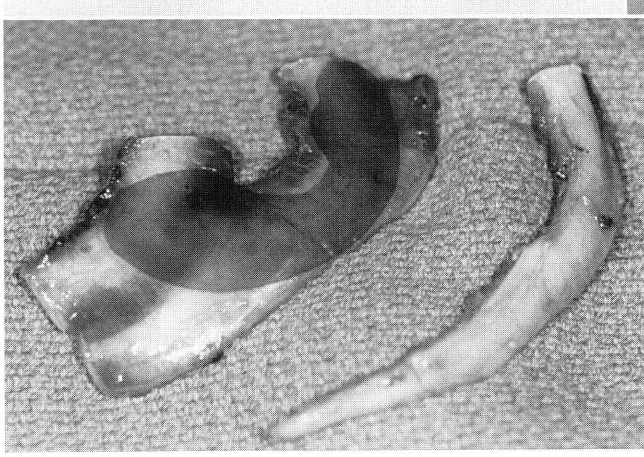

Fig. 28-8. The donor site. **A** to **C,** The contralateral chest is chosen for the donor site. The sixth, seventh, and eighth ribs and the synchondrosis between ribs 6 and 7 are depicted. The donor sites of the auricular framework and the helical rim are indicated.

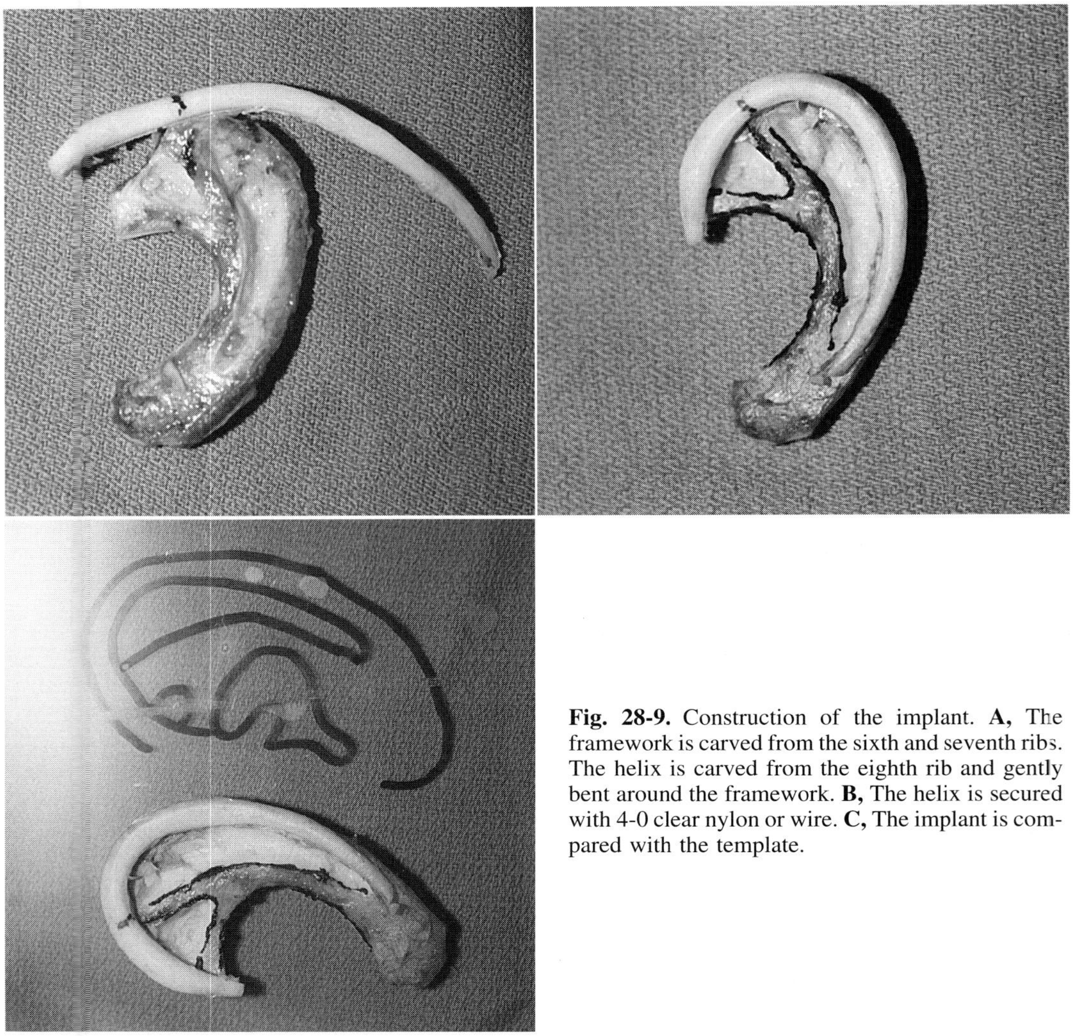

Fig. 28-9. Construction of the implant. **A,** The framework is carved from the sixth and seventh ribs. The helix is carved from the eighth rib and gently bent around the framework. **B,** The helix is secured with 4-0 clear nylon or wire. **C,** The implant is compared with the template.

intact. The entire cartilaginous portion of the floating rib (with the perichondrium intact) is removed; this typically reaches up to 9 cm in length. The donor site is checked for air leaks by flooding the area with saline and having the anesthesiologist apply positive ventilatory pressure. If a defect in the pleura is identified, a red rubber catheter is introduced into the pleural space and placed on continuous suction. The catheter is removed during positive-pressure ventilation, and the wound is closed with an airtight closure using 3-0 and 4-0 braided absorbable sutures. A flat suction drain is placed in the subcutaneous space after placement of intercostal bupivacaine blocks to reduce postoperative pain.

All incision planning should take into consideration future stages of reconstruction. The recipient incision is made vertically along the anterosuperior margin of the lobule. This incision site will be used for the second-stage lobule transfer. The rudimentary cartilage segment is meticulously removed, taking great care not to buttonhole or traumatize the flap. The recipient pocket is elevated over the mastoid in a subcutaneous plane, creating a thin flap to cover the cartilage framework. Using a headlight and fine scissors, the flap is trimmed to a uniform thickness. In the hair-bearing region, the skin is thicker because it becomes continuous with the scalp and contains a layer of galea. Dissection must be superficial to this layer of galea so that the flap remains uniformly thin and pliable. Hemostasis is obtained with bipolar cautery to minimize thermal trauma, and the sizing template is used to determine whether adequate undermining has been achieved. The pocket must be made so that the sizing template fits into the pocket with extra room to accommodate the thickness of the graft. The sizing template reduces the number of times that the reconstructed cartilage framework is transferred in and out of the pocket while adjustments are made. This helps reduce the amount of unnecessary handling and the risk of fracturing the framework.

The framework and helix are carved with the patient on a separate table using the X-ACTO carving instruments and #10, #11, and #15 blade scalpels. The $\frac{3}{8}$-inch gouge is used to create the triangular fossa, and the $\frac{3}{32}$-inch gouge is used to carve the scaphoid fossa. As much perichondrium as possible is left intact over the lateral surface to enhance revascularization and tissue fixation. Suture or wire fixation is needed occasionally to reinforce the synchondrosis and provide additional support to the framework. Additional cartilage grafts can be sutured to the posterior surface of the synchondrosis for more rigidity. The helix is carved from the eight rib using the thicker part of the graft for the root of the helix and the thin distal tip of the graft for the posterior helix. The graft is carefully thinned until it is pliable enough to bend around the framework and sutured in position with 4-0 clear nylon suture or wire. Additional thinning of the scaphoid and triangular fossa can be done after the helix is adequately fixated (Fig. 28-9).

The reconstructed framework with attached helix is then placed into the pocket in a rotational manner, beginning with the root of the helix and rotating the framework clockwise for the right side and counterclockwise for the left. The proper position of the implant is determined by using the positioning template. If the pocket is excessively tight and the overlying skin remains blanched with poor vascular refill, the implant is removed and the pocket enlarged. Once the graft is properly positioned, two small round drains are placed superficial and deep to the framework and are placed on suction while the wound is closed in two layers. Once the wound is sealed, the skin should conform to the framework and the details of the helix and antihelix should be clearly visible (Fig. 28-10). The concavities of the ear are packed with petroleum gauze, and a standard mastoid dressing is applied using fluffed gauze to avoid unnecessary pressure. The drains are placed on intermediate suction. One author (CSM) prefers continuous suction for 24 hours before placing the drains on bulb suction. The other (VQ) recommends continuous use of butterfly drains connected to vacuum-sealed red rubber top tubes.

A chest radiograph is obtained in the recovery room to rule out a possible pneumothorax. The chest drain is removed on the first postoperative day, and the ear drains are removed after 2 to 3 days when there is little or no drainage. The vascularity of the skin overlying the helix is inspected on a regular basis, and the mastoid dressing is removed at 24 to 48 hours. A Glasscock dressing is then applied for the next 2 weeks to protect the ear. The patient must refrain from strenuous activity for 4 to 6 weeks and is not allowed to participate in contact sports for 2 months to avoid injuring the donor rib site.

Stage II: lobule transfer

The lobule transfer is done 2 to 3 months after the stage I procedure. It is a simple transposition flap that transposes the lobule into the donor site along the inferior border of

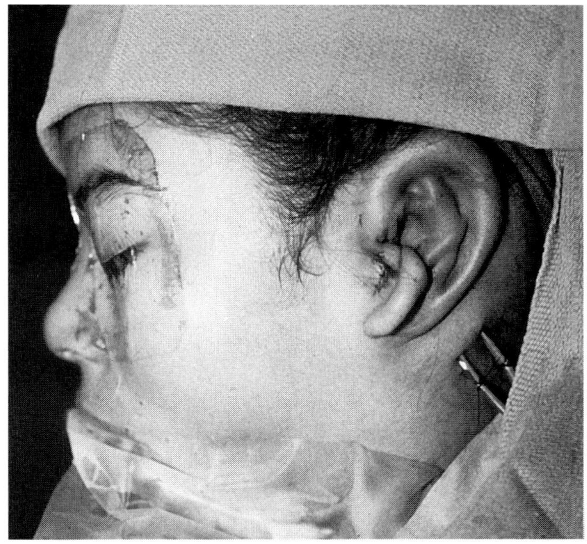

Fig. 28-10. Placement of the implant. The implant is placed into the pocket and positioned using the positioning template. One drain is placed over the surface of the implant as one is placed deep to the implant. The drains are then placed on suction. Note the contouring of the skin over the cartilaginous framework, with the drain traversing over the antihelix and into the scaphoid fossa.

the framework. The lobule is elevated and trimmed until it is symmetric with the contralateral ear. The inferior margin of the implant is dissected, taking care not to remove all of the soft tissue overlying the cartilage—which would expose the graft and increase the risk of devascularization and infection. The lobule is then wrapped around the posteroinferior margin of the cartilage framework (Fig. 28-11). Care is taken to evert the wound margins in an attempt to avoid a step-off at the junction of the lobule and framework. Occasionally a Z-plasty along the helical border is necessary to avoid scar contracture and a sharp demarcation from the lobule to the helix. The donor site is closed primarily after conservative mobilization of the surrounding skin.

There is often redundant skin that contours poorly over the surface of the framework despite removal of the rudimentary cartilage during the first stage. This extra skin is removed at this stage with simple excision and primary closure. Occasionally this extra tissue can be used to form a tragus. The ear is then covered with a Glasscock dressing for 1 week, and the wound is kept moist with an antibiotic ointment.

Stage III: postauricular skin grafting

The goal of the third stage of reconstruction is to create a postauricular sulcus and to project the ear away from the surface of the mastoid. This procedure is performed approximately 3 months after stage II with the patient under general anesthesia (Fig. 28-12). The position of the hairline is inspected, and in many cases there is hair over the superior

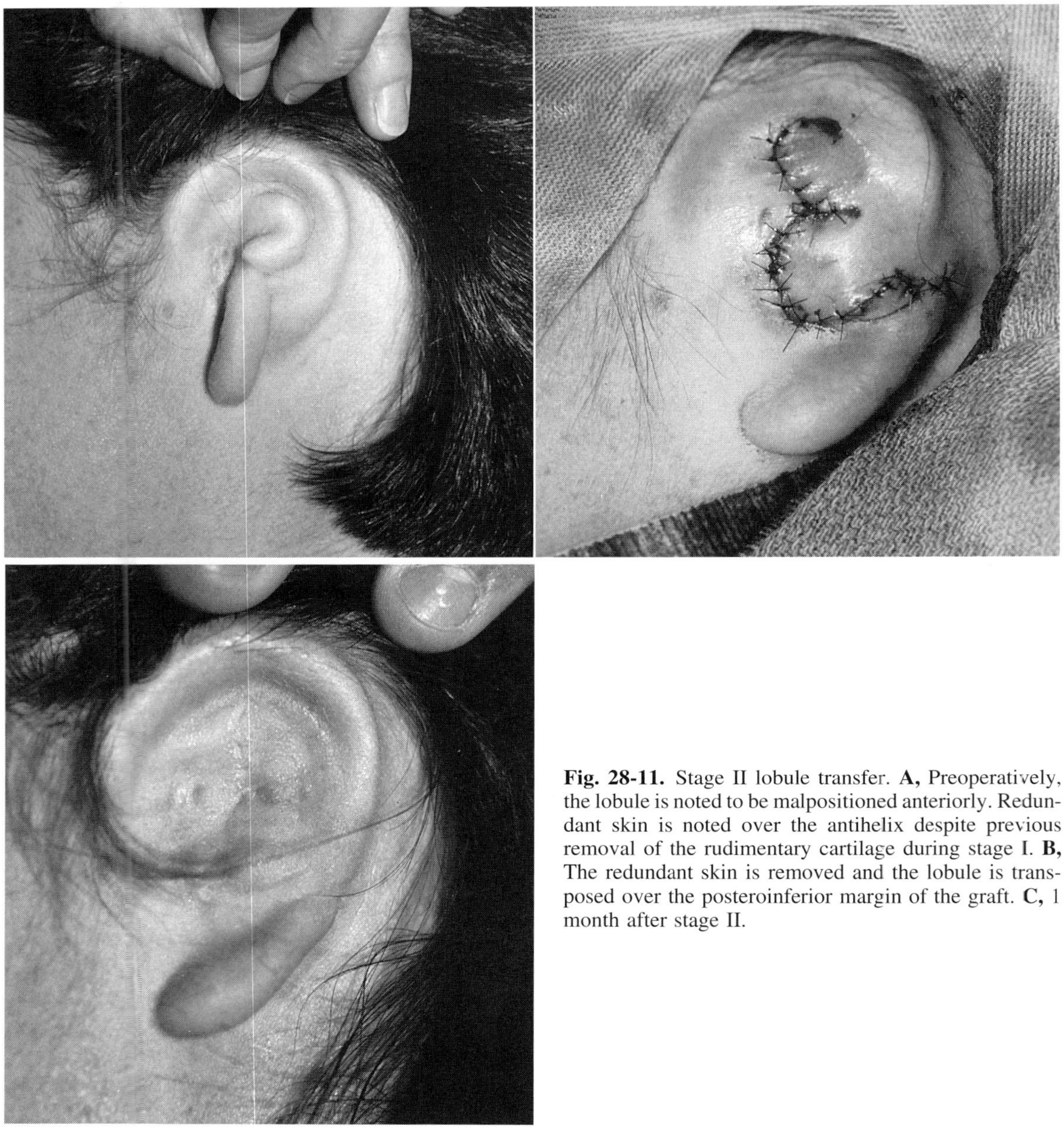

A B C

Fig. 28-11. Stage II lobule transfer. **A,** Preoperatively, the lobule is noted to be malpositioned anteriorly. Redundant skin is noted over the antihelix despite previous removal of the rudimentary cartilage during stage I. **B,** The redundant skin is removed and the lobule is transposed over the posteroinferior margin of the graft. **C,** 1 month after stage II.

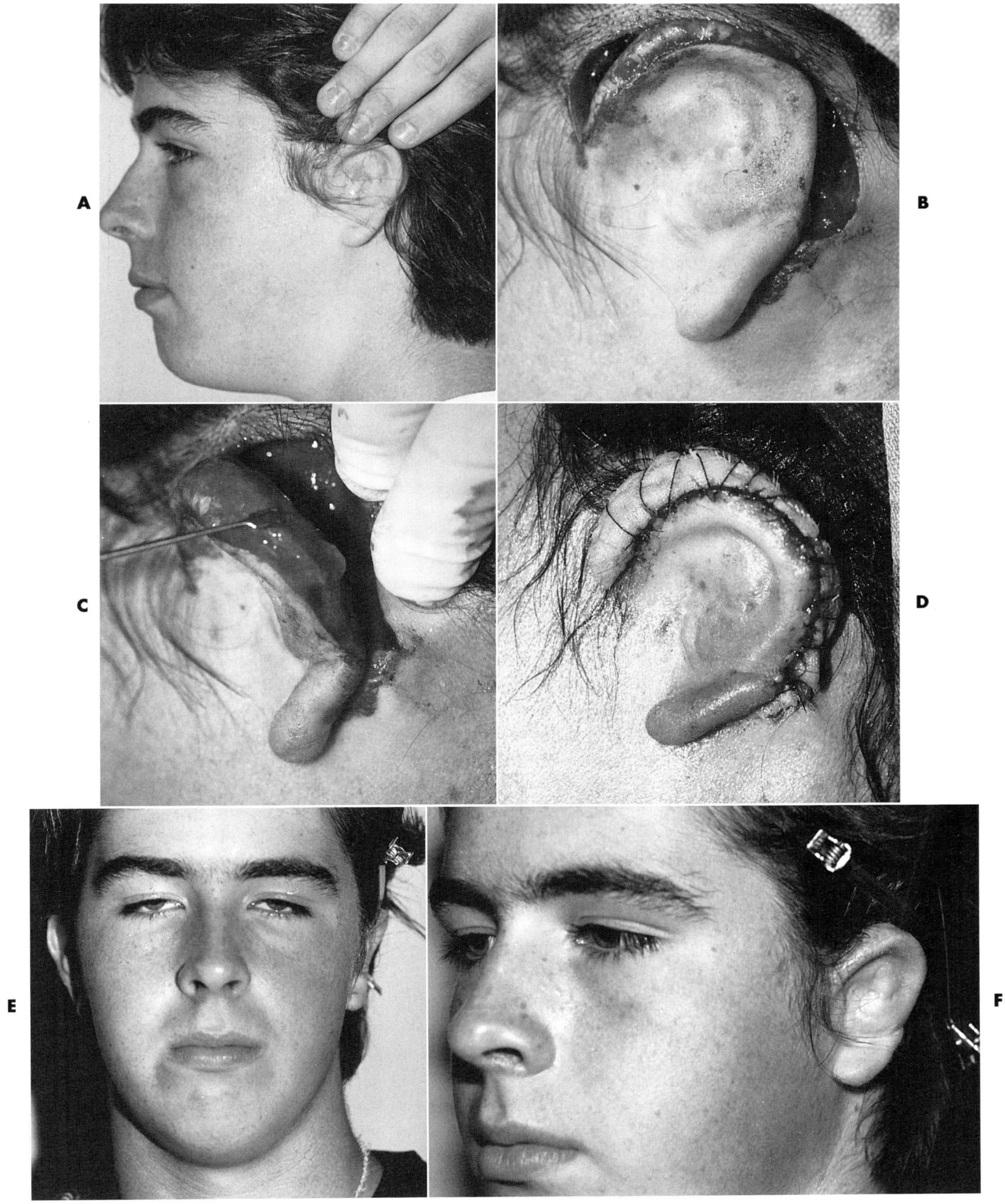

Fig. 28-12. Stage III skin grafting. **A,** Before the procedure. **B,** Release of the skin leaving the perichondrium intact. **C,** Dissection into the postauricular sulcus and advancement of the postauricular skin. **D,** Skin graft secured with a soft bolster. **E** and **F,** 2 months after the procedure.

and anterior margins of the helix. The incision is usually made along the superior margin of the helix from the anterior root of the helix to the lobule. However, if there is hair on the helix, the incision is made slightly lower on its lateral surface to eliminate some or all of this hair-bearing skin. The non–hair-bearing auricular skin is advanced 2 to 3 mm superiorly over the helical rim, and absorbable tacking sutures are placed between the subcutaneous tissue and the cartilaginous framework. The ear is released by dissecting into the postauricular sulcus and leaving the perichondrium intact to protect the cartilage graft. The postauricular skin over the mastoid is undermined and advanced into the postauricular sulcus. It is fixed with an absorbable suture, and the postauricular defect is measured. It usually measures 4 to 5 × 8 to 9 cm. An elliptic thick split-thickness graft is harvested freehand using a #15 blade scalpel from the left groin, lower abdomen, or buttock. The graft is secured into position in the postauricular sulcus with 4-0 chromic sutures and bolstered with petroleum gauze impregnated with an antibiotic ointment using 4-0 nylon. The ear is covered with a Glasscock dressing for protection for 1 to 2 weeks. The bolster is removed after 3 to 5 days, and the skin graft is kept moist with a topical moisturizer for 2 to 3 weeks. Advancement of postauricular skin into the postauricular sulcus helps to project the ear laterally away from the mastoid. If the ear requires further projection a small piece of cartilage can be inserted deep to the graft at a later date.

Stage IV: tragus reconstruction

The fourth stage of reconstruction is to form a tragus and conchal bowl. If the conchal bowl is well defined, a composite can be used to reconstruct the tragus. An elliptic composite graft is removed from the concha cymba of the contralateral healthy ear. An incision is made along the posterior border of the future tragus, and the composite graft is placed on the posterior surface to give the tragus some projection. The shadowing effect gives the illusion of an external auditory meatus. If the conchal bowl is not defined, an incision is made along the posterior border of the future conchal bowl and an anterior-based cutaneous circular flap is created. The conchal bowl is then debulked of scar tissue and any rudimentary skin and cartilage that might remain. Because of facial nerve anomalies a facial nerve monitor is recommended. The flap is folded onto itself to create a tragus then reinforced with a small piece of auricular or rib cartilage, and the surface of the conchal bowl covered with a small skin graft (Fig. 28-13). The bolster is removed in 3 to 5 days. Occasionally, an additional operation is needed to further elevate the reconstructed ear away from the mastoid using grafts of cartilage implanted medial to the framework.

ATYPICAL MICROTIA REPAIR

Second-degree dysplasia or atypical microtia presents a more difficult surgical challenge. As previously discussed, many components of the auricular structure are recognizable but there is a distinct tissue deficiency necessitating the transportation of cartilage and skin. The additional structure often eliminates the necessity for complete framework insertion. When the vertical height difference between the two ears is greater than 20 mm, consideration is given to using a rib framework. When the difference is less than 20 mm, the result is achieved by expanding the existing structure. This is done by a combination of unfurling, uncupping, and increasing the vertical height with the use of cartilage composite grafts[5] (Fig. 28-14). The helical root can also be advanced in a V-Y fashion into the helix to help augment the vertical height. Unlike classic microtia reconstruction, the use of vestigial remnants as a main framework does not lead to consistent results. Figure 28-15 shows a child with atypical microtia with an undeveloped lobule that was reconstructed by placing a cartilage implant harvested from the contralateral conchal bowl. This was followed by a staged skin graft with an advancement flap of postauricular skin.

COMPLICATIONS

Major complications are fortunately rare, although seemingly minor complications may lead to loss of the graft through infection or devascularization if they are not treated expeditiously. Immediate postoperative complications include hematoma formation, skin flap necrosis, infection, and pneumothorax. If a graft becomes exposed postoperatively secondary to breakdown of the overlying skin flap, the patient is placed on antibiotics to cover *Staphylococcus* and *Pseudomonas* infection and the exposed site is covered with moist continuous dressings. If the exposure is small (1 to 2 mm) and the perichondrium is intact, there is a small chance that the wound may granulate closed with local wound care alone. If cartilage is exposed, however, early coverage of the site with a local flap or a temporal–parietal fascia flap with an overlying skin graft should be considered. Once the perichondrium is gone and the cartilage exposed, it is difficult for the wound to granulate closed because the exposed cartilage quickly becomes devitalized and desiccated and destined to become infected. Prolonged antibiotic therapy after flap coverage is necessary to avoid progression of the infection and eventual collapse and resorption of the graft.

Minor complications include malpositioning, scar contracture or hypertrophy, and poor contouring. Generally, problems with scar formation and poor contouring improve with time if the cartilage has not become infected or undergone resorption. Minor scar revisions may be necessary when indicated, and the surgeon should be careful not to expose the cartilage graft. Problems with malposition are usually minor if proper template techniques were used and are commonly related to preexisting lobule asymmetry or generalized facial asymmetry caused by mild hemifacial microsomia. Major malposition problems are usually related to poor preoperative planning.

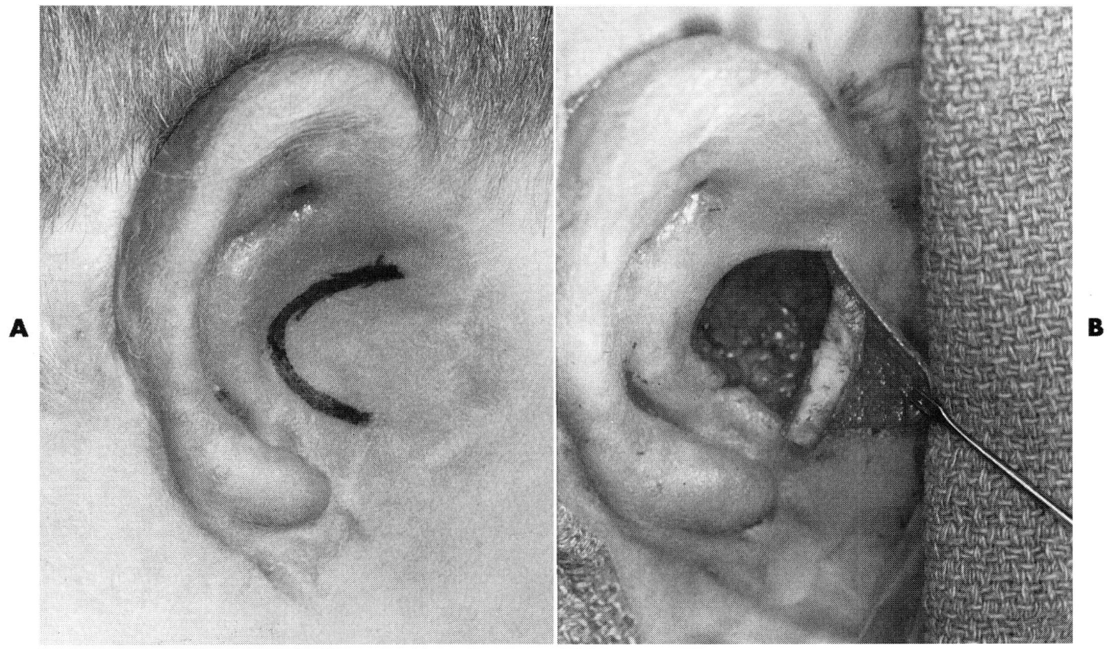

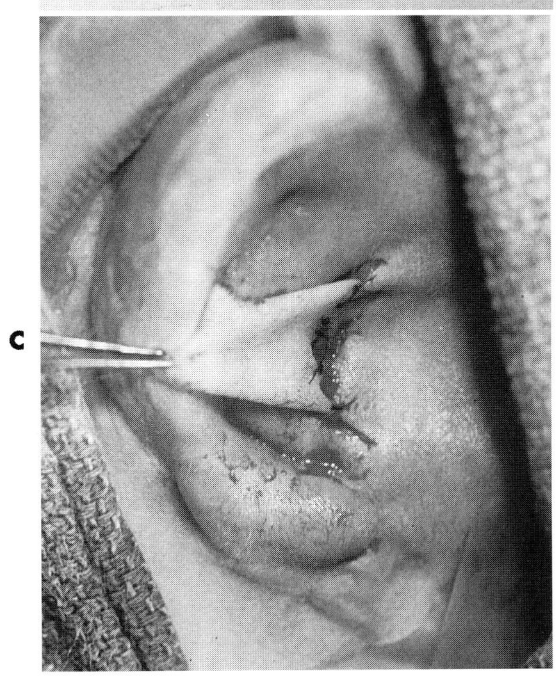

Fig. 28-13. Stage-IV tragus reconstruction. **A,** In bilateral microtia, tragal reconstruction is more difficult because both ears are reconstructed, thus normal concha cymba is not available for composite grafting. A longer flap must be elevated to provide both medial and lateral tragal lining. **B,** A free cartilage graft is placed to prevent contraction and is lined by the skin flap. **C,** The conchal bowl is deepened and lined with a skin graft. (From Quatela VC, Goldman ND: *Fac Plast Surg* 11: 257, 1995. With permission.)

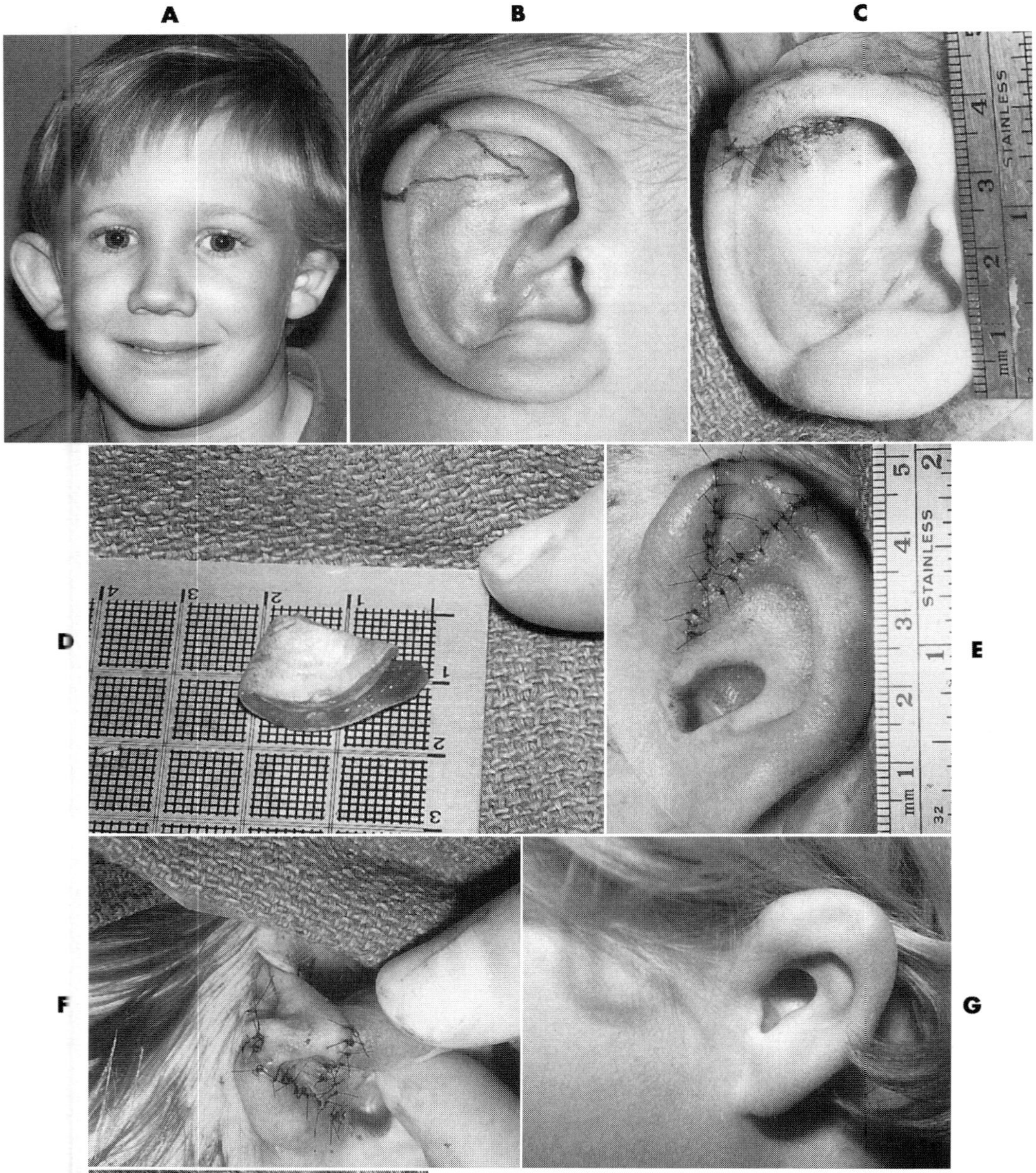

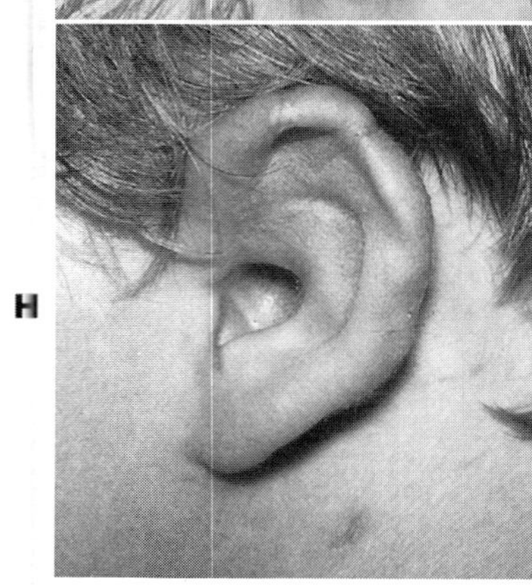

Fig. 28-14. Atypical microtia reconstruction. **A,** A congenital defect of the ear with more than 20 mm of vertical height compared with the contralateral healthy ear. **B,** The donor site composite graft is harvested to equal one half the size of the recipient defect, thereby reducing the disparity. The donor site is closed primarily, with the only resultant deformity being shortened vertical height, which is desirable in this patient's ear. **C,** The donor ear is shortened by 1 cm but retains good form. **D,** The composite graft. **E,** The composite graft sutured into position. Vertical height increased by approximately 1 cm. **F,** Epithelium is removed from the medial aspect of the composite graft, and the graft placed into a postauricular subcutaneous pocket. The medial skin is still attached at the rim as a hinge flap. The medial perichondrium is in contact with the retroauricular soft tissue. This will ensure maximum recipient contact for graft survival. Release is accomplished 2 weeks later, using the hinge flap skin for medial resurfacing. **G,** Before surgery. **H,** The final result at 1 year.

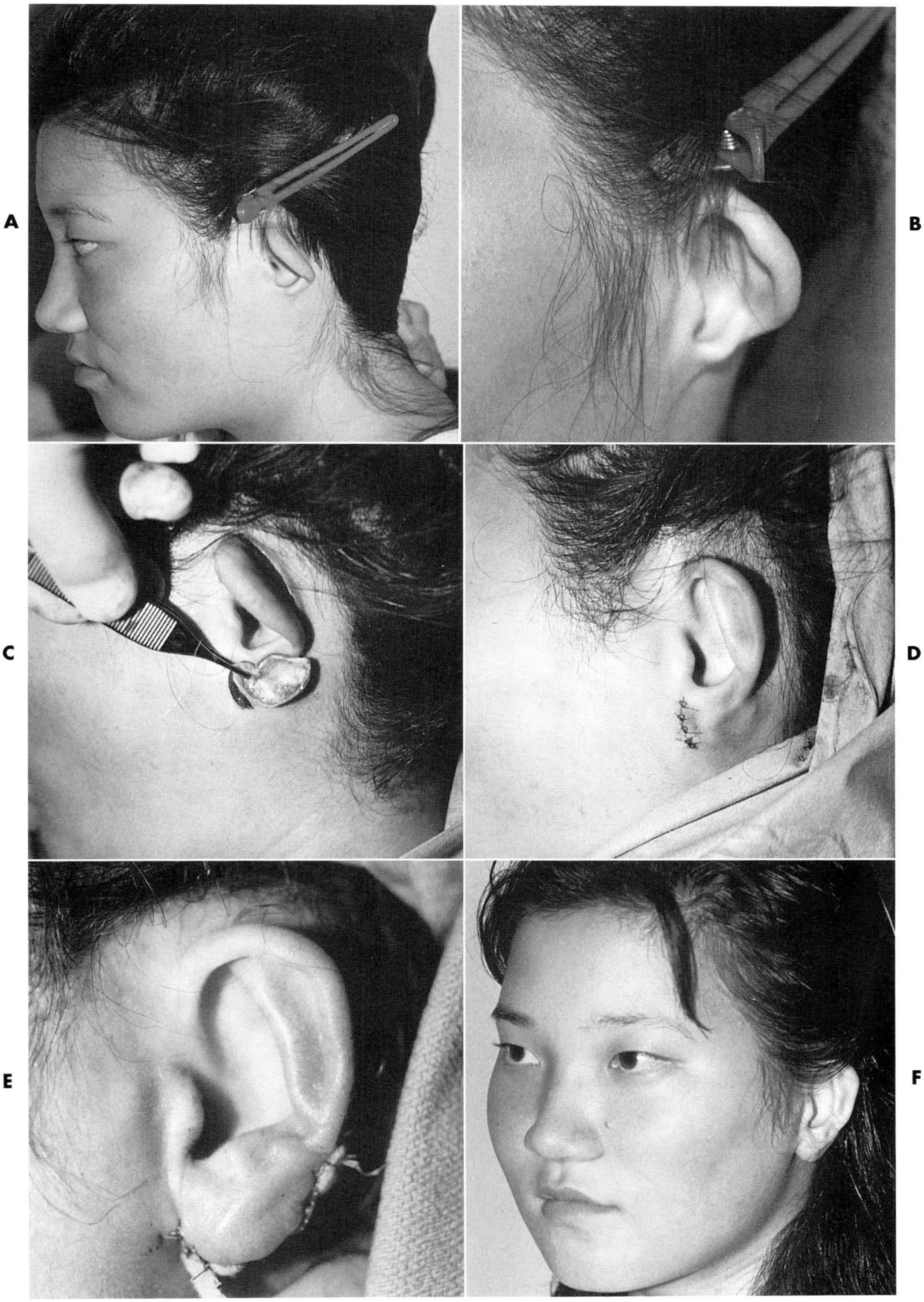

Fig. 28-15. **A** and **B,** Type II atypical microtia with a missing lobule and a dysmorphic helix and antihelix. **C** to **E,** Two-stage reconstruction required placement of a conchal cartilage graft followed by delayed release of the lobule, advancement of postauricular skin, and placement of a full-thickness skin graft that was secured with a bolster dressing. **F,** Final postoperative result at 1 year.

CONCLUSIONS

Managing patients with microtia can be a rewarding experience for both the patient and the surgeon if proper training, preparation, and planning are done. Each patient and each ear deformity are unique, making management of these patients a humbling, challenging, and perpetually stimulating problem. In many respects, microtia surgery is similar to rhinoplasty, in which the surgeon continually strives to achieve the elusive "perfect" aesthetic and functional result through meticulous planning and attention to detail.

REFERENCES

1. Aase JM, Tegtmeier RE: Microtia in New Mexico, *Birth Defects* 13: 113, 1977.
2. Aguilar EA: *Major congenital malformations of the auricle.* In Baily BJ and others, editors: *Head and neck surgery, otolaryngology,* Philadelphia, 1993, JB Lippincott.
3. Bennum RD and others: Microtia: a microform of hemifacial microsomia, *Plast Reconstr Surg* 76:859, 1985.
4. Brent B: Correction of microtia with autogenous cartilage grafts: I. Classic deformity, *Plast Reconstr Surg* 66:1, 1980.
5. Brent B: Correction of microtia with autogenous cartilage grafts: II. Atypical and complex deformities, *Plast Reconstr Surg* 66:13, 1980.
6. Brent B: The artistry of reconstructive surgery, St. Louis, 1987, CV Mosby.
7. Reference deleted in pages.
8. Farkas LG: Anthropometry of the normal and defective ear, *Clin Plast Surg* 17:213, 1990.
9. Fukuda O: Long-term evaluation of modified Tanzer ear reconstruction, *Clin Plast Surg* 17:241, 1990.
10. Gorlin RJ, Pindborg JJ, Cohen MM: *Oculoauriculovertebral dysplasia.* In *Syndromes of the head and neck,* New York, 1976, McGraw-Hill.
11. Granström G: Retinoid-induced ear malformations, *Otolaryngol Head Neck Surg* 103:702, 1990.
12. His W: Auf Stellung von Entwickelungsnormen zweiter Monat, *Anat Mensch Embryonen* Part II:55, 1883.
13. His W: Die Formentwickelung des äusseren ohres, *Anat Mensch Embryonen* Part III:21 , 1885.
14. Jarvis BL, Johnson MC, Sulik KK: Congenital malformations of the external, middle, and inner ear produced by isotretinoin exposure in mouse embryos, *Otolaryngol Head Neck Surg* 102:391, 1990.
15. Jones KL: *Smith's recognizable patterns of human malformation*, Philadelphia, 1988, WB Saunders.
16. Karmody CS, Annino DJ: Embryology and anomalies of the external ear, *Facial Plast Surg* 11:251, 1995.
17. Kaye CI and others: Microtia and associated anomalies, *Am J Med Genet* 34:574, 1989
18. Lammer E: Preliminary observations on isotretinoin-induced ear malformations and pattern formation of the external ear, *J Craniofac Genet Dev Biol* 11:292, 1991.
19. Lucente FE, Lawson W, Novick NL: *The external ear,* Philadelphia, 1995, WB Saunders
20. Marx H: Beitrag zur morholgie und genese der mittelohrmissbildungen mit gehorgangsatresie, *Z Hals Nasan Ohrenheilkd* 2:230, 1922.
21. Melnick M, Myrianthopoulos NC: *External ear malformations: epidemiology, genetics and natural history*, New York, 1979, Alan R. Liss.
22. Moore KL: *The developing human*, Philadelphia, 1977, WB Saunders.
23. Posnick JC, Al-Qattan MM, Whitaker LA: Assessment of the preferred vertical position of the ear, *Plast Reconstr Surg* 91:1198, 1993.
24. Rosa FW: Teratogenicity of isotretinoin, *Lancet* 2:513, 1983 (letter).
25. Skiles MS, Randall P: The aesthetics of ear placement: an experimental study, *Plast Reconstr Surg* 72:133, 1983.
26. Streeter GL: Development of the auricle in the human embryo, *Control Embryol* 14:111, 1922.
27. Sulik KK, Dehart DB: Retinoid-acid-induced limb malformations resulting from apical ectodermal ridge cell death, *Teratology* 37:527, 1988.
28. Tanzer R: Total reconstruction of the external ear, *Plast Reconstr Surg* 23:1, 1959.
29. Westerman ST, Gilbert LM, Schondel L: Vestibular dysfunction in a child with embryonic exposure to accutane, *Am J Otol* 15:400, 1994.

Auditory Canal and Tympanum

Antonio De La Cruz
Sujana S. Chandrasekhar

Congenital malformations of the temporal bone include aplasia or hypoplasia of the HAC, associated microtia (absence or deformity of the pinna) and middle-ear deformity, and occasional inner-ear abnormalities. Congenital aural atresia (CAA) occurs in 1 in 10,000 to 20,000 live births, is more often unilateral than bilateral, and preferentially affects boys and the right side of the face. CAA ranges in severity from a thin membranous canal atresia to a complete lack of tympanic bone, depending on the time of arrest of intrauterine development. The course of the facial nerve is usually abnormal. There is a relatively low (11% to 47%) incidence of inner-ear abnormality associated with CAA. Bony atresia of the EAC, which is more common than membranous atresia, is routinely associated with middle-ear deformities. Fusion of the malleus and incus is common, but because of its dual origin, the stapes footplate is usually normal. Generally, a more severe external deformity implies a more severe middle-ear deformity.

Surgical correction of CAA is one of the most challenging operations performed by otologists. It requires application of all modern lympanoplasty techniques, including canalplasty, meatoplasty, lympanic membrane grafting, and ossiculoplasty as well as a thorough knowledge of the surgical anatomy of the facial nerve, oval window and inner ear, and their congenital variants. The goal of surgery is to create a patent, skin-lined EAC and achieve closure of the air–bone gap to within 20 to 30 dB.

In 1883, Kiesselbach performed the first deep operation for atresia, with resultant facial nerve paralysis. There was a high incidence of complications and no middle-ear manipulation, so that CAA surgery was generally considered too dangerous to perform. Despite good outcomes reported in 1914 by Page[21] and in 1917[12] atresiaplasty did not come into favor until after 1947, when Ombredanne[20] in France and Pattee[22] the United States each reported a series of successful cases. Pattee[22] achieved better results with removal of the incus to "mobilize" the stapes; Ombredanne[20] added fenestration of the lateral semicircular canal (LSCC). When Wullstein and Zollner's techniques of tympanoplasty were added in the 1950's, interest and success rates in atresiaplasty rose.

In a landmark 1969 paper, Gill[13] reported a series of 83 cases. Ombredanne went on to report on over 600 "aplasia" cases by 1971 and 1600 cases of major and minor malformations by 1976. In the last two decades, large surgical series and excellent success rates have been reported by Crabtree,[8] Jahrsdoerfer,[15] Marques and others,[18] and De La Cruz and others.[9-11] Each of these authors modified their surgical techniques to add finesse to the procedure.

EMBRYOLOGY

Microtia is a result of first branchial cleft and pouch anomalies. The primitive auricle is fully formed by the end of the third month of gestation. The external auditory meatus develops from the first branchial groove. During the second month of gestation a solid core of epithelium migrates inward from the rudimentary pinna toward the first branchial pouch. This core is the precursor of the EAC and begins to hollow out and take shape in the sixth month of gestation. It canalizes in the seventh month, thus separating the mastoid and the mandible. Its subsequent posterior and inferior development carries the middle ear and facial nerve to their normal positions.

Meanwhile, the first branchial pouch grows outward to form the middle-ear cleft. The tympanic membrane is formed where the middle-ear cleft meets the epithelium of the EAC. The pouch forms the eustachian tube, tympanic cavity, and mastoid air cells, whereas Meckel's cartilage (of the first branchial arch) and Reichert's cartilage (of the second branchial arch) form the malleus, incus, and stapes superstructure. The stapes footplate has a dual origin from the second arch and the otic capsule. The ossicles attain their final shape by 4 months' gestation. By the end of the seventh to eighth month, the expanding middle-ear cleft surrounds the ossicles and covers them with a mucous membrane.

CLASSIFICATION SYSTEMS

Several modern atresiaplasty surgeons have devised classification schemes to grade atresia on the basis of degree of anatomic deformity. These classification systems are used for preoperative assessment of prognosis in elective atresiaplasty, surgical planning, patient counseling, and comparison of outcomes.

Altmann[2] categorized atresias into three groups—mild, moderate, and severe—based on the status of the EAC and tympanic cavity. Most surgical candidates fall into the second and third groups of this classification system. De La Cruz modified Altmann's system to offer more practical surgical guidelines. His modification uses only the moderate and severe classifications of Altmann's groups and divides abnormalities into "minor" and "major" categories. Minor malformations consist of normal mastoid pneumatization, a normal oval window, a reasonable facial nerve/oval-window relationship, and a normal inner ear. Major malformations include poor pneumatization, an abnormal or absent oval window, an abnormal course of the horizontal facial nerve, and abnormalities of the inner ear. Surgery in patients with minor malformations has a good possibility of yielding serviceable hearing, whereas with major malformations are frequently inoperable.

Jahrsdoerfer and others[18] devised a point-grading system based primarily on high-resolution CT (HRCT). The parameters are mastoid pneumatization, presence of oval and round windows, status of the ossicles and mesotympanum, facial nerve course, appearance of the external ear, and presence of the stapes. Each parameter receives one point, except for the stapes (which receives two points), for a total of 10 points. (In our experience, the presence of a stapes is less important than the presence of an oval window and a well-pneumatized mastoid.) In Jahrsdoerfer and others' grading system, a success rate of over 80% will be achieved in patients with a score of 8 or higher. A score of 7 implies a fair prognosis, 6 is marginal, and patients with lower scores are poor candidates.[16]

Schuknecht's[23] classification is based on both clinical and surgical observations. Type A (meatal) atresia is limited to the fibrocartilaginous portion of the EAC. Type B (partial) atresia has narrowing of both the fibrocartilaginous and bony RAC, but a patent dermal tract allows partial inspection of the tympanic membrane. Type B atresias are minor ossicular malformations in which hearing loss ranges from mild to severe. Type C (total) atresia includes all with a totally atretic ear but a well-pneumatized tympanic cavity. (This would be called a minor malformation in the De La Cruz classification system.) Type D (hypopneumonic total) atresia is total atresia with poor pneumatization; it is common in dysplasias such as Treacher Collins syndrome. These patients are not good surgical candidates.

PATIENT EVALUATION AND COUNSELING (Fig. 28-16)

When a newborn is noted to have aural atresia, several issues must be addressed promptly. Other congenital anomalies must be identified. Syndromic children with aural atresia and associated cephalic abnormalities (Treacher Collins syndrome; hemifacial microsomia; Crouzon's disease; vertebral, anal, tracheal, esophageal, and renal anomalies [VATER]; coloboma, hearing deficit, choanal atresia, retardation of growth, genital defects, and endocardial cushion defect [CHARGE]; drug teratogenicity; Pierre Robin syndrome) should be recognized. Evaluation of auditory function in both unilateral and bilateral atresia should be performed using ABR within the first few days of life. There have been occasional cases of total sensorineural hearing loss on the side of the normal-appearing ear in cases of unilateral atresia.

In unilateral cases in which the opposite ear hears normally, a hearing aid is not necessary, in bilateral cases, a bone-conduction hearing aid should be applied as soon as possible, ideally in the third or fourth week of life. Implantable hearing aids are not recommended in children because the surgical scars may preclude any future microtic repair. Syndromic children will require long-term bone-conduction hearing aids because surgical correction in these patients generally has poor results.

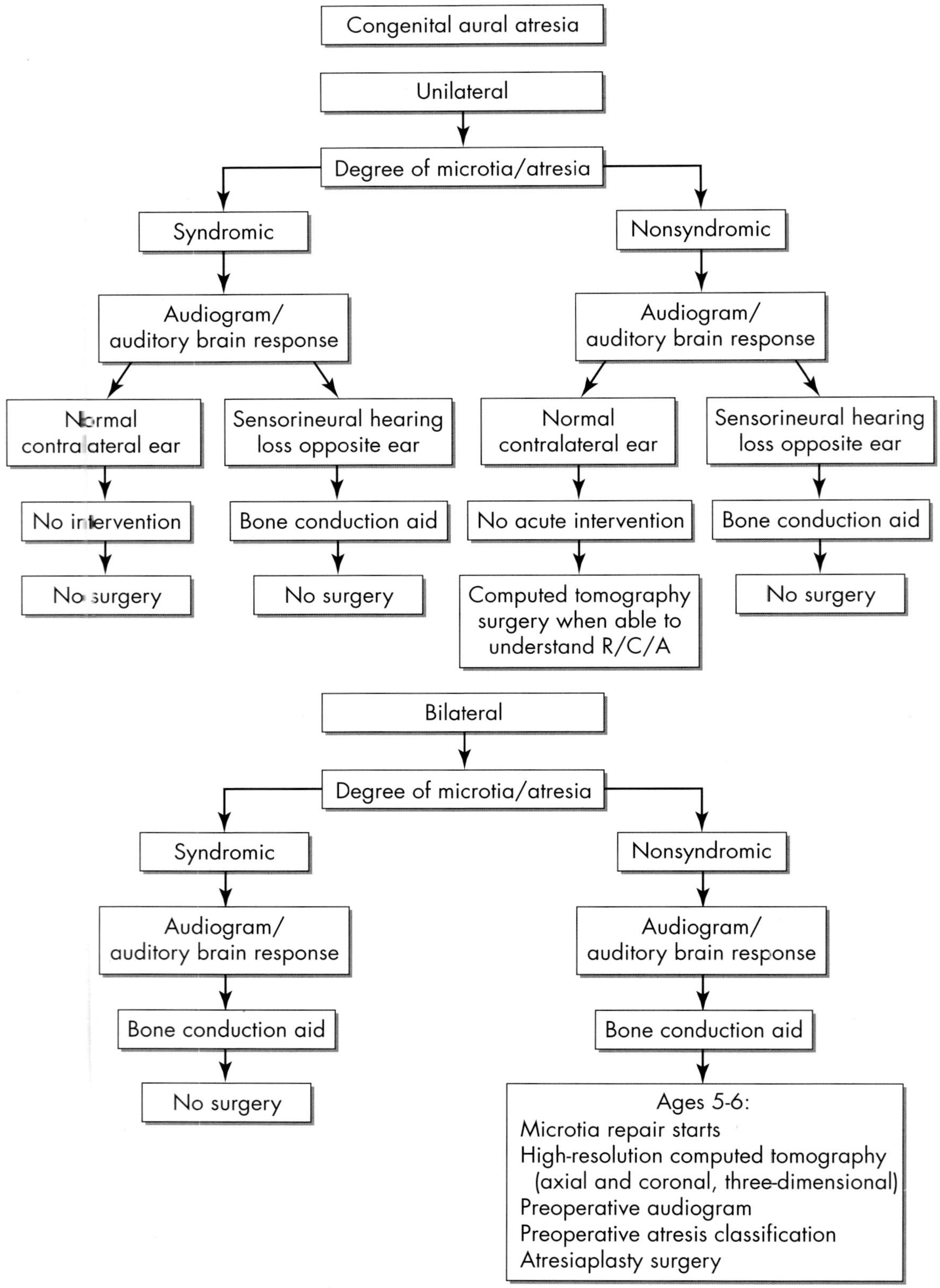

Fig. 28-16. The management of congenital aural atresia.

The parents of a child with sporadic (nonsyndromic) CAA should be counseled us follows. The risk of this problem in their subsequent children is no more than that in the general population; the child will probably require auricular reconstruction in the future; and, most importantly, the parents should understand that the patient requires proper hearing amplification to be instituted in a timely fashion in order to maximize speech and language acquisition and in preparation for "mainstreaming" the child into the regular classroom at the preschool age.

Radiologic and surgical evaluations are deferred until the child reaches 6 years of age. By this age, the costal cartilage has developed sufficiently to allow for harvesting and transplanting to create an auricle, and the mastoid has become as pneumatized as possible. The microtia repair is done first because the complex flaps and use of autologous rib grafts demand an excellent blood supply. Hearing restoration surgery is performed 2 months after the final stage of the microtia repair. Rehabilitation of severe auricular defects using tissue-integrated percutaneous mastoid implant prostheses with and without bone-conduction hearing aids has also been described.

In patients with unilateral atresia, atresiaplasty is delayed until the child is old enough to understand the significant risks to the cochlea, vestibular system, and facial nerve. The exception to this rule is a patient with a very thin unilateral atresia plate and normal pneumatization, ossicles, facial nerve, and inner ear. Surgery for this very minor atresia can be performed safely during childhood with the parent's consent.

Patients with CAA may present with an infected or draining ear and/or acute facial palsy; 14% have congenital cholesteatoma. Surgery in these cases is not elective but emergent, and the classification systems are not used for prognosticating outcome. Preoperative audiometry and CT are still necessary in these cases.

The only imaging modality acceptable for preoperative evaluation in patients with CAA is HRCT in both the axial and coronal planes. Three-dimensional CT is an interesting additional modality that has yet to prove its utility. The HRCT scan must be examined carefully by both the otologic surgeon and the otoradiologist. The four important imaging elements are the degree of pneumatization of the temporal bone, the course of the horizontal and vertical segments of the facial nerve, the existence of the oval window and the stapes footplate, and the status of the inner ear. CT also provides information on the thickness and form of the bony atretic plate, the size and status of the middle-ear cavity, the soft-tissue contribution to the atresia, and the presence of congenital cholesteatoma.

SURGICAL CAVEATS

The two requirements for elective surgery in CAA are radiographic evidence of an inner ear and audiometric evidence of cochlear function. In addition, it is preferable that the patient have a well-pneumatized mastoid and that there is a good facial nerve–oval window relationship. Fortunately, pneumatization is normal in the majority of cases. A clinical estimate of the size of the mastoid can be determined by palpation of the mastoid tip, the supramental spine of Henle (if present), the condyle, and the zygomatic arch. This is a useful measure because the new ear canal is constructed at the expense of the mastoid air-cell system. Depending on its severity, prolapse of the facial nerve over the oval window may prevent ossiculoplasty of the footplate. An absent oval window may necessitate either LSCC fenestration or creation of a neocanal and tympanic membrane and postoperative use of a conventional hearing aid.

There is significant potential for facial nerve injury in atresiaplasty. The nerve often ascribes a more acute angle than its usual 120° at the second surgical genu and often lies more lateral than usual. Even in atretic ears, where the facial nerve course is normal, the distances between the facial canal and the temporomandibular joint and the facial canal and the posterior wall of the cavum tympani are significantly reduced. Routine use of intraoperative needle electromyography of the facial nerve is indicated in all cases.

Use of the surgical laser to free the malleus–incus complex from its soft tissue attachments may result in less drill trauma transmitted to the inner ear and consequently less high-frequency sensorineural hearing loss. In addition, this technique may prevent delayed refixation of the ossicular mass.

Postoperative care is as important as proper surgical technique. Early identification of a narrowing meatus will allow for local dilation and restenting over a period of several months to 2 years, without the necessity for reoperation.

SURGICAL TECHNIQUE

General anesthesia is used in all cases. There is clear communication between the surgeon and the anesthetist to ensure that muscle relaxants are not used during the procedure, because this will negate the benefits of having placed a facial nerve monitor. The patient is in the otologic position with the head turned away from the surgeon. A large auricular area is shaved and prepared with iodine before the ear is draped in a sterile fashion. Additionally, the lower abdomen is shaved, prepared with iodine, and draped. Perioperative prophylactic cephalosporin antibiotics are used.

A postauricular temporo-occipital incision is made. When the patient has had prior microtia repair, it is imperative that the grafted costal cartilage not be exposed. The subcutaneous tissue and then the mastoid periosteum are elevated from the incision anteriorly to expose the temporomandibular joint space. Great care is taken not to inadvertently injure an anomalous facial nerve that may be exiting the temporal bone in this area. The temporomandibular joint space is explored to verify that the facial nerve or tympanic bone is not lying within it. A large piece of temporalis fascia is harvested and placed aside to dry.

Three approaches to the bony work necessary in atresiaplasty are described in the literature. Of these, the anterior and modified anterior approaches are the ones currently in use.

Anterior approach

If a remnant of tympanic bone is present, the new ear canal is begun through it; if there is no remnant drilling begins at the level of the lines temporalis, just posterior to the glenoid fossa. Dissection is carried out medially and anteriorly, keeping in mind the lack of landmarks in an atretic bone. The middle fossa plate is identified and followed to the epitympanum, where the fused malleus–incus mass is identified. The atresia plate is removed with diamond microdrills and curettes to completely expose the osicles. While dissecting inferiorly and posteriorly, an aberrant facial nerve can be encountered. The fibrous ligaments and bony adhesions now fixing the ossicular mass are vaporized with a CO_2 laser to avoid mechanical trauma to the inner ear. Although deformed, if the ossicular chain is intact it is kept in place rather than using a prosthesis. If the ossicular chain is not salvageable, a total or partial ossicular reconstruction prosthesis is used. Rarely is it necessary to drill out an obliterated oval window. Drilling is continued to create a new ear canal measuring about 1.5 times the normal size without exposing the temporomandibular joint space or an excessive number of mastoid air cells.

The previously prepared skin-graft donor site at the hypogastrium is exposed. A 0.012-inch 6-×-6–cm split-thickness skin graft is obtained. Hemostasis of the donor site is accomplished with pressure from a sponge wet with epinephrine 1:100,000 U and thrombin solution. When the donor site is dry, a sterile Opsite dressing is applied. One edge of the skin graft is cut in a zig-zag fashion such that four or five triangular points are created. The tip of each point and the two remaining 90° edges are marked with blue ink. The skin graft is kept moist and set aside.

The now-dry temporalis fascia is trimmed to a 20-× -1.5–mm oval. Small 3-×-5–mm "tabs" are cut into the anterior and superior aspects of the graft because it will be used for tympanic membrane grafting. If used, nitrous oxide is discontinued 20 minutes before grafting begins. The fascia is placed over the ossicular chain or over the cartilage covering the prosthesis, and the tabs are placed medially into the protympanum and epitympanum. All of these techniques are employed to prevent graft lateralization, the most common delayed cause of a poor hearing outcome.

The new ear canal is circumferentially lined with the skin graft. The zig-zags are placed medially to partially overlap the fascia. Because the points have been marked in blue, there is minimal risk of burying skin at this point. All bone of the EAC is covered. A single layer of antibiotic-soaked Gelfoam is used to hold the fascia and skin in place at the level of the new eardrum. A disk of 0.020-inch reinforced Silastic is placed over the tympanic membrane in order to reproduce the anterior tympanomeatal angle.

A 14-mm meatus is created because 30% of the diameter will reduce eventually as a result of the normal healing process. Care is taken not to expose or injure the cartilage of the microtia repair. The ear is turned and the lateral excess of skin graft is brought through the meatoplasty and sutured circumferentially to the meatal skin. A large Marocel ambrus ear wick is placed through the meatus into the EAC. This will apply diffuse pressure over the entire skin graft and allow for wide packing of the meatus. The postauricular periosteum is sutured back into place, and the incision is closed. The ear is dressed in the usual fashion.

Modified anterior approach

In patients with thick, bony atresia plates, maintaining orientation may be difficult during medial dissection. Because these mastoids have few air cells, landmarks are not easily identified and dissection too far in either the inferior or posterior direction risks inadvertent facial nerve or LSCC injury. Orientation is achieved in those cases with initial posterior dissection and limited exposure of the sinodural angle, enabling identification of the levels of the LSCC and the facial nerve. A new ear canal is created similarly to the anterior approach by following an "intact canal wall mastoidectomy" approach. The remainder of the surgery proceeds as described above.

Transmastoid approach

The transmastoid approach is no longer in use. Dissection is begun at the level of the linea temporalis, well posterior to the temporomandibular joint. The sinodural angle is identified and followed medially to the antrum. Mastoid air-cell exenteration and lowering of the facial ridge are performed, and the EAC is created as if in a canal wall–down mastoidectomy technique. The remainder of the operation proceeds as outlined above. The only additional step is bone pate or soft tissue obliteration of a large mastoid cavity before meatoplasty and canal skin grafting.

POSTOPERATIVE CARE

The patient is given a 5 day course of oral antistaphylococcal antibiotics. The mastoid dressing is removed on the first postoperative day. The clear dressing over the skin donor site is left on for 3 weeks because epithelization occurs under the plastic. The patient is seen 1 week postoperatively, during which the postauricular strips are removed as are the tacking ticron sutures at the meatus and the dried and crusted lateral end of the meatus pack. The patient is seen again in 2 weeks, at which time the dried portion of the pack is removed and the meatus is repacked with antibiotic-soaked Gelfoam. The patient is instructed to begin applying antibiotic suspension to the packing in the EAC twice daily. At the third postoperative visit, the Gelfoam and the Silastic disk are removed. The patient continues to use ear drops for

8 to 12 weeks. The first audiogram is obtained at 6 to 8 weeks. The patient is then seen at regular intervals in order to ensure that the canal does not restenose. Follow-up audiograms are obtained at 6 months, 1 year, and then yearly thereafter. Conscientious adherence to the postoperative routine on the part of both the patient and the physician is essential to ensure the best possible surgical outcome.

RESULTS

Chandrasekhar, De La Cruz, and Garrido[6] reviewed 92 atresiaplasty surgeries performed between 1985 and 1993. Of the cases studied, 37% were bilateral; of the unilateral cases, 77% affected the right ear. Eight ears were operated on emergently for acute infection; cholesteatoma was found in six cases and cholesterol granuloma in one. Long-term hearing results, which were available for 68 of the 92 cases, were very good. Of the primary operations ($n = 42$), 14% achieved closure of the air–bone gap to within 10 dB, 26% to within 20 dB, and 60% to within 30 dB. Of the revision surgeries ($n = 26$), 12% achieved closure of the air–bone gap to within 10 dB, 23% to within 20 dB, and 54% to within 30 dB. The stapes footplate was absent in four ears, three of which had an LSCC fenestration with good to excellent hearing. Absence of the incudostapedial joint was noted in 16%, and an ossicular replacement prosthesis was used in 22%. The facial nerve was in an abnormal position in 26% and was dehiscent in 23%.

Of the primary surgeries, 55% healed with no complications. The most common complications encountered included bony (12%) and soft tissue (10%) EAC stenosis and tympanic membrane lateralization (9%). Seventy-three percent of revision surgeries healed with no complications. At the time of revision surgery, the most common causes cited for failure of the primary surgery were lateralization of the tympanic membrane (42%), bony regrowth (35%), ossicular refixation (23%), granulation tissue (23%), soft tissue EAC stenosis (19%), and acquired cholesteatoma (8%). The most common complications following revision surgery were tympanic membrane lateralization (15%), bony EAC stenosis (12%), and epitheliitis (12%). Facial palsy was very uncommon, occurring once after primary surgery and once after revision surgery. One of these cases was a transient delayed palsy that recovered fully; the other was a lower-division palsy that developed secondary to a severe postoperative mastoid infection and only required surgical decompression.

A prior review of 302 atretic ears in 239 patients was done by De La Cruz, Linthicum, and Luxford[11] in 1985. Sixty-five patients underwent primary atresiaplasty. Hearing results were excellent, with 16% having an air–bone gap below 10 dB, 53% below 20 dB, and 73% below 30 dB. In six bilaterally atretic patients, the deformity was so severe that the procedure was terminated without hearing restoration. No patients had postoperative facial palsy. Twenty patients had revision surgery. Lateralization of the tympanic membrane was the cause of failure in 14 patients (22%). This is usually identified within 12 months. Five patients required reoperation for canal stenosis, and the other reason for revision surgery was persistent drainage. Eighteen of the 20 revision cases had had full-thickness skin grafting of the EAC initially. The change to split-thickness skin grafting has reduced the incidence of stenosis and the need for revision surgery. Nonetheless, hearing results following revision surgery have been very good: 10% closed the air–bone gap to within 10 dB and 60% closed the gap to within 20 dB. One patient had profound sensorineural hearing loss following a drillout for an absent oval window. There were no facial nerve injuries.[11]

Shih and Crabtree[24] reviewed 39 primary atresiaplasties and revealed long-term hearing results of 25 dB for mild atresia, 40 dB for moderate atresia, and 46 dB for severe atresia using a modification of the Altmann classification system. The two most common complications were stenosis (33%) and recurrent infections of the cavity and canal skin (31%); infrequently, lateralization or graft failure was encountered. Two cases of developmental cholesteatoma due to partial stenosis were encountered.

Jahrsdoerfer and others[11] reported postoperative speech reception threshold (SRT) in 86 ears with preoperative atresia grades of 5 through 9. Eight percent of ears had SRT scores of 10 dB or less; 63% had SRT scores between 15 and 25 dB; 22% had scores between 30 and 35 dB; and 7% had SRT scores higher than 35 dB. Over half of this least successful group had preoperative grades of 5 (poor) or 6 (marginal).

SUMMARY

The surgical management of CAA is a challenge. Early identification of hearing impairment, amplification, and speech and language therapy are crucial in bilateral cases. Cooperation with the auricular reconstruction surgeon will allow for both aesthetic and functional success. The use of strict radiologic and clinical criteria for surgical candidates is necessary. A logical classification system separating minor and major malformations should be used. The atresiaplasty surgeon should be an experienced otologist, have a thorough understanding of the embryologic maldevelopment, and adhere rigorously to the surgical principles of mastoidectomy, facial nerve dissection, and tympanoplasty in order to be able to offer patients optimal hearing restoration. Diligent postoperative office care is vital to maintaining the good results obtained at surgery. Patients should understand the possibility of requiring more than one procedure for an optimal outcome. When performed meticulously on appropriately selected patients by an experienced otologic surgeon, the results can be very rewarding.

REFERENCES

1. Aase JM: Microtia: clinical observations, *Birth Defects* 16:289, 1980.
2. Altman F: Congenital atresia of the ear in man and animals, *Ann Otol Rhinol Laryngol* 64:824, 1955.

3. Andrews JC and others: Three-dimensional CT scan reconstruction for the assessment of congenital aural atresia, *Am J Otol* 3:236, 1992.
4. Ars B, van Cauwenberge P, editors: *Middle ear structures: organogenesis and congenital defects*, Amsterdam/New York, 1991, Kugler Publications.
5. Brent B: Auricular repair with autogenous rib cartilage grafts: two decades of experience with 600 cases, *Plast Reconstr Surg* 90:355, 1992.
6. Chandrasekhar SS, De La Cruz A, Garrido E: Surgery of congenital aural atresia, *Am J Otol* 1995.
7. Chiossome E: *Surgical management of major congenital malformations of the ear.* Paper presented at the Politzer Society International Conference, Montreaux, Switzerland, September, 1983.
8. Crabtree JA: Tympanoplastic techniques in congenital atresia, *Arch Otolaryngol Head Neck Surg* 88:89, 1966.
9. De La Cruz A, Chandrasekhar SS: *Congenital malformation of the temporal bone.* In Brackmann DE, Shelton C, Arriaga M, editors: *Otologic surgery*, Philadelphia, 1994, WB Saunders.
10. De La Cruz A, Chandrasekhar SS: *Congenital malformations of the temporal bone.* In Lucente PE, editor: *Highlights of the instructional courses*, American Academy of Otolaryngology-Head and Neck Surgery, 1994.
11. De La Cruz A, Linthicum Jr FH, Luxford WM: Congenital atresia of the external auditory canal, *Laryngoscope* 95:421, 1985.
12. Dean LW, Gittens TR: Report of a case of bilateral, congenital osseous atresia of the external auditory canal with an exceptionally good functional result following operation, *Trans Am Laryngol Rhinol Otol Soc* 296, 1917.
13. Gill NW: Congenital atresia of the ear: a review of the surgical findings in 83 cases, *J Laryngol Otol* 83:551, 1969.
14. Granstrom G, Bergstrom K, Tjellstrom A: The bone-anchored hearing aid and bone-anchored epithesis for congenital ear malformation, *Otolaryngol Head Neck Surg* 109:46, 1993.
15. Jahrsdoerfer RA: Congenital atresia of the ear, *Laryngoscope* 88(suppl 13):1, 1978.
16. Jahrsdoerfer RA and others: Grading system for the selection of patients with congenital aural atresia, *Am J Otol* 13:6, 1992.
17. Kelemen G: Aural participation in congenital malformations of the organism, *Acta Otolaryngol (Stockh)* 321(suppl):1, 1974.
18. Marquet J and others: Congenital middle ear malformations, *Acta Otorhinolaryngol Belg* 1988.
19. Nager GT: Aural atresia: anatomy and surgery, *Postgrad Med* 29:529, 1961.
20. Ombredanne M: Chirurgie des (aplasies mineures): ses resultats dans les grandes surdites congenitales par malformations ossiculaires, *Ann Otolaryngol Chir Cervicofac* 81:201, 1964.
21. Page JR: Congenital bilateral microtia with total osseous atresia of the external auditory canals, operation and report of cases, *Trans Am Otol Soc* 13:376, 1914.
22. Pattee GL: An operation to improve hearing in cases of congenital atresia of the external auditory meatus, *Arch Otolaryngol Head Neck Surg* 45:568, 1947.
23. Schuknecht HF: *Congenital aural atresia and congenital middle ear cholesteatoma.* In Nado Jr JB, Schuknecht HF, editors: *Surgery of the ear and temporal bone*, New York, 1993, Raven Press.
24. Shih L, Crabtree JA: Long-term surgical results for congenital aural atresia, *Laryngoscope* 103:1097, 1993.
25. Van de Water TR, Maderson PFA, Jaskoll TF: The morphogenesis of the middle and external ear. *Birth Defects* 16:147, 1980.

Chapter 29

Acute Otitis Media and Otitis Media with Effusion

George A. Gates

Otitis media (OM) is the most common bacterial infection in children and the most frequent indication for antimicrobial or surgical therapy in this age group. It is also the leading cause of hearing loss in children. The morbidity associated with OM is substantial, and the costs of medical and surgical therapy for children 5 years of age and younger are estimated at $5 billion annually in the United States.[32] The number of operative procedures performed annually in the United States is estimated at about 600,000.[118] Given that prevention of OM by immunization is not widely available and that 85% of children experience at least one episode of OM, it is fair to say that this disorder is one of the most important, unresolved clinical problems in otolaryngology. Many factors predispose children to OM, but the impact of these factors is variable. Known risk factors are young age, male gender, bottle feeding, crowded living conditions (including multichild day care centers), smoking in the home, heredity, and a variety of associated conditions such as cleft palate, immunodeficiency, ciliary dyskinesia, Down syndrome, and cystic fibrosis. The genetic factors of OM have yet to be delineated, although it is well known that OM occurs more frequently in certain families.

Treatment of OM varies worldwide, with divergent results from numerous studies and clinical trials. The indications for therapy, particularly surgical therapy, remain controversial and often empiric. Although the widespread use of antimicrobial agents for OM has reduced the number of acute complications (most importantly intracranial extension of infection), the number of chronic complications, particularly hearing loss due to persistent middle-ear effusion (MEE), appears to be increasing. Because of the alarming increase in penicillin-resistant pneumococci,[17] attitudes about antibiotic use are changing. It is fair to say that acute OM (AOM) prophylaxis with long-term use of an antimicrobial agent, which has been the standard of practice in the United States for the past two decades, currently is discouraged.[88] It is likely that surgical therapy will be used more often in children with severe recurrent OM to reduce the number of new infections and to remove persistent effusion.

This chapter reviews current knowledge about OM based on contemporary clinical research. Emphasis is on treatment in the ambulatory setting within the context of the opposing forces of societal attitudes about cost containment and the continuing parental pressure for optimal care. As the chief providers of surgical care for children with OM, otolaryngologists frequently find their recommendations constrained by the policies of managed-care agents and their advisors who seek to control health-care costs by limiting surgical treatment, even though such therapy has been proven effective in reducing OM morbidity. Such policies typically examine only the short-term costs and fail to consider the long-term value. When the long-term impact of OM is considered, surgical therapy is more cost effective than medical therapy for severe cases.[32] With the welfare of patients as our primary concern, surgical therapy is selected from a rational, research-based, conservative protocol for patients for whom medical therapy fails and for whom there is no other choice for remediation of symptoms and correction of hearing loss.

BACKGROUND

Definitions

OM is used herein as a generic term for any inflammatory process in the middle-ear cleft beginning behind an intact tympanic membrane (TM). The two major classes of OM are AOM and chronic OM with effusion (COME). AOM is typified by the symptoms and signs of acute infection (fever, pain; a red, bulging TM; and MEE). COME indicates an MEE without pain, redness, or bulging of the TM. Equivalent terms are chronic secretory OM, chronic serous OM, and ''glue ear.'' MEE denotes a liquid in the middle-ear cleft regardless of etiology. Specifically excluded from this chapter are the various types of chronic suppurative OM associated with a permanent perforation of the TM or with cholesteatoma.

Clinical and functional anatomy

The middle-ear cleft is a continuous space that begins at the nasopharyngeal orifice of the eustachian tube and extends to the farthest mastoid air cells. The three main segments are the eustachian tube; the middle ear (tympanum); and the air cells of the mastoid, petrosa, and related areas. The middle-ear cleft is normally aerated and is highly variable in dimension, with each of the main segments delineated or constricted by narrow isthmi and subdivided by mucosal folds or by discrete, communicating cells. The physical characteristics of the TM that facilitate sound transfer also allow it to serve as a clinical window into the middle-ear cleft, one that permits inferences about the condition of the tympanum based on visible changes in the color, mobility, or position of the TM or from changes in the acoustic compliance of the middle-ear mechanism, as noted on immittance testing.

The mucosal lining of the middle-ear cleft varies from the thick, ciliated, respiratory epithelium of the eustachian tube and anterior tympanum to the thin, nonglandular cuboidal epithelium in the mastoid cells. Hyperplasia and an increase in the number of goblet cells are common findings in the middle ears of patients with OM.[106] These metaplastic changes, which predispose to the formation of effusion, are probably the result of the primary process. The tympanic mucous blanket is swept toward the nasopharynx by the coordinated action of the ciliated epithelium. This process clears secretions and particulate matter from the middle ear into the nasopharynx via the eustachian tube.

The normally closed eustachian tube opens briefly with swallowing and other maneuvers in which the tensor veli palatini muscle contracts (e.g., yawning). Equilibration of pressure in the middle ear to ambient pressure occurs during opening, provided the tubal lumen is unobstructed by inflammatory edema, secretions, or, rarely, neoplasm or trauma. Tubal opening is a reflex mediated by barosensors through Jacobson's nerve.[24] The closed eustachian tube protects the middle ear from the entry of unwanted materials, except during swallowing, when reflux of nasopharyngeal secretions may occur if the tube is patent and nasopharyngeal pressure rises substantially above that of the middle-ear cleft. The detailed morphology of the middle-ear cleft is described elsewhere.

EPIDEMIOLOGY

In a private pediatric practice in the southern United States, 84% of children had one episode of OM, 50% had three or more episodes, and 25% had six or more episodes; 9% of the children had 31% of the total episodes.[13] In the Greater Boston Otitis Media Study,[122] 93% of children had at least one episode of OM and 74% had three or more episodes. National statistics from the United States indicate an increasing prevalence.[129] The highest prevalence occurs in the first 2 years of life and decreases thereafter. OM is also most common in the first year of life in Finland, with 50% of first episodes occurring by the third year of life.[60] Howie, Ploussard, and Slayer[58] described the otitis-prone condition, noting that children with six or more episodes of AOM had in common onset of AOM before their first birthday and infection with *Streptococcus pneumoniae.*

OM is more frequent in the winter months regardless of climate, presumably due to crowding in schools and in large-group daycare centers during the upper-respiratory infection (URI) season. Henderson and others[51] confirmed the chronologic proximity of OM to URI in a daycare setting—regardless of time of year. Among the multiple risk factors for OM found to be statistically significant by Pukander, Karma, and Sipil,[99] attendance at a daycare center had the highest correlation.

Risk factors for OM identified by Teele, Klein, and Rosner[122] were male gender, bottle feeding, a sibling with OM, and early occurrence of OM. In addition to daycare, Pukander, Karma, and Sipil[99] found allergy, socioeconomic status, smoking by the mother, parental history of OM, and viral infections in the home to be significant risk factors; but birth weight was not significant and breast feeding was protective only until discontinued. The risk factors for AOM and COME are discussed together because they represent two stages of the same disorder, namely OM, and because in the studies in which the two are discussed separately the risk factors appear to be the same.

OM is more common in Native Americans than in whites. The incidence in blacks and whites is equal.[15] Differences in the size and angulation of the eustachian tube appear to be important in understanding racial predilection for or protection from OM.[23] However, submucous cleft palate and sinusitis are also more prevalent in Native Americans[124] and cannot be excluded as contributing factors to OM. Although impoverished living conditions have long been cited as a possible factor in OM, Shaw and others[112] found no variation in rates of OM in Arizona Native American children based on living conditions, number of persons in the home, sanitary conditions, method of infant feeding, distance to a healthcare facility, or mother's education.

The epidemiology of COME has been studied extensively in Denmark through several large-scale tympanometric serial screenings of children in different age groups.[126-127] These surveys showed that tympanometric evidence of COME was uncommon in newborns, that by 1 year of age 24% of ears had either a type-B (flat) or type-C2 (negative pressure < -150 daPa) tympanogram, and that the tympanometric patterns change spontaneously in the majority of examinations repeated at 3-month intervals. Improvement was noted more in the spring and summer months, and worsening was more prevalent in the winter months. The point prevalence of type-B tympanograms was greatest in 2- to 4-year-olds and declined after the age of 6 to 7 years.

PATHOPHYSIOLOGY

Historically, the pathophysiology of OM has been linked with abnormalities of eustachian tube function. The three classic functions of the eustachian tube are aeration, clearance, and protection of the middle ear. Early studies suggested that obstruction of the tube (i.e., underaeration) was the underlying problem. Newer work, however, has refined that concept to suggest that AOM is the result of bacterial entry into the middle ear (i.e., failure of protection). This entry is due to an abnormally patent (or compliant) tube rather than an obstructed one. Tubal obstruction along with failure of clearance, which are common findings in children with COME, may be secondary rather than primary processes. Evidence for these hypotheses is presented below.

Acute otitis media

That AOM is a bacterial disorder is beyond question. Worldwide, the same pathogens are cultured with remarkably similar frequency from the middle ears of children with AOM. Table 29-1 presents the results of cultures from children with AOM.[10] Viruses have been recovered from the middle ear in 20% of early cases, in some cases as the sole agent but more often with pathogenic bacteria.[65] Thus there is now evidence that respiratory viruses are important in AOM, both directly in the middle ear and indirectly as a cause of antecedent URI. Because the majority of cases of AOM have a bacterial etiology, it is logical to account for how the bacteria reach the middle ear. Although the evidence is indirect, it is reasonably persuasive. First, in usual cases of AOM, viral nasal infection precedes the ear infection.[51] Second, pathogenic bacteria subsequently appear and are found in the nasopharynges of 97% of patients with AOM, with correspondence to the organisms in the MEE in 69%.[57] Third, the adenoids of children with recurrent AOM contain pathogenic bacteria in clinically significant amounts.[12,21,96] Stenfors and Raisanen[119] noted a significant age correlation with middle-ear pathogens in the nasopharynges of clinically disease-free children; 57% of those under 2 years of age were culture positive compared with 40% of the 11- to 15-year-old children. Thus it appears that the adenoid is a bacterial reservoir in the nasopharynx in children with in AOM.

The most likely route of entry of nasopharyngeal microorganisms into the middle-ear cleft is via the eustachian tube. Reflux from the nasopharynx into the middle ear during swallowing has been demonstrated radiographically in OM-prone children by Bluestone and others.[9] Reflux is probably facilitated by nose blowing and closed-nose swallowing (i.e., Toynbee's maneuver)[63] or aspiration into the middle ear as a result of negative middle-ear pressure. One source of negative middle-ear pressure is sniffing.[2] Children with patulous eustachian tubes, in whom free flow of radiographic material into the middle ear occurs, have been shown by Bluestone and others[9] to be at high risk for OM. Bluestone, Beery, and Andrus[7] showed that young children have shorter, straighter, and more compliant eustachian tubes than do adults, which is an important factor in the pathogenesis of OM in children. Sade[106] was among the first to identify the open eustachian tube as a factor in AOM.

Table 29-1. Percentage of bacteria from middle-ear aspirates from children with acute otitis media from the United States, Finland, Denmark, and Japan

	United States* (n = 1,432 ears) 1980-1985	**Finland†** (n = 707 ears) 1977-1978	**Japan‡** (n = 1,227 ears) 1984-1986	**Denmark** (n = 147 ears) 1973
Streptococcus pneumoniae	29.8	33.8	45.9	19.1
Haemophilus influenzae	20.9	8.5	33.4	27.6
Branhamella catarrhalis	11.7	7.2	2.3	—
Streptococcus pyogenes	3.1	2.1	6.3	8.2
Staphylococcus aureus	1.6	5.0	5.0	17.1
Staphylococcus epidermidis	—	11.5	—	—
Other	19.1	3.0	3.9	—
No growth	19.6	39.3	7.2	—

From Bluestone CD and others, *Ann Otol Rhinol Laryngol* 99(suppl 149):43, 1990.
* From Rohn D, Wald ER, unpublished data, 1980-1985.
† From Karma P and others, unpublished data, 1986.
‡ From Takahara T and others, unpublished data, 1986.

During swallowing, the adenoid is elevated by the soft palate and, when large, may obstruct the posterior choanae and contribute directly to increased nasopharyngeal pressure and thus indirectly to reflux. Adenoid enlargement has long been postulated as a factor in OM,[91] but if reflux is indeed a sequela of adenoid enlargement, one would expect a greater prevalence of adenoid enlargement in children with OM. However, the evidence does not support this assumption. Adenoid size in children with OM did not differ from that of control children either radiographically[53] or by weight.[44] No difference was noted in the recurrence rate of effusion in children with large versus small adenoids, nor did the effect of adenoidectomy depend on adenoid size.[40,78,94]

The close proximity of the adenoid to the mouth of the eustachian tube has led many to presume the existence of a cause-and-effect relationship of adenoid-to–eustachian tube function. Under the working hypothesis that bacteria from the adenoid and nasopharynx enter the middle ear via the eustachian tube, it is unnecessary to postulate eustachian tube obstruction as a necessary precedent for AOM, as has been held since the time of Politzer.[97] Indeed, in the early stages of AOM, bulging of the TM and positive middle-ear pressure are common, yet there are no findings associated with eustachian tube obstruction. Furthermore, it has never been shown that the adenoid physically obstructs the eustachian tube; in fact, it has been shown that it does not. Honjo[56] studied 52 children with COME and compared eustachian tube function in those with a large adenoid, which appeared on fiberoptic endoscopy to obstruct the pharyngeal end of the eustachian tube, with those with a clearly open tube. No difference in the opening pressure or in positive-pressure equalization was noted between the two groups. Further, there was no difference in eustachian tube ventilation function before and after adenoidectomy. Therefore, Honjo concluded that the adenoid does not mechanically obstruct the eustachian tube.

Takahashi, Fujita, and Honjo[120] studied 10 adult patients with COME using a thin-pressure catheter and identified the site of eustachian tube obstruction in the distal part of the cartilaginous portion, 5 to 15 mm from the orifice, rather than at the orifice proper. Thus the role of eustachian tube obstruction as a precursor to AOM is called into question, and the locus of obstruction in chronic COME is likely to be within the eustachian tube rather than at its nasopharyngeal ostium.

The preceding findings suggest that eustachian tube dysfunction, which is clearly demonstrable in these children, may be the result of AOM rather than the cause of it. Thus the classic theories that the adenoid causes mechanical obstruction of the eustachian tube and that adenoidal enlargement is a factor in the pathogenesis of OM are not supported by current evidence. Improvement in eustachian tube function, however, does occur after adenoidectomy.[9,56] The exact mechanism for this effect is not clear, although relief from infectious stimulation may play a role (see the section on adenoidectomy).

Chronic otitis media with effusion

Although obstruction of the eustachian tube does not necessarily precede AOM, eustachian tube dysfunction is a nearly universal finding in children with COME. In addition, ligation of the eustachian tube in animal models invariably produces MEE. However, in humans the obstruction is probably secondary to the inflammatory process rather than the cause of it. The obstruction is usually functional in nature and is caused by edema, viscous secretions, or both.

There appear to be two broad categories of COME persistent MEE following an acute effusion and secretory OM. However, it is generally not possible to distinguish them on clinical grounds, except when the patient has been examined before onset.

In younger children at least, COME is most often the unresolved stage of AOM. In a long-term study of OM in infants and children, Teele, Klein, and Rosner[121] found persistent effusion (>30 days) in 40% of children after their first episode of AOM and continued effusion (up to 3 months) in 10%. Pathophysiologically this represents a failure of the middle-ear clearance mechanism. Factors that may be involved include ciliary dysfunction, mucosal edema and hyperplasia, viscosity of secretion, and possibly a middle-ear/nasopharyngeal-pressure gradient. Bacterial exotoxin causes a reversible paralysis of middle-ear cilia,[3] and inflammatory edema can obstruct middle-ear drainage. The high viscosity of MEE is well known to every otolaryngologist who has attempted to aspirate a middle ear. Any or all of these pathologic changes may functionally impede clearance of MEE. Negative middle-ear pressure may result from ciliary clearance of viscous secretions through the eustachian tube: as the bolus of secretion becomes impacted into the tube, the pressure decreases behind it, thereby drawing the TM inward. Fenestration of the TM, as with placement of a tympanostomy tube, relieves this negative pressure and aids clearance.

Many patients with COME, especially older children, have a silent onset without a clinically evident antecedent AOM, although most patients have a history of OM in earlier childhood. It is necessary, therefore, to postulate a second mechanism for the MEE in these cases. Secretion of fluid by the abnormal middle-ear mucosa (i.e., secretory OM) is held by many to be the origin.[105] Antigenic stimulation in an ear sensitized by prior infection may result in recurrent effusion in the absence of clinically identifiable acute infection.[105] The fluid in these cases is produced by the middle-ear mucosa in response to subclinical antigenic stimulation rather than by an overt acute inflammatory process. Many investigations have confirmed the finding of Senturia and others[110] that chronic MEE is not sterile, as previously hypothesized, and contains the same spectrum of microorganisms (Table 29-2) that is found in acute effusions. Thus

Table 29-2. Percentage of bacteria from middle-ear effusions from children with chronic otitis media with effusion from United States, Finland, and Japan

	United States (n = 4,483 ears) 1980-1985	**Finland (n = 510 ears) 1978-1984**	**Japan (n = 441 ears) 1984**
Haemophilus influenzae	14.7	8.0	20.2
Streptococcus pneumoniae	7.0	4.3	10.6
Branhamella catarrhalis	8.5	3.5	2.3
Streptococcus pyogenes	0.8	0.2	0.9
Staphylococcus epidermidis	—	7.5	—
Other	35.3	5.3	4.8
No growth	34.0	66.3	56.0

From Bluestone CD and others: *Ann Otol Rhinol Laryngol* 99:43, 1990.

the available evidence links chronic MEE, regardless of its clinical presentation, to bacterial infection.

Barotrauma is a known cause of MEE. When middle-ear pressure rapidly becomes lower than atmospheric pressure, a clear, watery transudate may form in the middle ear; this is known as serous OM. Serous OM is also seen sporadically in both children and adults, caused perhaps by viral infection and certainly by URI and acute eustachian tube dysfunction. The presence of negative middle-ear pressure in many people with URI and the subsequent formation of MEE led Politzer[97] to develop his hydrops *ex vacuo* theory as the source of MEE. Although the theory is attractive in its simplicity, the experimental data do not support the *ex vacuo* theory as the cause of COME (see the section on treatment of middle-ear inflation).

OM is nearly a universal finding in children with cleft palate, and the mechanisms and treatment have been studied extensively.[92] The principal defect is related to the function of the tensor veli palatini muscle, which, lacking its usual insertion into the soft palate, is unable to open the tube properly on swallowing. This creates a functional obstruction of the tube.

Histopathology of the temporal bone in cases of childhood OM shows vascular dilation and proliferation, mononuclear cell infiltration, thickening and metaplasia of the epithelium, gland formation, edema, and exudation. Sando and Takahashi[107] found eustachian tube malformation and inflammation in their patients with cleft palate and Down syndrome and a striking relationship of inflammatory changes in the middle ear to the degree of eustachian tube malformation.

Allergy has long been believed to be an underlying factor in the pathogenesis of OM. However, the evidence for and against this association is incomplete. It is not clear, for example, that the middle ear is an allergic target organ nor has the case been made that the observed findings are not simply the result of microbial-induced inflammation. Hurst[59] found a high prevalence of positive tests for allergy in children undergoing tympanostomy tube insertion as compared with a control group of a small number of adults without OM. It may well be the case that the immunologic findings in the MEEs of the children were specific for infectious OM, and the lack of these findings in the adult group merely reflects a different pathophysiologic disorder (i.e., eustachian tube dysfunction). Gates and others[40] found no higher prevalence of positive skin tests in children with OM than in the general community. Continued research is needed to clarify these contradictory data.

SEQUELAE

The adverse effects of COME on hearing and on the development of cognitive, linguistic, auditive, and communicative skills are of concern to parents and physicians alike. Although it is clear that severe hearing loss produces severe impairments, there is less agreement that mild hearing loss invariably produces mild impairment.

Research on both short-term and long-term consequences of OM with effusion has yielded mixed results.[26,29,37,100] Many children with recurrent OM with effusion show little or a very transient negative impact of the condition. However, there is considerable evidence that some children are especially at risk for negative consequences of OM with effusion for either environmental (e.g., low socioeconomic status) or biological reasons (children who are already late talkers for other, generally unknown, reasons).[34] In addition, certain aspects of language development appear to be especially vulnerable to the intermittent, fluctuating hearing loss caused by OM with effusion. These include articulation development, receptive vocabulary development, and phonologic awareness. Nittrouer[85] found that a group of 7 and 8 year-old children with histories of COME performed more poorly than a comparison group on measures of phonologic awareness. Thus phonologic awareness may be an important mediator of later academic difficulties for some children who experience recurrent OM with effusion as noted by Gravel and others.[47,48]

A number of studies have reported an adverse effect of OM on cognitive development. Holm and Kunze[54] were among the first to discuss this problem. In a study of 205 3-year-old children in Boston, Klein and others[66] found that in higher socioeconomic groups over 130 days of COME in early life is associated with significant language delays and lower intelligence quotient scores as compared with children with less than 30 days of COME. Thus there is evidence that COME has a retardive effect on development. What remains to be established, however, is the most effective strategy to counter this effect.

The differential effect of hearing loss on development (as opposed to just being chronically ill) needs to be established. Certainly, in many cases compensatory actions by the parents and teachers and, to an unknown degree, by the children themselves, may provide some remedy. Frequent or chronic illness of any type often has a deleterious effect on the child and family. Disruption of family life by an irritable, painful, or inattentive child plus the extra costs for physicians' services, time lost from work, and medications may place a financial and emotional strain on the family.

The otologic sequelae of OM are permanent perforation of the TM, chronic suppurative OM, tympanosclerosis, adhesive OM, ossicular necrosis, retraction pockets in the TM, cholesteatoma, and sensorineural hearing loss.[128] In social groups receiving prompt and effective medical therapy these sequelae are uncommon. In areas where health care is not readily available, however, these problems are common. With improved access to care the number of new cases of otologic sequelae decreased.[135]

DIAGNOSIS

The first step in diagnosis is usually the recognition of a problem by the child's caregiver. Older children will complain of earaches, but infants become fussy, sleep poorly, and often pull or tug at the affected ear. In infants, a fever often heralds the onset of AOM, but this sign may be absent in older children. Many parents are alerted by the URI that often precedes the AOM. Conversely, COME may be completely asymptomatic. Often the child is so accustomed to reduced hearing sensitivity that parents become aware of the problem only after the child turns up the volume of the radio or television or is not attentive during normal conversation.

Otoscopy

The normal TM is gray, concave, and translucent and moves briskly on pneumatic otoscopy. The classic signs of AOM are redness and bulging of the TM. In the beginning stages of AOM, the eardrum may bulge outward because of positive pressure in the middle ear, and it often moves normally. As effusion develops, drum mobility is decreased. In severe cases none of the usual landmarks may be visible. If the process continues to worsen, necrosis of the TM occurs and the effusion passes into the ear canal through a typically pinpoint perforation. Massive necrosis of the drumhead is rare, although necrotizing streptococcal infection is a known cause of permanent perforation.

In early or mild cases of AOM, considerable judgment must be used to differentiate subtle redness of the drumhead in crying children, whose struggles can result in vascular congestion of the TM that simulates OM. For this reason, assessment of TM mobility is vital to confirm the presence of MEE.

The pneumatic otoscope can be used to increase and decrease the pressure in the external auditory canal, and the TM should move inward and outward in synchrony with the pressure changes. In a healthy ear, pressures as low as 1 to 2 daPa result in detectable motion of the drumhead.[35] Use of the operating microscope improves the ability to make these subtle judgments. The best method to train the eye is to examine the ears just before myringotomy in the preoperative holding area. Comparing preoperatively recorded findings with the amount of MEE found at surgery is the surest way to develop good otoscopic discrimination for MEE. Most examiners quickly develop good sensitivity for the presence of effusion, but being confident about the absence of effusion (specificity) takes experience and practice.

A number of clinical variants of AOM are known and detectable otoscopically. Myringitis is an inflammation of the TM without MEE. The etiology and pathogenesis of myringitis are not well documented. In some cases, myringitis may represent the initial stages of bacterial AOM; in others, it may be due to a viral agent; in still others it may represent the effects of nose-blowing or sniffing. Because of the uncertainty of the clinical course of myringitis, most practitioners use the same treatment as for AOM. Bullous myringitis is seen in both adults and children. Early reports suggested an association with *Mycoplasma pneumoniae* infection. However, in most cases bullae on the TM are associated with the same pathogenic bacteria as AOM and should be treated similarly. Pain is an outstanding feature of bullous myringitis and is not relieved by opening the bulla(e). The classic findings of COME are a retracted, hypomobile or immobile TM and a dark, fluid-filled tympanum that obscures visualization of the long process of the incus. Negative middle-ear pressure is also associated with a retracted TM, but the membrane moves outward briskly when pressure in the ear canal is sharply reduced with the pneumatic otoscope. Judging the absence of MEE in the face of a retracted TM is often difficult.

Tympanometry

Tympanometry has an important place in the evaluation of children with middle-ear disorders. Ease of use, acceptance by patients, reproducibility of results, and availability of low-cost machines have led to widespread use of tympanometry in physicians' offices. By plotting the amount of energy reflected from the TM as the pressure in the external auditory canal is varied from −400 daPa to 100 daPa, a tympanogram is obtained, the shape of which provides considerable information about the status of the middle ear. When the tympanum is completely filled or impacted with effusion, compliance is low and the tympanogram is flat (i.e., does not vary with the pressure change). This shape was labeled type B by Jerger.[62] In air-containing ears the shape of the tympanogram is usually peaked, with the peak at −100 daPa (type A). Negative middle-ear pressure (i.e., below 150 daPa) with a sharp peak is labeled type C. Variants of these tympanogram types have been described for research purposes by Paradise, Smith, and Bluestone,[93] who pointed out that the ear canals of infants (<7 months) are hypercompliant, and normal tympanograms are possible in the presence of MEE. In these cases, the walls of the canals move with pressure, producing a ''canalogram'' rather than a tympanogram.

The type A tympanogram, which has a sharp compliance peak at ±100 daPa, suggests an aerated tympanum. Type B curves may be completely flat or have a very rounded compliance peak, which is often below −300 daPa. The type C tympanogram usually has a sharp peak between −150 and −200 daPa. Such tracings reflect negative middle-ear pressure and do not indicate effusion per se. When the pressure is below −250 daPa, the likelihood of MEE increases. Figure 29-1 shows the most common types of tympanometric curves seen in children with OM.

The acoustic reflex is often absent in children. As such, acoustic reflex testing has little usefulness in screening for OM or in making management decisions. However, if the tympanogram is normal, an absent reflex may indicate a sensorineural hearing loss.[19] Tympanometric screening should be considered for children in the early school grades, when OM is a frequent problem. The high sensitivity of tympanometry in screening programs often leads to overdiagnosis. Therefore, a modified protocol that restricts referrals to those with bilateral low-compliance tympanograms on two occasions 2 months apart appears to be a reasonable plan.[42]

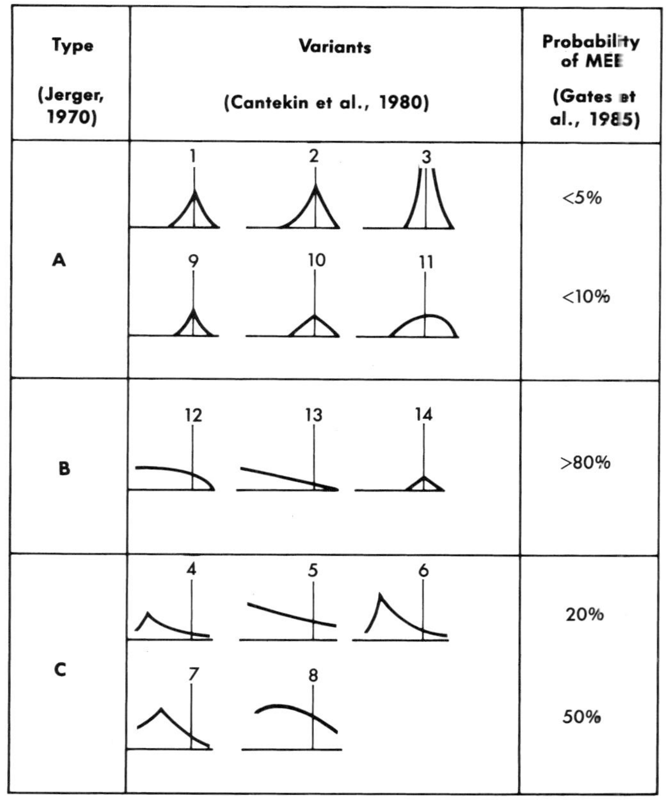

Fig. 29-1. Tympanometric patterns in otitis media. The vertical height of the pressure line is the same throughout only for comparison, as the units are arbitrary. Note that the shape of the curve (peaked or gradual), the height of the curve (proportional to the compliance of the middle ear), and the middle-ear pressure at peak compliance are all related to the classification and, in turn, to the likelihood of middle-ear effusion. The types correspond to Jerger's original classification;[62] the variants are adapted from Cantekin and others; and the likelihood of effusion is from Gates and others.[39]

Otoacoustic emissions

The active processes within the cochlea generate low-intensity sounds that may be recorded by a sensitive microphone in the ear canal. These emissions may be either spontaneous or induced by stimuli such as a click, a tone, or two tones of different frequencies. The latter stimuli result in a cubic distortion-product otoacoustic emission (OAE). The input/output function of the distortion-product OAE provides considerable information about the status of the middle ear and cochlea. Several commercial systems that record OAE are now available. However, the equipment and the distortion-product OAE measurement algorithms vary substantially; therefore one should be knowledgeable about these systems before investing in this technology. Distortion-product OAEs present at normal levels indicate a normally functioning cochlea and probably reflect the integrity of the outer hair cells, which are widely considered to be the source of the OAE. OAEs are easily concealed by middle-ear abnormalities; and in most patients with COME, distortion-product OAEs are absent because of a dual attenuation of both the stimulus and the response.

Audiometry

MEE that completely fills the middle-ear cleft usually results in a moderate conductive hearing loss. Small amounts of MEE may not alter hearing sensitivity. Many studies have shown the wide range of hearing loss in OM, with air-conduction thresholds averaging 27.5 dB.[28] Because of excellent cochlear sensitivity, as evidenced by bone-conduction thresholds less than audiometric zero in many children, even a significant MEE may not be detectable by audiometric screening methods. Therefore, school hearing screening programs are of limited value in detecting middle-ear disease. Because hearing loss due to MEE is a principal indication for surgical treatment of children with COME, audiometric testing is useful for validating the need for surgery in older children. In young children and infants with classic otoscopic and tympanometric findings, audiometry is unlikely to yield important new information that might alter clinical decisions.

The Agency for Health Care Policy and Research (AHCPR) guideline[117] for treatment of COME in young children recommends that audiometry be used in the decision algorithm for electing surgical drainage of the middle ear and that surgery should not be done if the pure-tone average is less than 20 dB. Unfortunately, audiometry is not always available, nor is it practical for 2-year-old children. Moreover, hearing levels may fluctuate frequently so that a normal pure-tone average on one day does not exclude abnormal thresholds on another. Thus the practicality of the audiometric recommendation of the AHCPR guideline may be limited. In older children, however, determination of hearing loss should be incorporated into the recommendations for surgery.

TREATMENT

Acute otitis media

Antimicrobial therapy

Antimicrobial therapy is the mainstay of treatment for AOM in the United States but not worldwide.[123] Modern agents are effective orally and are widely available, safe, and generally well tolerated. Due to the emergence of β-lactamase–producing strains of *Haemophilus influenzae* and the increasing role of *Branhamella catarrhalis* in OM,[114] it is important to consider using β-lactamase–resistant agents. In the past, only a minority of cases of AOM have been caused by β-lactamase–producing organisms, and it has not been cost-effective to use β-lactamase–resistant drugs, which are generally more expensive, as the first line of management. In many cities, however, the incidence of β-lactamase–producing organisms in AOM has risen to the point that amoxicillin may not be the best initial therapy.[84]

Duration of therapy is an important, unresolved issue. A 10-day treatment course is usually prescribed as a compromise between cost and adequacy of therapy. In children with AOM, comparable results were found by Meistrup-Larsen and others[80] after 2 versus 7 days of penicillin therapy and by Hendrickse and others[62] after 5 versus 10 days of cefaclor. The latter study noted a significantly higher failure rate with the 5-day treatment in children whose AOM resulted in a perforation; the authors recommend a full 10-day course for these more severe cases.

In communities where β-lactamase organisms are uncommon, amoxicillin is the first-line drug of choice in nonallergic patients. Trimethoprim–sulfamethoxazole and the combination of erythromycin estolate and sulfisoxazole (Pediazole; Ross Products Division of Abbott Laboratories, Columbus, Ohio) are appropriate alternatives except that the sulfas are not effective against the rare case of β-hemolytic streptococci.[131] If the inflammation does not show signs of response, the initial agent is discontinued and a second-line drug (e.g., cefaclor or amoxicillin–clavulanate) is used. Judgment and caution must be exercised if a short treatment course is chosen to ensure that the middle ear has been sterilized and that the infection is controlled. A 10-day course of treatment is generally used to ensure adequate therapy. Many cases would undoubtedly do well with a shorter course, but ensuring adequacy would increase costs because of the need for an interim physician visit. It is not possible with our current technology to predict which cases would do well with a shorter course of treatment. However, patients with severe AOM, especially those with spontaneous perforation, require full, if not prolonged, treatment.

Adjunct medical therapy

Because of the frequent association of OM and URI, use of a nasal decongestant to open the airway may be helpful, but antihistamines should be avoided because their atropine-like effect leads to drying of secretions. The combination of an antihistamine and decongestant was found not to affect the clearance of MEE.[14] Topical decongestants may be used for short periods, but prolonged use may actually worsen rather than improve the nasal airway because of rebound and sensitization of the nasal mucosa. A topical parasympathetic blocking agent that eliminates the problems associated with sympathetic agonists is now available in the United States. However, the utility of this treatment in children with sinusitis and OM remains to be explored.

Tympanocentesis

Knowledge of the specific organism is important for selection of therapy in cases of AOM occurring in premature newborns, immunocompromised patients, patients with progression of symptoms and signs while receiving an appropriate antimicrobial, patients with intracranial infection, and research subjects. The procedure is performed with an 18-gauge spinal needle attached to a 1-ml tuberculin syringe. No anesthetic is necessary. The needle is inserted into the anteroinferior quadrant of the TM, and the fluid is aspirated into the needle (Fig. 29-2). The fluid is then flushed out of the needle onto an agar plate containing appropriate media for middle-ear organisms. The needle hole closes too quickly for any significant drainage to occur, although the aspiration does temporarily decompress the middle ear.

Myringotomy

Although severe AOM has many of the clinical features of a closed-space abscess, incision and drainage (myringotomy) has proven to be of limited value. Myringotomy promptly relieves severe pain due to AOM in patients with severe pain[101] but adds little to either remission of infection or clearance of MEE in cases of AOM treated with amoxicillin–clavulanate.[25] In some European countries, myringotomy has been the mainstay of treatment of AOM,[22] with antibiotics being reserved for cases with persistent drainage.

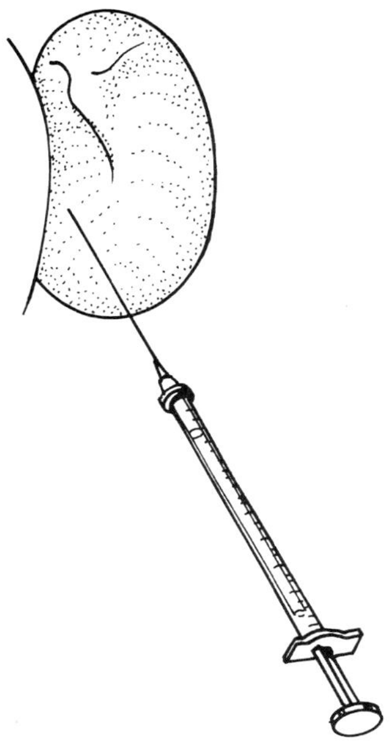

Fig. 29-2. Tympanocentesis. An 18-gauge spinal needle is attached to a 1-ml tuberculin syringe. Puncture of the tympanic membrane is performed in the anteroinferior quadrant, close to the anterior wall of the ear canal. The fluid is aspirated into the syringe and transferred onto an agar plate or into a transport medium.

van Buchem, Dunk, and Van't Hoff[130] have shown no difference in outcome of children with AOM whether antibiotic, myringotomy, both, or neither was used. However, the large number of methodologic flaws and the small number of subjects in each management group created substantial problems in interpretation. Although it appears that myringotomy does not offer sufficient benefit in the average case of AOM to justify its costs or risks, in complicated cases the procedure should be performed without delay to provide prompt drainage and material for culture. Such cases include AOM with facial paralysis, meningitis, or other central nervous system event; AOM not responding to antimicrobial therapy; and AOM in immunosuppressed individuals.

Follow-up

Follow-up examination is important for two reasons: to ensure that the infection is responding to the antimicrobial and to determine that the MEE has resolved. In infants and young children, follow-up is also important to exclude meningitis. In most of these cases, AOM and meningitis coexist rather than have a cause-and-effect relationship, but the signs of meningitis in infants may be subtle at first. Therefore, a 3-day check is often performed in infants for this reason and to determine whether the child is responding to the drug. A 2-week check is often performed to determine whether the MEE has cleared. The natural history of AOM indicates that only about half of the ears will have cleared at this point. Unfortunately, this is often taken as an indication for a second round of antimicrobial therapy, and it is not unusual to see asymptomatic children who have received four different antimicrobials for a single episode of AOM. There is little evidence to suggest that prolonged or repeated therapy is effective in the routine case of AOM. If the TM has ruptured, indicating a severe episode, it is prudent to continue the antimicrobial agent until drainage has ceased and the membrane has sealed.

Recurrent acute otitis media

Antimicrobial prophylaxis

Antimicrobial agents are effective in preventing AOM but they should not be used routinely because of the risk of promoting antimicrobial resistance in common pathogens. Several clinical trials have documented the efficacy of chemoprevention of AOM in children with frequently recurring ear infections[95,98a,131] Because of the risk of hypersensitivity reactions to the long-term use of sulfonamides, many practitioners use a single daily dose of amoxicillin (20 mg/kg) for 3 to 6 months to prevent recurrent AOM. Many use the fixed combination of trimethoprim–sulfamethoxazole even though the manufacturer's recommendations specifically prescribe against prolonged use for AOM prophylaxis. None of the studies has addressed the long-term consequences.

Barnett and Klein[4] expressed concern about the development of antimicrobial resistance in the common AOM pathogens from long-term antibiotic use, such as for AOM prophylaxis. Recent studies have compared modified regimens for prophylaxis. In a randomized, placebo-controlled study of 76 otitis-prone children 18 months of age and younger, Prellner and others[98] found that antimicrobial coverage with penicillin V during URIs reduced the number of episodes of recurrent acute OM with effusion (rAOME) by 50%. Berman and others[5] compared amoxicillin given twice daily for up to 4 months with intermittent amoxicillin during URI in 55 otitis-prone children. The continuous group ($N = 30$) had significantly fewer episodes of recurrent acute OM with effusion (eight) than did the intermittent prophylaxis group ($N = 25$, 12 episodes). Due to the worldwide emergence of resistant organisms, long-term use of antimicrobial prophylaxis is being questioned. Paradise[88] has argued against prophylaxis in most cases and earlier referral for tympanostomy tubes. Administration of an antibiotic in the early stages of URI reduces the number of new infections.[98] Short-term antimicrobial prophylaxis during the winter URI season has a long record of efficacy and is still being recommended in severely affected children.

Surgical prophylaxis

Surgical prophylaxis is being increasingly recommended for children with repeated episodes of AOM.[88] The efficacy of surgical prophylaxis has been established. Using a randomized, unblinded protocol, Gebhart[43] was the first to quantify the effectiveness of tympanostomy tube insertion in preventing recurrent AOM. Others showed a significant decrease in COME in patients undergoing tympanostomy tube placement versus placebo, but there was no difference between tympanostomy tubes and medical therapy. Casselbrant and others[16] demonstrated that tympanostomy tubes and antibiotic prophylaxis decreased the frequency of COME as compared with placebo but did not significantly reduce the incidence of recurrent acute OM with effusion. Le, Freeman, and Fireman[67a] compared unilateral tympanostomy tubes with unilateral myringotomy in treating 44 children with recurrent acute OM with effusion and 13 children with COME. The tubed ear had less infection while the tube was present, but the infection rate was the same for both ears after tube extrusion. Other studies[5a,73] in older children specifically addressed the impact of tympanostomy tubes on COME.

Adenoidectomy should logically also be an effective preventive treatment against recurrent AOM, but this hypothesis has not been adequately tested. In the San Antonio study,[40] the rate of new episodes of AOM in the two adenoidectomy groups did not differ from that of the two nonadenoidectomy groups.[40] However, these were older children in whom the rate of recurrent AOM is not great. In the Pittsburgh study,[94] there was a significant reduction in the number of episodes of AOM in each of the 2 years after adenoidectomy. These reports provide preliminary data about the efficacy of adenoidectomy in preventing AOM because this was not the primary research question. A clinical study of this question would be both appropriate and timely. Because logically there is little age difference in the outcome of surgical treatment, however, many otolaryngologists use adenoidectomy in the younger age group. The omission of adenoidectomy from the AHCPR recommendations was based on an age technicality that ignored the evidence of Paradise and others.[94]

Complications

The suppurative complications of AOM were not trivial in the preantibiotic era. Extension of the infection to involve the bone of the mastoid, soft tissues of the neck, meninges, and cerebral/cerebellar cortex was common. Today such problems are seldom seen except in areas where access to modern medical care is limited. The most likely patients seen by otolaryngologists today are those with postauricular tenderness and fullness in whom the diagnosis of mastoiditis is suspected. Because all severe cases of AOM have mucosal involvement of the mastoid, clouding of air cells on plain radiography or computed tomography is not unusual. These patients deserve prolonged antimicrobial therapy. The key sign of mastoid osteitis, namely demineralization of the air cell septae, lags behind the clinical findings. Once osteitis is diagnosed, mastoidectomy is generally warranted to remove the infected, often necrotic bone. In many of these cases, a subperiosteal postauricular abscess is present and surgery is performed for drainage of this pus and removal of the infected bone.

Intracranial complications are more common now in cases of chronic suppurative OM than in acute cases. Nonetheless, awareness of the possibility of meningitis, extradural abscess, or even brain abscess is an important part of the evaluation of patients with severe or neglected AOM.

Otitis media with effusion

Antimicrobial therapy

Otitis media with effusion, like AOM, is a bacterial disease, and the MEE is known to contain viable, pathogenic bacteria.[70] Antimicrobial therapy is a logical choice, and the efficacy of this therapy has been determined in several reports. In an uncontrolled study using the combination of erythromycin ethylsuccinate and sulfisoxazole (Pediazole), Gates and others[18,39] found that 45% of cases cleared by 1 month and 60% cleared by 2 months. In placebo-controlled trials by Healy[49] using trimethoprim–sulfisoxazole, by Mandel and others[73] using amoxicillin, and by Thomsen and others[127] using amoxicillin–clavulanate, the clear rates in the treated cases in each study were significantly greater than in the control groups. However, the magnitude of the difference was not great.[103]

The issue of antimicrobial treatment of COME has received much attention in the lay press because of overpublicized disputes among investigators. Williams and others[136] have clarified the issues and concluded that although there is statistical evidence of efficacy, the effectiveness of such therapy is slight. For children with asymptomatic COME discovered by screening or interval examination, a course of an appropriate antimicrobial, followed by at least a 1-month observation period, is recommended. If signs of improvement are noted by otoscopy or tympanometry, additional observation may be warranted. Surgical treatment may be considered if the effusion persists and is associated with hearing loss (see the section on surgical therapy).

Antihistamines and decongestants

To determine whether systemic medical therapy is of value in patients with COME, Cantekin and others[14] randomly assigned 553 infants and children with COME to receive either a decongestant–antihistamine or placebo. The clearance of COME did not differ between the two groups. As a consequence of this study, the routine use of decongestants in children with OM with effusion has been abandoned. However, specific nasal symptoms in patients with COME should be sought and treated as indicated. Moreover, acute and chronic sinusitis are not uncommon in children with OM. Therefore, symptoms of purulent rhinorrhea, nasal congestion, and cough should be followed up with appropriate investigation.

Middle-ear inflation

Because negative middle-ear pressure and retraction of the TM are common findings in patients with COME, middle-ear inflation has been used historically as a treatment option.[16] However, inflation, either by eustachian tube catheterization (Politzer's maneuver) or by autoinflation (Toynbee's maneuver), is not generally used in the United States, although inflation with nasal balloons is popular in Europe. Although transient aeration can be achieved, the long-term net effect is often to worsen the negative middle-ear pressure because the excess air injected into the middle ear passes out the eustachian tube, and the remaining oxygen is quickly absorbed through the middle-ear mucosa.[113] It is important to remember that the gas in the middle ear differs substantially from that in air, being hypercapnic and hypoxic, with gas tension values similar to those of arterial blood.[109] Therefore, middle-ear inflation with a different gas such as room air disturbs the equilibrium of the system and produces little lasting benefit. Transtympanic inflation of the middle ear with an inert gas or injection of mucolytic agents has been studied, but neither has proven to be practical.

The *ex vacuo* theory does not adequately explain negative middle-ear pressure without MEE. It has long been presumed that the oxygen in the middle ear is continuously absorbed until it is replenished by the ingress of nasopharyngeal air with swallowing. This effect would mean that middle-ear pressure would decrease during sleep or other states in which swallowing does not occur. However, it has been shown that resting middle-ear pressure in the morning is often slightly positive due to CO_2 retention.[71] Sniffing is a common practice in patients with a URI that may lead to negative middle-ear pressure.[55] Although the *ex vacuo* theory is probably valid in cases of barotrauma, in which there is a sudden drop in relative middle-ear pressure and formation of MEE from transudation due to capillary damage, it does not appear to play a role in AOM or COME.

Corticosteroids

The use of a short course of prednisone (1 mg/kg maximum dose) as a possible alternative to surgical therapy for the treatment of persistent COME was studied by Schwartz, Publese, and Schwartz,[103] who demonstrated a benefit, and by Lambert,[67] who did not. A randomized, double-blind, crossover experimental design was used in both studies with concomitant use of sulfisoxazole in the former and amoxicillin in the latter. Explanation and reconciliation of these contradictory results await further study. Although the risks of using a short course of corticosteroid are low in a child receiving an antimicrobial agent, the hazards of such therapy in the presence of a systemic viral infection should be kept in mind. For the moment, corticosteroid treatment of COME must be considered experimental. The AHCPR guideline did not recommend corticosteroid treatment.[102]

Surgical therapy

Although the efficacy of surgical therapy has clearly been established, there remains a wide range of opinions about its indications. The debate centers primarily on duration of effusion and whether persistent effusion, with its attendant mild conductive hearing loss, is harmful to the child's development. It is clear from the work of Klein and others[66] that even mild conductive hearing loss is a risk factor for impaired development. Gravel, Wallace, and Ruben[46] have shown long-lasting reductions in phoneme perception in children with documented frequent COME. It is undoubtedly true that this risk may be reduced through the compensatory measures of parents, teachers, and the children themselves; but this reduction is difficult to identify and quantify. Therefore, reduction of morbidity by surgical therapy remains an important option for parents of affected children, who often elect surgical treatment for prompt remediation of the hearing loss and avoidance of long-term sequelae. Surgical therapy does not cure patients with COME, but it does substantially reduce morbidity when medical therapy has failed.

For COME that persists more than 90 days despite adequate antimicrobial therapy, surgical treatment is an option for children with hearing loss and is recommended when the effusion and hearing loss persist for 4 to 6 months.[117] The uncertainty about duration of effusion criterion rests on the realization that effusions tend to resolve with time. Maw[76] however, has noted persistent effusion for up to 3 years in 40% of cases and for up to 5 years in 25% of cases (mean, 7.5 years). Thus a balance must be reached between the probability of spontaneous resolution versus the sequelae of prolonged morbidity and the risk of intercurrent infection. The time criterion is tempered by season. Surgery is recommended more often in the fall because of the high likelihood of exacerbation of the condition during the winter months; whereas in the spring, when otitis media and URIs are less prevalent, the effusion has a higher likelihood of spontaneous resolution and longer observation is warranted. Other, more urgent indications for surgical intervention, regardless of time of year, relate to structural abnormalities of the TM that may lead to ossicular erosion or cholesteatoma. These indications are retraction pockets in contact with the long process of the incus or the stapes or pockets in which epithelial debris accumulates, thus heralding an incipient cholesteatoma.

After a decision is made to treat the child surgically, a second decision remains about the type of procedure to be used. Historically, myringotomy, adenoidectomy, tympanostomy tubes, and even tonsillectomy have been advocated. Because tonsillectomy appears to have no additional effect on MEE over adenoidectomy alone in cases of COME,[74] it will not be discussed further.

Myringotomy. Evacuation of the MEE by myringotomy and suction aspiration has been studied as one type of therapy for COME. However, the results from this simple procedure have been disappointing.[37,72] Most investigators and clinicians agree that if a child is to receive an anesthetic for such treatment, then tympanostomy tubes should be inserted or an adenoidectomy performed (or both) because the cost: benefit ratio for myringotomy and aspiration is too low to justify myringotomy as an independent procedure.

Tympanostomy tubes. Modern tympanostomy tubes were introduced by Armstrong in 1954 and have become the therapeutic gold standard and the most widely used treatment option for COME.[1] Improved hearing and a decreased rate of recurrent AOM are predictable benefits of their use. The complications of tympanostomy tubes—purulent otorrhea, permanent perforation, and recurrent effusion—while minor, are a cause of concern, but most parents are willing to accept these small risks for the benefits accrued from improved hearing and freedom from OM while the tubes are in place. Nonetheless, the search continues for the most effective treatment strategy for children with COME.

Tympanostomy tubes are known by many different terms—pressure-equalizing tubes, grommets, bobbins, ventilating tubes—and are manufactured in a variety of shapes, sizes, and materials. Recent evidence suggests that the silver-oxide–impregnated tube has a significantly reduced rate of otorrhea.[18]

The two major types of tympanostomy tube are the short, generally grommet-shaped tubes and the long T-shaped tubes introduced by Goode.[45] Grommet-shaped tubes have retention times of a year or less, whereas the T-tubes may stay in place for several years. The risk of permanent perforation from the short-term tubes is about 1% and increases to a maximum of about 5% depending on the length of time the tube remains in place and the diameter of the tube. The larger T-tubes have longer retention times and a higher incidence of perforation. The factors that influence perforation have not been determined.

The rationale for using tympanostomy tubes is prolonged ventilation of the tympanum. Removal of the MEE and restoration of an aerated tympanum results in prompt return of hearing to preinfection levels in the vast majority of patients. Experimental evidence suggests that the mucosal hyperplasia of the tympanum will revert to a more normal condition with aeration.[106] Once the tubes are extruded, however, the clinical benefit appears to end.[40] Tubes appear to palliate the symptoms of middle-ear disease much as tracheostomy tubes bypass an upper-airway obstruction.

Many early investigators compared the effects of tympanostomy tubes in one ear and myringotomy in the opposite ear in children undergoing adenoidectomy.[64,68,69,111] The conclusions of these studies varied because the manifestations of OM may vary in the same child. Using a different design in which patients, not ears, were compared, Gates and others[40] found a significantly better outcome in terms of hearing, less time with MEE, longer time to recurrence, and fewer repeat operations in the children with tympanostomy tubes as compared with those undergoing myringotomy and aspiration. Similar conclusions were reached by Mandel, Bluestone, and Paradise.[72]

Paradise[40] and Paradise and Bluestone[91] argued that tympanostomy tubes should be used as the initial procedure of choice for patients with persistent COME, because tympanostomy tube placement is less involved and less expensive than adenoidectomy. They reserve adenoidectomy for cases of recurrent COME. Owing to the substantially higher rate of reoperation after tubes-only procedures, however, the greater initial expense of adenoidectomy may be negated by the cost of repeat intubation procedures, and the overall cost may be equivalent depending on hospital and physician charges.[41] In making such a decision, risks versus effectiveness should be considered in light of the needs of the child and family.

Technical considerations

Ototopic medications containing ototoxic agents are often used after tympanostomy tube insertion or later, if purulent otorrhea develops. Nonototoxic agents such as quinolone antibiotics are now available and should preclude the risk of possible sensorineural hearing loss and round-window absorption. Use of a silver-oxide–impregnated tube should reduce the incidence of postoperative otorrhea.[18,82]

Adenoidectomy

Adenoidectomy is being increasingly used again for the treatment of OM because recent studies have confirmed its effectiveness.[40,74,94] Adenoidectomy was once the principal surgical treatment for OM; with the widespread use of tympanostomy tubes, however, adenoidectomy was used far less often in the United States but not in other parts of the world.[83] Probable reasons for this difference were the following: adenoidectomy takes longer than tympanostomy tube insertion, adenoidectomy carries a risk of hemorrhage and other complications such as hypernasality, the mechanism of its effect on the middle ear is not well understood, and early studies failed to demonstrate its effectiveness.[27,104,133]

The adenoid (pharyngeal tonsil) forms the uppermost part of the ring of lymphoid tissue surrounding the oropharyngeal isthmus, described in 1884 by von Waldeyer.[132] Historically the term "adenoids" has been used loosely to indicate enlargement of the pharyngeal tonsil and does not mean that the adenoid is a bilateral structure. The adenoid is covered by respiratory epithelium that is rich in goblet cells and is plicated into numerous surface folds. Abundant lymphocytes are found within, especially on the crests of the folds. The adenoid develops as a midline structure by the fusion of two lateral primordia during early fetal life,[116] is fully developed during the seventh month of gestation, and increases in size until the fifth year of life, often causing some degree of airway obstruction. Thereafter the adenoid gradually atrophies, and with growth of the nasopharynx the airway improves.[61]

The adenoid is an important site of contact of inhaled microorganisms and other antigens with immunoreactive cells. The nasal mucociliary blanket carries material posteriorly across the adenoid. With the other components of Waldeyer's ring, the adenoid is important in the mucosal immunity of the upper aerodigestive tract, and like the palatine tonsil, the adenoid is regarded as a B-cell organ.

Rationale. The chief rationale for removal of the adenoid in children with OM has been enlargement, particularly that causing nasal obstruction and mouth breathing. Removal of a large adenoid that occludes the nasopharynx will open the airway and relieve the nasopharyngeal overpressure that occurs with closed-nose swallowing.[8] Removal should also lessen eustachian tube reflux. Although the proportion of children with OM caused by reflux is unknown, this rationale for adenoidectomy is logical. The association of enlargement with abnormality has been called into question, however, because adenoid and tonsil enlargement result from clonal expansion of immunocompetent cells.[31] This suggests that the large adenoid may be more immunocompetent than the small adenoid because chronic infection is associated with cellular depletion.[6] Brandtzaeg and Berdal[11] demonstrated a general decline in immunocytes in the tonsils of patients with recurrent tonsillitis. Thus current knowledge suggests that adenoid enlargement, a common phenomenon in 4- to 7-year-old children,[30] does not necessarily indicate abnormality. Basing the rationale for adenoidectomy in children with OM on size alone, therefore, has little scientific basis. Further, clinical evidence from three separate studies[40,75,94] indicates that the effect of adenoidectomy is independent of size. Removal of a large adenoid is a clinically attractive option because it offers symptomatic relief to a compromised airway; removing a small, chronically infected adenoid offers no obvious benefit except in controlling OM.

The other classic rationale for adenoidectomy is improvement in eustachian tube function. Honjo[56] showed improvement in equilibration of positive middle ear pressure following adenoidectomy but no change in the ability to equilibrate negative pressure and no change in the static opening pressure of the tube. Obstruction of the eustachian tube, either anatomic or functional, is a logical rationale for the procedure. Bluestone and others[9] showed that obstruction of the eustachian tube is unusual in most children with COME. The obstruction is functional in most cases. Eustachian tube function tests are not available except in research centers, and thus eustachian tube function is not routinely tested preoperatively. In children with hypercompliant eustachian tubes, adenoidectomy may increase reflux, particularly if the tissue in Rosenmüller's fossa is removed.[9]

The third and most current rationale is removal of the chronically infected adenoid to eliminate a nasopharyngeal source of infection.[36] Adenoidectomy should result in a smooth lining of the nasopharynx, which should decrease bacterial colonization of the nasopharynx and, indirectly, the middle ear. Further research is needed to develop the methodology to identify subgroups of children who might benefit the most from adenoidectomy for control of infection.

Efficacy. Recent studies of the efficacy of adenoidectomy have demonstrated consistent results even with variation in experimental design.[48,74,94] Several earlier studies, which showed a lack of effect of adenoidectomy,[27,104,133] were not sensitive enough to detect differences among the treatment groups that may have been clinically significant. Other older studies of adenoidectomy[77-79] are not reviewed here because of severe flaws in experimental design.[89]

Studies failing to demonstrate efficacy. Roydhouse[104] randomly assigned 100 children 3 to 14 years of age with COME to receive tympanostomy tubes with or without adenoidectomy. Otoscopy, which was performed annually, showed a slightly higher disease-free rate in the adenoidectomy group (82% versus 77% at 1 year, 85% versus 82% at 2 years, and 94% versus 84% at 3 years), but Roydhouse concluded that adenoidectomy was not effective.[104] Fiellau-Nikolajsen, Felding, and Fischer[27] observed 42 3-year-old children for 4 years who had been randomly assigned to receive bilateral myringotomy with or without adenoidectomy. No significant difference in outcome was noted at any assessment interval, even though nearly half the children had normal tympanograms preoperatively. The inclusion of a large proportion of patients destined to do well regardless of therapy may have decreased an already small sample size to the point that a clinically significant difference could not have been detected.

Widemar and others[133] nonrandomly assigned 59 children with mucoid effusion, selected from 78 patients with chronic OM undergoing myringotomy, to receive adenoidectomy or no adenoidectomy. After 2 years, otoscopy was normal in 13 of 24 patients (54%) who had adenoidectomy and in 13 of 35 patients (37%) who did not. They found this difference to be statistically insignificant but acknowledged that their limited sample size could not detect a difference of 30% or less between the groups.

Studies demonstrating efficacy. Maw[74] randomly assigned 103 children from 2 to 12 years of age (mean age, 5.25 years) with bilateral COME to one of three groups: adenotonsillectomy ($N = 34$), adenoidectomy ($N = 36$), or neither ($N = 33$). At surgery one ear was randomly assigned to receive a tympanostomy tube. The rate of clearance of MEE in the unoperated ear (as judged by otoscopy alone) was the criterion for success. At 3, 6, 9, and 12 months after surgery the clearance rates were 56%, 64%, 58%, and 72%, respectively, for adenoidectomy; 50%, 59%, 62%, and 62%, respectively, for adenotonsillectomy; and 22%, 26%, 19%, and 26%, respectively, for the control group. The difference between the two surgical groups and the control group at 12 months (71% versus 26%) was significant, but the difference between the adenoidectomy and the adenotonsillectomy groups (72% versus 62%) was not.

Gates and others[40] randomly assigned 491 4- to 9-year-old children with COME to surgical control, tympanostomy tube, adenoidectomy, or adenoidectomy plus tympanostomy tube. All children had failed on antimicrobial therapy, and none had prior tonsil or adenoid surgery. Bilateral myringotomy and suction aspiration of the middle ears were performed in all cases. Rosenmüller's fossa was not disturbed. The children in the two adenoidectomy groups experienced significantly less time with effusion and fewer repeat surgeries over the 2-year follow-up period than those who did not undergo adenoidectomy. There was no difference in time with abnormal hearing in the three surgical groups, regardless of whether tympanostomy tubes were placed. The reduction in morbidity (from control levels) in time spent with recurrent effusion was 29% with tympanostomy tube alone, 38% with adenoidectomy and myringotomy, and 47% with adenoidectomy and tympanostomy tube.

Paradise and others[44] examined the effect of adenoidectomy in two groups of children with COME recurring after prior tympanostomy tube placement. One group ($N = 99$) was randomly assigned; and the other ($N = 114$) was determined by parental choice for the procedure. In both groups, the outcomes for the adenoidectomized children were statistically better than for the control children for both follow-up years, with greater differences in the first than the second year. Adenoidectomy included routine curettage of Rosenmüller's fossa. In addition to significant reduction in time with effusion over time, the authors noted clinically significant reductions in AOM (28% and 35% in years 1 and 2, respectively) in the adenoidectomy group, which was statistically significant only in the second year.

These three recent randomized clinical trials, which had adequate sample size and frequent postoperative follow-up, have demonstrated statistically significant and clinically important effects from adenoidectomy in reducing morbidity in children with persistent COME. Thus the evidence supports the conclusion that adenoidectomy is effective in improving the natural history of COME in severely affected children 4 years of age and older.

Technical considerations. The goal of adenoidectomy is complete removal of the midline adenoid pad to achieve a smooth lining of the nasopharynx. Curettage of the tissue in Rosenmüller's fossa is performed by many who strive for complete removal of all upper pharyngeal tissue and not by others for fear of scar tissue formation and contracture, which may contribute to a patulous eustachian tube and reflux. In either case, care must be taken to avoid direct injury to the torus tubarius that might result in stenosis. From the authors' experience the latter complication is rare, whereas the incidence of the former is not known but is probably not uncommon.

Although the most common complication of adenoidectomy is postoperative bleeding, the incidence is low. Of 250 procedures performed by 13 surgeons, only one child required operative treatment for bleeding (0.4%) and none needed or received a blood transfusion.[40] Helmus, Grin, and Westfall noted that only four patients in 1000 (0.4%) bled after outpatient adenoidectomy, and all instances occurred in the first 6 postoperative hours and were managed without transfusion. Gates, Muntz, and Gaylis[23] showed the safety of adenoidectomy in young children (<3 years of age) undergoing surgery in a children's medical center; none of their 63 patients had postoperative bleeding.

Transient velopharyngeal insufficiency may occur after removal of a large adenoid but resolves quickly in the majority of cases. Persistent velopharyngeal insufficiency is the most feared complication because it requires either a prosthesis or a secondary procedure, such as a pharyngeal flap, for correction. Most cases of postoperative velopharyngeal insufficiency are caused by an undetected submucous cleft palate. Preoperative evaluation with fiberoptic nasopharyngoscopy is helpful in detecting an occult submucous cleft, which is often more obvious on the posterior than on the anterior surface of the palate.[20]

Reports regarding the immunologic consequences of tonsillectomy and adenoidectomy are conflicting, yet it is clear that no major systemic immunologic deficiencies result from these procedures.[115] Ogra[56] showed a threefold to fourfold drop in titers after tonsillectomy and adenoidectomy in children previously immunized with live poliovirus vaccine. Because adenoidectomy alone does not disturb the remainder of Waldeyer's ring, the likelihood of a major immunologic sequela developing from adenoidectomy alone is remote.

REFERENCES

1. Armstrong BW: A new treatment for chronic secretory otitis media, *Arch Otolaryngol Head Neck Surg* 69:653, 1954.
2. Aschan G, Ekvall L, Magnuson B: *Reverse aspiratory middle ear disease: a neglected pathogenic principle.* In Munker G, Arnold W, editors: *Physiology and pathophysiology of eustachian tube and middle ear*, New York, 1980, Thieme-Stratton.
3. Bakaletz LO and others: Effect of formalin-fixed *Haemophilus influenzae* and *Streptococcus pneumoniae* on dye transport by the chinchilla eustachian tube, *Acta Otolaryngol (Stockh)* 107:235, 1989.
4. Barnett ED, Klein JO: The problem of resistant bacteria for the management of acute otitis media, *Pediatr Clin North Am* 42:509 1995.
5. Berman S and others: Effectiveness of continuous vs. intermittent amoxicillin to prevent episodes of otitis media, *Pediatr Infect Dis J* 11:63, 1992.

5a. Bernard PA and others: Randomized controlled trial comparing long-term sulfonamide therapy to ventilating tubes for otitis media with effusion, *Pediatrics* 88:215 1991.

6. Bernstein J: *The tonsils and adenoid.* In Johnson J, editor: *American academy of otolaryngology-head and neck surgery instruction courses*, St Louis, 1990, Mosby.
7. Bluestone CD, Beery QC, Andrus WS: Mechanics of the eustachian tube as it influences susceptibility to and persistence of middle ear effusion in children, *Ann Otol Rhinol Laryngol* 83(suppl 11):27, 1974.
8. Bluestone CD, Cantekin EI, Beery QC: Certain effects of adenoidectomy on eustachian tube ventilatory function, *Laryngoscope* 85:113, 1975.
9. Bluestone CD and others: Eustachian tube function as related to adenoidectomy for otitis media, *Trans Am Acad Ophthalmol Otolaryngol* 76:1325, 1972.
10. Bluestone CD and others: Frequency of bacteria isolated from middle ear effusions of children from the United States, Finland, Japan, and Denmark, *Ann Otol Rhinol Laryngol* 99(suppl 149):42, 1990.
11. Brandtzaeg LS Jr, Berdal P: Immunoglobulin system of human tonsils. I. Control subjects of various ages: quantification of Ig producing cells, tonsillar morphometry and serum Ig concentration, *Clin Exp Immunol* 31:367, 1978.

12. Brook I: Aerobic and anaerobic bacteriology of adenoids in children: a comparison between patients with chronic adenotonsillitis and adenoid hypertrophy, *Laryngoscope* 91:377, 1981.
13. Brownlee RC and others: Otitis media in children, *J Pediatr* 15:636, 1969.
14. Cantekin RC and others: Lack of efficacy of a decongestant-antihistamine combination for otitis media with effusion ("secretory" otitis media) in children, *N Engl J Med* 308:297, 1983.
15. Casselbrant ML and others: Otitis media in a population of black American and white American infants 0-2 years of age, *Int J Pediatr Otorhinolaryngol* 33:1, 1995.
16. Casselbrant ML and others: Efficacy of antimicrobial prophylaxis and of tympanostomy tube insertion for prevention of recurrent acute otitis media: results of a randomized clinical trial, *Pediatr Infect Dis J* 11: 278, 1992.
17. Center for Disease Control: Prevalence of penicillin-resistant *Streptococcus pneumoniae*, Connecticut 1992-1193, *MMWR Morb Mortal Wkly Rep* 43:216, 1994.
18. Chole RA, Hubbell RN: Antimicrobial activity of Silastic tympanostomy tubes impregnated with silver oxide: a randomized, double-blind trial, *Arch Otolaryngol Head Neck Surg* 1215:62, 1995.
19. Cooper JC and others: An abbreviated impedance bridge technique for school screening, *J Speech Hear Disord* 40:260, 1975.
20. Croft CB and others: The occult submucous cleft palate and the musculus uvulae, *Cleft Palate J* 15:150, 1978.
21. DeDio RM and others: Microbiology of the tonsils and adenoids in a pediatric population, *Arch Otolaryngol Head Neck Surg* 113:763, 1988.
22. Diamant M, Diamant B: Abuse and timing of use of antibiotics in acute otitis media, *Arch Otolaryngol Head Neck Surg* 100:226, 1974.
23. Doyle WJ: *A functiono-anatomic description of eustachian tube vector relations in four ethnic populations: an otologic study*, doctoral dissertation, Pittsburgh, 1977, University of Pittsburgh.
24. Eden AR, Laitman JT, Gannon PJ: Mechanisms of middle ear aeration: anatomic and physiologic evidence in primates, *Laryngoscope* 100:67, 1990.
25. Englehard D and others: Randomised study of myringotomy, amoxicillin/clavulanate, or both for acute otitis media in infants, *Lancet* 2:141, 1989.
26. Feagans LV, Kipp E, Blood J: The effects of otitis media on the attention skill of day-care-attending toddlers, *Dev Psychol* 30:701, 1994.
27. Fiellau-Nikolajsen M, Felding J, Fischer H: *Adenoidectomy for eustachian tube dysfunction: long-term results from a randomized controlled clinical trial.* In Lim DL and others: editors: *Recent advances in otitis media with effusion*, Philadelphia, 1983, Mosby.
28. Fria TJ and others: Hearing acuity of children with otitis media with effusion, *Arch Otolaryngol Head Neck Surg* 111:10, 1985.
29. Friel-Patti S, Finitzo T: Language learning in a prospective study of otitis media with effusion in the first two years of life, *J Speech Hear Res* 33:188, 1990.
30. Fujioka M, Young LW, Girdany BR: Radiographic evaluation of adenoidal size in children: adenoidal-nasopharyngeal ratio, *Am J Radiol* 133:401, 1979.
31. Fujiyoshi T and others: Functional architecture of the nasopharyngeal tonsil, *Am J Otolaryngol* 10:124, 1989.
32. Gates GA: Cost-effectiveness considerations in otitis media treatment, *Otolaryngol Head Neck Surg* 114:525, 1996.
33. Gates GA, Muntz H, Gaylis B: Adenoidectomy; *Ann Otol Rhinol Laryngol* (suppl 155):24, 1992.
34. Gates GA: Workshop on effects of otitis media on the child: socioeconomic impact of otitis media, *Pediatrics* 71:648, 1983.
35. Gates GA: Differential otomanometry, *Am J Otolaryngol* 7:147, 1986.
36. Gates GA, Avery CA, Prihoda TJ: Effect of adenoidectomy upon children with chronic otitis media with effusion, *Laryngoscope* 98: 58, 1988.
37. Gates GA and others: Treatment of chronic otitis media with effusion: results of tympanostomy tubes, *Am J Otolaryngol* 6:249, 1985.
38. Gates GA and others: Medical treatment of chronic otitis media with effusion (secretory otitis media), *Otolaryngol Head Neck Surg* 94: 350, 1986.
39. Gates GA and others: Predictive value of tympanometry in middle ear effusion, *Ann Otol Rhinol Laryngol* 95:46, 1986.
40. Gates GA and others: Effectiveness of adenoidectomy and tympanostomy tubes in the treatment of chronic otitis media with effusion, *N Engl J Med* 317:1444, 1987.
41. Gates GA and others: Adenoidectomy and chronic otitis media, *N Engl J Med* 318:1470, 1988 (letter).
42. Gates GA and others: Diagnosis and screening, *Ann Otol Rhinol Laryngol* 98(suppl 139):39, 1989.
43. Gebhart DE: Tympanostomy tubes in the otitis media prone child, *Laryngoscope* 91:849, 1981.
44. Gerwat J: The structure and function of the lymphoid tissue with special reference to the etiology of secretory otitis, *J Laryngol Otol* 89:169, 1975.
45. Goode RL: T tube for middle ear ventilation, *Arch Otolaryngol Head Neck Surg* 97:402, 1973.
46. Gottschalk GH: Serous otitis: treatment by controlled middle ear inflation, *Laryngoscope* 72:1379, 1962.
47. Gravel JS, Wallace IF: Listening and language at 4 years of age: effects of early otitis media, *J Speech Hear Res* 35:588, 1992.
48. Gravel JS, Wallace IF, Ruben RJ: Early otitis media and later educational risk, *Acta Otolaryngol Stockh* 115:279, 1995.
49. Healy GB: Antimicrobial therapy of chronic otitis media with effusion, *Int J Pediatr Otorhinolaryngol* 8:13, 1984.
50. Helmus C, Grin M, Westfall R: Same-day-stay adenotonsillectomy, *Laryngoscope* 100:593, 1990.
51. Henderson FW and others: A longitudinal study of respiratory viruses and bacteria in the etiology of acute otitis media with effusion, *N Engl J Med* 306:1377, 1982.
52. Hendrickse WA and others: Five vs. ten days of therapy for acute otitis media, *Pediatr Infect Dis J* 7:14, 1988.
53. Hibbert J, Stell PM: The role of enlarged adenoids in the aetiology of serous otitis media, *Clin Otolaryngol* 7:253, 1982.
54. Holm VA, Kunze LH: Effect of chronic otitis media on language and speech development, *Pediatrics* 43:833, 1969.
55. Holmquist J: Eustachian tube function and upper respiratory tract infection, *Ann Otol Rhinol Laryngol* 94(suppl 120):41, 1985.
56. Honjo I: *Eustachian tube and middle ear diseases*, Tokyo, 1988, Springer-Verlag.
57. Howie VM, Ploussard JH: Simultaneous nasopharyngeal and middle ear exudate cultures in otitis media, *Pediatr Dig* 13:31, 1972.
58. Howie VM, Ploussard JH, Sloyer J: The "otitis prone" condition, *Am J Dis Child* 129:6768, 1975.
59. Hurst DS: Association of otitis media with effusion and allergy as demonstrated by intradermal skin testing and eosinophil cationic protein levels in both middle ear effusions and mucosal biopsies, *Laryngoscope* 106:1128, 1996.
60. Ingvarsson L and others: Epidemiology of acute otitis media in children, *Acta Otolaryngol Suppl (Stockh)* 388:1, 1982.
61. Jeans WD and others: A longitudinal study of the growth of the nasopharynx and its contents in normal children, *Br J Radiol* 54:117, 1981.
62. Jerger J: Clinical experience with impedance audiometry, *Arch Otolaryngol Head Neck Surg* 92:311, 1970.
63. Jorgensen F, Holmquist J: Otitis media and the blocked nose. In Lim DJ and others, editors: *Proceedings of the Fourth International Symposium on Recent Advances in Otitis Media*, Philadelphia, 1988, Mosby.
63a. Kemp D: Stimulated acoustic emission from the human auditory system, *J Acous Soc Am* 64:1386, 1979.
64. Kilby D, Richards SH, Hart G: Grommets and glue ears: two-year results, *J Laryngol Otol* 86:881, 1972.

65. Klein BS, Dollete FR, Yolken RH: The role of respiratory syncytial virus and other viral pathogens in acute otitis media, *J Pediatr* 101: 16, 1982.

66. Klein JO and others: *Otitis media with effusion during the first three years of life and development of speech and language.* In Lim DL and others, editors: *Recent advances in otitis media with effusion*, Philadelphia, 1983, Mosby.

67. Lambert PR: Oral steroid therapy for chronic middle ear effusion: a double-blind crossover study, *Otolaryngol Head Neck Surg* 95:193, 1986.

67a. Le CT, Freeman SW, and Fireman BH: Evaluation of ventilating tubes and myringotomy in the treatment of recurrent or persistent otitis media, *Pediatr Infect Dis J* 10:2, 1991.

68. Leek JH: Middle ear ventilation in conjunction with adenotonsillectomy, *Laryngoscope* 89:1760, 1979.

69. Lildholdt T: Unilateral grommet insertions and adenoidectomy in bilateral secretory otitis media: preliminary report of the results of 91 children, *Clin Otolaryngol* 4:87, 1979.

70. Liu YS and others: Chronic middle ear effusion: immunochemical and bacteriological investigation, *Arch Otolaryngol Head Neck Surg* 101:278, 1975.

71. Magnuson B, Falk B: Diagnosis and management of eustachian tube malfunction, *Otolaryngol Clin North Am* 17:659, 1984.

72. Mandel EM, Bluestone CD, Paradise JL: Myringotomy with and without tympanostomy tube insertion in the treatment of chronic otitis media with effusion, *Arch Otolaryngol Head Neck Surg* 115:1217, 1989.

73. Mandel EM and others: Efficacy of amoxicillin with and without decongestant-antihistamine for otitis media with effusion in children, *N Engl J Med* 316:432, 1987.

74. Maw AR: Chronic otitis media with effusion (glue ear) and adenotonsillectomy: a prospective randomized controlled study, *Br Med J* 287: 1586, 1983.

75. Maw AR: Age and adenoid size in relation to adenoidectomy in otitis media with effusion, *Am J Otolaryngol* 6:245, 1985.

76. Maw AR: *Glue ear in childhood: A prospective study of otitis media with effusion*, London, 1995, MacKeith Press.

77. Mawson SR, Adlington P, Evans M: A controlled study of adenotonsillectomy in children, *J Laryngol Otol* 81:777, 1967.

78. McKee WJE: A controlled study of the effects of tonsillectomy and adenoidectomy in children, *Br J Prev Soc Med* 17:49, 1963.

79. McKee WJE: The part played by adenoidectomy in the combined operation of tonsillectomy and adenoidectomy: second part of a controlled study in children, *Br J Prev Soc Med* 17:133, 1963.

80. Meistrup-Larsen KI and others: Two versus seven days penicillin treatment for acute otitis media: a placebo controlled trial in children, *Acta Otolaryngol (Stockh)* 96:99, 1983.

81. Meyer W: Adenoid vegetations in the nasopharyngeal cavity: their pathology, diagnosis and treatment, *Med Surg Trans* 53:191, 1870.

82. Morizono T: Toxicity of ototopical medications, *Ann Otol Rhinol Laryngol* 90(suppl 148):42, 1990.

83. Muenker G: Results after treatment of otitis media with effusion, *Ann Otol Rhinol Laryngol* 89(suppl 68):308, 1980.

84. Nelson JD: Emergence of *Branhamella catarrhalis* as a major cause of acute otitis media in Dallas, Texas, *Ann Otol Rhinol Laryngol* 99(suppl 149):41, 1990.

85. Nittrourer S: The relation between speech perception and phonemic awareness: evidence from low-SES children and children with chronic OM, *J Speech Hear Res* 39:1059, 1996.

86. Ogra PL: Effect of tonsillectomy and adenoidectomy on nasopharyngeal antibody responses to poliovirus, *N Engl J Med* 284:59, 1971.

87. Paul R, Lynn TF, Lohr-Flanders M: History of middle ear involvement and speech/language development in late talkers, *J Speech Hear Res* 36:1055, 1993.

88. Paradise JL: Managing otitis media: a time for change, *Pediatrics* 96: 712, 1995.

89. Paradise JL: Clinical trials of tonsillectomy and adenoidectomy: limitations of existing studies and a current effort to evaluate efficacy, *South Med J* 69:1049, 1976.

90. Paradise JL: On tympanostomy tubes: rationale, results, reservations and recommendation, *Pediatrics* 60:86, 1977.

91. Paradise JL, Bluestone CD: Adenoidectomy and chronic otitis media, *N Engl J Med* 318:1470, 1988 (letter).

92. Paradise JL, Bluestone CD, Felder H: The universality of otitis media in 50 infants with cleft palate, *Pediatrics* 44:35, 1969.

93. Paradise JL, Smith GC, Bluestone CD: Tympanometric detection of middle ear effusion in infants and children, *Pediatrics* 58:198, 1976.

94. Paradise JL and others: Efficacy of adenoidectomy for recurrent otitis media in children previously treated with tympanostomy-tube placement, *JAMA* 263:2066, 1990.

95. Perrin JM and others: Sulfisoxazole as chemoprophylaxis for recurrent otitis media, *N Engl J Med* 291:664, 1974.

96. Pillsbury HC III and others: Quantitative bacteriology in adenoid tissue, *Otolaryngol Head Neck Surg* 89:355, 1981.

97. Politzer A: *A textbook of diseases of the ear*, Philadelphia, 1883, Henry C Lea's Son.

98. Prellner K and others: Prevention of recurrent acute otitis media in otitis-prone children by intermittent prophylaxis with penicillin, *Acta Otolaryngol (Stock)* 114:182, 1994.

98a. Principi N and others: Prophylaxis of recurrent acute otitis media and middle-ear effusion. Comparison of amoxicillin with sulfamethoxazole and trimethoprim, *Am J Dis Child* 143:1414, 1989.

99. Pukander J, Karma P, Sipil M: Occurrence and recurrence of acute otitis media among children, *Acta Otolaryngol Stockh* 94:479, 1982.

100. Roberts J, Schuele M: Otitis media and later academic performance: the linkage and implications for intervention, *Top Language Disord* 11:43, 1990.

101. Roddey OF Jr, Earle R Jr, Haggerty R: Myringotomy in acute otitis media, *JAMA* 197:849, 1966.

102. Rosenfeld RM, Mandel EM, Bluestone CD: Systemic steroids for otitis media with effusion in children, *Arch Otolaryngol Head Neck Surg* 117:984, 199.

103. Rosenfeld RM, Post JC: Meta-analysis of antibiotics for the treatment of otits media with effusion, *Otolaryngol Head Neck Surg* 106:378, 1992.

104. Roydhouse N: Adenoidectomy for otitis media with mucoid effusion, *Ann Otol Rhinol Laryngol* 89(suppl 68):312, 1980.

105. Ryan AF and others: *Immunologically mediated models of chronic otitis media with effusion.* In Sade H, editor: *Acute and secretory otitis media*, Amsterdam, 1985, Kugler.

106. Sade J: Pathology and pathogenesis of serous otitis media, *Arch Otolaryngol Head Neck Surg* 84:297, 1966.

107. Sando I, Takahashi H: Otitis media in association with various congenital disease, *Ann Otol Rhinol Laryngol* 99(suppl 148):13, 1990.

108. Schwartz RH, Publese J, Schwartz DM: Use of a short course of prednisone for treating middle ear effusion: a double-blind crossover study, *Ann Otol Rhinol Laryngol* 89(suppl 68):296, 1980.

109. Segal J and others: *Mass spectrometric analysis of gas composition in the guinea pig middle ear-mastoid system.* In Lim DL and others, editors: *Recent advances in otitis media with effusion*, Philadelphia, 1983, Mosby.

110. Senturia BH and others: Studies concerned with tubotympanitis, *Ann Otol Rhinol Laryngol* 67:440, 1958.

111. Shah N: Use of grommets in glue ears, *J Laryngol Otol* 85:283, 1971.

112. Shaw JR and others: Observations of the relation of environmental and behavioral factors to the occurrence of otitis media among Indian children, *Public Health Rep* 96:342, 1981.

113. Shinkawa H, Ishidoya M, Okitsu T: Changes in tympanograms after middle ear inflation, *Arch Otorhinolaryngol* 247:125, 1990.

114. Shurin PA and others: Susceptibility of beta-lactamase-producing strains of *Branhamella catarrhalis* as important agents of acute otitis media, *Pediatr Infect Dis J* 2:34, 1983.

115. Siegel G: The influence of tonsillectomy on cell mediated immune response, *Arch Otolaryngol Head Neck Surg* 239:205, 1984.
116. Slipka J: The development and function of the pharyngeal tonsil in early ontogenesis, *Cesk Otolaryngol* 30:201, 1981.
117. Stool SE and others: *Otitis media with effusion in young children: clinical practice guideline technical report No. 12*, AHCPR Pub No 94-0622, Rockville, Md, 1994, Agency for Health Care Policy and Research, Public Health Service, US Department of Health and Human Services.
118. Stool SE, Field MJ: The impact of otitis media, *Pediatr Infect Dis J* 8:11, 1989.
119. Stenfors L-E, Raisanen S: Occurrence of middle ear pathogens in the nasopharynx of young individuals: a quantitative study in four age groups, *Acta Otolaryngol (Stockh)* 109:142, 1990.
120. Takahashi H, Fujita A, Honjo I: Site of eustachian tube dysfunction in patients with otitis media with effusion, *Am J Otolaryngol* 8:361, 1987.
121. Teele DW, Klein JO, Rosner BA: Epidemiology of acute otitis media in children, *Ann Otol Rhinol Laryngol* 89(suppl 68):5, 1980.
122. Teele DW, Klein JO, Rosner BA: The Greater Boston Otitis Media Study Group: Epidemiology of otitis media during the first seven years of life in children in Greater Boston: a prospective cohort study, *J Infect Dis* 160:83, 1989.
123. Thomsen J and others: Penicillin and acute otitis media, *Ann Otol Rhinol Laryngol* 89(suppl 68):271, 1980.
124. Thomsen J and others: Antibiotic treatment of children with secretory otitis media, *Arch Otolaryngol Head Neck Surg* 115:447, 1989.
125. Tos M, Poulsen G: Tympanometry in 2-year-old children: seasonal influence of frequency of secretory otitis and tubal function, *J Otorhinolaryngol Relat Spec* 41:1, 1979.
126. Tos M, Poulsen G, Hancke AB: Screening tympanometry during the first year of life, *Acta Otolaryngol (Stockh)* 88:388, 1979.
127. Tos M and others: Spontaneous course and frequency of secretory otitis in four-year-old children, *Arch Otolaryngol Head Neck Surg* 108:4, 1982.
128. Tos M and others: Spontaneous course of secretory otitis and changes of the eardrum, *Arch Otolaryngol Head Neck Surg* 110:281, 1984.
129. Vital and Health Statistics: *Series 10: Data from the National Health Survey No. 190*, Centers for Disease Control and Prevention, National Center for Health Statistics, US Department of Health and Human Services. DHHS Pub No 95-1518, Hyattsville, Md, 1994.
130. van Buchem FL, Dunk JHM, van't Hoff MA: Therapy of acute otitis media: myringotomy, antibiotics, or neither, *Lancet* 2:883, 1981.
131. Varsano I, Volvitz B, Mimouni F: Sulfisoxazole prophylaxis of middle ear effusion and recurrent acute otitis media, *Am J Dis Child* 139: 631, 1985.
132. von Waldeyer W: Uber den lymphatischen Apparat des Pharynx, *Dtsch Med Woschenschr* 10:313, 1884.
133. Widemar L and others: The effect of adenoidectomy on secretory otitis media: a 2-year controlled prospective study, *Clin Otolaryngol* 10:345, 1985.
134. Wiet RJ: Patterns of ear disease in the southwestern American Indian, *Arch Otolaryngol Head Neck Surg* 105:381, 1979.
135. Wiet RJ and others: Natural history of otitis media in the American native, *Ann Otol Rhinol Laryngol* 89(suppl 68):14, 1980.
136. Williams RL and others: Use of antibiotics in preventing recurrent acute otitis media and in treating otitis media with effusion: a meta-analytic attempt to resolve the brouhaha, *JAMA* 143:1414, 1993.

Chapter 30

Tympanostomy Tubes

Andrew F. Inglis, Jr.

Tympanostomy tube (TT) insertion is one of the most commonly performed surgeries in the United States, and the debate over its utility is proportional to the frequency with which it is performed. There are those who laud the procedure as one that restores hearing, decreases the morbidity of an illness that can be a tremendous drain on family resources, and may prevent persistent or permanent cognitive delays caused by longstanding early auditory deprivation. Others vilify the procedure as one that is unlikely to be beneficial even in the short-term and may be a potential cause of permanent damage to the tympanic membrane (TM) with an associated hearing loss. The stakes in this debate are extremely high based on resource consumption associated with otitis media (OM). Considering TT placement alone, an estimated 1.3 million operations were performed in 1988, with an overall OM prevalence rate of 1.3% in all children, and over 3% in children aged 2 years and under.[10]

Tympanostomy tubes improve middle-ear health during periods of eustachian tube dysfunction. A detailed description of eustachian tube function can be found elsewhere in this text. Briefly, the eustachian tube has three main functions for maintaining middle-ear health: aeration and pressure equalization, middle-ear drainage, and barrier protection. The first two functions are accomplished by the frequent brief openings of the eustachian tube valve, and the third function is achieved by maintaining appropriate closure of the eustachian tube valve. Most types of OM are caused by derangements of eustachian tube function (usually age-related, occurring most commonly in toddlers) along with an inadequate or inappropriate immune response (also usually age-related). TTs can be thought of as a form of ''eustachian tube bypass,'' and as such very effectively support the functions of aeration and drainage. Because eustachian tube dysfunction in children most often takes the form of an inadequate valve opening, restoring aeration and drainage often corrects the condition leading to OM. Conversely, TTs may promote OM in two ways. First, if the eustachian tube opens during periods of high intranasal pressure (e.g., nose-blowing), air may escape through the tube, allowing potentially infectious nasopharyngeal secretions to be blown into the middle ear. Second, the middle ear can be exposed to contaminants through the ear canal. Finally, TTs will in no way address an underlying immune immaturity or deficiency. Taken in balance, TTs generally greatly reduce the rate of OM in most patients.

The potential benefits of maintaining a small hole in the TM were recognized early on (dating back to the 1700s) by several practitioners. The modern era of TT placement began in 1954 with Armstrong's report[5] of successful, albeit brief, middle-ear ventilation with straight polyethylene tubes. Since that time, TTs have been made in an enormous variety of shapes and materials. Most fall into one of two types—grommet style tubes, which generally remain *in situ* for 6 months to a year, and the so-called ''permanent tubes,'' of which the T-tube is an example.

Rational indications for TT placement are drawn from a number of factors, including efficacy of the procedure compared with alternative management options; the drawbacks, risks, and potential complications of each form of management; costs; and expectations regarding the natural history and morbidity of the disease. Because TTs are effective in treating subsets of patients within the entire spectrum of OM disease states, it is impossible to draw a simple set of guidelines. The following discussion will include indications for TT placement, perioperative considerations, and potential complications.

Box 30-1. Conditions in which tympanostomy tube placement may be indicated

Recurrent acute otitis media
Chronic otitis media with effusion in healthy children
Otitis media or eustachian tube dysfunction coexisting with other medical conditions:
- Craniofacial anomalies
- Down syndrome
- Underlying sensorineural hearing losses
- Other (e.g., patients undergoing hyperbaric therapy)

Tympanic membrane abnormalities (e.g., severe retraction, atelectasis, impending ossicular chain erosion, or cholesteatoma)

Box 30-2. Factors influencing decisions about tympanostomy tube placement in "otitis-prone"* children

Factors making tympanostomy tube placement desirable:
- Severe pain with most bouts of acute otitis media (OM)
- Long (weeks or more) periods of OM with effusion following individual bouts of acute OM
- Hearing loss of 25 dB or more with OM with effusion
- Attendance in a large-group (six or more children) childcare setting
- Language or developmental delays
- Antibiotic allergies
- Poor response to medical therapy
- First bout of OM prior to 6 months of age
- Older siblings
- Craniofacial or syndromic anomalies predisposing to OM
- An underlying hearing loss
- Balance disorder with acute OM
- Pacifier use
- Other medical conditions whose management is complicated by OM

Factors making tympanostomy tube placement less desirable:
- Mild symptoms with acute stages of infection
- Good response to medical therapy
- Little or no hearing loss with OM with effusion

* A child with a history of four or more bouts of acute OM in the last 6 months, six or more bouts in the last 12 months, three or more months of bilateral OM with effusion, or 6 or more months of unilateral OM with effusion.

INDICATIONS

Situations in which TT placement may be indicated are listed in Box 30-1. TT placement does not "cure" the underlying conditions leading to OM, and thus these tubes are only effective for as long as they are in place and patent. The overall safety of TTs is quite good, acknowledging the complications listed below. Other drawbacks to TT usage include the need for long-term follow-up by a skilled otoscopist and the issue of water precautions. The following discussion outlines the natural history of the various pathologies, the efficacy of TTs for these pathologies, and reasonable guidelines for TT placement. Far and away the most common indications for TT placement are recurrent acute OM and OM with effusion; and while these entities are discussed separately, they frequently occur simultaneously in a given patient. Box 30-2 summarizes some of the factors to consider when deciding on a recommendation of TT placement in these children.

Recurrent acute otitis media

The severity of recurrent acute OM is affected by the presence of risk factors and by patient age. Children in group childcare settings are much more likely to be otitis-prone; and the larger the group, the higher the incidence of recurrent acute OM will be—with the rate doubling in groups of six or more children—as compared with their at-home counterparts.[1] As many as one in four infants or toddlers will have recurrent acute OM at a rate of six cases per 12-month interval at some point while in a group childcare setting. Although the course in an individual child is impossible to predict, certain generalizations can be made. Most otitis-prone infants and toddlers do not experience the seasonal variation of OM that the general, less severely affected population experiences.[64] The rate of recurrence generally does fall off dramatically in the ensuing year for the majority of otitis-prone children younger than 2 years of age. Overall, a reduction in the rate of recurrent acute OM by about 50% per year,[35] or 3.5 bouts fewer per year in the most severely affected children, can be expected.[49] Other factors contributing to an increased rate of recurrent acute OM in the general population include early age at onset of the first bout of acute OM, the presence of older siblings in the home, pacifier use, and possibly exposure to cigarette smoke.

Surprisingly few randomized studies have examined the use of TTs for the prevention of recurrent acute OM, and all studies can be criticized for design limitations that make extrapolation to the typical clinical population difficult. Casselbrant and others[12] randomized patients with recurrent acute OM into three groups comparing amoxicillin, TTs, and placebo. TTs did no better than amoxicillin in preventing the onset of new OM, defined as either acute OM behind an intact eardrum or otorrhea through a TT or TM perforation, but TTs did significantly reduce the time with OM of any type compared with amoxicillin. Both forms of management elicited significantly better results than placebo by both measures. Gebhart[24] randomized patients younger than 3 years of age who had three or more bouts of acute OM in the preceding 6 months to either TTs or observation and found the rate of acute OM in the surgical group to be less than half that of the control group. With similar entry criteria, Gonzalez and others[26] randomized patients to TTs, antibiotic prophylaxis, or placebo and defined management failure as two or more bouts of acute OM in less than 3 months.[26] They found failure rates of 23% in the TT group, 38% in the antibiotic group, and 60% in the placebo group. Differences between groups were statistically significant. In a model of bilateral OM in which one ear was intubated and the other served as a control, Le, Freeman, and Fireman[35] showed that TTs reduced the rate of recurrent acute OM by half as compared with the control ear.

In most of these studies the control group had a much less significant otitis burden on average during the management period. One difficulty in designing a good study mirrors the physician's paradox by the time a population of children has been declared "prone" to recurrent acute OM, a significant proportion has "outgrown" the problem. This decline in frequency of recurrent acute OM would make the issue of TT efficacy for preventing recurrent acute OM a moot point were it not for the significant minority (20% to 30%) of patients who continue to be severely affected and the larger subset that is at least moderately affected. Given the effectiveness of TTs in the setting of recurrent acute OM, it would be most useful to be able to predict which children will be otitis prone prior to the "season of crisis" or, lacking this, predicting which of the children who have been declared otitis-prone will continue to be so.

It is thus difficult to answer the following questions: How much reduction in morbidity of recurrent acute OM will TTs produce in a given child? Is this reduction worthwhile, given the risks and expense? Making a firm set of indications for TT placement for recurrent acute OM given the marked tendency for spontaneous improvement of the process is difficult. Although a good starting point would be three or more bouts of acute OM in the preceding 6 months or four or more bouts in the preceding 12 months,[3] the decision should not be based solely on some arbitrary number of bouts of acute OM per unit of time. A physician's recommendation should include a prediction of future rates of acute OM during the period the TTs are expected to remain in place. This prediction will be based on factors such as current patient age and age at onset of acute OM, group childcare attendance, and the presence of siblings. Other factors to consider are the degree of morbidity caused by a typical infection, the frequency and duration that each bout of acute OM is complicated by OM with effusion, the tolerance of and response to antibiotic therapy, and any other mitigating or extenuating factors that may be present. Some of these factors are outlined in Box 30-2.

One issue that has not been adequately addressed, but that undoubtedly will play a larger role in the future, is the extent to which the rapidly rising percentage of multidrug-resistant middle-ear pathogens, particularly *Streptococcus pneumoniae*, will alter the threshold of a recommendation for TT placement. A decrease in the prophylactic and therapeutic efficacy of first-line antibiotics has not yet been established in clinical trials, but this will likely change within the next few years. This development may make the recommendation for TT placement much more attractive in many instances.

Persistent otitis media with effusion

Otitis media with effusion is a common sequela of acute OM, and differing rates of spontaneous clearance have been reported. Various meta-analyses have reported short-term resolution rates between 16% and 32%.[49,63] Zielhuis, Rach, and van den Broek[65] reported long-term resolution rates of 65% at 3 months and 85% at 6 months. The main adverse effect of OM with effusion is hearing loss, which can be as little as 10 dB or as much as 30 dB or greater from 250 to 4000 Hz. Hearing loss in these cases can fluctuate between the two extremes. Losses of 20 dB or more will certainly hinder the child's understanding and appreciation of his or her surroundings; whether it will also lead to delays in short- or long-term speech and language acquisition or have lasting consequences for cognitive development is debatable. Some studies support the notion that the hearing loss during extended intervals of OM with effusion can lead to speech and language problems that persist at least into later childhood,[56] whereas others do not.[31,45]

Several studies have shown that TTs are highly effective in reversing the main adverse effect of OM with effusion—hearing loss.[7,8,11,58] In a prospective study, Gates and others[23] showed the percentage of time with a 20-dB hearing loss in the better ear in the 2 years following TT placement to be 19% in the "control" group (myringotomy only) and 10% in the TT group.[2] In all of these studies, the hearing improvement is limited to the length of time the tube is in place and patent. After 6 months, differences in the TT and control groups became less distinct as more TTs extruded, some of these ears reacquired a middle-ear effusion, and spontaneous clearance occurred in some control ears.

Given the uncertainty about whether hearing loss from OM with effusion in toddlers causes speech or language difficulties in school-age children, it is difficult to show that intervening with TTs will prevent short- or long-term speech and language delays for a significant number of affected children. The few small studies that have compared scholastic aptitude in children with unoperated OM with effusion with those who had TT placement do not show significant differences.[27,48]

Taking all this into consideration, TT placement should be seriously considered in cases of bilateral OM with effusion that has been present for 3 or more months if the hearing loss in the better ear is 20 dB or greater. This is appropriate purely for the short-term improvement in quality-of-life afforded by acquiring normal hearing, if not for cognitive advancement. The recommendation for TT placement is stronger when the child is having problems that may be exacerbated by a hearing loss such as speech and language delays or behavioral difficulties that may be borne of frustrations associated with not hearing well. Other symptoms that may be relieved are the intermittent otalgias or balance disorders that are sometimes present. If bilateral OM with effusion is present and TT placement is deferred because the hearing threshold is better than 20 dB in the better ear, prudence dictates frequent monitoring of the status of the TM, middle ear, and hearing to rule out evolving damage to the TM or progression to or persistence of a mild to moderate hearing loss. These indications are similar to those put forth by the Otitis Media Guideline Panel of the Agency for Health Care Policy and Research Clinical Practice Guidelines for children between 1 and 3 years of age.[43]

While this chapter focuses on management with TTs, it must be emphasized that adenoidectomy should be considered a mainstay of surgical management for OM with effusion, particularly in children older than 3 years of age. The efficacy of and indications for adenoidectomy are covered elsewhere in this text.

Frequent otitis media in patients with an underlying sensorineural hearing loss

The additional 10- to 30-dB hearing loss produced by a middle-ear effusion can significantly complicate efforts to take advantage of residual hearing in patients with an underlying hearing loss. A mild sensorineural hearing loss functionally becomes a moderate loss, a moderate loss becomes a severe loss, and a severe loss becomes a profound loss. Increasing levels of loss increase the magnitude of habilitative challenges, and the stable hearing level potentially afforded by TT placement in these patients is extremely desirable.

Cleft palate and other craniofacial abnormalities

The presence of a cleft palate per se is not an indication for TT placement, but severe eustachian tube dysfunction with longstanding OM with effusion and hearing loss is the norm in patients with cleft palate. Smith, DiRuggiero, and Jones[55] reviewed 81 cases and concluded that adequate recovery of eustachian tube function typically took 6 or more years following palatal repair; that 67% of ears without TTs but only 7.5% of ears with TTs demonstrated a greater than 20-dB hearing loss; and that short-acting TTs were associated with a much higher reintubation rate than long-acting TTs.

A multitude of other syndromes with associated craniofacial abnormalities is also associated with severe eustachian tube dysfunction as well as underlying conductive and sensorineural hearing loss. TT placement should be considered earlier and for a longer term in these patients because a fluctuating conductive hearing loss can make habilitative efforts in these children more challenging.

Suppurative complications of acute otitis media

Placement of at least a short-term TT may be warranted as an adjunctive measure when managing complications such as mastoiditis, facial nerve paralysis, or intracranial otogenic infections. TTs provide more consistent drainage of the middle ear than does simple myringotomy.

Severe tympanic membrane retraction with hearing loss, impending cholesteatoma formation, or ossicular chain erosion

Untreated TM atelectasis is frequently complicated by the difficult problems of cholesteatoma and erosion of the long process of the incus and eventual ossicular chain discontinuity. The former can lead to a host of devastating complications and the latter to a permanent conductive hearing loss. The preceding TT retraction/atelectasis can frequently be completely reversed by timely TT placement.

Hyperbaric oxygen therapy

Presswood and others[47] examined rates of middle-ear complications in patients managed with hyperbaric oxygen therapy. Of those undergoing hyperbaric oxygen therapy, 45% had middle-ear complications, including severe pain, hemotympanum, and OM with effusion. This rate increased to 94% of patients who required an artificial airway during therapy and presumably could not equalize middle-ear pressure during the ''dive.'' TT placement effectively prevents these difficulties and should be considered for routine use in these patients.

PERIOPERATIVE CONSIDERATIONS

Preoperative evaluation

An accurate history is obviously important, and a parent's narrative regarding the frequency and severity of the OM should be corroborated with the medical record because parents are prone to exaggeration when describing the level of otitis burden in their children.[2] Age-appropriate audiometry should be performed perioperatively in virtually all cases because there is a small but significant incidence of unsuspected sensorineural hearing loss in these patients.[38] Further, it stands to reason that confirmatory audiograms should be obtained preoperatively for all patients undergoing TT placement primarily for hearing loss, such as in otherwise uncomplicated OM with effusion, because the hearing loss produced by this condition can occasionally be negligible.

Anesthesia

Nearly all younger children and a large percentage of older children will require a general anesthetic for TT placement. A sedative premedication such as midazolam may be given to smooth out an inhalational anesthetic induction. A volatile agent (typically halothane) is used for induction. Sevoflurane, an agent recently approved for use in children in the United States, may lessen the need for premedication because it produces a very rapid induction and is not as noxious and thus is much better tolerated than halothane during nonpremedicated inhalational inductions. Avoidance of premedicating agents is desirable because it allows for faster emergence and a shorter stay in the recovery unit. An intravenous line is started at the option of the anesthesiologist. During the procedure, the patient's airway is typically maintained via a facemask and oral airway, although a laryngeal mask airway may be superior in terms of reducing episodes of hypoxia and producing a quieter field for the surgeon.[61] Recovery is generally quite rapid, and the procedure is routinely performed on an outpatient basis.

Some patients may be candidates for local anesthesia during TT placement. Prerequisites include a cooperative child who can lie still for several minutes and favorable ear anatomy, including a large ear canal and a TM that will not require much manipulation (as is sometimes necessary in cases of TM atelectasis). Because many adults and nearly all children will not tolerate subcutaneous infiltration of local anesthetics through even a very small needle, the procedure uses topical anesthesia. Topical anesthetic options include phenol, lidocaine delivered with iontophoresis, and a eutectic mixture of lidocaine and prilocaine (EMLA).

Concentrated phenol applied to the TM rapidly produces anesthesia and blanching. The TM can then be incised and the tube inserted. In the author's experience, the degree of anesthesia is often insufficient to allow for a painless myringotomy. Phenol may cause perforations in some cases.[36]

With the iontophoresis technique, a 60:40 mixture of 4% lidocaine and 1:1000 epinephrine is instilled into the ear canal. An electrode is applied to the ear canal, and a second grounding electrode is applied to an extremity. A small electric current supplied by a battery-powered device is applied for 10 minutes. Frequently an unpleasant tingling sensation occurs for the first few minutes; this is occasionally severe enough to require termination of the procedure. After 10 minutes the anesthesia is usually excellent unless the TM is acutely inflamed. TT tube placement proceeds in the usual fashion.

A third technique involves filling the medial-ear canal with EMLA and allowing it to sit for an hour. The cream is removed with suction and the tube inserted. A recent clinical trial suggested that this technique produced better anesthesia than did phenol.[36]

Tube selection

The ideal TT would be easy to insert, remain *in situ* as long as desired, be easily removed in the office without anesthesia, and be associated with few complications. The incomprehensible array of TTs currently on the market shows that such a tube does not exist; however, manufacturers will continue to tempt surgeons with TTs in a wide range of shapes, base materials, and coatings. Each ''breakthrough'' TT is brought to market with much fanfare, but rarely are clinical trials performed to support their claims of superiority. One example is the titanium TT. Titanium was touted to be a superior material because its light weight would produce fewer acoustic effects, and its surface could be highly polished, which would decrease bacterial and mucus adherence. When actually studied, however, titanium TTs were found to produce more infection and granulation tissue than did the less high-tech alternatives.[54] A notable exception that has undergone clinical testing is the silver-oxide–impregnated TT, which in a recent randomized trial showed significantly lower rates of otorrhea than did nonimpregnated tubes.[13]

Most TTs are variations of the grommet or the T-tube. Generally speaking, the larger and stiffer the flange, the longer the tube remains *in situ*. Small-flanged grommet tubes such as the Donaldson tube generally remain in place for 6 months to a year and are associated with a low rate of TM perforation (usually less than 5%). TTs of this genre should be considered for most cases of TT placement in otherwise healthy children in whom spontaneous improvement in otitis-prone status is expected within that time frame.

The T-tube deserves special mention. It will remain *in situ* for extended periods when designed with long, stiff flanges and is one of the few tubes that is easily removed in the office without an anesthetic. Thus T-tubes could potentially serve as either long- or short-term tubes. The big disadvantage of T-tubes is the high reported rate of perforation. The perforation rate can be reduced to less than 10% if a short-flanged T-tube of soft silicone is used, although the rate of spontaneous extrusion is somewhat higher with this configuration. Using a longer-lasting tube such as a T-tube may significantly reduce the necessity of reinsertion,[62] and this advantage may outweigh the drawback of a higher rate of perforation in some cases. T-tubes are appropriate for certain patients such as those with craniofacial anomalies in whom a long-term tube is desirable, as an ''emergency'' tube in patients with anatomically difficult ears if the flanges are trimmed to be very short, or even in young, severely affected children with many risk factors who are more likely to have long-term difficulties. T-tubes have a great advantage over other tubes in that they are easily removed in the office without an anesthetic.

Insertion technique

A binocular operating microscope is commonly used to insert TTs. A myringotomy is performed in the anterior portion of the TM to avoid the acoustically sensitive portion of the drum. Classic dogma states that a radial incision is less damaging to the TM and that TTs will be retained longer if placed in the anterosuperior quadrant. In a recent study Guttenplan and others[28] showed no difference in TM sequelae with radial or circumferential incisions and April and others[4] showed no difference in retention time based on location of incision. These studies are significant because it is sometimes easier to insert a TT using a circumferential incision, and TM perforation is more easily managed in the anteroinferior than the anterosuperior quadrant.

Antibiotic drops

Ototopic antibiotic drops can be considered in the immediate postoperative period in an effort to reduce postoperative otorrhea, particularly when a mucoid effusion was evident during TT placement.

Swimming

There is no consensus as to whether patients with TTs should be permitted to swim, and, if so, whether earplugs are necessary.[20] In a study consisting mostly of school-age children, Gates and others[22] found the incidence of otorrhea to be significantly higher in the summer months, possibly related to swimming. Prospective studies[6,15,44] found no difference in otorrhea rates in patients who did or did not swim or who swam with or without earplugs. These studies support the concept of abandoning the practice of requiring earplugs or avoiding swimming except in high-risk situations such as deep diving or water-skiing.

Follow-up

Patients with a hearing loss documented or suspected before surgery should have a follow-up hearing test to ensure a return to normalcy or to guide further intervention for the loss. Assuming there are no other problems, the ears should be examined at least twice yearly to assess TT and TM status. Given the risk for developing serious complications of the TM such as perforation, tympanic atelectasis, and cholesteatoma, ears should be checked by a physician who is skilled at recognizing these abnormalities and their significance at least yearly until the TT is out, the TM is healed, and healthy status of the TM and middle ear is confirmed.

Removal of tympanostomy tubes

There may be instances in which TT removal is desirable. Indications for removal include chronic otorrhea, granuloma formation, tube blockage, migration of the tube into the middle ear, and when external ventilation of the middle ear is no longer likely to be necessary.[16] This latter indication can be extremely difficult to determine. The T-tube can be removed easily without an anesthetic; removal of other TTs, particularly stiff-flanged grommet tubes, will require a general anesthetic in most children.

COMPLICATIONS

A summary of complications of TTs is presented in Table 30-1.

Anesthetic complications

The overwhelming majority of TTs are placed in children who require a general anesthetic, which carries some risk. While newer techniques, pharmacologic agents, and monitoring standards have made anesthesia administration safer and less traumatic, the potential for a catastrophic anesthetic-related incident is still around 1 in 40,000 cases.[57] The alternative is local anesthesia, which may be suitable for some older children. There is a risk of direct trauma to the ear with the use of local anesthetics if the patient moves unexpectedly, although the risk can be minimized with patience and experience.

Table 30-1. Complications of tympanostomy tubes

Complication	Study	Frequency (%)
Anesthetic catastrophe		None reported*
Otorrhea		
One or more episodes	Mandel Casselbrant, and Kurs Lasky[37]	50
	McLelland[42]	16.6
	Herzon[30]	21.4
Chronic	McLelland[42]	3.6
	Herzon[30]	3.5
Myringosclerosis	Bonding and Tos[8]	48
	Brown, Richards, and Ambegaokar[11]	42
	Pichichero, Berghash, and Hengerer[46]	52
Chronic perforations	Curley[17]	1
	Matt and others[39]	2 (grommet)
	McLelland[42]	3.1
	Matt and others[39]	13–18 (T-tube)
	Hawthorne and Parker[29]	30 (T-tube)
Focal atrophy	Brown, Richards, and Ambegaokar[11]	13
	Karma, Sipila, and Kokko[33]	18.4
Retraction pocket formation	McLelland[42]	1.6
Cholesteatoma	McLelland[42]	0.1
	Karma, Sipila, and Kokko[33]	1†
General anesthesia to remove tubes	Curley[17]	1
Grommet lost in middle ear	Curley[17]	0.1
	McLelland[42]	0.1

* Severe organ system damage, cardiac arrest, or death in children as a result of general anesthesia can be expected to occur at a rate of about 1 in 40,000 cases (Tiret and others[57]).
† This represented two cholesteatomas, neither of which occurred at the site of or as a result of tympanostomy tube placement.

Otorrhea

Otorrhea of variable duration is the most common complication following TT placement and will occur at some point during the life of the TT for as many as 50% of patients,[37] although others report lower rates.[30,32,42] Otorrhea is more likely to occur in children younger than 2 years of age and in this age group is more likely to follow an upper-respiratory infection.[18] Samuelson, Freijd, and Rynnel Dagoo[50] found a much higher risk of otorrhea following TT placement in children with nasopharyngeal *Haemophilus influenzae* colonization. Otorrhea usually has a trivial health impact and is easily managed, although Herzon[30] and McLelland,[42] in separate studies, reported about a 3.5% rate of persistent otorrhea.

Otorrhea can be classified as "early" or "late" depending on the time of onset. Early otorrhea occurs when TTs are inserted while the mucosa of the middle ear is in a hypersecretory phase, such as during an active infection. The results of randomized studies are mixed, but a recent meta-analysis suggested a decrease in the incidence of early otorrhea when antibiotic drops are applied topically in the postoperative period.[21] The incidence of early otorrhea does not seem to decrease when efforts are made to use sterile technique during insertion.[34,52] Late otorrhea is seen in at least 25% of patients following TT placement[22] and generally represents reinfection of the middle ear either as an ascending infection from the nasopharynx (often associated with an upper-respiratory tract infection), from nasopharyngeal reflux through a pathologically patent eustachian tube, or from contamination of the middle ear from the ear canal.

The bacteriology of otorrhea is age- and duration-related.[37,51] "Fresh" otorrhea in children younger than 3 years of age is usually associated with the same organisms that cause acute OM behind intact TMs: *Pneumococcus*, *Haemophilus,* and *Moraxella* spp. Persistent otorrhea and otorrhea in older children usually contain gram-negative bacilli such as *Pseudomonas* and gram-positive bacilli such as *Staphylococcus.* Initial management is usually empiric, consisting of an oral antibiotic for *Staphylococcus* spp. and a topical otic or ophthalmologic antibiotic preparation with activity against *Pseudomonas* spp.

Otorrhea that does not respond to one or more rounds of the usual therapies should be cultured after all antibiotics have been discontinued for a few days. If yeast is the predominant organism, antibacterial antibiotics should not be resumed and the ear can either be observed or topical anticandidal drops can be used. If no good oral agent is available for bacterial infections, topical agents can be instilled more vigorously with a displacement medicine dropper. If this fails, options include a course of intravenous antibiotics, removal of the TT, and simple mastoidectomy with antral catheter placement for antibiotic irrigation. Otorrhea may recur after any of these managements, and an evaluation for an immunodeficiency state should be considered in these instances.

Intravenous antibiotics are very effective, at least temporarily, and have the advantage of managing both ears if the process is bilateral. Drawbacks include the cost and the monumental burden of maintaining intravenous access and administering the medications (especially for a multidrug regimen requiring periodic serum concentration testing) for a 10-day to 2-week course, particularly for pediatric patients in the home setting.

Tympanostomy tube removal represents the least invasive alternative. The best candidates for this procedure are patients who develop otorrhea in a long-retained TT after an extended infection-free period. In these patients, the TT itself may have incited a foreign-body reaction with granulation tissue and infection. In other instances, tube removal runs the risk of converting a draining middle ear to one of the forms of intact-drum OM with all the attendant morbidities.

Simple mastoidectomy with catheter placement for antibiotic instillation represents a reasonable alternative to intravenous antibiotic therapy in terms of cost and convenience if the process is unilateral. The procedure can be performed on an outpatient basis, the catheter is easily maintained, and the process is generally well tolerated.[14] The disadvantages include the surgical risks and the perception that the procedure is more invasive than a course of IV antibiotics. An algorithm for managing otorrhea is presented in Figure 30-1.

Myringosclerosis

Several studies[8,11,46] have reported tympanosclerotic plaques within the TM in 40% to over 50% of TMs after TT placement—which is much higher than would be expected from a history of recurrent OM alone without TT placement. This has been used as an argument against the use of TTs, but a large series by Tos and Stangerup[59] showed that this finding did not significantly affect hearing. The formation of these plaques may be related to suction trauma to the TM during TT placement or to the increased oxygen tension in the middle-ear cleft following TT placement.[40]

Tympanic membrane perforation

The frequency of TM perforation varies with the type of tube and duration *in situ.* Generally speaking, smaller-flanged, briefly retained grommet-style TTs will have a perforation rate of between 1% and 3%,[17,39,42] whereas larger-flanged, longer-lasting TTs such as the large-flanged, stiff T-tube may have perforation rates as high as 30%[29] (although the softer, shorter-flanged T-tubes will have perforation rates under 10%).

Most perforations caused by TTs are small, produce a hearing loss of less than 10 dB, and are easily managed with a simple myringoplasty such as a fat patch.[19]

Tympanic membrane atrophy, retraction, and atelectasis

Focal thinning or atrophy of the TM is common following extrusion of the TT and healing of the membrane (occurring in as many as 40% of ears requiring repeated intubations[46] and in less than 15% of the more general population receiving tubes).[11] If there is enough support left in the TM and if eustachian tube function is good, focal atrophy is of little consequence. Occasionally, the TM will be extremely weak, eustachian tube function will be poor, or both, and the atrophic TM segment will retract into the middle-ear cleft, forming a permanent pocket. McLelland[42] reported that this process occurred in less than 2% of TT placements. Adhesions may form between the TM and promontory or other structures, and if the segment overlies the ossicular chain, erosion of the incus may occur. There usually is an accompanying hearing loss. The process may progress to cholesteatoma. Focal retractions may be followed clinically, but if progressive they should be excised.[53,60]

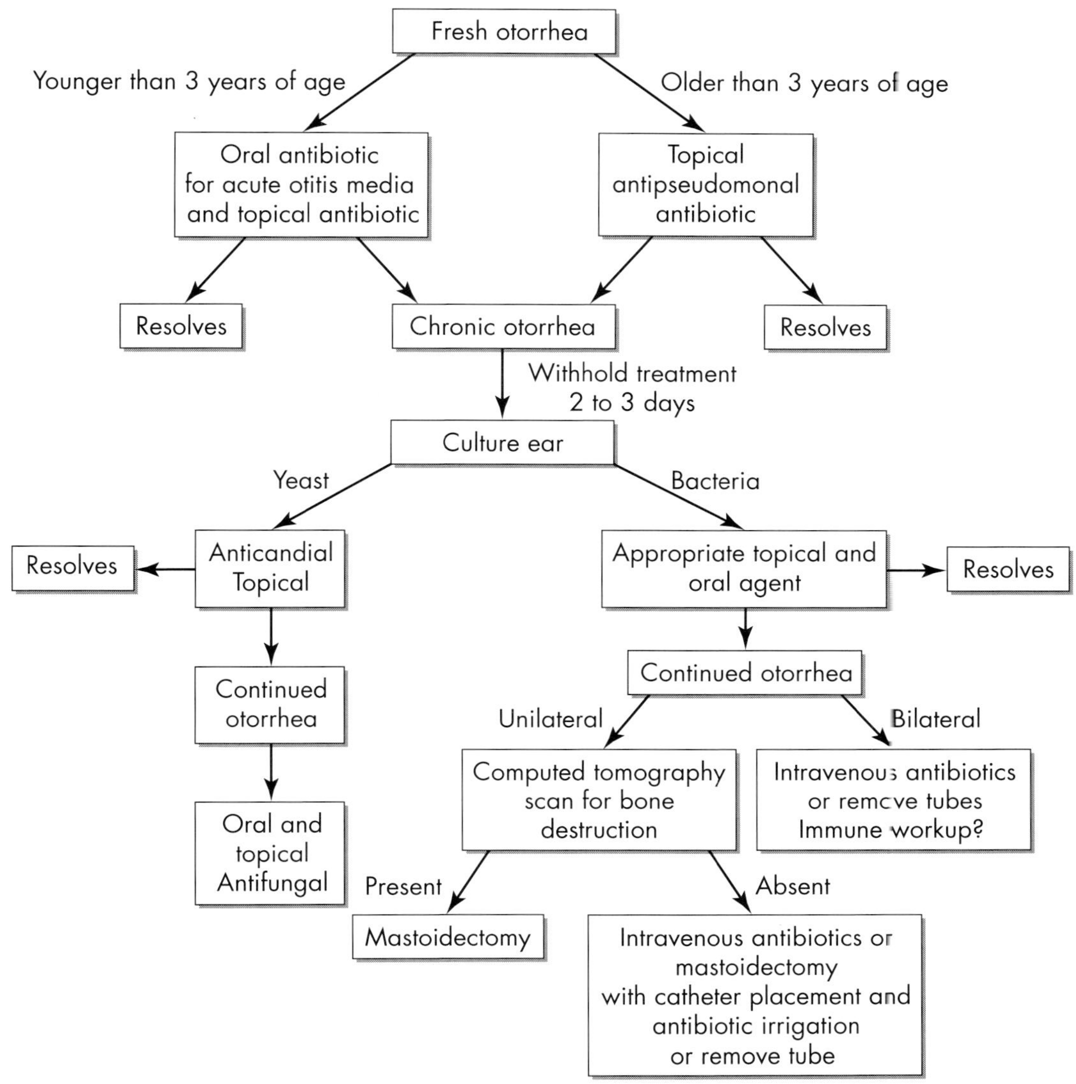

Fig. 30-1. The management of posttympanostomy tube otorrhea.

Focal retraction pocket formation should not be confused with severe, diffuse middle-ear atelectasis. The latter is no more likely to occur in ears treated for chronic OM with effusion with TTs than in those without.[41]

Cholesteatoma

Cholesteatoma may arise from several mechanisms in patients who have had TTs placed. It may arise independently of the TTs in patients with longstanding eustachian tube dysfunction and recurrent OM. It may also arise as a direct complication of TT placement, either in a retraction pocket that progresses to the point of debris accumulation or as the result of ingrowth or transplantation of keratinized epithelium into the middle-ear cleft. The frequency of this complication is uncertain, but rates between 0.1% and 0.5% can be expected as a direct result of TT placement,[42] and rates of up to 1% can be expected if cholesteatoma from concomitant disease is included.[33] The frequency may depend on the type of tube or the duration *in situ*,[39] with longer retention associated with higher rates of cholesteatoma formation. Prevention or early intervention is preferable to late intervention, so follow-up by an otoscopist capable of recognizing a problematic TM retraction or an early cholesteatoma should be routine in patients with TTs at some point shortly after tube extrusion, and ''at-risk'' ears should be regularly examined.

Tube removal requiring general anesthetic

A general anesthetic is usually required to atraumatically remove a grommet tube that has a stiff medial flange. Situations in which this may be desirable include prolonged retention and foreign body reaction or prolonged infection associated with the tube. Practice styles obviously vary, but Curley[17] reported a rate of 1.4% for TT removal with a general anesthetic. One advantage of the T-tube is the ease with which it can be removed in awake children.

Tympanostomy tube lost in the middle ear

Loss of the TT in the middle ear may occur at the time of insertion or later as an unusual complication of infection or external trauma. Efforts should be made to retrieve a tube lost at the time of surgery, but failure to do so rarely causes problems. Both Curley[17] and McLelland[42] reported this to occur in 0.1% of patients.

Early extrusion

The duration of TT retention is a function of the size and shape of the medial flange and the material of the TT. Even the most rapidly extruding grommets will typically last 6 to 9 months.[25] Very early extrusion may occur when an infected tide of mucus plugs and then pushes the TT out of the TM, often before a newly placed tube has the chance to "seat" itself in the healing membrane. Early extrusion may also occur occasionally when a flange of the TT is inadvertently inserted between the inner and outer layers of the TM. This situation may be difficult to recognize during surgery.

Plugging

Tympanostomy tubes may become obstructed with dried mucus, blood, or granulation tissue. Obstruction with dried mucus occurs following infection in a small number of cases and may sometimes be cleared with a pick or Rosen needle or with dilute hydrogen peroxide drops.[9] Granulation tissue may block a tube as a result of chronic infection and may require a prolonged course of topical steroid-containing antibiotic drops.

SUMMARY

TT placement can effectively relieve the sequelae of eustachian tube dysfunction in a large percentage of patients with this condition. Indications for insertion are imprecise in patients with recurrent acute OM and OM with effusion because of difficulties in predicting which patients will continue to be otitis-prone. Rising bacterial resistance to oral antimicrobial agents may greatly alter the indications for TT placement in the future. The beneficial effects of TTs are limited to the time in which the tubes are in place and patent, and the procedure is either not effective or produces significant complications in 5% to 10% of patients. The recommendation for TT placement warrants careful deliberation in most cases, and long-term follow-up by a skilled otoscopist is mandatory. Age-appropriate audiometric monitoring is highly desirable.

ACKNOWLEDGMENT

The author gratefully acknowledges the assistance that Taya Higgins, RN, and Judith Iwata provided in the preparation of this manuscript.

REFERENCES

1. Alho OP and others: Control of the temporal aspect when considering risk factors for acute otitis media, *Arch Otolaryngol Head Neck Surg* 119:444, 1993.
2. Alho OP and others: Which children are being operated on for recurrent acute otitis media? *Arch Otolaryngol Head Neck Surg* 120:807, 1994.
3. American Academy of Otolaryngology-Head and Neck Surgery: *Clinical indicators for otolaryngologic-head and neck surgery*, Alexandria, Va, 1992, American Academy of Otolaryngology-Head and Neck Surgery.
4. April MM and others: Tympanostomy tube insertion: anterosuperior vs. anteroinferior quadrant, *Otolaryngol Head Neck Surg* 106:241, 1992.
5. Armstrong B: New treatment for chronic secretory otitis media, *Arch Otolaryngol Head Neck Surg* 96:653, 1954.
6. Becker GD, Eckberg TJ, Goldware RR: Swimming and tympanostomy tubes: a prospective study, *Laryngoscope* 97:740, 1987.
7. Black NA and others: A randomised controlled trial of surgery for glue ear, *Br Med J* 300:1551, 1990.
8. Bonding P, Tos M: Grommets versus paracentesis in secretory otitis media: a prospective, controlled study, *Am J Otol* 6:455, 1985.
9. Brenman AK, Milner RM, Weller CR: Use of hydrogen peroxide to clear blocked ventilation tubes, *Am J Otol* 7:47, 1986.
10. Bright RA and others: The prevalence of tympanostomy tubes in children in the United States, 1988, *Am J Public Health* 83:1026, 1993.
11. Brown MJ, Richards SH, Ambegaokar AG: Grommets and glue ear: a five-year follow up of a controlled trial, *J R Soc Med* 71:353, 1978.
12. Casselbrant ML and others: Efficacy of antimicrobial prophylaxis and of tympanostomy tube insertion for prevention of recurrent acute otitis media: results of a randomized clinical trial, *Pediatr Infect Dis J* 11: 278, 1992.
13. Chole RA, Hubbell RN: Antimicrobial activity of Silastic tympanostomy tubes impregnated with silver oxide: a double-blind randomized multicenter trial, *Arch Otolaryngol Head Neck Surg* 121:562, 1995.
14. Clark SK, Richardson MA, Donaldson JA: A complete mastoidectomy with catheter insertion, *Laryngoscope* 98:582, 1988.
15. Cohen HA and others: Swimming and grommets, *J Fam Pract* 38:30, 1994.
16. Cunningham MJ and others: Tympanostomy tubes: experience with removal, *Laryngoscope* 103:659, 1993.
17. Curley JW: Grommet insertion: some basic questions answered, *Clin Otolaryngol* 11:1, 1986.
18. Debruyne F, Degroote M: One-year follow-up after tympanostomy tube insertion for recurrent acute otitis media, *J Otorhinolaryngol Relat Spec* 55:226, 1993.
19. Deddens AE, Muntz HR, Lusk RP: Adipose myringoplasty in children, *Laryngoscope* 103:216, 1993.
20. Derkay CS, Shroyer MN, Ashby J: Water precautions in children with tympanostomy tubes, *Am J Otolaryngol* 13:301, 1992.
21. Garcia P, Gates GA, Schechtman KB: Does topical antibiotic prophylaxis reduce post-tympanostomy tube otorrhea? *Ann Otol Rhinol Laryngol* 103:54, 1994.
22. Gates GA and others: Delayed onset post-tympanotomy otorrhea, *Otolaryngol Head Neck Surg* 98:111, 1988.
23. Gates GA and others: Chronic secretory otitis media: effects of surgical management, *Ann Otol Rhinol Laryngol Suppl* 138:2, 1989.
24. Gebhart DE: Tympanostomy tubes in the otitis media prone child, *Laryngoscope* 91:849, 1981.
25. Gibb AG, Mackenzie IJ: The extrusion rate of grommets, *Otolaryngol Head Neck Surg* 93:695, 1985.
26. Gonzales C and others: Prevention of recurrent acute otitis media: chemoprophylaxis versus tympanostomy tubes, *Laryngoscope* 96:1330, 1986.
27. Grievink EH and others: The effects of early bilateral otitis media with

effusion on language ability: a prospective cohort study, *J Speech Hear Res* 36:1004, 1993.
28. Guttenplan MD and others: Radial versus circumferential incision in myringotomy and tube placement, *Int J Pediatr Otorhinolaryngol* 21: 211, 1991.
29. Hawthorne MR, Parker AJ: Perforations of the tympanic membrane following the use of Goode-type 'long term' tympanostomy tubes, *J Laryngol Otol* 102:997, 1988.
30. Herzon FS: Tympanostomy tubes: infectious complications, *Arch Otolaryngol Head Neck Surg* 106:645, 1980.
31. Hubbard TW and others: Consequences of unremitting middle ear disease in early life: otologic, audiologic, and developmental findings in children with cleft palate, *N Engl J Med* 312:1529, 1985.
32. Jaffe BF: Are water and tympanotomy tubes compatible? *Laryngoscope* 91:563, 1981.
33. Karma P, Sipila M, Kokko E: Long-term results of tympanostomy tube treatment in chronic secretory otitis media, *Acta Otolaryngol Stockh* 94(suppl 386):163, 1982.
34. Kinsella JB and others: Tympanostomy tubes and early postoperative otorrhea, *Int J Pediatr Otorhinolaryngol* 30:111, 1994.
35. Le CT, Freeman DW, Fireman BH: Evaluation of ventilating tubes and myringotomy in the treatment of recurrent or persistent otitis media, *Pediatr Infect Dis J* 10:2, 1991.
36. Luotonen J and others: EMLA in local anaesthesia of the tympanic membrane, *Acta Otolaryngol Suppl Stockh* 492:63, 1992.
37. Mandel EM, Casselbrant ML, Kurs Lasky M: Acute otorrhea: bacteriology of a common complication of tympanostomy tubes, *Ann Otol Rhinol Laryngol* 103:713, 1994.
38. Manning SC and others: Incidence of sensorineural hearing loss in patients evaluated for tympanostomy tubes, *Arch Otolaryngol Head Neck Surg* 120:881, 1994.
39. Matt BH and others: Incidence of perforation with Goode T-tube, *Int J Pediatr Otorhinolaryngol* 21:1, 1991.
40. Mattsson C, Magnuson K, Hellstrom S: Myringosclerosis caused by increased oxygen concentration in traumatized tympanic membranes: experimental study, *Ann Otol Rhinol Laryngol* 104:625, 1995.
41. Maw AR, Bawden R: Tympanic membrane atrophy, scarring, atelectasis and attic retraction in persistent, untreated otitis media with effusion and following ventilation tube insertion, *Int J Pediatr Otorhinolaryngol* 30:189, 1994.
42. McLelland CA: Incidence of complications from use of tympanostomy tubes, *Arch Otolaryngol Head Neck Surg* 106:97, 1980.
43. Otitis Media Guideline Panel: Managing otitis media with effusion in young children, *Pediatrics* 94:766, 1994.
44. Parker GS and others: The effect of water exposure after tympanostomy tube insertion, *Am J Otolaryngol* 15:193, 1994.
45. Peters SA and others: The effects of early bilateral otitis media with effusion on educational attainment: a prospective cohort study, *J Learn Disabil* 27:111, 1994.
46. Pichichero ME, Berghash LR, Hengerer AS: Anatomic and audiologic sequelae after tympanostomy tube insertion or prolonged antibiotic therapy for otitis media, *Pediatr Infect Dis J* 8:780, 1989.
47. Presswood G and others: Effect of artificial airway on ear complications from hyperbaric oxygen, *Laryngoscope* 104:1383, 1994.
48. Rach GH and others: The effect of treatment with ventilating tubes on language development in preschool children with otitis media with effusion, *Clin Otolaryngol* 16:128, 1991.
49. Rosenfeld RM: What to expect from medical treatment of otitis media, *Pediatr Infect Dis J* 14:731, 1995.
50. Samuelson A, Freijd A, Rynnel Dagoo B: Treatment failure in otitis-prone children with prophylactic tympanostomy tubes is correlated with nasopharyngeal *Haemophilus influenzae* colonization, *Acta Otolaryngol Stockh* 111:1090, 1991.
51. Schneider ML: Bacteriology of otorrhea from tympanostomy tubes, *Arch Otolaryngol Head Neck Surg* 115:1225, 1989.
52. Scott BA, Strunk Jr CL: Posttympanostomy otorrhea: the efficacy of canal preparation, *Laryngoscope* 102:1103, 1992.
53. Sharp JF, Robinson JM: Treatment of tympanic membrane retraction pockets by excision: a prospective study, *J Laryngol Otol* 106:882, 1992.
54. Shone GR, Griffith IP: Titanium grommets: a trial to assess function and extrusion rates, *J Laryngol Otol* 104:197, 1990.
55. Smith TL, DiRuggiero DC, Jones KR: Recovery of eustachian tube function and hearing outcome in patients with cleft palate, *Otolaryngol Head Neck Surg* 111:423, 1994.
56. Teele DW and others: Otitis media in infancy and intellectual ability, school achievement, speech, and language at age 7 years: Greater Boston Otitis Media Study Group, *J Infect Dis* 162:685, 1990.
57. Tiret L and others: Complications related to anaesthesia in infants and children: a prospective survey of 40240 anaesthetics, *Br J Anaesth* 61: 263, 1988.
58. To SS, Pahor AL, Robin PE: A prospective trial of unilateral grommets for bilateral secretory otitis media in children, *Clin Otolaryngol* 9:115, 1984.
59. Tos M, Stangerup SE: Hearing loss in tympanosclerosis caused by grommets, *Arch Otolaryngol Head Neck Surg* 115:931, 1989.
60. Walsh RM and others: Management of retraction pockets of the pars tensa in children by excision and ventilation tube insertion, *J Laryngol Otol* 109:817, 1995.
61. Watcha MF and others: Laryngeal mask airway vs face mask and Guedel airway during pediatric myringotomy, *Arch Otolaryngol Head Neck Surg* 120:877, 1994.
62. Wielinga EW, Smyth GD: Comparison of the Goode T-tube with the Armstrong tube in children with chronic otitis media with effusion, *J Laryngol Otol* 104:608, 1990.
63. Williams RL and others: Use of antibiotics in preventing recurrent acute otitis media and in treating otitis media with effusion: a meta-analytic attempt to resolve the brouhaha, *JAMA* 270:1344, 1993.
64. Williamson HA Jr, DePra J, Sulzberger LA: Lack of seasonal variability for recurrent otitis media in very young children, *J Fam Pract* 33:489, 1991.
65. Zielhuis GA, Rach GH, van den Broek P: The natural course of otitis media with effusion in preschool children, *Eur Arch Otorhinolaryngol* 247:215, 1990.

Chapter 31

Education of the Hearing Impaired

Virginia W. Jenison
Barbara S. Stroer
Margaret W. Skinner
Christine Yoshinaga-Itano

The physician who diagnoses a child as hearing impaired is often the first professional to counsel parents on the management of their child. Often referred to as the *invisible handicap*, a hearing impairment can have devastating effects on educational, social, and vocational achievement.

When a child is identified as having a permanent hearing loss, parents often feel obliged to make immediate decisions that will have a lasting impact on the child's life. While grieving over the loss of their child's hearing, they are submerged in unfamiliar terminology, angered and frustrated by any delay in diagnosis, confused by the many educational methods, and frustrated by professionals who may disagree on what is best for the hearing-impaired child. Parents look to the diagnosing physician to provide comprehensive medical management and suggest the most appropriate rehabilitation and special educational services. This responsibility has significantly been affected by the increasing number of hearing-impaired children identified by infant hearing screening. As infant hearing screening programs become more widespread, the need for comprehensive systems for hearing screening, diagnostic and amplification services, and intervention services is critical. The interdisciplinary team (physician, audiologist, speech pathologist, deaf educator) provides parents with information to learn about their child's deafness and to make informed decisions about management. When a hearing loss occurs before basic language skills have been established, the subsequent communication deficit permeates the educational process. The child's mastery of language becomes the primary concern. During the preschool years, the focal point is habilitation of communication skills. At the elementary and secondary levels, the focus shifts to the application of language in the development of academic, social, and vocational skills. A continual effort should be made to develop the communication skills needed to take advantage of the educational, social, and vocational opportunities of the general populace. The issues of deaf education are complex, but with appropriate management, hearing-impaired children can become stable, independent, productive adults. This chapter highlights the history of deaf education and reviews educational guidelines, pertinent issues, and available resources for hearing-impaired children and their families.

EDUCATION OF THE DEAF

Misconceptions about the abilities of the deaf have influenced their educational, social, and legal status since early Greek, Hebrew, and Roman times. For hundreds of years, the relationship between hearing loss and the inability to speak was not recognized.[12,33] Because speech was the primary avenue for education and the deaf could neither speak nor understand speech, they were thought to be senseless and incapable of reason. The term *deaf and dumb* (a mistranslation of Aristotle's observation that those born deaf were also "speechless") came to be associated with mental deficiency. As a result, congenitally deaf persons had few rights and little or no social standing. They were banned from participating in religious and civic ceremonies, and only those from influential families received any education.

During the renaissance, teachers were usually physicians or clergy who took special interest in the care and management of a particular deaf person. The emphasis was most often on religious instruction rather than on pragmatic communication or integration into the hearing society. Girolamo Cardano (1501-1576) was one of the first physicians to recognize the deaf could be educated through associating written symbols with objects and pictures. In 1555, Pedro Ponce de Leon (1520-1584), a Spanish monk, used reading and writing to teach the deaf to speak. Juan Pablo Bonet (1579-1620) wrote the first book on education of the deaf, which described his methods of teaching speech and language through touch and vision supplemented with signs and a manual alphabet.

By the 18th century, Europe was divided on the issue of which method provided the best education for the deaf. The French priest Charles Michael de l'Pee (1712-1789) favored manual forms of communication. De l'Pee developed and expanded sign language as the more natural and more efficient means of instruction. He tried incorporating the teaching of speech by the methods of his predecessors but thought it was impractical. Samuel Heinicke (1729-1790), in Germany, believed that spoken language was the basis of thought and favored oral forms of communication, teaching language through speech and lip-reading. Both factions relied primarily on vision for instruction because, without hearing aids, the use of residual hearing was not feasible. Both methods were determined effective by the Zurich Academy in 1753. De l'Pee's success led to the establishment of the first public school for the deaf in Paris in 1775. His school served as a training program for teachers of his method. The specific oral techniques were often kept secret between the mentor and his disciples. Although Heinicke founded the first state-supported school for the hearing impaired in Germany in 1776, his methods had no disciples.

Deaf education in the United States is based on that in Europe. Thomas Hopkins Gallaudet (1787-1851) founded the first permanent public school for the hearing impaired in Hartford, Connecticut in 1817. Gallaudet's school, now known as the American School for the Deaf, served as the model for state schools for the deaf and promoted the use of sign language. Gallaudet had wanted to study the successful oral methods being used in England. He was discouraged, however, by the secrecy of those teachers and went to France to learn the manual methods of the Abbé Sicard, a disciple of de l'Pee. Efforts to establish an American oral school for the deaf were not successful until the Clarke School for the Deaf in Northhampton, Massachusetts and the Lexington School for the Deaf in New York City were founded in 1867.

The subsequent growth of deaf education in the United States occurred in public and private schools. Each state eventually established a public residential school. Special day schools were established in more populated areas, and by the 1940s several public school systems offered special services for hearing-impaired students.

Oral and manual methods have alternately been the preferred method of instruction. Although oral programs were most widely available until the mid-1970s, approximately 80% of the local school programs include manual sign language as a component of training.[3] Section 504 of Public Law:93-112, the Vocational Rehabilitation Act of 1973, began a trend toward equal rights for the disabled. In 1975, the United States Congress enacted Public Law:94-142: Education for All Handicapped Children Act (referred to as the civil rights act for the handicapped), which required public schools to provide for handicapped children. This legislation and later legislation support the special educational needs and human rights of hearing-impaired and other disabled persons in the United States.

LEGAL RIGHTS TO EDUCATION

United States Public Law:94-142 entitles all disabled children aged 5 to 21 years to (1) an education, (2) a free education, (3) an appropriate education, (4) an education in the least restrictive environment, (5) due process under the law, (6) confidentiality, and (7) evaluation using nondiscriminating tests. Federal funds are appropriated for direct teacher/child activities, teacher training programs, repositories of information, innovative programs, postsecondary education programs, and rehabilitation counseling.

PL:99-457—Education of the Handicapped Act amendments of 1986—extended the entitlement of PL:94-142 through the year 1994, mandated that by 1991 similar services be provided to children aged 3 to 5 years, and established the Part H program to assist states in the development of a comprehensive, multidisciplinary, and statewide system of early intervention services for infants and toddlers (birth to 3 years).

PL:101-476, The Education of the Handicapped Act amendments of 1990 renamed the act the Individuals with Disabilities Education Act (IDEA). This law reauthorized and expanded the original legislation. Parent-child services for the hearing impaired, offered since the 1940s and widely accepted since the 1960s, support the role of parents in facilitating speech, language, and auditory skills during the years considered most critical to their child's communication development (0 to 3 years). Services may be provided through home visits by a counselor/teacher or through parent/child visits to an instructional center.

Each state is required to implement the federal laws and to establish how federal funds are used within the local school systems. Specific guidelines for evaluation and program listings for each state are available from State Department of Education-Office of Special Educational Services. Because the federal laws offer special educational guidelines for specific disabling conditions, local programs have been planned and developed on the basis of category, degree, and incidence of impairment.

Eligibility criteria

To determine eligibility for special educational services under PL:94-142 and related legislation, the Rules and Regulations for Implementation of the Education for All Handicapped Children Act of 1975 provides specific definitions:[36]

Deaf means a hearing impairment so severe that the child cannot process linguistic information through hearing, with or without amplification, which adversely affects educational performance. (Most states also define *deaf* as unaided pure tone average of 500, 1000, and 2000 Hz of a 70-dB hearing level [ANSI] or more in the better ear.)

Hard of hearing means a permanent or fluctuating hearing impairment that adversely affects a child's educational performance but that cannot be defined as deaf. (Most states also define *hard of hearing* as an unaided pure tone average of 500, 1000, and 2000 Hz of 25- to 70-dB hearing level [ANSI] in the better ear.)

The generic term *hearing impaired* describes hearing loss that adversely affects a child's educational performance and includes deaf and hard-of-hearing children.

Evaluation process

Federal law requires that all school-aged children suspected of having a disability be evaluated by an interdisciplinary team and that children receiving special educational services be re-evaluated every 3 years. The evaluation should be completed in a timely fashion unless a justified written request for extension is made. Because an Individualized Educational Plan (IEP) is developed on the basis of the interdisciplinary evaluation results, it is necessary to include each developmental area in the evaluation. Areas typically included are academic, communication, intelligence, medical (including vision, hearing, and motor ability), and social/emotional behavior. Parents who disagree with the results of the evaluation conducted by the school system are entitled to an independent evaluation by an agency outside the school system.

The evaluation should be conducted using nonbiased evaluation procedures. Before this legislation was enacted, the use of standard verbal or written intelligence tests led to the placement of many hearing-impaired children into classes for the mentally retarded. The language level and overall communication ability of the hearing-impaired child potentially influence every aspect of evaluation. To obtain an accurate picture of the child's abilities, careful selection of appropriate tests, administration in the child's usual mode of communication, and critical interpretation of the results are necessary.

Individualized educational plan

An IEP should be developed for persons eligible for special educational services after the evaluation is completed. The IEP is a legal document jointly developed and agreed on by parents and representatives of the educational agency. Professionals from outside agencies may participate when appropriate. The IEP should specify the current status of the child, annual goals and short-term objectives for instruction, the educational and support services needed to meet these goals, the type of classroom in which the instruction will take place, the extent to which the child will participate in regular school activities, the evaluation plan, and the date the services will begin. To varying degrees, the specific methods for achieving these goals are described in the IEP.

Part H of IDEA requires that all infants, toddlers, and preschool-aged children have an Individualized Family Service Plan, which includes diagnostic evaluations every 6 months and goals and objectives for the child's education.

Due process

If the parents and school system cannot agree on an educational plan, the child is entitled to due process of law. Each school system should have written guidelines that describe the legal rights of parents, including procedures for requesting due process hearings. These written guidelines are available on request for use by professionals.

Least-restrictive environment

The decision as to where the child will receive the most appropriate instruction is part of the IEP. The least-restrictive environment allows for "separate schooling or removal of handicapped children from the regular educational environment . . . only when the nature or severity of the handicap is such that education in regular classes with the use of supplementary aids and services cannot be achieved satisfactorily."[36] That is, the most appropriate instruction is provided with the least degree of exclusion from the regular educational setting as possible. However, the term *least-restrictive environment* should not be considered synonymous with *mainstreaming* (participation in a class with normally hearing children). The least-restrictive environment for one child may be restrictive for another. Placement decisions should be based on the overall status of the child and the program goals.

A continuum of placement options is defined by PL:94-142. These options in many states reflect the type of services delivered and the degree to which the child participates in the regular instructional program; that is, the degree to which the child is "mainstreamed." These options are commonly described as follows:

- *Regular class with consultation* enrolls the child in a regular classroom. Support services may be offered to the classroom teacher regarding any special needs of the student.
- *Regular class with itinerant services* enrolls the child in a regular class with periodic special instruction as needed. The special educator may be responsible for providing services to students enrolled in several

schools and, therefore, may not be continually available at the school site.

- *Regular class with resource instruction* enrolls the child in a regular class, with special-education instruction in areas of special need provided for up to 3 hours per day.
- *Self-contained class with mainstreaming* enrolls the child in a special-education class, with participation in regular classroom instruction in areas of strength for up to 3 hours per day.
- *Self-contained class on regular campus* enrolls the child in special-education class for the entire school day. The classes are located on a regular school campus, which allows for interaction with nondisabled children for activities outside the classroom.
- *Self-contained class in special school* enrolls the child in a special school for disabled children for the entire school day where the child receives specialized instruction and related services.
- *Hospital/homebound* students receive special instruction at home or in a hospital when health or other factors preclude their participation in instruction with other children. This placement is used most often for children with health impairments.
- *Residential placement* enrolls the child in a special school on a 24-hour basis. Educational services are provided on campus, and extracurricular activities consider the special needs of the students.

COMMUNICATION METHODS OF THE DEAF

Improving communication and academic achievement is the common goal of all educational programs and teaching methods for hearing-impaired children.

Neither severity of hearing loss nor method of communication predict language abilities of deaf and hard-of-hearing children.[11,16] However, age of identification of hearing loss may predict later language abilities.[39]

Many believe that oral skills enhance the ultimate life options available to a child; however, not every deaf child can achieve intelligible spoken language or be educated exclusively through spoken language. The development of intelligible speech in deaf or hard-of-hearing children relates to hearing levels. Children with hearing levels of 70 dB or better show intelligible or very intelligible speech, whereas approximately 50% of those whose hearing levels are 71 to 90 dB and approximately 23% of those whose hearing levels are greater than 91 dB HL have very intelligible or intelligible speech.[13] Speech intelligibility ratings vary highly in children with hearing levels exceeding 70 dB.

Philosophic divisions continue between (1) those who believe that speech should be the "first language" of the hearing-impaired child and (2) those who believe that visual (sign) language should be developed first and used as the basis for teaching other forms of communication.

Oral methods

The goals of any oral program are for the child to learn to speak, to understand speech, and to function in a world in which people communicate through spoken language. The underlying premise is that spoken language is an innate, human capacity and that hearing-impaired children have the same biologic predisposition for language learning as does any child. Oral programs focus on the acoustic and visual codes of spoken language. Depending on the particular technique advocated, access to these codes may be provided through audition, vision, touch, or proprioception.

The traditional oral approach primarily emphasizes speech reading for learning. Tactile cues provide additional information about the differences in the production of speech features lost to the visual sense (e.g., voicing, nasality). This approach continues to be used with children who have limited or no auditory ability. With advances in hearing aids and other assistive listening devices, more emphasis has been placed on the role of residual hearing in conjunction with these traditional oral training techniques.

Auditory/oral describes programs that emphasize residual hearing and speech reading for learning spoken language. Hearing aids and assistive listening devices are used in conjunction with the traditional techniques of speech reading, writing, and direct touch to facilitate development of auditory perceptual skills and spoken language. Cochlear implants and vibrotactile or electrotactile devices may be used as alternatives to conventional hearing aids when adequate auditory responses are not achieved.

Auditory/verbal programs emphasize the exclusive use of hearing to facilitate spoken language through the normal sequential stages of receptive auditory skills development. The child is encouraged to interpret the many aspects of speech and environmental sounds accomplished only through hearing. To varying degrees, the training is conducted without speech reading or other visual cues.

Cued speech was developed as an aid to speech reading and speech development. Eight handshapes in four positions near the speaker's face differentiate among speech sounds, two thirds of which look the same on the lips (Fig. 31-1).[6] Hand signals differentiate speech sounds that look alike on the lips. A common misconception is that cued speech is a form of sign language; however, because the cues are meaningful only when used in conjunction with spoken language, cuing is considered an oral method.

Manual methods

Manual methods use various forms of sign language to develop communication competency. The underlying premise is that visual language is the natural language of the deaf and is the most efficient avenue for communication. A brief description of the forms of manual communication commonly used in the United States follows.

American Sign Language (ASL or Ameslan) is regarded

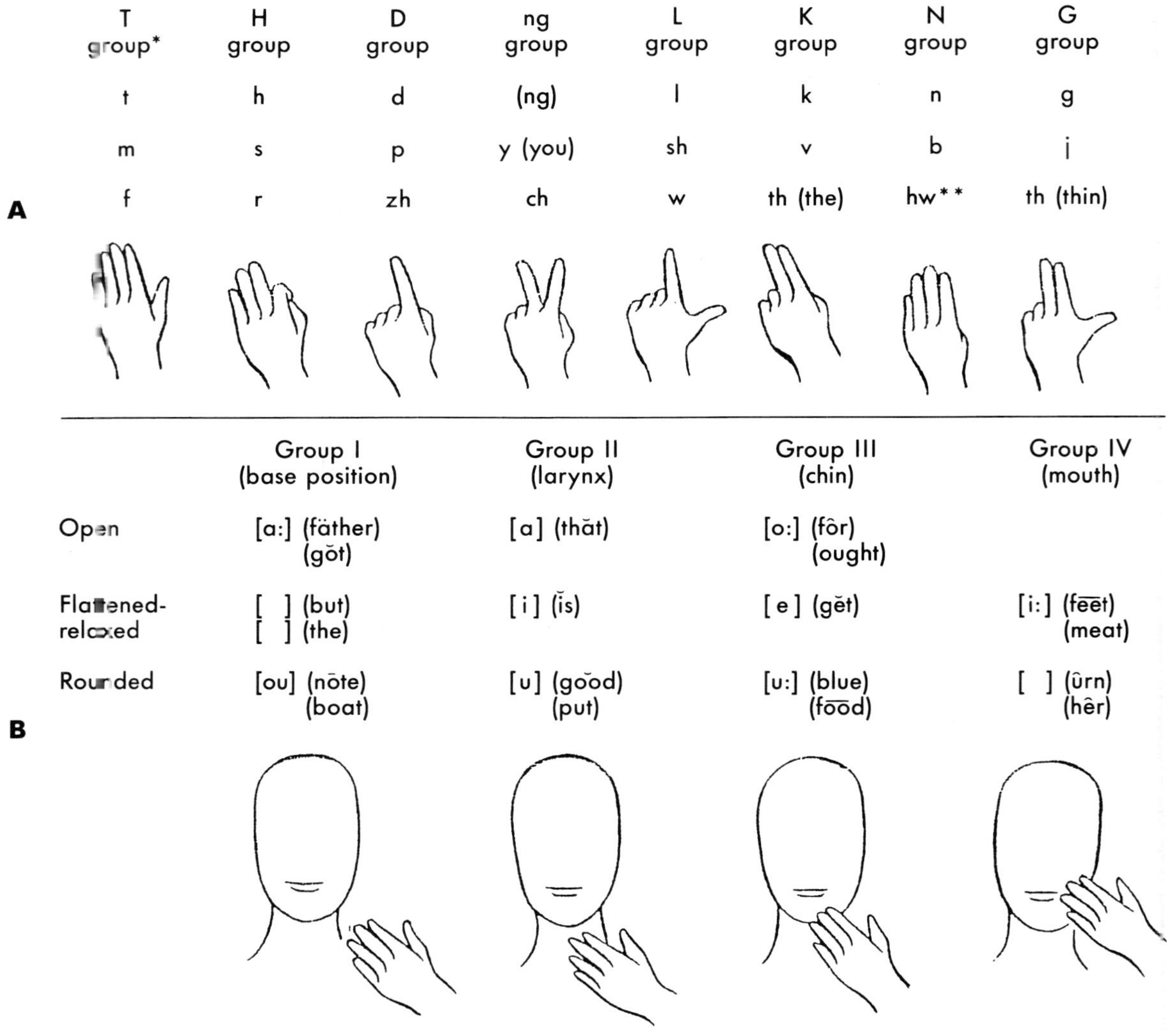

Fig. 31-1. **A,** Cues for English consonants. **B,** Cues for English vowels. (From Cornett RO: Cued speech, *Am Ann Deaf* 112:3, 1967.)

by many to be the natural language of the deaf. The meaning of a sign is determined by its position, configuration, direction of the palms, and specific hand or body movements. Many signs are iconic and can be understood by most people. ASL is recognized as a formal language consisting of unique vocabulary, grammar, syntax, morphology, and expressions that are distinct from other recognized languages, including English. As a result, manually coded English systems have been developed to more closely represent English. Whether English should be taught as the primary language or as a secondary language to ASL is debated.

Signed English maintains English syntax and grammar using the vocabulary (i.e., signs) of ASL. Special markers may be used with a sign to designate plurality, possessives, and verb tense. This form of manual communication had been endorsed by the National Association of the Deaf as the preferred language of instruction because it eases the transition from the expressive form of language to the written forms of the English language.

Seeing Essential English uses literal translations of English morphology rather than conceptually based signs. Signs represent each word as it would occur in spoken English, and a system of signed markers identifies articles, verbs, verb tenses, numbers, roots, prefixes, and suffixes. Because signs are translated literally, they do not always resemble the ASL signs on which they are based. For example, the word butterfly is expressed by using the sign for *butter* followed by the sign for *fly* rather than using one sign to express the concept for the insect. Therefore, proficiency in ASL does not guarantee comprehension of Seeing Essential English 1.

Signing Exact English was developed to make Seeing Essential English more intelligible to those using ASL and yet maintain the syntax of English. English rules of grammar

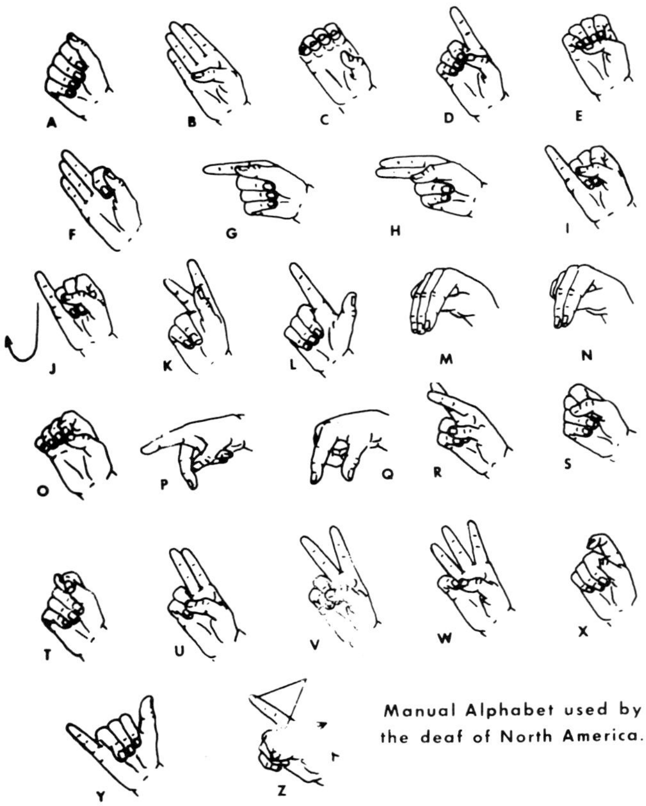

Fig. 31-2. American manual alphabet.

and syntax are applied to the conceptually based signs of ASL with the signed markers of Seeing Essential English used to clarify specific words.

Fingerspelling is a manual alphabet system with a hand shape and movement to represent each letter of the alphabet (Fig. 31-2). Each word in a message is spelled. Fingerspelling is most often used with other forms of manual communication to convey specific ideas for which there are no signs.

Total communication

The principal goal of total communication is to develop a language system as early as possible to enhance all developmental areas. Manual signs, auditory training, and speech reading mutually reinforce language development. A skill established in one modality can facilitate skills in another. To provide better quality models in one modality, some programs advocate sequential rather than simultaneous presentation.

The Rochester method was one of the first combined methods developed to provide simultaneous presentation of spoken language and a visible manual form. This visible speech method consists of fingerspelling each word as it is spoken. Its major disadvantage is difficulty in maintaining a good spoken language model while fingerspelling at the slower rate.

The contemporary total communication method uses a form of manually coded English (sign and fingerspelling); auditory training with hearing aids, cochlear implants, assistive listening devices, vibrotactile aids, or electrotactile devices; speech; speech reading; reading and writing; and a combination of visual/proprioceptive/tactile cues. The signing system should be decided on and consistently used. Periodic evaluation of the child's use of language through each modality helps determine how much emphasis to place on the auditory/oral and manual program components. Similar to other methods, programming for the child using total communication is designed based on critical factors.

ACADEMIC ACHIEVEMENT

The traditional teacher-as-lecturer style used in most schools assumes that a school-aged child has acquired the communication skills necessary for formal instruction. The most powerful predictor of reading skill of deaf and hard-of-hearing students is their vocabulary development. The ability to apply these skills to academic, social, and vocational matters determines the child's ultimate educational success. The challenge to deaf educators is how to bring the academic performance of the hearing impaired to a level comparable with that of their hearing peers. Without comparable skills, expectations for job opportunity and life earning for the hearing impaired will continue to lag behind those for the general public. Despite advances in each of the many professional fields serving hearing-impaired students, this challenge is unmet for many students.

For more than three decades, the Center for Assessment and Demographic Studies at Gallaudet University's Research Institute has examined the demographic profiles and academic performance of hearing-impaired students in special-educational programs across the United States. Results of their Annual Survey of Hearing Impaired Children and Youth and the normative data collected from the Stanford Achievement Test Revised for the Hearing Impaired provide the most extensive information available on this population. The survey results[2] represent 60% to 70% (over 55,000 students) of school-aged, hearing-impaired children and youth and include part-time and full-time special-education students in public, private, residential, and day school programs. Results of the Center for Assessment and Demographic Studies Testing Program reflect the academic trends of hearing-impaired students in the United States.

The two areas of achievement are reading comprehension (most influenced by language ability and critical to all subject areas) and mathematics computation (least influenced by language ability). A comparison of the test results collected in 1974 with those in 1983 suggests several trends regarding achievement levels (Fig. 31-3).[2,30] The achievement levels of hearing-impaired students are less than those of their hearing peers for reading comprehension and mathematic computation, with the deficit in reading comprehension being more substantial. An unexplained trend in the

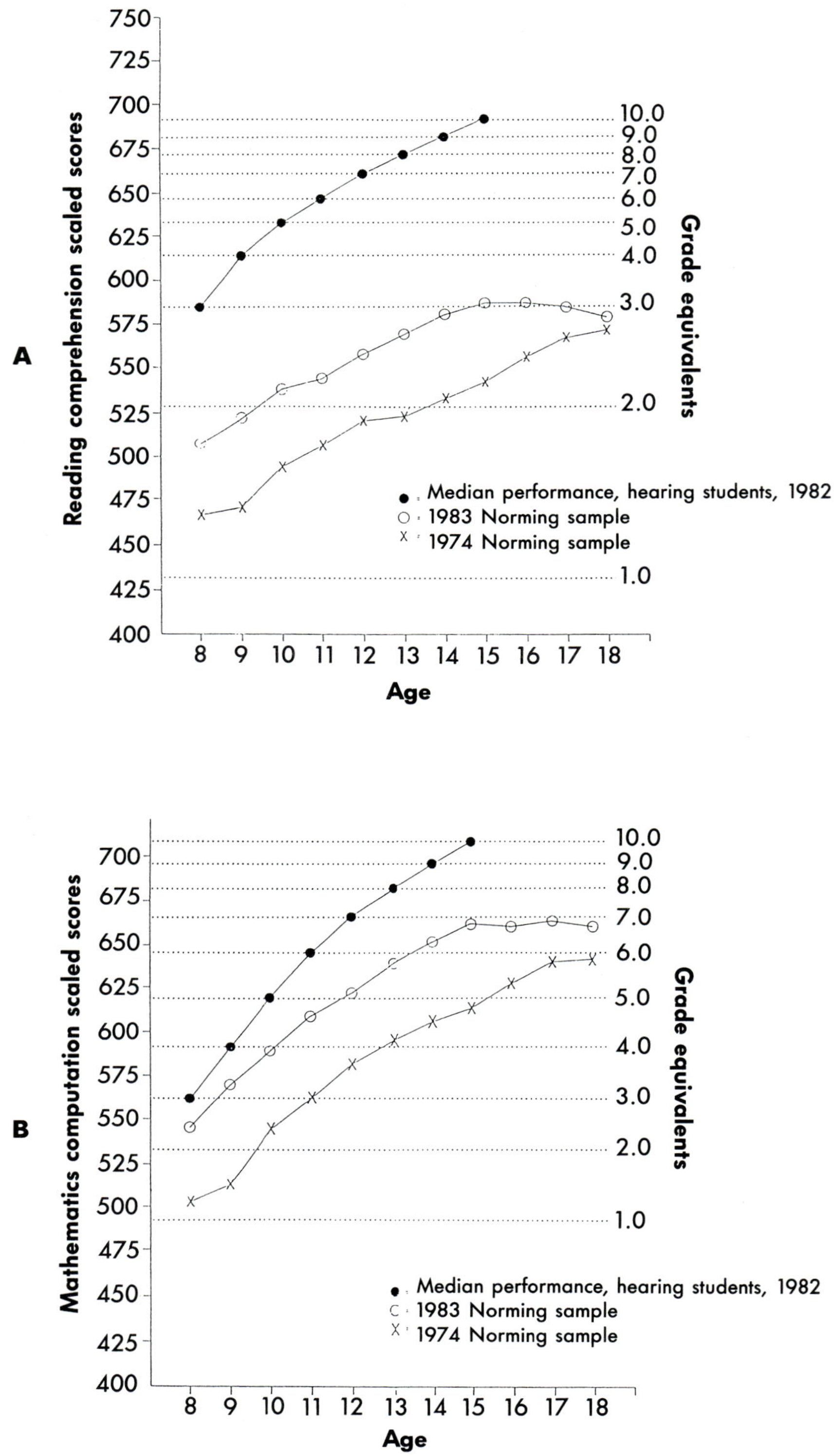

Fig. 31-3. A, Mean reading comprehension and **B,** mean mathematics computation scaled scores for 1974 and 1983 hearing-impaired normal samples according to age (plotted with median performance of hearing students). (From Allen T: *Patterns of academic achievement among hearing-impaired students: 1974 and 1983.* In Schildroth A, Karchmer M, editors: *Deaf children in America,* San Diego, 1986, College-Hill Press.)

performance of the hearing-impaired group in 1984 is a noticeable plateau in achievement, which appears to occur at the third-grade level for reading and at the seventh-grade level for mathematics. The nature of the study (cross-sectional rather than longitudinal) and the various changes in demographics between 1974 and 1983 make it difficult to account for this trend. However, for both data collection periods, less than one grade level was achieved in reading comprehension between ages 10 and 18. Although the 1983 results showed improved overall performance when compared with the 1974 results, the average 18-year-old hearing-impaired student had slightly less than a third-grade reading comprehension level for both study periods. The 1990 norming sample shows a slight increase in reading comprehension scores over the 1983 sample. This sample indicates that 17- and 18-year-olds achieved between a middle third- and fourth-grade reading level. However, these results still represent about 1 year of development from ages 11 to 18 years (Fig. 31-4).[14]

FACTORS THAT INFLUENCE COMMUNICATION AND EDUCATION

Results of the Center for Assessment and Demographic Studies survey and other reports have identified multiple factors that influence communication and education of the hearing impaired in the United States. Specifically, these factors affect the child's ability to acquire competency in English as the language of instruction in American schools. In February 1988, the United States Federal Commission on Education of the Deaf submitted a report entitled *Toward Equality: Education of the Deaf*, which emphasized the need for a higher level of competence in the English language among deaf persons.[5] A study by Geers and Moog[11] suggested that such mastery of English is the predominant predictor of reading achievement. The degree to which the hearing-impaired child masters language depends on several patient and program variables.[23]

Patient variables

Type and degree of loss

Several attempts have been made to define degree of hearing loss in a way that will predict educational needs. In general, the greater the hearing loss, the greater the impact on communication as the basic skill for learning. The child should be able to hear the range of frequencies and intensities of normal conversational speech for normal language to develop. This range of frequencies and intensities can be represented on the audiogram as the speech banana (Fig. 31-5).[18] The relationship between the child's unaided hearing thresholds and the speech banana is a general indicator of the amount of speech information that is detected without a hearing aid. Although a child may be classified as deaf or hard of hearing on the basis of unaided pure tone average, this classification may unduly influence the expectations of parents and teachers because it does not reflect how the child will perceive speech with a well-fitted hearing aid.

To avoid the many misconceptions associated with the terms *hard of hearing* and *deaf*, consideration should always be given to how the child functions when using amplification. For example, many children with hearing losses of 90 or 100 dB consistently use their hearing aids to enhance their overall communication. Thus, the term *hearing impaired*, which encompasses all degrees of hearing loss (mild to profound), is preferred when the child's ability to use residual hearing has not been determined. The preferred use of terms such as *deaf*, *hard of hearing*, or *hearing impaired* may differ widely among adults with significant hearing losses.

It is difficult to predict the effects of unilateral and fluctuating conductive losses on auditory skill development, language development, and subsequent educational performance. Until recently, unilateral hearing was believed to be adequate for speech and language development with little or no impact on educational achievement. However, an estimated 35% of children with unilateral hearing loss have failed at least one grade during their educational career, and 13% have needed some type of special educational services.[3] Learning-disabled children with central auditory processing deficits reportedly have a history of recurrent otitis media at a significantly higher rate (46.3%) than learning-disabled children with no central auditory processing deficits (22%).[8] Although most agree that the presence of a conductive hearing loss resulting from otitis media alters the child's ability to perceive speech and language, the long-term effects on language ability and educational achievement have not been well established.

Age of onset

The first 3 years in a child's life are critical for learning normal speech and language. The normally hearing child acquires basic communication skills by listening to speech and language models. By trial and error, the child learns to understand and produce spoken language; no formal training is usually required. A hearing loss disrupts this normal chain of events. Terms such as *prelinguistic* (before language acquisition), *perilinguistic* (during the normal language acquisition years), *postlinguistic* (after language acquisition), and *prevocational* (after language acquisition, but before vocational training is complete) attempt to describe the level of language development or educational status at the onset of the hearing loss. Such terminology implies a certain level of ability or expected level of performance. Although each group requires special attention for optimal achievement, each has programmatic issues. For example, the existing language skills of the prevocationally deafened child serve as a tool for rehabilitation, whereas the acquisition of language skills will be a continual goal of the program for the prelinguistically deafened child.

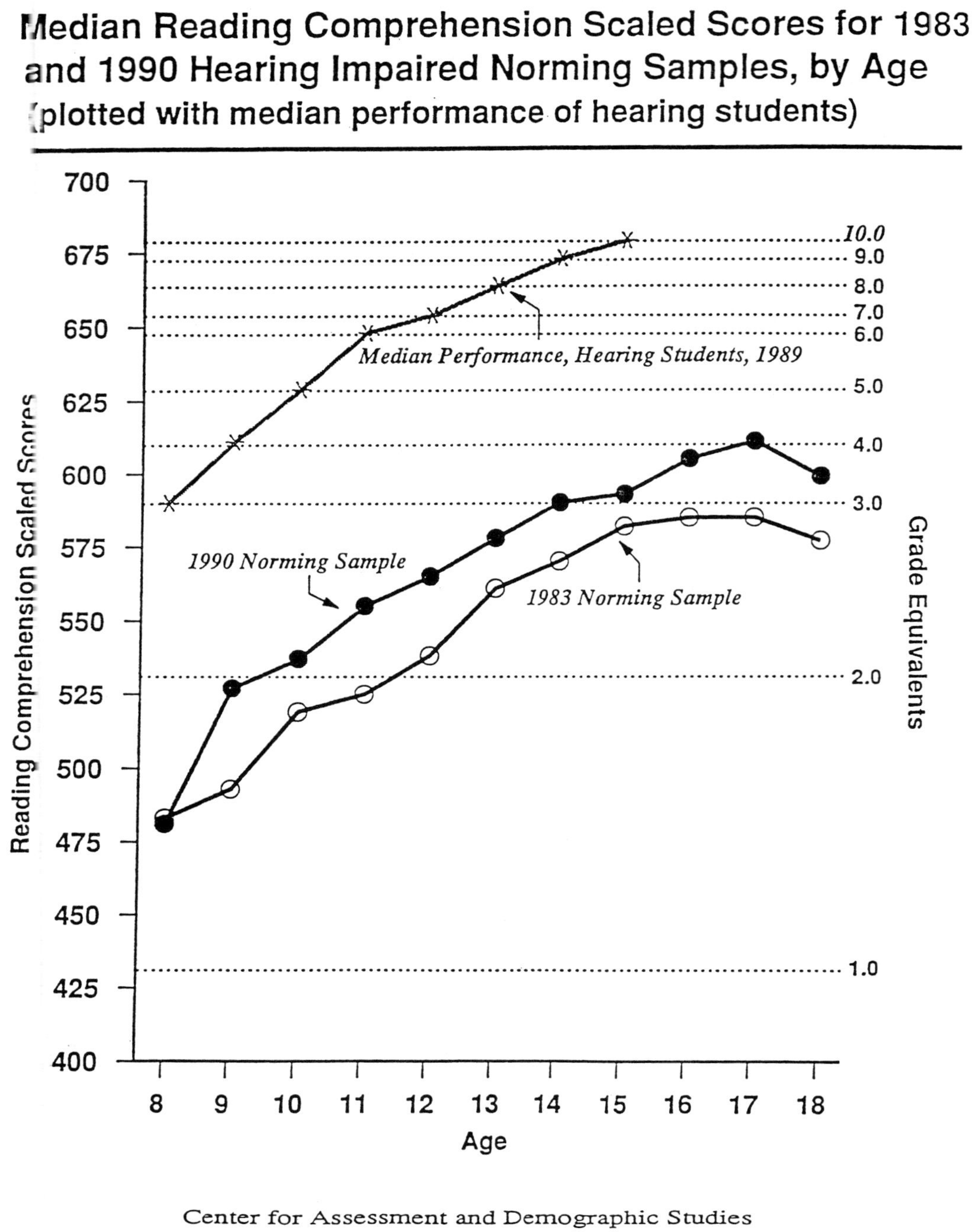

Fig. 31-4. Median reading comprehension scaled scores for 1983 and 1990, hearing-impaired normal samples according to age. (From Karchmer M: *Educational outcomes and achievement levels*, Presented at the Joint National Association of State Directors of Special Education (NASDE) Conference of Executives of Schools for the Deaf (CEASD), "Status of Education of the Deaf in the United States," Las Vegas, Nev, 1991.)

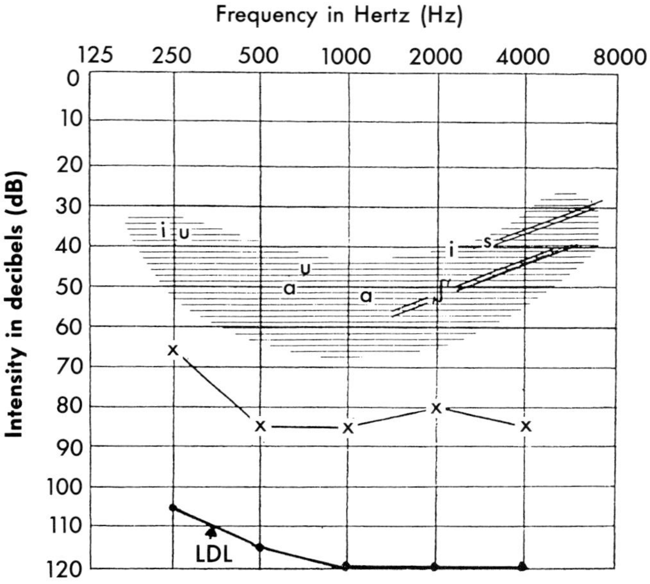

Fig. 31-5. An audiogram shows the relative intensity levels (*HL*) of the main components of five sounds /u/, /a/, /i/, /ʃ /, /s/ spoken at 2 yards. By calculating how much amplification is required to increase these sounds so that they fall between the child's threshold of hearing and loudness discomfort level (*LDL*), the approximate gain provided by a hearing aid can be calculated. (From Ling D, Ling AH: Aural habilitation: the foundations of verbal learning in hearing-impaired children, Washington, DC, 1978, The Alexander Graham Bell Association for the Deaf.)

Length of deprivation, age of identification, age at start of intervention

Children whose hearing deficit is identified early and who are enrolled immediately in special education are more likely to develop better communication skills. Early intervention is critical to parent education and adjustment and to avoiding lost time during the critical learning period. Yoshinaga-Itano and Apuzzo[39] and Yoshinaga-Itano and others[41] report that the expressive and receptive language skills of children between the ages of birth and 3 years diagnosed with hearing loss prior to 6 months of age are significantly higher than those of children diagnosed with hearing loss after 6 months of age. This significant developmental difference is present at all testing ages between 12 and 36 months, irrespective of degree of hearing loss. Some evidence suggests that periods of sound deprivation cause permanent physiologic changes in the auditory pathways of the brainstem[37]; however, the impact of these changes on human speech perception needs further investigation.

Response to amplification

The functional gain (i.e., the difference between un-aided and aided audiometric thresholds) is most often the first measure used to judge whether the hearing aid is providing appropriate amplification. Ling's speech banana (see Fig. 31-5), which represents the spectrum of normal speech frequencies and intensities, is commonly used as the target for aided thresholds. Unless a child can detect speech sounds at comfortable loudness levels, development of higher level auditory perceptual skills cannot be expected. In addition to aided detection, speech perception skills, such as pattern perception and word identification, should be evaluated using standard or modified test materials with systematic observation for younger children. If expected levels of auditory perceptual skills are not achieved with training, an alternative to conventional amplification, such as a cochlear implant or tactile device, may provide more information and greater benefit.

Family support

The issue of family support is significant when addressing the increasing probability that infants with congenital hearing loss may be identified through newborn infant hearing screening in the well-baby nursery. Because the hearing loss may be diagnosed shortly after birth, parents deal with a new set of emotional issues. Appropriate follow-up and delivery of information are critical for the emotional well-being of the family. However, data suggest that referral for hearing testing within 24 hours after birth and diagnosis of hearing loss within the next few months can be accomplished without undue emotional trauma to the family.[1] Appropriate follow-up, including diagnosis, fitting of amplification, and enrollment in an intervention program, is critical for optimal outcomes.

Parents active in their child's management are more likely to accept a life-style that promotes effective communication consistent with the method chosen. The status of the parent's hearing is an important factor in how the family accepts and copes with the child's hearing loss. Deaf children of deaf parents have the advantage of early exposure to visual forms of communication and their parents' acceptance of deafness. The parents as role models enhance the child's self-esteem and feelings of acceptance.[24] The reaction of the 90% of parents with normal hearing is often grief and dismay. The parents' ability to take an active role in the initiation of rehabilitative services is often impeded by their emotional reaction to the diagnosis. Professionals should recognize and accept that parents experience the Kubler-Ross stages of grieving (denial, guilt, depression, anger, anxiety, and coping) as described by Tanner.[35] Those counseling parents at the time of diagnosis should be aware that terminology used to describe a child's hearing may affect parent-child interactions, expected standards of achievement, determination of educational placement, and expected response from amplification.[27] Follow-up counseling with the physician or audiologist scheduled within 1 week allows the parents time to adjust to their emotional reaction before they have to consider specific recommendations for follow-up care. Although the grieving process is most evident after the initial diagnosis, it typically recurs, albeit with lesser intensity, when the child reaches school age, pubescence, high school graduation age, and the age of expected independence and when the parents reach retirement age. These recurrences should be viewed as normal processes of acceptance. However, referral for psychologic counseling may be appropriate when parents experience difficulty coping.

Etiology and other disabilities

Although the number of more severely hearing-impaired children is decreasing, the percentage of those with additional handicaps has increased. The many hearing-impaired children from the 1964 rubella epidemic have passed through the educational system; however, advances in medical technology have made it possible for more children to survive complicated births and illnesses. Any additional disabling condition, especially those related to vision or motor ability, should be considered when programs and program components are selected.

Program variables

Availability of support services

Audiologic support services, speech therapy, note taking, and interpreter services are typically associated with education of the hearing impaired. With the increasing numbers of hearing-impaired children with additional disabling conditions, other types of support services are more frequently needed (e.g., occupational therapy, physical therapy, adaptive physical education). Special schools for the hearing impaired often offer stronger support services to their students than do schools with normal hearing children. Because of the number of students enrolled in these special schools, services can be provided by professionals with expertise in the unique needs of the hearing impaired. Although special-education programs are available for 90% of deaf children, less than 25% of hard-of-hearing children receive adequate support services.[20] Although more children with mild-to-severe degrees of hearing loss wear hearing aids, their school programs may offer only speech therapy and no other support services.[9]

Parent education and training

Effective parent education programs expedite the parents' acceptance of their child's condition, promote proficiency in the instructional method of choice, and engage the parents as the principal managers of the child's rehabilitation program. These programs are needed most after initial diagnosis, when information is most critical to the emotional stability of the family and to the acquisition of appropriate services for the child. The program should include knowledge of hearing impairment, its effects on communication, care of amplification, instruction in specific communication techniques, behavior management, legal rights, educational placement options, and information about various associations for the hearing impaired. Individual Family Service Plans, which are required for the families of disabled infants and toddlers by PL:99-457: Education of the Handicapped Act Amendments of 1986, are likely to become more common within the next few years as a mechanism for implementing family support services.[28] The parents' ability to fully participate will depend on the quality of education and training they receive. Parent education and training programs should be designed to accommodate a changing society, particularly in view of the number of working and single parents, and to prepare parents to take an active role in the child's intervention.

State of hearing aids

Despite technologic improvements and suggested maintenance programs, the past 20 years have seen little or no improvement in the functioning of amplification. Repeated studies indicate that less than half of the hearing aids used by children in school are functioning properly.[4] As the primary tool for auditory training, a proper functioning hearing aid is essential. Programs that offer audiologic services in support of auditory training are more likely to successfully monitor the hearing aid and intervene when repair is needed.

Recognizing residual hearing

The degree to which a child can use residual hearing has the strongest impact on the rehabilitation process. The more residual hearing available (aided or unaided), the easier the process. Prognosis improves if the child takes advantage of the hearing when available and seeks other means of instruction when not. Failure to recognize a lack of residual hearing results in inappropriate teaching techniques or failure to consider alternative devices that would provide better information from sound.

Expertise of teacher

The strength of any deaf education program depends on the caliber of the teacher and the degree to which available support services are used. The teacher's knowledge of and commitment to the method of choice is the most important factor in the quality of implementation. Professional training in deaf education includes instruction in the various communication methods used to teach the hearing impaired. The practical aspects of training, however, usually occur in a facility that uses a particular methodology. Proficiency in one method of communication does not guarantee proficiency in another. The level of proficiency of the teacher determines the quality of the language model given the child. For example, Pidgin sign, a combination of English and ASL, is commonly used by those less proficient at sign language. Because it is neither English nor ASL, Pidgin sign is comparable with the broken English of a person for whom English is a second language. Such language is less than optimal for the child who is required to apply language to reading and writing. Likewise, those involved in the auditory training aspects of rehabilitation should be versed in speech acoustics, amplification, and speech and language development.

Consistency of use of the method of choice

For the communication method to be effective, it should become a way of life for the child and family. Most parents will be unfamiliar with techniques needed to facilitate communication and will require instruction to apply those techniques in the home. In addition, the communication methods used among the professionals working with the child should also be consistent. The advantage of special school settings is that the personnel are familiar with the method and provide an enriched communication environment for the child.

Acoustic environment

The noise levels and reverberation in classrooms may make it impossible for a child using a hearing aid to hear. Average noise levels of 50 to 70 dB sound pressure level (SPL) are typical for regular classrooms. It has been suggested that the acceptable noise level during academic instruction—when the use of hearing aids is most critical—is 30 to 35 dB SPL; during nonacademic instruction (e.g., art, physical education), the noise should be no greater than 45 dB SPL.[4] Preferential seating of the child near the teacher is not practical throughout the school day and does not consistently meet the signal-to-noise ratio needed for satisfactory speech perception. The recommended signal-to-noise ratio of +20 dB can be easily achieved with the use of FM auditory training units or other assistive listening devices. The microphone (used near the teacher's mouth) reduces the level of background noise and transmits the teacher voice via FM to the child's hearing aid at a level 15 to 30 dB above the background noise.

BASIS FOR CHOOSING A COMMUNICATION METHOD

Families with infants whose hearing deficit was diagnosed before 4 months of age should establish trust with the parent facilitator and may not be ready to make decisions about communication method until their child is older. To facilitate this decision-making, Stredler-Brown and Yoshinaga-Itano[34] recommend the use of comprehensive diagnostic evaluations, which include parent questionnaires and videotape analyses of parent-child interaction every 6 months. These data will help parents understand the impact of a variety of variables on their child's developmental progress. To provide unbiased professional input, in-service training of the parent facilitators is vital to ensure that nonjudgmental interaction with parents and families is maintained. Such interactions will encourage the parents and families to make decisions about their child's educational future.

One of the first questions usually posed by the parents of a hearing-impaired child after acquiring information about hearing loss is whether to use sign or spoken language. An auditory/oral method is usually appropriate for less severely hard-of-hearing children with properly fitted and well-maintained hearing aids. However, there is more controversy concerning the most appropriate method for educating severely and profoundly hearing-impaired children. No technique predicts the most appropriate method of communication for a hearing-impaired child. The method is frequently chosen based on the availability of programs and bias of the parents' counselor at the time of diagnosis. Decisions about appropriate method of communication should be based as much as possible on objective criteria and developmental data.

For most hearing-impaired children whose hearing losses were identified at around 2 years of age, diagnostic teaching enables parents and professionals to assess the effects of patient and program variables on the child's communication ability. With this information, the child's strengths and weaknesses can be determined, and the program methods or the emphasis on program methods can be changed. The child's needs should be emphasized rather than the rate of success of a particular communication method. Because each method has its benefits and each its failures, a lack of progress should not be viewed as a failure on the part of the child or parents but as identification of the need for a more appropriate teaching method for the child.

Two scales have been proposed to determine the likelihood of a child's ability to acquire spoken language (i.e., appropriateness of oral education). The Deafness Management Quotient designed by Northern and Downs[22] and the Spoken Language Predictor developed by Geers and Moog[10] weigh the most important factors in the acquisition of spoken language. The Deafness Management Quotient uses a point system to weigh the factors of unaided pure tone findings, central auditory system intactness, intelligence, family support, and socioeconomic status. The Spoken Language Predictor, developed to improve the Deafness Man Quotient, considers aided speech perception skills, language competence, nonverbal intelligence, family support, and the child's speech communication attitude the most important factors in predicting a child's potential for developing spoken language.

Those working with a deaf child should provide parents with a realistic profile of the child's strengths and weaknesses and an unbiased account of the strengths and weaknesses of all methods. The parents can then select the communication method that best serves the needs of the child and the family. In practice, the low incidence of hearing-impaired children often precludes the availability of many options in a given geographic area. Families may relocate to access programs of choice and to allow the child to continue living at home.

ISSUES RELATED TO PROGRAM PLACEMENT

The current federal mandates regarding the education of disabled children have supported some of the most significant advances in the history of special education. As a result, the trend has been toward parental preference for local school enrollment to preserve the family unit and access regular (normally hearing) educational programs. Although these mandates afford more appropriate education for most children with all types of disabling conditions, they also have negative aspects. Issues of compliance with the law, documentation, extreme interpretations of mainstreaming, and fear of litigation by the local school systems have complicated the issues of child learning, educational philosophy, and sound teaching practices. The issues of least-restrictive environment, civil rights, and human rights have become associated with placement. Nevertheless, PL:94-142 has made local school placement a viable alternative for many hearing-impaired children. One of the most difficult aspects of program placement is inability to objectively determine adequate and appropriate placement and least-restrictive placement. To make placement decisions primarily based on objective criteria rather than solely on personal testimony, individual experience, or availability of programs, the Colorado service providers developed the Colorado Individual Performance Profile and Preschool Colorado Individual Performance Profile. The Colorado system provides a suggested means of evaluating whether children with educationally significant hearing losses are making adequate academic progress.[40]

Local public schools

An increasing number of students are enrolled in the special education programs of local public school systems; however, because hearing impairment has a low incidence, many school systems do not have a sufficient number of children of appropriate age to offer many communication methods or support services. The total communication approach is often considered more likely to meet the needs of more children within public school. As a result, 80% of public school programs use total communication as the preferred instructional method for deaf children.[3] Some local school systems form cooperative programs to provide high-quality education. Some children travel considerable distances to benefit from these cooperatives. When there are sufficient numbers of children to form a special class (maximum age range of 3 years for a given class), the schools may offer total communication and auditory/oral programs. In most cases, children classified as hard of hearing are recommended for the oral program.

In the local school systems, access to regular educational programs is more readily available. This trend toward mainstreaming is a result of (1) benefits of early intervention; (2) public school cooperative programs for low incidence; (3) preference by the parents for regular classes rather than special-education programs; (4) a shift from a medical model to an educational model of management for the disabled; (5) better use of residual hearing by technologic advancement; and (6) development of support services within regular educational programs.

Considerable efforts to successfully mainstream hearing-impaired students have included strategies such as team teaching (combining classes of hearing and hearing-impaired students using one teacher of the deaf and one regular education teacher) and reverse mainstreaming (having normally hearing students attend special schools). Although there are no guidelines for identifying who will benefit from mainstreaming, successful students share certain characteristics: (1) maximized use of residual hearing; (2) full-time use of hearing aids; (3) an academic performance level comparable with that of class members; (4) competence in communication; (5) a self-directed personality; (6) use of appropriate support services within the school; (7) parental support; and (8) available assistive listening devices.[7]

State schools for the deaf

Most students at state schools for the deaf reside at the school; however, some persons may attend as day students. The advantage of the state school is the availability of support services specific for the hearing impaired. In adolescence, when the need for developing social competence intensifies and vocational preparation is more focal to the educational program, the advantages of the support offered in a special environment may be more evident to the child and family. The major disadvantage is the restricted opportunity to interact with normally hearing children. More recently, however, many state schools are working cooperatively with local school systems to provide these opportunities.

Private school alternatives

Many parents choose private auditory/oral schools as an alternative to the total communication programs in the public schools. The administrators of several of these schools formed the OPTION association in 1981 to promote quality oral education for the hearing impaired. Twenty-four option-affiliated facilities offer oral education as an alternative to the public school total communication trend by providing day and residential oral educational programs.

Postsecondary education

Until the 1960s, Gallaudet University, established in 1864, was the only postsecondary institution for the deaf in the world. Other established programs, particularly vocational technical programs such as the National Technical Institute for the Deaf, received financial support from federal legislation and offered specialized training for the hearing impaired. In addition, more state and private colleges and universities offer support services to disabled students.

STEPS FOR THE REFERRING PHYSICIAN

The physician who identifies a child with a hearing loss has a key role in directing the parents toward appropriate special-educational services. Referral should be expeditious.

1. Refer immediately any child at risk for hearing loss or whose parents express concern over the child's re-

sponse to sound or speech and language development to an audiologist experienced in and specially equipped for pediatric testing. Auditory brainstem response testing makes assessment of the peripheral auditory system possible, even in newborns, and can be ordered for young children who cannot participate in behavioral testing. Referral will reassure concerned parents about the status of the child's hearing or result in early identification for appropriate and timely intervention.
2. Give medical clearance for fitting hearing aids as soon as possible.
3. Refer the parents to the child's local school system or State Department of Education–Office of Special Educational Services for information about legal rights and the location of special-educational services.
4. Keep a list of the available programs for the hearing impaired and encourage parents to investigate each for strengths and weaknesses.
5. Provide ongoing medical identification and management of any condition that would interfere with, complicate, or restrict rehabilitation (e.g., allergies to earmolds, outer or middle ear disease, visual difficulties).
6. Encourage parents to reassess the child's progress periodically to determine the benefits of the hearing aid and effectiveness of the educational program.
7. Encourage parents to contact the local chapter of the association for the deaf and the local support group for parents of hearing-impaired children.

Physicians who provide sensitive guidance help parents cultivate a positive attitude and pursue appropriate services. The following counseling techniques are common to parents who have a positive working relationship with their child's physician:

1. Information is presented in simple, nonthreatening terms. The reasons for tests are presented and the results interpreted in a positive manner.
2. The child is managed as a whole person. Parents are most comfortable with the physician who expresses concern for the child's total development, the progress of the rehabilitation, and the effects of the disability on the child and family.
3. The physician takes time to listen. Given time, parents begin to more fully grasp the implication of a hearing impairment and may develop a positive outlook toward their child's future. The parents' outlook may interfere with their interaction with the child, their self-confidence in making decisions for their child, and their ability to follow through on instructions.
4. The physician directs parents toward appropriate information services and respects their decisions as parents.

SUMMARY

The presence of a hearing loss changes a child's relationship with the environment. As a result, issues related to education of the hearing impaired are complex. Despite the changes in educational services resulting from federal mandates, the academic performance of the hearing impaired suggests that considerable improvement of services is needed. To be successful, rehabilitation techniques should be implemented as early as possible and extend beyond the educational setting as a way of life for the child and family.

Which method of teaching is best has been debated. Although the intensity of this debate may be difficult to understand, it fosters quality care and promotes alternatives for a population with many needs. The successful method acknowledges the needs of the child and family and fosters suitable communication for social, academic, and vocational pursuits.

The physician's role includes making the initial diagnosis of the hearing loss, counseling and directing parents toward services that best meet the needs of their child, monitoring the status of the child's hearing, and assisting parents in the ongoing assessment of the child's management. Although the ultimate outcome for a given child cannot be predicted, many critical criteria for success have been identified and, when met, result in quality education.

ACKNOWLEDGMENTS

The authors thank Gary L. Jenison, MD; Roanne K. Karzon, PhD; and Beverly T. Fears, MS, for contributing their ideas and editorial comments to the preparation of this chapter.

INFORMATION SOURCES

Alexander Graham Bell Association for the Deaf (A G Bell)
3417 Volta Place NW
Washington, DC 20007
Phone: (202) 337-5220 (voice or telephone device for the deaf [TDD])

American Speech-Language-Hearing Association (ASHA)
10801 Rockville Pike
Rockville, MD 20852
Phone: (301) 897-5700

National Association for Speech and Hearing Action
Phone: 800-638-8255 (helpline for consumers)

BEGINNINGS for parents of Hearing Impaired Children
1316 Broad Street
Durham, NC 27705
Phone: (919) 286-9797 or 800-541-HEAR (parents only)

Boys Town National Research Hospital
555 30th Street
Omaha, NE 68131
Phone: (402) 498-6511

Cochlear Implant Club International
PO Box 464
Buffalo, NY 14223-0464
Phone: (716) 838-4662 (voice or TDD)

Children's Center
House Ear Institute
2100 W 3rd Street
Los Angeles, CA 90057
Phone: (213) 353-7005 (voice) or (213) 484-2642 (TDD)

Infant Hearing Resource
Oregon Health Sciences University
3930 SW Macadam Avenue
Portland, OR 97201
Phone: (503) 279-4206

International Hearing Dog, Inc.
5901 E 89th Avenue
Henderson, CO 80640
Phone: (303) 287-3277 (voice or TDD)

National Association for the Deaf
814 Thayer Avenue
Silver Spring, MD 20910
Phone: (301) 587-1788

National Captioning Institute, Inc.
1900 Gallows Road
Vienna, VA 22182
Phone: (703) 917-7600

The Cued Speech Center
304 E. Jones Street
Raleigh, NC 27601
Phone: (919) 823-1218 (voice or TDD)

National Technical Institute for the Deaf (NTID)
One Lomb Memorial Drive
PO Box 9887
Rochester, NY 14623-0887
NTID Bookstore
Phone: (716) 475-2504

National Information Center on Deafness
Gallaudet University
800 Florida Avenue NE
Washington DC 20002
Phone: (202) 651-5253 (voice) or (202) 651-5976

Gallaudet University Press
Phone: 800-451-1073

OPTION
% Principal
St. Joseph Institute for the Deaf
1809 Clarkson Road
Chesterfield, MO 63017-5065
Phone: (314) 532-3211 (voice or TDD)

Self-Help for Hard of Hearing People, Inc. (SHHH)
7800 Wisconsin Avenue
Bethesda, MD 20814
Phone: (301) 657-2248 (voice) or (301) 657-2249 (TDD)

John Tracy Clinic
806 W Adams Boulevard
Los Angeles, CA 90007
Phone: (213) 748-5481

REFERENCES

1. Abdala de Uzcategui C, Yoshinaga-Itano C: Parents reactions to newborn hearing screening, *Audiology Today* 9:24, 1997.
2. Allen T: *Patterns of academic achievement among hearing-impaired students: 1974 and 1983.* In Schildroth A, Karchmer M, editors: *Deaf children in America*, San Diego, 1986, College-Hill Press.
3. Bess FH, Humes LE: *Audiology: the fundamentals*, ed 2, Baltimore, 1995, Williams & Wilkins.
4. Bess FH, McConnel FE: *Audiology, education, and the hearing impaired child,* St Louis, 1981, Mosby.
5. The Commission on Education of the Deaf: *Toward equality: education of the deaf a report to the Congress of the United States,* Washington DC, 1988, United States Department of Health, Education and Welfare.
6. Cornett RO: Cued speech, *Am Ann Deaf* 112:3, 1967.
7. Davis JM, Hardick EJ: *Rehabilitative audiology for children and adults,* New York, 1981, John Wiley & Sons.
8. Downs MP: *Contribution of mild hearing loss to auditory language learning problems.* In Roeser RJ, Downs MP, editors: *Auditory disorders in school children,* ed 2, New York, 1988, Thieme.
9. Flexer C: Audiological rehabilitation in the schools, *ASHA* 32:44, 1990.
10. Geers AE, Moog JS: Predicting spoken language acquisition of profoundly hearing-impaired children, *J Speech Hear Disord* 52:84, 1987.
11. Geers A, Moog J: Factors predictive of the development of literacy in profoundly hearing-impaired adolescents, *Volta Review* 91:69, 1989.
12. Harper-Bardach P: *Education of the deaf.* In Cummings CW and others, editors: *Otolaryngology—head and neck surgery,* vol 4, St Louis, 1986, Mosby.
13. Jensema CJ, Karchmer MA, Trybus RJ: *The rated speech intelligibility of hearing-impaired children: basic relationships*, Washington DC, 1978, Gallaudet College Office of Demographic Studies.
14. Karchmer M: *Educational outcomes and achievement levels*, Presented at the Joint National Association of State Directors of Special Education (NASDE) Conference of Executives of Schools for the Deaf (CEASD), "Status of Education of the Deaf in the United States," Las Vegas, Nev, 1991.
15. Katz J, editor: *Handbook of clinical audiology*, ed 4, Baltimore, 1994, Williams & Wilkins.
16. Levitt H, McGarr NS, Geffner D, editors: *Development of language and communication skills in hearing-impaired children: ASHA monograph #26*, Rockville, Md., 1987, ASHA.
17. Ling D, editor: *Early intervention for hearing impaired children: total communication options*, Boston, 1984, College-Hill Press.
18. Ling D, Ling AH: *Aural habilitation; the foundations of verbal learning in hearing-impaired children*, Washington DC, 1978, The Alexander Graham Bell Association for the Deaf.
19. Luterman DM: Audiological counseling and the diagnostic process, *ASHA* 32:35, 1990.
20. Moores JM, Moores DF: *Educational alternatives for the hearing impaired.* In Schow RL, Nerbonne MA, editors: *Introduction to aural rehabilitation,* ed 2, Austin, 1989, ProEd.
21. Reference deleted in pages.
22. Northern JL, Downs MP: *Hearing in children*, ed 3, Baltimore, 1984, Williams & Wilkins.

23. Nowell RC: *Psychology of hearing impairment.* In Katz J, editor: *Handbook of clinical audiology*, ed 3, Baltimore, 1985, Williams & Wilkins.
24. Prinz PM: *Language and communication development, assessment and intervention in hearing-impaired individuals.* In Katz J, editor: *Handbook of clinical audiology*, ed 3, Baltimore, 1985, Williams & Wilkins.
25. Rodel MJ: *Children with hearing impairment.* In Katz J, editor: *Handbook of clinical audiology*, ed 3, Baltimore, 1985, Williams & Wilkins.
26. Roeser RJ, Downs MP, editors: *Auditory disorders in school children*, ed 2, New York, 1988, Thieme.
27. Ross M, Calvert D: The semantics of deafness, *Volta Review* 69:644, 1967.
28. Roush J: Expanding the audiologist's role, *ASHA* 33:47, 1991.
29. Roush J, McWilliam RA: A new challenge for pediatric audiology: public law 99-457, *J Am Acad Audiol* 1:196, 1990.
30. Schildroth A, Karchnmer M, editors: *Deaf children in America*, San Diego, 1986, College-Hill Press.
31. Schildroth A: Recent changes in the educational placement of deaf students, *Am Ann Deaf* 133:61, 1988.
32. Schow RL, Nerbonne MA, editors: *Introduction to aural rehabilitation*, ed 3, Boston, 1996, Allyn & Bacon.
33. Silverman SR: *From Aristotle to Bell and beyond.* In Davis H, Silverman SR, editors: *Hearing and deafness*, ed 4, New York, 1978, Holt, Rinehart & Winston.
34. Stredler-Brown A, Yoshinaga-Itano C: *The FAMILY assessment: a multidisciplinary evaluation tool.* In Roush J, Matkin N, editors: *Infants and toddlers with hearing loss*, Baltimore, 1994, York Press.
35. Tanner DC: Loss and grief: implications for the speech language pathologist and audiologist, *ASHA* 22:916, 1980.
36. United States Department of Health, Education, and Welfare: Rules and regulations for implementation of the education for all handicapped children act of 1975, Fed Regis 42:45 CFR, Part 121,a et. seq., August 23, 1977.
37. Webster DB, Webster M: Effects of neonatal conductive hearing loss on brain stem auditory nuclei, *Ann Otol Rhinol Laryngol* 88:684, 1979.
38. Withrow MS: *The federal role in services to hearing-impaired people.* In Roeser RJ, Downs MP, editors: *Auditory disorders in school children*, ed 1, New York, 1981, Thieme-Stratton.
39. Yoshinaga-Itano C, Apuzzo M: Early identification of infants with significant hearing loss and the Minnesota Child Development Inventory, *Seminars in Hearing* 16:2, 1995.
40. Yoshinaga-Itano C, Ruberry J: The Colorado Individual Performance Profile, *Volta Review* 94:2, 1992.
41. Yoshinaga-Itano C and others: *The effect of early identification on the development of deaf and hard-of-hearing infants and toddlers*, Poster session at the National Convention of the Academy of Audiology, Fort Lauderdale, Fla. 1996.

SUGGESTED READINGS

Alpiner JG, McCarthy PA, editors: *Rehabilitative audiology: children and adults*, Baltimore, 1987, Williams & Wilkins.

Amon C: *Meeting state and federal guidelines.* In Roeser RJ, Downs MP, editors: *Auditory disorders in school children*, ed 1, New York, 1981, Thieme-Stratton.

Berg FS: *Educational audiology: hearing and speech management*, New York, 1976, Grune & Stratton.

Calvert DR: *Physicians' guide to the education of hearing-impaired children*, Washington DC, 1986, Alexander Graham Bell Association for the Deaf.

Clark JG: Counseling in a pediatric audiologic practice, *ASHA* 24:521, 1982.

Domico WD: The 1986 education of the handicapped act and judicial decisions relating to the child who is hearing impaired, *ASHA* 31:91, 1989.

Katz J, editor: *Handbook of clinical audiology*, ed 4, Baltimore, 1994, Williams & Wilkins.

Ling D, editor: *Early intervention for hearing impaired children: oral options*, Boston, 1984, College-Hill Press.

Ling D, editor: *Early intervention for hearing impaired children: total communication options*, Boston, 1984, College-Hill Press.

Rodel MJ: *Children with hearing impairment.* In Katz J, editor: *Handbook of clinical audiology*, ed 3, Baltimore, 1985, Williams & Wilkins.

Roeser RJ, Downs MP, editors: *Auditory disorders in school children*, ed 2, New York, 1988, Thieme.

Roush J, McWilliam RA: A new challenge for pediatric audiology: public law 99-457, *J Am Acad Audiol* 1:196, 1990.

Schildroth A, Karchnmer M, editors: *Deaf children in America*, San Diego, 1986, College-Hill Press.

Schildroth A: Recent changes in the educational placement of deaf students. *Am Ann Deaf* 133:61, 1988.

Schow RL, Nerbonne MA, editors: *Introduction to aural rehabilitation.* ed. 3, Boston, 1996, Allyn & Bacon.

Withrow MS: *The federal role in services to hearing-impaired people.* In Roeser RJ, Downs MP, editors: *Auditory disorders in school children.* ed 1, New York, 1981, Thieme-Stratton.

Chapter 32

General Sensorineural Hearing Loss

Patrick E. Brookhouser
Kenneth M. Grundfast

Hearing loss in infants and children may be sensorineural, conductive, or mixed; unilateral or bilateral; symmetric or asymmetric; syndromic (involving other identifiable features) or nonsyndromic (isolated hearing loss); congenital or postnatal; prelingual, perilingual, or postlingual (i.e., onset before, during, or after speech or language acquisition); and genetic or nongenetic. It may range in severity from mild to profound, be characterized by stable or unstable auditory thresholds, and be coexistent with one or more independent developmental disabilities (e.g., a learning disability, mental retardation).

Early identification of significant sensorineural hearing loss (SNHL) in infants and young children was designated a national health priority in the 1990 United States (US) Health and Human Services document *Healthy People 2000: National Health Promotion and Disease Prevention Objectives*, which established a goal of reducing the average age of identification of infants with significant hearing loss from 24 to 30 months (typical in 1990) to no more than 12 months. Early rehabilitation, as required by the Americans with Disabilities Act, is essential for development of age-appropriate speech and language (necessary for literacy) by school age. Research supports the existence of a critical period in the first years of life for optimal acquisition of speech and language. The absence of adequate auditory stimulation in the infant may impede full development and maturation of central auditory pathways. Emerging data from longitudinal studies of children with congenital or early-onset hearing loss show a significant advantage in communicative skill development over time among infants of equal cognitive abilities whose hearing losses are identified and intervention instituted before 6 months of age compared with infants identified later.[90]

Without obvious ear, head, or neck deformities, congenital hearing loss may not be recognized until an infant fails to achieve expected communicative milestones. Persistent, congenital, or early-onset hearing loss that is moderate to profound (41 to 100 dB) distorts the child's perception of attempts at speech production and the speech of others. If significant bilateral hearing loss is undetected during the first years of life, impaired receptive and expressive speech or language development can impede acquisition of literacy skills, school achievement, and social or emotional development.[9,44,60,87] Persistent moderate-to-profound unilateral hearing loss was regarded as developmentally innocuous in a school-age child if appropriate compensatory strategies (e.g., preferential classroom seating) were implemented. Follow-up studies, however, link unilateral SNHL to poor academic performance, increased likelihood of repeating a grade, and school behavior problems.[8,18] Children with unilateral SNHL can experience impaired speech perception when background noise is presented to the better ear. Background noise in most elementary schools approaches 50 to 70 dB sound pressure level (SPL), and unfavorable sound reverberation compounds problems in open classrooms.

In developed countries, 1 to 2 of 1000 school-age children exhibit bilateral SNHL of 50 dB or worse, including 0.5 to 1 of 1000 whose bilateral losses exceed 75 dB.[22] Data from the United Kingdom[29] indicate that 1 of 943 newborns followed longitudinally until school age had SNHL or mixed hearing loss. Children who had been in the neonatal intensive care unit (NICU) had an increased risk for hearing loss (1 of 174 NICU infants versus 1 of 1278 non-NICU infants). Infants and children with less persistent hearing loss (i.e., hard of hearing versus deaf) are 5 to 10 times more common than those with severe-to-profound losses.[89] Unilateral SNHL of 45 dB or worse among US school-age children has a prevalence of about 3 in 1000.[6] If the hearing loss criterion is 26 dB instead of 45 dB, the prevalence increases to 13 in 1000. No reliable prevalence data are available for infants and preschoolers because unilateral losses are generally discovered later in life than are bilateral impairments (mean age in one study, 8.78 years).[18]

The 1993 National Institutes of Health (NIH) Consensus Statement on Early Identification of Hearing Impairment in Infants and Young Children[37] reported an average age of 2.5 years for diagnosis in children with congenital or early-onset hearing loss. Previous early identification initiatives, such as public awareness campaigns, mass screening questionnaires for newborns, and various neonatal hearing screening techniques (e.g., cribogram), were prohibitively expensive or failed for other reasons to gain widespread acceptance. The Joint Committee on Infant Hearing (JCIH), established in 1969, is a multispecialty body that includes pediatricians, otolaryngologists, audiologists, educators of the hearing impaired, and public health specialists. The JCIH generated serial position statements to facilitate identification of neonates at sufficiently increased risk for permanent hearing loss to warrant hearing screening. The 1982 JCIH Position Statement[50] recommended seven criteria for identifying infants at risk for hearing impairment. 1990 Recommendations expanded the risk criteria to include neonates (birth to 28 days) and infants (29 days to 2 years). As many as 2% to 5% of neonates at high risk have moderate-to-severe SNHL. Recommendations were made regarding optimal audiologic screening protocols and early intervention strategies for hearing-impaired infants and their families. Such focused screening programs, however, fail to identify significant hearing loss in as many as 50% of children of elementary school age. Renewed interest in universal hearing screening of newborns in the US has resulted from the availability of reliable objective techniques using evoked otoacoustic emissions (EOAEs) and automated auditory brainstem responses (ABRs). The 1993 NIH Consensus Statement on Early Identification of Childhood Hearing Loss recommended in-hospital hearing screening for all infants admitted to NICUs and all other infants within the first 3 months of life. EOAE measures were recommended for initial screening followed by rescreening with ABR for all EOAE failures. Infants failing rescreening should be promptly referred for comprehensive audiologic evaluation.

The 1994 JCIH Position Statement[49] endorsed universal detection of infants with hearing loss as early as possible. The importance of identifying infants with SNHL onset after 3 months of age is stressed. The JCIH also advocated continued use of risk indicators in clinical settings in which universal screening has not been implemented.

The 1994 Position Statement includes an expanded list of indicators associated with SNHL or with conductive hearing loss to help identify neonates in need of early hearing screening and to determine which infants should undergo rescreening or periodic monitoring of hearing.

The 1994 indicators include:

For use with neonates (birth to 28 days) when universal screening is unavailable:

1. Family history of hereditary childhood SNHL
2. *In utero* infection, such as cytomegalovirus (CMV), rubella, syphilis, herpes, and toxoplasmosis
3. Craniofacial anomalies, including those with morphologic abnormalities of the pinna and ear canal
4. Birth weight less than 1500 g (3.3 lbs)
5. Hyperbilirubinemia at a serum level requiring exchange transfusion
6. Ototoxic drugs including but not limited to aminoglycosides used in multiple courses or in combination with loop diuretics
7. Bacterial meningitis
8. Apgar scores of 0 to 4 at 1 min or 0 to 6 at 5 min
9. Mechanical ventilation lasting 5 days or longer
10. Stigmata or other findings associated with a syndrome known to include an SNHL or conductive hearing loss

For use with infants (29 days to 2 years) who develop certain health conditions requiring rescreening:

1. Parent or caregiver concern regarding hearing, speech, language, or developmental delay
2. Bacterial meningitis and other infections associated with SNHL
3. Head trauma associated with loss of consciousness or skull fracture
4. Stigmata or other findings associated with a syndrome known to include an SNHL or conductive hearing loss
5. Ototoxic medications including but not limited to chemotherapeutic drugs or aminoglycosides used in multiple courses or in combination with loop diuretics
6. Recurrent or persistent otitis media with effusion for at least 3 months

For use with infants (29 days to 3 years) who require periodic monitoring (at least every 6 months until age 3 years and at appropriate intervals thereafter) of hearing to detect delayed-onset SNHL or conductive hearing loss:

1. Family history of hereditary childhood hearing loss
2. *In utero* infection, such as CMV, rubella, syphilis, herpes, or toxoplasmosis
3. Neurofibromatosis type II and neurodegenerative disorders
4. Persistent pulmonary hypertension in the newborn period

5. Recurrent or persistent otitis media with effusion
6. Anatomic deformities and other disorders that affect eustachian tube function
7. Neurodegenerative disorders

Additional universal newborn screening requirements are viewed with a healthy skepticism by neonatologists and others responsible for implementing screening programs. Test sensitivity and specificity are important considerations for a low incidence disorder such as hearing loss. The failure rate for initial screening should be manageable to allow for rescreening and prompt elimination of false-positives, minimizing the need for unnecessary and more costly comprehensive audiological evaluations. The JCIH Position Statement identifies EOAEs and automated ABRs as acceptable screening techniques, and a multicenter clinical trial has been funded by the National Institute on Deafness and Other Communication Disorders to compare efficacy of these methods (1997). In carefully monitored programs, failure rates requiring referral can be kept in the 3% range. Approximately 120 hospital-based newborn hearing screening programs had been established by 1995, and the Bureau of Maternal and Child Health has funded initiatives to help additional programs. The Center for Disease Control and Prevention is developing a national database to monitor prevalence data and the effectiveness of state programs. The availability of facilities and staff to institute appropriate follow-up and plan individualized programs for each newly identified hearing-impaired child is essential in the cost-benefit analysis of any early identification program.

EVALUATION OF THE HEARING-IMPAIRED CHILD

Comprehensive evaluation of a child with significant hearing impairment requires the coordinated efforts of a multispecialty team that includes an otolaryngologist experienced with children, a pediatric audiologic team competent with behavioral and electrophysiologic testing, a pediatrician skilled in detecting subtle findings associated with hearing loss syndromes, a genetic counselor, a pediatric ophthalmologist with competence in electroretinography, a psychologist to assess the child's cognitive abilities, an educator of the deaf with expertise in early intervention, and a speech and language pathologist to assess oral motor function and linguistic development. Consultation in pediatric neurology and neuroradiology also should be easily accessible.

A thorough case history provides the foundation for the remainder of the evaluation. In addition to a detailed prenatal, birth, and postnatal history for the child, a complete family history should be obtained, which includes hearing loss; speech or language disorders; ear, nose, and throat disorders; craniofacial deformities; and such syndromic features as kidney disorders, sudden death at a young age, thyroid disease, intracranial tumors, progressive blindness, and café au lait spots. Because most genetic hearing loss is recessive, it is very important to rule out marital consanguinity in the family history. If a family history of hearing loss is identified, an exhaustive pedigree should be constructed, including at least three generations. Many families with genetic deafness fail to recognize the heritable nature of the disorder because family tradition ascribes each case to an extrinsic cause such as mastoid disease, head trauma, or noise damage.

A careful physical examination should involve assessment of the ears and a search for subtle findings (e.g., preauricular or branchial pits, heterochromia irides, blue sclerae, dystopia canthorum, facial asymmetry, café au lait spots). No physical finding should be disregarded until genetic consultation has been obtained. Ophthalmologic evaluation is critical because the visual system assumes an even more important neurosensory role in a child with impaired auditory acuity. Additionally, early detection of coexisting retinitis pigmentosa with electroretinography can influence rehabilitative decisions. An electrocardiogram should be obtained on all SNHL children who do not have a documented nongenetic cause for their hearing loss. A family history of syncopal spells or sudden death at an early age demands exclusion of a potentially fatal yet manageable cardiac conduction defect, which can be associated with early-onset hearing loss.

Basic laboratory studies should include complete blood count with differential and sickle cell prep, if indicated; basic blood studies: chemistries, lipids, blood sugar, creatinine, blood urea nitrogen, and thyroid studies; and urinalysis. If hematuria is present (''red diaper'' in infants), additional renal studies (e.g., ultrasound) should be undertaken. Serologic tests to detect congenital syphilis and toxoplasmosis, which are potentially manageable, are advisable. The rubella vaccination status of the mother should determine the necessity for these tests. CMV accounts for a significant percentage of childhood deafness; confirmation of true congenital infection should be based on positive serology early in life, probably within the first 2 or 3 weeks. Antibodies to perinatally or postnatally acquired CMV can obscure the diagnosis. The role of autoimmunity in the etiology of progressive SNHL in children is unclear, and judgment regarding the cost-effectiveness of routine clinical studies aimed in detecting such disease processes should await evidence regarding their prevalence. In addition, management of this disorder in adults—extended high-dose corticosteroids and cytotoxic drugs—would have to overcome serious ethical and health-related concerns regarding complications before being judged safe for administration to a child or adolescent. The usefulness of temporal bone imaging studies for assessing profoundly deaf children for cochlear implant candidacy has resulted in increased use of this diagnostic modality. Discovery of inner ear anomalies, such as Mondini malformation, can also have important prognostic and counseling implications.

Pediatric audiologic evaluation should determine the type

of hearing loss (i.e., conductive, sensorineural, or mixed); the degree of loss (i.e., mild, moderate, severe, profound, and anacusic); the audiometric configuration and symmetry of the impairment; and finally, with serial assessment, the stability or progression of the loss. Behavioral thresholds cannot be compared precisely with threshold information obtained by electrophysiologic methods such as ABR. Although ABR thresholds correlate best with high-frequency behavioral thresholds, they are not as sensitive. Behavioral thresholds for click stimuli, which are commonly used in ABR testing, typically occur at 30- to 36-dB peak SPL, yet few normal-hearing patients show ABRs to such low-level stimuli in the usual clinical test paradigm. Vestibular dysfunction may coexist with hearing loss having a genetic etiology (e.g., Usher's syndrome type I) and with hearing loss having a nongenetic cause, such as bacterial meningitis and ototoxic drugs and chemicals. The availability of computerized rotational testing has facilitated vestibular system evaluation in young children, which may be important in determining the cause of delayed gross motor skill development (e.g., sitting unsupported, walking, standing on one foot). Progressive and fluctuating SNHL, with or without vertigo, in children raises the specter of possible perilymphatic fistula or other manageable disorder; more extensive work-up is indicated in these cases. Even intensive multidisciplinary evaluation and intervention, which may entail corticosteroids or exploratory ear surgery to search for a perilymphatic fistula, may fail to arrest threshold fluctuation or gradually decreasing auditory acuity in many of these children. The likelihood of progressive SNHL in an affected child's ear is generally estimated at 2% to 6%, but some authors project a substantially higher risk of threshold deterioration.

Serial auditory threshold behavior in children with SNHL may be influenced by intrinsic and extrinsic factors, apart from an actual change in auditory sensitivity over time. Exposure to sufficiently intense sound, including overamplification with hearing aids, may cause a temporary threshold shift. The young patient may learn to tune in more attentively to soft sounds, thus achieving better thresholds not reflective of an actual change in auditory acuity. Different examiners may use diverse criteria to assess a young child's conditioned response (e.g., head turn in visual reinforcement audiometry) to an auditory stimulus. This type of error is particularly common in multiply handicapped, hearing-impaired children with limited response. The best protection against inadvertent errors resulting from methodologic differences is to arrange for the same audiologists to evaluate a particular child's hearing over time. Any errors would be consistent in this instance. In general, threshold variation at 250 Hz should be ascribed less relative importance because background conditions in the test environment can affect low-frequency responses. Interest is greater in variation of thresholds at 8000 Hz outside the allowable 10-dB envelope (i.e., ± 5 dB). In contrast, significant threshold change at the four middle test frequencies (500, 1000, 2000, and 4000 Hz) should elicit greater clinician concern. Fluctuation or deterioration of thresholds (absent middle ear dysfunction) frequencies by 15 dB or more should prompt careful reevaluation of the hearing-impaired child.

In one series of 229 SNHL children with threshold variation over time (normal middle ear function), fluctuation with or without progressive deterioration was more common than pure progressive loss.[21] The probability of contralateral threshold fluctuation was 0.91, whereas the probability of contralateral progressive threshold deterioration was 0.67. A companion study examined 95 of 229 children who sustained a 20-dB or greater decrement in auditory acuity at one or more frequency.[18] Children who had undergone medical or surgical intervention were excluded from this retrospective review. A 20-dB or greater drop at any target frequency was designated an *episode*; 429 episodes were identified in 138 ears that met the criteria. Frequency-specific serial thresholds obtained during the 6 months after each episode were classified as stable (± 5 dB), improved (10 dB or more), or worse (10 dB or more). These data confirm a significant tendency (i.e., approximately 50%) for spontaneous improvement of auditory acuity over the 6 months after a 20-dB decrement at any frequency. A 10-dB or greater improvement was observed after 52.4% of the episodes, threshold stability occurred after 31%, and additional loss (10 dB or more) occurred in 16.6% of cases. Of the episodes, 80% at 4000 Hz and 88.5% at 1000 Hz were followed by threshold stability or improvement. Further hearing loss was observed most often at 4000 Hz (20%) and least often at 1000 Hz (11.4%). Episodic losses occurred in both ears in 45% of 95 children, but these losses were not necessarily simultaneous or symmetric. Of the 95 study children, 65 experienced sufficiently severe decrements during 110 episodes to sustain a 20-dB or greater deterioration of the three-frequency average (i.e., 500-, 1000-, and 2000-Hz thresholds). An improvement of 10 dB or more in the three-frequency average, without management, was documented in 50% of these cases; the three-frequency average remained stable in 45%, and a 10-dB or greater decline occurred in only 4% during 6 months of follow-up. Recovery to pre-episodic levels occurred after only 14% of these episodes, although at least 20-dB improvement was observed 24% of the time. These observations of the natural history of the disorder provide a benchmark against which the efficacy of therapeutic intervention in fluctuating and progressive childhood SNHL can be compared.

Genetic and nongenetic etiologies merit diagnostic consideration in children with fluctuating and progressive SNHL. Nonsyndromic, hereditary, progressive SNHL was categorized by Konigsmark and Gorlin[55] according to age at onset, involved frequencies (i.e., low, mid, and high), and mode of inheritance (i.e., dominant, recessive, and X-linked).

Syndromic disorders associated with fluctuating and progressive SNHL include features such as anhidrosis, ataxia, branchial fistulas, optic atrophy, piebald trait, and preauricular pits. Acoustic neuromata associated with neurofibromatosis, particularly type 2, can present in younger patients. Inner ear anomalies such as Mondini's aplasia and enlarged vestibular aqueduct, detectable by temporal bone imaging, have been linked with fluctuating and progressive SNHL in children and are often exacerbated by minimal head trauma. The differential diagnosis also should include drugs and chemicals; noise trauma; ear or head trauma; mumps; and congenital infections (e.g., rubella, CMV, toxoplasmosis, and syphilis; bacterial meningitis; hyperlipidemia, thyroid dysfunction, diabetes, and hypercoagulability state; sickle cell disease, leukemia, and autoimmune inner ear disease; perilymphatic fistula).

The role of possible perilymphatic fistulas in children with fluctuating and progressive hearing loss has been debated in the literature. The unavailability of a sensitive and specific diagnostic technique to confirm the presence of a perilymphatic fistula preoperatively has necessitated invasive procedures (middle ear exploration, myringotomy with oto-endoscopy) to assess the integrity of the perilymphatic compartment. Definitive surgical confirmation of a perilymphatic fistula is also problematic, prompting an ongoing search for perilymph-specific biochemical markers to differentiate perilymph from other clear middle ear fluids in the clinic or operating room. Although preoperative confirmation of perilymphatic fistula remains elusive, a monitored fistula test seems reasonable in these cases. A positive fistula test may be helpful, whereas a negative result should be considered inconclusive on the basis of reported series. Temporal bone imaging is helpful in identifying middle ear anomalies in children with conductive or mixed losses and inner ear or internal auditory canal anomalies or lesions in cases of SNHL that might predispose the child to fistula formation and progressive hearing loss.

A diligent search for etiology of SNHL in a child using state of the art techniques will prove inconclusive in 30% to 40% of cases. With the declining incidence of nongenetic etiologies (e.g., prenatal rubella, measles, mumps, *Haemophilus influenzae* meningitis), genetic hearing loss will affect more newly identified cases. Many parents are anxious to determine the etiology of their child's loss for prognostic and family planning considerations. Clinicians should address a family's concerns regarding the lack of a definitive diagnosis.

Several detailed etiologic classifications of SNHL in children have been suggested. Terminology such as *genetic versus acquired* and *congenital versus acquired* can be confusing. It would seem most helpful to classify SNHL cases as genetic versus nongenetic and congenital versus delayed (i.e., postnatal) onset. Many genetic hearing losses are not congenital, and certain nongenetic hearing impairments (e.g., rubella deafness) are present at birth. Rapidly expanding knowledge regarding genetic hearing loss should lead to techniques for the prenatal or early postnatal diagnosis of these disorders even if clinical manifestations are delayed for months or years.

GENETIC HEARING LOSS

Based principally on retrospective review of student records at schools for the deaf, it has been estimated that about 50% of childhood SNHL is caused by genetic factors; 20% to 25% of cases are attributable to identifiable environmental causes, occurring prenatally, perinatally, or postnatally; and 25% to 30% are sporadic cases of uncertain etiology, undoubtedly including some nonsyndromic genetic losses. These estimates may vary depending on the specific population being studied. Reports during the rubella epidemic in the US between 1964 and 1966 attributed only 18% of new SNHL cases to heritable factors because of the disproportionate number of newly identified congenital rubella hearing loss.[12,13] In contrast, of many nongenetic infectious SNHL etiologies should favor genetic causes in future cohort studies.

Heritable forms of hearing loss may be congenital or delayed in onset, progressive or nonprogressive, unilateral or bilateral, symmetric or asymmetric in audiogram configuration, and syndromic (involving other identifiable traits) or nonsyndromic (isolated hearing loss). At least 400 genetic syndromes involving hearing loss have been identified; they are typically classified on the basis of other organ systems involved: craniofacial or cervical, skeletal, integumentary, ocular, neurologic, renal, metabolic, and other. Classification of nonsyndromic hearing impairments (i.e., hearing loss only) is generally based on audiologic characteristics (e.g., frequencies involved), presence or absence of progression, age of onset, and mode of inheritance. Approximately 75% to 80% of genetic hearing loss is generally attributed to autosomal recessive genes and 18% to 20% to autosomal dominant genes, with the remainder classified as X-linked, or chromosomal disorders. In males, 5% to 6% of SNHL may be attributable to X-linked inheritance. Approximately half of all genetic losses involve recognizable syndromes. More accurate estimates of hearing loss etiologies should result from emerging techniques for identifying single cases of nonsyndromic SNHL, particularly recessive losses.

BASIC GENETIC PRINCIPLES

Human genes are arranged linearly on 22 two pairs of autosomes and one pair of sex chromosomes. Each pair of chromosomes carries a distinctive set of gene loci for which there may be several alternative codes or alleles. For any trait, the genotype may be comprised of two identical alleles (homozygous) or two different alleles (heterozygous). Physical expression of the trait is called the *phenotype*, which is determined by the nature and interaction of the two alleles, which were each inherited from one parent. An autosomal dominant allele is phenotypically expressed in the homozygous or heterozygous state, whereas an autosomal recessive allele is expressed only in the homozygous state. An X-

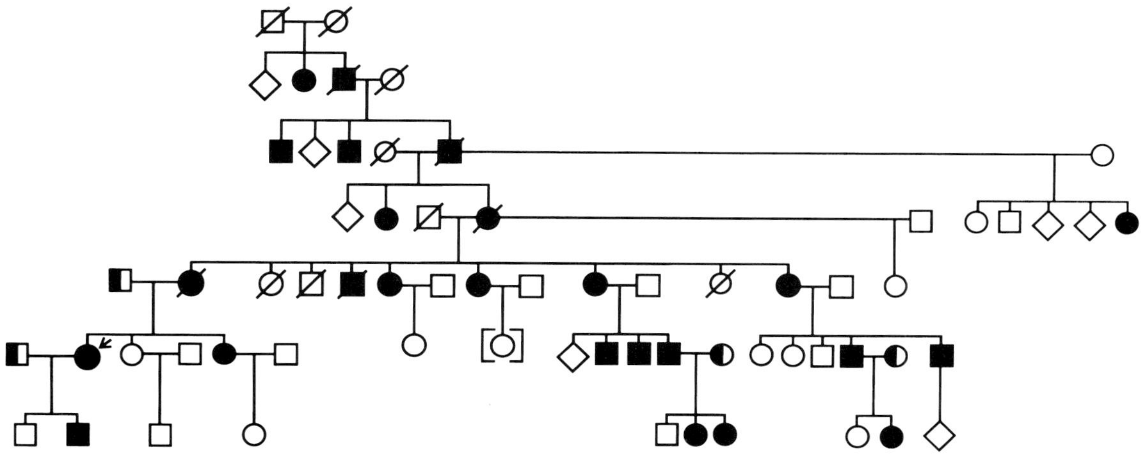

Fig. 32-1. Dominant pattern of inheritance.

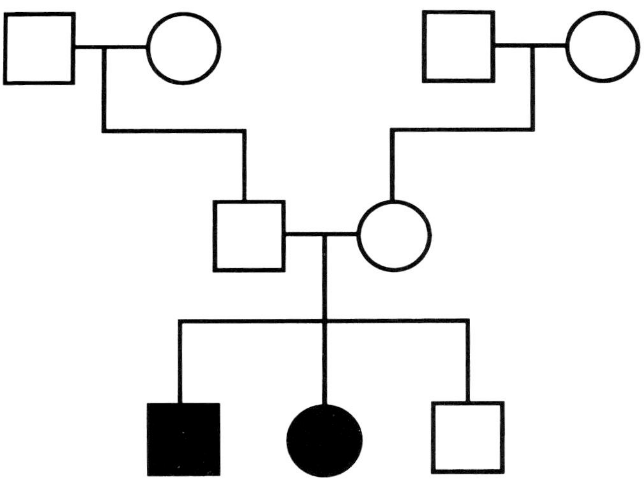

Fig. 32-2. Recessive pattern of inheritance.

linked (i.e., sex chromosome–linked) recessive gene is expressed in the hemizygous condition in the male because the Y chromosome does not carry a complementary allele. A parent who is heterozygous for an autosomal dominant gene has a 50% chance of transmitting it to each child. (Fig. 32-1). Offspring of heterozygotic carriers of an autosomal recessive gene have a 25% recurrence risk (Fig. 32-2). An X-linked recessive trait is not usually expressed in a heterozygous female, but each male child has a 50% chance of inheriting the gene, which would be phenotypically expressed. There is a 50% chance that each of a female carrier's daughters would inherit the gene, but 100% of the daughters of an affected male will inherit his only X chromosome and thus the abnormal gene. None of an affected male's sons inherit his X chromosome or the abnormal gene. The hallmark of X-linked inheritance is the absence of male-to-male transmission.

Dominant genes may not be phenotypically expressed in all persons heterozygous for the gene, a phenomenon called *decreased penetrance*. Different family members may show diverse manifestations of the gene, which is characteristic of dominant disorders. Phenotypic expression may be modified by environmental influences or interaction with other genes.

Chromosomal abnormalities involving autosomes result from extra or deficient chromosomal material being present in each cell; the phenotypic expression may be severe or even fatal. Phenotypes associated with abnormalities of sex chromosomes are generally less severe. In patients with trisomy, three copies of a given chromosome are present: trisomy 21 or Down syndrome is the least severe, whereas trisomy 13 (Patau's syndrome) and trisomy 18 (Edward's syndrome) are less common and more severe. Other autosomal trisomies are almost always fatal, as is the presence of a single chromosome, monosomy. Chromosomal deletions (absent segments) or duplications (extra material) may be present, with the nature and severity of each phenotype depending on the amount and origin of the material involved. Newer techniques using high-resolution chromosomal banding and fluorescent *in situ* hybridization allow microscopic identification of small abnormalities, which may help localize involved genes.

Mitochondria, cytoplasmic organelles, contain 2 to 10 copies of a small ring-shaped piece of nonnuclear deoxyribonucleic acid (DNA), each of which contains about 16 kb. This mitochondrial DNA includes genes that encode messenger, ribosomal, and transfer ribonucleic acid (RNA) active in the synthesis of mitochondrial-produced proteins. It is hypothesized that during evolution some mitochondria DNA migrated to become nuclear DNA, which interacts with the remaining mitochondrial genome to facilitate energy production through adenosine triphosphate (ATP) synthesis and oxidative phosphorylation. Because mitochondrial genome mutations can impact energy production, tissues with high energy requirements (e.g., muscle) are particularly vulnerable. A less effective DNA repair mechanism in the mitochondria results in a higher rate of mutation than is observed with nuclear DNA. Involvement in patients with mitochondrial disorders is graded because only a fraction of all mitochondria in a cell may harbor a particular mutation at a given time. A typical mitochondrial disorder may gradually worsen. Because sperm transmit few, if any, mitochondria, maternal transmission of mutations is the rule. All offspring of a mother who is homoplasmic for a mitochondrial mutation will be affected.

GENE LINKAGE ANALYSIS

Genetic linkage analysis determines the precise chromosomal location of a specific gene as a prelude to fine mapping, cloning, and translation of the gene. In linkage analysis, genetic material may be randomly exchanged (i.e., crossover) between two members of a chromosome pair during cell meiosis, and two genetic loci are linked when their alleles are transmitted together more frequently than expected by chance. If two genetic loci are sufficiently separated on the same chromosome so that crossovers occur 50% of the time, they are not linked and will be transmitted by random assortment. If the chromosomal location of one gene is known (a marker gene), the linked locus can be determined. The likelihood that two loci are linked is expressed in terms of the lod score (i.e., logarithm of the odds of linkage) which, by convention, should be 3 or higher to accept the hypothesis of linkage for the loci under study. A trait is genetically heterogeneous if linkage with a marker locus is proven in some families, whereas other families fail to show linkage to the same marker or are linked to a different remote marker. Usher's and Waardenburg's syndromes show genetic heterogeneity within subtypes that cannot be differentiated clinically. Nonsyndromic hearing loss is also heterogeneous and may involve more than 100 genes, many of which are rare in the population. To help overcome the challenge of heterogeneity in recessive disorders, inbred or isolated study populations have been used, whereas large kindreds with multiple affected persons aid the study of dominant disorders.

In the past, the only available markers for linkage studies were genes for several hundred phenotypic features (e.g., blood type), which were distributed sporadically throughout the genome. A new era of linkage analysis began with the discovery of DNA markers based on inherited variations (i.e., restriction fragment length polymorphisms) in DNA sequence rather than on gene product. Partially stimulated by the Human Genome Project, these polymorphic markers are becoming so pervasive and strategically placed throughout the genome that they can serve as useful markers for essentially any gene locus being studied. In addition to libraries of DNA sequences from expressed genes, homologous genes from animals such as mice have been useful candidates in the final stages of gene identification. The ultimate criterion for identifying a particular gene as the causal gene for a specific disorder is the presence of mutations in the gene in all patients and absence of mutations in unaffected patients (Tables 32-1 through 32-4). The exact nature of the mutation disrupting a gene's function may not be identical among families.

INNER EAR STRUCTURAL MALFORMATIONS

By week 9 of gestation, the cochlea reaches full growth (2 3/4 turns). Arrest in normal development (agenesis) or aberrant development (dysgenesis) of inner ear structures may result in hearing impairment. Studies using modern temporal bone imaging reveal subtle or severe anomalies of the inner ear in about 20% of children with congenital SNHL, with about 65% being bilateral and the remainder unilateral. Depending on the timing and nature of the developmental insult, a range of inner ear anomalies can result. The most widely used classification scheme is based on the findings of temporal bone histopathologic studies; premortem confirmation through imaging studies of anomalies limited to the membranous labyrinth is not feasible.

Complete agenesis of the petrous portion of the temporal bone occurs in Michel aplasia although the external and middle ear may be unaffected. Because of the severity of the malformation, an insult prior to the end of the third gestational week has been postulated. This would correspond to the period when the otic placcode is formed on the lateral surface of the neural tube. Temporal bone imaging confirms the diagnosis, although labyrinthitis ossificans, which occurs after meningitis, has a similar appearance. Affected ears are anacusic because of the absence of sensory and neural inner ear structures. Vibrotactile devices have been of some benefit in these patients, but conventional amplification and cochlear implantation are ineffective. Safe and effective brainstem level implants, which stimulate the cochlear nucleus, may offer hope for patients. Mouse genetic studies indicate that several genes may cause Michel aplasia. Although inheritance has been documented to be autosomal dominant, it may also be recessive.

In Mondini aplasia, the basal coil of the cochlea can be identified, but the interscalar septum is absent in the upper coils, which assume a cloacal form. The endolymphatic duct also is typically enlarged. It is postulated that the deformity results from developmental arrest at approximately the sixth week of gestation. The anomaly can be inherited in an autosomal dominant fashion, may not be bilateral, and has been described in several disorders including Pendred's, Waardenburg's, Treacher Collins and Wildervaank's syndromes. Nongenetic etiologies such as congenital CMV infection have also been associated with Mondini deformity. Aggressive early intervention with conventional amplification is advisable in cases with residual neurosensory structures.

Table 32-1. Genes causing dominant nonsyndromic hereditary hearing loss

Locus name	Type of loss	Location	Gene	Study
DFNA1	Progressive	5q31	Unknown	Leon and others, 1992
DFNA2	Progressive	1p34	Unknown	Couke and others, 1994; Chaib and others, 1994
DFNA3	Congenital	13q12	Unknown	Kelsell and others, 1997
DFNA4	Progressive	19q13	Unknown	Chen and others, 1995
DFNA5	Progressive	7p15	Unknown	Van Camp and others, 1994
DFNA6	Progressive	4p16.3	Unknown	Lesperane and others, 1995
DFNA7	Progressive	1q21-q23	Unknown	Granebjaerg and others, 1995
DFNA8	Congenital	11q22-24	Unknown	Kirschhofer and others, 1995
DFNA9	Progressive	14q12-q13	Unknown	Manolis and others, 1996
DFNA10	Progressive	6q22-q23	Unknown	O'Neill and others, 1996
DFNA11	Progressive	11q12.3-q21	Unknown	Tamagawa and others, 1996
DFNA12	Progressive	11q22-q24	Unknown	Verhoeven and others, 1997
DFNA13	Not available	6p21	Unknown	Brown and others, 1997
DFNA14	Not available	4p16	Unknown	Van Camp, unpublished
DFNA15	Not available	5131	Unknown	Avraham, unpublished

Table 32-2. Genes causing recessive nonsyndromic hereditary hearing loss

Locus name	Type of loss	Location	Gene	Study
DFNB1	Congenital	13q12	Unknown	Guilford and others, 1994; Kelsell and others, 1997
DFNB2	Congenital	11q13.5	Unknown	Guildford and others, 1994
DFNB3	Congenital	17p11.2	Unknown	Friedman and others, 1995
DFNB4	Congenital	7q31	Unknown	Baldwin and others, 1995
DFNB5	Congenital	14q12	Unknown	Fukushima and others, 1995
DFNB6	Congenital	3p14-p21	Unknown	Fukushima and others, 1995
DFNB7	Congenital	9q13-q21	Unknown	Jain and others, 1995
DFNB8	Congenital	21q22	Unknown	Veske and others, 1996
DFNB9	Congenital	2p22-p23	Unknown	Chaib and others, 1996
DFNB10	Congenital	21a22.3	Unknown	Bonne-Tamir and others, 1996
DFNB11		9q13-21q	Unknown	Scotte and others, 1996
DFNB12	Congenital	10q21-22	Unknown	Chaib and others, 1996
DFNB13		7q34-36	Unknown	Mustapha and others, in press
DFNB15		3q21-q25 19p13	Unknown	Chen and others, 1997
DFNB16		15q21-q22	Unknown	Campbell and others, in press
DFNB17		7q31	Unknown	Greindwald and others, in press
DFNB18		11p14-15.1	Unknown	Jaine and others, 1997
DFNB19		18p11	Unknown	University of Iowa

Table 32-3. Genes causing X-linked nonsyndromic hereditary hearing loss

Locus name	Type of loss	Location	Gene	Study
DFN1	Progressive	Xq22	*DDP*	Tranebjaerg and others, 1995
DFN2	Congenital	Xq22	Unknown	Tyson and others, 1996
DFN3	Progressive mixed (gusher)	Xq21.1	*POU3F4*	de Kok and others, 1995
DFN4	Congenital	Xp21.2	Unknown	Lalwani and others, 1994
DFN6	Progressive	Xp22	Unknown	del Castillo and others, 1996

Table 32-4. Genes that cause hearing loss

Disorder	Inheritance	Linkage	Gene	Study
Albinism deafness syndrome	X-linked	Xq		Shiloh, 1990
Alport's syndrome	Autosomal recessive	Xq22	*COL4A5*	Barker and others, 1990
Alport's syndrome	Autosomal recessive	2q36-q37	*COL4A3, COL4A4*	Mochizuki, 1994
Bronchia-oto-renal syndrome	Autosomal dominant	8q	*EYA1*	Abdelhak and others, 1997; Vincent and others, 1997
Crouzon syndrome	Autosomal dominant	10q	*FGFR2*	Reardon, 1994
Insley syndrome, OSMEDq	Autosomal recessive	6p	*COL11A2*	Vikkula and others, 1995
Jervell and Lange-Nielsen 1	Autosomal recessive	11p	*KVLQT1*	Neyroud and others, 1997
Jervell and Lange-Nielsen 2	Autosomal recessive	21q	*KCNE1 (IsK)*	Tyson and others, 1997; Schultze-Bahr and others, 1997
Neurofibromatosis type II	Autosomal dominant	22q	*NF2, SCH*	Rouleau, 1993
Norrie's disease	X-linked	Xp11.3	*Norrin*	Berger and others, 1992; Chen and others, 1992
Osteogenesis imperfecta	Autosomal dominant	17q	*COL1A1*	Sykes and others, 1990
Osteogenesis imperfecta	Autosomal dominant	7q	*COL1A2*	Sykes and others, 1990
Pendred's syndrome	Autosomal recessive	7q21-34	*Pendrid*	Everett and others, 1997
Stickler syndrome (also Kneist, SED)	Autosomal dominant	12q	*COL2A1*	Ahmed and others, 1991
Stickler syndrome	Autosomal dominant	6p	*COL11A2*	Brunner and others, 1994
Treacher Collins syndrome	Autosomal dominant	5q32-q33.1	*TREACLE*	Dixon and others, 1996
Usher's syndrome type IA	Autosomal recessive	14q32		Kaplan and others, 1992
Usher's syndrome type IB	Autosomal recessive	11q13.5	*MYO7A*	Kimberling and others, 1992
Usher's syndrome type IC	Autosomal recessive	11p15.1		Smith and others, 1992
Usher's syndrome type ID	Autosomal recessive	10q		Wayne and others, 1996
Usher's syndrome type IE	Autosomal recessive	21q		Chaib and others, 1997
Usher's syndrome type IF	Autosomal recessive	10		Wayne and others, 1997
Usher's syndrome type IIA	Autosomal recessive	1q41		Kimberling and others, 1990
Usher's syndrome type III	Autosomal recessive	3q21-q25		Sankila and others, 1995
Waardenburg's syndrome type I	Autosomal dominant	2q35	*PAX3*	Tassabehji and others, 1992
Waardenburg's syndrome type II	Autosomal dominant	3p14.1-p12.3	*MITF*	Tassabehjii and others, 1994
Klein-Waardenburg syndrome	Autosomal dominant	2q35	*PAX3*	Hoth and others, 1993
Waardenburg-Shah syndrome	Autosomal recessive	13q22	*EDNRB*	Attie and others, 1995
Waardenburg-Shah syndrome	Autosomal recessive	20q13.2-113.3	*EDN3*	Edery and others, 1996
X-Linked mixed deafness, deafness with stapes fixation, and perilymphatic gusher	X-linked	Xq21.1	*POU3F4*	De Kok and others, 1995

The bony labyrinth and superior portion of the membranous labyrinth, including the utricle and semicircular canals, are normally differentiated in patients with Scheibe aplasia. Corti's organ is generally poorly differentiated with a deformed tectorial membrane and collapsed Reissner's membrane. An autosomal recessive nonsyndromic trait, Scheibe's is the most common aplasia and has also been observed in temporal bones from patients with Jervell and Lange-Nielsen, Refsum's, Usher's, and Waardenburg's syndromes and in congenital rubella infants. Conventional amplification with habilitative intervention is beneficial in many of these children.

In Alexander aplasia, cochlear duct differentiation at the level of the basal coil is limited with resultant effects on Corti's organ and ganglion cells. High-frequency hearing loss is the rule in these patients, with enough residual low-frequency hearing to warrant the use of properly fitted amplification.

An enlarged vestibular aqueduct, observed radiographically, has been associated with early-onset SNHL, which is usually bilateral and often progressive and may be accompanied by vertigo or incoordination. Initial hopes that endolymphatic sac surgery in these patients might be beneficial proved incorrect, and such intervention is contraindicated. Although some surgeons advocate prophylactic labyrinthine window grafting to prevent suspected perilymphatic fistula formation, definitive evidence that this procedure conserves hearing has not been forthcoming. Family studies suggest autosomal dominant inheritance, but a recessive pattern of transmission has been observed, as has an association with Pendred's syndrome.

Beginning in the sixth gestational week, formation of the semicircular canals commences with the superior semicircular canal and terminates with the lateral semicircular canal. Although isolated lateral semicircular canal anomalies are the most commonly identified inner ear malformation in temporal bone imaging studies, superior semicircular canal deformities also involve the lateral semicircular canal.

AUTOSOMAL DOMINANT DISORDERS

An autosomal dominant syndrome might be expected to be easily identified by a positive family history of classic dominant inheritance and by a recognizable phenotype. However, variation in expressivity may be reflected in different phenotypic characteristics in affected family members. An obligate carrier may not have any detectable phenotypic expression because of decreased penetrance. If a new mutation has occurred, the family history might be negative although the disorder is transmitted in a dominant fashion.

Variable expressivity is observed with Waardenburg's syndrome, which includes unilateral or bilateral SNHL in 20% of type I and more than 50% of type II patients; pigmentary anomalies, such as white forelock (20% to 30% of cases), heterochromia irides, premature greying, and vitiligo; and craniofacial features, such as dystopia canthorum broad nasal root and synophrys. Clinically, there are two types of Waardenburg's syndrome, based on the presence (type I) or absence (type II) of dystopia canthorum; hearing loss is more frequent in type II. Lateral displacement of the medial canthi may not be obvious, and normative objective indices based on distances between landmarks (e.g., medial canthi, pupils, and lateral canthi) may be helpful in reaching a diagnosis. Essentially all cases of type I are caused by a mutation of the *PAX3* gene on chromosome 2q37, which is homologous with a mouse gene for a condition called splotch, involving pigmentary and ocular abnormalities; however, only murine homozygotes are deaf and have severe neural tube defects.[80] About one fifth of type II cases are caused by a mutation of the *MITF* gene (microphthalmia transcription factor) on chromosome 3p.[79]

Features of Stickler syndrome may include a small jaw, often with a cleft palate (Robin sequence); myopia, which may be accompanied by retinal detachment or cataracts; hypermobility and enlargement of joints with early adult-onset arthritis; and occasional spondyloepiphyseal dysplasia. Educationally significant SNHL or mixed hearing loss, which may be progressive, is present in about 15% of cases, whereas hearing loss of lesser severity may be present in up to 80%. Stickler manifests variable expressivity traceable to allelic and genetic heterogeneity. Most cases are attributable to a range of mutations of the type II collagen gene (*COL2A1*) on chromosome 12.[74] Other mutations of the same gene result in the more severe syndromes of Kneist and congenital spondyloepiphyseal dysplasia, which include progressive SNHL.

In bronchia-oto-renal (BOR) or Melnick-Fraser syndrome, ear pits (possibly tags) or cervical fistulae are present, as are renal findings ranging from agenesis with renal failure to minor asymptomatic renal dysplasia, detectable by ultrasound or intravenous pyelography. The hearing loss may be sensorineural, conductive, or mixed. BOR is thought to affect about 2% of children in schools for the deaf in the US. The gene for BOR, which has been identified on chromosome 8q, is the human homologue of the developmental *Drosophila* gene eyeless.[1]

The craniofacial features of Treacher Collins syndrome (mandibulofacial dysostosis) may include microtia, aural meatal atresia, and conductive hearing impairment about 30% of the time. SNHL and vestibular dysfunction may also be present. Malar hypoplasia, with underdeveloped zygomatic arches, downward slanting palpebral fissures, coloboma of the lower eyelids, and a hypoplastic mandible, characterize the face of patients. Symmetric facies and bilateral eyelid coloboma differentiate Treacher Collins from Goldenhar's syndrome and other oculo-auricular-vertebral syndromes that involve similar, but unilateral, microtia and craniofacial abnormalities. Although ossicular malformations are common in Treacher Collins patients with conductive hearing loss, surgical correction can be technically challenging. The oculo-auriculo-vertebral spectrum is sporadic and thought to be multifactorial, whereas Treacher Collins syndrome is autosomal dominant with high penetrance. Because a new mutation may be present in as many as 60% of cases of Treacher Collins syndrome, genetic counselors should differentiate this disorder from oculo-auriculo-vertebral syndrome. *TCOF1*, the gene responsible for Treacher Collins syndrome, is located on chromosome 5q and produces a protein named *treacle*, which is operative in early craniofacial development.[35] The variable expressivity between and within families suggests that other genes may modify expression of the treacle protein.

Persons affected by neurofibromatosis (NF) may present with café au lait spots (light brown, variable-sized pigmented spots) and multiple fibromatous tumors. Cutaneous tumors are most common, but the central nervous system (CNS), peripheral nerves, and viscera may also be involved. Mental retardation, blindness, and SNHL may result from CNS lesions. Two forms have been identified clinically, the more common being NF1 (von Recklinghausen's disease), with an incidence of about 1:3000 persons, which generally includes many café au lait spots, cutaneous neurofibromas, plexiform neuromas, pseudoarthrosis (e.g., tibia), Lisch nodules of the iris and optic gliomas; however, acoustic neuromas (typically unilateral) occur in only 5% of cases. The expressed phenotype may vary from a few café au lait spots to multiple disfiguring neurofibromas. Lesions within the CNS may result in mental retardation, blindness, or hearing loss. Careful audiologic and neurologic follow-up of children with this disorder is essential. A mutation of a nerve growth factor gene located on chromosome 17 has been implicated in NF1.[72]

Bilateral acoustic neuromas (vestibular schwannomas) are present in 95% of cases with NF2, which is genetically distinct from the classic form. Presenting signs and symptoms of the bilateral lesions may not be noted until early adulthood. There are fewer café au lait spots and cutaneous neurofibromas in NF2 than in NF1, and neither optic gliomas nor Lisch nodules have been observed in NF2. As with NF1, NF2 is autosomal dominant with high penetrance but variable expressivity. NF2 is caused by mutation of a tumor-suppressor gene on chromosome 22.[67]

Otosclerosis appears to be transmitted in an autosomal dominant pattern with decreased penetrance, so only 25% to 40% of gene carriers show the phenotype; the preponderance of affected females suggests a possible hormonal influence. Genetic heterogeneity is likely, and certain involved genes may be more penetrant than others. Recent statistical studies suggest a role for the gene *COL1A1* in otosclerosis, and measles viral particles have been identified within the bony overgrowth in otosclerotic foci, raising the possibility of interaction with this viral genome. Delayed-onset conductive or mixed hearing impairment may begin in childhood but usually presents in adulthood. Although stapedotomy or stapedectomy can alleviate the conductive component of the hearing loss, otic capsule involvement (i.e., cochlear otosclerosis) with the otosclerotic process may result in gradual worsening of the SNHL.

Osteogenesis imperfecta (OI) is characterized by bone fragility, blue (clear) sclerae, hearing loss (conductive, mixed, or sensorineural), and hyperelasticity of joints and ligaments. The disorder is transmitted as an autosomal dominant with variable expressivity and incomplete penetrance. Two genes for OI have been identified, *COL1A1* on chromosome 17q and *COL1A2* on chromosome 7q.[78] A severe congenital type may present with intrauterine fractures severe enough to threaten fetal viability. The age at which the more common tarda variety becomes clinically apparent is variable. van der Hoeve's syndrome is a subtype of osteogenesis imperfecta in which progressive hearing loss begins in early childhood. Although some investigators have postulated a relationship between OI and otosclerosis, histopathologic studies of stapedial footplates in each disorder show significant differences. Minimal peripheral fixation of a markedly thickened stapedial footplate is present in a typical case of OI hearing loss. In view of the recent evidence for a possible role in otosclerosis for *COL1A1* that has been implicated in OI, the two conditions may represent different phenotypes associated with different mutations.

NONSYNDROMIC AUTOSOMAL DOMINANT HEARING LOSS

Dominant progressive hearing loss is a type of nonsyndromic, noncongenital SNHL that varies in age of onset and rate of progression and is autosomal dominant. Idiopathic, it differs from otosclerosis by the absence of ossicular and otic capsule involvement and from presbycusis by the earlier age of onset. Many types of dominant progressive hearing loss eventually progress to severe or profound hearing loss, but initial frequency involvement and the rate of progression vary among families. Konigsmark and Gorlin[55] defined four types of dominant progressive hearing loss: early onset, high frequency, midfrequency, and low frequency. Heterogeneity has been documented for each subtype as exemplified by four types of high-frequency dominant progressive hearing loss identified by audiogram configuration within family groups. More than 12 genes causing dominant progressive hearing loss have been localized. Previous estimates of the frequency of dominant progressive hearing loss among the general population have been rendered inaccurate by failure of studies to differentiate it from otosclerosis and other (e.g., nongenetic) causes of congenital hearing loss.

Recessive disorders

SNHL and retinitis pigmentosa characterize Usher's syndrome, which has an estimated frequency of 3/100,000 in Scandinavia and 4.4/100,000 in the US. This disorder, initially recognized by von Graefe[84] but intensively studied as an hereditary disorder by Usher,[82] affects about one half of the 16,000 deaf and blind persons in the US. Three clinical subtypes are differentiated on the basis of severity or progression of hearing loss and extent of vestibular involvement. Patients with type I present with congenital bilateral profound hearing loss and absent vestibular function, whereas those with type II have moderate hearing loss and normal vestibular function (Fig. 32-3). Type III, found principally among Norwegians, combines progressive SNHL and variable vestibular function. Early estimates of the relative prevalence of the Usher subtypes, based on reviews of student records at schools for the deaf, tended to overestimate the prevalence of type because these children had profound hearing loss, making their enrollment in deaf schools more likely. Recent reports of large clinical series reflect near equality between the numbers of type I and type II cases. Linkage analysis studies have localized five genes for type I and at least two genes for type II.* Thus far, only one gene has been localized for type III.[69] Ophthalmologic evaluation is an essential part of the diagnostic work-up, and subnormal electroretinographic (ERG) patterns have been observed in children as young as 2 to 3 years of age, before retinal changes are evident funduscopically.

In the autosomal recessive disorder Pendred's syndrome, SNHL is associated with abnormal iodine metabolism resulting in a euthyroid goiter, which usually becomes clinically detectable at about 8 years of age. The perchlorate discharge test shows abnormal organification of nonorganic iodine in these patients; exogenous thyroid hormone is the therapy of choice. Hearing loss in Pendred's syndrome may be profound at birth or may present with lesser degree of loss with subsequent progression. Temporal bone imaging studies in most cases of Pendred's syndrome reveal Mondini aplasia or enlarged vestibular aqueduct. Recessive inheritance is seen in many families, whereas others show a dominant pattern with variable expression. One gene for Pendred's syndrome has been localized to chromosome 7q in families with

* Refs. 24, 52, 54, 73, 85, 86.

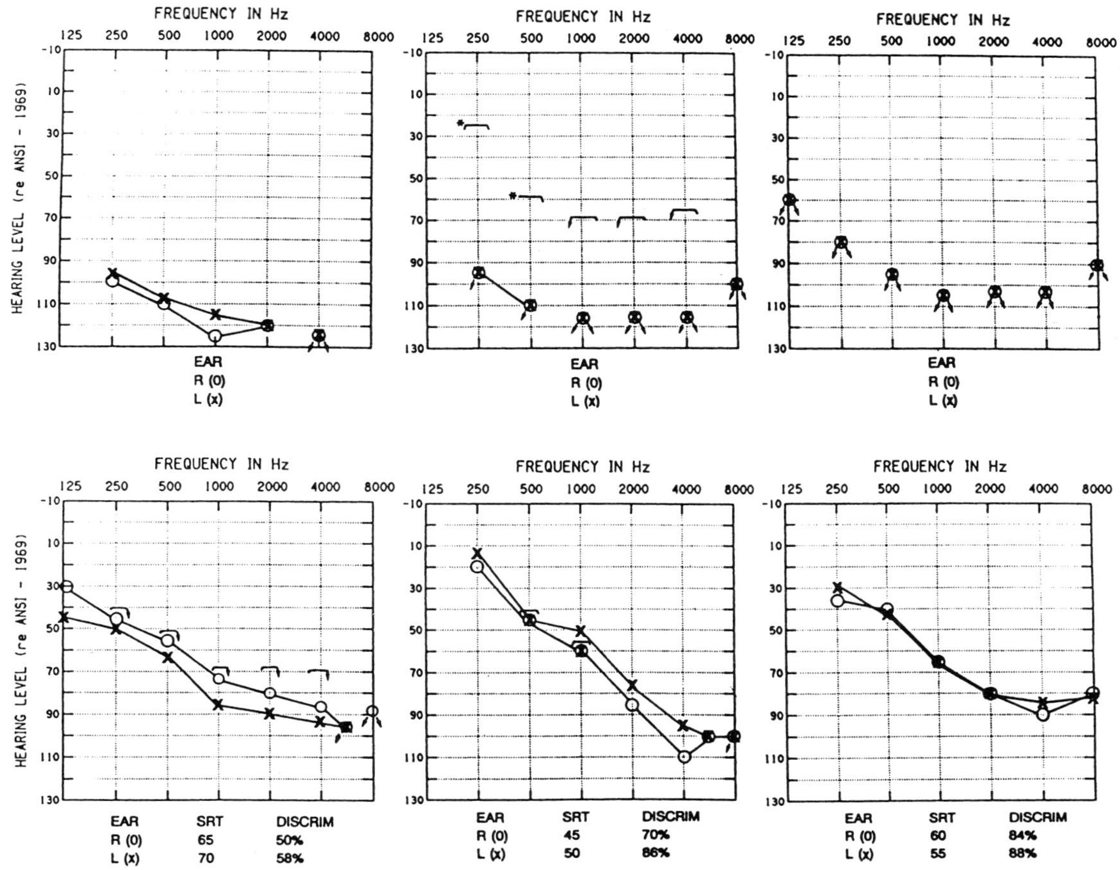

Fig. 32-3. Typical hearing loss in patients with Usher's syndrome type I (upper) and type II (lower). (From Moller CG and others: Usher syndrome: an otoneurologic study, *Laryngoscope* 99:73, 1989.)

a consistent autosomal inheritance pattern.[26,71] Further studies may confirm heterogeneity in this disorder.

In patients with Jervell and Lange-Nielsen syndrome,[48] severe congenital SNHL is inherited in a recessive pattern together with a cardiac conduction defect that can produce syncopal episodes and even sudden death as early as the second or third year of life. The syndrome is rare, with an estimated incidence of 1.6/6 cases. Electrocardiographically, large t waves and prolongation of the QT interval are observed, so that electrocardiography should be performed on all children with early-onset hearing loss of uncertain etiology. Syncope results for torsade de pointes, ventricular tachycardia, and ventricular fibrillation. β-adrenergic blockers (e.g., propranolol) effectively manage the cardiac component of the disorder. Clinically, the syncopal events may be mistaken for seizures; some patients have been managed inappropriately and ineffectively with anticonvulsants. Genetic studies attribute one form of Jervell and Lange-Nielsen syndrome to homozygosity for mutations affecting a potassium channel gene (*KVLQT 1*) on chromosome 11p15.5, which are thought to result in delayed myocellular repolarization in the heart.[83] Other mutations of the same gene have been implicated in the dominantly inherited Long QT syndrome (Romano-Ward syndrome), which is more common than Jervell and Lange-Nielsen syndrome and is not associated with hearing loss or other phenotypic abnormalities. Because parents and siblings of a patient with Jervell and Lange-Nielsen syndrome may manifest dominantly inherited Romano-Ward syndrome with attendant risk of sudden death, all family members should undergo electrocardiography.

Konigsmark and Gorlin[55] described three subtypes of nonsyndromic recessive SNHL: congenital severe-to-profound; congenital moderate; and early onset, which usually progresses rapidly from onset at age 1.5 years to profound loss by age 6. The congenital severe-to-profound type is most prevalent, and genetic heterogeneity is confirmed by the high likelihood that offspring of parents with clinically identical recessive hearing loss will have normal hearing. Genetic linkage studies have identified at least 15 gene loci for recessive nonsyndromic hearing loss. The gene *DFNB2* on chromosome 11q may be the most common and has been identified as connexin 23.[42] Although many genes may be implicated in recessive nonsyndromic hearing loss, it is likely that most of them are rare, affecting one or a few inbred families. It should soon be possible to conduct laboratory screening tests to rule out more common genetic causes for this disorder in the diagnostic challenging singleton hearing loss cases of uncertain etiology.

SEX-LINKED DISORDERS

Approximately 6% of nonsyndromic profound losses in males may be attributable to sex-linked disorders. In Norrie syndrome, congenital or rapidly progressive blindness, development of pseudoglioma, opacification, and ocular degeneration resulting in microphthalmia are observed. Progressive SNHL with onset in the second or third decade, affects approximately one third of persons with this sex-linked disorder. Some families also manifest progressive mental deterioration. A gene for Norrie syndrome has been localized to chromosome Xp11.4, where cytogenetic studies have detected deletions involving contiguous genes, including the monamine oxidase genes, which may account for mental deficiency in certain families.[7]

Characteristics associated with oto-palato-digital syndrome may include hypertelorism, craniofacial deformity involving supraorbital area, flat midface, small nose, and cleft palate. Patients are short in stature with broad fingers and toes that vary in length, with an excessively wide space between the first and second toe. An associated conductive hearing loss usually results from an ossicular malformation. Although affected males manifest the full spectrum of syndromic features, females may show mild involvement. Gene localization studies place the gene on chromosome Xq28.[10]

Wildervaank's syndrome is comprised of the Klippel-Feil sign involving fused cervical vertebrae, SNHL or mixed hearing impairment, and cranial nerve VI paralysis causing retraction of the eye on lateral gaze. Isolated cranial nerve V paralysis is called *Duane's retraction syndrome*. Wildervaank's syndrome is almost always observed in females because of the high mortality associated with the X-linked dominant form in males. Hearing impairment is observed in about one third of patients with isolated Klippel-Feil sign, but this form is rarely familial. Less than 10% of patients with Duane's syndrome also may have an associated hearing loss.

In Alport's syndrome, SNHL is associated with renal impairment of varying severity. The progressive hearing impairment may not become clinically evident until the second decade of life. The renal disease may cause hematuria in infancy (e.g., "red diaper") but generally remains asymptomatic for several years before onset of renal insufficiency. Renal involvement is especially severe in males, and death from uremia before age 30 was the rule before the availability of renal dialysis and kidney transplantation. Genetic heterogeneity has been confirmed for Alport's syndrome, although most cases are the X-linked form attributable to a collagen gene (*COL4A5*) on the X chromosome. Autosomal type IV collagen gene mutations result in an autosomal dominant inheritance pattern, but males are still more severely affected.[4,59]

Two types of nonsyndromic, X-linked severe SNHL have been described: early onset rapidly progressive and moderate slowly progressive. At least six gene loci for nonsyndromic hearing loss on the X chromosome have been determined.

A progressive mixed hearing loss with apparent stapes fixation is observed in patients with X-linked stapes fixation with perilymphatic gusher. Attempted stapedotomy or stapedectomy in these patients carries a high risk of significant postoperative SNHL resulting from a perilymphatic gusher. C-bone imaging, which should be considered preoperatively in any young boy, may detect suggestive findings, such as an enlarged internal auditory canal with thinning or absence of bone at the base of the cochlea. Although males are more severely affected, female carriers may have a mild degree of gene expression. The responsible gene, *POU3F4*, is located on Xq21, which is closely linked to a gene for choroideremia. Deletion of these genes results in the contiguous gene syndrome of choroideremia, hearing loss, and mental retardation.[31]

MULTIFACTORIAL GENETIC DISORDERS

Some genetic disorders appear to result from a combination of genetic factors interacting with environmental influences. Such multifactorial disorders associated with hearing loss include clefting (i.e., cleft lip and palate) syndromes, involving conductive hearing loss, and the microtia/hemifacial microsomia/Goldenhar spectrum. Findings in the latter may include preauricular tags or pits, vertebral anomalies such as hypoplastic or hemivertebrae in the cervical region, epibulbar dermoids, and coloboma of the upper lid. Goldenhar's syndrome (oculo-auriculo-vertebral dysplasia) has been described as autosomal dominant in some families, although this may simply represent fortuitous clustering.

AUTOSOMAL CHROMOSOMAL SYNDROMES

Middle ear and mastoid disease are often observed in Down syndrome children. Significant SNHL has been documented in patients with trisomy 13 who survive the newborn period, during which most patients die. Turner's syndrome, monosomic for all or part of one X chromosome, presents generally in females as gonadal dysgenesis, short stature, and often a webbed neck or shield chest. Sensorineural, conductive, or mixed hearing loss, which may be progressive, may be the first diagnostic clue to Turner's syndrome in prepubertal females.

MITOCHONDRIAL DISORDERS

Hearing loss can occur as an additional symptom in a range of mitochondrial syndromes.[41,64] Kearns-Sayre syndrome includes progressive external ophthalmoplegia (PEO) and retinopathy that are usually evident before the age of

10 with delayed onset of heart block or cerebrospinal fluid (CSF)-protein elevation. SNHL can occur as part of the phenotype. No relationship has been found between the proportion of abnormal mDNA in muscle and clinical severity. Myoclonic epilepsy and ragged red fibers are characterized by myoclonus, epilepsy, and ataxia with less frequent occurrence of optic atrophy, dementia, and varying degrees of hearing loss. Maternal transmission has been definitively shown in some families. MELAS (myopathy, encephalopathy, lactic acidosis, and stroke-like episodes), often associated with short stature, encompasses a range of clinical signs and symptoms, including hearing loss in approximately 30% of patients. Diabetes mellitus type II and SNHL associated with mitochondrial mutations have been documented in several families, the most frequently detected mutation being at position 3243, which is also found in MELAS. The mutation has been found in a few diabetic patients.

Few families with nonsyndromic hearing loss have shown a mitochondrial mutation (e.g., nucleotide 1555 in a large Arabic kindred) and a recessive mutation in a nuclear gene, which apparently interact to produce the disorder. This identical mitochondrial mutation and several others produce enhanced sensitivity to ototoxic effects of aminoglycosides in therapeutic doses. Relatives of carriers of this mutation may manifest less degrees of hearing loss before being exposed to aminoglycosides; screening of maternal relatives of patients could prove beneficial. Gradual worsening of a mitochondrial disorder over time, as many mitochondria with a given mutation accumulate in affected tissues, has stimulated interest in a possible mitochondrial role in presbycusis, but additional studies should be completed before such a relationship could be confirmed.

GENETIC EVALUATION AND COUNSELING

Genetic counseling should be tailored to provide information to parents about their child's hearing loss etiology and about the expected pattern of inheritance of any genetic disorder. Family histories often involve many marriages between patients, with hearing losses of uncertain etiology. Specific information should be sought about the age of onset; type, severity, and stability of any reported hearing loss; and known syndromic features such as ear pits. Previous audiologic evaluation results for all affected family members should be reviewed and a pedigree constructed to include third-degree relatives. Family tradition may incorrectly attribute hearing losses in multiple generations to nongenetic causes so that all family members with a hearing loss should be initially included in the pedigree. An important step in diagnosis of recessive disorders is exploration of consanguinity, which is more likely among geographically isolated populations and cohesive religious or ethnic groups in which multiple intermarriages may be identified. Reasonable criteria for obtaining cytogenetic studies would be the presence of two major malformations or one major malformation with two or more minor malformations. The etiology of a hearing loss may remain uncertain after an intensive, often expensive evaluation.

A complete genetic evaluation should consider prognosis and recurrence risk. The usual pattern of penetrance of a gene should be considered in counseling regarding recurrence risks for autosomal dominant disorders. If full penetrance is characteristic of the gene, the children of a patient have a 50% chance of inheriting the gene and expressing the disorder, whereas decreased or nonpenetrance affects only the likelihood of expression, not gene inheritance. Heterozygotic carriers of a recessive gene may have a low recurrence risk (about 1 : 100) depending on the frequency with which a specific recessive gene is found in the general population. Offspring of two heterozygous carriers of the same autosomal recessive gene have a 50% chance of being a carrier but only a 25% chance of having the disorder. Gender-specific rules govern the inheritance patterns of X-linked and mitochondrial disorders. The recurrence risk for multifactorial disorders may be low because most cases are sporadic. If both parents have normal karyotypes, the recurrence risk of a chromosomal disorder in future offspring would also be low.

The recurrence risk in deaf marriages depends on the etiology of the deafness. For example, if both parents have identical recessively inherited deafness, the recurrence rate would be 100%; however, if parents have disparate etiologies, the risk may be small.

Bieber and Nance[11] developed empiric risk tables based on an "averaged" risk, taking into account various possibilities, including the number of affected and unaffected children in the family. For instance, the risk of recurrence in future offspring in a family whose only child has an unexplained hearing impairment is 10% to 16%. Each normal-hearing child born to such a family reduces the probability of a genetic etiology, with a consequent decrease in estimated recurrence risk.

If a normal-hearing person marries a patient with SNHL of uncertain etiology, the risk of having a hearing-impaired child ranges from negligible (nongenetic or uncommon recessive) to 50% if the gene is a fully penetrant dominant. The averaged empiric risk for such a couple is 6%, which would decrease with each unaffected child born to them. When both husband and wife have hearing losses of uncertain etiology, most counselors assign an empiric risk for a deaf child of about 10%. The risk declines with the birth of each hearing child but increases to 62% if the firstborn is hearing impaired.

Some deaf parents may view having a deaf child as positive, and counselors should be sensitive to this point of view. Because American sign language may be the primary communication modality of adult deaf parents, a qualified interpreter should be available. Boughman and Shaver[16] developed specific signs to communicate genetic terminology to deaf persons.

INFECTIOUS DISEASES

Congenital and neonatal infections

Infections acquired during the prenatal, perinatal, or neonatal period occur in about 10% of all live births. In most instances, these infections are asymptomatic or present nonspecific findings. New diagnostic techniques, including fetal ultrasound, sampling of peripheral umbilical blood, and polymerase chain reaction technology, hold promise for more specific diagnostic capability in the future.

Viral infections

Several viruses have been implicated as etiopathogenic agents for congenital and acquired hearing loss. Pathogens that access the inner ear may originate in the bloodstream, middle ear, or CSF. CMV has been isolated from human labyrinthine fluids. Seroconversion studies and virus isolation from urine and nasopharyngeal secretions have confirmed an association of labyrinthitis with rubella, rubeola, mumps influenza, varicella-zoster, Epstein-Barr, poliomyelitis, variola, and adeno- and parainfluenza viruses. Before advent of an effective vaccine, mumps was a common etiology of acquired profound unilateral SNHL in childhood. Effective immunization programs for rubella, rubeola, and mumps in developed countries have decreased their importance in the etiology of childhood hearing loss, but these infections continue to play a significant role in the third world.

Animal studies confirm an inflammatory response in the cochlea as early as 48 hours after viral inoculation, but inflammatory cells may be slow to clear from the cochlear duct leaving behind a matrix, which may undergo calcification with obliteration of cochlear spaces. Histopathologic studies of temporal bones from patients who were affected by prenatal rubella, mumps, rubeola, or CMV reveal evidence of an endolymphatic labyrinthitis with pathologic changes limited to the cochlear duct, saccule, and utricle. These findings are consistent with a blood-borne spread of infection, most likely through vessels of the stria vascularis. Measles, mumps, and CMV also may present with a meningoencephalitis, permitting direct spread along meningeal and neural structures into the perilymphatic spaces where inflammatory changes may later progress to fibrosis. Bordley and Kapur[15] studied temporal bones of patients with acute smallpox, varicella (chicken pox), or measles and found the most severe pathologic changes in the middle ears, although two measles patients also revealed histopathologic evidence of endolabyrinthitis.

Davis and Johnson[30] showed selective vulnerability of inner ear structures of experimental animals to specific viruses. In newborn hamsters, influenza virus infected mesenchymal cells in the perilymphatic system, whereas mumps virus infected principally endolymphatic structures. Rubeola and vaccinia viruses infected perilymphatic and endolymphatic cells, whereas herpes simplex involvement was essentially limited to the sensory cells of the labyrinth.

Cytomegalovirus infection

CMV are members of the herpes virus group that are widely prevalent in developed and developing countries. Congenital CMV infection is the most common human intrauterine infection. Annually, 30,000 to 40,000 infants are born in the US with congenital CMV infection (i.e., approximately 1% of all newborns), of whom 6000 to 8000 have or will develop CMV-related disabilities. Human CMV appears to be species specific with no known external reservoirs or animal vectors involved in transmission. CMV may be transmitted vertically (i.e., from mother to child) or horizontally, and primary infection is accompanied by viral shedding in all secretions, including saliva, urine, semen, and cervical or vaginal fluids, which may persist for months to years. Seronegative organ transplant recipients may acquire infection from organs from seropositive donors, including blood donors. Reinfection with one of several antigenically distinct CMV strains is possible even after primary infection with another strain, especially in immunocompromised patients. Transplacental passage of CMV to the fetus occurs during maternal viremia, giving rise to hematogenous spread through the fetus to target organs such as the CNS, eyes and liver. The virus has an affinity for neurons of cranial nerve VIII and ependymal cells lining the ventricles of the brain. Congenital CMV infection differs from rubella and toxoplasmosis in that the virus can be transmitted *in utero* in the course of primary maternal infection and infection resulting from reactivation of latent virus in immune women. Although CMV antibodies in the expectant mother do not completely protect against transmission to the fetus, they reduce the transmission rate and mitigate the sequelae. The probability that a newborn will have a harmful congenital CMV infection is about nine times less likely in a mother with recurrent infection than in a mother who has had a primary infection. Women with recurrent infections rarely give birth to infants with symptomatic congenital CMV infection.

In populations of higher socioeconomic status, approximately 55% of women of childbearing age are CMV-immune; 45% are susceptible to primary CMV infection. In lower socioeconomic status groups, 85% of fertile women show immunity. About 1% to 4% of susceptible women will experience primary CMV infection during pregnancy, with a resultant fetal infection rate of 40%. Higher socioeconomic status women with evidence of CMV immunity at conception have infants with congenital infection in 0.15% of cases, whereas the congenital infection rate among offspring of immune lower socioeconomic status mothers varies from 0.5% to 1% (Fig. 32-4). Although Hardy[46] found that the gestational age of the fetus is the most important factor determining the extent and long-range consequences of congeni-

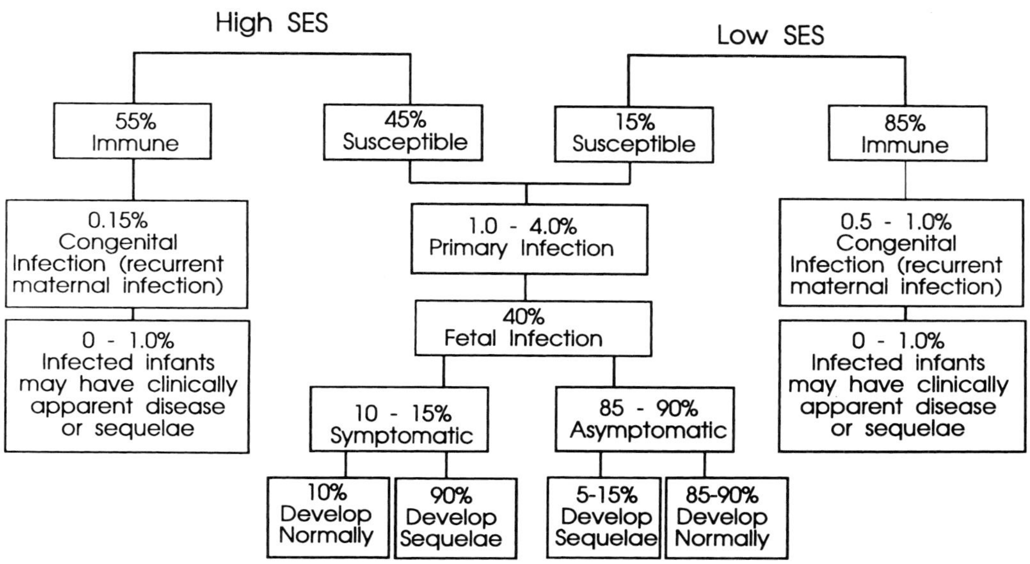

Fig. 32-4. Cytomegalovirus during pregnancy. SES—Socioeconomic status.

tal viral infections, the time of greatest susceptibility for CMV is unknown.

The overall CMV infection rate in the US is about 2% per year, but higher rates occur among women being managed in sexually transmitted disease (STD) clinics (35%) and among workers in daycare centers. CMV infection is endemic in daycare centers, and transmission of the virus from young children who acquire CMV at such centers to their pregnant mothers is important epidemiologically. Daycare studies reveal that 25% of children younger than 3 years excrete CMV.[2] In one population of seronegative mothers, 15% had children younger than 3 years who excreted CMV; 40% of these seronegative mothers became seropositive during 1 year's follow-up. The annual seroconversion rate among daycare center workers is 11% compared with 2.2% in the general population. Among populations studied at STD clinics, sexually active adolescent females showed a seroconversion rate of 34% per year, with the highest rates in female teenagers with multiple sex partners. The congenital CMV infection rate is markedly increased (20% to 25%) for lower socioeconomic status mothers younger than 20 years, most of whom are unmarried (80% in one study) and about half of whom are primiparous. Maternal age does not correlate strongly with congenital CMV infection in mid–socioeconomic status mothers.

Congenital CMV infection, which is definitively diagnosed by isolation of the virus from neonates in the first few weeks of life, is the most common cause of intrauterine infection, occurring in approximately 1% of all live births. An additional 4% to 10% of infants acquire the infection through cervical virus shedding, virus in breast milk, or blood transfusions. Most mothers excreting the virus during pregnancy do so in the course of a recurrent rather than primary infection. About 40% to 60% of seronegative infants who are breast-fed for more than 1 month by a seropositive mother will convert. Infections that occur peripartum may be associated with pneumonitis, slow weight gain, adenopathy, rash, jaundice, anemia, and atypical lymphocytosis. The diagnosis of congenital CMV infection is confirmed by isolation of the virus from urine or saliva (often with polymerase chain reaction techniques) within the first 2 weeks of life because all congenitally infected infants shed the virus in urine or saliva in high titers. Perinatally infected infants usually begin to excrete virus between 3 and 12 weeks of age, making early viral isolation studies essential to the diagnosis of a true congenital infection. Of congenitally infected infants, 10% to 15% are symptomatic; of these, 90% show typical cytomegalic inclusion disease (CID), characterized by involvement of the CNS and reticuloendothelial system, commonly presenting with hepatosplenomegaly, petechiae, and jaundice. Microcephaly, intrauterine growth retardation, and prematurity also characterize the CID population, which may experience a mortality rate as high as 30%. As many as 90% of children with true CID develop severe mental and perceptual deficits by 2 years of age, including severe to profound SNHL and ocular abnormalities such as chorioretinitis and optic atrophy in 25% to 30% of cases.

Before current viral isolation techniques were available, speculation regarding the dire outcome of congenital CMV infection was based solely on data from the 10% of congenitally infected infants who were symptomatic. Investigators were unaware of the many asymptomatic infected neonates

Such subclinical infections, which account for 90% of congenitally infected infants, may become apparent months to years after birth. Although prognosis for normal neurologic development among these infants is better, approximately 10% to 15% will develop significant mild to profound SNHL. SNHL is the most common irreversible sequela of congenital CMV infection, with an estimated 30% to 50% incidence in symptomatic cases and 10% to 15% in asymptomatic infants with congenital infection. It is bilateral in about 50% of cases, varying in magnitude from 50 to 100 dB. Stagno and others found that nearly 25% of SNHL develops or increases in severity after the first year of life, reiterating the need for longitudinal screening programs during the preschool years. Searching for related findings that might predict delayed-onset CMV hearing loss, several investigators found a higher likelihood of hearing loss in infants with periventricular radiolucencies or calcifications on computed tomography (CT). Two studies reported that mothers of infants born with asymptomatic CMV infection and hearing loss had significantly higher titers of envelope glycoprotein gB antibodies throughout the pregnancy, possibly reflecting prolonged antigenic stimulation, than did mothers of non–hearing-impaired infants. With the vaccine-related decline in congenital rubella, congenital CMV infection is the most common cause of nongenetic congenital deafness and early-onset SNHL in developed countries. Whereas rubella occurs in epidemic cycles, CMV infection is recurrent in newborns.

In an attempt to find a safe and effective management for symptomatic congenital CMV, a clinical trial has been initiated with ganciclovir, an acyclic nucleoside analogue of acyclovir, which acts to inhibit herpes viruses. Preliminary reports confirmed a decrease in virus excretion during management followed by a recurrence of excretion after drug withdrawal. Higher dosage schedules have been advocated by some investigators in an attempt to produce more lasting benefit. Strategies to prevent congenital CMV infection have been focused on development of a safe and effective vaccine for widespread use. The Towne vaccine is an attenuated live-virus vaccine capable of inducing antibodies to CMV and cellular immunity. It is used in immunosuppressed adults, but public health officials believe that it lacks sufficient immunogenicity to produce lasting immunity in some populations and that its live viral component may cause latent infection and carcinogenicity. An alternative approach to achieve enhanced immunity involves use of a vaccine that uses noninfectious viral subunits, the most promising of which is a portion of the viral envelope consisting of a glycoprotein gB. Early clinical trials of CMV gB protein vaccine have shown its ability in a three-dose regimen to induce neutralizing antibody titers equivalent to those observed after wild-type virus exposure. Because of the greater risk for primary maternal and consequently congenital infections of adolescent mothers in the US, a major immunization effort aimed at prepubertal girls may impact incidence of congenital CMV infection. Because much nongenetic early-onset SNHL is attributable to CMV, such a public health initiative may impact the future of hearing-impaired children. Histopathologic study of temporal bones of infants dying of CID has revealed characteristic inclusion bodies in the superficial cells of the stria vascularis, Reissner's membrane, limbus spiralis, saccule, utricle, and semicircular canals. Although no inclusion-bearing cells were present in the organ of Corti, cristae, or ganglia, endolymphatic hydrops was present in at least a portion of each cochlear duct.

Congenital rubella

During the Australian rubella epidemic of 1941, the ophthalmologist Gregg[45] first recognized the teratogenic potential of prenatal maternal infection, and Swan and others[77] first described deafness as a component of the rubella triad, along with congenital cataracts and heart defects. Initial estimates of fetal damage after first-trimester maternal rubella ranged from 16% to 59%. After isolation of the rubella myxovirus, an enveloped RNA virus, in 1962, serologic and viral isolation techniques to confirm infection became feasible. Laboratory-based case identification permitted documentation of subclinical rubella infection in expectant mothers and confirmation of congenital rubella infection in infants who did not manifest all components of the classical rubella syndrome. During the 1963 to 1965 rubella epidemic in the US, laboratory confirmation of the presence and timing of rubella infection led to the description of rubella-related disorders in addition to the classical triad. Included in the expanded rubella syndrome are deafness, eye defects (cataracts, glaucoma, microphthalmia), congenital heart defects (patent ductus, pulmonary artery stenosis), microcephaly, mental or motor retardation, newborn hepatosplenomegaly, thrombocytopenia, radiolucencies in long bones, interstitial pneumonitis, encephalitis, and low birth weight. Prospective studies were carried out on paired sera samples obtained from pregnant women, thus pinpointing the exact timing of clinical or subclinical maternal rubella infection.[14] Maternal rubella is confirmed by a fourfold rise in immunoglobulin G (IgG) antibody as shown by hemagglutination inhibition, enzyme-linked immunosorbent assay (ELISA), or fluorescent antibody assays. Immunofluorescence techniques can also detect rubella-specific immunoglobulin M (IgM) antibody.

The risk of fetal infection is approximately 90% during first-trimester maternal infection; most of these infants have detectable disabilities. The risk of fetal infection declines to about 50% between 12 and 20 weeks' of gestation, and only one third of these infants are damaged. There is a risk of congenital infection later in pregnancy but with little likelihood of lasting effects. Among congenital rubella infants asymptomatic at birth, most will develop sequelae within the first 5 years of life. Of 165 laboratory-documented cases of maternal rubella in one study, 49% were clinically apparent, whereas 51% were subclinical. Maternal rubella during the first trimester of pregnancy was most severe on the fetus, but some offspring of mothers with second-trimester infection had deafness, microcephaly, cataracts, and mental-motor retardation. Infants with only one or two components of the rubella triad were clearly victims of congenital rubella infection.

Hearing loss was the most common deficit in the laboratory-documented congenital rubella population and the only defect in 22% of cases. Among infants from whom rubella virus was isolated, 57% were hearing impaired; 41.5% of infants in whom only serologic confirmation could be obtained were hearing impaired. Approximately 30% of babies born of mothers with subclinical but laboratory-confirmed infection had hearing loss. The hearing loss was typically SNHL, ranged in severity among patients, and had some asymmetry in individual patients. Some patients showed no response at any frequency, but the most frequently observed audiometric curves were of the ''cookie-bite'' type with greatest loss in the middle frequencies between 500 and 2000 Hz. Serial audiograms showed progressive decrease of auditory acuity in 25% of cases.

Essentially all congenital rubella babies shed virus from the nasopharynx; viral shedding may persist as long as 1 year, particularly among infants who are progeny of mothers with first-trimester infection and who continued to fail to thrive. Viral excretion can be hazardous to rubella-susceptible health care and child care personnel interacting with infected babies. A general miniaturization of organs from rubella-infected fetuses and infants was noted at autopsy, and histopathologic examination revealed hypocellularity. Highly specialized cells, such as fiber cells in the lens of the eye, appear to become more susceptible to the effects of intracellular virus with increasing cellular specialization. As a consequence, gradual progression in cataract formation was noted in the postnatal period.

Temporal bone histopathologic findings in rubella infants include Scheibe-type cochleosaccular changes, although the utricle, semicircular canals, and spiral ganglion are unaffected. Partial collapse of Reissner's membrane with adherence to the stria vascularis and organ of Corti was observed in several cases. In some sections, the tectorial membrane was found to be rolled and lying in the internal sulcus. Saccular collapse with histologic evidence of recent acute inflammation was documented in several temporal bones. The organ of Corti was relatively unaffected, but the stria vascularis was smaller than normal and areas of cystic dilatation were observed at the junction of Reissner's membrane and the spiral ligament.

Before the availability of an effective rubella vaccine, epidemics in most developed countries occurred at 6- or 9-year intervals. Up to 60% of newly identified deafness in infants and young children was attributed to prenatal rubella in epidemic years, falling to less than 1% in nonepidemic years. Widespread and, in some instances, mandatory administration of the rubella vaccine to children and nonpregnant women of childbearing age in the US has decreased the incidence of rubella by more than 99%. In some parts of the world, however, prenatal rubella still poses a threat to hearing, and it should be considered an etiologic possibility in immigrant children with SNHL.

Herpes simplex encephalitis

Herpes simplex encephalitis (HSE) is uncommon, but 25% to 30% of cases involve the pediatric age group and the neonatal infection rate has paralleled the rising incidence of genital herpes infection among women of childbearing age. The neonatal herpes simplex virus (HSV) infection rate varies from 1:2500 to 1:20,000 live births in published reports. Intrapartum or postpartum exposure is more common than intrauterine transmission, which accounts for only 5% of neonatal infections. Many HSV-infected neonates are born prematurely to young, often nulliparous mothers. Neonatal HSV patients may present with mucocutaneous involvement or disseminated infection, and one fourth to one third of the infants are also affected by meningoencephalitis. However, up to 20% of newborns with HSV infection never manifest cutaneous involvement. The route by which the HSV reaches the brain during primary infection is unclear, although hematogenous dissemination, direct spread from the nasopharynx via the cribriform plate, and retrograde spread from infected ganglia have been postulated. The infection has shown a predilection for the temporal and frontal areas of the brain.

Herpes simplex meningoencephalitis, which has an incubation period up to 4 weeks, most likely occurs in the second or third postpartum week. Epidemiologically, only 50% of neonatal HSV infections can be related by history to a definite maternal or paternal infection, so the absence of a positive history does not exclude the disease. Nonspecific clinical findings, including fever and an altered mental state, are accompanied by abnormal CSF findings in more than 90% of patients. Electroencephalography, CT, and magnetic resonance imaging (MRI) help detect focal meningoencephalitis. Brain biopsy, which is positive in 33% to 55% of HSE cases, represents the only definitive means of diagnosing HSE and excluding other disease processes that may mimic the condition. Chemotherapy for HSE involves the antiviral drug acyclovir for 10 to 14 days. Clinicians caring for a child with undiagnosed focal encephalitis should introduce broad-spectrum antimicrobial therapy in addition to acyclovir until definitive diagnostic tests have been completed. Effective management of HSE requires the involvement of neurologists, neurosurgeons, pulmonologists, intensivists, and infectious disease specialists.

Congenital toxoplasmosis

Toxoplasmosis is spread by the ingestion of oocysts on food contaminated by cat feces, by ingestion of tissue cysts in undercooked meat products, or by congenital transmission. The prevalence of tissue cysts in the US meat supply is 25% to 40% for pork, about 20% for lamb, and less for beef. The cat is the definitive natural host for the intracellular protozoan parasite *Toxoplasma gondii*, excreting about 10,000,000 oocysts per day during active infection; ingested feline fecal material containing oocysts leads to the liberation of organisms that invade human intestinal mucosa and are widely disseminated. Cysts may be formed in all tissues, including the human placenta, through which fetal infection occurs. Except in immunocompromised mothers, fetal infection is usually the result of primary maternal infection during gestation, with an overall rate of transmission of 30% to 40%. Although the incidence of fetal infection is greatest if maternal infection occurs during the third trimester (60%), greater fetal damage follows first-trimester infection. Most infants (75%) with congenital *Toxoplasma* infections are asymptomatic at birth, 15% are born with only ocular lesions, and the remaining 10% have more extensive involvement. Two clinical forms are recognized: the more common neurologically dominant type and a disseminated variant with multiple organ system involvement. Clinical presentation of congenital *Toxoplasma* infection may include chorioretinitis, hydrocephalus, generalized intracranial calcifications, microcephaly, thrombocytopenia, hepatosplenomegaly, and jaundice. Such infants have a very poor prognosis for normal development. Subclinical infection should be confirmed by laboratory studies because unmanaged infants run a high risk of subsequent chorioretinitis with decreasing visual acuity, progressive CNS involvement with decreased intellectual function, deafness, and precocious puberty.

French investigators conducted extensive studies of pregnancies at risk for congenital toxoplasmosis, and compulsory programs for the identification of seronegative women early in pregnancy have been implemented in that country.[27,32,34,76] Maternal infection is confirmed by the appearance of specific IgG in a previously seronegative patient or a rising IgG titer after 3 weeks or longer. Prompt and intensive maternal management with a combination of pyrimethamine plus a sulfonamide of the sulfapyrimidine type (sulfadoxine or sulfadiazine) is advocated as a means of decreasing the likelihood and mitigating the effects of fetal infection. French experience with spiramycin administered to infected mothers during pregnancy significantly reduced the rate of transplacental transmission. Fetal infection is diagnosed prenatally by acquisition of amniotic fluid through amniocentesis and fetal blood samples from the umbilical cord under ultrasound control. Inoculation of fetal blood and amniotic fluid into mice, IgM immunosorbent assays, and quantitative maternal and fetal IgG studies document the presence of fetal infection. The availability of polymerase chain reaction techniques for recovering traces of the organism from amniotic fluid should lead to safer fetal screening methods when maternal infection is suspected. In the French studies, which included prenatal management of maternal infection, congenital infection occurred in 0.6% of cases with documented maternal infection during the preconceptual and early pregnancy period, in 3.7% of fetuses carried by mothers who were infected from the sixth to the sixteenth week of gestation, and in 20% of infants born after maternal infection during the sixteenth through the twenty-fifth week of pregnancy. The relatively low incidence of fetal infection among the 16- to 25-week group was 70% less than reported in previous studies, showing that adequate management of primary maternal infection during pregnancy reduces the likelihood of transmission to the fetus. Extended management for up to 1 year is advocated for congenitally infected infants, in the form of alternating courses of pyrimethamine and sulfonamide (sulfadiazine), coupled with folinic acid to prevent pyrimethamine complications. Infected infants should receive careful follow-up, including CT to assess CNS status and ophthalmologic examination for chorioretinitis. French investigators found that management of congenitally infected infants, begun at birth, reduced the frequency of chorioretinitis from 60% to 10%. All of these drugs, however, have poor activity against the encysted form of *Toxoplasma*, and delayed onset of chorioretinitis has been observed in managed cases. Initial reports from a Chicago-based series of managed infants suggest a substantial decline in congenital toxoplasmosis–related hearing loss with no losses detected in 57 infected infants followed with longitudinal ABR and behavioral tests.[75] Histopathologically, temporal bones of two infected infants have shown calcified scars, predominantly in the stria vascularis, comparable with those observed in the CNS.

Accurate incidence figures for congenital toxoplasmosis in the US are elusive, with estimates ranging from 1:1000 to 1:8000 live births. Previous reports estimated 3000 *Toxoplasma*-infected infants are born annually and about 15% to 25% of inadequately managed infants eventually develop SNHL. As many as 85% to 90% of American women of childbearing age may be uninfected and consequently at risk for primary infection. The most effective strategy for control of fetal damage is prevention of maternal infection by careful attention to hygienic measures, including cleaning of fruits and vegetables and thorough cooking of meat products. Expectant mothers should be careful when cleaning cat litter boxes. Immunization strategies have focused on developing an anti-*Toxoplasma* vaccine for administration to feline carriers rather than to susceptible females of childbearing age. Careful serologic testing of women concurrently with initial confirmation of pregnancy and during prenatal visits will facilitate accurate identification of seroconverters and prompt institution of maternal management during pregnancy. Prenatal and neonatal evaluation of the fetus and infant can confirm congenital infection so that postnatal management can be instituted as early as possible. Longitudinal follow-up studies in France should further show the effectiveness of recommended management regimens in preventing sequelae, including deafness.

Syphilis

Congenital syphilis, resulting from transplacental transmission of the causative organism *Treponema pallidum* to the fetus after the fourth month of gestation, may manifest at birth or may be inapparent until as late as the fifth decade of life. Infection of the fetus may occur during any stage of maternal disease, although it is most likely during primary syphilis (70% to 100%) and least likely (30%) in the late stages. After a rapid increase over the past decade, the number of acquired and congenital syphilis cases appears to be leveling off. Concurrent human immunodeficiency virus (HIV) infection in patients with acquired syphilis may increase the likelihood of early progression to neurosyphilis and may be associated with failure to respond to penicillin therapy. Although SNHL has been reported in patients with primary, secondary, and later acquired syphilis, the primary concern in children is congenital infection.

Fetal death occurs in about 25% of cases of unmanaged fetal infection, and another 25% to 30% of these infants die perinatally. About one third of surviving neonates with congenital syphilis manifest physical findings at birth. Classical signs of congenital syphilis, which may not present until after the first 2 years of life, include SNHL, interstitial keratitis, Hutchinson's teeth (notched incisors), nasal septal perforation and saddle deformity, and frontal bossing. Early findings may include osteochondritis and periostitis of long bones, hepatosplenomegaly, maculopapular rash on hands and feet with desquamation, and low birth weight. Prevalence estimates of hearing loss among patients with congenital syphilis range from 3% to 38%; about 37% of cases present before age 10, 51% present at age 25 to 35 years, and 12% present even later in life. Few affected infants present with SNHL during the neonatal period, so longitudinal audiologic screening is mandatory and, in some instances, SNHL may be the only presenting symptom. A commonly reported audiometric configuration is a bilateral, flat SNHL, which may present in children as a sudden, bilateral profound impairment, usually without vertigo. In late congenital syphilis, hearing loss may be sudden, asymmetric, fluctuating, or progressive, and often accompanied by episodic tinnitus and vertigo. Speech discrimination scores tend to be poorer than expected from the audiometric configuration, loudness recruitment severe, and caloric responses weak to absent. A positive labyrinthine fistula test may be present (Hennebert's sign) and Tullio's phenomenon, dysequilibrium in response to loud sounds, may be observed.

Because any attempt to carry out direct darkfield examination of perilymph for *T. pallidum* would present an unacceptable risk of additional hearing loss, serological tests present the best alternative means for diagnosing otosyphilis. *T. pallidum* infection gives rise to nonspecific reagin antibody and specific antitreponemal antibodies. Nonspecific tests are used for screening many patients from low-incidence populations, such as state-required tests of cord blood from all newborns. However, reports from large otologic centers indicate a prevalence of 570/100,000 of presumed otosyphilis among otologic referrals, justifying the use of more expensive *Treponema*-specific procedures. The most widely used Treponema-specific test is the fluorescent *Treponema* antibody absorption test (FTA-ABS) with a high sensitivity rate to all stages of syphilis and a low rate of false-positives; the specificity rate approaches 98% in large studies. Most false-positive results involve autoimmune or drug-induced collagen vascular diseases, such as systemic lupus erythematosus. Other *Treponema*-specific tests used to confirm FTA-ABS are the microhemagglutination–*T. pallidum* (MHA-TP) and the *T. pallidum* inhibition test, a complex and costly but highly specific (99%) procedure. Because *Treponema*-specific tests may remain positive after adequate management, Birdsall and others (1990) introduced a western blot assay to identify antitreponemal antibody isotype and determine whether the infection remains active. In the presence of active infection, antitreponemal IgM and IgG antibodies are present. After successful management, only IgG antibodies persist. All offspring of seropositive mothers should be followed at 1, 2, 4, 6, and 12 months of age with nontreponemal antibody tests. Stable or rising titers by 6 months of age warrant reevaluation and management. Infants with neurologic involvement should have serial lumbar punctures with CSF examination at 6-month intervals until the CSF is normal.

High-dose parenteral penicillin is the management of choice in nonallergic patients with a presumptive diagnosis of otosyphilis; consideration should be given, in dosage determination, to the potential limits on penicillin diffusion posed by the blood-CSF and blood-perilymph barriers. The discovery that treponemes may lie dormant for as long as 90 days between replications in late congenital syphilis cases dictates the necessity for longer term management schedules than formerly recommended. Current recommendations for dosage and management may be found in publications from the Center for Disease Control and Prevention.

As an adjunct to adequate antimicrobial therapy, systemically administered corticosteroids (generally oral prednisone) have stabilized or improved hearing in approximately 50% of patients with syphilitic deafness. Greater improvement is usually observed in speech discrimination scores than in pure tone thresholds. The mechanisms of corticosteroid action in these cases are uncertain but may involve nonspecific reduction of vasculitis, suppression of immune reaction to spirochetal antigens, or enhancement of penicillin diffusion into the perilymph. Relative contraindications to corticosteroid therapy include lack of immunity to varicella, recent vaccination, hypertension, diabetes mellitus, glaucoma, pregnancy, and peptic ulcer disease. Fatal cases of varicella have been reported in young children receiving corticosteroid therapy; careful case selection is essential. Corticosteroids, initially administered in a gradually tapered dosage regimen, are usually discontinued after 4 to 8 weeks if hearing does not improve. However, long-term maintenance therapy may be required to sustain hearing improvement. Alternate-day dosage appears to carry less risk of sequelae, such as cataract formation, bone growth disturbance, and adrenal suppression.

Temporal bone histopathologic features in cases of congenital otosyphilis include obliterative endarteritis, mononuclear cell infiltrates, osteitis of the otic capsule, and varying degrees of tissue necrosis. Early congenital syphilis may involve the labyrinth, as well as cranial nerve V, with round cell infiltration or may present as a meningolabyrinthitis. Osteitis of the temporal bone with secondary involvement of the membranous labyrinth can also be found in late congenital otosyphilis. Atrophy of the organ and involvement of the stria vascularis, spiral ganglion, and cranial nerve VIII fibers have been reported. Gummatous changes may be found in all bones of the ear, including the ossicles, which may add a conductive component to a preexisting SNHL.

Neonatal sepsis

Neonatal sepsis, characterized by signs of infection and septicemia in the first month of life, carries a mortality rate of 10% to 50%, with an inverse relationship to the age and weight of the child. The bacterial pathogens involved may vary, but group B streptococci and gram-negative enteric bacilli are most commonly observed. Meningitis is a common outcome of bacteremia in these infants, and uncommon organisms such as *Listeria monocytogenes* may play a significant role in such cases. Postmeningitic deafness should be suspected in all survivors of neonatal meningitis, and appropriate evaluation with techniques such ABR should be undertaken.

Later onset infections

Mumps and measles

Measles and mumps immunization as part of standard well-baby care has effected a 90% to 95% decrease in the incidence of these diseases in the US. Mumps is caused by a paramyxovirus spread by infected droplets or material contaminated by infected saliva. The highest incidence of the disease was typically between 5 and 15 years of age and rarely before 2 years of age. Before the availability of an effective vaccine for mumps, the most common otologic sequela attributed to this virus was unilateral profound SNHL or unilateral anacusis without vertigo or vestibular impairment. Hearing loss is observed in about 5/10,000 patients with mumps, is usually sudden in onset during the course of the infection, and may be accompanied by tinnitus, vertigo, nausea, and vomiting.

Two distinct pathogenetic mechanisms have been implicated in SNHL as a sequela of measles or mumps. In cases of SNHL without signs of meningoencephalitis, the virus appears to access the inner ear through the stria vascularis during viremia. Sluggish strial circulation, coupled with an intraepithelial capillary network, predisposes to the onset of inflammation in this structure, which is followed by degeneration and scarring. The resultant change in the volume and constitution of endolymph explains subsequent degeneration of the stria vascularis, the organ of Corti, the tectorial membrane, and peripheral cochlear neurons, proceeding from the cochlear base to the apex. Collapse of Reissner's membrane with adherence to underlying structures has also been described. The perilymphatic system, the vestibular sensory organs, and the internal auditory canal contents are generally uninvolved. These histopathologic changes are also compatible with findings in cases of SNHL caused by prenatal rubella.

Temporal bone findings in patients who suffered meningoencephalitis in conjunction with measles or mumps are substantially similar to those associated with meningogenic bacterial labyrinthitis. It appears that direct extension of the viral inflammatory process occurs along the nerves and vessels in the internal auditory meatus into the inner ear. Findings compatible with a transmeatal route of infection include severe degeneration of neural elements in the modiolus in contrast to lesser degrees of involvement of neural structures in the cochlear duct. Temporal bones from infants who died during acute meningoencephalitis show lymphocytic infiltration along nerves and vessels in the internal auditory canal without concurrent involvement of the stria vascularis. Intralabyrinthine fibrosis and osteoneogenesis in perilymphatic spaces were found in patients who had survived the acute disease process.

Bacterial meningitis

Bacterial meningitis in young children was associated with a 90% to 100% mortality rate during the preantibiotic era. By 1986, clinical investigators reported a mortality rate of 2% to 3% among children older than 1 month with adequately managed bacterial meningitis. In cases of neonatal meningitis, *Escherichia coli* and group B β-hemolytic streptococci are the most common causative organisms. Most childhood meningitis cases in the US occur in children 6 to 9 months of age; before the availability of an effective vaccine against *H. influenzae B, H. influenzae, Neisseria meningitis*, and *Streptococcus pneumoniae* collectively accounted for 84% of cases. *H. influenzae* was typically the most commonly isolated pathogen, but early widespread use of the *H. influenzae B* vaccine has reduced the incidence by more than 90%. Clinical vaccine trials are underway aimed at preventing both meningococcal and pneumococcal meningitis.

The dramatic decline in mortality rates was not accompanied by a concomitant decrease in the incidence of immediate and long-term sequelae among meningitis survivors. Seizures are experienced by 28%-40% of meningitis patients before or during their hospital stay, and at least one handicap was detected during 1 year's follow-up in 57% of pneumococcal meningitis survivors and 14.5% of children in whom *H. influenzae* is the etiologic agent. Apart from SNHL, meningitis sequelae may include mental retardation, hydrocephalus, seizure disorders, motor abnormalities (e.g., hemiparesis, diplegia, quadriplegia, cerebral palsy), vestibular deficits, speech defects, language disorders, hyperactivity, poor impulse control, visual impairment, and learning disabilities. CT of the CNS in children with severe sequelae reveals evidence of brain infarction, arterial occlusion, and brain or spinal cord necrosis.

The reported incidence of SNHL after meningitis has varied from 3% to 40%, with most reports clustered in the 15% to 20% range. In one series of 280 meningitis survivors, 89% of those who suffered postmeningitic hearing loss contracted the disease before their third birthday.[17] Most patients with postmeningitic hearing loss sustain permanent, bilateral, severe-to-profound SNHL, but in a series of 64 carefully documented cases, 38% had bilateral, asymmetric SNHL and 11% exhibited a unilateral SNHL. Some reports have documented improved hearing acuity in a few cases followed longitudinally, whereas hearing losses fluctuated or progressed in others. These reports can be broadly classified into those using behavioral audiologic tests and those using primarily ABR.

Several observations can be drawn from these studies. The onset of hearing loss associated with bacterial meningitis usually occurs early in the course of the disease, and no particular regimen of antibiotic therapy appears to offer any degree of protection against this sequela. These findings are consistent with recent observations regarding the role of the host's initial inflammatory response in damage sustained by neural tissue. Direct spread of the infection from the middle ear to the labyrinth during otitis media is much less likely than (1) the penetration of bacteria and toxins along the cochlear aqueduct or internal auditory canal leading to a suppurative labyrinthitis or perineuritis or neuritis of cranial nerve VIII; (2) serous or toxic labyrinthitis constituting a sterile inflammatory response; (3) septic thrombophlebitis or embolization of small labyrinthine vessels; and (4) hypoxic insult to cranial nerve VIII or central auditory pathways.

Meningitis patients who exhibit normal ABR after the first few days of hospitalization and antibiotic therapy are unlikely to develop SNHL. A prospective study of hearing loss in 124 British children with meningitis using otoacoustic emissions, ABR, and tympanometry confirmed that all cases of hearing loss were apparent at initial testing 6 hours after hospital admission.[65,66] Late-onset SNHL, after discharge from the hospital, is distinctly uncommon. Some patients whose ABR results are abnormal early in their hospital course may have a normal ABR by the time of discharge or in follow-up evaluation. EOAE supports a cochlear site of lesion in most cases. In some cases, the resolution of a coexisting conductive loss caused by middle ear effusion may contribute to overall improvement in auditory acuity. Most patients with postmeningitic losses who show improvement of auditory thresholds over time show mild or moderate, rather than severe or profound, SNHL. Thresholds in patients who exhibit improvement, deterioration, or fluctuation of auditory acuity often require 1 year or more after meningitis to stabilize. Some patients with improving thresholds continue to exhibit absent vestibular responses. The likely pathophysiologic explanation for changing bone conduction thresholds during and after an episode of bacterial meningitis has traditionally been attributed to serous labyrinthitis, but recent histopathologic results suggest the possibility of reversal in milder suppurative labyrinthitis. All meningitis survivors should have careful evaluation of auditory function, initially by ABR in younger children followed by behavioral audiologic testing when the child's condition permits. Because postmeningitic hearing losses may assume many audiometric configurations, click-evoked ABR, which assesses hearing sensitivity primarily in the high frequency region (2000 to 4000 Hz), may lead to erroneous conclusions regarding auditory acuity at lower frequencies. Careful longitudinal follow-up of postmeningitic children will avoid diagnostic errors.

Neurologic sequelae of bacterial meningitis, including SNHL, may be attributable to direct bacterial action on nervous tissue, the host's inflammatory response, or both factors. Studies of the progression of events at the molecular level during an episode of bacterial meningitis confirm that significant injury to the CNS occurs during the first hours of antibiotic therapy. Experimental animal models show that bacterial surface components, including endotoxin and cell wall structures, can produce the symptom complex of meningitis even in the absence of viable bacteria. Bacterial disintegration resulting from antibiotic action produces a veritable flood of cell wall antigens and endotoxins stimulating an intense immunologic response by the host. Damage attributable to such an inflammatory reaction was first seen in animal studies of pneumococcal meningitis and later in gram-negative pathogens. Reports involving neonates and young children with meningitis have also documented a rapid host inflammatory response after antibiotic-induced release of bacterial components. It is hypothesized that inflammatory exudate, a result of meningeal invasion by bacteria, is potentially harmful and is not critical for containment of the infection. By studying paired CSF samples drawn at admission and 18 to 30 hours later, clinical investigators found a correlation between the intensity of inflammation and subsequent clinical outcome. Poorer outcome in neonates receiving intraventricular gentamicin rather than intravenous antibiotics may be attributable to the patient's response to an additional load of bacterial degradation products in the CSF.

Local production of interleukin-1β (IL-1β) and tumor necrosis factor (TNF) in response to CNS tissue interacting with bacterial breakdown products is thought to be the first step in a complex series of molecular events resulting in inflammation and tissue destruction. Based on the hypothesis that down-modulation of the host inflammatory response could ameliorate the severity of postmeningitic sequelae, corticosteroids have been used as adjunctive therapy to bactericidal antibiotics. Corticosteroids inhibit the activity of phospholipase with consequent decrease in prostaglandin-E_2, thromboxane, and leukotriene formation. Dexamethasone decreases the production of IL-1β and TNF. In double-blind, placebo-controlled trials with bacterial meningitis patients, CNS indices of infection severity, such as decreased glucose levels, elevated protein, and increased lactate levels, were significantly less pronounced after 24 hours of therapy with antibiotics and dexamethasone than with antibiotics alone. In one study of 200 infants and two studies of older children, patients receiving dexamethasone became afebrile earlier and were less likely to suffer moderate to severe SNHL than controls.[5,33] Of patients in the placebo group, 14% had severe or profound hearing loss, whereas only 1% of the corticosteroid-managed group were affected. Another prospective, multicenter, placebo-controlled clinical trial involving early audiologic evaluation and follow-up on 143 infants and children who survived bacterial meningitis found that dexamethasone did not significantly improve audiologic, neurologic, or developmental outcome. Hearing loss was already evident for all but one affected child as detected by ABR within 24 hours of hospital admission, which is consistent with a multicenter British study documenting the presence of hearing loss as early as 6 hours after admission.[65,66] A Finnish study comparing the efficacy of oral glycerol (an osmotic diuretic) and dexamethasone in preventing neurologic and audiologic sequelae of meningitis found that 7% of glycerol-managed patients suffered sequelae as compared with 19% of those not given glycerol.[53] The efficacy of oral glycerol was greater than intravenous dexamethasone among the 122 infants and children in the study. Because some clinicians will not administer corticosteroids in the face of a potentially life-threatening infection and because of controversy regarding their efficacy, other strategies for down-modulating host response to the infection are being explored.

In a histopathologic study of the temporal bones of 41 patients[58] who died of acute bacterial meningitis, suppurative labyrinthitis was found in 20 specimens (49%). The cochlea was affected in all patients, whereas vestibular involvement, primarily affecting the lateral semicircular canal, was present in only 50%. The inflammatory response was confined to perilymphatic spaces in all but one case; the scala tympani were consistently involved, whereas the scala vestibuli was affected only half the time. A pattern of eosinophilic staining in the absence of any inflammatory cells, thought to be the pathologic correlate of serous labyrinthitis, was described in 14 of the remaining 21 temporal bones, affecting primarily vestibular components including the superior (100%) and posterior (86%) semicircular canals. Cochlear involvement primarily scala tympani, was noted in only 40% of specimens. The endolymphatic and perilymphatic compartments demonstrated eosinophilic staining with about the same frequency, whereas suppuration, was confined to the perilymph. The cochlear aqueduct and modiolus were confirmed as routes of ingress of the infection into the inner ear, but the perivascular and perineural channels in the modiolus were most often involved. In cases with confirmed modiolar spread, neural damage preceded hair cell involvement, whereas the converse was true with aqueductal spread. Structural integrity of sensory and neural structures was noted in most bones from the suppurative labyrinthitis and eosinophilic staining groups, raising future possibilities for preventive intervention to mitigate resulting SNHL. In only 12% of all temporal bones was severe degeneration of spiral ganglion cells present, but these findings could have important implications for cochlear implant candidacy in some children with postmeningitic SNHL.

OTOTOXIC DRUGS AND CHEMICALS

As a result of more accurate reporting of adverse drug effects mandated by federal regulations, more potentially ototoxic drugs and chemicals are being identified. Some drugs, such as thalidomide, taken early in pregnancy produce severe embryopathic effects, including deformities of the external, middle, or inner ear with associated SNHL. Other ototoxic drugs and chemicals produce more profound effects after the sensory endorgan of the inner ear has reached a greater degree of differentiation later in pregnancy.

A partial listing of drugs and chemicals with ototoxic potentials includes:

Antibiotics
Streptomycin
Dihydrostreptomycin
Neomycin
Gentamycin
Kanamycin
Vancomycin
Polymyxin B
Erythromycin
Chemicals
Carbon monoxide
Mercury
Gold
Lead
Arsenic
Aniline dyes
Loop Diuretics
Ethacrynic acid
Furosemide
Other Drugs
Cisplatin
Quinine
Chloroquine
Salicylates
Polybrene
Nitrogen mustard
Thalidomide

Aminoglycosides

Aminoglycosides are bactericidal antibiotics administered parenterally because they are poorly absorbed from the gastrointestinal tract, with only 3% actually entering the bloodstream. Normal serum half-life is about 2 hours in patients with unimpaired renal function. This class of antimicrobials is not metabolized in the body and is excreted almost entirely by glomerular filtration so that urinary concentrations can approach 100 times serum levels if renal function is impaired. Hemodialysis and peritoneal dialysis lower serum levels in renal compromised patients. It was previously believed that comparable aminoglycoside concentration occurred in the inner ear fluids, but studies have confirmed that inner ear levels never rise above serum levels even in the face of suboptimal renal function. Nor is the differential toxicity to cochlear and vestibular structures correlated with tissue levels in those organs. Schacht[70] showed that the drugs are transmitted into hair cells by an energy-dependent process involving binding to the phospholipid phosphatidylinositol biophosphate. A relationship has been shown between binding affinity of various aminoglycosides and the drug's ototoxic potential. Although outer hair cells, observed *in vivo* or in tissue culture, sustain damage from exposure to gentamicin, Brownell[23] and others showed that isolated outer hair cells do not sustain damage even if exposed to high concentrations unless the drug has been enzymatically pretreated. Schacht[70] confirmed the existence of a cytotoxic gentamicin metabolite (gentatoxin) and provided a basis for developing preventive strategies. Attempts to block the toxicity of gentatoxin initially centered on glutathione, which has an antioxidative role and protects isolated outer hair cells against cytotoxicity from activated gentamicin. An observation that gentamicin promotes the production of free radicals in the presence of iron salts suggested activity as a chelator, which could facilitate irocatalyzed oxidation and free radical formation. Recent interest has been centered on the possible use of competitive, less toxic iron chelators (e.g., deferoxamine) to mollify gentamicin's ototoxicity without impairing, sometimes enhancing, its antimicrobial properties.

Histopathologic evidence of injury has been observed in the stria vascularis, suprastrial spiral ligament, pericapillary tissues in the spiral prominence, the outer sulcus, and Reissner's membrane. Cochlear damage usually proceeds from the basilar turn toward the apex, with initial destruction being observed in the inner row of outer hair cells. Although the remaining rows of outer hair cells may also be destroyed, inner hair cells are usually spared except in cases of overwhelming toxicity. In the vestibular system, type I hair cells of the crista ampullaris appear to be more sensitive to damage by streptomycin, kanamycin, and gentamicin than are type II cells. Supporting cells are largely spared, and regeneration of vestibular hair cells after damage has been documented in some experimental animals.

Although the reported incidence in most clinical studies ranges from 10% to 15%, there is wide variation. Neomycin is the most ototoxic, whereas netilmicin and sisomicin appear to be much less toxic. Streptomycin, gentamicin, and tobramycin are primarily vestibulotoxic, whereas kanamycin and amikacin are principally cochleotoxic. Fee[39] observed that gentamicin was significantly more vestibulotoxic than tobramycin, the toxicity being further potentiated by high hematocrit, elevated creatinine clearance, criticality of illness, and duration of therapy beyond 10 days. The margin between therapeutically effective blood levels and potentially toxic concentrations for aminoglycosides is relatively small, so careful monitoring of peak serum levels (30 minutes after intravenous administration) and trough levels (immediately before the next intravenous dose) is essential. Dosage levels should be appropriately adjusted downward in patients with renal dysfunction. In addition to compromised renal function, other factors thought to predispose to aminoglycoside ototoxicity include pre-existing hearing loss, temporarily related noise exposure, age, duration of therapy, prior use of aminoglycosides, nutritional status, and concomitant use of additional ototoxic drugs such as other aminoglycosides and loop diuretics (e.g., ethacrynic acid, furosemide). The greatest ototoxic synergy between these drug classes is observed if the aminoglycoside is administered first.

Transplacental passage of aminoglycosides has been confirmed in animals, but the risk to a developing fetus if the mother receives these drugs has been debated. Aminoglycosides are used regularly to manage serious infections in neonates and young infants, but controversy exists as to the inherent risk posed to hearing and balance function. On the basis of extensive studies, Finitzo-Hieber, McCracken, and Brown[40] concluded that aminoglycosides at appropriate dosage levels pose little risk of ototoxicity in children. Eviatar and Eviatar,[38] however, conducted controlled prospective studies of infants receiving aminoglycosides for neonatal sepsis, evaluating such parameters as acquisition of head control and nystagmus induced by position change, perrotatory stimulation with a torsion swing, and caloric irrigations. Nearly 10% of infants who received aminoglycosides showed vestibular abnormalities and delay in acquisition of head control as would be compatible with vestibulotoxicity Prolonged administration of the drugs (i.e., 25 to 45 days) increases the risk of damage as does concomitant administration of other ototoxic drugs. Serial audiometric screening, including frequencies above 12,000 Hz, and vestibular evaluation may provide early warning of impending damage. Some investigators report partial return of vestibular function after an initial deficit has been shown during extended gentamicin therapy, but in other cases further deterioration has occurred after cessation of therapy.

Each mitochondrion contains mtDNA chromosomes consisting of 16,569 base pair double-stranded circles, which encode messenger, ribosomal, and transfer RNA to produce 13 specific proteins necessary for intracellular oxidative phosphorylation. In China, where aminoglycoside use is widespread, some families appeared to be exquisitely sensitive to their ototoxic effects. Point mutations (1555 A-G in the mitochondrial 12S ribosomal RNA) were identified in several affected Asian families. Recently, unrelated, ethnically diverse American patients and families with hearing loss after aminoglycoside exposure were screened for mitochondrial RNA mutations; 17% showed the nucleotide 1555 A-G mutation, whereas no controls harbored the mutation. Family history of drug-related hearing loss should be reviewed before aminoglycoside therapy is instituted, and if necessary, screening for mitochondrial mutations can be accomplished to minimize avoidable ototoxicity in these patients.

Loop diuretics

Powerful loop diuretics, such as ethacrynic acid and furosemide, promote the rapid excretion of large amounts of iso-osmotic urine. Early clinical observations of a transient ototoxic effect associated with the use of these drugs were followed by reports of permanent ototoxicity, particularly when these diuretics are used concurrently with apparently safe levels of aminoglycosides. Matz[57] estimated the incidence of ototoxic effects with this class of drugs as 0.7% with ethacrynic acid to 6.4% with furosemide. Temporal bone histopathology in animals managed with toxic levels of these drugs reveals changes in the stria vascularis and significant hair cell loss. Rybak, Whitworth, and Scott[68] postulate that furosemide and ethacrynic acid have different mechanisms of action on the cochlea. Because of the synergy between the ototoxic effects of loop diuretics and aminoglycosides, dosages of these medications should be carefully adjusted when they are administered concurrently, and the order of administration should be adjusted to minimize the risk.

Erythromycin

The ototoxic potential of erythromycin became evident with the relatively large intravenous dosage levels used to manage pneumonia caused by *Legionella pneumophila*. Bilateral SNHL, often accompanied by tinnitus and vertigo, was noted in adults with erythromycin dosages of 2 g/day, particularly in patients with concomitant renal hepatic failure. Blood levels at which ototoxic effects were observed ranged upward from 63 mg/l. Animal studies suggest a cochlear site of lesion, and a transient effect on the stria vascularis has been postulated.

Salicylates

High therapeutic doses of salicylates (exceeding 20 mg/dl) are associated with reversible hearing loss and tinnitus. Hawkins[47] showed that salicylates in the perilymph can reduce transaminases, cochlear adenosine triphosphate levels, and cochlear blood flow. Changes in cochlear function have been attributed to a salicylate-mediated increase in the membrane conductance of outer hair cells. Decreased levels of perilymphatic prostaglandins and elevated leukotrienes have been linked with toxic effects in animal models, raising the possibility that corticosteroid management might minimize the deleterious effects. The association of the ingestion of therapeutic doses of salicylate in young febrile children with Reye's syndrome has led to a marked decrease in the use of this class of drugs in the pediatric and adolescent age groups without strict indications.

Vancomycin

Nephrotoxicity and ototoxicity have been reported in patients receiving vancomycin, particularly if blood levels exceed 45 mg/L. Adults have described tinnitus at slightly lower serum levels, which could be an early warning of impending damage. Matz[57] reports that premature infants are more susceptible to the ototoxic effects than full-term babies because they have larger volumes of distribution of the drug, which has a longer half-life in these neonates.

Cisplatin

Cisplatin, which is used for managing many neoplasms, has been implicated as an ototoxic drug, with the potential for permanently affecting cochlear and vestibular function. The drug's cytotoxic effects result from inter- and intrastrand cross-linking of DNA. Side effects include myelosuppression, neurotoxicity, and nephrotoxicity, but irreversible ototoxic effects impose dose limits. Studies using serial high-frequency audiometry show that hearing loss usually begins in the 10,000- to 18,000-Hz range and gradually involves frequencies below 8000 Hz if management continues. Audiometric screening at 12,000 and 14,000 Hz helps early identification of ototoxicity. The pathophysiologic mechanism by which damage occurs involves drug-mediated blockade of outer hair cell transduction channels, coupled with a decrease in adenylate cyclase. Histopathologically, outer hair cell loss is observed, particularly in the basal turn of the cochlea with gradual involvement of inner hair cells proceeding in an apical direction. Atrophy of the stria vascularis and Reissner's membrane collapse have also been described.

Estimates of the risk of ototoxicity posed by cisplatin vary with the audiometric frequencies evaluated. Early estimates placed the risk at 20% or less. In a study evaluating thresholds from 8 to 20 kHz, Dreschler, Hulst, and Tange[36] used conservative criteria for damage, including deterioration of 20 dB or more at one frequency, 15 dB at two frequencies, or 10 dB at four frequencies. They found that 46% to 83% of patients in the various study groups showed some degree of loss, principally at higher frequencies. Of these losses, 80% were bilateral with the remainder having unilateral involvement. Most investigators agree that dosage levels exceeding 3 to 4 mg/kg of body weight carry a definite risk of ototoxicity. In one report of 54 cases, no ototoxic changes were noted in patients in whom the peak plasma concentration of cisplatin did not exceed 1 μg/l. Children are at considerable risk for cisplatin-related SNHL because of the widespread use of the drug for the management of solid tumors such as osteogenic sarcoma and neuroblastoma. Cisplatin reportedly induced high-frequency hearing loss (40 dB or greater at 1000 Hz and above) in about half of children managed with a standard therapeutic dose (60 to 100 mg/m^2 per course). Davidson, Hyde, and Alberti[28] reported that permanent bilateral high-frequency SNHL was detected in 88% of children receiving cisplatin doses over 450 mg/m^2. Cochlear damage, which was related to cumulative doses exceeding 279 mg/m^2, was inversely proportional to the age of the child. Animal studies have confirmed that the ototoxic effects of noise exposure (85 dB SPL or greater) and cisplatin are synergistic, producing greater hair cell loss and hearing impairment at high frequencies than is observed with either agent alone. Although conclusive studies addressing this issue are not available, prudence would dictate avoidance of exposure to potentially damaging sound levels (e.g., amplified music at high volume) during cisplatin therapy.

Quinine and chloroquine

The antimalarial drugs quinine and chloroquine phosphate, a synthetic quinolone derivative, have shown ototoxic potential. Mothers receiving quinine during pregnancy may give birth to infants with severe to profound hearing impairment. Retinopathy and hearing loss have been observed in offspring of pregnant mothers managed with chloroquine. The pathophysiologic mechanism involved with both drugs appears to be a vasculitis and ischemia in the inner ear, with subsequent degenerative changes of the stria vascularis, organ of Corti, and neuronal elements.

Retinoids

Retinoids, such as isotretinoin, used to manage severe recalcitrant cystic acne, administered systemically to a pregnant woman have been linked to spontaneous abortion or severe malformation including CNS, cardiovascular, and respiratory anomalies; cleft lip; cleft palate; and external ear defects, which may include canal agenesis.

ANOXIA AND HYPOXIA

Anoxia and hypoxia during the perinatal period, resulting from such factors as cord compression and neonatal seizures, are strongly correlated, statistically, with subsequent SNHL in young infants. Objective evidence of anoxia and hypoxia in the neonatal history can include meconium staining, primary apnea, a history of resuscitation at birth, low Apgar scores at 1 and 5 minutes, postnatal apnea, and the need for prolonged postnatal ventilatory assistance. Histopathologic evidence shows that anoxic damage occurs in the brainstem reticular formation and cochlear nuclei, which show decreased cell numbers and volume in proportion to the length and severity of oxygen deprivation. Some infants with perinatal anoxia may have multiple high-risk factors, making the precise role of oxygen deprivation in the etiology of hearing loss unclear. However, recent studies of neonates with chronic hypoxemia resulting from persistent fetal circulation revealed a 20% incidence of SNHL, 75% of which was moderate to severe and 25% profound.

HYPERBILIRUBINEMIA

A causal relationship between elevated bilirubin levels in neonates, with associated kernicterus, and SNHL has been appreciated for decades. Whether resulting from inadequate conjugation, impaired albumin binding, or increased unconjugated bilirubin production, bilirubin that crosses the blood-brain barrier may be deposited in the basal ganglia, particularly the ventrocochlear nucleus, resulting in neurologic sequelae, including SNHL. Histopathologically, the middle and inner ears are generally free of abnormality. Improved prenatal care, including the introduction of Rh immunoglobulin, exchange transfusions, and phototherapy have markedly decreased the incidence of kernicterus detected at autopsy. However, studies have shown reversible ABR changes (absence of the wave IV-V complex) in about one third of neonates with bilirubin levels of 15 to 25 mg/dl, suggesting a transient encephalopathy. Jaundice develops in more than half of full-term infants; about 6% will have serum bilirubin concentrations exceeding 12.9 mg/dl. Although neonatal hyperbilirubinema is one of the most common indications for readmission to the hospital in the first weeks of life, some authors have criticized the aggressive use of "bililights" in these infants. Exchange transfusion is also associated with complications such as hyperkalemia, hypocalcemia, hypothermia, blood pressure fluctuations, and acidosis. About 50% of infants who develop kernicterus will die, and survivors may have cerebral palsy, mental retardation, and hearing loss. Measurement of breath carbon monoxide was recently introduced for identifying infants with increased bilirubin production secondary to hemolysis who may require more aggressive prevention. Another promising advance is represented by heme-oxygenase inhibitors (e.g., tin-mesoporphyrin), which bind to heme-oxygenase more aggressively than heme itself, thus retarding access of the natural substrate to the binding site and retarding heme degradation and bilirubin production.

PREMATURITY AND FULL-TERM LOW BIRTH WEIGHT

Although several high-risk factors, such as perinatal hypoxia, sepsis, and kernicterus, may be present in premature and dysmature neonates, prematurity itself constitutes a reliable risk indicator. Admission to an NICU is standard care for these small infants, and NICU outcome studies reveal that premature infants may be as much as 20 times more likely to be severely hearing impaired than infants of normal weight and gestational age. As many as 2% of infants with birth weight of 3 pounds or less manifest significant SNHL. Audiologic evaluation and habilitation of these hearing-impaired infants may be further complicated by the presence of additional handicaps.

RECURRENT OTITIS MEDIA AND MASTOID DISEASE

Conductive hearing loss is the usual sequela of recurrent otitis media and mastoiditis, but early retrospective studies by Paparella and others[62,63] suggested that otitis-prone children were more likely to have coexisting SNHL than would be predicted by incidence figures for the general population. Preliminary results from a more recent prospective study[56] found that extended high-frequency (250 to 8000 Hz) acuity in children who had positive histories for recurrent otitis media was poorer than that in a group of children without otitis media. Results also suggest a relationship between the severity of otitis media and degree of extended high-frequency loss. Multifrequency tympanometry was carried out to assess the potential contribution of middle ear dysfunction to high-frequency loss. Study children with normal 226-Hz tympanograms and normal multifrequency tympanometry, who were least likely to have residual mechanical disturbances of the middle ear, had poorer hearing than normal counterparts at all extended high frequency. Possible causes include penetration of the labyrinthine windows (particularly the round window membrane) by infectious byproducts or toxins, topical drugs with ototoxic potential, or both. Because inner ear structures involved in frequency coding for high frequencies are located along the portion of the basilar membrane nearest to the round window, these frequencies might be expected to be affected before lower frequencies. Animal experiments of round window permeability suggested a greater risk for penetration by middle ear contents into the inner ear than observed empirically in humans. It has been postulated that edema and granulation tissue, which accompany middle ear infection, may help prevent transmission of unwanted substances through the round window membrane.

EAR AND HEAD TRAUMA

Middle ear and inner ear trauma can result from diverse etiologies, including a slap on the ear, a foreign body (e.g., cotton swab) inserted in the external canal, impact against water while diving or water skiing, and skull trauma, which may include temporal bone fracture. An infant's foreshortened ear canal can predispose to transcanal injury, whereas head trauma is a more common etiology in older children and adolescents. Youngsters may report symptoms such as acute pain, bloody otorrhea, hearing loss, tinnitus, and possibly vertigo. Mild-to-moderate conductive hearing loss is the most common audiometric finding, but intralabyrinthine injury may produce a concurrent, usually high-frequency, sensorineural component. More severe conductive impairment suggests possible ossicular damage, whereas labyrinthine membrane disruption, including perilymphatic fistula, should be suspected in patients with fluctuating or progressive SNHL. Large traumatic tympanic membrane perforations, particularly if accompanied by ossicular injury, may require surgery, but most heal with little scarring.

Motor vehicle accidents; mishaps involving bicycles, skateboards, and roller skates; and falls are among the common etiologies for temporal bone fractures in children and adolescents. Such fractures are broadly classified as longitudinal or transverse with respect to the long axis of the temporal bone; the longitudinal variety accounts for 70% to 90% of these injuries. Longitudinal fractures are associated with middle ear and ossicular damage, usually sparing inner ear and internal canal structures. Transverse fractures often disrupt labyrinthine integrity or transect neural structures in the internal auditory canal, leading to permanent SNHL, facial nerve paralysis, or vertigo.

Temporal bone fractures reportedly occur in 7% of children admitted to the hospital after head injury; 13% of these patients sustained SNHL. In a group of 324 children and adolescents with unilateral SNHL, 10.8% of losses were attributed to head trauma, which in 35% of cases had been sustained at or before age 6 years.

NOISE-INDUCED HEARING LOSS

Sounds of sufficient loudness and duration produce ear damage resulting in temporary or permanent hearing loss, often accompanied by tinnitus. Irreversible inner ear damage from loud sounds is cumulative, can occur at any age, and is not presently amenable to medical or surgical management. An important consequence of typical noise-induced hearing loss (NIHL) is difficulty understanding speech sounds, which could impair classroom performance. NIHL is entirely preventable except in rare cases of accidental exposure.

About 10,000,000 Americans have hearing losses at least partly attributable to damage from loud sounds. More than 20 million Americans, including children and adolescents, are regularly exposed to hazardous sound levels, which could result in hearing loss. Much of this noise exposure occurs in the workplace, but the proliferation of potentially harmful noise sources at home, on farms, and in recreational environments has placed more children and adolescents at risk (Table 32-5).

Current US Department of Labor regulations set the boundary between acceptable and damaging noise in the workplace at 85 dB(A) for continuous exposure. Because the decibel scale is exponential, a change of a few decibels can represent a significant change in loudness; e.g., a 20-dB sound is 10 times as loud as a 10-dB sound. The "A" refers to a type of sound filter used in a sound level meter when measuring potentially damaging sound. These devices can measure continuous loud noise (e.g., by amplified music) and intermittent, short-duration noises with very loud peak components (e.g., gunfire, firecrackers). Susceptibility to the damaging effects of loud sounds varies, so it is difficult to predict the magnitude of hearing loss resulting from expo-

Table 32-5. Causes of noise-induced hearing loss*

Noise level (dB)	
140	Firecrackers, gunshot, jet engine
130	Jackhammer
120	Boom cars, band practice, headphones, rock concerts
110	Shouting in ear, disco, chainsaw
100	Snowmobile, subway, woodworking
90	Traffic, lawnmower, motorcycle, orchestra
85	
80	Alarm clock, hair dryer, assembly line
70	Restaurant, vacuum cleaner, sewing machine
60	Conversation, air conditioner
50	Average home, refrigerator
40	Principal's office
30	Quiet library, soft whisper

* Levels greater than 85 dB are potentially dangerous.

sure to a potentially damaging sound. Damage risk criteria are based on the average responses of many persons.

Ear damage resulting from hazardous noise levels may be classified as acoustic trauma or NIHL. The pattern of damage resulting from exposure to a particular sound source depends on the frequency, intensity (i.e., loudness), duration, and scheduling (i.e., continuous or intermittent) of the exposure and the susceptibility of the ear involved. Exposure to intense sounds (>140 dB[A]) of short duration, such as gunfire or an explosion, can produce immediate, severe, and permanent hearing loss, termed *acoustic trauma*. By means of direct mechanical destruction, such high-intensity sound waves can disrupt virtually any structure in the ear, ranging from the tympanic membrane and ossicles to the organ of Corti.

Moderate exposure to less intense but potentially damaging sounds may cause a temporary threshold shift (TTS). With additional exposure, NIHL gradually becomes permanent, initially involving frequencies of 3000 to 6000 Hz as reflected in a characteristic ''notch'' audiometric configuration. Experimental evidence indicates that hair cells of the inner ear are most vulnerable to damage, and outer hair cells are initially affected. Disruption of intracellular organelles, including endoplasmic reticulum, lysosomes, nucleus, and mitochondria, has been observed with electron microscopy, as have disorganization, fusion, and loss of stereocilia. The stereocilia rootlet structure, which anchors it into the top of the hair cell, appears to be affected first. Degeneration of damaged hair cells may lead to eventual loss of auditory nerve fibers and changes in auditory areas of the CNS. With repeated exposure, hair cell loss will continue to increase; there is no evidence that degenerated hair cells are replaced in mammals. Recent studies in birds, however, showed some hair cell regeneration after initial loss after noise exposure. The anatomic and physiologic changes in the inner ear during a TTS are subtle and may be limited to swelling of hair cells and underlying afferent nerve fiber terminals, which resolves during a rest period from loud sounds. Acute changes in stereocilia rootlets might alter cochlear micromechanics, whereas vascular spasm and metabolic exhaustion may also play a role in TTS.

Impulse noises (e.g., gunfire, firecrackers) are characterized by short duration and very high sound intensity levels, 132 to 170 dB(A) during the initial acoustic pulse of a typical gun discharge. Large caliber rifles and shotguns are particularly hazardous and can produce immediate and permanent injury to sensitive inner ear structures. Sound levels produced by toy weapons measured at a distance of 50 cm showed mean peak values from 143 to 153 dB(A), whereas firecrackers produced peak levels of 125 to 156 dB at 3 meters. Adolescents who work in noisy environments may worsen occupational hearing loss by shooting or setting off firecrackers.

Although an explosion risks hearing loss in an unprotected ear, other potentially damaging environmental sounds may be less readily apparent. Parents and public policy makers have expressed concern about hearing risks resulting from exposure to rock music, boom cars, motorcycles, and personal casette players.

Average sound levels in a typical disco are 95 dB(A) and at a rock concert are 105 to 115 dB(A), well above the discomfort level for most people. In addition to the audience, rock musicians, stagehands, ushers, and concessionaires are at risk for NIHL after prolonged exposure to these very high sound levels. Most children and youth can attend a typical concert without suffering a permanent hearing loss, but practically everyone exposed to such sound levels will experience TTS often accompanied by tinnitus.

Personal cassette players can produce sound levels in excess of 110 to 115 dB(A). Because these electronic devices are portable and often drown out loud background noises exposure time can be long. A child may unwittingly compensate for a TTS by turning up the volume to even more hazardous levels. Surveys reveal that about 80% of elementary school children own or use personal cassette players, and 5% to 10% listen for extended periods at potentially dangerous volumes. A child who experiences a full feeling in the ear, muffled hearing, or tinnitus after personal cassette player use should be cautioned to modify listening habits to avoid NIHL. Sound levels in many boom cars, which have very powerful stereo amplifiers and speakers, may exceed 120 dB(A). All persons, including children, exposed to such high ambient sound levels for prolonged periods risk permanent NIHL.

Brookhouser, Worthington, and Kelly[20] reported results of a study of 114 children and adolescents (age 19 and younger) diagnosed with NIHL on the basis of history and audiometric configuration. In 42 children, the loss was unilateral, whereas bilateral losses were present in 72. The gender distribution of the sample was consistent with the findings of other investigators in that 90.3% of the affected children were males. The mean age of referral for evaluation was 12.7 years (range, 1.2 to 19.8 years; standard deviation, 4.21 years), but 26% of these losses were diagnosed in children 10 years or younger. Parents or guardians were asked to identify the potentially damaging noise sources to which their child was exposed. Among 70 children for whom very reliable information was available, fireworks or firearms were identified as the sole noise source in 21 of 58 children (36%) with bilateral losses and 8 of 12 children (67%) with unilateral losses. Histories of 14 of 19 children (74%) with exposure to multiple noise sources also noted fireworks or firearms. Consequently, noise exposure histories on 43 of 94 children (46%) included exposure to impulse sounds produced by fireworks or firearms. Although cap pistols and noisy toys have been identified in the literature as possible hazardous noise sources, none of the histories mentioned either. Such an omission may reflect a lack of caregiver awareness of the noise levels produced by such devices. Live or amplified music was identified in 11 of 94 cases (12%) as the principal source of noise exposure.

The age of identification of the hearing loss in relation to the type of noise source implicated in the history was also examined (Table 32-6). Although the loud music category contained only youth aged 10 years or greater, all other categories included youngsters in the preschool and early elementary age groups. The noise exposure histories were replete with descriptions of children riding with a parent on a recreational vehicle (e.g., motorcycle, snowmobile), assisting a parent in a home workshop, or accompanying a parent on a hunting trip or a visit to a target range. Eight of forty-seven children (17%) for whom serial audiometric test data were available showed progression of their hearing loss, including involvement of additional frequencies in some cases, over a mean follow-up of 2 years and 1 month.

The 1990 NIH Consensus Statement on Noise and Hearing Loss[25] recommended development and dissemination of a comprehensive education program aimed at school-aged children and their parents that focuses on the causes and prevention of NIHL.

Table 32-6. Age of hearing loss diagnosis versus source of noise

	Age (yr)	
	Bilateral hearing loss	**Unilateral hearing loss**
Fireworks	1.1-17.7	9.4-14.4
Firearms	6.7-19.7	5.1-18
Music	10.2-19.8	10
Recreational vehicle	5.6-12	—
Power tools or equipment	4.2-18.4	16.2
Multiple sources	6.4-18.3	13.3-15.6
Unspecified	4.8-15	10.7-19.3

From Brookhouser PE and others: Noise induced hearing loss in children, *Laryngoscope* 1022:645, 1992.

REFERENCES

1. Abdelhak S and others: A human homologue of the Drosphilia eyes absent gene underlies branchio-oto-renal (BOR) syndrome and identifies a novel gene family, *Nature Genet* 15:157, 1997.
2. Adler SP: Cytomegalovirus transmission and child daycare, *Adv Pediatr Infect Dis* 7:109, 1992.
3. American Academy of Pediatrics: Position statement 1982: Joint Committee on Infant Hearing, *Pediatrics* 70:496, 1982.
4. Barker DF and others: Identification of mutations in the COL4A5 collagen gene in Alport syndrome, *Science* 248:1224, 1990.
5. Belsey MA, Hoffpauir CW, Smith MHD: Dexamethasone in the treatment of acute bacterial meningitis: effect of study design on the interpretation of results, *Pediatrics* 44:503, 1969.
6. Berg FS: *Educational audiology: hearing and speech management*, New York, 1972, Grune & Stratton.
7. Berger W and others: Isolation of a candidate gene for Norrie disease by positional cloning, *Nat Genet* 1:199, 1992.
8. Bess FH, Klee T, Culbertson JL: Identification, assessment and management of children with unilateral sensorineural hearing loss, *Ear Hear* 7:43, 1986.
9. Bess FH, Paradise JL: Universal screening for infant hearing impairment: not simple, not risk-free, not necessarily beneficial, and not presently justified, *Pediatrics* 93:330, 1994.
10. Biancalana V and others: Oto-palato-digital syndrome type I: further evidence for assignment of the locus to Xq28, *Hum Genet* 88:228, 1991.
11. Bieber FR, Nance WE: *Hereditary hearing loss.* In Jackson LG, Schimke RN, editors: *Clinical genetics: a source book for physicians*, New York, 1978, John Wiley & Sons.
12. Bordley JE, Alford BR: The pathology of rubella deafness, *Int Audiol* 9:58, 1970.
13. Bordley JE, Alford BR: The pathology of rubella deafness, *Int Audiol* 9:58, 1970.
14. Bordley JE and others: Prenatal rubella, *Acta Otolaryngol (Stockh)* 66: 1, 1968.
15. Bordley JE, Kapur YP: The histopathological changes in the temporal bone resulting from acute smallpox and chickenpox infection, *Laryngoscope* 82:1477, 1972.
16. Boughman JA, Shaver KA: Genetic aspects of deafness: understanding the counselling process, *Am Ann Deaf* 393, 1982.
17. Brookhouser PE, Auslander MC, Meskan ME: The pattern and stability of postmeningitic hearing loss in children, *Laryngoscope* 98:940, 1988.
18. Brookhouser PE, Worthington DW, Kelly WJ: Unilateral hearing loss in children, *Laryngoscope* 10:1264, 1991.
19. Brookhouser PE, Worthington DW, Kelly WJ: Fluctuating and/or progressive sensorineural hearing loss in children, *Laryngoscope* 104:958, 1994.
20. Brookhouser PE, Worthington DW, Kelly WJ: Noise-induced hearing loss in children, *Laryngoscope* 102:645, 1992.
21. Brookhouser PE, Worthington DW, Kelly WJ: *The natural history of progressive fluctuation SNHL in children.* Presented at American Society of Pediatric Otolaryngology Annual Meeting, Palm Beach, Fla, May 12, 1994.
22. Brookhouser PE: *Incidence and prevalence.* Presented at National Institutes of Health Consensus Development Conference on Early Identification of Hearing Impairment in Infants and Young Children, Bethesda, MD, March 1-3, 1993.
23. Brownell WE and others: Evoked mechanical responses of isolated cochlear outer hair cells, *Science* 227:194, 1996.
24. Chaib H and others: A newly identified locus for Usher syndrome, USH1E, maps to chromosome 21q21, *Hum Mol Genet* 6:27, 1997.
25. Consensus Conference: Noise and hearing loss, *JAMA* 263:3185, 1990.

26. Coyle B and others: Pendred syndrome (goitre and sensorineural hearing loss) maps to chromosome 7 in the region containing the nonsyndromic deafness gene DFNB4, *Nature Genet* 12:421, 1996.
27. Daffos F and others: Prenatal management of 746 pregnancies at risk for congenital toxoplasmosis, *N Engl J Med* 318:271, 1988.
28. Davidson J, Hyde ML, Alberti PW: Epidemiological patterns in childhood hearing loss: a review, *Int J Pediatr Otorhinolaryngol* 17:239, 1989.
29. Davis A, Wood S: The epidemiology of childhood hearing impairment: factors relevant to planning of services, *Br J Audiol* 26:77, 1992.
30. Davis LE, Johnson RT: Experimental viral infections of the inner ear: I. Acute infections of the newborn hamster labyrinth, *Lab Invest* 34: 349, 1976.
31. de Kok YJ and others: Association between x-linked mixed deafness and mutations in the POU domain gene POU3F4, *Science* 3:685, 1995.
32. Decoster A and others: IgA antibodies against P30 as markers of congenital and acute toxoplasmosis, *Lancet* 2:1104, 1988.
33. DeLemos RA, Haggerty RJ: Corticosteroids as an adjunct to treatment in bacterial meningitis: a controlled clinical trial, *Pediatrics* 44:30, 1969.
34. Desmonts G, Couvreur J: Congenital toxoplasmosis: a prospective study of 378 pregnancies, *N Engl J Med* 290:1110, 1974.
35. Dixon J and others: Positional cloning of a gene involved in the pathogenesis of Treacher Collins syndrome, *Nature Genet* 12:130, 1996.
36. Dreschler WA, Hulst RJAM, Tange RA: The role of high-frequency audiometry in early detection of ototoxicity, *Audiology* 24:387, 1985.
37. *Early identification of hearing impairment in infants and young children*, National Institutes of Health Consensus Statement, March 1-3, 1993.
38. Eviatar L, Eviatar A: Development of head control and vestibular responses in infants treated with aminoglycosides, *Dev Med Child Neurol* 24:372, 1982.
39. Fee WE: Aminoglycoside ototoxicity in the human, *Laryngoscope* 90 (suppl):1, 1980.
40. Finitzo-Hieber T, McCracken GH Jr, Brown KC: Prospective controlled evaluation of auditory function in neonates given netilmicin or amikacin, *J Pediatr* 106:129, 1985.
41. Fischel-Ghodsian N and others: Mitochondrial mutation associated with nonsyndromic deafness, *Am J Otolaryngol* 16:403, 1995.
42. Guilford P and others: A YAC contig and an EST map in the pericentromeric region of chromosome 13 surrounding the loci for neurosensory nonsyndromic deafness (DFNB1 and DFNA3) and limb-girdle muscular dystrophy type 2C (LGMD2C), *Genomics* 29:163, 1995.
43. Reference deleted in pages.
44. Greenberg MT: Family stress and child competence: the effects of early intervention 128:407, 1983.
45. Gregg NM: Congenital cataract following German measles in the mother, *Opthal Cos Aust* 3:35, 1941.
46. Hardy J: Fetal consequences of maternal viral infections in pregnancy, *Arch Otolaryngol Head Neck Surg* 98:218, 1973.
47. Hawkins JE Jr: Ototoxic mechanism: a working hypothesis, *Audiology*, 12:383, 1973.
48. Jervell A, Lange-Nielsen F: Congenital deaf-mutism, functional heart disease with prolongation of the Q-T interval and sudden death, *Am Heart J* 54:59, 1957.
49. Joint Committee on Infant Hearing: 1994 Position statement, *ASHA* 36:38, 1994.
50. Joint Committee on Infant Hearing: Position statement, *ASHA* 24:1017, 1982.
51. Joint Committee on Infant Hearing: 1990 Position statement, *ASHA Suppl* 33:3, 1991.
52. Kaplan and others: A gene for Usher syndrome type I (USH1A) maps to c 14q, *Genomics* 14:979, 1992.
53. Kilpi T and others: Oral glycerol and intravenous dexamethasone in preventing neurologic and audiologic sequelae of childhood bacterial meningitis: the Finnish Study Group, *Pediatr Infect Dis J* 14:270, 1995.
54. Kimberling W and others: Localization of Usher syndrome type II to chromosome 1q, *Genomics* 7:245, 1990.
55. Konigsmark BW, Gorlin RJ, editors: *Genetic and metabolic deafness*, Philadelphia, 1976, WB Saunders.
56. Margolis RH and others: Effects of otitis media on extended high frequency hearing in children, *Ann Otol Rhinol Laryngol* 102:1, 1993.
57. Matz GJ: Clinical perspectives on ototoxic drugs, *Ann Otol Rhinol Laryngol* 99:39, 1990.
58. Merchant SN, Gopen Q: A human temporal bone study of acute bacterial meningogenic labyrinthitis, *Am J Otol* 17:375, 1996.
59. Miyamoto RT and others: Contemporary management of neurofibromatosis, *Ann Otol Rhinol Laryngol* 100:38, 1991.
60. Mochizuki T and others: Identification of mutations in the alphae 4(IV) collagen genes in autosomal recessive Alport syndrome, *National Genetics* 8:77, 1994.
61. Otolaryngology Clinical Trials Cooperative Group, Grant #1 U01 DCO 3209-01, NIH-NIDCD, 4/15/97–3/31/02.
62. Paparella MM, Brady DR, Hoell R: Sensorineural hearing loss in chronic otitis media and mastoiditis, *Trans Am Acad Ophthalmol Otolaryngol* 74:108, 1970.
63. Paparella MM and others: Sensorineural hearing loss in otitis media, *Ann Otol Rhinol Laryngol* 93:623, 1984.
64. Reardon W, Harding AE: Mitochondrial genetics and deafness, *J Audiol Med* 4:40, 1995.
65. Richardson MP and others: Hearing loss during bacterial meningitis, *Arch Dis Child* 76:386, 1997.
66. Richardson MP and others: Hearing loss during bacterial meningitis, *Arch Dis Child* 76:134, 1997.
67. Rouleau GA and others: Alternation in a new gene encoding aputative membrane-organizing protein causes neurofibromatosis type 2, *Nature* 363:515, 1993.
68. Rybak P, Whitworth C, Scott V: Organic acids do not alter the cochlear effects of ethacrynic acid, *Hear Res* 46:95, 1990.
69. Sankila EM and others: Assignment of an Usher syndrome type Ii (USH3) gene to chromosome 3q, *Hum Mol Genet* 4:93, 1995.
70. Schacht J: Molecular mechanisms of drug-induced hearing loss, *Hear Res* 48:297, 1986.
71. Sheffield VC and others: Pendred syndrome maps to chromosome 7q21-34 and is caused by an intrinsic defect in thyroid iodine organification, *Nat Genet* 12:424, 1996.
72. Shen MH, Harper PS, Upadhyaya M: Molecular genetics of neurofibromatosis type 1 (NF1), *J Med Genet* 33:2, 1996.
73. Smith RJH and others: Localization of the gene for branchiootorenal syndrome to chromosome 8q, *Genomics* 14:841, 1992.
74. Snead MP and others: Masked confirmation of linkage between type 1 congenital vitreous anomaly and COL2A1 in Stickler syndrome *Graefes Arch Clin Exp Ophthalmol* 234:720, 1996 (letter).
75. Stein LK, Boyer KM: Progress in the prevention of hearing loss in infants, *Ear Hear* 15:116, 1994.
76. Stepick-Biek P and others: IgA antibodies for diagnosis of acute congenital and acquired toxoplasmosis, *J Infect Dis* 162:270, 1990.
77. Swan C and others: Congenital defects in infants following infectious diseases during pregnancy with special reference to relationship between German measles and cataracts, deaf-mutism, heart disease and microcephaly and to period of pregnancy in which occurrence of rubella is followed by congenital abnormalities, *Med J Aust* 2:201, 1943.
78. Takahashi H, Sando I, Takagi A: Computer-aided three-dimensional reconstruction and measurement of the round window niche, *Laryngoscope* 99:505, 1989.
79. Tassabehji M, Newton VE, Read AP: Waardenburg syndrome type 2 caused by mutations in the human microphthalmia (MITF) gene, *Nat Genet* 8:251, 1994.
80. Tassabehji M and others: Waardenburg's syndrome patients have mutations in the human homologue of the Pax-3 paired box gene, *Nature Genet* 355:635, 1992.
81. United States Department of Health and Human Services, Public Health

Service: *Healthy people 2000: national health promotion and disease prevention objectives*, Washington DC, 1990, Government Printing Office.

82. Usher CH: The Bowman lecture: on a few hereditary eye afflictions, *Trans Ophthalmol Soc UK* 55:164, 1935.
83. Vincent GM: Genetics and molecular biology of the inherited long QT syndrome, *Ann Med* 26:419, 1994.
84. von Graefe A: Vereinzelte beobachtungen und bemerkungen: exceptionelles verhalten des geischtsfeldes bei pigmentenartung der netzhaut, *Albrecht von Graefes Arch Klin Ophthalmol* 4:250, 1858.
85. Wayne S and others: Localization of the Usher syndrome type ID gene (USH1D) to chromosome 10, *Hum Mol Genet* 5:1689, 1996.
86. Weil D and others: Defective myosin VIIA gene responsible for Usher syndrome type 1B, *Nature* 374:60, 1995.
87. Weisel A: Early intervention programs for hearing impaired children: evaluation of outcomes, *Early Child Dev Care* 41:77, 1990.
88. Weller TH, Neva FA: Propagation in tissue culture of cytopathic agents from patients with rubella-like illness, *Proc Soc Exp Biol Med* 3:215, 1962.
89. White KR, Maxon AB: Universal screening for infant hearing impairment: simple, beneficial, and presently justified, *Int J Pediatr Otorhinolaryngol* 32:201, 1995.
90. Yoshinaga-Itano C: *The impact of age of identification upon the development of deaf and hard of hearing children.* Presented at the 1997 Conference on Develops in Pediatric Audiology: Current Issues in Assessment and Management, Omaha, NE, October 17-19, 1997.

Index

Note: Page numbers set in italic indicate figures; those followed by *t* indicate tables; those preceded by *P* indicate material found in the Pediatric volume.

A

B

C

F

G

H

I

J

K

L

M

N

O

P

T

U

V